Maxillofacial Trauma
and Esthetic Facial
Reconstruction

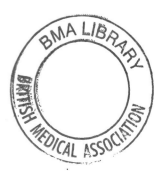

Commissioning Editor: **Alison Ashmore**
Project Development Manager: **Tim Kimber**
Project Manager: **Susan Skinner**
Illustration Manager: **Mick Ruddy**
Design Manager: **Andy Chapman**

Maxillofacial Trauma and Esthetic Facial Reconstruction

Edited by

Peter Ward Booth FDS, FRCS

Consultant Maxillofacial Surgeon
Department of Maxillofacial Surgery
The Queen Victoria Hospital
East Grinstead
UK

Barry L Eppley MD, DMD

Associate Professor of Plastic Surgery
Division of Plastic Surgery
Indiana University School of Medicine
Indianapolis, Indiana
USA

Rainer Schmelzeisen MD, DDS

Professor and Chairman,
Department of Oral and Maxillofacial Surgery
Albert-Ludwigs-University and Hospital
Freiburg
Germany

CHURCHILL
LIVINGSTONE

Edinburgh London New York Philadelphia St Louis Sydney Toronto

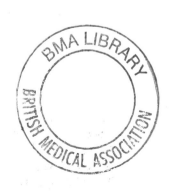

First published 2003

ISBN 0 443 07124 1

British Library Cataloguing in Publication Data
A catalogue record for this book is available from the British Library

Library of Congress Cataloging in Publication Data
A catalog record for this book is available from the Library of Congress

Notice
Medical knowledge is constantly changing. Standard safety precautions must be followed, but as new research and clinical experience broaden our knowledge, changes in treatment and drug therapy may become necessary or appropriate. Readers are advised to check the most current product information provided by the manufacturer of each drug to be administered to verify the recommended dose, the method and duration of administration, and contraindications. It is the responsibility of the practitioner, relying on experience and knowledge of the patient, to determine dosages and the best treatment for each individual patient. Neither the Publisher nor the editors assume any liability for any injury and/or damage to persons or property arising from this publication.

The Publisher

your source for books,
journals and multimedia
in the health sciences
www.elsevierhealth.com

Printed in Spain

The
publisher's
policy is to use
**paper manufactured
from sustainable forests**

Contents

Contributors

Lisa Alexander DClin Psy, BSc(Hons), Dip Hyp
Clinical Psychologist
Department of Psychology
The Queen Victoria Hospital
East Grinstead, UK

Peter Ayliffe FRCS(Eng), FRCS, OMFS(Eng),
MBBS(Lond), FDSRCS(Eng), BDS(Lond)
Consultant Maxillofacial Surgeon
Department of Maxillofacial Surgery
Great Ormond Street Hospital for Children
University College NHS Trust
London, UK

Nicholas J Baker FDSRCS, FRCS, FRCS(Maxfac)
Consultant Oral and Maxillofacial Surgeon
Maxillofacial Unit
Southampton General Hospital
Southampton, UK

Amardip Bhuller MD, FRCSI
Chief Resident
Division of General Surgery
Indiana University School of Medicine
Indianapolis, IN, USA

Stephen E Bond MBBS, FDSRCS, FRCS
Specialist Registrar
John Radcliffe Hospital
Oxford, UK

Rudolf RM Bos DMD, PhD
Professor in Oral and Maxillofacial Surgery
Department of Oral and Maxillofacial Surgery
University Hospital Groningen
Groningen, The Netherlands

Nicholas B Bowley MBBS, DMRD, FRCR
Head of Department and Consultant Radiologist
X-Ray Department
The Queen Victoria Hospital
East Grinstead, UK

Henk J Busscher PhD, MSc
Professor and Chairman of the Department of
Biomedical Engineering
Faculty of Medical Sciences
University of Groningen
Groningen, The Netherlands

Malcolm Cameron FDS, FRCS
Specialist Registrar
Queen Victoria Hospital
East Grinstead, UK

Alex Clarke DPsych, MSc, BSc(Hons), AFBPsS
Consultant Clinical Psychologist
Department of Plastic and Reconstructive Surgery
Royal Free Hospital
London, UK
(formerly Adult Specialist, Changing Faces,
London, UK)

John J Coleman MD
James E Bennett Professor of Surgery,
Chief of Plastic Surgery
Division of Plastic Surgery
Indiana University School of Medicine
Indianapolis, IN, USA

Bernard J Costello DMD, MD
Assistant Professor of Oral and Maxillofacial
Surgery, Pediatric Dentistry and
Pediatric Surgery
Cleft and Craniofacial Center
University of Pittsburgh Medical Center
and Children's Hospital of Pittsburgh
Pittsburgh, PA, USA

John Crossman FRCS
Specialist Registrar in Neurosurgery
Department of Neurosurgery
Newcastle General Hospital
Newcastle upon Tyne, UK

M Devlin MBBS, BDS, FRCS, FDSRCS
Specialist Registrar in Maxillofacial Surgery
Department of Maxillofacial and Oral Surgery
Southern General Hospital
Glasgow, UK

Gordon N Dutton MD, FRCOphth
Consultant Ophthalmologist
Tennent Institute of Ophthalmology
Gartnavel General Hospital
Glasgow, UK

Barry L Eppley MD, DMD
Associate Professor of Plastic Surgery
Division of Plastic Surgery
Indiana University School of Medicine
Indianapolis, IN, USA

Barry T Evans FRCS (Eng & Edin),
FDSRS (Eng), FFDRCS (Ire)
Consultant Oral & Maxillofacial Surgeon
Oral and Maxillofacial Surgery
Southampton General Hospital
Southampton, UK

Miriam A Farley LLB(Hons)
Assistant Solicitor
Kennedys
London, UK

Nils-Claudius Gellrich MD, DMD
Associate Professor
Department of Oral and Maxillofacial Surgery
Albert-Ludwigs-University and Hospital
Freiburg, Germany

Mark M Hamilton MD
Clinical Assistant Professor
Department of Otolaryngology Head
and Neck Surgery
Indiana University School of Medicine
Indianapolis, IN, USA

Stefan Hassfeld MD, DMD, PhD
Senior Lecturer
Maxillofacial and Craniofacial Surgery
Heidelberg University Hospital
Heidelberg, Germany

Jarg-Erich Hausamen MD, DDS, PhD
Professor and Chairman
Klinik und Poliklinik fur Mund-, Kiefer - und
Gesichtschirurgie
Medizinische Hochschule Hannover
Hannover, Germany

C Michael Hill MSc, FDSRCSEd, BDS, MDSc
Consultant Oral and Maxillofacial Surgeon
Department of Oral and Maxillofacial Surgery
University of Wales College of Medicine
Cardiff, UK

Alistair Jenkins MD, FRCS(Ed)
Consultant in Neurosurgery
Department of Neurosurgery
Newcastle General Hospital
Newcastle upon Tyne, UK

David Carl Jones FRCS, FDSRCS
Consultant Maxillofacial Surgeon
Regional Maxillofacial Unit
University Hospital Aintree
Liverpool, UK

David A Koppel MBBS, BDS, FRCS, FDSRCS
Cranio-Maxillofacial Surgeon
Department of Maxillofacial and Oral Surgery
Southern General Hospital
Glasgow, UK

Alexander C Kübler MD, DMD, PhD
Professor and Consultant
Department of Craniomaxillofacial Plastic Surgery
University of Cologne
Cologne, Germany

Dorothy A Lang FRCS
Consultant Neurosurgeon
Wessex Neurological Centre
Southampton University Hospitals Trust
Southampton, UK

Richard A Loukota BDS, MBBS, FDSRCS, FRCS
Consultant Oral and Maxillofacial Surgeon
Department of Oral and Maxillofacial Surgery
Leeds Dental Institute
Leeds, UK

David W Macpherson MBBS, FDSRCS, FRCS
Consultant Maxillofacial Surgeon
The Maxillofacial Unit
St Richard's Hospital, Chichester and
Worthing Hospitals
Chichester, UK

Patrick J McCann MB, BCh, BAO, BDS, FDSRCSEng,
FRCSI
Specialist Registrar Oral & Maxillofacial Surgery,
Department of Oral & Maxillofacial Surgery
Leeds Dental Institute
Leeds, UK

Jeremy D McMahon MBChB, FRACDS, FRCS
Maxillofacial Head and Neck Surgeon
Royal Hallamshire Hospital
Sheffield Teaching Hospitals NHS Trust
Sheffield UK

Shawn McPartland MD, JD
Yosha, Krahulik and Levy
Indianapolis, IN, USA

Khursheed F Moos OBE, MBBS, BDS, FRCS, FDSRCS
Cranio-Maxillofacial Surgeon
Oral Surgery
Glasgow Dental Hospital
Glasgow, UK

Joachim Mühling MD, DMD, PhD
Head, Maxillofacial and Craniofacial Surgery
Heidelberg University Clinic
Heidelberg, Germany

G Neil Dwyer MS (Lon), FRCS (Eng), FRCS (Edin)
Department of Neurosurgery
Wessex Neurological Centre
Southampton University Hospitals Trust
Southampton, UK

Justin Nissen FRCS
Consultant in Neurosurgery
Department of Neurosurgery
Newcastle General Hospital
Newcastle upon Tyne, UK

Chi Wang Peter Pang MBChB(CUHK), FRCS Edin,
FCSHK, FHKAM(Surgery)
Medical and Health Officer
Specialist in Plastic Surgery
Department of Surgery
The Prince of Wales Hospital
Shatin
New Territories
Hong Kong SAR

Parkash Ramchandani MB, BCh, FDSRCS, FRCS
Specialist Registrar in Oral and Maxillofacial
Surgery
Maxillofacial Department
Poole General Hospital
Dorset, UK

David Richardson FRCS, FDSRCS
Consultant Maxillofacial Surgeon
Regional Maxillofacial Unit
University Hospital Aintree
Liverpool, UK

Ramon L Ruiz DMD, MD
Assistant Professor, Oral/Maxillofacial Surgery
and Pediatrics
Associate Director, Pediatric Oral/Maxillofacial
Surgery
University of North Carolina at Chapel Hill
Chapel Hill, NC, USA

Henning Schliephake MD, DDS, PhD
Oral Maxillofacial Surgeon, Facial Plastic Surgeon
Department of Oral and Maxillofacial Surgery
George-Augusta-University
Göttingen, Germany

Rainer Schmelzeisen MD, DDS
Professor and Chairman
Department of Oral and Maxillofacial Surgery
Albert-Ludwigs-University and Hospital
Freiburg, Germany

Ralf Schön DDS, MD
Assistant Professor
Consultant Maxillofacial Surgeon
Department of Oral and Maxillofacial Surgery
Albert-Ludwigs-University and Hospital
Freiburg, Germany

Alexander Schramm DDS, MD
Assistant Professor
Consultant Maxillofacial Surgeon
Department of Oral and Maxillofacial Surgery
Albert-Ludwigs-University and Hospital
Freiburg, Germany

Kenneth J Sneddon BDS, MBBS, FDSRCS, FRCS
Consultant Oral & Maxillofacial Surgeon
Department of Oral & Maxillofacial Surgery
The Queen Victoria Hospital
East Grinstead, UK

Rajiv Sood MD, FACS
Associate Professor of Plastic Surgery
Indiana University School of Medicine
Indianapolis, IN, USA

Leo F A Stassen FRCS (Ed), FDSRCS, MA
Consultant Maxillofacial Surgeon
Sunderland Royal Hospital
Sunderland, UK

David W Thomas FDS, MScD, PhD
Professor of Oral Surgery
Department of Oral and Maxillofacial Surgery
University of Wales
Cardiff, UK

Edward Wai Hei To FRCS(Eng) FFDRCS(Ire)
Consultant Oral and Maxillofacial Surgeon
Oral and Maxillofacial Surgery Center
St Teresa's Hospital
Kowloon , Hong Kong
and Honorary Clincial Associate Professor
Department of Surgery
The University of Hong Kong
Hong Kong, SAR

Man Kwong Tung MBBS(HKU), FRCS(Glasg),
FRCS(Edin), FCSHK, FHKAM(Surgery)
Consultant Plastic Surgeon
Specialist in Plastic Surgery
Department of Surgery
Princess Margaret Hospital
Kowloon, Hong Kong SAR

Anthony G Tyers FRCS(Eng), FRCSEd, FRCOphth
Consultant Ophthalmologist and Ophthalmic
Oculoplastic Surgeon
Department of Ophthalmology
Salisbury District Hospital
Salisbury, UK

Peter Ward Booth FDS, FRCS
Consultant Maxillofacial Surgeon
Department of Maxillofacial Surgery
The Queen Victoria Hospital
East Grinstead, UK

Richard R Welbury MBBS, BDS(Hons), PhD,
FDSRCS(Eng), FDSRCPS(Glasg)
Professor of Paediatric Dentistry
Department of Child Dental Health
Glasgow Dental School and Hospital
Glasgow, UK

Alan W Wilson MB, BCh, FDSRCS, FRCS
Consultant Maxillofacial Surgeon
St Richard's Hospital
Chichester and Worthing Hospitals
Chichester, UK

Joachim E Zöller MD, DMD, PhD
Professor and Head of Department
of Craniomaxillofacial Plastic Surgery
University of Cologne
Cologne
Germany

Preface

Hard and soft tissue facial trauma is one of the three major areas of maxillofacial surgery. Along with cancer of the face and mouth, and facial deformities, facial trauma is subjected to ever-changing scenarios of 'disease' and treatment. For example, whilst increasing patterns of 'disease' (in this case trauma) occur through inter-personal violence, we see a reduction in other areas such as road traffic accidents. As physicians we can do little about these factors, except document these changes.

In contrast, however, changes in treatment are very much in our hands. As maxillofacial surgeons our most important role is to critically understand innovation and hopefully extend our evidence base for all our therapies. As always there is a fine line between waiting for 'gold standard' evidence and depriving our patients of new, potentially better treatments. A similar line must be drawn between the innovation and support provided by industry, and blindly accepting seductive and subtle marketing. One can only be impressed by the comparative studies by, for example, Ed Ellis in Dallas. In contrast one must be wary of the many non-comparative studies which dominate the literature, in which highly profitable devices, apparently offering little therapeutic benefit, are reported in terms seemingly plucked from manufacturers' brochures.

In recent years there have been many innovations, particularly in the field of small plate osteosynthesis, popularised by Maxime Champy. His system, marked by critical evaluation, ushered in a new concept of esthetic trauma treatment, where simply uniting the bones was replaced by accurate open reduction and functional repair. This mirrors in many ways the work of James Brown and his colleagues in Liverpool, in 'rehabilitation' after oncological resection.

This book brings together experts from around the world to demonstrate how facial trauma can be managed and aims to stress the importance of not only returning normal function, but also reconstructing facial esthetics.

The Editors thank all our contributors for their tremendous enthusiasm and support, and are indebted to the large team at Elsevier for their help.

Peter Ward Booth

Section 1
Principles

1 Etiology and Prevention of Craniomaxillofacial Trauma

C Michael Hill, Barry L Eppley, David W Thomas, Stephen E Bond

Introduction

Injuries to the face, head and neck are relatively common and yet, in the overall trauma literature, the etiology of maxillofacial injuries has received relatively little attention. Virtually all injuries result from some form of trauma, which (in terms of surgery) may be defined as 'a physical force resulting in injury'. Injuries may also be the result of chemical, thermal or even radiation trauma but these occur far less commonly than physical trauma.

Despite the frequency of facial injuries there has also been relatively little research until recently into their etiology, treatment and prognosis. This despite the fact that such injuries are clinically important for several reasons.

- The soft tissues and bones of the face give anterior protection to the cranium.
- Facial appearance is a major (if not the most significant) factor in 'appearance'.
- The whole anatomical region is associated with several important functions of daily life including sight, smell, eating, breathing and talking. If any of these suffer significant impairment, it has potentially serious effects on the patient's lifestyle and quality of life.

Trauma has traditionally been classified according to anatomical site. Whilst this is logical in terms of an approach on which to base treatment, in terms of developing strategies to prevent injury it is more informative to consider etiology and the applied forces which produce injuries of differing types. Patterns of injury can be described that relate to certain types of accident and, in relation to forensic evidence, it is important to understand these. In addition, strategies to reduce the injuries being sustained need to be developed since the cost of treatment of maxillofacial injuries can be quite high.

The response of the body to trauma is dependent on the nature of the assault and the response of the victim. The concept of applied force and the extent of injury following trauma is therefore dependent upon several factors. The kinetic energy (or potential to inflict damage) is calculated as the mass of the object striking the face or head multiplied by the velocity squared (usually represented by the formula: $K=MV^2$). Sometimes the situation is the opposite and the momentum is generated by the movement of the head striking a static object, e.g. in a fall. In all cases, however, it is the velocity rather than the mass of an object that has the greater proportional effect because of the kinetic energy generated. This is clearly demonstrable in road traffic accidents where the severity of injuries associated with collisions at speeds over 20 mph (30 kph) is increased compared with those at lower speeds. In such situations, the risk of serious or fatal injury rises disproportionately. The same is evident with high-velocity semi-automatic weapons when compared with rifle or gunshot injuries, which superficially may appear to be more damaging but which seldom cause the same severity of injury.

In most cases, the applied force is predetermined but there are four other variables which affect the type and severity of injury sustained.

- The *position of strike*: the anatomical region where the force is applied.
- The *area of strike*: the wider the area, the more dissipation of force.
- The *resistance*: whether there is any movement of the head or the soft tissues; any restriction of movement potentially increases the severity of injury.
- The *angulation of strike*: a glancing blow causes a less serious injury.

The strength of the soft tissues and underlying bone also plays a part in the extent of any injury but there has been little work to assess susceptibility to injury in these terms.

Classification of Facial Trauma

The classification of maxillofacial trauma is usually related to outcome (i.e. type of injury sustained). It can also be considered with respect to etiology under a variety of headings including assaults, falls, industrial injuries, road traffic accidents (RTAs), animal bites, sports injuries, burns and war injuries. The list is not exhaustive, however, and other categories could be included (e.g. iatrogenic, self-inflicted, etc.). In all published studies, industrial injuries only represent a small percentage of the overall total although it is possible that there is underreporting of such injuries. Many of these are the result of falls at work but equipment breakages also account for a significant proportion.

In reviewing the literature several difficulties exist in comparing published work, due to variations in both data collection and classification of injuries.[1] Soft tissue injuries, nasal bone fractures, dental injuries and dentoalveolar fractures are presented in different ways between centers and, in some studies, they are completely omitted. True comparison of published studies is also made difficult by the frequent use of different selection criteria of injuries and the reporting of retrospective, poorly collected data (which are commonly restricted to either types of injury or etiology). Even so, the existing data have been useful in helping to promote changes in legislation and practise in order to try and reduce the number and extent of maxillofacial injuries.

Attempts to standardize the recording of injury pattern and severity have also been made.[1] With respect to assessing the injury severity associated with maxillofacial trauma, a number of injury severity scales have been described. These have three important uses.

- They promote targeted care, e.g. the Glasgow Coma Scale.[2]
- They help to predict the likely outcome, e.g. the Abbreviated Injury Scale[3] and the Injury Severity Score.[4]
- They encourage the accurate assessment of critically injured patients, e.g. APACHE II.[5]

Whilst it is well recognized that scoring systems are useful for determining the extent of maxillofacial trauma, they do have a number of drawbacks. For example, whilst the International Classification of Diseases (ICD) describes diagnostic codes for most injuries,[6] in practise the coding for patients with multiple craniofacial injuries may be complex[7] and data recovery almost certainly introduces bias in retrospective studies. There can be little doubt, therefore, that the prospective, systematic collection of data is always to be preferred in considering the etiology of facial injuries.

Assault

From a forensic viewpoint, assault can be defined as the perceived threat of an imminent attack. Any act of physical violence is legally referred to as 'battery' although in medical parlance, the word 'assault' has become synonymous with the act of violence itself. The comparative study of the prevalence of maxillofacial trauma as a result of assault (battery) is not easy. This is again due to the fact that relatively few studies have considered consecutive, non-selective data to estimate the pattern of injuries sustained, the actual treatment delivered or the resulting demand for services. It is well accepted, however, that there is an increasing incidence of maxillofacial trauma associated with the rise in interpersonal violence in much of Western society (Fig. 1.1). Whilst in the developed world there has been a pattern of increasing violence in urbanized settings since the Second World War,

figures for the developing nations suggest that this is less evident. With the increase in interpersonal violence in Western society (coupled with the improvements in road safety and car design), assaults are replacing RTAs as the most common etiological factor in maxillofacial trauma[8,9] (Table 1.1) whilst in the Third World this is not yet the case. This trend has been observed in many countries including the USA, UK, Scandinavia, Australia and New Zealand.[10-14] The pattern in other societies is, however, different with RTAs often remaining the most common cause of maxillofacial trauma.[15-17] In Holland RTAs still predominate but this is due to the number of bicycle accidents that occur.

When considering interpersonal violence, the frequency with which the face is involved in assaults has been shown by one study to be approaching half of all reported cases. Indeed, approximately 40% of attendances at casualty departments relating to assaults had facial injuries in that study and almost 30% of assault victims had fractures. Eighty three percent of these fractures affected the facial skeleton.[18] The inexorable rise in interpersonal violence has therefore directly increased the trauma workload, particularly for oral and maxillofacial surgeons especially with regard to the more serious facial injuries.[19]

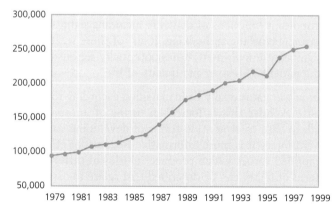

Fig. 1.1: The increasing incidence of violence in the United Kingdom as demonstrated by government statistics.

Table 1.1 The etiology of facial injuries in different studies around the world

	Australia	NZ	Japan	Norway	UK	USA	India	Nigeria	Tanzania
Assaults	52	32	15.5	49	52	49	25	43	14.5
RTAs	19	30	38.5	14	16	43	40	27	81
Sports	16	20	16.5	8	19	4	4	9	<2
Falls	10	9	28.5	15	11	3.5	24	18	<2
Industrial	1.5	~	0.3	9	2	0.5	1.3	3	1
Others	1.5	9	0.7	4	~	~	1.2	~	~
Reference	7	12	15	22	81	83	16	38	13

In assault cases (with the exception of the sex of the assailant which is usually male), the single most important etiological factor appears to be alcohol consumption. This may be the case for both the assailant and/or the victim. Almost 50% of patients are found to have increased blood alcohol (>100 mg/dL) and alcohol abuse has been described as a contributing factor to assault in almost all independent studies.[20,21] It is, of course, difficult to get accurate figures of the numbers of assailants who have consumed alcohol since so many escape. It is, however, widely reported and the fact that so many assaults take place in or around locations where alcoholic beverages are supplied gives further confirmation to this hypothesis. In the British Association of Oral and Maxillofacial Surgeons' survey of facial injuries (an intensive multicenter study), 55% of assaults were related to alcohol consumption and 24% of the facial injuries recorded were caused by assaults, but this study still is incomplete and formal testing of all involved was not possible.

The victims of trauma from assaults are most frequently young adult males in the 18–25 age group and they are most commonly assaulted by an unknown assailant.[8] The individuals affected tend to be employed in manual labor, leading to a suggestion that there may be a causal link between social deprivation and aggression. This has not been confirmed in other studies, however.[22] Facial injuries typically occur in a bar or a public place within close proximity and frequently late at night.[18,23] The relative effects of cumulative alcohol consumption compounded by the effects of tiredness have not been independently studied but they would appear to offer a simple reason why this should be the case. In particular, the relationship between alcohol and assault seems to be even clearer in the UK study which showed that in those over 15 years of age, alcohol consumption was associated with 90% of facial injuries occurring in bars, 45% in the street and 25% in the home situation. Nearly a quarter of all facial injuries in all age groups were related to alcohol consumption within 4 hours of the injury.

Studies within large cities show that assaults often occur within a relatively limited geographical area and that they tend to be focused in areas adjacent to licensed premises.[24] Interestingly, assaults make up a slightly larger proportion of facial injuries in A&E departments in cities (26%) than in county towns (21%).

Whereas males are more commonly assaulted by unknown assailants, the converse is true of female victims. The location is also different with a typical example being a partner or ex-partner assaulting them in or around the home. In addition, a greater percentage of women are assaulted at home in county towns (52%) compared to cities (38%), whilst fewer females are assaulted in public bars in county towns. The number of injuries caused by female assailants is small but there is some evidence that it is growing. Again, alcohol appears to be the main factor in the etiology of such attacks.

The pattern of injury sustained depends largely on the 'implement' used. Whilst studies on maxillofacial trauma have often considered bony injury in isolation, a number of studies have shown that soft tissue lacerations are, in fact, the most common maxillofacial injuries sustained.[25,26] Despite

their frequency, soft tissue injuries are often overlooked in studying trauma epidemiology. It should be remembered, however, that over 66% of the injuries sustained in assaults are lacerations and almost 40% of *all* assault victims have facial lacerations.[18] Interestingly, this figure rises to 95% of victims in domestic violence.[27] Soft tissue injuries are most frequently inflicted by direct, blunt trauma and although stab injuries to the face are uncommon,[28] the use of broken glass or blades was responsible for 11% of facial injuries in one study.[18]

A number of studies have considered hard tissue injuries in isolation. Fractures occur most frequently following assaults, in descending frequency, in the nasal bones, the mandible, zygoma and midface. This finding is in contrast to the pattern of injury observed in RTAs, where injuries principally affect the midface (see below). The pattern of injury will be affected greatly by the weapon selected. In the past the use of fists, feet, blunt instruments and broken glass has been common. More recently, the increased use of baseball bats and automatic and semi-automatic weapons in premeditated assaults, principally in the US, has had a considerable impact on the extent and pattern of injuries presenting for treatment in some studies.[29–31] Despite attempts to reduce the incidence of injuries due to assault[32] (including education about alcohol consumption, the introduction of drinking glasses made of toughened safety glass in licensed premises, increased policing and improved street lighting) the available data suggest that the rise in maxillofacial trauma due to assaults and interpersonal violence will unfortunately probably continue for some time yet.

Medicolegal Description of Injuries

Bruises or contusions

A bruise is the result of subcutaneous bleeding following impact from a blunt object. Bruises may be seen adjacent to lacerations or abrasions but they frequently occur without the skin being ruptured. The extent of any bruising is a factor of the severity of the impact, the laxity of the tissues, the individual's propensity to bruising and age (older people and children being most susceptible). Particular care needs to be taken, therefore, in trying to correlate severity of a blow with the extent of bruising, particularly in older patients where bruising can be disproportionately excessive.

Abrasions

An abrasion is a superficial wound, which does not fully penetrate the dermis. The point at which an abrasion may be termed a laceration is not always easy to determine since deeper abrasions frequently bleed (sometimes excessively) and must, therefore, have penetrated the dermis. This is especially noticeable after a RTA where the head may have skidded over a gravel surface. Careful examination of abrasions will often reveal a 'heaping' of skin at the distal end of impact. This raised skin or small skin tags can indicate the direction of impact and can thus be useful in helping to establish possible causes. In addition, deeper wounds are often accompanied by foreign bodies – wood splinters, road dirt, paint specks and the like – all of which can be used to provide forensic evidence. It is clearly good medical practice to clean wounds before repair or dressing but few practitioners collect any debris from a wound, a practice which could be of considerable legal benefit.

Lacerations

A laceration is a full-thickness wound of the skin caused by compressing the skin against the bone with a blunt object. This may be a blunt weapon (e.g. a fist or bat) but it may be the result of the head hitting a blunt object such as may result from a fall. There is no way of distinguishing the cause with certainty unless the wound contains foreign matter. On occasion it can also be difficult to distinguish a laceration from an incision although the former usually shows mild inversion of the wound edges on close examination, a feature not seen in wounds caused by sharp objects. Lacerations may bleed profusely but they frequently do not due to the retraction of the blood vessels that were compressed during the creation of the laceration.

Incisions

An incision is a full-thickness skin wound caused by a sharp instrument. If the length of the wound exceeds its depth it is referred to as a slash wound and if the converse is true, a stab wound. The clinical appearance of a slash wound is affected by the muscular pull and the crease lines of the skin. Such wounds may bleed profusely and it is not always easy to identify and occlude vessels that have been cut. From a forensic point of view, it is not easy to glean much information from a slash wound although the deeper end of the incision tends to be the origin. Ragged edges may suggest a blunter implement but the actual type of implement used cannot be categorized with any certainty. Although stab wounds to the face are less common they do yield more forensic information and good close-up photographs of such wounds should be taken before suturing. Multiple stab wounds in the region of the neck should also lead the clinician to consider a possible diagnosis of attempted suicide although the use of other areas of the body (chest, wrists) remains more common.

Road Traffic Accidents

Motor car accidents

RTAs are a major health problem which, in the US alone, account for an estimated 50 000 deaths and over 3 million injuries annually. Although RTAs are frequently associated with severe maxillofacial injuries the majority of injuries are facial lacerations. The 15 years following the Second World War comprised the greatest source of maxillofacial trauma in many studies in Western countries (Table 1.1).[33] Whilst in the developing world RTAs still account for the majority of maxillofacial trauma,[34-37] the introduction of seat-belt and drink-driving legislation, as well as improvements in car

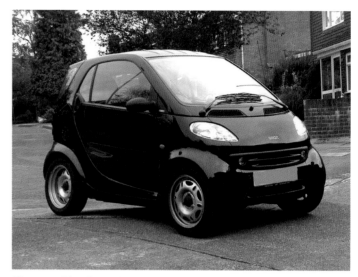

Fig. 1.2: The 'Smart' microcar – small in size but big in safety features.

design (see below), has greatly decreased the incidence of fatalities and RTA-associated maxillofacial trauma.[38,39] This serves to illustrate not only the progress of car design but also the benefits of studying the detailed etiology of facial trauma. The most important factor in determining the extent of injury which patients sustain in RTAs is the direction of the collision, i.e. drivers involved in head-on collisions have an 18% increase in survival.

In the last 30 years modern cars have developed an impressive array of safety features to reduce the risk of serious injury (Fig. 1.2). Some improvements are principally design features in the car itself such as crumple zones, collapsing steering wheels and side impact bars. Others have involved the development of new technologies (often adopted from the aviation industry), including improved seat restraint, laminated windscreens, airbags, computerized warning systems and anti-lock and assisted braking systems.[40] Improvements can also be made to the environment such as improved road design, better signposting and lighting as well as innovations like rumble strips and bright 'cats' eyes'.

External support devices for prevention

Technical support and/or protective devices play a significant role in either preventing facial injuries or significantly reducing the magnitude of the facial damage. Such devices can be differentiated between protective devices that are installed as part of vehicles or sporting equipment and those devices that are carried or worn by the individual.

The decrease in maxillofacial trauma associated with RTAs has been dramatic. In the UK, figures demonstrate how in the past 20 years, whilst car ownership increased rapidly, the total incidence of facial fractures associated with RTAs has decreased by a third.[41] Most encouragingly, however, the percentage of all facial fractures associated with RTAs decreased from 46.8% in 1948 to 18.6% over the same period.[33] Furthermore, not only has the incidence of maxillofacial trauma diminished but the severity of injuries has also decreased from 54% of the midfacial injuries being at Le Fort II and III levels in 1948–1955 to 8.6% in 1987–1993.[33] These dramatic improvements have followed the introduction of drink-drive legislation in the 1970s and compulsory seat-belt wearing which was introduced in the UK in 1983. This reduced the incidence of facial injuries in patients involved in RTAs from 21% to 6% in less than 2 years.[42] Similar findings have been noted in several other countries although in Japan, Tanaka et al[15] reported that seat-belt legislation had not made a great difference to the pattern of facial injuries. In another Japanese paper, Imai et al concluded that the number of mid-facial fractures was significantly reduced.[43] It is difficult to postulate why these findings differ and whether the perceived lack of improvement may have been due to poor compliance or an already low incidence. Compliance with seat-belt legislation is another area where there is consider-able national variation. Despite the proven benefits of seat-belts, it is interesting to note that almost 70% of individuals involved in RTAs were not using any form of restraint whatsoever. Particularly alarming was the finding in a study of pediatric facial trauma in RTAs in the US, which demon-strated that only 138 of 412 children with facial trauma were restrained at the time of impact.

Seat-belts and lap-belts

Seat-belts work in three separate ways. The first, and perhaps most obvious, is the restraint of the person within the vehicle, thereby preventing evulsion through the windscreen. Secondly, they spread the area over which the energy of impact is dissipated and thirdly they are made of a fabric that has a slight degree of elasticity. This spreads the time over which the energy of impact is dissipated.

The current three-point combination lap and diagonal belt positioned across the pelvis and rib cage was developed by a Swedish aircraft engineer and was introduced in 1959. This provides a strong three-point harness with a simple pendulum and ratchet mechanism that locks the belt in sudden-stop situations. The lap-belt spreads crash forces across the strong pelvic bone and keeps the passenger from being tossed around the car, while the shoulder harness spreads forces across the rib cage and prevents the upper body from jack-knifing forward. In the United States, this three-point system has been mandatory in automobiles since 1974 and saves thousands of lives every year.[44]

It is universally accepted that seat- and lap-belt use is asso-ciated with a lower risk of serious injury, particularly to the head and face (Fig. 1.3). The difference in injury rates is so significant that their use by passengers is mandated by law in

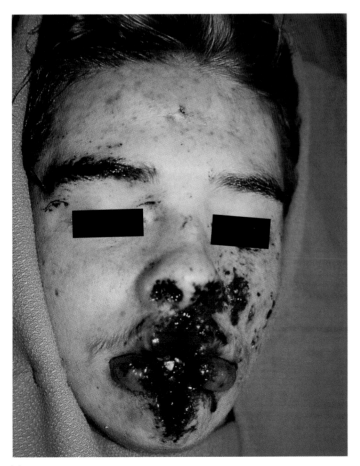

(a)

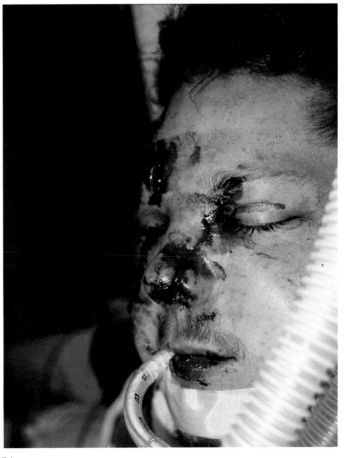

(b)

Fig. 1.3: The combination of seat-belts and lap-belts prevents the face from either 'eating the steering wheel' if you are the driver or direct impact onto either the dashboard or back of the seat if you are a passenger. (**a**) Unrestrained driver in motor vehicle accident. (**b**) Unrestrained passenger in motor vehicle accident.

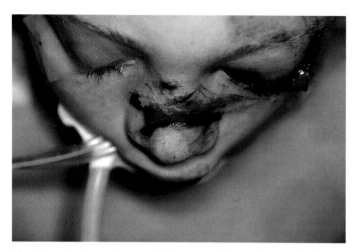

Fig. 1.4: Pediatric (4-year-old) female with nasal and orbital fractures who was not restrained in a car seat.

every state in America and is punishable by monetary fines when the driver is found in violation. Despite these recognized safety facts, it is appalling how frequently they are not used (up to 33% of front seat occupants), particularly when looking at trauma registry records.

In pediatric motor vehicle trauma, the restraint rate is improved over adults (78%) from the latest National Pediatric Trauma Registry information from 92 centers reporting throughout the United States. This is typically higher than that seen in adults, probably due to the effects of pediatric education campaigns and the requirement by law of their use up to the age of 4 or 40 lbs in weight (Fig. 1.4).

Despite its craniofacial protection, severe systemic injuries still do occur in belted individuals.[45,46] Certain specific injuries do occur with belt use, the so-called seat-belt syndrome, and have included cervical, lumbar and intra-abdominal injuries. With the exception of sternal fractures, however, more recent critical analysis suggests that injuries

previously associated with the seat-belt syndrome occur in similar proportions of belted and unbelted patients.

Airbags

Like seat-belts and lap-belts, the airbag has proven to be effective in reducing injury and fatalities in motor vehicle accidents.[47,48] They work best when combined with a belted driver, reducing fatalities by more than 50%. In an unbelted driver, fatalities are reduced by up to one-third and the decrease in facial injuries is obvious given the prevention of direct facial impact onto the steering wheel, dashboard or seat (Fig. 1.5). Airbags probably provide the single best protection of all automotive safety devices for the driver, preventing lacerations and facial fractures. Among passengers, interestingly, airbags have been reported to reduce the incidence of facial lacerations but not of fractures.

The airbag is a round inflatable nylon bag which is slightly larger than the steering wheel and less than 1 foot in thickness at its central section when fully inflated. It is deployed when sudden longitudinal deceleration occurs through sensors located within the forward portion of the vehicle. The deployment is nearly instantaneous, becoming fully inflated in about 0.01 second and coming out of the dashboard at rates up to 200 miles per hour, faster than the blink of an eye. This provides a temporary cushion which is then deflated over several seconds by the release of hot gases through exhaust ports on the back of the airbag. Its use has been mandated by the United States Congress with the requirement of dual airbags in all new passenger cars since 1997 and in all vans, trucks and utility vehicles since 1998.

While severe facial trauma is clearly reduced by airbags, some facial injuries still occur. The rapid deployment is caused by a combustion process which releases a significant amount of heat. It is possible that this heat can burn a patient's face but the exhaust ports are positioned such that they blow away from the driver. More commonly, burns attributed to airbags are minor and are frictional in nature

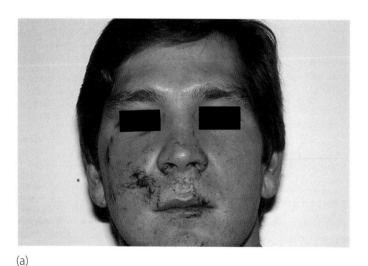

(a)

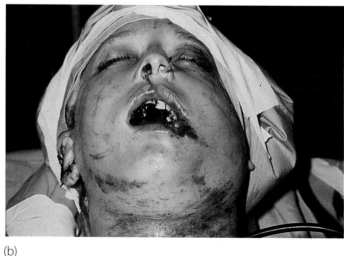

(b)

Fig. 1.5: The deployment of airbags significantly reduces the magnitude of facial injuries from motor vehicle accidents. (**a**) Minimal facial injuries (abrasions, small lacerations) with the use of an airbag in a restrained driver. (**b**) Significant facial injuries (Le Fort fractures) affecting an unrestrained driver with no airbag.

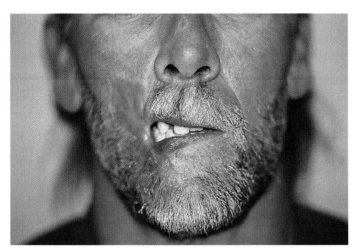

Fig. 1.6: Airbags can cause some minor injuries, particularly friction burns. This 35-year-old male suffered significant burns from an airbag, sustaining full-thickness injury to the right commissure and cheek with resultant severe contracture.

due to high-velocity fabric impact to the face, chin and neck (Fig. 1.6). More serious, however, is the potential for alkali burns to the eye due to the fine aerosol byproducts of combustion including sodium hydroxide, sodium carbonate and other metallic oxides.[49] This risk as well as frictional burns can be decreased by positioning the driver's seat as far back as possible when driving to decrease the force of the airbag deployment onto the face. In addition, the risk of injury to children can be prevented by never having an infant in the front seat of a vehicle with an airbag and children under 12 should always be properly restrained in a child safety seat or safety belt and ride in the back seat.

Side impact airbags have also been developed and are currently available on more expensive models.

Some controversy remains over the influence of airbags on the pattern of injury sustained in RTAs. Recent data, however, conclusively show that the deployment of a driver's airbag in a collision significantly prevents facial fractures although the protective benefit for patients against facial lacerations was unproven[48]. Abbreviated injury Scale (AIS) scores in another US study showed an AIS of 1.13 for the airbag group plus seat-belt, AIS 1.29 for seat-belt only and AIS 1.46 for unrestrained groups.

Other safety features

Of other safety features in cars, the introduction of laminated safety glass for windscreens has virtually eliminated the multiple penetrating facial and frontal injuries that were regularly seen in casualty departments after RTAs.

Summary

Injuries resulting from RTAs typically affect males in the 18–25 year age group.[7] The fractures incurred in these accidents are due to rapid deceleration and direct impact of the head usually with the steering wheel, frame of the car or dashboard. Numerous studies have shown that the typical injuries are commonly midfacial, principally affecting the nasal bones, zygoma and maxilla. The incidence and severity of maxillofacial injury vary greatly in different parts of the world and in some countries there is still evidence that RTAs represent the most common cause of maxillofacial fractures.[15,34–37,44]

Motorcycle accidents

Motorcycle accidents only account for approximately 50% of all traffic-related injuries. Studies have shown that most of the remaining injuries are related to motor and pedal cycles with relatively few pedestrian accidents. The incidence and severity of head injuries associated with motorcycle accidents have been reduced drastically with the mandatory introduction of crash helmets and drink-driving legislation.[45] The reduction in the risk of death when wearing a crash helmet has been shown to be almost 30%. Consequently, crash helmets are compulsory even for pedal cyclists in parts of Australia.[7] In some countries, however, they are not even compulsory for motorcycle riders and in regions of China (where helmet wearing is rare) almost 60% of head injuries relate to motorcycling accidents.

The incidence of facial injuries in motorcycle and foot-powered cycling accidents is predictably significant. Average numbers range from one-third to one-half of all such accidents resulting in facial trauma which obviously varies dependent upon the hospital setting, the study population and the case identification methods. The magnitude of the facial trauma is understandably higher in motorcycles as opposed to cycles due to the higher speeds involved and open traffic conditions in which they occur.

Helmets

The scientific evidence that helmets protect against head, brain and facial injuries from motorcycle and pedal cycling accidents has been well established by multiple well-designed case-controlled studies.[51,52] Helmet use in motorcycle riders not only decreases the risk of facial injuries by more than 50% compared to riders without helmets but is also associated with fewer fractures and a decreased number of moderate and severe systemic injuries (Fig. 1.7). Studies have also shown a lower incidence of facial injuries among those riders who used a full-face helmet compared with open-face and jet helmets.

Facial injuries to non-motorized cyclists occur at a rate comparable to head injuries. Helmets are protective against trauma to the upper and midfacial regions, reducing injuries by two-thirds. A well-fitting helmet only covers the forehead but the midface gets some protection, probably through a shadow effect. Historically, the use of protective headwear amongst cyclists was quite low throughout the world. Helmet use has risen dramatically recently in many areas of the world due to community-wide helmet campaigns and legislative efforts. As cycle speed is an independent risk factor for injury, it should be compulsory that recreational riders as well as the serious competitor use helmets.

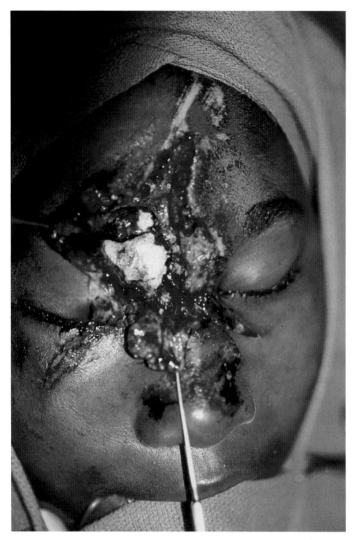

(a)

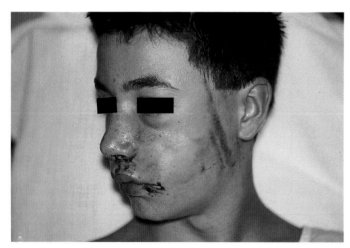

(b)

Fig. 1.7: The lack of any safety gear in low-velocity motorized vehicle accidents is a frequent source of facial injuries in young patients. (**a**) Eight-year-old female with open frontal sinus fractures from a head-on collision with a pole while driving a moped. (**b**) Fourteen-year-old male with zygomaticomaxillary fractures sustained while driving a motorbike.

Despite the incontrovertible evidence, it is alarming to note that a large number of car occupants and motorcyclists involved in RTAs failed to wear either safety belts or crash helmets. These findings may be partially explained by the association of injuries with alcohol[50] and/or drugs.[51] The other factor that significantly affects the injury severity is the speed at which an accident occurs. Because of the concept of applied force/kinetic energy ($K=\frac{1}{2}MV^2$), even small increases in speed result in disproportionate intensification of injury. The converse is inevitably true: small reductions in speed reduce the seriousness of injuries sustained.

Cycling injuries

Cycling has seen a rise in popularity in recent years and much attention has been given to the prevention of head injury in cyclists.

In the UK, as in the US, at present there is no legal requirement to wear protective helmets. A 2-year case-controlled trial in the US reported serious facial injuries to 20.7% of patients attending A&E following cycling accidents.[53,54] After adjustments for age, sex, speed and surface, it was concluded that helmets reduced the risk of lacerations and fractures to the upper and middle face by 65% but had no effect in preventing serious injury to the lower face. One recommendation is that consideration is given to the fitting of chin protection, which may decrease the risk to the lower face. A prototype helmet of this kind has recently been developed (Fig. 1.8). Its

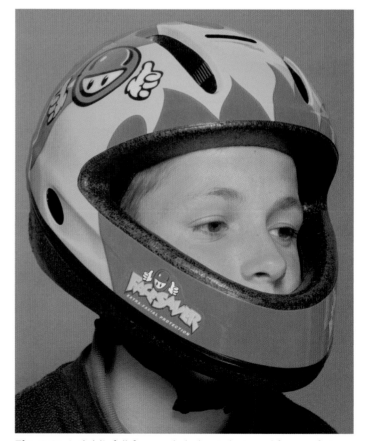

Fig. 1.8: A child's full-face cycle helmet designed for comfort and better facial protection.

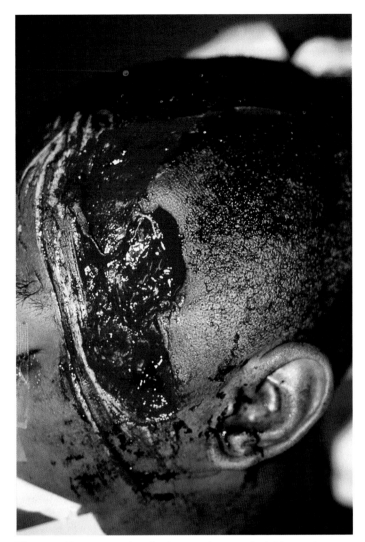

Fig. 1.9: Teenage male who incurred severe facial lacerations from a tree branch while falling from a mountain bike.

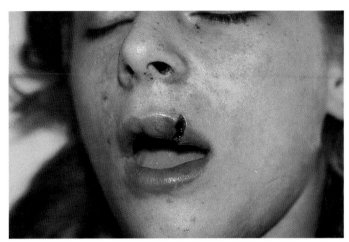

Fig. 1.10: Facial laceration sustained while falling from roller blades and striking the face on a mailbox.

acceptance will depend on creating an ethos within the younger age group that encourages use of helmets rather than resenting them, as is largely the case at present.

The epidemiology of maxillofacial injuries observed in pedestrians is in marked contrast to those of drivers with more severe cranial fractures and increased AIS scores. Injuries to pedestrians more frequently affect children and complex craniomaxillofacial trauma represents an important cause of mortality and morbidity in the community.[52]

Mountain bike-related accidents show a different profile of facial injuries, probably reflecting the terrain in which they are ridden (Fig. 1.9). Cycling accidents result in a higher percentage of facial fractures, especially severe midfacial fractures, and more associated systemic injuries. This strongly suggests that the addition of face guards to helmets, particularly in this specialty riding group, should be considered.

Two more recent additions to recreational activities for non-athletes that pose facial injury risks are in-line skating (roller blading) and skate boarding. In the past decade, roller blading has generated great participation and is a good aerobic

workout. However, it is not without risk and between 1993 and 1995, nearly 100 000 skaters were injured enough to require emergency care. Nearly 20% of roller-blading injuries were to the head, face or chin (Fig. 1.10). Of these injured skaters, nearly half (46%) were wearing no safety equipment and only 7% of those hurt were fully outfitted, including a helmet. In contrast, the traditional form of skate boarding in which jumping and aerobatic manuevers are done has always been associated with safety wear due to the more obvious risk exposure (Fig. 1.11). A most recent variation of this activity has been the advent of the 'scooter' form of skate boarding in which an upright handle has been added to the front of the board (sometimes known as a 'razor scooter'). This now enables the very young and inexperienced to enjoy this form of street boarding. Due to the small size of the front wheel beneath the handle, injury risk is also significant as it can easily get caught in small depressions and flip the rider. The presence of the upright handlebar puts the face at more risk than in traditional skate boarding and safety equipment should always be used.

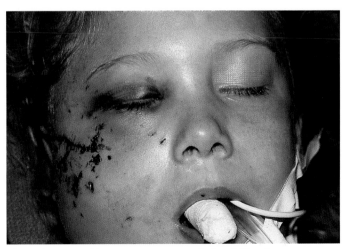

Fig. 1.11: Facial lacerations sustained after falling from a skateboard and being struck by the tip of the board on the way down.

Gun and War Injuries

War has been a feature in some part of the world for almost the whole of the 20th century. In addition to conventional war, the rise of terrorism has added yet another dimension to the potential for war-like injuries. Where prevalent, it is an important cause of facial injuries, previous studies having shown that 16% of all such injuries were to the head and neck. The pattern and extent of war injuries have changed with the development of armaments technology and the use of anti-personnel devices. Correspondingly, the role of the maxillofacial surgeon in the treatment of these injuries has developed from providing a small amount of technical assistance to being pivotal in the management of injured personnel. Studies of US servicemen showed that the principal cause of injury at all sites in wartime was shrapnel from exploding armaments, represented some 60% of Second World War injuries and 75% of all injuries in the Vietnam conflict.[55,56] Despite these figures, Dobson *et al* were unable to demonstrate any evidence of increases in the overall numbers of maxillofacial injuries associated with wars over the past 80 years.[56]

Injuries sustained as a result of high-velocity bullets to the head and neck are frequently fatal due to the dispersal of energy distant to the entry site. Whilst in past wars, young adult males have been principally affected, recent conflicts have shown dramatic rises in the numbers of females and children wounded.[57]

Although the incidence of war injuries obviously varies throughout the world, in Western societies gunshot wounds are becoming more common at the present time and are most likely to be the result of violent crime or attempted suicide rather than a result of war/terrorism.[7]

Modern warfare has considerably changed the pattern of facial injuries and this can clearly be seen in the evolution of the literature on maxillofacial injuries of this etiology. In the US, shotgun injuries are more common in both assault and attempted suicide.[58] Despite figures showing that the US has an eightfold higher incidence in gun fatalities than all its economic counterparts combined, the gun lobby in the States remains a powerful and vocal body, presenting gun ownership as a human rights issue. It is salutary to realize that over 30 000 people die annually in the US alone from gunshot wounds, of whom approximately half are suicides.

Sports Injuries

Participating in sports has become increasingly popular in recent years and this has focused attention on the epidemiology of sports injuries. A limited number of studies have investigated the type and etiology of maxillofacial injuries associated with sports.[59] Workers have investigated both the overall distribution and severity of sports trauma and that associated with individual sports.[60–63] It must be remembered, however, that the treatment of such injuries relates not only to the repair of maxillofacial and dentoalveolar fractures but also to the treatment of soft tissue injuries.

There are differing ways of classifying generalized sports injuries but they have commonly been classified as acute or repetitive. In terms of maxillofacial injuries, however, the vast majority of such injuries in most published surveys of maxillofacial trauma are acute. The etiology of sports-related trauma varies throughout the world according to the type of sports played in a particular country. Consequently, the reporting of sports injuries varies considerably between studies and countries and also within sports.[59,61,62] Whilst the face is the most frequently affected area of the body in some studies, in others the limbs are more commonly affected.[61] A prospective UK study demonstrated that almost 80% of injuries solely affect the soft tissues, confirming that investigating facial fractures alone or dentoalveolar injuries associated with sports does not accurately indicate maxillofacial service demand.

Predictably again, the majority of injuries occur in young males in the 18–25 year age range. In virtually all sports played by both genders, there is always a positive male:female ratio which has varied in various studies from 1.2:1 to 3:1. The seasonal presentation of patients with sports injuries in the UK is interesting, the incidence of these injuries being highest at the beginning of the main sporting season (late August through to October). This presumably results from a low level of general fitness and the lack of timing that follows a long period of rest. A decreased incidence of sports injuries has previously been noted in fit, professional athletes. When type of sport was considered, rugby was the sport most commonly associated with facial injuries in the UK, a finding previously published in studies of facial fractures in both the UK and Japan where rugby is increasing in popularity.

Studies in both the UK and the US have shown how prevention has decreased the number of dental/dentoalveolar injuries.[64] The reason for the reduction may be the increased use of mouthguards and protective headgear but it may also be due to better safety awareness in general.[64] The relatively low incidence of facial injuries in contact sports may reflect the wearing of mouthguards and protective headgear but it may also be a result of under reporting.

Several other factors can be identified in relation to risk, including a 5 mm+ overjet, being left-handed and parental attitude. Another obvious factor is the relative prevalence of any particular sport. For example, skiing injuries are self-evidently unknown in countries without snow. However, in those countries where skiing is a national pastime, skiing or ice sport-related injuries may be a significant proportion of the overall workload of the oral and maxillofacial surgeon.

Falls

The etiology of injuries sustained as a result of falls is somewhat different to other facial injuries since they usually result from impact onto a static object of variable size and density. Whereas maxillofacial trauma associated with assaults, RTAs and sports is found predominantly in the 17–26 year age group, a bimodal age distribution can be identified in the pattern of fall injuries. The initial peak occurs in the first 10 years and the second (as frailty increases) in patients over 65.[66] In the younger age group males are predominantly affected, whereas in the older age groups females have a somewhat higher incidence of fractures. The reasons for this are not entirely clear but probably relate to changes in bone density.

The distribution and severity of maxillofacial injuries sustained following a fall are dependent on the terminal velocity and mass of the victim and the density, mobility and area of contact of the object that has been struck. There are two distinct patterns of fall injuries: tripping whilst walking or running or falling from a height. The latter is more common in the developing world where lack of safety measures and design inadequacies frequently contribute to accidents particularly amongst children. In the majority of published series from the developing world, falls are usually the second most frequent cause of maxillofacial injuries, accounting for up to 40% of injuries in some studies, although 15–20% is more common.

The actual injury pattern in this type of accident is affected by the ability (or otherwise) of a victim to cushion the fall with outstretched arms and to involuntarily rotate the head as it approaches its target. In high-speed falls, the central section of the face is more vulnerable with a tendency to sustain dentoalveolar injuries, avulsed teeth, fractured nasal bones and abrasions. If the arms are pushed forwards, there is usually rotation of the body and head so that the injury pattern is more often unilateral with the zygoma and mandible more frequently involved. For some reason, the left side of the face is slightly more commonly affected than the right side. The younger patients tend to have higher rates of distal extremity injuries on falling whereas the elderly tend to have a more central type of injury, including to the face and scalp possibly due to diminished protective reflexes. Repeated falls in the elderly should be thoroughly investigated to determine whether there is a treatable medical or social cause for the falls.[66]

It is obviously impossible to eliminate the incidence of falls completely but, as mentioned earlier, many can be prevented. In the developing world, working and living on mountainous terrain, inadequate or absent railings and open-plan windows all increase the risk of falls occurring. All these situations are readily amenable to safety improvements (at a comparatively low cost) and are relatively rarely reported as places of injury in developed countries, where legislation and fear of litigation often dictate safety design features.

Prevention

Medical prevention

Medical prevention primarily involves the use of numerous medications to treat various abnormal physiologic conditions that may result in traumas by falling. These include such medical problems as circulatory disturbances and vasovagal reactions, transient ischemic attacks from intracranial and carotid vessel arteriosclerosis and adequate insulin replacement in severe diabetes, to name a few. This is a pharmaco-

logic approach to prevent the side effects that may occur from loss of consciousness and subsequent falls.

One of the most common traumatic effects from facial accidents is dental injury. Tooth fracture, luxation and avulsion can be partially prevented in some patients by proper and regular dental care and maintenance. The preservation of alveolar bone height by long-term tooth retention and periodontal care will prevent complete tooth avulsion in some cases and may make it more likely that splinting loose teeth

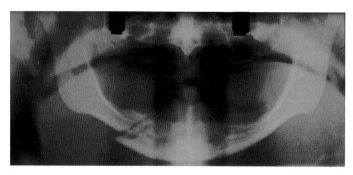

(a)

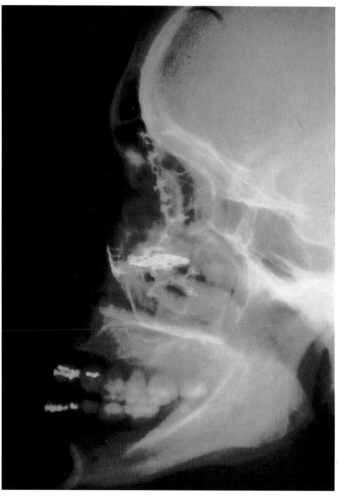

(b)

Fig. 1.12: Significant loss of alveolar bone (edentulous) weakens the jaw bones and predisposes them to fracture. (**a**) Fracture of mandibular body. (**b**) Repair of severe zygomaticomaxillary fracture in edentulous maxilla.

will be successful. In addition, some facial injuries will be avoided by better maxillomandibular bone stock preservation which can absorb and transfer more force without fracture (Fig. 1.12).

Orthodontic and/or orthognathic correction of severe malocclusions, particularly those in which the anterior teeth are in a proclined position, can help decrease the number of traumatized teeth. Early removal of impacted third molars and subsequent replacement by bone decreases the risk of suffering a mandibular angle fracture later in life although this is not an indication for prophylactic removal of wisdom teeth.

Prevention through external support devices

Mouthguards/protectors

With the increased participation and competitiveness of athletics around the world, sports-related injuries are occurring more frequently than ever before. In particular, orofacial trauma to the teeth, gums and lips is more prevalent. Fractured, partially avulsed and completely knocked out teeth are common, with associated lacerations to the gums, tongue and lips (Fig. 1.13). In the United States, the National Youth Sports Foundation estimates that more than 5 million teeth will be knocked out and over 200 000 other oral injuries will occur in sporting activities each year. Fortunately, many orofacial injuries can be prevented through the use of a mouthguard.[65]

Although mouthguards have been used in boxing for almost a century and have been advocated by the American Dental Association in football and hockey for several decades, many participants in other sports such as basketball, soccer, baseball and rugby have been reluctant to wear them. The benefits of wearing a sports mouthguard have been well documented. In football where mouthguards are mandatory, for example, less than 1% of all injuries involve the teeth and mouth. Conversely, in basketball where mouthguards are not routinely worn, more than one-quarter of all player injuries involve the teeth, tongue and lips. Mouthguards provide a number of advantages to the amateur and professional athlete alike. The most obvious advantage is the protection of the teeth which is achieved by the separation of the dental arches by a plastic interface. They protect against oral lacerations and contusions by holding the lips and cheek tissues away from the teeth. In addition, by absorbing and distributing the force of the impact, the risk of mandibular angle and condylar fractures is decreased. When properly fitted, mouthguards are comfortable to wear and provide no obstruction to breathing.

Mouthguards come in two basic types: stock, which are typically found in stores ('boil' and bite'), and custom fabricated which are made by a dentist. In comparing the two types, stock mouthguards do not fit as accurately as custom guards, are often uncomfortable and frequently interfere with breathing and speaking. In addition, stock guards provide a false sense of protection due to a dramatic decrease in interocclusal thickness when one bites it into place in the

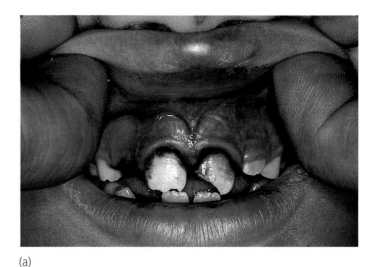

(a)

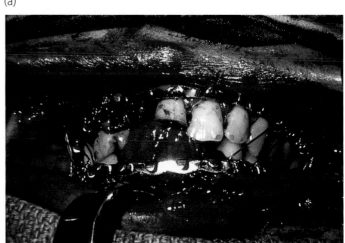

(b)

Fig. 1.13: Dentoalveolar injuries are common in sporting events and can be reduced by wearing a mouthguard. (**a**) Loose teeth and crown fracture from a mouth injury in soccer. (**b**) Multiple avulsed/fractured teeth and a mandible fracture sustained in a rugby match.

softened state. Given that the total replacement cost for a single knocked-out tooth is more than 20 times the cost for a custom-fabricated mouthguard, it makes sense that every person should wear one if the sport involves contact or the possibility of falling. This is specially true in sports such as football, hockey, basketball, boxing, rugby, lacrosse, martial arts, soccer, skating and cycling.

Whilst the overall severity of maxillofacial sports injuries tends to be less serious than those sustained in assaults or RTAs, facial bone fractures remain common.[58] Research into the etiology of sports injuries has shown how the numbers and severity of these injuries can be reduced with appropriate rule changes and improved protective clothing where necessary. Vacuum-formed mouthguards are particularly effective at preventing dental injuries and the newer, bimaxillary mouthguards (Fig. 1.14) give added support to the mandible. Whether they decrease the risk of injury to the mandible or maxilla is uncertain but they are popular with players once they have got used to them. Overall,

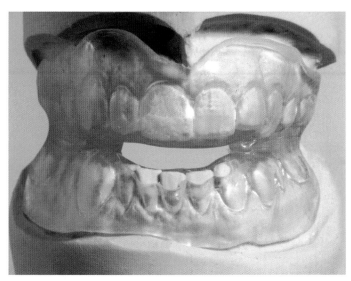

Fig. 1.14: A bimaxillary mouthguard, protecting the teeth and possibly the jaws (design and photograph courtesy Mr P Millward, Cardiff).

however, attitudes to mouthguards remain problematic with evidence that both players and coaches sometimes do not support their use. Despite all the published studies supporting the effectiveness of mouthguards, large numbers of players are still not convinced about their effectiveness and personal desirability. It is difficult to know how far sport's governing bodies should be encouraged to enforce protective measures but the medical profession could clearly do more to promote the messages of effectiveness of such measures in preventing injury. The cost to society as a whole of not reducing sporting injury rates will be considerable and the balancing of individual freedom against corporate responsibility is not easy. What is certain, however, is that good protective measures are effective (see, for example, Castaldi's paper[64] about the effect of protective measures in hockey) and can be promoted wholeheartedly to try and induce societal change.

Eye protection

Sports injuries are a common mechanism of ocular trauma and typically occur in ball-related events. The curved shape of any surface of a small-sized ball is capable of bypassing the surrounding protruding orbital rims to make direct contact with the globe. It is estimated that more than 100 000 sport-related eye injuries occur annually in the United States that will require physician evaluation or treatment. Baseball players are particularly at risk with roughly 10–20% of all injuries in the sport occurring in the face and accounting for nearly one-third of all sports-related eye injuries. Other ball-related sports with significant ocular trauma risk are handball, racquetball and basketball.

Virtually all ocular injuries should be preventable with the appropriate protection. Protective eyewear such as goggles should be composed of shatter-resistant plastics that wrap around the lateral rim of the orbit for maximal globe protection (Fig. 1.15). Failure to use safety wear is largely due to

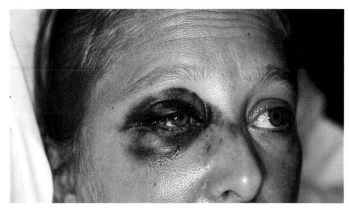

(a)

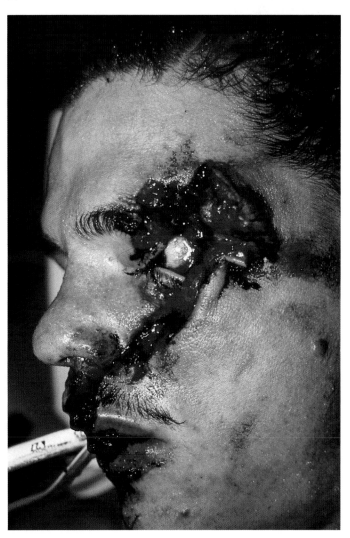

(b)

Fig. 1.15: The potential injuries from orbital trauma can be reduced by proper safety eyewear. (**a**) 27-year-old female with orbital floor blow-out fracture after being struck in the eye with a softball. She was not wearing protective eyewear. (**b**) 25-year-old unprotected male who suffered severe facial lacerations and orbital fractures from being struck by the loose cable of a chainsaw.

lack of perceived risk by the participant as well as comfort considerations.

Protection Through Education

Education in all aspects of life in which the face is exposed to trauma is important, whether it be in motorized or pedaled transportation or other outdoor activities. In most of these exposures, the face is known to be at risk and protective devices are recommended and commonly used. Sport activities, for example, represent a source of facial trauma. In examining different sports, facial injury occurrence rates compared to other body locations varied from 26% in ice hockey, 36% in wrestling, 11% in basketball, 7% in baseball, 7% in handball and 4% in skiing. Numerous other risk exposures, however, are not as easily recognized.

One such risk exposure deserves special mention as it is often a source of severe facial disfigurement and scarring, that of dog bites, in which education is the only means of prevention. Dog bites commonly occur in small children and teenagers in whom the evidence of the repaired facial injuries will remain for the rest of their lives. In the United States, the frequency of dog bites is alarming with several million people bitten per year. Over 300 000 of these dog-bite injuries will require emergency room treatment with over

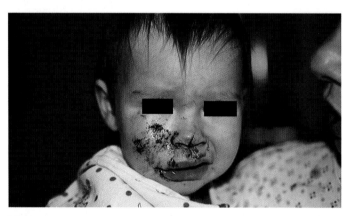

(a)

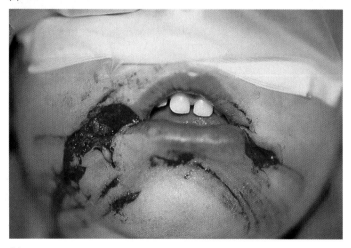

(b)

Fig. 1.16: Dogbites are common sources of facial injuries in young children. (**a**) Multiple puncture marks in a 2-year-old male which occurred while playing with the neighbor's dog (unsupervised). (**b**) Severe facial lacerations in a 3-year-old which occurred while trying to kiss an unknown dog.

6000 reconstructive surgeries and hospitalizations needed. Every 40 seconds, someone in the United States is bitten and nearly 20 people a year die in the US from such injuries. Total medical costs are expected to exceed $250 million per year and there can be no cost estimates on the associated human suffering.

Unfortunately, over 60% of the victims are children and those under the age of 15 have the highest incidence of dog bites, frequently being bitten in the face, neck and head (Fig. 1.16). A 10-year retrospective internal review of all dog bites from the trauma registry at the Riley Hospital for Children in Indianapolis (143 cases) revealed several interesting and underappreciated findings. In the overwhelming majority of cases (84%), the dog was either a family pet or well known to the victim (belonging to a neighbor or relative). Most dog bites occur when the dog is on the owner's property (89%). A significant number of the dog-bite patients are infants and children under the age of 5 (72%). The three most common breeds identified for biting are pit bull terriers, chows and rottweilers, which made up 64% of the identified dogs.

While dogs provide a wonderful source of companionship and pleasure, one must be aware that dogs are not human and may not always respond to certain situations in a completely predictable manner. This is particularly true around children who often do not appreciate that their behavior may be unsettling to the dog. Preventive measures through education, therefore, can be helpful in reducing the risk of dog-bite injuries and those endorsed by the American Society of Plastic Surgeons include:

- never approach an unfamiliar dog
- never run from or scream at a dog
- don't disturb a dog while it is eating, drinking, sleeping or caring for puppies
- if a dog knocks you over, roll into a ball and stay still
- never allow a child to play with a dog unless supervised by an adult
- don't stare a dog directly in the eyes
- don't touch a dog without allowing it to see you and sniff you first.

Another preventable facial injury that is unique to the pediatric patient is the electrical commissure burn. This low-voltage electrical injury occurs in infants and children from chewing or sucking on the live end (female end) of an electrical cord (Fig. 1.17). The combination of a violation of the plastic covering with the electrolyte-rich saliva from the mouth completes an electrical circuit as an arc burn. This can generate temperatures as high as 2500°C which causes extensive local tissue damage at the corner of the mouth with eventual sloughing, scar replacement and subsequent contracture and microstomia. While the lip injury can be initially treated with oral splints or a secondary surgical commissuroplasty, it can be completely prevented by covering of electrical outlets, replacement of old appliances and lights and curbing the curiosity of toddlers who are prone to oral investigation.

The incidence of injuries to the head, neck and face is quite high in cases of domestic violence (DV) and women are the

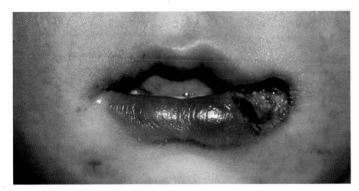

Fig. 1.17: Typical commissure burn from chewing on an electrical cord in an 18-month-old male.

predominant victims (Fig. 1.18). Current research indicates that approximately two-thirds of these women suffer injuries about the face and they can be used as a diagnostic marker in the emergency room. This anatomic location of DV injuries is so significant that a woman presenting for evaluation of facial injuries is 7.5 times more likely to have experienced domestic violence than a woman with injuries limited to other locations. This suggests that any woman who presents to the emergency room for evaluation of non-motor vehicle or sports accidents be considered at high risk for being a victim of domestic violence. Most of these injuries are from blunt trauma and commonly consist of facial bruising and abrasions as well as lip lacerations and nasal fractures. Education and counseling remain the only preventive modalities for this etiology of facial injury.

Shifting Etiological Factors

Oral and craniomaxillofacial surgery has emerged as one of the most progressive specialties of recent years. This has led to an increased awareness of the role of dental occlusion, modern repair methods of bony fractures and the treatment of complex orbital and soft tissue injuries all of which have raised the profile of trauma to the face and the importance of specialist treatment.

There are several factors which suggest that the pattern of injuries will continue to change on a global scale, although it is difficult to predict the extent of such change. At the start of a new millennium for Western society, despite improved safety design, increased legislation and the absence of an 'epidemic' of war, there are two important factors that will probably increase the need for maxillofacial trauma services in the next century. The first of these is the continuing rise in interpersonal violence; although Western society may well address the problems caused by excessive alcohol consumption (as with cigarette smoking, excessive drinking is starting to become more socially unacceptable), other drug-related injuries and crime are likely to continue rising. In association with this, the growth of legal (forensic) medicine will probably continue unabated and clinicians will require more training in forensic techniques.

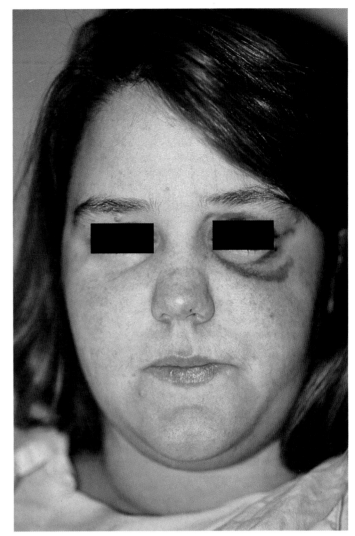

(a)

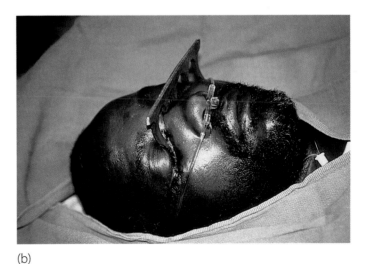

(b)

Fig. 1.18: Domestic violence is a frequent source of facial trauma, particularly in women. (**a**) A zygomaticomaxillary fracture in a young female from a punch thrown by a male companion. (**b**) A rake in the face of a 42-year-old male that was implanted while he was sleeping after a domestic argument.

Secondly, the increasing age of the population will probably result in an increased number of fractures in the older age group – fractures which are more difficult to treat and slower to heal. Research into aging and healing processes may offer advances in this area but change is unlikely to be rapid.

Increasing globalization and population drift through immigration and emigration also make the future difficult to predict. With diverse cultures aspiring to move closer together, whilst at the same time retaining their own identity, it is conceivable that there could be some 'convergence' of the etiological patterns of maxillofacial trauma in the Western and developing worlds. Although the West tends to feel the subject of too much Health and Safety regulation, the challenges facing the developing world are to implement safety and design legislation in order to minimize RTAs and falls and to act simultaneously to prevent injuries relating to violent crime and assault replacing them, as has occurred in Western postmodern society. Here, the changing pattern of injuries places a considerable demand on those responsible for the planning of healthcare. There is a need not only to plan service provision and manpower requirements but also to be aware of the continually changing incidence and nature of the injuries sustained. Prospectively monitoring the etiology, severity and treatment outcomes of maxillofacial trauma must assume a higher profile if accurate service planning is to take place. Information on these factors then needs to be shared more widely. If these things occur, it should be possible to balance the provision of healthcare with service demand in the most optimal way.

References

1 Ali T, Shepherd JP 1994 The measurement of injury severity. British Journal of Oral and Maxillofacial Surgery 32: 13–18

2 Teasdale G, Jennet B 1974 Assessment of coma and impaired consciousness: a practical scale. Lancet 1: 81–84

3 Society for the Advancement of Automotive Medicine 1990 Abbreviated Injury Scale. Des Plaines, Illinois

4 Baker SP, O'Neill B, Haddon W et al 1974 The injury severity score: a method for describing patients with multiple injuries and evaluating emergency care. Journal of Trauma 14: 187–196

5 Knaus WA, Zimmermann JE, Wagner DP et al 1981 APACHE Acute physiology and chronic health evaluation: a physiology based classification system. Critical Care Medicine 9: 591–597

6 World Health Organization 1977 Manual of the international statistical classification of diseases and related health problems, tenth revision (ICD-10). WHO, Geneva

7 Simpson DA, McLean AJ 1995 Epidemiology. In: Simpson DA, David D (eds) Craniomaxillofacial trauma. Churchill Livingstone, London

8 Brickley MR 1993 The circumstances and aetiology of urban violence. MScD thesis, University of Wales

9 Cohen LE, Felson M 1979 Social change and crime rate trends: a routine activity approach. American Sociological Review 44: 588–608

10 Dimitroulis G, Eyre J 1991 A 7-year review of maxillofacial trauma at a central London hospital. British Dental Journal 170: 300–302

11 Brook I, Wood N 1983 Aetiology and incidence of facial fractures in adult. International Journal of Oral and Maxillofacial Surgery 12: 293–298

12 Hammond KL, Ferguson JW, Edwards JL 1991 Fractures of the facial region in the Otago region 1979–1985. New Zealand Dental Journal 87: 5–9

13 Moshy J, Mosha HJ, Lema PA 1996 Prevalence of maxillo-mandibular fractures in mainland Tanzania. East African Medical Journal 73: 172–175

14 Telfer M, Jones GM, Shepherd JP 1991 Trends in the aetiology of maxillofacial fractures in the UK (1977–1987). British Journal of Oral and Maxillofacial Surgery 29: 250–255

15 Tanaka N, Tomitsuka K, Shionoya K et al 1994 Aetiology of maxillofacial fractures. British Journal of Oral and Maxillofacial Surgery 32: 19–23

16 Naik BK, Paul G 1986 Incidence and aetiology of fractures of the facio-maxillary skeleton in Trivandrum: a retrospective study. British Journal of Oral and Maxillofacial Surgery 24: 40–44

17 Thomas DW, Sageman M, Shepherd JP 1995 Trends in the management of fractured mandibles. Health Trends 26: 113–115

18 Shepherd JP, Shapland M, Scully C, Leslie IJ 1990 Pattern, severity and aetiology of injury in assault. Journal of the Royal Society of Medicine 83: 75–78

19 Thomas DW, Smith AT, Walker R, Shepherd JP 1994 The provision of oral and maxillofacial surgery services in England & Wales 1984–1991. British Dental Journal 176: 215–219

20 Heather N 1981 Relationship between delinquency and drunkenness amongst Scottish young offenders. British Journal of Alcohol and Alcoholism 16: 150–161

21 Torgerson S, Tornes K 1992 Maxillofacial fractures in a Norwegian district. International Journal of Oral and Maxillofacial Surgery 21: 335–338

22 Tarling R 1982 Social deprivation and violence in London. Home Office Research Bulletin. HMSO, London

23 McClintock FH, Wilkstrom POH 1992 The comparative study of urban violence and criminal violence in Edinburgh and Stockholm. British Journal of Criminology 32: 505–520

24 Shepherd JP, Robinson L, Levers BGH 1990 Roots of urban violence. Injury 21: 139–141

25 Hocking D 1989 Assaults in SE London. Journal of the Royal Society of Medicine 82: 283–284

26 Key SJ, Thomas DW, Shepherd JP 1995 The management of soft tissue facial wounds. British Journal of Oral and Maxillofacial Surgery 33: 76–85

27 Ochs HA, Neuenschwander MC, Dodson TB 1996 Are head, neck and facial injuries markers of domestic violence? Journal of the American Dental Association 127: 757–761

28 Cascarini L, Bleetman T 1995 Head and neck stabbing injuries. British Journal of Oral and Maxillofacial Surgery 33: 63

29 Hussain K, Wijetunge DB, Grubnic S, Jackson IT 1994 A comprehensive analysis of craniofacial trauma. Journal of Trauma 36: 34–47

30 Berlet AC, Talenti DP, Carroll SF 1992 The baseball bat: a popular mechanism of urban injury. Journal of Trauma 33: 167–170

31 Stone JL, Lichtor T, Fitzgerald LF, Barret JA, Reyes HM 1995 Demographics of civilian cranial gunshot wounds: devastation related to escalating semiautomatic usage. Journal of Trauma 38: 851–854

32 Shepherd JP, Farrington DP 1993 Assault as a public health problem: discussion paper. Journal of the Royal Society of Medicine 86: 89–92

33 Vincent-Townend JPL, Shepherd JP 1995 The epidemiology of maxillofacial trauma. In: Williams JLL (ed) Maxillofacial trauma. Churchill Livingstone, London

34 Adekeye EO 1980 The pattern of fractures of the facial skeleton in Kaduna, Nigeria. Oral Surgery 49: 491–495

35 Abiose BO 1986 Maxillofacial skeleton injuries in the Western States of Nigeria. British Journal of Oral and Maxillofacial Surgery 19: 268–271

36 Khalil AF, Shaladi OA 1981 Fractures of the facial bones in eastern regions of Libya. British Journal of Oral and Maxillofacial Surgery 19: 300–304

37 Adeloye A, al-Kuoka N, Semabatya-Lule GC 1996 Pattern of acute head injuries in Kuwait. East African Medical Journal 73: 253–258

38 Homel R, Castledene D, Kearns I 1988 Drink-driving counter measures in Australia. Alcohol, Drugs and Driving 4: 33–44

39 Tunbridge R 1990 The long-term effect of seat-belt legislation on road-user injury patterns. Health Bulletin 48: 347–349

40 Huelke DF, Moore JL, Ostrom M 1992 Air bag injuries and occupant protection. Journal of Trauma 33: 894–898

41 Telfer M, Jones GM, Shepherd JP 1991 Trends in the aetiology of maxillofacial fractures in the UK. British Journal of Oral and Maxillofacial Surgery 29: 250–255

42 Perkins CS, Leyton SA 1988 The aetiology of maxillofacial injuries and seat-belt law. British Journal of Oral and Maxillofacial Surgery 26: 353–363

43 Imai Y, Toyohashi M, Sakamoto H et al 1991 A clinical study of maxillo-facial fracture (1). Journal of the Japanese Stomatological Society 40: 826–829

44 The science of seat belts. Progressive.com website 2/24/2001

45 Porter RS, Zhao N 1998 Patterns of injury in belted and unbelted individuals presenting to a trauma center after motor vehicle crash: seat belt syndrome revisited. Annals of Emergency Medicine 32:418–424

46 Tufts University School of Medicine, Rehabilitation and Childhood Trauma 2000 National Pediatric Trauma Registry, Phase 3. Tufts University, Boston

47 Barry S 1999 The effectiveness of airbags. Accident Analysis and Prevention 31:781–787

48 Murphy RX Jr, Birmingham L, Okunski WJ, Wasser T 2000 The influence of airbag restraining devices on the patterns of facial trauma in motor vehicle collisions. Plastic and Reconstructive Surgery 105:516

49 Baruchin AM, Jakim I, Rosenberg L, Nahlieli O 1999 On burn injuries related to airbag deployment. Burns 25:49–52

50 Brown RD, Cowpe JG 1985 Patterns of maxillofacial trauma in two different cultures. A comparison between Riyadh and Tayside. Journal of the Royal College of Surgeons of Edinburgh 30: 299–302

51 Muellman RL, Milinek EJ, Collicot PE 1992 Motorcycle crash injuries and costs: effect of a re-enacted comprehensive helmet use law. Annals of Emergency Medicine 21: 266–272

52 Evans L, Frick MC 1988 Helmet effectiveness in preventing motorcycle driver and passenger fatalities. Accident Analysis and Prevention 20: 447–458

53 McDermott FT 1992 The effectiveness of helmets in the prevention of bicyclist head injuries. World Journal of Surgery 16: 379–383

54 Lee MC, Chiu WT, Chang LT, Liu SC, Lin SH 1995 Craniofacial injuries in un-helmeted riders of motor bikes. Injury 26: 467–470

55 Sastry MS, Sastry MC, Paul BK et al 1995 Leading causes of facial trauma in the major trauma outcome study. Plastic and Reconstructive Surgery 95: 196–197

56 Dobson JE, Newell MJ, Shepherd JP 1989 Trends in Maxillofacial injuries in wartime 1914–1986. British Journal of Maxillofacial Surgery 27: 441–450

57 Taher AA 1993 Pediatric facial injuries in Tehran: a review of 87 patients. Journal of Craniofacial Surgery 4: 21–27

58 Haugh RH 1998 Gunshot wounds of the face in attempted suicide patients. British Journal of Oral and Maxillofacial Surgery 56: 933–934

59 Hill CM, Burford K, Martin A, Thomas DW 1998 One-year review of maxillofacial sports injuries treated at an accident and emergency department. British Journal of Oral and Maxillofacial Surgery 36(1): 44–47

60 Hill CM, Crosher RF, Mason DA 1985 Dental and facial injuries following sports accidents: a study of 130 patients. British Journal of Oral and Maxillofacial Surgery 23: 268–274

61 Schatz JP, Joho JP 1994 A retrospective study of dento-alveolar injuries. Endodontics and Dental Traumatology 10: 11–14

62 Tanaka N, Hayashi S Suzuki K et al 1992 Clinical study of maxillofacial fractures sustained in sports. Journal of the Stomatological Society (Jpn) 59: 571–577

63 Kujala UM, Taimela S, Antti-Poika I, Orava S, Tuominen R, Myllynen P 1995 Acute injuries in soccer, ice hockey, volleyball, basketball, judo and karate: analysis of national registry data. British Medical Journal 311: 1465–1468

64 Castaldi C 1986 Sports-related oral and facial injuries in the young athlete: a new challenge for the pediatric dentist. Pediatric Dentistry 19: 455–460

65 Guven O 1992 Fractures of the maxillofacial region in children. Journal of Cranio Maxillofacial Surgery 20: 244–247

66 Chew DJ, Edmondson HD 1996 A study of maxillofacial injuries in the elderly resulting from falls. Journal of Oral Rehabilitation 23: 505–509

2 Medicolegal Implications of Facial Injuries

Shawn McPartland, Barry L Eppley, Miriam A Farley

Introduction

As many societies become increasingly more litigious, there is a considerable likelihood that a surgeon treating patients who have sustained facial injuries will become a participant in the litigation process. The prominent visibility of the face and its importance to each individual ensures that its physical characteristics and emotional perspective are both highly valued and guarded.

Most likely, this participation will be in the form of a treating physician in a civil action in which the patient is taking action against the 'offender': the driver of a car, an employer or the owner of a dog. From this perspective, the physician is providing information as to the extent of the wounds, the care provided and potentially needed and an assessment of permanent injury (e.g. scars and dysfunction). As medical insurers become increasingly vigilant and more financially restrictive, the physician may not only participate in the care of the facial wound alone but also in aiding the patient's legal representative in obtaining the maximal medical benefits due to them under the guidelines of their health policy. Lastly, the specter of being a named defendant in a medical liability suit is an ever-present consideration, albeit the most unpleasant one.

If there is one caveat that the treating surgeon should bear in mind when treating an individual with a facial injury, it is that one must be aware that when a medical record is being created, a legal record is simultaneously being formed. The recording of patient information through emergency room records, hospital charts, office notes or operative reports is establishing unchangeable evidence of what occurred and how the patient was medically treated. Being every bit as meticulous in clinical record keeping as one would be in the treatment of the patient will always serve the physician well.

Several aspects of the legal system are worth reviewing so that the treating physician may have some perspective on the medicolegal process. Furthermore, this information is useful as it relates to how these issues may directly impact on the care delivered and how such events may be interpreted in the future. It should be noted that this chapter is written from the perspective of the legal system in the United States. It is acknowledged that many countries have different medicolegal laws that are variably enforced.

Tort Law

Tort law is the branch of the law in which an aggrieved individual seeks compensation to right a wrong which was done to him in a civil context, usually the wrongful act of another. However, the failure to act when there is a legal duty to do so (e.g. physicians) may also subject the wrongdoer to liability for his omissions. Some wrongful acts may also be criminal in nature (e.g. battery) as well as a civil tort. If the wrongdoer is prosecuted criminally, he may also be subject to civil liability without running foul of the issue of double jeopardy.

The most common tort for which a facial reconstructive surgeon will become involved in litigation is negligence. While the surgeon treating facial injuries need not be overly concerned with the legal proof of negligence, it is defined as follows.

1. The existence of a duty
2. Breach of the duty
3. Causation (between the breach of duty and harm suffered)
4. Damages.

Negligent operation of a motor vehicle may be the most common type of tort for which an individual suffers a facial injury. This usually occurs when an individual suffers injuries from being hit by another driver. More rarely, an action may originate from an injured passenger against the driver of the motor vehicle in which the person was riding. Animal bites, particularly in children, are a particularly obvious injurious circumstance in which litigation rates are high per occurrence of injury (Figs 2.1–2.3). Unsafe maintenance of premises, the manufacture of defective products and intentional torts, such as battery, are also commonly encountered in clinical practice.

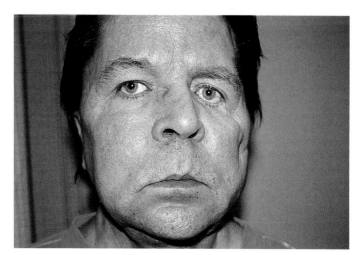

Fig. 2.1: Secondary facial deformity secondary to untreated zygomatico-maxillary fracture.

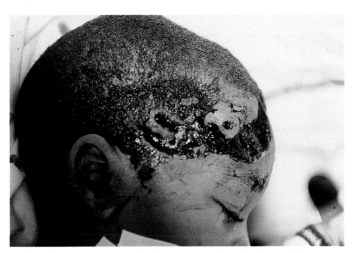

Fig. 2.2: Forehead and facial nerve transection (frontal branch) due to dogbite injury from a neighbor's pet.

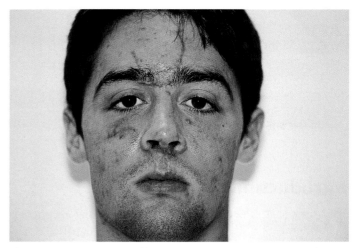

Fig. 2.3: Resultant scars from extensive facial lacerations after being hit by a drunk driver.

The Treating Physician and Litigation

When a physician encounters a patient with a facial injury in which there is some suspicion that tort litigation may result, he should be thinking of his potential role in any lawsuit.

Documentation is of the utmost importance. This means that records should be complete, accurate and without editorial comment. The events which resulted in the facial injury should be recorded in the patient's medical record. The presence of underlying medical conditions, such as acute drug or alcohol intoxication, is a very important part of the initial medical record. However, if the physician is going to document the use of illicit drugs or alcohol, he must not speculate and there should be confirmatory medical tests to support these comments.

Documentation of a facial injury should go beyond a written chart note or dictated operative report. Exact measurement of all lacerations should be taken and recorded, either in the emergency room note or as part of the operative report. Such wound measurements are often taken anyway as the billing of wound closures (CPT codes) is done based on length and depth of the wound. Diagrams may be helpful but preoperative and postoperative photographs are absolutely invaluable and should be taken whenever possible. Slide and print film has been the mainstay of photographic documentation in the past but the more recent introduction of digital photography will soon set a new standard. This photographic medium is important not so much for the improved image quality but for the ability to rapidly view, transmit and store the image information (Fig. 2.4).

There is no aspect of medical care in which photographs are more widely helpful than in the treatment of facial injuries. The establishment of visual documentation in the medical record has numerous merits in the present and potential future care of the patient. Thorough documentation

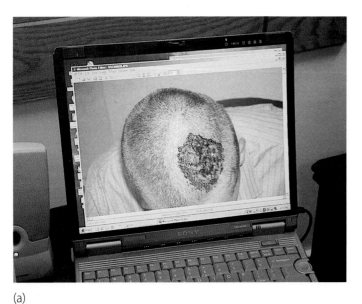

(a)

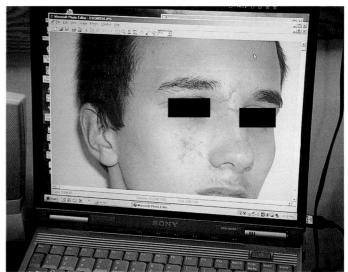

(b)

Fig. 2.4: Facial trauma patients whose photos were taken with a digital camera and immediately downloaded to a laptop for storage **(a)** partial scalp avulsion, **(b)** facial scars from lacerations. These images can be easily sent by e-mail or burned onto a disk.

of facial injuries creates a record for the patient to review in the future. This serves to educate the patient about the severity of their initial injuries. This is very useful as many facially injured patients will need subsequent reconstructive surgeries or scar revisions. An appreciation of their original problem may help them understand why this is often necessary. Furthermore, if a physician is going to become involved in any resulting litigation, either willingly or reluctantly, good photographic documentation of the facial wounds will likely lead to both parties understanding the nature and severity of the injuries and make settlement before trial, or sometimes before filing suit, more likely to occur.

The more ambiguous the nature and extent of the injuries appear in the medical record, the more room the attorneys will have for arguing a position that is favorable to their client, leaving the treating physician in the middle of a legal tug-of-war in which he is not likely to be an enthusiastic participant.

The Litigation Process

The treating physician may likely expect litigation if the patient has suffered severe, extensive and/or disfiguring injuries in a setting of potential negligence. The first concrete indication of a lawsuit on the horizon, however, is a request for medical records by a plaintiff's attorney. Each state has its own statutes for handling medical records requests and it would be prudent to be familiar with the laws in the state in which you practice. Under no circumstances should original records be provided; copies should be sent, with the original records kept in your office at least as long as your state requires. Medical records should not be purged from your files when the statutory time for maintenance of medical records has elapsed, if your patient is involved in litigation. Additionally, a patient's confidential medical record should never be duplicated and forwarded in the absence of a properly executed release form, signed by the patient or his guardian.

Occasionally, the physician's involvement in litigation will go no further than providing medical records but this usually will not be the end of the physician's involvement in the underlying legal matter. The pace of personal injury litigation is most often driven by the plaintiff's attorney; therefore, your first contact with a lawyer is likely to be the one who is representing your patient. Depending upon the attorney's style and practice habits, you may be asked to meet with him in an informal conference. Frequently, the plaintiff's attorney will ask for a narrative statement to record in writing the content of your conference. Typically, you will be asked to respond to very specific questions regarding causation, history and physical examination findings, treatment and prognosis. Some plaintiffs' attorneys will forego the conference, especially if there is not sufficient funding for the case and just ask for a narrative report.

Many physicians do not like to become involved in litigation, even if they are not a party to it. Unfortunately, the physician may always be subpoenaed to testify at a deposition or trial, so this task cannot be completely avoided. In general, cases are far more likely to settle in advance of trial if both sides have reasonable expectations and know as much information as possible about liability and damages. If your response to a request for a narrative report is both clear and complete, the prospects for early settlement are better. However, there may be matters and issues beyond your control, which cause some cases to proceed towards trial, despite your full co-operation in providing the medical information that is available to you.

Deposition and Trial Testimony

There are two types of depositions in the litigation process – discovery (or evidentiary) depositions and trial depositions.

Discovery depositions

The purpose of a discovery deposition is to learn what the deponent's testimony will likely be at trial. Discovery depositions are usually taken by defense counsel. Since all depositions are taken under oath, under the penalty for perjury, defense counsel will seek to build a record which may be used at trial to impeach the deponent's credibility, if there are inconsistencies or inaccuracies.

The attorney conducting the deposition will ask a series of questions which usually begin by asking the deponent-physician about his medical education and training. After the preliminary questions have been asked and answered, the substance of the legal case will be explored. Unlike examination at trial, leading questions are permissible on direct examination. Objections may be made by the plaintiff's attorney but the custom in most jurisdictions is for the attorney to state his objection and have the deponent answer, unless advised otherwise. The admissibility of the objection to questions and answers at trial will be decided upon by the trial judge at a later date. If the plaintiff's attorney and the defense attorney disagree as to whether a particular question should or should not be answered, they may seek to contact the trial judge for an impromptu ruling or skip the question for the time being and have the deponent answer the question at a later date, if that is in accordance with the trial judge's ruling.

In most jurisdictions, deposition testimony in one matter may be admissible in another. If there is a significant chance of a subsequent medical malpractice action arising from the care rendered to the plaintiff, it would be wise to seek counsel prior to attending any depositions. While medical negligence laws vary from state to state, a showing of negligent care generally has to be present, if the medical malpractice plaintiff is to prevail. A mere unsatisfactory outcome in the absence of negligence will not typically suffice. However, the requirements for filing a medical malpractice action are not as burdensome as sustaining the charges of negligence, so any physician may be a medical malpractice defendant, even if the suit is largely without merit.

Trial depositions

The other type of deposition is a trial deposition. Most jurisdictions allow for some depositions to be conducted outside the court room and either be read into evidence at trial or recorded on audiotape or, most commonly, on videotape. A common setting for a trial deposition to be conducted in this fashion is when the witness is a physician, whose schedule does not permit him to testify live at trial. Typically, the plaintiff's attorneys will prefer live testimony from treating physicians, because it holds the jury's attention better than a videotape. The plaintiff's attorney usually seeks to have the treating physician play the role of a teacher for the laypeople on the jury, taking the medical evidence and making it easily understandable. In certain cases, especially when a medical device (e.g. metal plate and screws) has been used on the plaintiff, the plaintiff's attorney may bring a similar device into the court room, have the treating physician explain its function, admit it into evidence and perhaps pass it to the jury for inspection.

A good attorney will prepare his witnesses in advance of trial testimony. The attorney would like the answers to be responsive to the questions asked, without going too far afield. Testimony should give the appearance of being thoughtful and complete, without looking rehearsed or staged. In cases involving facial injuries, the plaintiff's attorney might seek your guidance about the use of demonstrative aids. Photographs, diagrams or illustrations are commonly used, especially when the damages are severe or the anatomy is complicated (Fig. 2.5). Sometimes the attorney will request several conferences with the testifying physician in advance of trial to make the presentation smooth and to anticipate the questions which are likely to arise on cross-examination by defense counsel. If liability is either admitted by the defendant or clearly apparent, it is likely that the treating physician will be the main witness and the focus of attention for the trial.

The same caveat applies to trial testimony as to deposition testimony. Any statement made by the physician in the course of trial testimony is made under oath, under the penalties for perjury, and may be admissible evidence in other matters. Variations or departures from the truth are to be strictly avoided.

The Physician as an Expert Witness

While the most common setting for the physician treating individuals with facial injuries will be that of a treating physician, there are other circumstances in which testimony might be given. The term 'expert witness' sometimes implies a physician who is called to testify on the basis of his specialized knowledge, even when not involved in the treatment of the individual. However, most treating physicians are deemed to be expert witnesses as well. Jurisdictions vary as to the evidence required to designate a physician as an expert witness but the role of the expert is largely the same, regardless of the jurisdiction. Rule 702 of the Federal Rules of Civil Procedure states the following as it relates to expert testimony:

> If scientific, technical, or other specialized knowledge will assist the trier of fact to understand the evidence or to determine a fact in issue, a witness qualified as an expert by knowledge, skill, experience, training, or education, may testify thereto in the form of an opinion or otherwise, if (1) the testimony is based upon sufficient facts or data, (2) the testimony is the product of reliable principles and methods, and (3) the witness has applied the principles and methods reliably to the facts of the case.

The role of the expert is to explain to the jury what is outside the range of the knowledge of the ordinary layperson. Unlike lay witnesses, expert witnesses may give their opinions and are not restricted to a recitation of facts. Furthermore, expert witnesses may testify as to their opinion on ultimate issues, even though the trier of fact will make the final determination.

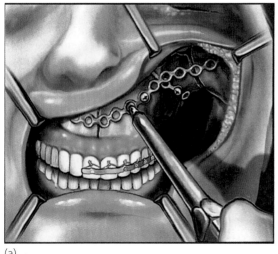

(a)

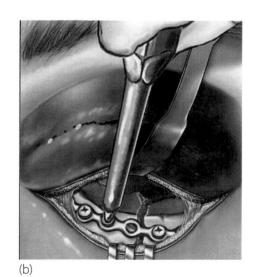

(b)

Fig. 2.5: Actual artistic renderings made of the intraoperative repair of a patient's facial injuries which were used for illustration to a jury **(a)** zygomatico-maxillary repair, **(b)** orbital repair.

A common source of referrals for physicians to serve as expert witnesses in cases where they did not render care is from law firms which practice insurance defense law. Most jurisdictions allow for an 'independent medical examination' by a physician chosen by defense counsel for this purpose. A physician who is engaged in independent medical examinations will typically review the plaintiff's medical records, imaging studies and any other data that are relevant to the issues of causation or damages. The rules of trial procedure in most jurisdictions require personal injury plaintiffs to submit to independent medical examinations, since the plaintiff is putting his medical status into the controversy. The independent medical examiner is expected to write a report of findings, including conclusions, a copy of which will be delivered to the other attorney, upon request.

Similar to the treating physician, the independent medical examiner may be subject to being deposed at a discovery deposition and perhaps at trial. Most jurisdictions allow for questioning of the independent medical examiners regarding their prior testimony and the income derived from it. Experts who derive a substantial portion of their income from testifying in court, particularly if it is usually for the same side, appear to have diminished credibility and may be perceived as a 'hired gun'.

Medical Malpractice

Virtually every practicing physician has had a malpractice concern, be it real or imagined, at one time or another. Typically, a physician is concerned in situations in which there was a less than desirable outcome. It is well known that the best safeguard against being a named defendant in a medical malpractice suit is to be an effective communicator with your patients and their families. Poor or suboptimal outcomes can occur even when the appropriate surgical principles and techniques are used. This is particularly true in severe facial injuries where the surgeon is left to deal with traumatized tissues which will often not heal in an ideal manner. The physician who is available to speak to his patients and, more importantly, actually listen to the patient is less likely to be the target of a lawsuit than those who do not communicate effectively.

Ultimately, the optimization of patient–physician rapport through the establishment of trust is the single most important factor in how patients feel about their surgical outcomes. The factors involved in obtaining a patient's trust are numerous but include a belief in the physician's honesty, effort and concern. In short, if the patient feels that his physician cares about his problem and has made his best effort, satisfaction with the end result usually occurs.

While most physicians believe that they know what constitutes medical negligence, they are frequently incorrect. Medical negligence or medical malpractice is a legal term of art, not a medical one. The elements of medical negligence are similar to those discussed earlier in the context of general negligence: duty, breach, causation and damages. However, for a prima facie case of professional negligence, there must also be a showing of a doctor–patient relationship. As it relates to negligence that is the result of an affirmative act,

the relationship may be inferred. However, when the negligence alleged is one of omission or failure to act, the doctor–patient relationship must be proven to exist for the claim to succeed.

Medical malpractice law is different from jurisdiction to jurisdiction. While there is not one definition of medical negligence that will exactly fit the laws of each state, it generally consists of rendering treatment which is 'below the standard of care'. The standard of care is an amorphous legal concept. As an example, Indiana law defines the standard of care that a physician owes to a patient as 'that degree of care, skill and proficiency exercised by reasonably careful, skillful, and prudent practitioners in the same class to which he belongs, acting under the same or similar circumstances'. Typically, medical care need not result in a perfect outcome to avoid the attachment of liability and physicians are generally not held liable for errors in judgment if they were made in good faith. The fact that another physician in the same specialty might have treated a given patient differently from the defendant physician does not mean that the care rendered was negligent.

The majority law was that a particular physician's medical care was judged by a community standard. This means that a physician's care is not compared to a textbook standard but rather to the standard of care in his particular medical community ('the locality rule'). Many jurisdictions have supplanted this doctrine with the 'modified locality rule' which allows for a physician's care to be judged by a standard in a similar community, not necessarily the same community in which he practices. Since medical negligence cases require an expert opinion, it was found to be difficult in smaller communities to find a plaintiff's expert to testify critically about the care given by another member of the same medical community.

Due to advances in technology, the abundance of seminars and written materials, some jurisdictions are moving towards a national standard of care. If this trend progresses, it would be detrimental to practitioners in a smaller community with less sophisticated medical resources, who currently are not held to the same standard as their large urban center counterparts. This is a developing area in medical negligence law, whose progress should be carefully monitored by American physicians and organized medicine.

Controversies

While few physicians relish participating in the medicolegal process, treating the patient with facial injuries will likely lead to multiple interactions with attorneys and the courts. This is inevitable and should not be viewed as controversial or undesirable. It is an inherent part of helping the patient recover from his facial injuries. It is not as glamorous or as appealing as surgical reconstruction but is very important for many patients who will be scarred, deformed or suffer some lifelong orofacial dysfunction.

The acquisition of imaging data, whether it be in print or slides or more recently digital formats, can be a two-edged sword. While every patient has a legal right to his own imaging information, whether it be preoperative, intraoperative or postoperative photographs, the question frequently arises as to how much of this information should be voluntarily given to the patient. Many patients are aware that some or all of it exists and will frequently request it. Increasingly, patients are asking for their photographic file to be e-mailed to them. Often this contains intraoperative images of procedures and very explicit illustrations of open facial anatomy. Whether patients or their families can emotionally handle or should be exposed to such dramatic images of themselves is debatable. This situation creates an obvious ambiguity between what the patient is legally entitled to see and what the physician thinks is appropriate for patient viewing. Recognizable images of the patient and any use thereof are clearly within the release discretion of the patient. Unrecognizable images of intraoperative procedures, even if of the patient, are often felt to be within the province of the physician. The exact legal precedence on these issues remains to be established.

Conclusion

Facial injuries frequently result in medicolegal concerns due to the potential for resultant disfigurement and dysfunction. Most commonly, the treating physician becomes involved as a source of medical information to chronicle the history of care provided from the initial injury to the present time as well as the potential need for future reconstructive surgeries. In this role, the physician's involvement is as the patient's ally in his effort to receive legal and financial recovery from his injuries. More infrequently, the treating physician may become involved in an adversarial role in which his care is questioned or felt to be a contributory factor in the less than desirable outcome. Fortunately, in traumatic injuries, such physician involvement is usually rare. In either case, proper medical documentation, both written and photographic, is an invaluable asset.

With these potential roles in mind, the creation of written notes and dictated operative reports should be as thorough as possible and they should never be altered subsequently. The objective medical facts should be recorded and comments about the etiology of the facial injury kept to what can be substantiated. Facial photographs should be obtained prior to the initiation of any care, in either slide or print formats. The recent introduction of digital imaging is altering how we currently acquire, store and transfer patient facial records and will undoubtedly play an expanded role in the future.

The English Legal System

Miriam A Farley

Introduction

Legal systems vary around the world and it is not possible to explore all these variations. This part of the chapter looks at the legal system in England, which is predominantly involved with working with doctors involved in the state-run National Health Service (NHS).

The circumstances in which a clinician may be brought before the courts in the United Kingdom are similar to those which pertain in the United States; that is, to give evidence in a civil or criminal action. In either of these situations clinicians may be asked to give factual evidence or to give evidence and opinion as a medical expert. Whilst factual evidence is limited to the nature and extent of injury and the observed course of recovery, expert evidence further gleans the opinion of the expert as to the likely mechanism of the injury as well as the potential for partial or complete recovery in the future.

In a civil action, the clinician may be called upon to give factual or expert evidence about possible clinical negligence. Such cases of alleged negligent treatment may be brought by patients either against an NHS trust in the public sector or against a clinician or one of his colleagues in the independent healthcare sector.

The Clinician's Role in the Legal Process

The criminal case

A clinician who treats an individual who has suffered facial trauma may be asked to give factual or expert evidence in a criminal action if the trauma was the possible result of a criminal act. This usually follows an allegation of physical assault, although other common causes are road traffic accidents, attacks by animals and occasionally accidents at work. The evidence required from the clinician will relate to the extent of injury at presentation, an opinion about the possible cause of the injury and any relationship to the alleged criminal act. In criminal law, the evidential standard is higher than in civil law and the case must be proved without reasonable doubt.

The civil case

In order to prove negligence in a civil action, the court has to be satisfied that there was a duty of care owed to the individual by the defendant, that that duty was breached and that the breach resulted in loss or damage to the individual that was not so remote as to have been unforeseeable by the defendant. As already stated, the evidential standard is lower than that which is required in criminal law and is proved on a balance of probabilities, i.e. is more likely than not.

Allegations of negligence in a civil action may be against one or more of the following:

- an employer, if the individual was injured at work
- another individual, for example if the claimant was involved in a road traffic accident or an accident on another person's property
- the manufacturer of a defective product
- the owner of an animal that has caused injury
- an NHS trust
- a clinician treating patients in the independent healthcare sector.

In relation to the first four of these, the clinician will be asked either to give factual evidence about the nature and extent of injury sustained or to give expert evidence about the probable mechanism of that injury. The extent to which it has affected the claimant and the expert's opinion on the potential for recovery as well as future effects on quality of life may also be requested.

In relation to the last two, the clinician may also be asked to give factual evidence about the medical treatment the individual received following the injury and his role in that treatment if he was personally involved. As an expert the clinician may also be asked to give an opinion on the standard of that treatment and upon its appropriateness in the particular circumstances.

The most common allegations relating to clinical negligence are that:

- inappropriate medical or surgical treatment was given (e.g. wrong or unnecessary surgery)
- there was a delay in diagnosis and treatment
- there was incorrect prescription or administration of medicines or other preparations
- there was a lack of informed consent about the risks of treatment and that those risks ultimately materialized
- the treatment was not performed to the standard expected from a reasonable body of practitioners working in the same field.

Considerations for the treating clinician

Clinicians should consider the possibility of future litigation during every consultation with patients who have sustained facial injury. In the current atmosphere of an increasingly litigious society, clear and concise documentation of the nature and extent of injury is vital. The patient's version of the history of the injury is obviously extremely important. Diagrams and photographs, where appropriate and where resources allow, are usually invaluable. They are particularly useful where facial scarring could result in a future allegation that the cosmetic result falls below the standard expected of a reasonably competent surgeon. Photographic evidence may also avoid a later dispute about the extent of the presenting injury.

The Anatomy of the Litigation Process

The first indication of an impending claim is usually a letter detailing a complaint or requesting access to the patient's medical records. This may come from the patient or from his solicitor.

The Data Protection Act 1998 governs the 'obtaining, holding, use or disclosure of information'. It makes provision for regulating the processing of information about individuals and recognizes the individual's right to be told what information is being processed about him and to have it disclosed. Under the Act 'data subjects' (in this case patients) have the right to be told by any 'data controller' (in this case the doctor, the health authority or the trust) whenever there are personal data about them that are being processed. The term 'process' is defined widely to cover every possible act relating to the data. The request for access must be made in writing and the data controller must disclose the relevant information within 40 days of receiving the request. However, the data may be withheld:

- if there has not been a reasonable interval since the individual last had access
- if disclosure would be likely to cause serious harm to the physical or mental health or to the condition of the patient or any other individual[1]
- if disclosing the records would mean giving information about a third party.

The NHS has a complaints procedure policy operating within trusts to deal with letters of complaint from patients before solicitors are involved.[2] The Department of Health places great emphasis on resolving complaints as quickly as possible.[3] This may be through a swift informal response from the clinician involved or prompt action to open further investigations and seek conciliation. A properly handled complaints procedure can result in local resolution of many grievances and avoid expensive litigation. It should be remembered that the complaints file is disclosable to the claimant (patient) or his solicitors in any subsequent litigation unless it can be argued that it has been specifically created for the purposes of the litigation when it attracts privilege from disclosure.

If the claimant is not satisfied upon completion of the internal complaints procedure or any internal investigation concludes that the standard of treatment was unacceptable, he may instruct solicitors to pursue the complaint.

If the patient does decide to proceed, a letter detailing the claim will be sent to the trust's legal department or solicitors or the defendant's solicitors in the independent sector. This letter of claim is the first step in the legal process and is termed the 'pre-action protocol'. This sets out the steps to be taken by both the patient and the defendant to attempt to resolve the dispute if at all possible before proceedings are issued in court. The aim is to encourage openness between the parties and to reduce delay, costs and the need for litigation. The letter of claim must set out the allegations and the alleged causal link and indicate the likely damages claimed. A letter of response must be provided within 3 months. If there is no merit in the allegations, the claim may be denied, giving clear and detailed reasons, and further legal proceedings may not be brought by the claimant.

If an agreement cannot be reached between the two parties, the claimant can then issue a formal court document to begin legal proceedings. He must submit particulars of the claim, detailing the specific allegations and the damage caused. If the clinician has been involved in the complaints procedure and/or the pre-action protocol stage of proceedings, he will be asked to comment upon the particulars of the claim. At this stage a barrister (known legally as counsel) will become involved and the clinician may be asked to attend a conference with counsel to examine the evidence obtained so far and to assess the probability of defending the claim successfully. Another clinician may be instructed to give an expert opinion at this stage.

The role of the factual witness

In a civil action, the treating clinician may be approached by either the patient's solicitors or the solicitors for the defense to act as a factual witness since there is no property in a factual witness. It is important to discover the exact nature of the proposed litigation immediately since any potential for a clinical negligence claim will require early advice from the solicitors acting for the trust or a defense organization.

As a factual witness, the clinician is likely to be asked to give details of the extent of the initial injury or complaint. This will be in the form of a witness statement. The clinician should only provide information about facts that are within his scope of knowledge, although such information may include a statement relating the patient's version of the etiology of the injury. He should be clear and accurate and where there is no direct recollection of events, he should state that the evidence is based on the contemporaneous recordings in the notes. He should refrain from giving an expert opinion. If for any reason he refuses to give evidence he may be subpoenaed and if he still refuses he may be held in contempt of court, which can attract a fine or even a penal sentence.

If the allegations are in respect of the quality of the treatment given to the patient then the factual witness is most likely to be approached by the trust's solicitors or by those retained by a defense organization. There is a duty under his contract with the NHS to assist with any such litigation. The evidence should be submitted as above, i.e. only related to facts within his knowledge or related in the medical records. He may also comment on his usual clinical practice at the time if this helps to clarify the evidence.

The process of giving evidence in England and Wales is different from that in the United States. The US legal process frequently involves depositions, often given on video where questions from the lawyers acting for both parties are answered. In England and Wales the witness statement is written down in a specific format required by the court and there are no questions from the opposing lawyers until the witness appears in court. The factual witness submits a written statement setting out the facts within his knowledge, which are relevant to the allegations being made. He concludes by signing a statement of truth, which appears at the end, and he can be held in contempt of court if the statement is later proven to be false. The statement is disclosed to the claimant and stands as the evidence of the factual witness at trial, although counsel for the defense may, with leave from the trial judge, raise some additional questions about it. The witness will be cross-examined by the opposing Counsel who may attempt to discredit the accuracy of the evidence submitted. This can be prevented in part by good medical documentation and in some instances by photographic evidence. The trial judge may also ask the witness questions, particularly for the purposes of clarifying any part of the evidence.

The clinician as a factual witness should consider the questions carefully and give answers accordingly. Answers should only be given where the information is within his knowledge and the response should be unhurried. Answers are always addressed to the judge and speech should be slow and clear to give the judge time to take a note of the evidence.

The role of the expert witness

The expert witness has a duty directly to the court and *not* to those instructing him. He should be entirely independent according to Part 35 of the Civil Procedure Rules 1998, which sets out the rules that apply to expert evidence.

Wherever practical, the courts will direct the use of a single joint expert witness instructed by both parties to the litigation. This is most appropriate where the expert is asked to comment on the present condition of the claimant as well as the prognosis of the injury sustained. In a case of clinical negligence the expert will also be asked to comment on any breach of duty and causation. Although a single joint expert may still be appropriate in some cases, most defense solicitors will be concerned that the expert is being asked to arbitrate, which would be inappropriate. It must be remembered that the legal test to be satisfied is whether a responsible body of doctors practicing in the same field would support the treatment given. It is not difficult to imagine that whilst one expert might be a proponent of the treatment in question, another might not. This obviously raises difficulties in using a single expert to represent both sides because it may be important for the judge to hear contrary views in order to decide whether the allegations of breach of duty and causation can be sustained. It remains usual practice, subject to court approval, to use separate experts to represent each side.

Once expert evidence has been obtained, the next procedural step is for the solicitors acting for both parties to simultaneously exchange their reports. Each expert may become involved again at this stage since both parties may submit written questions directly to the other party's expert within 28 days of this exchange for the purpose of clarifying the evidence contained therein. The expert witness receiving questions directly from the patient's solicitor may need to refer to his own solicitor for advice and clarification of the questions posed. For example, if a question relates to the factual evidence, it will be appropriate to decline to give a response since the expert will not have been there at the time of the alleged incident.

Following the exchange of expert evidence and supplementary written questions, the court will direct the experts to meet in an attempt to narrow the areas in dispute and reduce the time of any subsequent trial. Even at this late stage it may still be possible to resolve the matter altogether. A written statement must be produced following the meeting, which should set out the areas of agreement and disagreement between the experts and the reasoning behind any remaining disagreement.

All the statements and reports are signed and must contain a statement of truth. At trial, the expert's report should stand as his submission of evidence, although he may be taken through the report by counsel in order to summarize and clarify its contents for the benefit of the judge. As with the factual witness, experts should take time to consider the questions posed carefully and give unhurried answers based within the limits of knowledge. Answers are always given to the judge and should be slow and clear to allow the judge time to record the evidence.

Conclusion

Many practicing clinicians will have encountered a complaint from a patient and the more unfortunate may have become involved in the processes outlined above. In facial trauma this is most likely to involve allegations relating to the cosmetic result. As in the United States, excellent documentation and good communication with the patient and relatives will serve the treating clinician well in the avoidance of litigation. However, the increase in public expectations and a tendency to resort to litigation have resulted in a relentless rise in medical litigation.

Except for minor procedural differences in Scotland and Wales, the principles of law relating to clinical negligence are consistent throughout the UK, without the variations which occur between states in the USA. For a claim to be successful, the patient must prove, on the balance of probabilities:

- that the doctor owed a duty of care
- that there was a breach of that duty of care

- that foreseeable harm followed as a result of that breach of duty of care.

The standard of care is the standard of a responsible body of doctors practicing in the same field. However, it does *not* have to be the standard of the majority. This is known as the *Bolam test*.[4] Although this has been challenged in the case of *Bolitho v Hackney Health Authority*,[5] it remains essentially intact. Since Bolitho, a doctor needs to demonstrate that other doctors would not only have acted in a similar way but that in addition, it was a reasonable course of action in the circumstances. There is no equivalent of 'the locality rule' used in the United States.

With the further use of audit and clinical governance the standard of treatment administered throughout the UK will inevitably become more regulated and as a consequence less varied, although there is always likely to be a range of techniques for different procedures, all of which are appropriate. However, whether this will mean that legal tests will be easier to satisfy with reference to national standards remains to be seen.

References

1 Data Protection (Subject Access Modification) (Health) Order 2000
2 The Hospital Complaints Procedure Act 1985
3 http://www.doh.gov.uk
4 *Bolam v Friern Hospital Management Committee* [1957] 1 WLR 582
5 *Bolitho v City and Hackney Area Health Authority* [1998] AC 232

3 Immediate Care (Emergency Room)

David W Macpherson, Alan W Wilson, Parkash Ramchandani

Introduction

Fifty percent of all trauma deaths occur, within minutes, at the site of the accident. However, for every trauma death, 200 other patients sustain injuries requiring medical attention and of these 24 will need admission to hospital. In the USA, every year there are 150 000 deaths from injury, three times as many patients suffer permanent disability and over 25 million people will sustain an injury that requires at least 1 day off work. The cost of trauma in the USA is estimated to be $400 billion per year.

Since the full financial cost – rather than just the emotional and physical suffering – has been realized, major reviews of trauma management have been carried out to endeavor to improve the quality of service and reduce the mortality and morbidity. These reviews have encompassed both national strategic planning and also the more local provision of care.

Once the trauma has occurred, with resulting injuries, the aim of the healthcare services must be to transfer injured patients as rapidly and safely as possible to an appropriately staffed and equipped hospital. The ideal hospital is a Level 1 trauma center where all medical specialties with full back-up services are on site, but these hospitals are an extremely expensive resource and are therefore centered in urban areas of high population. By definition, considerable volumes of trauma occur a significant distance from such a facility and comprehensive transport arrangements are necessary if these centers alone are to directly receive all major trauma.

In the UK, the majority of trauma victims are treated at the local district general hospital, designed to serve a population of between 250 000 and 400 000, where most acute services are on site but the patient may need to be transferred to specialized units, which are far more thinly spread around the country, if neurosurgical, burns or cardiothoracic care is needed.

It is essential therefore that trauma services are thoroughly planned and funded to ensure that the most efficient and effective service is provided to meet the predictable needs of the population served, within the capital budget available.

In the UK this has resulted in a number of initiatives including the upgrading of the role of the ambulance service to enable resuscitation to be started at the scene and during transfer to the hospital, the appropriate resourcing of accident and emergency departments and back-up services and the widespread dissemination of training, such as the Advanced Trauma Life Support (ATLS) course, which has become the gold standard and 'common language' of trauma management.

Box 3.1 Aim of trauma care

- High-quality care provided by well-trained personnel with comprehensive facilities and equipment.
- Minimize delays in care pathways at all stages (seamless care).
- Do no further harm.

The whole ethos of management of the patient, from the arrival of the first emergency personnel at the scene through the entire patient care continuum to their complete rehabilitation and discharge, must be to **do no further harm** and appropriately trained personnel must therefore provide care.

Prehospital

All the emergency services personnel – police and fire fighters in addition to ambulance – are trained in basic life support techniques. The aim of the ambulance crew is to transfer the patient to the nearest appropriate hospital without delay and with the provision of whatever emergency support can be provided.

Ambulance crews attending trauma scenes are specifically trained 'paramedics' who, in addition to providing basic life support, are able to assess the patient and carry out more advanced supportive techniques, concentrating on airway maintenance, respiratory support, immobilization of the patient and control of external bleeding and shock during any delay that occurs in freeing and transporting the patient to hospital.

Paramedical crews importantly liaise with the hospital, ensuring that the hospital is able to receive the patient(s). In addition, advance warning is given of the nature of the incident: the number, age and sex of the patients; the patients' complaints, priorities and injuries; airway, ventilatory and circulatory status; the level of consciousness, and the estimated time of arrival. Frequently now they have Polaroid cameras, taking photos which come with the patient, as a visual picture of the scene carries enormous value in assisting the 'index of suspicion' of injuries incurred (Fig. 3.3).

Triage

Triage is the sorting of patients based on the need for treatment and the available resources to provide that treatment.

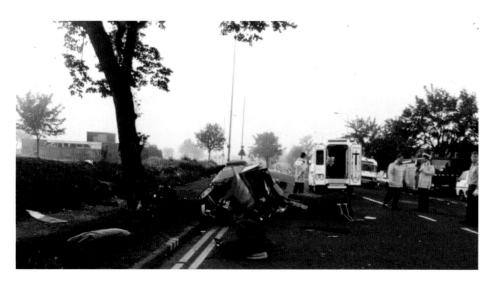

Fig. 3.1: Road traffic accident scene. Emergency services are clearing up. The road will remain closed until the Accident Investigation team have assessed the scene fully.

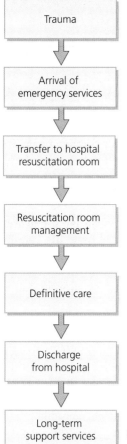

Fig. 3.2: Seamless trauma care continuum.

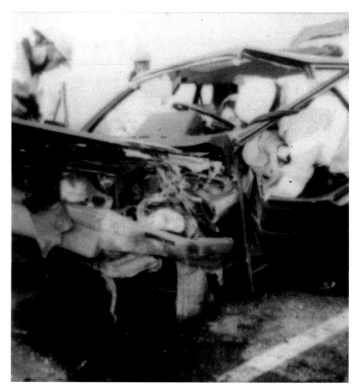

Fig. 3.3: Typical Polaroid photograph brought in with the patient, taken by the paramedics at the scene. Although out of focus, the severity of the accident can be pictured and enables the 'Index of suspicion' to be more focused.

Prehospital trauma scoring may be helpful in determining which patients are to be transported to a trauma center. There are two types of triage. 'Multiple casualties' is the term used when the number of patients and the severity of their injuries do not exceed the ability of the facility to provide care. Patients with life-threatening problems and those sustaining multiple-system injuries are treated first. 'Mass casualties' is the term used to describe the situation where the number of patients and the severity of their injuries exceed the capability of the facility and the staff. Those patients with the greatest chance of survival with the least expenditure of time, supplies, equipment and personnel are managed first.

Preparation at the receiving hospital

Each hospital is only capable of managing a limited number of patients and if the number exceeds the ability of that hospital, then a 'Major incident' is called and a pre-prepared and practiced action plan is implemented whereby neighboring hospitals are involved. Natural incidents such as floods, hurricanes and tidal waves still account for most of the deaths

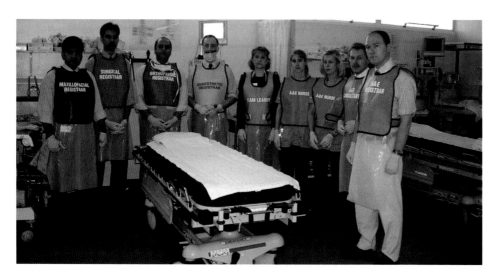

Fig. 3.4: Full trauma team lined up in the resuscitation room, prior to the arrival of the patient. Telephoning ahead by the paramedical team in the ambulance enables the team to be fully prepared for the victim's arrival. Medical and nursing staff work together as a team.

worldwide but man-made incidents as a result of technological or other human interactions are more common, especially in the urban setting.

However, under most circumstances the receiving hospital should be capable of receiving the victims. The hospital must have a fully equipped and staffed resuscitation room with comprehensive back-up of all the necessary support teams, such as radiology, blood bank, ITU, etc.

A formally constituted 'trauma team', ideally comprising specialist anesthetic, surgical and orthopedic components in addition to the accident and emergency staff, should be immediately available (Fig. 3.4) and a method to summon extra medical assistance if necessary should be in place. The involvement of the maxillofacial surgeons in the trauma team has significant benefits in terms of training and in the early identification and optimal management of craniofacial trauma. As a member of the trauma team, the maxillofacial surgeon must be skilled in trauma life support techniques, capable of dealing not only with specialty-specific problems but also other life-threatening conditions.

The team should assemble in the resuscitation room and put on protective clothing. The absolute minimum is rubber latex gloves, plastic aprons and eye protection, because all blood and body fluids should be considered to be infected with HIV and hepatitis viruses. In addition, all the members of the team should be immunized against tetanus and the hepatitis B virus. Staff who undress the patients should initially wear more robust gloves, since trauma patients often have glass and other debris in their clothing and ordinary surgical gloves give no protection against this.

The team leader should brief the team and assign specific duties, so that each member knows the task for which he or she is responsible, such as airway and circulation. To avoid chaos no more than six people should be touching the patient at any one time. A final check of the equipment by the appropriate team members can then be made. Only minimum preparation of the resuscitation room should be necessary, as it should be kept fully stocked and ready for use at all times.

Once the patient arrives in the resuscitation room a stop clock is started so that accurate times can be recorded. The patient should be transferred from the stretcher to the trolley in a co-ordinated fashion to avoid injury to the spinal column or exacerbation of pre-existing injuries. The lines and leads should be checked so that they do not become tangled or disconnected.

Initial assessment of the patient

Deaths following trauma follow a trimodal distribution (Fig. 3.5). The first peak, at the scene, has already been discussed. Within seconds or minutes of the injury, deaths generally result from lacerations of the brain, brain stem, high spinal cord, heart, aorta and other large blood vessels. Very few of these patients survive because of the severity of their injuries. Only prevention can significantly reduce this peak of trauma-related deaths. The second peak constitutes those patients who arrive alive in the resuscitation room but who succumb to their injuries within minutes or hours. Deaths in this period are usually due to severe chest injuries with hemothorax or cardiac tamponade, abdominal trauma with ruptured spleen or lacerations of the liver, or fractures, particularly pelvic and/or other multiple fractures associated with significant blood loss. The third peak represents patients who succumb days or even weeks later from causes such as

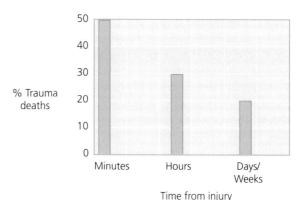

Fig. 3.5: Trimodal death distribution. About 50% of victims die at the scene of the accident and the remainder succumb soon after arrival in hospital (c. 30%) or subsequently (c. 20%).

multiple organ failure, respiratory distress or sepsis. Care provided during each of the preceding periods impacts on patient outcome during this stage.

Causes of death

- *Deaths at the scene*: brain stem injury, airway obstruction, heart or major vessel injury
- *Early deaths:* airway obstruction, uncontrolled blood loss, extra- or subdural hematoma
- *Late deaths*: multiple organ failure, respiratory distress, sepsis

The immediate assessment and early management of the trauma patient is comprehensively covered by the ATLS course. ATLS focuses on the second peak, where appropriate and timely intervention in the resuscitation room will not only save lives but also minimize morbidity, thereby also reducing the third peak in the subsequent definitive care period in the coming days or weeks.

Primary Survey and Resuscitation

The patient is transferred to the emergency (resuscitation) room where a rapid primary survey is carried out. Care must follow the safest pathway, diagnosing and simultaneously treating life-threatening injuries in the order in which they would otherwise kill the patient. As each most pressing killer injury is treated, more resuscitation time is created to deal with the next most pressing problem.

Each patient should be assessed in the same way and the appropriate tasks performed automatically and simultaneously by the team. To facilitate this, the primary survey of the patient follows a strict sequential protocol: ABCDE.

A   **Airway with Cervical Spine Control**
B   **Breathing and Ventilation**
C   **Circulation and Hemorrhage Control**
D   **Disability = Neurological Status**
E   **Exposure + Environment** – completely undress the patient but prevent hypothermia

Frequent reassessment must be made.

If a number of teams are available to manage the patient then they can be assigned to address specific elements, such as A, B, or C concurrently, but if only one team is available then the strict order must be maintained. Emphasis must be placed on the team working together in the resuscitation room.

It is essential to ensure that the prehospital personnel provide a comprehensive account of the accident scene. In addition to patient details, other important information such as the time of the accident, weather conditions, ambient temperature, other factors such as fires, explosions, hazardous chemicals, and injuries sustained by other victims must all be gathered.

Maxillofacial injuries are only addressed at this stage if they have an impact on the airway, breathing and circulation. Comprehensive assessment and definitive management of maxillofacial injuries occur later, away from the resuscitation room setting.

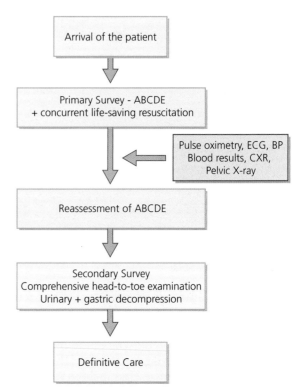

Fig. 3.6: Management of the trauma patient.

Priorities for the care of the pediatric patient are the same as those for adults and priorities for the care of the pregnant woman are similar to the non-pregnant patient. Pregnancy should be identified early by palpation of the abdomen for a gravid uterus and laboratory testing for HCG and early fetal assessment is important for maternal and fetal survival. Trauma is the fifth most common cause of death in the elderly. Co-morbidities such as cardiac, respiratory and metabolic diseases are more common and, together with the aging process, reduce the ability of the patient to respond to injury. The chronic use of medication may also alter the usual physiological response to injury. The narrow therapeutic window frequently leads to over- or underresuscitation in the elderly and early invasive monitoring is valuable.

A   Airway and cervical spine control

There should be a high index of suspicion for cervical spine injury in the patient with maxillofacial injuries or multisystem trauma, if the patient has an altered level of consciousness or if there is a history of a high-speed impact. Approximately 15% of patients with supraclavicular injuries will have a cervical spine injury and 5% of head-injured patients will have some form of associated cervical, thoracic, lumbar or sacral spinal injury. Although the majority of spinal injuries occur in the cervical region, 45% of injuries affect the remaining spine and in 10% there may be a second and distinctly separate spinal injury. Therefore, while assessing and managing a patient's airway great care should be taken to prevent excessive movement of the cervical spine. The overriding management principle should be '**do no further harm.**'

Box 3.2 Cervical spine – assume injury

- **Blunt trauma above the clavicles**

- **Head injury** – any patient with altered level of consciousness, **trauma, alcohol, drugs**

- **Maxillofacial trauma**

- **Multiple trauma** – injury above and below the clavicles

- **Therefore manage patient on the assumption of a cervical spine problem**

Assessment must rapidly be made as to whether the patient can maintain and protect his own airway. The team leader should talk to the patient while the neck is kept manually in a neutral position, without longitudinal compression or distraction. This can be achieved simply and quickly by placing one hand on either side of the patient's head and holding the head in a neutral position, taking care not to cover the ears. If the head is twisted to one side, it should be carefully straightened, ensuring that the neck is not extended or flexed in the process. In the motorcyclist the neck should be supported from below while an assistant carefully expands the helmet laterally and removes it from above. Removal of the helmet using a cast cutter while stabilizing the head and neck minimizes cervical spine motion in a patient with a known cervical spine injury. The neck is then splinted with an appropriate size rigid collar to grip the chin.

Supplemental oxygen delivered through a well-fitted reservoir (rebreathing) mask, at a rate of 15 litres per minute to achieve maximum oxygenation of the tissues, should be given to every trauma patient.

Definitive cervical spine control requires the application of semirigid cervical collar, sandbags placed on either side of the head and tapes over the forehead and chin, immobilizing the head and neck to the trolley. Alternatively, a commercially available long spine board with head blocks can be used. If these need to be removed temporarily, the head and neck should be immobilized by manual in-line immobilization. In the restless and agitated patient, immobilizing the head and neck while allowing the rest of the body to move can damage the cervical spine and here just a semirigid collar is acceptable. Stabilization should be maintained until cervical spine injury is excluded. Cervical spine X-rays may be obtained to confirm or exclude injury once potentially life-threatening injuries have been addressed.

As long as the patient's spine is protected, full evaluation of the spine and exclusion of spinal injury may be safely deferred, especially in the unstable patient.

If the patient is able to communicate verbally, the airway, at least for the time being, is patent but repeated assessment is prudent. If the patient gives an appropriate and coherent response, it suggests that the breathing and ventilation are sufficiently effective to deliver enough oxygen into the circu-

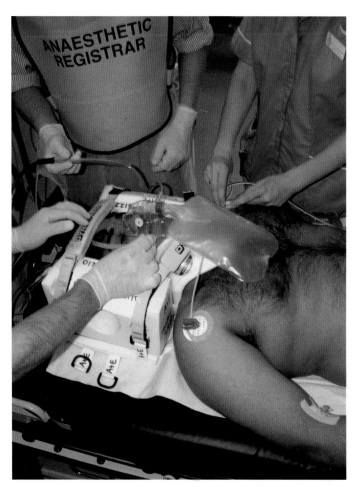

Fig. 3.7: C-spine immobilization. Semi-rigid cervical collar with head-blocks and tapes. Supplementary oxygen being supplied by mask with reservoir bag.

lation, which is functioning sufficiently to transport the oxygen to the brain, which in turn is working sufficiently to comprehend and respond. If there is no reply the patient's mouth should be opened and any solid foreign objects such as fractured teeth, fillings and dentures removed with Magill forceps and fluid sucked out.

If the patient vomits, the patient's head should not be moved to one side unless a cervical spine injury has been excluded clinically and radiologically. If the patient is secured on a spinal board, however, the whole board can be turned. In the absence of a spinal board, the whole trolley should be tipped head down and the vomit sucked away with a rigid sucker.

As always, clinical assessment should follow **Look, Listen and Feel**.

- **Look** to see if the patient is agitated or obtunded. Agitation suggests hypoxia and obtundation suggests hypercarbia. Cyanosis indicates hypoxemia and can be seen in the lips and nailbeds. Look for retractions and the use of accessory muscles of ventilation.

    Look for facial burns, singed eyebrows, facial hair, nasal vibrissae, soot around the lips, in the mouth or in the sputum – indicating burns injury, inhalational burns and possible impending airway obstruction.

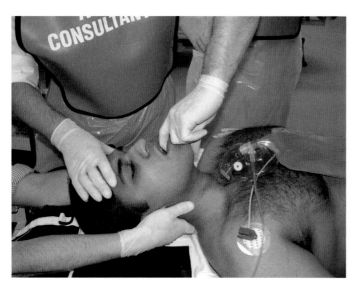

Fig. 3.8: Chin lift with assistant performing in-line C-spine immobilization.

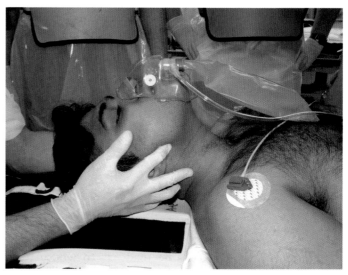

Fig. 3.9: Jaw thrust – performed by one person also carrying out in-line immobilization.

■ **Listen** for abnormal sounds. Noisy breathing is obstructed breathing. Snoring, gurgling and crowing noises (stridor) may be associated with partial obstruction of the pharynx or larynx. Hoarseness implies functional laryngeal obstruction. The abusive or belligerent patient may be hypoxic and should not be presumed to be intoxicated.

■ **Feel** for location of the trachea and quickly determine if it is in the midline.

The tongue can often fall back and obstruct the airway in unconscious patients and in these a simple chin lift or jaw thrust maneuver can be used to correct the tongue position and open the airway. Those patients with a gag reflex can maintain their own airway and as the use of oropharyngeal (Guedel) airways in these patients can precipitate vomiting, neck movement and a rise in intracranial pressure, a nasopharyngeal airway is preferred, provided there is no evidence to suggest a base-of-skull fracture.

Chin lift should be performed without hyperextending the neck. The mandible is gently lifted upward using the fingers of one hand placed under the chin. The thumb of the same hand lightly depresses the lower lip to open the mouth (Fig. 3.8).

Jaw thrust is performed by grasping the angles of the mandible with one hand on each side and displacing the mandible forward. When this method is used with the face-mask of a bag-valve device, a good seal and adequate ventilation are achieved (Fig. 3.9).

The **oropharyngeal airway** must not be used in the conscious patient, in whom it may induce coughing, gagging, vomiting and aspiration. During its insertion care must be taken not to push the tongue backward and block rather than clear the airway. It is introduced upside-down, so that its concavity is directed upwards until the soft palate is encountered. At this point, with the device rotated 180°, the concavity is directed caudad and the device is slipped into place over the tongue.

Alternatively, it can be introduced directly but using a tongue spatula to depress the tongue, again ensuring that the tongue is not displaced backwards as the tube is inserted. This method should be utilized in children to avoid knocking out loose primary teeth and potentially displacing them into the oropharynx.

The well-lubricated **nasopharyngeal airway** is inserted in the nostril that appears to be unobstructed and passed gently into the posterior oropharynx. It is preferred to the oropharyngeal airway in the responsive patient because it is better tolerated and less likely to induce vomiting. If obstruction is encountered during introduction of the airway, stop and try the other side.

Maxillofacial injuries

Up to 5% of patients attending A&E may have facial injuries and some of these may present with airway compromise. Maxillofacial trauma demands aggressive airway management and it may be appropriate for the maxillofacial surgeon to assist the anesthetist in assessing and securing the airway. The following problems may be encountered.

■ The midface consists of a series of bony struts passing upwards from the upper teeth to the base of skull (Fig. 3.10). These bone struts may fracture with severe impact and the middle third of the face can be sheared off the cranial base and forced downwards and backwards along the inclined plane formed by the frontal and sphenoid bones. It should be disimpacted by exerting upwards and forward traction on the maxilla with the index and middle fingers of one hand inside the mouth behind and above the soft palate, with the palm of the other hand braced against the forehead applying countertraction.

■ Voluntary tongue control is lost only when the patient's level of consciousness is depressed and consequently it is only in these circumstances that the tongue constitutes a threat to the airway. In these patients, a deep traction suture (0 black silk) can be inserted through the dorsum of the tongue and taped to the side of the face or

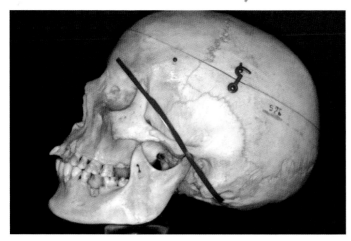

Fig. 3.10: Skull showing the plane of the cranial base. With severe midface trauma, the facial bones shear off from the cranial base and are pushed down and backwards.

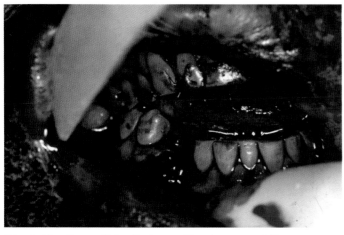

Fig. 3.11: Gagged bite. Patient suffered severe midface trauma, displacing the maxilla backwards down the cranial base, gagging the bite open.

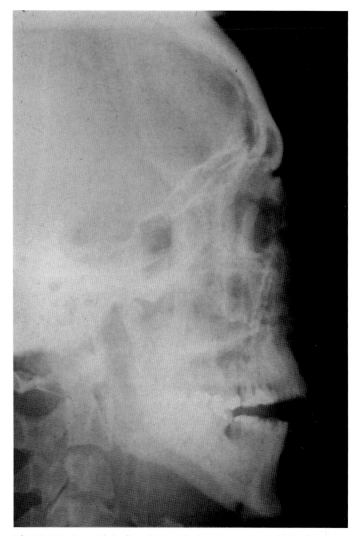

Fig. 3.12: Lateral skull radiograph showing gagged bite (patient in Fig. 3.11). Multiple midface fractures impacting the maxilla down the plane of the cranial base.

alternatively the tongue may be pulled forward using a towel clip. However, both of these techniques may cause additional bleeding and insertion of an oropharyngeal airway or a definitive airway, if necessary, is preferable.

It is often said that in patients with bilateral symphyseal or parasymphyseal anterior mandibular fractures, the tongue may lose its anterior insertion and then, under the influence of the genial muscles, drop back in the supine patient, blocking the oropharynx. In fact, this is not the case, as the tongue is still firmly attached to the hyoid bone, which in turn remains connected to the mandible by the posterior parts of the mylohyoid muscle. In addition, the intrinsic muscles of the tongue continue to exert control.

In elderly patients it is not unusual to see bilateral fractures of the body of the edentulous mandible each occurring near the posterior attachment of the mylohyoid diaphragm. Under these circumstances extreme downward and backward angulation of the anterior part of the mandible may occur under the influence of the digastric and mylohyoid muscles, which may compromise the airway. This 'bucket handle' displacement should be reduced manually to unblock the airway.

- Teeth, dentures, vomitus, hematoma and other foreign bodies may block the airway at any point from the oral cavity to the bronchi, with the right main bronchus being particularly susceptible. Early in the primary survey, the oral cavity should be cleared using a finger sweep followed by aspiration using a rigid sucker. It is important to record any missing teeth, crowns, bits of denture, etc. and to check on the chest X-ray that they have not been aspirated.
- Hemorrhage may result from several causes to obstruct the airway. Bleeding from vessels in open wounds can be controlled by pressure with gauze swabs. The fractured nose may need to be packed as a result of damage to the anterior or posterior ethmoidal vessels or the maxillary artery. Many patients with facial fractures will be conscious and be able to maintain their own airway when upright (Fig. 3.13), but lose their airway when forced to remain supine.
- Soft tissue swelling and edema resulting from trauma to the oral cavity may compromise the airway.

Rarely, maxillofacial trauma may be associated with injuries to the larynx and trachea. Any neck swelling,

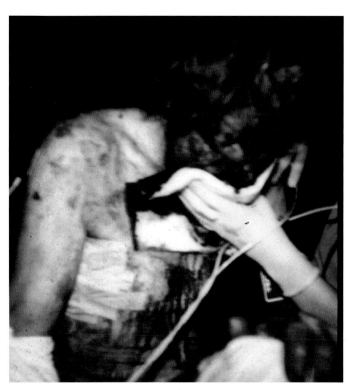

Fig. 3.13: Polaroid photo taken in the resuscitation room. The patient has had his lower face and anterior jaw shot away by shotgun form above but is maintaining his own airway by sitting up, head down and tongue hanging loose.

dyspnea, voice alteration or frothy hemorrhage should be noted and the neck palpated for surgical emphysema, tenderness and laryngeal or tracheal crepitus at the fracture site. Penetrating trauma to the neck may result in vascular injury with significant hemorrhage, which may cause displacement or obstruction of the airway. Endotracheal intubation should be attempted and if this is impossible an urgent surgical airway may be necessary. Blunt or penetrating injury to the neck may cause disruption of the larynx or trachea, resulting in airway obstruction or severe bleeding in to the tracheobronchial tree. A definitive airway is again urgently required.

Laryngeal fractures – indicated by hoarseness, subcutaneous emphysema and palpable fracture – although rare, can present with acute airway obstruction. If the patient's airway is totally obstructed, an attempt at intubation is warranted. Flexible endoscopic intubation may be helpful but only if it can be organized quickly. If unsuccessful, emergency tracheostomy is indicated, followed by operative repair. However, tracheotomy performed under these conditions can be difficult, associated with profuse bleeding and may be time consuming. Under these circumstances, surgical cricothyroidotomy may be a life-saving option. If the injury is in the trachea below the potential tracheostomy site, the thoracic surgeons should be involved.

Definitive airway

This provides oxygen-assisted ventilation via a cuffed tube present in the trachea with the cuff inflated and the tube secured in place with a tape. Definitive airways are of three types: orotracheal tube, nasotracheal tube and surgical airway (cricothyroidotomy or tracheostomy). A definitive airway should be considered when there is:

- apnea
- inability to maintain a patent airway by other means
- need to protect the lower airway from blood or vomit
- potential compromise of the airway, e.g. following inhalational injury, facial fractures, retropharyngeal hematoma or sustained seizure activity
- the presence of a closed head injury requiring assisted ventilation (GCS </= 8)
- inability to maintain adequate oxygenation by facemask oxygen supplementation.

Patients without a gag reflex should be intubated with an appropriately sized endotracheal tube with a low-pressure cuff, so that ventilation can be carried out safely. Attempts at ventilation with a bag and mask in these patients may lead to

---

Box 3.3   Airway – patients at risk

1. **Altered level of consciousness**
   - Hypoxia
   - Head injury
   - Alcohol
   - Drugs
2. **Maxillofacial injuries** – patient in supine position
   - Profuse bleeding
   - Displaced teeth, dentures, etc.
   - Facial fractures
3. **Burns** – inhalational injury → impending obstruction
4. **Penetrating neck injury** → compression of airway from closed hemorrhage
5. **Direct laryngeal trauma**

Box 3.4   Decision to provide definitive airway

- Presence of apnea

- Inability to maintain a patent airway by other means

- Need to protect the lower airway from blood or vomit

- Impending or potential compromise of the airway, e.g. following inhalational injury – burns or chemical, facial fractures, retropharyngeal hematoma or sustained seizure activity

- The presence of a closed head injury requiring assisted ventilation (GCS </= 8)

- Inability to maintain adequate oxygenation by facemask oxygen supplementation

gastric distension with air and can precipitate vomiting. Orotracheal intubation with cervical in-line immobilization is recommended, rather than blind nasotracheal intubation, especially if a base-of-skull fracture is suspected. If this proves to be difficult then a surgical airway is considered. A laryngeal mask airway is not a substitute for a cuffed tube in the trachea and is not yet proven in the emergency setting.

The most important determinant of whether to proceed with orotracheal or nasotracheal intubation is the experience of the doctor. Nasotracheal intubation should not be attempted in an apneic patient nor undertaken if fracture of the base of the skull is suspected.

The route of choice for securing the airway depends on several factors: 5–10% of patients with blunt trauma of the head and neck have an associated fracture of the cervical spine. Laryngoscopy and orotracheal intubation are generally considered to be safe procedures and can be performed with minimal changes in the position of the neck, when performed by a competent operator while an assistant immobilizes the patient's head. Visualization of the cords may require aids such as the gum elastic bougie. Another skilled assistant must provide pressure on the cricoid to protect the patient from aspirating gastric contents. Indeed, the stomach may already have been emptied by the passage of a nasogastric tube. Fiberoptic endoscopy may facilitate difficult orotracheal or nasotracheal intubation if the patient's condition permits.

Rapid-sequence induction with anesthetic agents, neuromuscular blocking drugs and esophageal occlusion by cricoid pressure is best carried out by the anesthetist, who is experienced in the use of these drugs. Before embarking on intubation the equipment must first be checked. Anesthetics with duplicate ampoules should be ready in labeled syringes and vasoactive drugs such as atropine should be to hand in case untoward bradycardia complicates extended laryngoscopy. A skilled assistant applies pressure to the cricoid while another assistant stabilizes the neck. Secure venous access and a pulse oximeter are essential.

Patients with an intact gag reflex require induction of anesthesia and muscle paralysis for the airway to be secured by an oral or a nasotracheal tube. Preoxygenation is essential and while an assistant maintains pressure on the cricoid, neuromuscular blockade is produced with suxamethonium and intubation proceeds with the onset of paralysis.

In deeply unconscious patients with a head injury, intubation should be preceded by the administration of a cerebral sedative and a muscle relaxant, thereby avoiding dangerous increases in cerebral blood volume and intracranial pressure during laryngoscopy.

Orotracheal intubation

In-line immobilization of the head must be maintained by an assistant to ensure no extension of the cervical spine occurs. This is contrary to normal anesthetic practice in the non-trauma patient where extension of the neck makes visualization of the vocal cords, and therefore intubation, easier.

The laryngoscope, held in the left hand, is inserted into the right side of the patient's mouth, thereby displacing the tongue to the left. While observing the back of the tongue, the curved blade of the laryngoscope is advanced until the epiglottis comes into view. Taking care not to move the neck, the whole lower jaw is moved anteriorly as the tip of the blade is moved anterior to the epiglottis. Under direct vision, the anesthetist then advances the endotracheal tube through the vocal cords. If a gum elastic bougie is used an endotracheal tube of the appropriate size is 'rail-roaded' into the trachea. A size 8 tube is usually suitable for women and a size 9 tube for men. The cuff is then inflated, producing an airtight seal.

Proper placement of the tube is suggested but not confirmed by hearing equal breath sounds bilaterally on auscultation in both axillae and detecting no breath sounds in the epigastrium. An end-tidal carbon dioxide monitor will rapidly confirm the presence of the endotracheal tube in the airways. Pressure on the cricoid can only now be released and the tube secured with tapes. Proper position of the tube is best confirmed by a chest X-ray once the possibility of esophageal intubation has been excluded.

End-tidal CO_2 detectors are colorimetric devices that use a chemically treated indicator strip to reflect the CO_2 level. The indicator changes color from purple at low levels of CO_2, such as atmospheric air, to yellow at higher levels. A tan color indicates levels of CO_2 that are generally lower than those found in the exhaled tracheal gases. Patients with gastric distension may have elevated CO_2 levels in their esophagus, which clear rapidly after several breaths, and here care should be taken to avoid assessing the results until after at least six breaths. If the colorimetric device still shows an intermediate range, six additional breaths should be taken or given.

After intubation, the patient is appropriately ventilated. To facilitate respiratory support sedation and analgesia may need to be maintained by intravenous administration of benzodiazepines or anesthetic inducing agents and opiates together with neuromuscular blocking drugs for muscle paralysis. Although capnography and pulse oximetry may provide immediate non-invasive assessment of oxygenation and the adequacy of ventilation, arterial blood gas tension should be analyzed at the first opportunity.

Nasotracheal intubation

This is useful when urgency of airway management precludes a cervical spine X-ray. Blind nasotracheal intubation requires spontaneous breathing and is therefore contraindicated in the apneic patient. The deeper the patient breathes, the easier it is to follow the air into the larynx. Facial fractures, frontal sinus fracture, base-of-skull fractures and cribriform plate fractures are relative contraindications and are suggested clinically by nasal fractures, 'panda' eyes (Fig. 3.14), Battle's sign (Fig. 3.15) and the suggestion of CSF leaks.

It is important to be aware that endotracheal tubes can easily become displaced when patients are transported and so patients who arrive in hospital with an endotracheal tube in place must have the proper position of their tube confirmed.

Inability to intubate the trachea orally or nasally is a clear indication for creating a surgical airway. When edema of the glottis, fracture of the larynx or severe oropharyngeal hemorrhage obstructs the airway and an endotracheal tube cannot

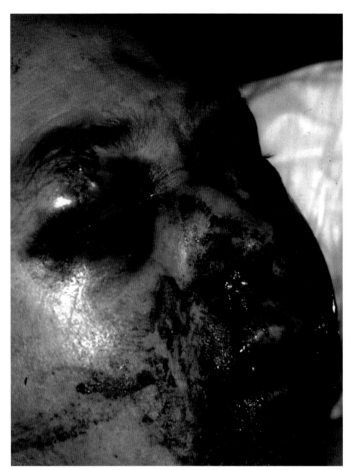

Fig. 3.14: Severe facial trauma results in enormous facial swelling, 'football face,' and bilateral 'panda' (raccoon) eyes, associated with middle-third facial fractures.

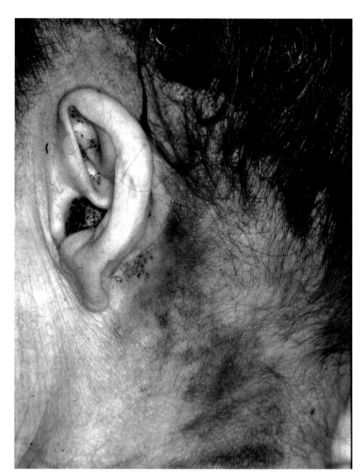

Fig. 3.15: Battle's sign – bruising over the post-auricular and mastoid area – usually indicates a base of skull fracture. It may take some hours before it becomes evident.

be placed through the cords, a surgical airway is performed. A surgical cricothyroidotomy is preferable to a tracheostomy for most patients. It is easier to perform, is associated with less bleeding and requires less time to perform than an emergency tracheostomy.

Surgical airway

Life-saving oxygenation can be provided by **needle cricothyroidotomy** with a large-bore (12–14G) cannula connected to wall oxygen at 15 litres/minute with a Y-connector or a side hole in the tubing attached between the oxygen source and the cannula. Intermittent insufflation, 1 second on and 4 seconds off, can be achieved by occluding the open end of the Y-connector or the side hole of the oxygen tubing.

Although needle cricothyroidotomy can provide a life-saving supply of oxygen, there are associated problems.

■ Ventilation is not adequate and there is a gradual rise in pCO_2. The patient can only be ventilated by this technique for a maximum of 30–45 minutes. Jet insufflation must also be used with caution when obstruction by a foreign body is suspected in the glottic area. Although high pressure may expel the impacted material into the hypopharynx where it can be readily removed, significant barotrauma may occur, including

pulmonary rupture with tension pneumothorax. Low flow rates (5–7 litres per minute) should be used when a persistent glottic obstruction is present. During the 4 seconds that the oxygen is not being delivered under pressure, some exhalation occurs. Because of the inadequate exhalation carbon dioxide slowly accumulates and limits the use of this technique, especially in head-injured patients.

■ Cases in which a surgical airway is needed may often have a head injury and a rise in pCO_2 must be avoided as this will result in cerebral vasodilatation, a rise in cerebral blood flow and possibly intracranial pressure.

■ Needle cricothyroidotomy does not protect the airway and in cases of severe maxillofacial trauma, with disruption of the normal anatomy and profuse bleeding, orotracheal intubation may fail and a surgical airway may be necessary.

Needle cricothyroidotomy should therefore be looked upon only as an immediate life-saving procedure and as soon as it has been completed arrangements should commence to perform a surgical cricothyroidotomy to effect a definitive and secured airway. Indeed, an experienced surgeon may elect to carry out a surgical cricothyroidotomy rather than a needle in the first place.

Technique for needle cricothyroidotomy

1. Universal precautions against crossinfection.
2. Prepare skin quickly with antiseptic.
3. Attach syringe to Venflon with 1 ml of air in syringe.
4. Identify cricothyroid membrane.
5. Immobilize trachea with finger and thumb.
6. Insert Venflon in midline, through skin and membrane, at 45°, aiming caudad.
7. Eject air from syringe and aspirate through syringe – if air comes back, cannula must be in trachea.
8. Remove syringe and trocar.
9. Connect O_2 supply via tubing with Y-connector.
10. Jet insufflate – 1 second occluding the Y, 4 seconds off.
11. Prepare for surgical cricothyroidotomy and call for experienced surgeon to perform if possible.

Surgical cricothyroidotomy is performed by making a skin incision that extends through the cricothyroid membrane. Ideally a tracheal dilator should be inserted to open up the incision, separating the thyroid and cricoid cartilages, enabling visualization of the trachea, suction with a Yankuer-type tube and insertion of the tracheostomy tube under direct vision. A curved hemostat may be used if a tracheal dilator is not available. A small endotracheal tube or a tracheostomy tube (preferably 5–7 mm) should be inserted to avoid tearing the trachea or damaging the cricoid cartilage. Care must be taken especially with children to avoid damage to the cricoid cartilage, which is the only circumferential support to the upper trachea.

Percutaneous tracheostomy is not a technique designed for the emergency situation. For this, the patient's neck must be extended to properly position the head to perform the procedure safely. Percutaneous tracheostomy involves the use of a guidewire and multiple dilators (Seldinger technique), which is time consuming and fiddly and is not advocated when a safer, more rapid technique is available.

Tracheostomy is rarely indicated as an emergency procedure. Severe distorting injury to the structures above or at the level of the larynx can render endotracheal intubation impossible, but cricothyroidotomy is preferred to emergency tracheostomy in this setting. Emergency tracheostomy has a high mortality and morbidity, often with profuse hemorrhage, and cricothyroidotomy is quicker, easier and safer to perform.[1,2]

Technique for surgical cricothyroidotomy

1. Universal precautions.
2. Prepare skin with antiseptic.
3. Infiltrate local anesthetic – allow time for vasoconstrictor to work.
4. Check equipment – connections fit, cuff inflates.
5. Immobilize trachea between finger and thumb.
6. Remove jet insufflation Venflon.
7. 3 cm horizontal incision through skin so skin edges part, using hole from Venflon to identify the level.
8. Stab vertically down with scalpel through cricothyroid membrane and incise 1 cm cut.
9. Insert tracheal dilator and spread – separating thyroid and cricoid cartilages, creating an airway.
10. Insert suction to remove blood, etc., view trachea (+/− apply O_2), keeping tracheal dilator spread.
11. Insert tracheostomy tube, under direct vision remove tracheal dilator, remove introducer from tube.
12. Inflate cuff.
13. Connect O_2 supply via Ambu-bag.
14. Auscultate chest.
15. Secure tracheostomy tube with tapes or stitches.
16. Monitor O_2 saturation and end-tidal CO_2.
17. If insertion fails, reinsert Venflon, reoxygenate and reassess.

B Breathing and ventilation

Once the airway has been secured, breathing and ventilation must be assessed. Ventilation may be compromised not only by airway obstruction but also altered ventilatory mechanics or central nervous system depression. Therefore, if breathing is not improved by clearing the airway other factors must be considered.

- Direct trauma to the chest, especially with rib fractures, causes pain with breathing and leads to rapid shallow breathing and hypoxemia. Elderly patients and those with pre-existing pulmonary pathology are particularly vulnerable.
- Intracranial injury may cause abnormal patterns of breathing and compromise the adequacy of ventilation.
- Cervical spinal cord injury may result in diaphragmatic breathing and interfere with the ability to meet increased oxygen demands. Complete cervical cord transection which spares the phrenic nerves (C3–4) results in abnormal breathing and paralysis of the intercostal muscles. Assisted ventilation may be required.

Thoracic injuries that are immediately life threatening include **tension pneumothorax, flail chest with pulmonary contusion, massive hemothorax, open pneumothorax** and **cardiac tamponade.** These should be identified in the primary survey. The simple mnemonic ATOM FC reminds us that they are:

- **A**irway obstruction
- **T**ension pneumothorax
- **O**pen pneumothorax
- **M**assive hemothorax
- **F**lail chest
- **C**ardiac tamponade.

Simple pneumothorax or hemothorax, fractured ribs and pulmonary contusion may compromise ventilation to a lesser degree and are usually identified in the secondary survey.

Since ventilation requires adequate function of the lungs, chest wall and diaphragm each component must be examined and evaluated rapidly.

All the clothes covering the front and sides of the patient's chest must be removed. The respiratory rate, effort and symmetry should be recorded, because these are sensitive indicators of underlying pulmonary contusion, hemothorax, pneumothorax and fractured ribs. At the same time both sides of the chest should be inspected and then palpated for

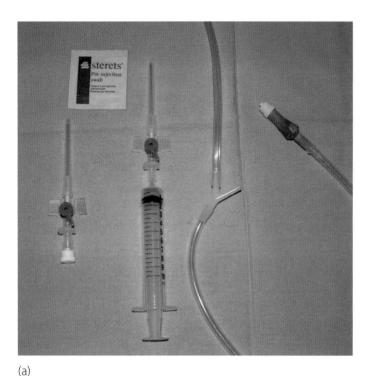

(a)

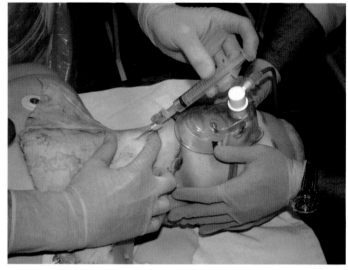

(b)

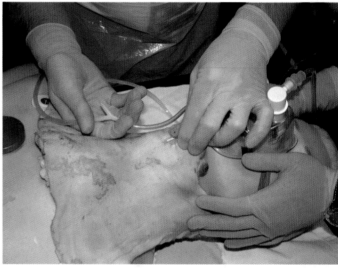

(c)

Fig. 3.16: Technique of needle cricothyroidotomy.

(a) Equipment – alcohol wipe, 12–14G I.V. cannula with 10 ml syringe, with 1 ml of air, and I.V. tubing with Luer lock connection to cannula and Y-connector.

(b) Insert cannula through the cricothyroid membrane, 45° caudad, eject air from syringe and aspirate. Air indicates correct placement.

(c) Remove syringe and needle while fully inserting the cannula. Connect tubing to cannula, other end to oxygen supply and run at 12–15 litres per minute, 1 second occluding the Y-connector, 4 seconds off.

Box 3.5   Needle cricothyroidotomy – equipment required

- Source of oxygen – to run at 12 litres / minute
- Connecting tube with either Y-connector or hole in side of tube
- 10 ml syringe
- 12–14 G Venflon and spare

---

bruising, abrasions, open wounds and evidence of penetrating trauma. Cardiac tamponade is usually associated with a penetrating injury. Paradoxical breathing is seen with a flail chest only if the segment is large or central or when the patient's muscles become fatigued. After inspection and palpation, the chest should be auscultated and percussed to assess symmetry of ventilation and resonance.

Listening over the anterior chest detects air moving mainly in the large airways and listening in the axillae gives an accurate assessment of pulmonary ventilation. This aids in the diagnosis of a tension pneumothorax or a massive hemothorax. A tension pneumothorax should be relieved immediately by needle thoracocentesis and the insertion of a chest drain. A pneumothorax or a hemothorax should be treated by the insertion of a chest drain with a gauge of >28 in the fifth intercostal space just anterior to the midaxillary line. This allows blood and air to be drained but should always be preceded by intravenous lines. During examination of the chest the patient should be attached to a pulse oximeter. This gives information regarding the patient's oxygen saturation and peripheral perfusion but does not assure adequate ventilation. ECG leads should also be attached.

Pulse oximetry monitoring

The pulse oximeter measures oxygen saturation and the pulse rate in the peripheral circulation. A microprocessor calculates

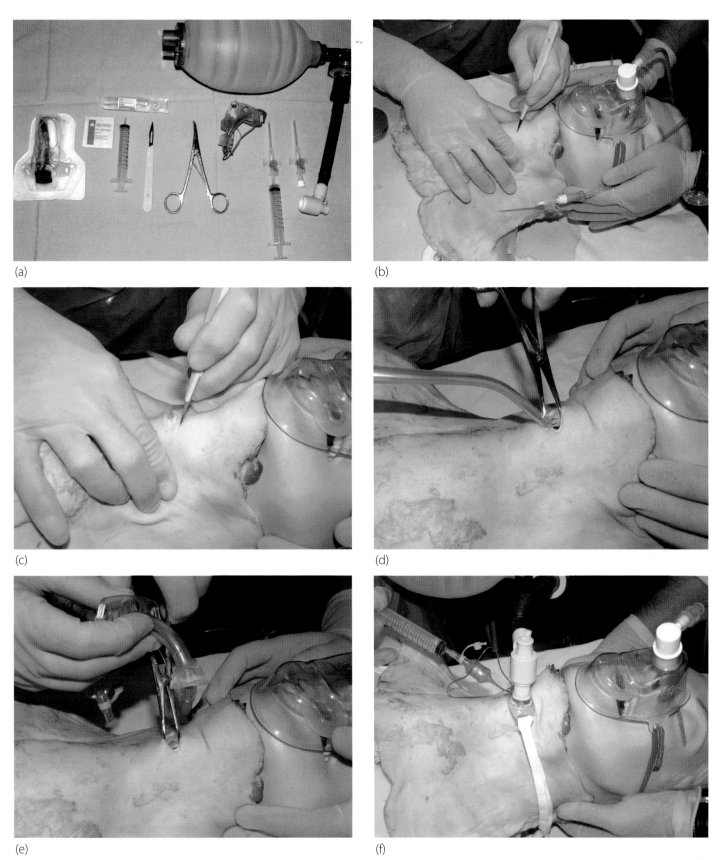

Fig. 3.17: Technique of Surgical Cricothyroidotomy. **(a)** Equipment – local anaesthetic with lidocaine (lignocaine) and adrenaline (epinephrine) for both anaesthesia and vasoconstriction. **(b)** In-line immobilization of head by assistant. 3 cm horizontal incision through skin over membrane (having removed the cannula if needle cricothyroidotomy has been performed). **(c)** Stab vertically down through membrane and make 1 cm incision. **(d)** Insert tracheal dilator horizontally and open, separating the thyroid and cricoid cartilages. Suck out trachea with Yankeurs sucker. **(e)** Having checked that the cuff inflates, insert the tracheostomy tube into the trachea. **(f)** Remove introducer, inflate the cuff and connect to oxygen supply via Ambu-bag. Reassess and monitor O_2 saturation, end-tidal CO_2 and auscultate both sides of the chest for air-entry.

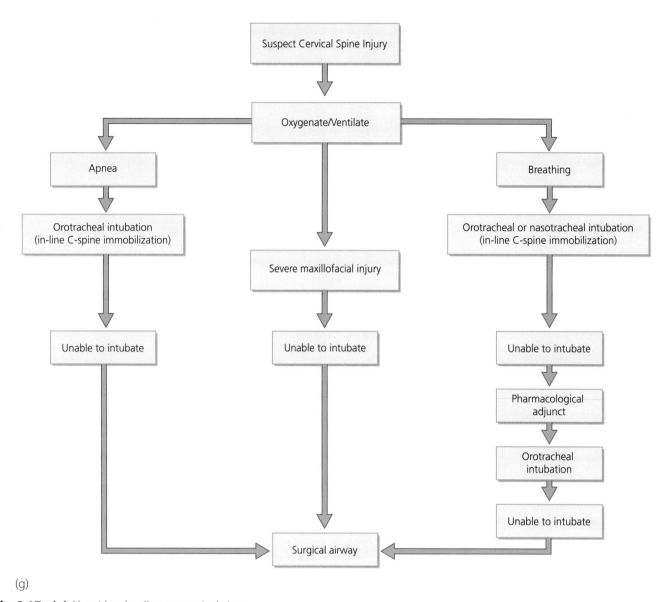

(g)

Fig. 3.17: (g) Algorithm leading to surgical airway.

the percentage saturation of oxygen in each pulse of arterial blood that flows past a sensor and also calculates the heart rate at the same time. Two thin beams of light, one red and the other infrared, are transmitted from a light-emitting diode (LED) to a photodiode through blood and body tissue, which absorb a portion of this light. The photodiode measures that portion of the light that passes through the blood and body tissue. The relative amount of light absorbed by oxygenated hemoglobin differs from that absorbed by deoxygenated hemoglobin and the microprocessor evaluates these differences in the arterial pulse and reports the values as a calculated oxyhemoglobin saturation (% SaO_2). The accuracy is unreliable when there is poor peripheral perfusion. This may be due to vasoconstriction, hypotension, a blood pressure cuff that is inflated above the sensor, hypothermia and other causes of poor blood flow. Severe anemia and high levels of carboxyhemoglobin or methemaglobin may cause abnormalities and circulating dye (methylene blue) may interfere with the measurement. Excessive patient move-

ment, other electrical devices or intense ambient light may also cause malfunction of the device.[3]

Tension pneumothorax

A tension pneumothorax develops when a 'one-way valve' air leak occurs either from the lung or through the chest wall. Air is forced into the thoracic cavity, between the parietal and visceral pleura, without any means of escape, completely collapsing the affected lung. As ventilatory effort increases to overcome the increasing dyspnea, the mediastinum is displaced to the opposite side, decreasing venous return and compressing the opposite lung.

The most common cause is positive pressure ventilation in the patient with a visceral pleural injury. However, a tension pneumothorax can complicate a simple pneumothorax following penetrating or blunt chest trauma in which a parenchymal lung injury has failed to seal or even as a complication of subclavian or internal jugular vein line insertion. It is

<table>
<tr><td>

Box 3.6   Surgical cricothyroidotomy – equipment required

- Local anesthetic – lidocaine (lignocaine) + adrenaline
- Scalpel
- Suction – rigid (Yankuer-type) tube
- Tracheal dilator
- Two size 6 cuffed tracheostomy tubes (1 spare)
- 10 ml syringe
- Two 12–14 G Venflons (1 spare)
- Ambu-type bag
- O_2 supply
- Stethoscope

</td></tr>
</table>

a clinical diagnosis and treatment should not be delayed by waiting for radiological confirmation. A tension pneumothorax is characterized by chest pain, air hunger, respiratory distress, tachycardia, hypotension, tracheal deviation, unilateral absence of breath sounds, neck vein distension and cyanosis as a late manifestation. It may be confused initially with cardiac tamponade, although a hyperresonant percussion note and absent breath sounds over the affected hemithorax distinguish a tension pneumothorax from cardiac tamponade.

It requires immediate decompression by inserting a large-bore needle into the second intercostal space in the midclavicular line of the affected hemithorax. Definitive treatment requires the insertion of a chest drain into the fifth intercostal space (nipple level) between the anterior and midaxillary lines.

Needle thoracocentesis

1. Universal precautions.
2. Assess the patient's chest and respiratory status.
3. Administer high-flow oxygen and ventilate as necessary.
4. Identify the second intercostal space in the midclavicular line on the side of the tension pneumothorax. Find the angle of Louis and move out laterally.
5. Surgically prepare the chest.
6. Place the patient in an upright position if a cervical spine injury has been excluded.
7. Attach a 10 ml syringe, with 1 ml of air in it, to a large-bore (12–14G) over-the-needle catheter.
8. Insert catheter into the skin and direct the needle just over the rib into the intercostal space.
9. Puncture the parietal pleura.
10. Eject air from syringe into chest, ejecting plug of skin from the catheter, remove plunger from syringe.
11. Listen for a sudden escape of air when the needle enters the parietal pleura, indicating that the tension pneumothorax has been relieved.

12. Remove the needle. Leave the plastic catheter in place and secure it. Attach a three-way valve. Apply a small dressing over the insertion site.
13. Prepare for a chest drain insertion. The chest drain should be inserted at the nipple level anterior to the midaxillary line of the affected hemithorax.
14. Connect the chest drain to an underwater seal device and remove the catheter used to relieve the tension pneumothorax initially.
15. Obtain a chest X-ray.

Open pneumothorax

Large defects of the chest wall which remain open result in an open pneumothorax. Equilibration between intrathoracic pressure and atmospheric pressure is immediate. If the opening in the chest wall is approximately two-thirds the diameter of the trachea, air passes preferentially through the chest defect with each respiratory effort. Effective ventilation is thereby impaired, leading to hypoxia and hypercarbia.

Initial management is by promptly closing the defect with a sterile occlusive dressing large enough to overlap the wound's edges that is taped securely on three sides, which provides a flutter-type valve effect. A chest drain should be placed remote from the site as soon as possible. Definitive surgical closure of the defect may be required later.

Chest drain insertion

1. Universal precautions.
2. Identify the insertion site – usually the nipple level (fifth intercostal space) anterior to the midaxillary line on the affected side. A second chest drain may be used for a hemothorax.
3. Prepare and drape the chest.
4. Administer local anesthetic with adrenaline to the skin and rib periosteum.
5. Make a 3 cm transverse incision at the predetermined site and bluntly dissect through the subcutaneous tissue just over the top of the rib.
6. Puncture the parietal pleura with the tip of a clamp and perform a finger sweep with a gloved finger through the incision, to avoid injury to other organs and to clear adhesions and clots.
7. Remove the trocar from the chest drain.
8. Clamp the proximal end of the thoracostomy tube and advance the tube into the pleural space to the desired length.
9. Look for 'fogging' of the chest tube with expiration or listen for air movement.
10. Connect the end of the thoracostomy tube to an underwater seal.
11. Suture the tube in place.
12. Apply an occlusive dressing and tape the tube to the chest.
13. Obtain a chest X-ray.

Flail chest

This occurs when a segment of the chest wall loses bony continuity with the rest of the thoracic cage, usually as a result of trauma associated with multiple rib fractures. The presence of a flail chest segment results in severe disruption of the normal chest wall movement. Although chest wall instability leads to paradoxical movement with inspiration and expiration, this alone does not cause hypoxia. Serious hypoxia may result when there is a significant injury to the underlying lung (pulmonary contusion). Associated pain with chest wall movement and underlying lung injury add to the patient's hypoxia.

Flail chest may not be apparent initially because of splinting of the chest wall. The patient moves air poorly and movement of the thorax is asymmetrical and unco-ordinated. Palpation of abnormal respiratory motion and crepitus of rib or cartilage fracture aid diagnosis. A chest X-ray shows multiple rib fractures and arterial blood gases show respiratory failure with hypoxia.

Initial treatment includes adequate ventilation, administration of humidified oxygen and fluid resuscitation. In the absence of hypotension, fluid resuscitation should be carefully controlled to prevent overhydration. The definitive treatment is to re-expand the lung, ensure oxygenation as completely as possible, administer fluids judiciously and provide analgesia to improve ventilation. Some patients can be managed without the use of a ventilator. However, prevention of hypoxia is important and a short period of intubation and ventilation may be necessary.

Massive hemothorax

This results from a rapid accumulation of more than 1500 ml blood in the chest cavity. It is most commonly caused by a penetrating wound that disrupts the systemic or hilar vessels but can also result from blunt trauma. The neck veins may be flat due to severe hypovolemia but they may be distended if there is an associated tension pneumothorax or cardiac tamponade. It is discovered when shock is associated with the absence of breath sounds and/or dullness to percussion on one side of the chest.

It is initially managed by a simultaneous restoration of blood volume and decompression of the chest cavity. If 1500 ml is drained immediately, it is highly likely that the patient will require an early thoracotomy. Additionally, those patients who initially lose less than 1500 ml but continue to bleed may also require a thoracotomy. This decision, however, is based not so much on the rate of blood loss (200 ml per hour for 2–4 hours) but more on the patient's physiological status.

Penetrating anterior chest wounds medial to the nipple line and posterior chest wounds medial to the scapula should alert the examiner to the possible need for thoracotomy, because of the possible damage to the great vessels, hilar structures and the heart, with the associated potential for cardiac tamponade. Thoracotomy is not indicated unless a surgeon qualified by training and experience is present.

Cardiac tamponade

Cardiac tamponade results commonly from penetrating injuries, but blunt injury may also cause the pericardium to fill with blood from the heart, great vessels or pericardial vessels. The human pericardial sac is a fixed fibrous structure and only a relatively small amount of blood is required to restrict cardiac activity and interfere with cardiac filling. Removal of small amounts of blood, as little as 15–20 ml by pericardiocentesis, may result in immediate improvement.

The diagnosis can be difficult.

- The classic diagnostic Beck's triad consists of venous pressure elevation, decline in arterial pressure and muffled heart sounds. However, muffled heart sounds may be difficult to assess in a noisy resuscitation room; distended neck veins may be absent due to hypovolemia; and hypotension is most often caused by hypovolemia.
- Pulsus paradoxus (normal physiological decrease in systolic blood pressure during inspiration) greater than 10 mmHg is another sign of cardiac tamponade but this may also be absent in some patients and may be difficult to assess in the emergency setting.
- Tension pneumothorax on the left side may mimic cardiac tamponade.
- Kussmaul's sign (a rise in venous pressure with inspiration when breathing spontaneously) is a true abnormality associated with cardiac tamponade.
- Pulseless electrical activity (PEA) in the absence of hypovolemia and tension pneumothorax suggests cardiac tamponade.

A high index of suspicion in association with a patient who is unresponsive to resuscitation is all that is necessary to initiate pericardiocentesis by the subxiphoid method. The use of a plastic sheathed needle or the Seldinger technique insertion of a flexible catheter is ideal, but the urgent priority is to aspirate blood from the pericardial sac. ECG monitoring is mandatory and may identify traumatic (or pre-existing) and needle-induced dysrhythmias. Because of the self-sealing qualities of the injured myocardium, aspiration of pericardial blood alone may relieve symptoms temporarily. However, all patients with positive pericardiocentesis resulting from trauma will require open thoracotomy for inspection of the heart.

Pericardiocentesis may not be diagnostic or therapeutic because the blood in the pericardial sac may have clotted and open pericardiotomy may be life saving, but is indicated only in the presence of a qualified surgeon.

Pericardiocentesis

1. Universal precautions.
2. Monitor the patient's vital signs and ECG before, during and after the procedure.
3. Surgically prepare the xiphoid and subxiphoid area if time allows.
4. Administer local anesthetic if necessary.
5. Using a 16–18G, 6 inch or longer over-the-needle catheter, attach a 20 ml empty syringe with a three-way stopcock.

6. Assess the patient for any mediastinal shift that may have caused the heart to shift significantly.
7. Puncture the skin 1–2 cm inferior to the left of the xiphochondral junction, at a 45° angle to the skin.
8. Carefully advance the needle cephalad, aiming towards the tip of the left scapula.
9. If the needle is advanced too far, penetrating ventricular muscle, an injury pattern known as the 'current injury' appears on the ECG monitor (extreme ST changes and widened or enlarged QRS complexes). This indicates that the needle should be withdrawn until the previous baseline ECG tracing appears. Premature ventricular contractions may also occur, secondary to irritation of the ventricular myocardium.
10. When the needle enters the blood-filled pericardial space, withdraw as much non-clotted blood as possible.
11. During the aspiration the epicardium approaches the inner pericardial surface, as does the needle tip. Subsequently an ECG current injury pattern may reappear. Again, this indicates that the needle should be withdrawn slightly. If the pattern persists withdraw the needle completely.
12. After aspiration, leave the catheter in place, remove the syringe and needle and attach a three-way stopcock, leaving the stopcock closed. Secure the catheter in place.
13. If the cardiac tamponade symptoms persist, the stopcock may be opened and the pericardial sac reaspirated. The plastic pericardiocentesis catheter can be taped in place with a small dressing to allow for continued decompression en route to surgery.[4]

Resuscitative thoracotomy

Closed heart massage for PEA or cardiac arrest is ineffective in the hypovolemic patient. Patients with penetrating thoracic injuries who arrive pulseless but with myocardial electrical activity may be candidates for immediate resuscitative thoracotomy. A qualified surgeon gains access by a left anterior thoracotomy, while restoration of intravascular volume is continued in the intubated and ventilated patient.

The following can be accomplished with resuscitative thoracotomy:

- evacuation of pericardial blood causing tamponade
- direct control of intrathoracic hemorrhage
- open cardiac massage
- cross-clamping of the descending aorta to slow blood loss below the diaphragm and increase perfusion to the brain and heart.

Despite the value of these maneuvers, multiple reports confirm that A&E thoracotomy for patients with blunt trauma and cardiac arrest is rarely effective.

C Circulation with hemorrhage control

Shock is defined as an abnormality of the circulation that results in inadequate organ perfusion and tissue oxygenation.[5] If unchecked, this will lead to end-organ dysfunction.

Most injured patients in shock are hypovolemic, but other forms of shock include cardiogenic, neurogenic and septic. Additionally tension pneumothorax and cardiac tamponade can reduce venous return and produce shock. Neurogenic shock results from extensive injury to the CNS or the spinal cord. For all practical purposes shock does not result from isolated brain injuries. Patients with spinal cord injury may initially present with shock from both vasodilatation and relative hypovolemia. Septic shock is unusual but must be considered for patients whose arrival is delayed by many hours. Hemorrhage is the most common cause of shock in the injured patient.

Recognition of shock

Hemorrhage is the main cause of postinjury deaths that are preventable by rapid treatment in the hospital setting. Hypotension following injury must be considered to be hypovolemic in origin until proved otherwise. The sequelae of profound circulatory shock, namely hemodynamic collapse, inadequate perfusion of the skin, kidneys and CNS, are easy to recognize. However, after the airway and breathing have been stabilized, careful and rapid evaluation of the patient's circulatory system is important to identify the early manifestations of shock.

- *Central pulse* (femoral or carotid artery) should be assessed bilaterally for quality, rate and regularity. Full slow and regular pulses are usually signs of relative normovolemia in a patient who has not been taking β-blockers. A rapid thready pulse (caused by catecholamine release) is a sign of hypovolemia. An irregular pulse is usually a warning of impending cardiac dysfunction. Absent central pulses signify the need for immediate resuscitative action to restore depleted blood volume and effective cardiac output if death is to be avoided.
- *Skin color*: a patient with pink skin, especially in the face and extremities, is rarely critically hypovolemic after injury. Conversely, the ashen gray skin of the face and the white skin of the exsanguinated extremities are ominous signs of hypovolemia.
- *Level of consciousness*: when circulating volume is reduced, cerebral perfusion may be critically impaired, resulting in confusion, aggression, drowsiness or coma. However, a conscious patient may also have lost a significant amount of blood.
- *Respiratory rate*: the patient may be tachypneic due to hypoxia and acidosis.
- *Weakness*: the patient may be generally weak due to hypoxia and acidosis.
- *Urinary output*: this may be reduced due to reduced renal perfusion.

It must be remembered that healthy elderly patients have a limited ability to increase their heart rate in response to blood loss and their tachycardia, one of the earliest signs of volume depletion, may not reflect their true volume loss. Also, blood pressure has little correlation with cardiac output in this age group. Children, on the other hand, usually have

Table 3.1 Classifications and signs of hypovolemic shock[6] (in an adult, assuming a 70 kg patient with normally 5 litres of circulating volume)

	Class I	Class II	Class III	Class IV
Blood loss				
Volume (ml)	750	800–1500	1500–2000	>2000
Percentage	<15	15–30	30–40	>40
Blood pressure				
Systolic	Unchanged	Normal	Reduced	Very low
Diastolic	Unchanged	Raised	Reduced	Unrecordable
Pulse (beats/min)	Slight tachycardia	100–120	120 (thready)	120 (very thready)
Capillary refill	Normal	Slow (>2 s)	Slow (>2 s)	Undetectable
Respiratory rate	Normal	Tachypnea	Tachypnea (>20/min)	Tachypnea (>20/min)
Urinary flow rate (ml/h)	>30	20–30	10–20	0–10
Extremities	Color normal	Pale	Pale	Pale, cold, clammy
Complexion	Normal	Pale	Pale	Ashen
Mental state (if otherwise unaffected)	Alert	Anxious or aggressive	Anxious, aggressive, drowsy	Drowsy, confused or unconscious

abundant physiologic reserve and often demonstrate few signs of hypovolemia even after severe volume depletion. When deterioration does occur it is precipitous and may be catastrophic. The well-trained athlete has similar compensatory mechanisms, is normally bradycardic and does not demonstrate the usual level of tachycardia with blood loss.

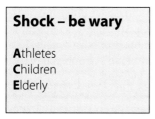

Shock – be wary

Athletes
Children
Elderly

Hemorrhage

Hemorrhage is an acute loss of circulating blood volume. The normal adult blood volume is approximately 7% of the body weight. Classes of hemorrhage based on percentage of acute blood volume loss have been described. Volume replacement should be directed by the response to initial therapy rather than by relying solely on the initial classification. It is dangerous to wait until the trauma patient fits the precise physiologic classification of shock before initiating aggressive volume restoration. Fluid resuscitation must be initiated when early signs and symptoms of blood loss are apparent not when the blood pressure is falling or absent.

- *Class I hemorrhage*: up to 15% blood volume loss. This is equivalent to an individual donating a unit of blood. Minimal tachycardia may be seen. No measurable changes occur in blood pressure, pulse pressure or respiratory rate. For healthy individuals this amount does not require replacement. Blood volume is restored within 24 hours.

- *Class II hemorrhage*: 15–30% blood volume loss. In a 70 kg man this represents 750–1500 ml blood. Clinical symptoms include tachycardia, tachypnea and a decrease in pulse pressure, thereby making the pulse less palpable. The latter is mainly related to a rise in the diastolic component due to an increase in the circulating catecholamines. Despite the significant blood loss and cardiovascular changes, urinary output is only mildly affected – usually 20–30 ml per hour in the adult. Some of these patients may eventually require a blood transfusion but may be stabilized initially with crystalloid solution.

- *Class III hemorrhage*: 30–40% blood volume loss. This is approximately 2000 ml in an adult and can be devastating. Patients present with the classic signs of inadequate perfusion, including marked tachycardia and tachypnea, changes in the mental status and a measurable fall in systolic pressure. This is the least amount of blood loss that consistently causes a drop in systolic blood pressure. Patients almost always require transfusion.

- *Class IV hemorrhage*: more than 40% blood volume loss. This is immediately life threatening. Symptoms include marked tachycardia, significant fall in systolic blood pressure and a narrow pulse pressure. Urinary output is negligible and mental status markedly depressed. The skin is cold and pale. These patients require rapid transfusion and immediate surgical intervention. Loss of more than 50% of the patient's blood volume results in loss of consciousness, pulse and blood pressure.

It is important to remember that up to 30% loss of blood volume produces tachycardia and reduced pulse pressure but the blood pressure may remain within normal limits. There is a consistent fall in the systolic blood pressure only when more than 30% of the blood volume has been lost.

Initial management of hemorrhagic shock

After airway and breathing, the initial treatment of shock is directed toward restoring cellular and organ perfusion with adequately oxygenated blood. In hemorrhagic shock this means increasing preload, rather than restoring the patient's blood pressure and pulse rate to normal. Vasopressors are contraindicated as significant hemorrhage will require surgical intervention.

The priority is to **control the source of hemorrhage**. **External hemorrhage** is identified and controlled by direct manual pressure on the wound. Tourniquets should not be used (except in unusual circumstances like traumatic amputation of an extremity) because they crush tissue and cause distal ischemia. The use of hemostats is time consuming and surrounding structures like nerves and veins can be injured. **Occult hemorrhage** into the thoracic or abdominal cavities, into the soft tissues surrounding a major long bone fracture, into retroperitoneal space from a pelvic fracture or as a result of penetrating torso injury require immediate surgical intervention. A fractured tibia or humerus can be associated with the loss of as much as 1.5 units (750 ml) of blood loss. Twice that amount (up to 1500 ml) is commonly associated with femoral fractures and several litres of blood may accumulate in a retroperitoneal hematoma associated with a pelvic fracture.

Two short, wide-bore (14–16G) peripheral lines must be inserted, preferably in the antecubital fossa. The rate of flow is proportional to the fourth power of the radius of the cannula and is inversely related to its length (Poiseuille's Law). If this is impossible venous access should be gained by a venous cut-down, 2 cm anterior and superior to the medial malleolus into the greater saphenous vein, or by inserting a short, wide-bore central line into the femoral or subclavian vein, using the Seldinger technique. If a subclavian approach is used and a chest drain is already in place, the central line must be inserted on the same side. In children younger than 6 years, the placement of an intraosseous needle should be performed before central line insertion.

Twenty millilitres of venous blood should be drawn off for group, type or full crossmatch, full blood count, urea and electrolyte, blood sugar, clotting screen and a pregnancy test for females of child-bearing age. Venous blood should also be taken for toxicology – alcohol and drugs. An arterial blood sample should also be taken for blood gas and pH. The blood pressure and the rate, volume and regularity of the pulse should also be recorded. A blood pressure monitor and an ECG should be attached to the patient.

Fluid replacement

The aim of fluid management in hypotensive resuscitation should be to restore critical organ perfusion until hemorrhage that is amenable to surgery is stemmed. Therefore in a standard adult trauma victim, 2 litres of warmed crystalloid, preferably Ringer's lactate, should be given[7] and then the patient reassessed.

In reassessing the circulatory state one of three responses is seen.

- *Responder*: the vital signs return to normal. In this case the patients have lost less than 20% of their circulating volume and are not actively bleeding.
- *Transient responder*: the vital signs initially improve but then deteriorate. These patients are actively bleeding and have usually lost more than 20% of their blood volume. They require transfusion with typed blood and the source of the bleeding must be controlled which usually requires an operation.
- *Non-responder*: the vital signs do not improve at all. This implies that either the shock is not due to hypovolemia or that the person is bleeding faster than the blood is being transfused. History, mechanism of injury and physical findings will help to distinguish between these. Central venous pressure measurements may assist in the diagnosis.

Patients with hypovolemia whose vital signs do not improve at all have lost more than 40% of their blood volume. The source of the bleeding requires immediate operation and is usually located in the thorax, abdomen or pelvis.

Crystalloid versus colloid

The ATLS teaches that if a patient needs colloid, i.e. an agent that replaces intravascular loss and remains intravascular, thereby increasing circulating volume, then blood should be given as it is the only agent in general use that improves oxygen-carrying capacity.

Crystalloids such as Ringer's lactate are isotonic electrolyte solutions and pass freely between the intravascular and interstitial spaces and therefore need a greater volume, three to four times, to produce a similar hemodynamic effect to colloids. Crystalloids, however, are cheap and safe.

Colloids are generally iso-oncotic and can be used to replace blood loss on a 1:1 volume basis but, of course, do not directly improve the oxygen-carrying capacity. Polygelatins such as Hemaccel and Gelofusine are reasonably cheap, have relatively low anaphylactic risk and have an intravascular half life of 6–8 hours. With this, care must be taken not to fluid overload the patient if blood transfusion is subsequently necessary. Hetastarch is more expensive, has a

---

Box 3.7   Urgent blood tests

- Full blood count
- Urea + electrolytes
- Blood sugar
- Group + crossmatch
- Clotting screen
- Pregnancy test
- (Toxicology – alcohol + drugs)

longer half life (about 12 hours) but still a relatively low anaphylactic risk.

However, a systematic review comparing the mortality rates of fluid resuscitation using colloid and crystalloid solutions in critically ill patients showed that resuscitation with colloids was associated with an increased absolute risk of mortality and 'does not support the continued use of colloids for volume replacement in critically ill patients'.[8]

As stated above, restoration of oxygenation to the tissues is essential to prevent metabolic acidosis and organ failure. Research is therefore under way to produce synthetic fluids with oxygen-carrying capacity such as diaspirin cross-linked human hemoglobin solution (DCLHb) but these are expensive, still under trial and therefore not clinically available yet. With limited blood supplies, limited shelf life of blood and the risks of cross-infection, a synthetic, sterile alternative will have a valuable role.[9]

Blood replacement

Packed red blood cells versus whole blood therapy

Either whole blood or packed cells can be used to resuscitate the trauma patient. To maximize blood product availability, most blood centers currently provide only component therapy. The main purpose in transfusing blood is to restore the oxygen-carrying capacity of the intravascular volume. Volume resuscitation itself can be accomplished with crystalloids.

Crossmatched, type-specific and type O blood

Fully crossmatched blood is preferable but this takes 1 hour in most blood banks. For patients who stabilize rapidly, crossmatched blood should be obtained and should be available when indicated.

Type-specific blood can be provided by most blood banks within 10 minutes. This is compatible with ABO and Rhesus blood types, but incompatibilities of other antibodies may exist. It is preferred for patients who are transient responders. If it is required, completion of the crossmatching should be performed by the blood bank.

If type-specific blood is unavailable, type O packed cells are indicated for patients with life-threatening hemorrhage. To avoid sensitization and future complications Rh-negative cells are preferred for women of child-bearing age. For life-threatening blood loss the use of unmatched, type-specific blood is preferred over type O blood. This is true unless multiple unidentified casualties are being treated simultaneously and the risk of inadvertently administering the wrong unit of blood to a patient is great.

Hypothermia

Hypothermia is a potentially lethal complication in the trauma patient and aggressive measures should be taken to prevent the loss of body heat and to restore body temperature to normal. It may be present when the patient arrives or it may develop quickly in the emergency department in the uncovered patient and by the rapid administration of room temperature fluids and refrigerated blood. The most efficient way to prevent hypothermia in any patient receiving massive volumes of crystalloid is to heat the fluid to 39°C before using it. The fluid can be stored in a warmer or a microwave oven can be used. Blood products should not be warmed in a microwave oven, but can be heated by passage through intravenous fluid warmers. In addition, the temperature of the resuscitation area should be increased to minimize the loss of body heat.[10]

Coagulopathy

This is a rare problem in the first hour of treatment of the multiply injured patient. Massive transfusion with resultant dilution of platelet and clotting factors along with the adverse effect of hypothermia on platelet aggregation and the clotting cascade are the usual causes of coagulopathies in the injured patient.

Prothrombin time (PT), partial thromboplastin time and platelet count are valuable baseline studies to obtain in the first hour, especially if the patient has a history of a coagulation disorder, takes medication that alters coagulation or if a reliable bleeding history cannot be obtained. Transfusion of platelets, cryoprecipitate and fresh frozen plasma should be guided by these coagulation parameters, including fibrinogen. Routine use of these products is not warranted. Patients with a major closed head injury are particularly prone to the development of coagulation abnormalities as a result of substances, especially tissue thromboplastin, released by damaged neural tissue. These patients should have their coagulation parameters closely monitored.[11]

Hypotensive resuscitation

When acute blood loss occurs, causing hypotension, baroreceptors in the carotid sinus release catecholamines which cause peripheral vasoconstriction, a narrowing of pulse pressure, increased myocardial contractility and tachycardia. This tachycardia and increased myocardial contractility result in increased oxygen demand from the myocardium and there is preferential perfusion to the vital organs at the expense of skin and peripheral tissues. The myocardium, cerebrum and kidneys receive this preferential flow.[12] Continuing uncontrolled hemorrhage results in shock – inadequate organ perfusion and oxygenation – anaerobic metabolism and metabolic acidosis, causing further end-organ dysfunction.

The initial aim of fluid resuscitation in the hypotensive patient is therefore to restore tissue oxygenation to the vital organs.

Animal studies have suggested that aggressive fluid resuscitation, restoring blood pressure and volume to normal before the hemorrhage is controlled, may result in increased blood loss and greater mortality. The most important step is to stop further blood loss.[13,14]

Classic teaching in the management of hypovolemic shock requires aggressive fluid resuscitation to endeavor to return vital signs, particularly blood pressure, to normal pretrauma parameters. It may be, however, that in some situations this may be detrimental to the patient. Certainly in the prehospital setting, where immediate surgical intervention to 'turn the tap off' is not available, better results may be produced by 'hypotensive resuscitation' in which the aim is only to resuscitate to a level where the cerebral, myocardial and renal perfusion is satisfactory.

A systolic BP of 90 mmHg should ensure adequate vital organ perfusion for the average adult. Children have a greater degree of hemodynamic compensation than adults but elderly patients, who may have a higher pretrauma BP anyway, do not tolerate hypotension well and a relatively higher BP should be the target.[15]

In line with this, further research is under way to determine whether a moderate degree of planned hypothermia during resuscitation may improve mortality statistics.[16] Animal studies are also looking at preventing the metabolic acidosis caused by anaerobic metabolism by using perfluorocarbon, an oxygen-carrying agent, to improve oxygen delivery to the tissues.[17]

The ideal may be to manage airway and breathing immediately at the scene and then circulation with hypotensive resuscitation until the patient reaches a hospital where hemorrhage can be properly controlled and definitive treatment commenced. The concept of hypotensive resuscitation is appropriate for the prehospital setting or when there may be delay in definitive surgical intervention to stop continuing hemorrhage. If these concepts are to be formally implemented, then it is essential that comprehensive training must be provided for all parties involved in emergency medical care.

Maxillofacial aspects

Despite the good blood supply to the head and neck, lacerations in this area rarely produce life-threatening hemorrhage. If this does occur it usually involves a moderate-sized artery such as the facial artery or the superficial temporal artery. Initially, direct pressure should be applied to control the hemorrhage. The facial artery can be compressed against the lower border of the mandible just anterior to the masseter muscle. The superficial temporal artery can be compressed against the cranium just anterior to the ear.

Significant hemorrhage can also occur in patients with closed injuries to the bony structures of the middle third of the face – that is, the maxilla, nose and the ethmoids. This presents as a steady flow of blood from the nose and oral cavity and bleeding into the soft tissues of the face. The two main problems are failure to realize the extent of blood loss and the subsequent development of a coagulopathy, and inability to define the source of the bleeding – fractures of the middle third of the face are usually bilateral with disruption of the nasal septum so that hemorrhage from one side manifests as bleeding from both nostrils.

In the intubated patient, palpate the posterior pharyngeal wall with the index finger through the mouth, feeling for tears and fractures, which can be the source of profuse bleeding. Disimpact the maxilla, place mouth props between upper and lower molars then insert and inflate Epistats to splint the maxilla between the base of skull and the mandible. The mandible is supported by the cervical collar. If Epistats are not available use anterior and posterior nasal packs.[18]

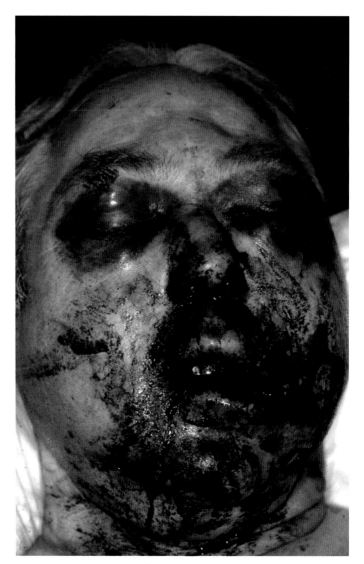

Fig. 3.18: Severe maxillofacial trauma. In the resuscitation room the patient has already developed a 'football face' and 'panda' eyes. There is bilateral epistaxis with CSF rhinorrhea.

Procedure for anterior and posterior nasal packing[19]
If the maxilla is mobile first place mouth props between the upper and lower molars on both sides otherwise the balloons cannot exert tamponade.

Using Epistats

- Insert an Epistat into each nostril, aiming for a fingertip inserted into the mouth to the back of the soft palate, so that the posterior cuff is resting in the nasopharynx.
- Inflate the posterior cuff with up to 10 ml saline.
- Withdraw the Epistat until resistance is felt at the nasopharyngeal wall.
- Inflate the nasal (anterior) cuff with up to 30 ml saline.
- Suction catheters can be inserted through the central lumen to aid in cleaning debris from the nasopharynx.
  Procedure in the absence of Epistats
- Insert a 12–14G Foley catheter with 20 ml balloons into the nose, aiming for a fingertip inserted through the mouth to the back of the soft palate.

- Inflate the balloons when the tip of the catheter is in the postnasal space.
- Pull back on the catheter until the balloon occludes against the choana at the back of the nose.
- Tie the catheters together after passing behind the head, catheter from the right alar to go round the left side of the head, and release periodically to prevent ischemic necrosis.
- Insert bismuth iodoform paraffin paste 5 cm ribbon gauze packs into the nose in front of the balloons and Foley catheter.

In patients with a base-of-skull fracture there is a significant risk of entering the cranial cavity and so the Foley catheter or Epistat should be directed caudally. Massive bleeding can be controlled by compression of the maxilla against the cranial base with head splints. Mandibular fractures should be repositioned using wire that is fixed around the adjacent tooth. This prevents pain and stabilizes the mandible.

D Disability (neurological evaluation)

A rapid evaluation is performed at the end of the primary survey and this establishes the level of the patient's consciousness, as well as pupillary size and reaction. A simple mnemonic is AVPU:

A Alert
V responds to Vocal stimuli
P responds to Painful stimuli
U Unresponsive to all stimuli

The Glasgow Coma Scale (GCS) is more detailed and is quick, simple and predictive of patient outcome. This can be done in lieu of AVPU. If not done in the primary survey, it should be performed in the secondary survey.

A decrease in the level of consciousness may indicate decreased cerebral oxygenation and/or perfusion or may be due to direct cerebral injury. An altered level of consciousness indicates an immediate need for re-evaluation of the patient's oxygenation, ventilation and perfusion. Alcohol and/or other drugs may also alter the patient's level of consciousness. However, if hypoxia and hypovolemia are excluded changes in the level of consciousness should be considered to be of traumatic central nervous system origin until proven otherwise. Note that the lucid interval associated with acute extradural hematoma is an example where the patient may talk yet subsequently die. Frequent re-evaluation will minimize this problem, by allowing early detection of changes. It may be necessary to return to the primary survey to confirm that the patient has a secure airway, adequate ventilation and oxygenation and adequate cerebral perfusion. Early consultation with a neurosurgeon may also be necessary to guide additional management efforts.

E Exposure and environment

The patient should be completely undressed, usually by cutting off the garments with large sharp scissors to facilitate thorough examination and assessment. Thorough examination must involve a formal controlled logroll to assess the back of the head, neck, torso and lower limbs. After the assessment is completed it is important to cover the patient with warm blankets or an external warming device to prevent hypothermia in the emergency department. Intravenous fluids should be warmed before infusion and a warm temperature should be maintained.

Adjuncts to primary survey and resuscitation

ECG monitoring of all trauma patients is required. Dysrhythmias may indicate blunt cardiac injury. Pulseless electrical activity may suggest tension pneumothorax, cardiac tamponade or profound hypovolemia. When bradycardia, aberrant conduction and premature beats are present, hypoxia, hypoperfusion or hypothermia should be suspected immediately.

Urinary and gastric catheters should be placed as part of the resuscitation process and a urine specimen should be sent for routine laboratory analysis.

Urinary output is an important indicator of the volume status of the patient and reflects the renal perfusion. An indwelling bladder catheter should be inserted but is contraindicated in patients in whom urethral transection is suspected, i.e. if there is:

- blood at the penile meatus
- perineal bruising
- scrotal hematoma (Fig. 3.19)
- high-riding, non-palpable prostate
- a pelvic fracture.

Therefore the urinary catheter should not be inserted before an examination of the rectum or genitalia. A retrograde urethrogram can be used to confirm a urethral injury prior to inserting the catheter.

A gastric tube should be used orally or nasally to reduce stomach distension and decrease the risk of aspiration. For the tube to be effective it must be placed on suction. Blood in the gastric aspirate may represent swallowed blood, traumatic insertion or actual injury to the upper digestive tract. If a fracture of the cribriform plate is present or is suspected, the gastric tube should be inserted orally to prevent potential intracranial passage.

Adequate resuscitation is suggested by improvement in physiologic parameters, pulse rate, BP, pulse pressure, respiratory rate, arterial blood gases, body temperature and urinary output. Actual values for these should be obtained as soon as possible after completing the primary survey and repeated re-evaluation is mandatory.

X-rays should be used judiciously and should not delay resuscitation. The AP chest film and AP pelvis may provide information that can guide resuscitation in a patient with blunt trauma. Chest X-rays may detect potentially life-threatening injuries that require treatment and pelvic films may show pelvic fractures that indicate the need for early blood transfusion. A lateral cervical spine X-ray that shows an injury is an important finding, whereas a negative or an inadequate film does not exclude cervical spine injury. These films can be taken in the resuscitation area, usually with a portable X-ray unit, but should not interrupt resuscitation. Essential diagnostic X-rays should not be avoided in the pregnant patient.[20]

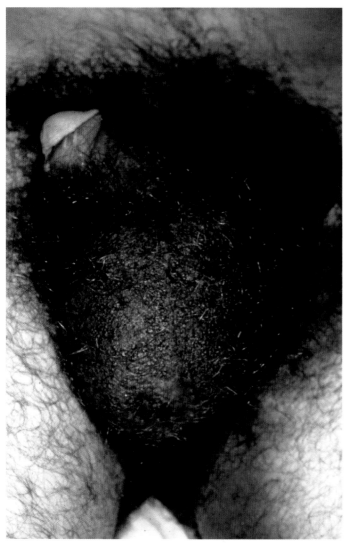

Fig. 3.19: Scrotal hematoma may be indicative of urethral injury and per-urethral urinary catheterization is contra-indicated until urethral trauma has been excluded. Supra-pubic cathetherization should be performed instead.

Diagnostic peritoneal lavage (DPL) and abdominal ultrasound can quickly detect intra-abdominal bleeding. These techniques should be performed by a skilled and experienced doctor and certainly the DPL by the surgeon who would be taking the patient to the operating theatre.

During the primary survey and resuscitation phase it may become clear that the patient should be transferred to another facility for more specialized services such as neuro-surgery, cardiothoracic or burns. Administrative personnel, at the direction of the examining doctor, may initiate the process but once the decision to transfer has been made, doctor-to-doctor communication between the centers is essential.

Secondary Survey

This does not begin until the primary survey has been completed and the patient stabilized. It is a head-to-toe and front-to-back evaluation of the trauma patient. A thorough history

and physical examination, including a reassessment of all vital signs, are carried out and each region of the body is completely examined. The potential for missing an injury is great, especially in the unresponsive patient. The secondary survey has been described as 'tubes and fingers in every orifice'.

History

A thorough history should be taken from the patient, prehospital personnel and family. The **AMPLE** history is a simple useful mnemonic for this:

A Allergies
M Medications currently used
P Past illnesses/pregnancy
L Last meal
E Events/environment related to the injury

Physical examination

Broadly speaking, injury is classified as either blunt or penetrating.

- *Blunt trauma* results from road traffic accidents, falls, sporting and occupation-related injuries. In relation to road traffic accidents, important factors in the history include seat-belt usage, steering wheel deformation, direction of impact, damage to the vehicle in terms of major deformation or intrusion into the passenger compartment (Fig. 3.20) and ejection of the occupants from the vehicle. The latter, in particular, suggests a major injury.
- *Penetrating trauma* includes injuries from firearms, stabbings and impaling objects and is increasing. The type and extent of injury and subsequent management depend upon the region of the body injured, the organs in proximity to the path of the penetrating object and the velocity of the missile. With firearm injuries, knowledge of the velocity, caliber, presumed path of the bullet and the distance from the weapon to the wounded provide important clues to the extent of the injury.

Scalp

Examine the entire scalp and head for lacerations, contusions and signs of fractures. Examination of the occiput will have to wait until the patient is turned. Fractures may be seen in the base of the lacerations but wounds should not be probed blindly as this may result in further damage to the underlying structures. Digital pressure should be used to control major bleeding.

Neurological state

Head injuries form 10% of the workload of an accident and emergency department. Most attenders are only mildly injured but head injuries have a reputation for being treacherous. In patients who present with persistent impaired consciousness (<5%) correct diagnosis and assignment of priorities can be life saving. The limited availability of special-

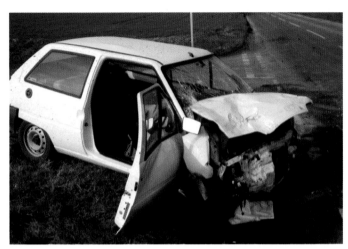

Fig. 3.20: Modern cars have an engine compartment crumple zone to absorb the force of the impact. Intrusion of the passenger compartment is indicative of more severe trauma. Note the 'bulls-eye' on the windscreen indicating risk of head injury for the driver.

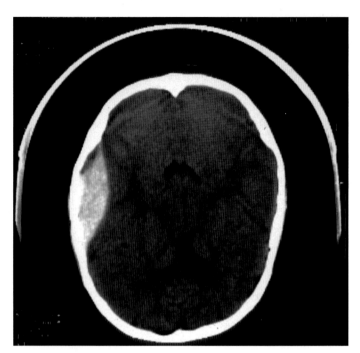

Fig. 3.21: CT scan showing extradural (epidural) hematoma, characterized by biconvex appearance.

ist neurosurgical facilities in the United Kingdom means that only 1% of patients with head injuries who attend hospital are admitted to the neurosurgical unit.

The principal aims of management are:

- to provide the best conditions for recovery from any brain damage already sustained
- to prevent or treat complications leading to secondary brain damage.

Mechanisms of brain damage include the following.

- *Diffuse damage*: the brain is poorly anchored within the skull and its soft consistency renders it liable to move within the skull in response to rapid acceleration or deceleration. Contact between the surface of the brain and the interior skull causes contusions, particularly at the frontal and temporal poles. Distortion of the brain caused by internal shearing forces leads to stretching and tearing of axonal tracts within the white matter.
- *Focal impact damage*: skull fractures are less common in children than in adults because of their more elastic skulls. A compound depressed fracture results when a violent sharp blow lacerates the scalp and drives bone fragments into the intracranial cavity, sometimes tearing the dura and exposing the surface of the brain. This injury may result in intracranial infection and requires prompt surgical elevation and debridement. A depressed fracture is also a powerful cause of epilepsy but the risk of this complication is not influenced by surgical treatment. A linear fracture is important as an indicator of the force applied to the cranium and therefore the risk of intracranial damage.[21]
- *Extradural (epidural) hematoma*: extradural hematomas most often occur in the temporal or temporoparietal region, usually from tearing of the middle meningeal artery, where it runs immediately below the bone, as a result of a fracture. Since they are located outside the dura but within the skull they are typically biconvex or

lenticular in shape. Although relatively uncommon (0.5% of all head-injured patients and 9% of those that are comatose), they should always be treated rapidly. They can be associated with little primary brain damage and optimal management should minimize mortality and morbidity caused by secondary cerebral compression. If treated early, the prognosis is usually excellent but delay in treatment can cause irreversible brain damage. Patients may present with the classic 'lucid interval' and 'talk and die'. Although suspicion of such an injury will be based on the history and examination, CT scan makes the definitive diagnosis. The need for an operation should be established by a neurosurgeon.

- *Intradural hematoma*: subdural and intracerebral hematomas are four times more common than extradural hematoma and are seen in approximately 30% of severe head injuries. They result from tearing of cerebral veins or from lacerations of the brain's surface, or both. The associated primary brain damage is usually far greater than that associated with an extradural hematoma and the prognosis is proportionately much worse. The mortality may be reduced by early neurosurgical intervention.
- *Hypoxia and ischemia*: permanent ischemic neuronal damage occurs within a few minutes if perfusion is reduced below a critical threshold. The brain regulates its own blood supply to maintain constant perfusion, despite variations in systemic blood pressure, but when injured it loses this capacity and is particularly vulnerable to ischemic damage when hypotension or hypoxia occur. A mean arterial blood pressure below 60–80 mmHg, especially when intracranial pressure is raised, may cause ischemic neuronal damage if sustained for more than a few minutes.

- *Raised intracranial pressure*: about 70% of patients persistently in coma (GCS 8 or less) after severe head injury have raised intracranial pressure. The intracranial compartment has a finite volume, limited by the surrounding bony box. As the brain has a fixed volume, any expanding hematoma results in a compensatory reduction in intracranial cerebrospinal fluid (CSF). This protects the brain by maintaining a normal intracranial pressure (ICP) – about 10 mmHg.

However, if the hematoma continues to expand, then the compensatory mechanism will eventually be unable to maintain a normal ICP and this will rise precipitately with only small increases in the volume of the hematoma.

CPP	=	MAP	–	ICP
Central perfusion pressure	=	Mean arterial pressure	–	Intracranial pressure

This jeopardizes cerebral perfusion pressure because cerebral perfusion pressure is equal to the mean arterial pressure minus the intracranial pressure. As the pressure continues to rise brain shifts occur within the cranial cavity. The most important of these is uncal transtentorial herniation or 'coning'. This causes impairment of the conscious level, development of an ipsilateral fixed dilated pupil and brain stem compression with cardiovascular and respiratory abnormalities.

The fixed dilated pupil occurs because the parasympathetic constrictor pupillae fibers travel intracranially with the oculomotor nerve, which is compressed by uncal herniation, leaving unopposed sympathetic dilator pupillae activity.

Management of head injuries

Head injuries should be assessed using the **Glasgow Coma Scale** (GCS), **pupillary response** and the presence of any **lateralizing signs**.

The GCS score quantifies neurological findings and by allowing uniformity in description of patients with head injury, it not only allows monitoring of the patient's level of consciousness but also facilitates communication of this with colleagues.

Coma is defined as the inability to obey commands, utter words and open the eyes. No single score within the range 3–15 defines the cut-off point for coma. However, 90% of patients with a score of 8 or less, and none of those with a score of 9 or more, are found to be in coma according to the above definition. Therefore a GCS of 8 or less has become the generally accepted definition of coma. Somewhat arbitrarily, head-injured patients with a GCS score of 9–13 have been categorized as 'moderate' and those with a GCS of 14–15 have been designated as 'mild'. It should be noted that in assessing GCS, it is important to use the best motor response in calculating the score.

If there is any deterioration in the GCS score, it is important to exclude hypoxia and hypovolemia before considering intracranial injury. For patients with a depressed level of consciousness, therefore, the priorities are to establish a clear airway and provide neck control and stabilize respiration and circulation to prevent further cerebral damage.

A rise in pCO_2 causes cerebral vasodilatation and an associated potential rise in ICP. Head-injured patients should therefore be intubated and ventilated to maintain the pCO_2 between 3.3 and 4.0 kPa. Early communication with the neurosurgical unit is essential.

Traumatic tetraplegia should be excluded by response to painful stimuli, by supraorbital nerve compression if limb responses are absent. Priorities for management depend on whether the patient can talk. If he or she cannot do so intracranial and extracranial complications are more likely. Life-threatening airway, respiratory and circulatory conditions should be treated as soon as they are identified. Urgent blood tests include blood glucose, arterial blood gases and a coagulation screen. In patients who can talk, document their history, duration of both pre- and posttrauma amnesia, mechanism of injury, previous medical and surgical history and previous intake of drugs and alcohol. Tetanus prophylaxis should be given if indicated, when the secondary survey is completed.

Indications for endotracheal intubation in patients with severe head injury include:[22]

- absent gag reflex when oropharyngeal intubation is attempted in unconscious patients
- when airway protection is needed, e.g. when there is oropharyngeal bleeding, facial fracture or vomitus that cannot be easily cleared by the patient
- when ventilation or blood gas tension or both are too poor to allow spontaneous ventilation (PaO_2 <9 kPa breathing air or <13 kPa when receiving supplemental oxygen; $PaCO_2$ >5.3 kPa). Exclude pneumothorax on the basis of the chest radiograph
- to allow controlled hyperventilation when a patient's condition is deteriorating because of raised intracranial pressure.

Table 3.2 Glasgow Coma Scale

Assessment Area	Score
Eye Opening (E)	
Spontaneous	4
To speech	3
To pain	2
None	1
Best Motor Response (M)	
Obeys commands	6
Localizes pain	5
Normal flexion (withdrawal)	4
Abnormal flexion (decorticate)	3
Extension (decerebrate)	2
None (flaccid)	1
Verbal Response (V)	
Orientated	5
Confused conversation	4
Inappropriate words	3
Incomprehensible sounds	2
None	1

GCS = (E+M+V): best possible score = 15; worst possible score = 3
Coma = 8 or less: eyes, 1; motor response, 5 or less; verbal, 2 or less

Skull X-rays are of little value in the early management of patients with obvious head injuries, except in cases of penetrating injuries. The unconscious patient should have skull X-rays only if A, B and C are under control and continuing reassessment can be assured. Physical examination is usually more valuable than skull X-rays.

Basal skull fractures require CT scanning with bone windows for identification. The base of skull extends from the mastoid process to the orbits, so that fractures of the base of skull can produce signs along this line. The presence of clinical signs, including panda (racoon) eyes, Battle's sign, CSF leaks and seventh nerve palsy, should increase the index of suspicion.

As a rule, fragments depressed more than the thickness of the skull require surgical elevation. Open or compound skull fractures have a direct communication between the scalp laceration and the cerebral surface because the dura is often torn and these require early surgical repair.

A linear vault fracture increases the likelihood of an intracranial hematoma by about 400 times in a conscious patient and by 20 times in a comatose patient, in whom the risk of hematoma is already higher.

Sedation and analgesia can be difficult in patients with a head injury; they may be in pain and nauseous, yet strong opiate analgesics and drugs with respiratory depressant effects must be avoided as they may cause iatrogenic deterioration in conscious level and respiratory depression. For adults, intravenous or oral analgesia and antiemetics may be given. Hypoxia must be excluded and paracetamol or dihydrocodeine preparations such as DF118 or Co-codamol are useful, with metoclopramide for nausea. For children paracetamol suspension is suitable.

The choice of antibiotic for an established infection should be guided by identification of the causative organism and its sensitivity. The value of **prophylactic antibiotics** is controversial because of the risk of developing resistant infection and advice from the local neurosurgeon should be sought.

Mannitol is a powerful osmotic diuretic and may be life saving. It should be used in consultation with a neurosurgeon, to 'buy' time while the patient is being prepared for transfer to the nearest neurosurgical center.

There is no clear evidence supporting the use of **steroids** (even at high doses) in patients with head injury.

Restless patients should not be sedated without excluding hypoxia, hypotension, metabolic derangement, a full bladder or pain from other injuries.

If a patient shows **secondary deterioration** in their level of consciousness, it is important to exclude hypoxia, ischemia, metabolic derangement, missed intracranial hematoma, seizures and meningitis.

The use of **exploratory burr holes** in the management of head injury is controversial. It is said that even experienced neurosurgeons miss one-third of intracranial hematomas and may start bleeding and worsen brain damage. Burr holes should only be carried out by an experienced neurosurgeon, in a previously alert patient who deteriorates rapidly and develops a fixed dilated pupil that is ipsilateral to a skull fracture and in patients whose transfer to a neurosurgical center is likely to take 2 hours or more.

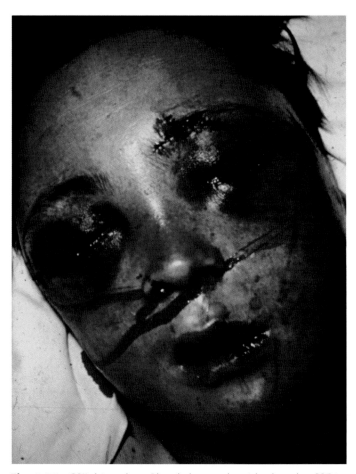

Fig. 3.22: CSF rhinorrhea. Blood clots at the sides but the CSF in the middle doesn't clot, producing the 'rail-track' appearance.

If interhospital transfer is being considered, telephone consultation supplemented by image transfer should precede transfer of the patient and should help decision making if there is uncertainty.

Computed tomography (CT) scanning

CT scans should be performed urgently within 2–4 hours of admission and the 24-hour service must be available. A neurosurgical opinion with regard to scan interpretation is always valuable. Units should have direct telecommunication link with the neurosurgeon, enabling distant viewing of the CT scan.

The indications for urgent CT in a head-injured patient are:[23]

- coma persisting after resuscitation
- deterioration of consciousness or progressing neurological signs
- fracture of skull with any of the following:
  — confusion or worse impairment of consciousness
  — epileptic seizure
  — neurological symptoms or signs
- open injury:
  — depressed compound fracture of the skull vault
  — fracture of the base of the skull
  — penetrating injury.

Additional indications are:

- skull fracture or after a fit
- confusion or neurological signs persisting after initial assessment and resuscitation
- unstable systemic state precluding transfer to neurosurgery
- uncertain diagnosis
- tense fontanelle or suture diastasis in a child.

When a CT scan is urgently performed for investigation of a head injury, radiologists have historically often been reluctant to extend the scan to include the facial bones, firstly because this may significantly increase the time taken for the scan and secondly that if orbital floor views, necessitating coronal slices, were needed, this would further extend the time that the patient spends in an inherently less safe environment.

However, with the advent of spiral and multislice scanners, the additional time required to include the facial bones is minimal and the scanner can reformat the information to any plane required. Also, if the patient has sustained head and facial injuries, then scanning the cervical spine may also be necessary.

Interhospital transfer

Adequate preparation for interhospital transfer can reduce morbidity and mortality. Problems are caused by:

- delay in arranging transfer
- inadequate resuscitation before transfer
- inadequate preparation for journey
- inadequate care during the journey
- inadequate communication between transferring and receiving units

Hypovolemic patients not fully resuscitated may develop profound hypotension on an ambulance journey. A patient in a coma should be intubated and accompanied by an experienced doctor.

Cervical spine and neck

Patients with maxillofacial or head trauma should be presumed to have an unstable cervical spine injury and the neck should be immobilized until such an injury has been excluded. The absence of neurological deficit does not exclude injury to the cervical spine.

As always, clinical examination proceeds along the lines of inspection, palpation and auscultation. Cervical spine tenderness, subcutaneous emphysema and laryngeal fracture should be elicited. Suspicion of an injury to the upper cervical spine may be aroused by a retropharyngeal hematoma seen through the open mouth. In this case the trachea may be deviated. Angiography or duplex ultrasound scanning may be required to exclude occlusion or dissection of the carotid artery.

Extreme care needs to be exercised when removing motorbike helmets.

Penetrating injuries to the neck have the potential of injuring several organ systems. Wounds extending through the platysma should not be explored manually or probed in A&E by personnel not trained to deal with such injuries. A surgeon should evaluate these injuries either operatively or with specialized diagnostic procedures. Active arterial bleeding, expanding hematoma, arterial bruit or airway compromise usually requires surgical operative evaluation.

A radiograph of the lateral cervical spine, showing all seven cervical vertebrae and the junction with the first thoracic vertebra, is essential in patients with multiple injuries and may have been carried out in the primary survey. This can usually be achieved by applying downward traction to both arms, but pain in the neck and exacerbation of neurological symptoms must be avoided. If the lower cervical vertebrae are still not adequately shown, a 'swimmer's view' and, if necessary, conventional or computed tomograms can be requested. This view, however, can still miss 15% of fractures, so an anteroposterior radiograph and odontoid peg views or a CT scan are required for a more complete evaluation of the cervical spine. These can be delayed until the secondary survey has been completed.

The lateral radiograph may show fractures, subluxations and dislocations. Unifacet dislocation is associated with forward vertebral displacement of less than half the diameter of the vertebral body. Displacement of more than half the vertebral width normally indicates bifacet dislocation. A chip fracture of the lower and anterior margin of the vertebra ('tear drop' fracture) is associated with an unstable flexion injury. This may produce widening of the interspinous gap, loss of normal cervical lordosis and minor subluxations. There may be a prevertebral hematoma, which is indicated by an increased gap between the nasopharynx or trachea and the cervical spine. The retropharyngeal space at C2 should not exceed 7 mm in adults and children, whereas the retropharyngeal space at C6 should not exceed 22 mm in adults and 14 mm in children.

The open mouth odontoid view may detect Jefferson fractures of the atlas as well as odontoid fractures.

The anteroposterior cervical spine radiograph allows visualization of fractures of the upper thoracic vertebrae and the first two ribs. It also shows alignment of spinous processes, which may be displaced laterally at sites of unilateral facet dislocation.

Chest

The priority is to identify potentially life-threatening conditions. Anterior and posterior inspection of the chest identifies open pneumothorax and large flail segments. Palpate the entire chest wall, including the clavicles, ribs and sternum. Contusions and hematomas suggest the possibility of occult pulmonary or cardiac injury.

Pain, dyspnea and hypoxia may suggest significant chest injury. Evaluation includes auscultation of the chest wall and chest X-ray. Breath sounds are auscultated high on the anterior chest wall for pneumothorax and posterior bases for hemothorax. Distant heart sounds and narrow pulse pressure may suggest cardiac tamponade. Distended neck veins may suggest cardiac tamponade or tension pneumothorax, although associated hypovolemia may minimize this finding. Decreased breath sounds, hyperresonance to percussion and shock may be the only findings in tension pneumothorax.

The chest X-ray, which may have been done in the primary survey, confirms the presence of hemothorax or simple pneumothorax. Rib fractures may also be seen. A widened mediastinum or deviation of the gastric tube to the right may suggest an aortic rupture.

Abdomen

A specific diagnosis is not as important as recognizing that an injury exists and that surgical intervention may be necessary. Close observation and frequent re-evaluation are important, preferably by the same observer.

An intra-abdominal bleed should be suspected if there are fractures of the ribs (5–11) that overlie the liver and the spleen, the patient is hemodynamically unstable or there are marks caused by seat-belts or tyres over the abdomen (Fig. 3.23). Patients with unexplained hypotension, neurological injury, impaired sensation secondary to alcohol and/or other drugs and equivocal abdominal findings should be considered for diagnostic peritoneal lavage (DPL), abdominal ultrasound or, if hemodynamically normal, CT of the abdomen. Fractures of the pelvis or the lower rib cage causing guarding also may hinder accurate diagnostic examination of the abdomen. Ideally DPL should be done by the surgeon who will be responsible for any subsequent laparotomy. There is no indication for DPL if laparotomy is already deemed necessary.

Injury to the retroperitoneal organs such as the pancreas may be difficult to identify even with the use of CT scan.

Perineum/rectum/vagina

Examine for contusions, hematomas, lacerations and urethral bleeding. A rectal examination should always be carried out before placing a urinary catheter. Assess for the presence of blood within the rectum, a high-riding prostate, the presence of pelvic fractures, the integrity of the rectal wall and the quality of the sphincter tone.

A vaginal examination is an essential part of the assessment in female patients. Look for the presence of blood in the vaginal vault and vaginal lacerations. In addition, pregnancy tests should be performed on all women of childbearing age.

Musculoskeletal

Each limb must be inspected for bruising, wounds and deformities and examined for vascular and neurological defects. The viability of the skin overlying fractures or dislocations must be assessed before and after the deformity has been corrected. The examiner must palpate all the bones in the limbs. Swabs should be taken for microbiological analysis from sites of open fractures. The wounds should then be covered with sterile dressings. Splinting of broken limbs is important because it reduces further damage to the soft tissues, pain and possibly the production of fat emboli. A Polaroid picture or digital image taken before covering an open fracture will avoid the need for repeated inspection and reduce the risk of infection.

Pelvic fractures are suggested by:

- ecchymosis over the iliac wings, pubis, labia or scrotum
- pain on palpation of the pelvic ring in the alert patient
- mobility of the pelvis in response to gentle anteroposterior pressure in the unconscious patient.

Assessment of the peripheral pulses enables identification of vascular injuries.

Significant limb injuries can exist without fractures being evident on examination or X-rays. In particular, ligament ruptures produce joint instability and muscle-tendon injuries interfere with active motion of the affected structures.

Impaired sensation and/or loss of voluntary muscle contraction strength may be due to nerve injury and/or to ischemia, including that due to compartment syndrome.

Spinal cord assessment

A detailed neurological examination, which includes testing for cranial nerves, sensation to fine touch and pinprick, proprioception, power, tone, co-ordination and reflexes, is carried out at this stage to identify abnormalities in the peripheral nervous system. The patient should have a urinary catheter in place, because spinal injury may result in urinary retention. Immobilization of the patient using a long spinal board and a semirigid collar must be maintained until spinal injury is excluded. The common mistake of immobilizing the head and freeing the torso allows the cervical spine to flex with the body as a fulcrum. Any evidence of sensory or motor loss suggests major injury to the spinal column or peripheral nervous system and should never be disregarded no matter how unimportant it may seem at the time.

The patient may complain of electrical shock-like pain radiating down the spine or into the limbs due to nerve root compression. In patients with partial cord lesions, some neurological function may be spared distal to the level of the injury (for example, the sacral segments) and this may suggest a vascular lesion. The acute urinary retention seen in paraplegic and tetraplegic patients may not be seen when

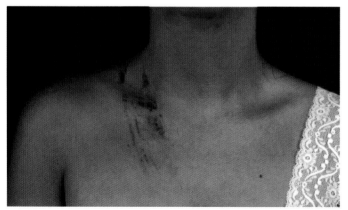

Fig. 3.23: Seat belt bruising. Bruising over the shoulder may overlie a fractured clavicle and over the abdomen may warn of intra-abdominal trauma.

there is sacral sparing. In patients with central cord syndromes, the zone of injury lies centrally and encroaches on the cervical segments of the long tracts, producing a flaccid weakness in the arms. Anterior contusions are associated with weakness and impaired pain and temperature sensation. Posterior injury results in loss of vibration sense and proprioception. In the Brown–Sequard syndrome, trauma is confined to one side of the cord, producing ipsilateral weakness and impaired contralateral pain and temperature sensation.

In the unconscious patient there are no truly pathognomonic features of spinal cord injury, but important signs are flaccid paralysis, diaphragmatic breathing, priapism and upward movement of the umbilicus on tensing the abdomen. If the cord has been transected above the level of the sympathetic outflow, neurogenic shock results, in which hypotension, without a corresponding tachycardia, is observed.

Thoracic and lumbar spinal fractures and/or neurological injuries must be considered based on physical findings and mechanism of injury. If a spinal injury is suspected the patient should be moved only by a well co-ordinated logrolling technique. The back should be examined from the occiput to the heels. After palpating the spinous processes and the paraspinal muscles a rectal examination should be carried out to assess anal sphincter tone and the prostate. The patient can then be logrolled back to the supine position.

Good-quality radiographs are essential in diagnosing spinal injuries. Anteroposterior and lateral radiographs are the standard views of the thoracolumbar spine. Unlike a cervical hematoma, a paravertebral hematoma in this area is best seen in an anteroposterior radiograph and may appear as mediastinal widening that may resemble aortic dissection. Subluxations, burst fractures or potentially unstable injury affecting the posterior vertebral ligaments or bone may be seen on the lateral radiograph. Instability requires at least two of the three columns of the spine to be disrupted. The upper thoracic spine is usually difficult to assess and if indicated, CT should be considered.

Investigations that require transportation of the patient to other areas of the hospital should only be sanctioned after the patient has been fully examined and deemed hemodynamically stable.

In some patients, decubitus ulcers may develop quickly over the sacrum, heels and other pressure areas following immobilization on a rigid spine board or from a cervical collar. Efforts to exclude the possibility of spinal injury and remove these devices should be initiated as soon as practical. Removal can usually be achieved at the end of the secondary survey, when debris can also be removed from the back. If further radiographs have to be taken in the radiology department, the board provides a useful means of transfer to the X-ray table. Patients should not be transferred to a tertiary center on a spinal board.

Maxillofacial

Definitive management of maxillofacial trauma can usually be deferred until after the airway has been secured and hemor-

rhage stemmed and after life-threatening neurosurgical, thoracic and abdominal and neurovascular limb injuries have been dealt with. Maxillofacial examination then proceeds as follows.

- The affected area should be exposed adequately and all wounds cleaned with Savlon.
- Examine the scalp for swelling, lacerations and bruises and palpate for bony steps, not forgetting the back of the scalp if it is possible to move the patient.
- The eyes should be examined as a matter of some priority before swelling makes it more difficult to do so. In particular, examine and document the following.
  — Visual acuity is checked using a standard Snellen chart at 6 metres. If the chart cannot be read at 1 metre, can the patient count fingers? If they cannot, can they detect hand movements? It may be that they can only perceive light.
  — The patient may have restriction of eye movement, diplopia or unequal pupillary levels following trauma to the orbital floor or medial wall, with entrapment of periorbital tissues.
  — Pupillary size, direct, consensual and accommodation reflexes are an effective way of checking the integrity of the visual pathways. They may help detect a rise in intracranial pressure but false-positive findings can be caused by trauma to the globe, resulting in posttraumatic mydriasis and retrobulbar hemorrhage. The latter also causes proptosis, pain and decreasing visual acuity and is a surgical emergency requiring immediate maxillofacial attention; treatment with acetazolamide, mannitol and steroids buys time while arranging theatre for surgical decompression of the hematoma.
  — Proptosis suggests hemorrhage within the confines of the orbital walls.
  — Enophthalmos suggests fracture of the floor or medial wall of the orbit.
  — Periorbital swelling and ecchymosis implies a fracture of the maxilla or zygoma.
  — Subconjunctival ecchymosis suggests direct trauma to the globe or a fractured zygoma (Fig. 3.24).
  — The anterior chamber of the eye and fundus should be examined for signs of direct trauma and raised intracranial pressure.
  — A ruptured globe must be excluded in all patients with trauma to the head and neck and if necessary, the ophthalmologist should be contacted. A painful eye as a result of blepharospasm suggests damage to the globe.
- Examine the nose for deformity, pain, mobility and difficulty in breathing, which suggest bony or cartilaginous fractures. A septal hematoma may cause nasal obstruction, appearing as swellings on both sides of the septum; if left untreated there is a risk of cartilage necrosis and nasal collapse and therefore the blood clot should be immediately evacuated.
- Epistaxis and in particular CSF rhinorrhea may suggest an anterior cranial fossa fracture at the cranial base. If the

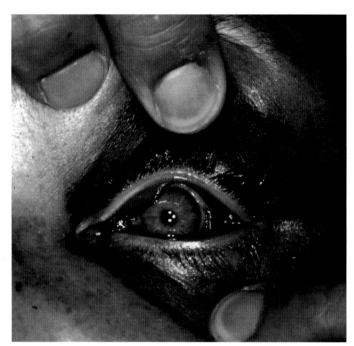

Fig. 3.24: Subconjunctival hemorrhage may strongly suggest a fractured zygoma. If severe the conjunctiva may herniate through the closed eyelids.

patient is lying supine on a trolley, CSF may be trickling posteriorly into the nasopharynx rather than onto the face. If present, do not pass a nasotracheal tube or nasogastric tube. Measure the intercanthal distance and if it is more than 35 mm suspect a nasoethmoid fracture.

- Examine the ears for hemotympanum and CSF otorrhea and if present, give prophylactic antibiotics.
- Look for sensory (fifth nerve) impairment, e.g. upper or lower lip and motor (seventh nerve) deficit.
- Pooling of tears and leakage from the eye may indicate damage to the nasolacrimal apparatus.
- Venous engorgement of the face suggests trauma to the major vessels in the neck.
- Surgical emphysema around the eyes and on the face suggests facial fractures. The patient should be instructed not to blow his nose if this complication is suspected. If present, prophylactic antibiotics should be given.
- Examine the face for lengthening, bilateral facial swelling and circumorbital ecchymosis ('panda eyes') and dish face deformity, which suggest bilateral maxillary fractures (Fig. 3.25).
- Palpate the orbits and zygomas for steps, particularly at the frontozygomatic (FZ) and zygomaticomaxillary (ZM) sutures, and the zygomatic arch. Step deformity with point tenderness is pathognomonic of a fracture. Isolated zygomatic arch or body of zygoma fractures can cause a restriction in mandibular excursions. Palpate the mandible for tenderness, step defects and crepitus.
- A sublingual hematoma indicates a mandibular fracture. Also inspect intraorally for lacerations, bleeding, loose teeth, broken teeth and dentures, mobile bone segments, abnormal alignment of the jaw, step defects and teeth meeting prematurely. If possible, ask the patient to bite

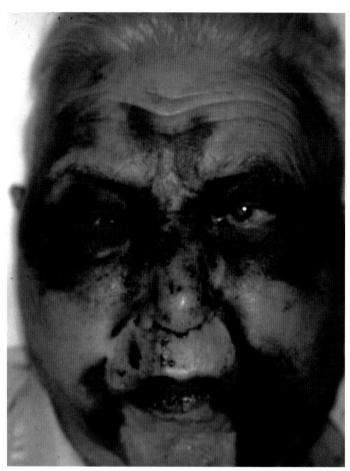

Fig. 3.25: Bilateral circumorbital ecchymosis ('panda' eyes) is suggestive of midfacial fractures although it can occur in the elderly in the absence of bony injury.

together on his back teeth. Do his teeth meet evenly? If teeth lost as a result of trauma are not accounted for, then a chest X-ray is mandatory.

- Gripping the anterior maxillary teeth with one hand (with the thumb in front and the index finger on the palatal side), while applying the other hand across the forehead, followed by simple manipulation, will confirm whether the nose or cheekbones move, indicating a maxillary fracture at the Le Fort I, II or III level. Any combination of Le Fort fractures can be present on one or both sides. Gagging of the occlusion often occurs and gross displacement of the maxillary and mandibular midlines may be apparent. Articulation may be impaired. Percussion of the maxillary teeth may produce the 'cracked cup' sound.

Imaging and investigation are only helpful in definitive planning and treatment.

Records and the Legal Consideration

It is important to keep meticulous contemporaneous notes, including times. This is especially important in the trauma setting when, by its very nature, legal proceedings are frequently taken and multiple doctors can be caring for the patient over a short period of time. Polaroid or digital photographs of injuries are ideal; alternatively clear accurate drawings, particularly in relation to facial injuries, must be made.

Consent for treatment

In simple terms, consent is sought before treatment if possible. If not possible, as in life-threatening injuries, treatment should be given first and formal consent obtained later.

Forensic evidence

Sometimes injury is thought to be due to criminal activity and in these circumstances it is important to preserve all the evidence. Clothes and bullets should be saved for the police. In addition, laboratory determination of blood alcohol and other drugs may be relevant.

Conclusion

Initial management of trauma patients requires a team approach in which each member is allocated a specific task, the overall aim being to identify and treat life-threatening conditions collectively. The ABC approach provides the doctor with one acceptable method for safe immediate management in which life-threatening injuries are identified and treated in the order in which they would otherwise kill the patient. Once the patient has been stabilized, a full assessment is carried out in which an AMPLE history is taken and the patient examined from top to toe, front to back and side to side. Throughout this process the emphasis is on continuous assessment and re-evaluation, so that the response to any therapy can be monitored and if there is any deterioration, the primary survey is repeated.

Maxillofacial injuries may be the source of significant airway compromise and/or life-threatening hemorrhage and maxillofacial surgeons have a crucial role to play as part of the trauma team. Their detailed knowledge of the anatomy of the head and neck and their familiarity with practical procedures put them in the front line in trauma management.

References

1 Boyd AD, Conlan AA 1979 Emergency cricothyroidotomy: is its use justified? Surgical Rounds 12: 19–23

2 Kress TD, Balasubramaniam S. 1982 Cricothyroidotomy. Annals of Emergency Medicine 11(4): 197–201.

3 Committee on Trauma, American College of Surgeons 1997 ATLS manual. ACS, Chicago p 79

4 Committee on Trauma, American College of Surgeons 1997 ATLS manual. ACS, Chicago p 155

5 Committee on Trauma, American College of Surgeons 1997 ATLS manual. ACS, Chicago p 99

6 Committee on Trauma, American College of Surgeons 1997 ATLS manual. ACS, Chicago p 98

7 Committee on Trauma, American College of Surgeons 1997 ATLS manual. ACS, Chicago pp 106–107

8 Schierhout G, Roberts I 1998 Fluid resuscitation with colloid or crystalloid solutions in critically ill patients: a systematic review of randomised trials. British Medical Journal 316: 961–964

9 Schultz SC, Hamilton IN, Malcolm DS 1993 Use of base deficit to compare resuscitation with lactated Ringer's solution, Haemaccel, whole blood and diaspirin cross-linked haemoglobin following haemorrhage in rats. Journal of Trauma 33: 417–423

10 Committee on Trauma, American College of Surgeons 1997 ATLS manual. ACS, Chicago p 32

11 Committee on Trauma, American College of Surgeons 1997 ATLS manual. ACS, Chicago pp 101–102

12 Hyde JAJ, Rooney SJ, Graham TR 1996 Fluid management in thoracic trauma. Hospital Update 22: 448–452

13 Bickell WH, Bruttig SP, Millnamow GA et al 1991 The detrimental effects of intravenous crystalloid after aortotomy in swine. Surgery 110: 529–526

14 Stern SA, Dronen SC, Wang X 1995 Multiple resuscitation regimens in a near-fatal porcine aortic injury haemorrhage model. Academic Emergency Medicine 2: 89–97

15 Hyde JAJ, Rooney SJ, Graham TR 1998 Hypotensive Resuscitation. In: Greaves I, Ryan JM, Parker KM (eds) Trauma. Edward Arnold, pp 177–185.

16 Shoemaker WC, Peitzman AB, Bellamy R 1996 Resuscitation from severe haemorrhage. Critical Care Medicine 24(suppl): 12–23

17 Stern SA, Dronen SC, McGoran AJ et al 1995 Effect of supplemental perfluorocarbon administration on hypotensive resuscitation of severe uncontrolled hemorrhage. American Journal of Emergency Medicine 13: 269–275

18 Driscoll P, Skinner D, Earlam R, 2000 (eds) ABC of Major Trauma. BMJ Publishing Group, London, p 44

19 Driscoll P, Skinner D, Earlam R, 2000 (eds) ABC of Major Trauma. BMJ Publishing Group, London, p 44

20 Committee on Trauma, American College of Surgeons 1997 ATLS manual. ACS, Chicago p 34

21 Driscoll P, Skinner D, Earlam R, 2000 (eds) ABC of Major Trauma. BMJ Publishing Group, London, p 34

22 Driscoll P, Skinner D, Earlam R, 2000 (eds) ABC of Major Trauma. BMJ Publishing Group, London, p 37

23 Driscoll P, Skinner D, Earlam R, 2000 (eds) ABC of Major Trauma. BMJ Publishing Group, London, p 38

4 Management of Head Injury

John Crossman, Justin Nissen, Alistair Jenkins

Introduction

Head injury is a major cause of preventable death in the Western world in adults under 45 years and in those who survive a significant head injury, a leading cause of chronic disability. The victims of head injury are responsible for a large cost in terms of manpower and resources. The aims of those involved in the management of head-injured patients must be:

- to prevent or reduce the number of head injuries suffered
- to provide optimium care for those unfortunate enough to suffer a head injury, preventing secondary brain injury from further compounding primary brain injury
- to produce an optimum environment in which rehabilitation from head injury can occur.

This chapter discusses the causes and mechanisms of head injury, the associated pathophysiology, the grading of the severity of injury and management of minor, moderate and severe head injury.

Epidemiology of Head Injury

About 200 per 100 000 individuals in the Western world suffer a head injury each year. These range from a minor knock on the head without loss of consciousness or lasting neurological sequelae to a head injury that leads directly to death. Collection of accurate data about the cause and seriousness of head injuries is difficult in the UK for several reasons.

- Many head injuries are minor and as such, are unreported to medical attendants.
- Many head injuries are part of a spectrum of serious injuries sustained during polytrauma, and are classified as such.
- No single international disease classification exists for head injuries; instead patients are classified under categories such as S00 – superficial injury of the head, S02 – fracture of the skull and facial bones. Whilst these diagnoses are suggestive of brain injury, the underlying injury is not described.[1]

Most studies of the epidemiology have therefore had to rely on a classification based on disposal of the patient, which within the UK is usually split into:

- A&E attender, but not admitted
- admitted for observation
- transferred to regional neurosurgical unit
- operated on in neurosurgical unit.

Clearly this does not include those patients with very severe injuries who may die before reaching hospital and those with apparently insignificant head injuries. Additional confounding factors include differences in the management of head injuries between different neurosurgical units, in that some units may transfer most or all serious head injuries whilst others may elect to manage at a distance those in whom neurosurgical intervention is not indicated.[2]

Most head injuries occur following falls, vehicular road accidents, pedestrian road accidents and assaults. Cause of accident varies amongst different age groups. Young children and the elderly are most commonly injured by falls, whilst young males are more commonly victims of assault. Sports and other leisure activities are also an increasingly important cause of head injury.

Two peaks are observed in the incidence of death following head injury: between 10 and 30 years old and greater than 70 years old. Hospital admission rates follow a similar pattern. Men have a higher incidence of mortality and hospital admission following head injury than women and more head injuries following assault are admitted at weekends. Admission and death rates have been shown to be affected by ethnicity.

Alcohol is undoubtedly an important factor in head injury. In studies where the influence of alcohol was assessed, it was shown that high levels are associated with assault and road traffic accidents.

As a consequence of the studies of the cause of head injury, many Western countries have introduced legislation to enforce the wearing of seat-belts and motorcycle crash helmets and have reduced vehicle speed limits. These preventive measures have contributed to a downward trend in the number of severe head injuries. However, in the developing world an increasing number of head injuries is occurring as road traffic increases.

Measurement of Injury Severity and Outcome

Glasgow Coma Scale

The Glasgow Coma Scale (GCS) is the scale most widely used to assess consciousness following a head injury.[3] Prior to its development, a series of loosely defined terms such as obtunded, lethargy, stupor and coma were employed to categorize the degree of unconsciousness.

A standardized method of scoring the level of consciousness, such as the GCS, is important in the management of

Table 4.1 Glasgow Coma Score: motor component

Action	Description	Score
Obeys commands	Patient obeys spoken commands	6
Localizes	Brings up arm(s) to painful stimulus applied in area of sensation supplied by cranial nerves	5
Withdrawal	Purposeful withdrawal from nailbed painful stimulus	4
Flexion	Flexion of the elbow on nailbed painful stimulus	3
Extension	Extension of the elbow on nailbed painful stimulus	2
None	No motor response to adequate painful stimulus	1

Table 4.2 Glasgow Coma Score: verbal component

Speech	Description	Score
Orientated	Knows time, place, location	5
Confused	Talks in complete sentences but does not know time, place, location	4
Words	Answers or uses only words	3
Sounds	Utters incomprehensible sounds	2
None	No speech	1

Table 4.3 Glasgow Coma Score: eye component

Eye opening	Stimulus	Score
Spontaneously	Eyes normally open	4
To speech	Eyes open only to speech	3
To pain	Eyes open only to pain	2
None	No eye opening	1

head injuries for several reasons. A substantial number of head injuries present to hospitals without resident neurosurgical support and a standardized scale of consciousness, together with image linking of the CT scan, allows a rapid evaluation of the severity of the injury to be made by the neurosurgeon and a decision made on whether transfer to the neurosurgical unit is required. The GCS also has been shown to have prognostic value about the eventual outcome of the injury.[4,5]

The development of the GCS permitted a reliable and reproducible assessment, with little interobserver variability across all classes of healthcare workers. The actual level of consciousness and deterioration in this level are more clearly identifiable when regular GCS assessments are performed.

The GCS consists of three parts – a motor response, a verbal response and an eye response. The motor component responses are given in Table 4.1. The motor response is scored as the best limb response. Failure of the patient to obey commands requires the observer to determine the patient's response to a painful stimulus, either pressure on the supraorbital nerve or the nailbed as detailed in the table. Usually the best response is elicited in the upper limbs and an asymmetrical response indicates a focal lesion of the central nervous system.

The verbal response is assessed as indicated in Table 4.2. Lack of a verbal response in an otherwise awake patient usually indicates damage to the speech center. The eye response (Table 4.3) assesses the integrity of the brain's arousal mechanisms. The eye response to pain should be elicited by limb stimulus as reflex eye opening may occur in response to facial stimulation. Also vital is the pupillary response to light and pupillary size and these should be assessed with the GCS in head-injured patients.

The severity of a head injury is usually classified according to the best postresuscitation GCS. A minor head injury is classified as a GCS score of 15, mild 13–14, moderate between 9 and 12 and severe between 3 and 8. Coma is defined as not obeying commands, no intelligible speech and no eye opening (M5V2E1). This classification is used to guide management and is prognostic of the eventual outcome.[6]

Glasgow Outcome Scale

In order to compare outcome following a head injury and to compare the beneficial effect or otherwise of interventions during the management of head injury, a standardized outcome measure has to be employed. The Glasgow Outcome Scale was developed in order to measure global brain functioning, rather than to specifically assess a particular mental or physical outcome.[7]

Improvement often occurs up to 6 months following head injury and may continue to occur for up to 1–2 years and so assessment of outcome should not be performed before 6 months after the injury.

The GOS assesses outcome based on the level of dependence or independence of the patient. There are five possible outcomes, shown in Table 4.4 and described below.

Good recovery implies the patient is able to resume previous employment, with possible existing neurological sequelae, but able to maintain an independent existence. *Moderate disability* indicates the patient is independent at home and can travel by public transport, but often has significant persisting physical or mental neurological deficits. A patient with a *severe disability* is conscious but dependent on the assistance of another person each day. *Persistent vegetative state* (PVS) allows normal respiration and sleep/wake states. A patient with PVS may occasionally follow a moving object or look to a bright light or loud sound and also withdraws from a painful limb stimulus. The final category is *death*. The scale is often abbreviated to favorable outcome – good recovery, moderate disability – and unfavorable outcome – severe disability, PVS, death.

As with the GCS, criticisms can be made of the GOS, in that it is too global an assessment and that a significant disability, either mental or physical, can exist despite an apparent favorable outcome, and that different levels of recovery are required to return to high-level professional or managerial employment than to lower level manual work, which may alter the outcome category.

Table 4.4 Glasgow Outcome Scale

Category	Description	Score
Good outcome	Resumption of normal life, despite minor neurological/psychological deficits	5
Moderate disability (disabled but independent)	Independent in daily life; however, often significant disability remains, e.g. dysphasia, hemiparesis and cognitive dysfunction	4
Severe disability (conscious but disabled)	Patients who are dependent on support for physical and/or mental activities	3
Persistent vegetative state	This is a difficult diagnosis; however, such patients often remain unresponsive following brain injury and may develop sleep/wake cycles	2
Death		1

Physiology of Head Injury

An understanding of the concepts of cerebral blood flow, cerebral perfusion pressure and intracranial pressure is essential to comprehend the pathophysiology and management of head injury.

Cerebral blood flow, intracranial pressure and cerebral perfusion pressure

The brain receives approximately one-fifth of the total cardiac output – about 1 l per minute at rest. This is equivalent to a mean cerebral blood flow in gray matter of 49 ml per 100 g of brain per minute. The brain has little capacity to store either glucose or oxygen and is therefore dependent on continuous blood flow. Reduction in cerebral blood flow to between 25 and 39 ml/100 g/min causes confusion and sometimes loss of consciousness. Reduction to 15 ml/100 g/min causes loss of measurable neuronal electrical activity and flow less than 8 ml/100 g/min causes neuronal death.[8]

Cerebral blood flow

Flow of a Newtonian fluid through a rigid vessel is described by Poiseuille's equation:[9]

$$Q = \text{pressure gradient} \cdot \text{pi} \cdot r^4 / 8 \cdot \text{length} \cdot \text{viscosity}$$

Clearly in the physiological situation, the importance of the pressure gradient and vessel diameter on blood flow can be seen. The pressure gradient is usually calculated as the mean arterial pressure minus the venous pressure and is known as the cerebral perfusion pressure (CPP):

$$CPP = \text{mean arterial pressure} - \text{venous pressure} \quad (1)$$

Because of the high compliance of the cerebral veins within the subarachnoid space, the venous pressure is usually approximated to the intracranial pressure and in practice (1) is approximated to the following:

$$CPP = \text{mean arterial pressure} - \text{intracranial pressure} \quad (2)$$

If the resistance component of the Poiseuille equation is defined in terms of cerebrovascular resistance (mmHg/ml/100 g/min), then the cerebral blood flow (CBF) can be calculated as:

$$CBF = \text{cerebral perfusion pressure/cerebrovascular resistance} \quad (3)$$

Intracranial pressure

The Monro–Kellie principle states that since the skull is a rigid structure and the skull contents of brain, cerebrospinal fluid and blood are incompressible, an increase in any one or several of these, or development of a mass lesion such as a hematoma, will cause an increase in intracranial pressure.

Measurement of intracranial pressure

Intracranial pressure can be measured by inserting a pressure transducer into the ventricular system, subarachnoid space, subdurally or intraparenchymally. The gold standard measurement is that of ventricular pressure. The pressure is normally measured in centimeters of water relative to the foramen of Munro. Normal adult intracranial pressure ranges from 0 to 15 cmH$_2$O.

Autoregulation

This is defined as maintenance of a constant cerebral blood flow over a range of cerebral perfusion pressures. Constant blood flow is maintained through variation in arterial diameter, the arterial diameter increasing as the perfusion pressure falls and decreasing as perfusion pressure increases.

When the autoregulatory mechanism is exhausted or deficient, as may be the case following head injury, the cerebral blood flow is dependent on the cerebral perfusion pressure and therefore in turn on the blood pressure. Low blood pressure will therefore decrease cerebral blood flow and cerebral ischemia occurs as the cerebral perfusion pressure falls below 50 mmHg. Following brain injury, loss of autoregulation is usually patchy within the brain and areas of the brain retain normal autoregulation. Flow 'steal' may then occur when blood vessels in normally functioning areas of brain dilate and therefore have a lower carebrovascular resistance than the blood vessels in the abnormal area of brain.[5]

Biomechanics and Pathology of Head Injury

Brain injury is usually classified into primary and secondary groups.[8,10] Primary brain injury is that which occurs at the time of the injury and is regarded as irreversible. Secondary brain injury occurs following the primary insult and it is the aim of head injury management to prevent or reduce damage

Table 4.5 Complications of head injury

Primary	Secondary	Extracranial
Scalp injury	Intracranial hematoma	Electrolyte disturbance
Skull fractures	Cerebral swelling	Chest sepsis
Perforating/penetrating wounds	Cerebral herniation	Thromboembolism
Focal brain injury	Cerebral ischemia	Gastrointestinal bleeding
Diffuse brain injury	Infection	

occurring as a consequence of secondary brain injury. The mechanisms of secondary brain injury are:

- hematoma formation
- brain swelling and cerebral herniation
- cerebral infection
- extracranial complications such as hypotension, hypoxia and metabolic complications leading to cerebral ischemia and hyponatremia (Table 4.5).

Primary brain injury

The forces that cause primary brain injury can be categorized as *inertial* or *contact*, although there is overlap between the groups. Most brain injury is a consequence of direct trauma to the skull, although facial injuries can result in brain injury.

Inertial brain injury

Inertial forces are a consequence of differential acceleration within the brain and between the brain and skull, usually following a glancing blow to the head. Such a blow results in deformation of the brain substance and shear stresses throughout the brain, causing axonal injury. Inertial injuries usually affect the whole of the brain and are termed *diffuse axonal injury* and may also cause rupture of bridging veins and pial vessels with consequent hematoma formation. The center of the brain is most affected by the rotational forces and consequently, it is the brain stem, corpus callosum and other central brain areas in which the diffuse injury is most marked.

Diffuse axonal injury

The shearing force causes stretching of the nerve fibers and this results in axonal damage. In the early stages of injury, this is represented pathologically by axonal bulbs or retraction balls, seen particularly in the central stuctures such as the corpus callosum, the white matter either side of the ventricle and regions of the brain stem. Over time, atrophy and degeneration of the long white matter tracts take place and patchy microglial formation occurs. Macroscopically in the early stages, small hemorrhagic lesions are seen in the locations of maximal stress. Rupture of the fornix may cause intraventricular hemorrhage. Later, brain matter atrophy with ventricular dilatation is the major finding.

The clinical consequence of this brain injury is a poor GCS from the outset, with a lack of lucid interval, low association

with skull fractures and, if survival occurs, often a high degree of residual brain dysfunction because of the widespread structural damage.

Contact brain injury

Contact injuries are usually the result of a direct blow to the skull and result in skull fractures and contusions of the brain both at the site and at a distance from the location of the injury. A blow to the skull results in inward movement of the skull at the point of impact, a fracture occurring if the degree of deformity exceeds the critical amount the skull is able to deform. The morphology of the fracture is dependent on the size of the contact area of the impact with the skull, a small area usually resulting in a relatively smaller depressed fracture whilst a larger area with a greater dissipation of the force will usually result in a relatively larger linear fracture.

Cerebral contusions

Cerebral contusions result from trauma to the brain causing localized hemorrhagic swelling. Typically cerebral contusions are found on the undersurface of the frontal lobes and temporal lobes and occur when these areas of the brain are damaged by the rough bone edges found in the region of the anterior and middle cranial fossae. The contusions may swell over several days, causing raised intracranial pressure, or bleeding into a contusion may result in the development of an intracranial hematoma.

Skull fractures

Fractures are a discontinuity of the bones forming the skull surrounding the brain. A fracture usually occurs following a contact injury, when a large displacement of the bone at the point of impact has occurred and exceeded bone plasticity. Fractures may occur in the calvarial region and base of the skull.

A stellate skull fracture, with fracture lines radiating from the point of impact, occurs as a result of a blow which contacts only a small area of the skull surface, such as a hammer or missile. A linear fracture tends to occur following a blow during which the force was spread over a greater area of the skull surface. Stellate fractures occur only rarely in the skull base because of the protection afforded by the occipitocervical musculature, pharynx and facial skeleton. Figure 4.1 demonstrates the intraoperative appearance of a linear skull fracture.

A skull fracture is compound if there is a continuity from the external environment through either a scalp laceration or paranasal sinus. This represents a route through which intracranial infection may occur, leading to abscess, empyema or meningitis.

A depressed skull fracture occurs when the fracture fragment lies deep to the surrounding bone, usually greater than the thickness of the surrounding bone. Depression of the fracture to this degree implies a dural laceration and therefore a potential route of infection. Depressed fractures may be closed or compound and may be linear or stellate.

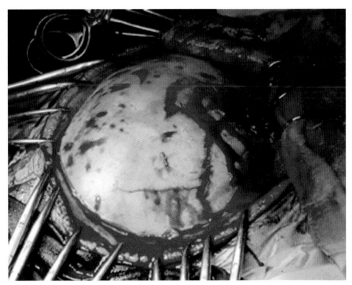

Fig. 4.1: Intraoperative appearance of a linear skull fracture. This patient's CT scan is illustrated in Figure 4.2 and the intraoperative appearance of the extradural hematoma in Figure 4.5.

Fractures may occur through the skull base and cause disruption of the vessels and nerves passing though the region of the fracture. CSF fistulae may occur with fractures through the frontal, sphenoidal or ethmoidal sinuses or through the cribriform plate. CSF leakage through temporal bone fractures may present as rhinorrhea, if the fluid leaks into the nasopharynx through the middle ear and eustachian tube, or otorrhea if leakage occurs through a perforated eardrum into the external auditory canal.

Elevation of a depressed skull fracture does not appear to alter the incidence of posttraumatic epilepsy.

Penetrating and perforating brain injury

Penetrating injury refers to those injuries caused by missiles or gunshot wounds, whilst perforation implies a puncture or stab wound by a knife or a nail. This type of injury results in a skull fracture with a tract hematoma. The severity of the injury is dependent on the area of brain damaged. The most common complications of perforating injury are infectious – brain abscesses and meningitis – and hemorrhagic. Vascular injury occurs in approximately one-third of brain wounds and may lead to the formation of traumatic aneurysms.

Secondary brain injury

Secondary brain injury is the most important cause of preventable morbidity and mortality.

Hematoma formation

Hematoma formation or the formation of a lesion with mass effect, i.e. causing a rise in intracranial pressure, represents a neurosurgical emergency.

The type of hematoma occurring following a head injury is dependent on the mechanism of the injury.

Extradural hematoma

A focal injury associated with the formation of a skull fracture may result in the development of a hematoma in the extradural space. Typically, this occurs in the region of the temporal bone and results from damage to the middle meningeal artery but extradural hematomas may also form in the frontal, parietal or occipital regions and in the posterior fossa from lacerations to dural arteries or from bleeding from the fracture itself. Because the source of the hematoma is usually arterial, these hematomas are usually under high pressure and cause mass effect. Typically the size of the hematoma is limited by the dura being tightly bound to the skull at the cranial sutures. Figure 4.2 illustrates the CT appearance of an extradural hematoma.

Acute subdural hematoma

An acute subdural hematoma is usually the consequence of a widespread superficial cortical injury, with multiple resultant bleeding points. Occasionally, rupture of a cortical bridging vein between the brain and the cerebral venous sinus, as it passes through the potential subdural space between the dura and arachnoid membranes, can result in a subdural hematoma. The bridging veins are most vulnerable when placed on stretch, as is the case in the young child and in those with an atrophic brain such as the elderly. Figure 4.3 illustrates the CT appearance of an acute subdural hematoma.

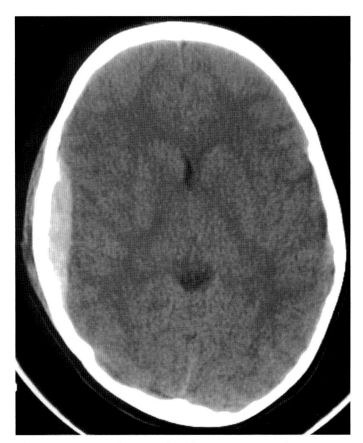

Fig. 4.2: CT scan of an extradural hematoma. Note the asymmetry of the lateral ventricles and minor degree of midline shift, indicating that the hematoma has mass effect.

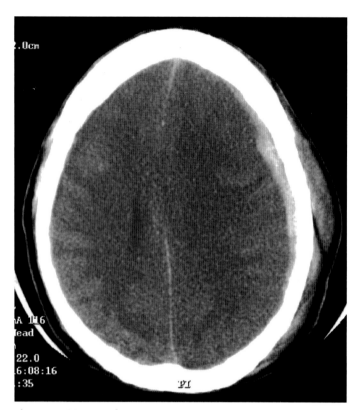

Fig. 4.3: CT scan of an acute subdural hematoma.

A rotational injury causing differential shearing between the skull and brain causes the veins to stretch beyond capacity and therefore rupture, with bleeding then occurring into the subdural space. The arachnoid and dura are only tightly bound at the cerebral sinuses and blood is therefore able to track within the subdural space more extensively than occurs with an extradural hematoma. Because these hematomas usually result from venous bleeding and because of the larger potential space in which to spread, they are usually low pressure and conform to the surface of the brain.

Chronic subdural hematoma

A chronic subdural hematoma also occurs in the space between the dura and the brain and is also found usually in the elderly. The origin of the hematoma is uncertain but most probably arises following minor and often repeated insignificant head injury. With time the volume of the hematoma enlarges, either through repeated episodes of bleeding or because the high osmotic potential of the blood attracts water. Within the hematoma, the blood liquefies over about 10 days during which the hematoma consists of a mixture of fluid blood and organizing clot. This stage is often referred to as a subacute subdural hematoma. After about 3 weeks, the collection has usually liquefied. A fresh bleed can occur into a chronic subdural hematoma and may result in a rapid rise in the intracranial pressure, with consequential neurological deterioration, which may prompt diagnosis of the previously unrecognized hematoma.

Often a chronic subdural hematoma can grow to a substantial size and result in mass effect, leading to compression of the ipsilateral cerebral hemisphere and midline shift, with

relatively little neurological deficit. This is because the rise in intracranial pressure occurs over days rather than within minutes and hours, as is the case with an extradural or acute subdural hematoma, and this allows intracranial compensation to occur.

Intracerebral hematoma

Intracerebral hematomas arise from two distinct mechanisms in relation to head injury. Deep-seated hematomas, usually within the basal ganglia, arise from rotational injury and are therefore indicative of diffuse axonal injury. They are often small and do not usually require surgical intervention. A hematoma may also occur in relation to a contusion, as discussed above. Such a hematoma may swell progressively over several days, develop mass effect and raise the intracranial pressure.

Burst lobe

A burst lobe is distinct from an intracerebral hematoma, in that the hematoma occurs in continuity with the overlying contused brain, which is in contact with an acute subdural collection. This injury occurs most frequently in the frontal and temporal lobes.

Intraventricular hemorrhage

This is a rare occurrence following head injury. The origin of the intraventricular blood is usually a tear of a central midline intraventricular structure such as the fornix and as such, indicates that the brain has suffered a major rotational injury. Hence, intraventricular blood is usually associated with severe diffuse axonal injury. It is important to consider whether the intraventricular bleed occurred as part of a primary event such as rupture of a cerebral aneurysm, particularly if there is associated subarachnoid blood, and the head injury occurred as a result of a collapse.

Traumatic subarachnoid hemorrhage

Traumatic subarachnoid hemorrhage results from injury to cerebral vessels as they cross the subarachnoid space. Extensive subarachnoid hemorrhage can occur, with subsequent vasospasm. The distribution of the blood in traumatic subarachnoid hemorrhage is usually easily distinguishable from that of aneurysmal subarachnoid hemorrhage but if uncertainty exists, cerebral angiography may be required to distinguish between the two causes.

Brain swelling

Brain swelling may be caused by an increase in the brain water content, such as occurs in cerebral edema, or increased blood due to cerebral hyperemia or development of an intracerebral mass lesion.

There are two main forms of cerebral edema. *Vasogenic* cerebral edema occurs when the blood–brain barrier has been disrupted and extravasation of water, sodium and protein molecules into the extracellular space occurs. *Cytotoxic* cerebral edema occurs when the neurons lack energy to maintain the ionic gradient across the cell membrane and water passes into the cells, which causes them to swell.

Cerebral hyperemia is more common in children than in adults. The causative mechanism is unknown but the arterioles appear to dilate and blood passes directly to the capillary bed.

As discussed above, brain swelling causes a rise in the intracranial pressure and, in the absence of intact autoregulation, leads to a reduction in the cerebral blood flow.

Brain herniation

The skull is divided into compartments by the infolding of the dura to form the cerebral falx and cerebral tentorium. Development of a mass lesion, such as an intracerebral or extradural hematoma, creates a pressure gradient across the different compartments. Brain herniation occurs in response to the pressure gradient.

Several different forms of herniation have been described. *Subfalcine herniation* occurs when a unilateral supratentorial mass lesion causes brain to herniate under the falx. Compression of the anterior cerebral arteries is a possible consequence, but clinical symptoms and/or signs related to this are rare.

Lateral tentorial herniation is also a consequence of a unilateral supratentorial mass lesion. The medial edge of the ipsilateral temporal lobe is forced medially and compresses the third cranial nerve. Clinically this causes the pupil to dilate and become non-reactive to light. The brain stem can also become displaced and compressed with deterioration of conscious level and compression of the ipsilateral cerebral peduncle causing contralateral hemiparesis.

Central tentorial herniation occurs as a consequence of diffuse supratentorial swelling, when the contents of the supratentorial compartment are forced vertically through the tentorial hiatus. Pressure on the tectum causes loss of upgaze. Further downward movement of the brain stem leads to a deterioration in conscious level, pupillary abnormalities and eventually, as traction injury to the pituitary stalk occurs, diabetes insipidus.

A hematoma in the infratentorial compartment can cause the cerebellar tonsils to herniate through the foramen magnum and upwards herniation of the cerebellum through the tentorial hiatus.

Cerebral infection

Compound fractures represent a potential route of infection, through which organisms may track and cause meningitis. Meningitis results in a purulent exudate, which spreads throughout the subarachnoid space. Cerebritis and brain abscess formation may follow. The infection leads to vascular thrombosis, causing infarcts, and occasionally obstruction of CSF flow results in hydrocephalus.

Extracranial complications

Many extracranial complications may occur, such as hyponatremia, respiratory complications and gastrointestinal hemorrhage. These compromise brain blood flow and oxygenation to the detriment of the patient.

Management of Head Injuries

The overriding aim of the management of a patient who has suffered a head injury is to minimize the morbidity and mortality related to secondary brain injury. This requires rapid evaluation and triage of patients presenting with head injuries. Guidelines for the initial management of head injuries were published in 1984 and revised in 1998.[11,12] These guidelines advise on the appropiate triage of patients to:

- observation at home with a responsible adult
- observation in hospital

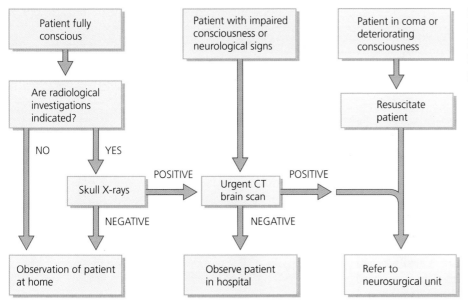

Fig. 4.4: Guidelines for the initial triage of head injuries (from Bartlett J, Kett-White R, Mendelow AD et al 1998 British Journal of Neurosurgery 12(4):349–352, with permission).

- urgent CT at presenting hospital and/or discussion with a neurosurgical unit
- referral to a neurosurgical unit.

Figure 4.4 illustrates the triage categories and initial management. Patients are usually transferred to the neurosurgical unit for specialized monitoring and observation or because an operation is indicated.

Initial management of head injuries

The initial management of any head injury is to ensure adequate resuscitation of the patient. Whilst the majority of minor head injuries do not require resuscitation, in a patient with a severe head injury it is vital to ensure the airway is clear and adequate respiration and circulation are established prior to dealing with the head injury.

Following resuscitation and stabilization of the patient, the history of the injury should be determined. In the case of a minor injury, this will be gained from the patient whilst in a more severe injury, witness accounts should be sought. The most important information to determine is the initial GCS, pupillary reaction and size, whether the patient's condition is improving or deteriorating, the blood pressure and pulse rate and the presence of other associated injuries. Other factors include period of unconsciousness, the period of posttraumatic amnesia, whether a seizure has occurred and the presence or absence of a focal neurological deficit. The events surrounding the injury should also be determined, such as the degree of damage to the vehicle in a motor accident and number of other people and their injuries, as this information can be used to gauge the seriousness of the accident.

The patient should then be examined. Obviously the conscious level of the patient will affect the examination performed but in general, the following should be assessed:

- the conscious level of the patient, using the Glasgow Coma Score
- presence or absence of lateralizing signs, i.e. pupillary abnormalities and hemiplegia/paresis, paraparesis
- external evidence of head injury
- evidence suggesting a base-of-skull fracture, such as raccoon eyes, subconjunctival hemorrhage or Battle's sign
- presence of a CSF leak
- presence of spinal and other extracranial injuries.

Investigations such as CT brain scanning, referral to the local neurosurgical unit or skull X-rays may then be indicated, as per the head injury management guidelines, and management decisions should be as indicated in the guidelines.

Surgical evacuation of intracranial hematomas

Mass lesions within the skull, such as intracranial hematomas, may cause a rise in the intracranial pressure and therefore a reduction in the cerebral perfusion pressure. Locally raised pressure around the hematoma may also cause cerebral herniation. In order to minimize secondary brain damage, any hematoma with significant mass effect should be removed. Hematomas without significant mass effect may be treated conservatively with serial observation of the patient's condition. Invasive monitoring of the intracranial pressure may be required. Persistent elevation of intracranial pressure or a decline in the conscious level indicates the need for a further CT brain scan in order to determine whether the hematoma has increased in size and requires operative removal. Exploratory burr holes are very seldom performed.

Extradural hematoma

Extradural hematomas most commonly arise from the tearing of a middle meningeal artery in the region of the squamous temporal bone. A craniotomy is performed over the site of the hematoma. The hematoma, which usually consists of a mixture of coagulated blood with some fresh blood, is aspirated and washed away and the bleeding vessel found and diathermied. If necessary, the middle meningeal artery is coagulated as proximally as required. Hitch stitches are then placed around the edges of the dura and the bone flap replaced and fixed into position. If the intracranial pressure is markedly elevated, the bone may be simply placed back in the skull defect and allowed to ride, although this is rarely the case with an extradural hematoma.[6] Figure 4.5 illustrates the operative appearance of an extradural hematoma.

Acute subdural hematoma

Acute subdural hematomas are often more extensive in size than extradural hematomas and accompanied by extensive brain swelling. The hematoma lies between the dura and cortical surface. Bleeding is usually the result of a widespread superficial cortical contusion, with multiple bleeding points, or occasionally the result of a ruptured parafalcine or sylvian fissure cortical vein. A craniotomy is performed in the usual manner over the center of the clot. The dura is then opened and the clot washed away. Once hemostasis has been

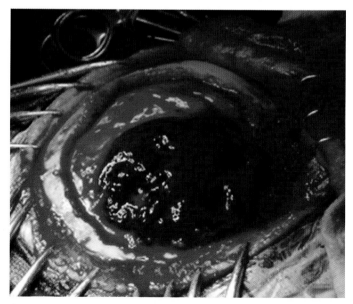

Fig. 4.5: Intraoperative appearance of an extradural hematoma.

achieved, the bone should be replaced as described above and the wound closed in the usual manner.[6]

Management of skull fractures

Most skull fractures do not require operative treatment. The indications for elevation of a depressed skull fracture are related to the presence of a dural tear and cosmesis. Fractures that are displaced beyond the inner table of the surrounding cortical bone indicate the presence of a dural tear and in the presence of a scalp wound, debridement and elevation of the fracture are required. Fractures outwith the hair line are usually elevated for cosmesis.

Elevation of a depressed skull fracture

In the case of a compound depressed skull fracture, the depressed fragments of bone are isolated from the skull and extracted from the fracture. The wound and bone fragments are then cleaned and dural tear repaired. The bone is then replaced if not too contaminated. The wound is then closed and the patient given a course of intravenous antibiotics.

Treatment of perforating/penetrating head injury

Penetrating injury is usually a result of a gunshot wound. Several factors affect the degree of damage caused to the brain by a gunshot, the most important being the projectile velocity, as the kinetic energy is related to the square of the velocity. As the projectile passes through the brain, a pulsating cavity, often many times larger than the projectile diameter, is created which undergoes cyclical dilatation and collapse several times. Shock waves created by the projectile impacting against the skull also produce rapid and sudden compression and re-expansion of brain adjacent to the site of impact.

Penetrating and perforating injuries should be treated with prophylactic antibiotics and if the patient's condition warrants, he should undergo a cerebral angiogram and wound debridement. Traumatic aneurysms are more likely to rupture than congenital aneurysms and should be managed operatively.

Subsequent management of moderate and severe head injury

Avoidance of secondary brain injury is of vital importance following the initial management of the head injury, if the brain is to be given maximum potential for recovery and rehabilitation. Following control of ICP, the sedation is gradually reduced and the patient is extubated when his conscious level is good enough to maintain his airway and respiration. At this stage, the patient may still not be awake enough to obey commands or may have focal deficits related to cerebral damage as a result of the trauma, such as dysphasia. Some patients require continued ventilation, either because of extracranial injuries, such as chest trauma or chest infections, or in order to control the intracranial pressure.

During this time, it is important to continue patient monitoring – blood pressure, oxygen saturation, intracranial and cerebral perfusion pressure – in order to prevent secondary brain injury.

Control of cerebral perfusion pressure and intracranial pressure

In order to minimize cerebral ischemia, an important cause of secondary brain injury, the brain must have an adequate blood flow. Cerebral blood flow is difficult to measure continuously on a routine basis and in most centers the cerebral perfusion pressure is measured as a surrogate. Cerebral blood flow is related to cerebral perfusion pressure as discussed above, although it should be recalled that the autoregulation mechanism is often disrupted following brain injury.

That clinical outcome is related to intracranial pressure and/or cerebral perfusion pressure is debated. The ideal ICP and CPP following a head injury are unknown but several studies have examined outcome in relation to CPP and most authorities accept that an ICP below 20–25 mmHg and a perfusion pressure greater than 70 mmHg are required for optimal management. Hyperventilation is rarely used in the management of head injury because it leads to vasoconstriction and therefore a reduction in the CPP.[6,13]

Ischemic brain injury is found in about 90% of patients who die following head injury and a single episode of hypotension is associated with an 85% increase in mortality. Experimental animal work has suggested that higher perfusion pressures are beneficial in the presence of mass lesions and reductions in perfusion pressure significantly increase the risk of brain-stem ischemia.

Autoregulation maintains a constant blood flow to the brain over a wide range of cerebral perfusion pressures and is therefore important in the prevention of cerebral ischemia. At cerebral perfusion pressures of less than 50 mmHg, cerebral arteriole vasodilatation is exhausted and the vessel collapses, with consequent cerebral ischemia. The upper limit of cerebral perfusion pressure autoregulation is 140 mmHg. Above this level, cerebral perfusion pressure increases with blood flow, causing damage to the blood–brain barrier and subsequently brain swelling. Following head injury, the autoregulatory mechanism is often damaged and experimental studies suggest that a perfusion pressure of between 60 and 70 mmHg is required to achieve autoregulation.

Persistently elevated intracranial pressure is managed by:

- surgical evacuation of mass lesions
- head elevation
- control of $PaCO_2$
- maintenance of a CPP greater than 70 mmHg
- increasing sedation and paralysis
- mannitol infusion or bolus
- ventricular drainage
- decompressive craniectomy.

The initial measures are elevation of the head to about 30°, with maintenance of the head in neutral position to increase venous return, maintenance of the CPP greater than

70 mmHg and ensuring the $PaCO_2$ is about 4 kPa. If these measures are unsuccessful in lowering the intracranial pressure, further measures are instituted as listed above.

Failure to control the ICP is an indication for a repeat CT scan, as a traumatic hematoma may develop or enlarge with time; contusions or swelling may also worsen. If the ICP remains elevated, surgical decompression should be considered. In the absence of a mass lesion, the brain may be decompressed by a frontal or temporal lobectomy or by a decompressive craniectomy.

Barbiturates

Barbiturates are rarely used for ICP control because of their deleterious effect on blood pressure and hence cerebral perfusion pressure. Episodic rises in intracranial pressure may be caused by seizure activity and this should be treated with an anticonvulsant drug.

Hyperventilation

Chronic hyperventilation in the management of intracranial pressure is no longer practiced as it has a tendency to decrease the cerebral perfusion pressure. Conversely, Muizelaar[14] demonstrated that patients maintained at normocapnia, compared to those with hypocapnia, had a better outcome at 3 and 6 months although not at 1 year. Cerebral blood flow is usually most severely decreased in the 24 hours immediately following head injury and hyperventilation during this time is most harmful.

Neuroprotective agents

Trials involving steroids, free radical scavengers and NMDA receptor antagonists have not shown any benefit to patient outcome, although the search continues.

Management of extracranial complications

Extracranial complications are common in head-injured patients. The most common are respiratory complications. If a patient remains intubated for more than 10 days a tracheostomy should be considered. Chest infection should be treated with antibiotics, guided by microbiological culture of sputum, suctioning as required and physiotherapy. Nutritional support via nasogastric tube feeding should be commenced as soon as is possible and converted to a percutaneous gastrostomy if nutritional support is required for a period of time. Hyponatremia may be caused by the syndrome of inappropriate secretion of antidiuretic hormone (SIADH) or by cerebral salt wasting. The best way to determine the cause is to measure the volume status. The dehydrated patient with hyponatremia due to cerebral salt wasting can be treated by sodium and volume replacement. Hyponatremia secondary to SIADH is normally responsive to fluid restriction. Hypernatremia is less common than hyponatremia and is usually a consequence of hypothalamic or pituitary injury causing diabetes insipidus. This is treated with desmopressin if required.

Deep vein thrombosis and pulmonary emboli occasionally occur and should be treated with anticoagulants. In the immobile patient consideration should be given to heparin prophylaxis.

Posttraumatic Seizures

Posttraumatic seizures are a common accompaniment to head injury and are of serious consequence to recovery, in that driving is disallowed and the side effects of anticonvulsant medication may delay cognitive recovery. Prevention of posttraumatic seizures and satisfactory management when they occur is essential for optimum management.

Not all seizures occurring following a head injury are related to the head injury per se. Seizures can occur as a consequence of alcohol or illicit drug withdrawal, hypoxia or therapeutic drugs.

Classification

Jennett defined early seizures as those occurring within 1 week of the injury and late seizures as those occurring thereafter. Others have added an additional category of immediate seizures, although this adds little to prognosis and management.[15]

Early seizures

Early seizures occur in about 2% of unselected series of head injury. In pediatric series, the incidence approaches 7–9%. Risk factors for early seizures include skull fractures, especially depressed fractures, hematoma formation, contusions, a prolonged period of unconsciousness, focal signs and young age.

One-third of seizures occur within 1 hour, another third between 1 and 24 hours and the final third between 1 and 7 days. Seizures tend to occur later in adults than in children. The majority of early seizures are focal and about 10% of adults and 20% of children under 5 develop status epilepticus.

Late seizures

Between 2% and 5% of patients suffer from late seizures following civilian head injury. The major risk factors are a penetrating missile wound, hematoma formation, depressed skull fracture and early seizures. The risk of a late seizure is highest initially and decreases slowly with time, although following missile head injury, seizures may occur up to 10–15 years later. The majority of the seizures are either primary generalized or secondary generalized following focal onset.

Management of posttraumatic seizures

Recurrent early seizures are usually managed with a loading dose of an anticonvulsant, usually valproate or phenytoin, followed by regular oral or intravenous doses.

If status epilepticus occurs, despite adequate anticonvulsant doses, serum electrolytes, glucose, calcium and magnesium should be estimated and corrected. Further seizure activity requires intubation, sedation and ventilation, usually with propofol in an intensive care unit, ideally with continuous EEG monitoring. An intracranial pressure monitoring device may also be inserted and the patient should undergo a CT brain scan in order to exclude development of a treatable surgical cause. Continued epileptiform activity on EEG monitoring whilst intubated, ventilated and sedated requires specialist advice.

Following control of early seizures, anticonvulsant medication is usually continued for 6 weeks and the dose tailed off thereafter, providing no further fits have occurred.

Patients who suffer from two or more late seizures are usually commenced on long-term anticonvulsant medication. This may be continued for some years before a gradual reduction is considered, prior to stopping the anticonvulsant drug.

Prophylaxis

Despite several randomized controlled trials of anticonvulsant drugs following head injury, no clear benefit or consensus opinion concerning their use has emerged.

Postconcussion Syndrome

The hallmarks of the postconcussion syndrome are a minor head injury, a normal neurological examination and a variety of symptoms, usually out of proportion to the severity of the injury, most of which are difficult to substantiate.[16] The symptoms are variable but in the main consist of headache associated with dizziness and memory difficulties. A full list of symptoms is given in Box 4.1.

Epidemiology

Postconcussion syndrome occurs almost exclusively in those patients who have suffered from a minor head injury. Different studies have reported different incidences, possibly because of assessment at different times following injury. Rimel and colleagues followed a group of patients for 3 months.[17] The inclusion criteria for the study were a hospi-

tal admission lasting less than 48 hours, with mild head injury, i.e. GCS score between 13 and 15, and a period of unconsciousness lasting less than 20 minutes. This group found that 79% complained of persistent headaches, whilst 59% complained of ongoing memory problems. Return to work was more likely in the professional, business and managerial groups and litigation was apparently not an important factor. Postconcussion syndrome is far less commonly observed in children, when compared to adults.

Pathophysiology

Elucidation of the pathophysiology of this disorder is difficult because of the vague nature of the symptoms, and because the head injury is minor, little formal neuropathological information is available. It is likely the syndrome is a consequence of microscopical structural changes, probably with related changes in neurotransmitter balance.

Clinical assessment and investigation

A formal history, with full information about the accident and the patient's premorbid personality, is required. The symptom complex should be carefully delineated. Additional information may be provided by family members. A full neurological examination should be performed and any abnormality apparent on clinical assessment should be confirmed with formal investigations.

Radiological imaging is important to exclude structural abnormality and may reveal chronic subdural hematoma, atrophy, especially of the frontal lobes, and hydrocephalus. Magnetic resonance imaging may provide further evidence of subtle brain injury. Electroencephalography should be performed in those patients whose symptoms could conceivably be caused by seizure activity.

Psychological assessment, using the Paced Auditory Serial Addition Task, has demonstrated an impairment in the rate of information processing, which improved with clinical improvement in the symptoms. Other tests have demonstrated problems with memory recall.

Management

In most cases, reassurance that there are no abnormal findings on examination and investigation and education of the patient and the family about the syndrome help the symptoms to resolve, usually by 1 year post injury. Symptomatic treatment of headache is indicated, as is treatment of proven seizures. If psychological testing demonstrates impaired processing, development of coping strategies is appropriate.

Box 4.1   Symptoms following minor head injury

Headaches
Dizziness
Vertigo
Tinnitus
Visual blurring
Reduced/absent taste and smell
Irritability
Anxiety
Depression
Fatigue
Memory problems
Impaired concentration
Light/noise sensitivity

References

1 Jennett B 1998 Head injury. In: Martyn C, Hughes RAC (eds) Epidemiology of head injury. BMJ Books, London
2 Jennett B, MacMillan R 1981 Epidemiology of head injury. British Medical Journal 282: 101–104
3 Jennett B, Teasdale G 1974 Assessment of coma and impaired consciousness: a practical scale. Lancet ii: 81–83

4 Signorini DF, Andrews PJD, Jones PA, Wardlaw JM, Miller JD 1999 Predicting survival using simple clinical variables: a case study in traumatic brain injury. Journal of Neurology, Neurosurgery and Psychiatry 66: 20–25

5 Mendelow AD, Teasdale G, Jennett B, Bryden J, Hessett C, Murray G 1983 Risks of intracranial hematoma in head injured adults. British Medical Journal 287: 1173–1176

6 Kelly DF, Nikas DL, Becker DP 1996 Diagnosis and treatment of moderate and severe head injuries in adults. In: Youmans JR (ed) Neurological surgery WB Saunders, Philadelphia, pp 1618–1718

7 Jennett B, Bond M 1975 Assessment of outcome after severe brain damage: a practical scale. Lancet i: 480–484.

8 Liau LM, Bergsneider M, Becker DP 1996 Pathology and pathophysiology of head injury. In: Youmans JR (ed) Neurological surgery WB Saunders, Philadelphia, pp 1549–1594

9 Miller JD 1987 Normal and increased intracranial pressure. In: Miller JD (ed) Northfield's surgery of the central nervous system Blackwell Science, Oxford, pp 7–57

10 Adams JH, Graham DI 1994 Trauma. In: An introduction to neuropathology Churchill Livingstone, Edinburgh, pp 133–156

11 Briggs M, Clarke P, Crockard A 1984 Guidelines for the initial management after head injury in adults. British Medical Journal 288: 983–985

12 Bartlett J, Kett-White R, Mendelow AD, Miller JD, Pickard J, Teasdale G 1998 Guidelines for the initial management of head injuries: recommendations from the Society of British Neurological Surgeons. British Journal of Neurosurgery 12: 349–352

13 Juul N, Morris GF, Marshall SB, Marshall LF 2000 Intracranial hypertension and cerebral perfusion pressure: influence on neurological deterioration and outcome in severe head injury. Journal of Neurosurgery 92: 1–6

14 Muizelaar JP, Marmarou A, Ward JD 1991 Adverse effects of prolonged hyperventilation in patients with severe head injury: a randomized clinical trial. Journal of Neurosurgery 75: 731–739

15 Temkin NR, Haglund MM, Winn HR 1996 Post traumatic seizures. In: Youmans JR (ed) Neurological surgery WB Saunders, Philadelphia, pp 1834–1839

16 Miller JD, Ward BA, Alexander LF 1996 Post traumatic syndrome. In: Youmans JR (ed) Neurological surgery WB Saunders, Philadelphia, pp 1825–1833

17 Rimel RW, Giordani B, Barth JT et al 1981 Disability caused by minor head injury. Neurosurgery 9: 221

5 Radiographic Assessment

Nicholas B Bowley

Introduction

Very thorough clinical appraisal, preferably by a specialist, should always precede imaging. Some facial injuries require no imaging at all, others need quite complex image investigation. Many factors are involved in the process, from presentation of the facially injured patient through imaging, to the final report of the images. This process is heavily dependent on good teamwork between surgeons, nursing staff, radiographers and radiologists.

Three important aspects moderate many of the decisions in this process:

- radiation cost (to the individual and to the community)
- financial cost (to the individual or the community)
- risk that a particular image process may delay more urgent treatment for the patient.

Initial Assessment

Tailoring the imaging to the immediate, early and late evolving scenario is essential in achieving a balance between identifying all important lesions and minimizing radiation exposure. The presentation of the patient varies enormously, from a 'walk-in' alert patient who has received a minor blow to a severely injured comatose multitrauma patient who may have extremity, abdominal, thoracic, spinal and central nervous system injury in addition to the facial fracture.

The stable patient

There is nearly always adequate time (hours, if not days) to take a measured view in assessing the facially injured patient. Stable patients comprise the vast majority and, as Johnson has put it, 'Attempts at extensive plain radiographic evaluation under the direction of busy emergency room personnel often will not yield optimal results'.[1]

In the majority of cases fractures will be adequately demonstrated on a few plain films and/or panoramic tomography; this is true of most isolated injuries to the zygoma and nearly all mandibular injuries.

If any radiographic view is felt necessary for evaluation of midface injury in the early stages, a single occipitomental 10° or 15° view (Figs 5.1, 5.2) is sufficient as a screening tool. This screening view is recommended where the clinical diagnosis is uncertain and there is no cervical injury. For suspected injuries to the mandible a panoramic view (OPG) and a posteroanterior (PA) view of the mandible (Figs 5.3

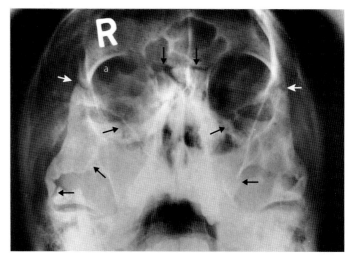

Fig. 5.1: Fractures through the Le Fort II and III lines of weakness on an occipitomental 10° projection (black arrows). There is slight separation of the frontozygomatic sutures (white arrows). Step deformities are present at both inferior orbital margins. The pattern appears incomplete as no fracture is evident in the left arch on this view. However, note the decreased gap between the coronoid process tip and the buttress of the malar bone on the left side when compared to the right side. The ethmoidal air cells and the maxillary antra are opacified, with a fluid level in the left antrum. Air is present in the right orbit (a).

and 5.4) suffice in most cases but again, as with the midface, specialist advice is preferable before imaging.

Certain injuries either do not require imaging at all or only in very specific situations. There is, for example, no evidence that patients with uncomplicated (isolated) nasal trauma benefit in any way from imaging. Patient management is determined purely on the basis of clinical examination and patient preference (i.e. a desire for improvement in function or appearance of the nose). The correlation between radiographic findings and external nasal deformity or the need for surgical reduction is poor. Indeed, some 20–25% of patients requiring some form of reduction of nasal fracture or dislocation will have negative radiology. Similarly, there is no place for a very urgent evaluation of most patients with diplopia and suspected blow-out fractures with entrapment (this is discussed in more detail below).

The multiply injured patient

The initial management of a multiply injured patient is guided by the ABCD (airway, breathing, circulation and

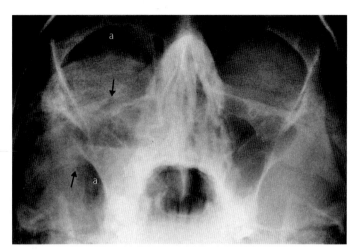

Fig. 5.2: Fracture of the zygoma on an occipitomental 15° projection. Note a fracture with a step deformity at the inferior orbital margin and at the medial part of the buttress (arrows). There is a double shadow to the medial aspect of the arch (arrowheads). Frontozygomatic suture separation is not evident. There is a fluid level in the right antrum. Air is present in the orbit and lateral to the antral wall (a). The soft tissues of the cheek and lower lid are swollen.

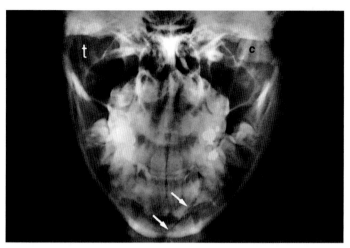

Fig. 5.4: Posteroanterior projection of the mandible: illustrating a left condylar neck fracture and a left parasymphysis fracture (arrows). The fracture at the condylar neck is not itself seen but is evident from the displaced and rotated condylar head (c). This is the classic condylar displacement and on this radiographic projection the lucent triangle (t) bounded by the skull base, the zygomatic arch and the posterolateral antral wall should always be closely inspected on both sides.

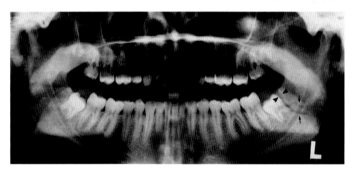

Fig. 5.3: Fracture of the mandible on a panoramic tomograph. There is a lucent fracture line crossing the left angle of the mandible, involving the lamina dura of the third molar tooth. Slight separation of the fragments has caused apparent widening of the distal periodontal ligament (arrowheads). Note that the fracture line appears to diverge into two limbs (arrows). These lines join together at both ends. The lower line is the fracture through the lingual cortex. This breaches the walls of the inferior dental canal, whereas the fracture through the buccal cortex (upper line) does not. The patient also sustained a fracture of the left zygoma: note the deformed arch on this side.

disability) of resuscitation. Airway, breathing and circulation take precedence over neurological damage (disability), as an oxygenated supply of blood to the brain is essential. CT imaging of the brain, and for that matter radiographs and CT of the face, should not therefore be undertaken in the inadequately ventilated or hemodynamically unstable patient, whatever his neurological status.

Certain other plain radiographs may be appropriate in the early stages of care. If clinical appraisal or history suggests the possibility of thoracic injury (e.g. if there is blood loss/shock without obvious cause) a chest X-ray should be obtained.

Mediastinal emphysema, pneumothorax, hemothorax, flail chest and diaphragmatic rupture may all be apparent. If no cause for hidden blood is found in the chest or on abdominal peritoneal lavage, a pelvic X-ray may reveal fractures.

Injury to the cervical spine must be considered present in all patients who have depressed consciousness, are intoxicated or have signs or symptoms related to the cervical spine. All such patients should have a cross-table lateral view of the cervical spine. Unwise attempts to intubate or otherwise maneuver the patient can have catastrophic results.

In the patient with suspected neurological damage a brow-up cross-table lateral skull view may give useful information (Fig. 5.5). Apart from such situations, no other imaging should take place until there is an adequate airway and ventilation and the patient is hemodynamically stable.

Suspected intracranial injury

A skull X-ray series is commonly acquired in patients suspected of having skull fractures or intracranial injury. There is, however, very little indication for this and very little evidence that it is of benefit to the patient, except in a few very well-defined situations. Masters et al[2] reviewed 22 058 cases from a number of studies and found that only 3% had any fractures detected on skull X-rays. Of these, 91% had no evidence of any associated intracranial injury; indeed, only 0.6% of the 22 058 cases had any intracranial injury and 51% of those with intracranial injury did not have a skull fracture. The detection of a fracture on a skull radiograph altered patient management only if there was significant fragment depression, involvement of the skull base or extension to a paranasal sinus. All three of these findings were uncommon in their series and in the 'low-risk' category, no depressed or basilar fractures were found. Clinical findings associated with

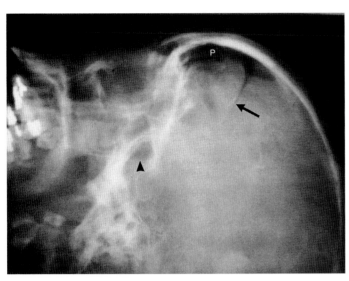

Fig. 5.5: Horizontal beam lateral skull radiograph (brow-up lateral skull). There is fracturing of the frontal calvarium (arrow), a pneumocephalus (p) and a fluid level in the sphenoid sinus (arrowhead). Note also a fluid level in the maxillary antrum.

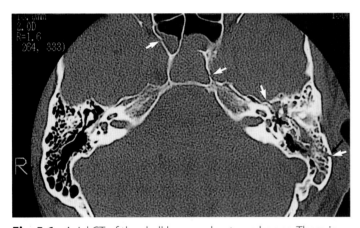

Fig. 5.6: Axial CT of the skull base and petrous bones. There is longitudinal petrous fracture on the left side. This runs across the mastoid air cells, the middle ear cavity and anterior to the petrous apex, eventually crossing the walls of the sphenoid sinus (arrows). Note soft tissue shadow (blood/CSF) in the mastoid air cells, the middle ear cavity and sphenoid sinus. Soft tissue swelling is present over the left mastoid. The normal right petrous bone structures help to demonstrate the asymmetry.

a skull fracture were altered level of consciousness, focal neurological deficit, signs of a basilar skull fracture (e.g. Battle's sign, otorrhea) and palpable diastasis or depression of calvarial fragments. Most of these findings put a patient in a 'high-risk' group and such patients should therefore be evaluated using CT scanning rather than a skull X-ray (Fig. 5.6).

Skull X-rays still have some importance in documenting child abuse and also in some patients with penetrating injury, where they may help in deciding whether emergency angiography is required. In general, they rarely change management and are performed on too many injured patients.

The counterargument (again using Masters' figures) suggests that 9% of those with a fracture will have intracranial injury

and 49% of those with intracranial injury will have a skull fracture and that some method of clinically selecting patients for skull X-ray may be more appropriate in order to reduce their use. With this in mind, a regimen may allow a skull X-ray for trauma if one or more of the following criteria are met.

- Any loss of consciousness
- Posttraumatic amnesia exceeding 10 minutes
- Neurological signs, including disorientation or confusion
- Leaking of blood or CSF from the nose or ear
- Suspected penetrating injury
- Significant scalp hematoma (>10 cm)
- Significant scalp laceration (>10 cm)
- Assessment difficult (the young, epileptic, intoxication)
- Previous craniotomy with shunting tube in place

Admission and observation are alternatives to skull radiography but the financial cost of this is far greater than providing radiographs.

The inclusion of 'the young' in this list requires further comment. There are significant differences between a head injury in a child and one in an adult. Although a large number of adults with intracranial hemorrhage will have a fracture, this is not so in children – most don't. However, depressed fractures are more common in children (Fig. 5.7). These may be impossible to detect clinically and such fractures are important. Jennett,[3] reporting on 28 depressed skull fractures, found 19 (67%) had no immediate skull radiograph or the skull radiograph was not reported in time to influence management. Of these, eight developed major complications. Heiskanen[4] reported on 224 depressed skull fractures and found that 7% eventually developed infection and that the risk of this complication was greater if surgery was delayed beyond 24 hours from injury. Laceration of the scalp should also be taken seriously, as delayed recognition of a compound fracture may have profound consequences.

CT scanning of the brain is performed whenever there is a likelihood of remediable intracranial injury (that is, secondary brain injury). The timing depends on the state of the patient and the evolution of the signs and symptoms. In a patient who has clinical evidence of transtentorial herniation and who is rapidly deteriorating neurologically, it may be necessary to perform an emergency burr hole exploration. Such situations are very rare and normally, if the patient demonstrates progressive brain stem deterioration, CT imaging is carried out immediately.

CT scanning, done as an emergency, should be considered in the following situations:

- A GCS ≤ 8
- Depressed skull fracture >1 cm
- Acute pupillary inequality >1 mm (excluding orbital trauma, medication or prior surgery)
- Persistent neurological deficit
- A decrease in the GCS of 3 or more, regardless of absolute score
- Known bleeding diathesis or anticoagulant therapy

Such an emergency scan can be performed prior to any treatment of non-neurological injuries, provided the patient is

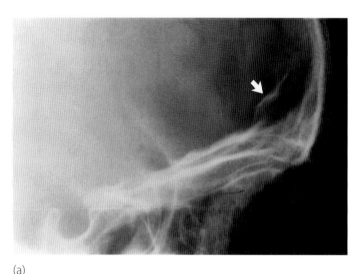

(a)

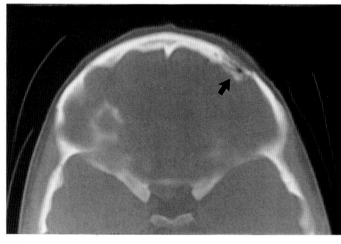

(b)

Fig. 5.7: Depressed skull fracture. **(a)** Part of a lateral skull projection showing a linear density caused by the depressed fragments (arrow). **(b)** Axial CT of the same patient showing depressed fragments (arrow).

not in shock and is adequately ventilated. The patient who is in shock is at risk of dying in transit and performing a CT is rarely worth the risk.

In cases where time and the patient's condition permit, the brain CT scan examination can be usefully expanded to include other areas of interest. It is often appropriate to include the rest of the face, some of which will in any event be visible on the brain scan. Head-injured or multiply injured patients requiring endotracheal intubation are difficult to assess clinically because facial features are obscured and distorted by tubes and tapes and because response to painful stimuli is blunted or erased. Indeed, McAuley et al found that 16% of missed fractures involved the facial skeleton and 21% of all missed injuries were accounted for by an impaired sensorium.[5]

The cervical spine (Fig. 5.8)

The fact that a patient walks into the A&E department does not preclude serious cervical injury and if there is any doubt, all cases, especially those in road traffic or other high-velocity accidents, should be given a collar until injury has been excluded. On the other hand alert, co-operative, non-intoxicated patients with a cervical spine injury *always* complain of pain or discomfort.

Routine cervical spine X-ray in all patients with isolated mandibular fractures is inappropriate, as the 'pick-up' rate of cervical injury is likely to be negligible. Indeed, the majority of facial trauma patients will have no cervical injury and it is obviously preferable to be selective and not expose large numbers of patients to unnecessary radiation. Velmahos et al have looked at this problem in relation to the alert asymptomatic blunt trauma victim.[6] In a series of 549 alert, oriented, clinically non-intoxicated blunt trauma victims with no neck symptoms, no injury was missed when a careful three-step clinical examination was used. In such patients, if there is no report of neck symptoms and no tenderness to palpation or on neck motion, the collar can be left off and no radiographic studies are necessary.

An unconscious, sedated or otherwise non-alert patient, a patient with suspected neck injury and those with overt cord or root symptoms should have a horizontal beam (cross-table) lateral view of the cervical spine taken as soon as possible and this should be done with the cervical collar on. Extreme caution should be used in maneuvering the patient. If other injury has to take precedence the patient must wear the collar until cervical injury can be ruled out. Because most injuries occur in the lower cervical spine, especially the C7–T1 level, the spine must be visualized down to these levels. It may be necessary to supplement with a 'swimmer's' view or trauma oblique views (without turning the patient). If this still fails then CT or MRI must be performed. An AP view of the cervical spine and an open-mouth, odontoid peg view should also be obtained if possible.

Second fractures occur in 5% of patients with spinal injury and very subtle changes may be a sign of major injury. Missed cervical spine injury can occur in 15–30% of patients. Plain lateral views give a false-negative rate of 26–40%. In equivocal clinical cases CT imaging is recommended; more fractures are identified and it is more accurate in identifying and locating the position of bone fragments. Beirne therefore recommends CT in all unconscious patients with neck trauma and all alert conscious patients who complain of neck pain and spasm after high-velocity injuries.[7]

However, CT imaging is not good at identifying ligamentous injury in the cervical spine. Although ligamentous injury can be identified on flexion/extension lateral views, this is a potentially hazardous procedure and must be done under medical supervision and then only in alert co-operative patients with minimal spasm who have no evidence of a potentially unstable fracture on plain X-ray or CT imaging. Such views are best done under fluoroscopic control. It should also be remembered that spinal cord injury can occur without a fracture in about 0.7% of cases.

MRI, however, can identify ligamentous and cord injury and should be considered if the above investigations remain unhelpful or cannot be undertaken. Ideally all patients sustai-

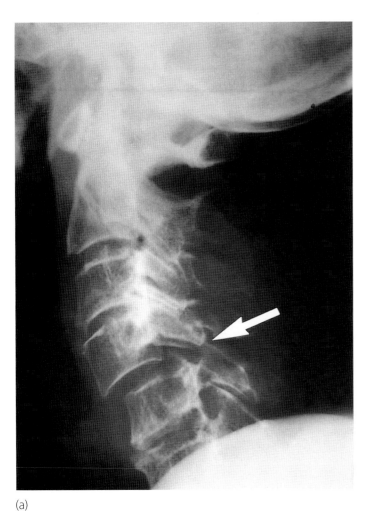

(a)

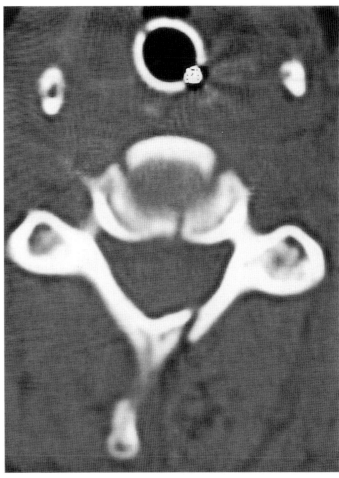

(b)

Fig. 5.8: Injury to the cervical spine. **(a)** Lateral cervical spine showing locked facets at C5–6 (arrow). **(b)** Axial CT of the cervical spine showing a burst fracture of the vertebral body and fracture of the vertebral lamina.

ning significant spinal injury should have MRI, but for practical purposes this is not possible. However, MRI in the acute phase should be mandatory in those patients demonstrating neurology, but in whom no fracture is seen on plain radiographs (to assess cord and soft tissue injury), and also in patients who have ascending neurology (to exclude an epidural hematoma). Furthermore, it should also be performed after a set period of time on patients in whom clinical evaluation remains impossible. MRI is also indicated if the neurological state is fluctuating or if the degree of neurological deficit appears out of proportion to the bony injury. In addition, it can assist in differentiating spinal cord edema (which has a greater capacity for neurological recovery) from cord hemorrhage and it may be helpful in the later stages if there is further neurological deterioration.

Bleeding

In most hemodynamically unstable facial trauma patients the site of blood loss will be located outside the face, this site being either overt or occult.

Nevertheless, bleeding related to the facial injury may rarely either contribute to, or be, the sole cause of shock. Such bleeding may be presentational or may be delayed in onset, even occurring after fixation of facial fractures. Such bleeding is most common following the more severe transfacial or panfacial fractures. It may originate from disruption of the anterior or posterior ethmoidal vessels or the terminal branches of the maxillary artery. Nasal packing, clipping or ligation of obvious bleeding points and arterial ligation may all be used. A few cases may need urgent temporary external reduction or fixation of their facial fractures. A small group will be resistant to such treatments or recurrent and in these, arteriography and selective embolization should be considered. Angiography should also be considered in situations where there is penetrating injury to the neck, particularly where this is above the mandibular angle.

More rarely, a mandibular fracture can cause a complete transection of the inferior alveolar artery and if spasm and spontaneous arrest of bleeding do not occur, considerable hemorrhage may take place, requiring urgent temporary fixation with a bridle wire.

Visual loss

Visual loss may result from a lesion anywhere along the path from the globe to the visual cortex. Loss that is instantaneous (at the moment of trauma) is usually considered irreversible and is not imaged. However, difficulty arises in patients who have been rendered unconscious for a period of time, as instantaneous loss cannot then be determined.

Causes arising within the globe, such as gross rupture and hemorrhage, are usually clinically obvious or can be investigated with ultrasound. CT done for other reasons, such as fracture assessment, may provide useful information: rupture of the globe, lens dislocation, hemorrhage and retinal detachment may be evident. Optic nerve damage at the canal level can occur, but assessment by imaging in this situation will depend much on local practice, as surgery here is controversial. Fractures at the canal are rare, but compression by bony fragments may be seen on CT images. Visual loss may also occur due to lesions further forward in the extraocular intraorbital compartment. Bone fragments, foreign bodies or a penetrating injury may involve the optic nerve and may be identified on CT. Optic nerve avulsion or transection may be detectable on CT or MRI, but blindness will be permanent. Optic nerve hemorrhage (as opposed to optic nerve sheath hemorrhage) cannot reliably be identified at present. Together with osseous compression of the optic nerve, these all form the direct forms of traumatic optic neuropathy. Visual evoked potentials (VEP) using flashlight goggles provide valuable additional information on optic nerve injuries (see Chapter 10).

The indirect forms are much more common and may be due to: contusion of the optic nerve leading to edema and compression of the vascular supply to the optic nerve, hemorrhage into the optic nerve sheath, shearing of the nutrient vessels or increase in intraorbital pressure. Nutrient vessel shearing is untreatable. Hemorrhage into the optic nerve sheath can be identified using CT or MRI but is rare: it is often accompanied by fundal appearances of central retinal vein occlusion and can be amenable to decompression. However, the most common treatable problem is increased intraorbital pressure due either to bleeding or to the presence of air (see below). Patients with trauma involving the optic nerve (traumatic optic neuropathy) can therefore benefit from imaging but in some circumstances it is useless and in others harmful. The danger is that imaging will delay urgent treatment. Careful patient selection is therefore essential.

Imaging Modalities and Techniques

Plain radiographs and tomographic techniques

Plain radiographs provide the foundation of imaging. They may be sufficient on their own or may need to be complemented by other modalities, such as CT scanning. The general rule (anywhere in the body) is that fractures should be imaged in at least two planes, preferably at right angles to one another. However, although this is true in many circumstances in facial injury, and is also true for locating foreign bodies, it is not a universal rule in the face.

None of the plain film techniques (see Appendix) require the use of a specialized skull X-ray unit, although this is helpful. Most can be quite adequately obtained using an

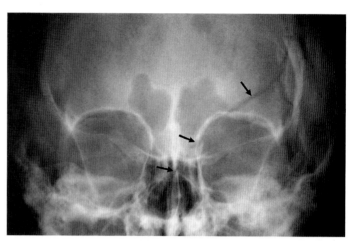

Fig. 5.9: Caldwell projection in a patient with a fracture of the frontal bone extending down to the superior orbital rim and crossing to the medial orbital wall in the region of the frontal sinus ostium to involve the upper nasal septum (arrows).

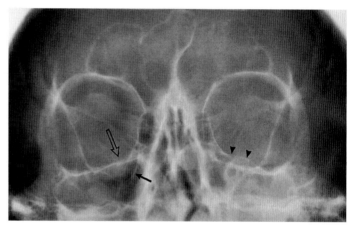

Fig. 5.10: Modified Caldwell projection illustrating a blow-out fracture of the orbital floor. There is absence of the right orbital floor medial to the infraorbital groove and fissure (open arrow). The corresponding segment of floor on the left is intact and normal in position (arrowheads). There is a depressed fragment of bone on the right side (closed arrow) and mucosal thickening in the antrum on this side. The opacification in the left antrum is due to coexisting and unrelated inflammatory disease. Note also the air in the right upper orbit.

upright bucky apparatus with overhead gantry tube, provided the patient can sit up or stand.

For reasons of classification and convenience, the face is often divided into upper, middle and lower thirds and the middle third is further divided into central and lateral components. Suspected fractures of the upper third of the face require a Caldwell (Fig. 5.9) or, preferably, a modified Caldwell view (Fig. 5.10) and a lateral projection. Middle third injuries require occipitomental 10° (Figs 5.1, 5.2) and 30° views (Fig. 5.11), which can be supplemented by a lateral projection if the central middle third is involved (Fig. 5.12). Lower third injuries require a PA mandible and panoramic tomography (OPG) or, if the latter is not available, lateral oblique views of both sides (see Appendix). These views should be taken with the patient erect whenever possible, not

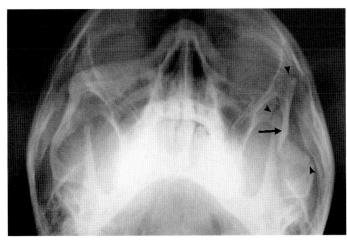

Fig. 5.11: Occipitomental 30° projection showing a depressed left zygomatic arch fracture. Note the rotated anterior arch fragment (arrow), the fracture in the posterior arch and a fracture crossing the zygomatic buttress to reach the frontozygomatic suture (arrowheads).

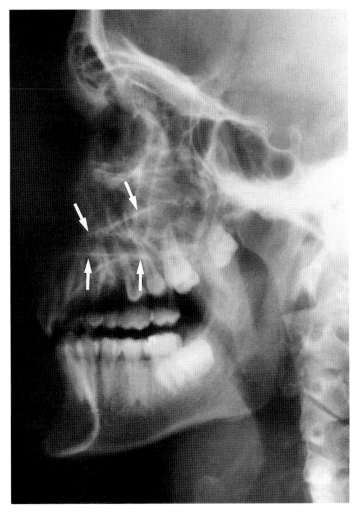

Fig. 5.12: Lateral projection of the face in a patient with a unilateral Le Fort I type fracture. The dentition on each side of the mandible superimpose, whereas the left upper dental arch is displaced upwards and backwards. The two halves of the split palate are widely separated and at an angle to one another (arrows).

only for his comfort but to show fluid levels in the sinuses. Such plain film views may not be necessary if CT has to be (or has been) done as an emergency or if there are adequate radiographs available from a primary referring hospital. Other projections (see Appendix) are rarely needed.

Computed tomography (CT)

This has supplanted non-panoramic tomography almost entirely. It has the advantage of providing images of thin slices of the facial skeleton, overcoming the problem of the superimposition of structures that inevitably occurs on plain radiographs. Furthermore, the digital acquisition of information, as opposed to the analogue information of plain films, allows electronic manipulation of the data by altering the settings to provide images either at bony window levels or for optimal soft tissue evaluation. This increased contrast sensitivity also provides improved visualization of a wide variety of foreign bodies. In addition, slice information obtained in one plane can be reconstructed to provide images in alternative planes, where such alternative image planes are not obtainable directly.

A small field of view should be used and the scanning performed with high-resolution bone algorithm. Soft tissue windows can then be obtained from these data. Generally, a slice thickness of 2–4 mm is adequate in assessing facial trauma and has the advantage that the examination is faster than when acquiring thinner slices. However, if reformatting is needed, very thin (e.g. 1.5 mm) slices are best.

In nearly every case coming to CT scanning, axial slice images are obtained (Figs 5.6, 5.7, 5.13). The standard

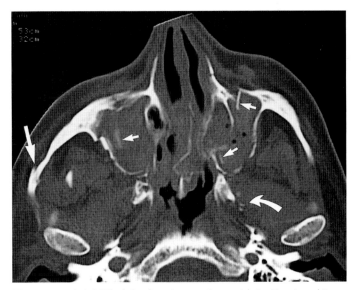

Fig. 5.13: Axial CT of the face in a patient with Le Fort I and II level injuries and a right zygomatic fracture. There is extensive fracturing involving all the walls of the maxillary antra with several bone fragments displaced into the antra (small arrows). There is fracturing of the left nasal plate of the maxilla, fracturing and submucosal hemorrhage in the posterior nasal septum and a fracture with lateral bowing of the right zygomatic arch (large arrow). The maxillary antra are opaque from blood. There are fragments of bone avulsed from the left pterygoid plates (curved arrow).

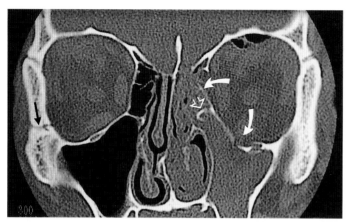

Fig. 5.14: Coronal CT of the face in a patient with medial wall and orbital floor blow-out fractures (curved arrows). The left nasal cavity, ethmoidal air cells and antrum are opaque from blood. There is air beneath the left orbital roof. The orbital floor fracture involves the inferior orbital canal. The major fragments of both fractures are hinged at the junction with the ethmomaxillary plate (open arrow). The lucent line crossing the base of the frontal process of the right zygoma (black arrow) is the canal for the zygomaticotemporal nerve and is not a fracture.

position for axial (transverse) slices is with the slice plane parallel to the anthropological baseline. This position is easy for the patient and landmarks are easy to identify on the initial scanogram view. However, CT scanning protocols vary considerably with clinical circumstances. Coronal images are particularly helpful in orbital examination (Fig. 5.14) but are also useful in other situations. Coronal imaging has the benefit of visualizing the horizontal 'struts' or plates of bone, which in standard axial slices lie parallel to the slice plane and are therefore poorly visualized. Such horizontal plates include the orbital roof, cribriform plate, orbital floor and hard palate.

Direct coronal imaging is ideally performed in the true coronal plane but two factors may require the gantry angle to be adjusted. First, many patients, particularly the elderly and those with a rigid spine, may not be able to extend their neck sufficiently. Indeed, in some patients direct coronal scanning cannot be done at all (or, if the cervical spine is still under suspicion, should not be done). Second, dental amalgam and other fixed prosthodontic devices can produce serious streak-like artefacts which seriously diminish the image quality.

The development of spiral / multislice CT scanning gives a number of advantages:

- the acquisition of data is much faster – these techniques can acquire a volume data much larger than conventional CT scanning in the same time
- high-quality reconstruction is available in any plane
- CT angiography is a more realistic goal
- three-dimensional applications are enhanced.

Data are obtained volumetrically and so slices can be reconstructed at any interval greater than 1 mm, allowing variable degrees of overlap. However, the potential for acquiring large numbers of slices with such techniques has financial and ionizing radiation costs.

When to perform CT imaging of facial injuries

Although it may be convenient and sensible to expedite CT of the face in those patients having a CT of the brain, the majority of facially injured patients can be managed quite adequately without CT scanning. The decision to perform CT imaging depends upon both the initial radiographic evaluation and the clinical findings. If plain radiographs are negative, with no evidence of fracture, no fluid levels, no mucosal thickening of the sinuses, no orbital or soft tissue emphysema, and there is no evidence of penetrating injury, then the chance of finding a significant midface fracture on CT imaging is negligible. However, *all* patients with upper third fractures or suspected fractures should receive CT evaluation. There is a very high incidence of intracranial damage in such patients and there are important questions relating to the posterior wall of the frontal sinus, the nasofrontal duct and the orbital roof, the answers to which affect the surgical approach and indeed long-term outlook. These questions are not reliably addressed by plain radiographs.

Many patients with central middle third fractures require CT evaluation, although mild injury to the nasomaxillary complex (that is, injury confined to the nasal bones and the nasal plates of the frontal process of the maxillae) does not, and the utility of CT in the patient with a Le Fort I level injury is highly debatable. Lateral middle third injuries seldom require CT imaging unless there is severe displacement or extension to the external angular process of the frontal bone or to the sphenoidal and temporal calvarium. There is no doubt that CT shows displacement well, particularly displacement of the zygomatic arch, but careful evaluation of unrotated PA, OM 10° and 30° radiographs is nearly always sufficient for management, although the uncommon lateral bowing injury of the arch may be difficult to appreciate. Some orbital injuries require CT evaluation but this should be guided clinically. Most patients with penetrating injury to the lids or conjunctiva should at least be considered for CT: the risk of missing a foreign body in the orbit or anterior cranial fossa is significant. CT may also be needed later for evaluation of *some* patients with suspected blow-out injury (see below) and for evaluation of enophthalmos and other malpositions of the globe.

Neither CT, nor plain radiographs, nor MRI should be used to evaluate severe retrobulbar hemorrhage. This is an emergency and orbital exploration should be carried out as soon as possible.

In the lower third of the face (the mandible and hyoid) CT imaging is virtually never needed, except in some cases of suspected condylar head fracture. Such suspicion should only arise if a condylar fracture is not clinically or radiographically evident, but where there is otorrhagia or an apparent Battle's sign. It is then done primarily to exclude a petrous fracture. A significant number of patients with a condylar fracture will have otorrhagia and Battle's sign can be mimicked by seepage of blood back from the injury to the external auditory canal, caused by a condylar fracture.

Three-dimensional CT (3D CT)

In the vast majority of patients with facial injuries the normal 2D CT imaging is quite sufficient for diagnosis and treatment. A few of the more severe and complex injuries may nevertheless benefit from 3D CT and there is no doubt about the utility of 3D CT in the management of complex posttraumatic malformation and defects.

Magnetic resonance imaging (MRI)

Certain atomic nuclei behave like spinning magnets. In the human body one of the most widespread of these is hydrogen. When a patient is placed in a magnetic field these hydrogen nuclei align their magnetic axes parallel to that field.

Energy can be introduced into the patient by use of a specific radiofrequency pulse, which will rotate the magnetization into a different plane. When the pulse is discontinued, the nuclei return to their original orientation in the general magnetic field and in so doing, emit the absorbed energy. This change in orientation results in the originally rotated magnetization cutting receiver coils and inducing a signal. A variety of pulse sequences can be used and a cross-sectional image can be built up, much as can be done with CT.

This technique does not depend on X-rays, which is an advantage over CT. A disadvantage is that the demonstration of fine bone detail in the face remains inferior to CT. Furthermore, ferromagnetic material in (or indeed outside) the patient, such as iron filings in the globe of the eye and some intracranial aneurysm clips, may move, with disastrous consequences. Such material can also produce spectacular artefacts, degrading the images. In addition, poor access and difficulty with some forms of monitoring equipment make MRI less attractive than CT in acute maxillofacial injury.

However, MRI does have growing application in a number of specific areas. The most important of these is its ability to detect CSF fistulae and leaks (see below), and its superior demonstration of posttraumatic meningoceles and encephaloceles (Fig. 5.15). It has increasing application in the orbit for injuries to the globe and optic nerve sheath complex and has a place in evaluating post blow-out repair problems. It can also be used to demonstrate acute soft tissue injury in the temporomandibular joint, although there is no conclusive evidence that such demonstration affects the early management of patients and it is probably best reserved for those with persistent joint symptoms. MRI is also of assistance in estimating the vascularization of hydroxyapatite orbital implants following exenteration for trauma.

Other modalities

A number of other modalities, e.g. angiography (including therapeutic maneuvers), dacryocystography, sialography, arthrography, very occasionally play a part in the management of the maxillofacial patient. Angiography may be required in the acute phase and sialography has a place in evaluating suspected parotid duct transection. The others, however, are usually reserved for assessing the delayed sequelae to trauma. Ultrasound has been used to demonstrate facial fractures, but although it can demonstrate some fractures in superficial bone structures, it does not generally help the management of the patient and is unlikely to be of any widespread appeal. On the other hand, it does have application in assessing the globe, particularly the posterior elements when anterior opacification (blood or cataract) prevents direct vision, and also for assessing intraocular foreign bodies. Ultrasound can detect foreign bodies in soft tissues with high accuracy.

Recognition and Interpretation of Facial Injury

Introduction

The skeletal anatomy of the face is the most complex in the body. The maximum amount of information will be gleaned from the radiographs and images if a few rules are followed and there is a methodical approach to searching the image

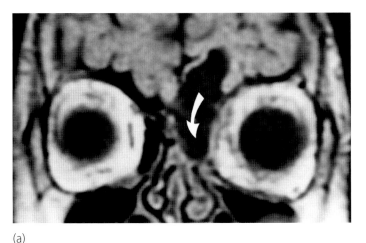
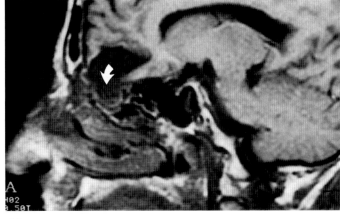

(a)　　　　　　　　　　　　　　　　　　　　(b)

Fig. 5.15: MRI of a patient with an encephalocele. Encephalomalacic brain tissue (darker than normal brain on image) originating from the rectus gyrus, and part of the medial orbital gyrus, has herniated through the left ethmoidal roof (arrows). **(a)** Coronal reconstruction. **(b)** Parasagittal reconstruction (courtesy Dr BG Conry).

for information: you see what you look for! A number of approaches to image assessment in the context of facial injury are suggested and described below, as are specific signs that should be sought.

Every film of the face should be examined, including any that may have been sent from a referring hospital or clinic. Radiographs made elsewhere should always be obtained – they may hold important information, even if badly done, and may obviate the need to obtain some or all of the radiographs one would normally acquire. Some patients are habitual attenders: their previous radiographs should be reviewed. Every image should be checked for the date it was obtained, for the patient's name and for orientation (left or right) markers. X-ray packets have an uncanny habit of acquiring other patients' films, even in the best-regulated departments!

Search patterns and reminders

McGrigor & Campbell have described a search pattern of four lines which the eye should follow when examining the frontal view (occipitomental 10° projection).[8] These are known as Campbell's lines or sometimes as McGrigor's lines. A fifth line is known as Trapnell's line[9] (Fig. 5.16). Using these lines allows one to examine all those parts of the face where fractures and other signs are most likely to be found and reduces the chance of missing a fracture.

The first of these lines runs across the frontozygomatic sutures, the superior margins of the orbit and the frontal sinuses. The second passes along the zygomatic arches, the zygomatic body, the inferior orbital margin and the nasal bones. The third crosses the condyles, the coronoid processes and the maxillary sinuses. The fourth crosses the mandibular ramus and the bite line (occlusal plane of the teeth) and the fifth runs along the inferior border of the mandible from angle to angle.

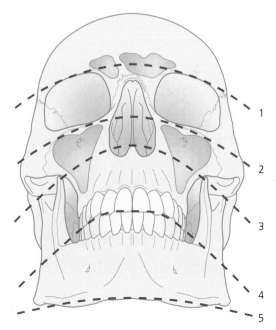

Fig. 5.16: Campbell's and Trapnell's lines.

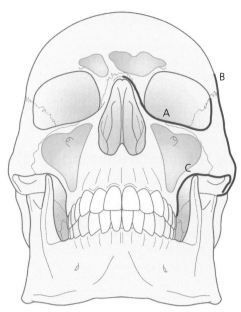

Fig. 5.17: Dolan's lines for the occipitomental projection. **A** Orbital line. **B** Zygomatic line. **C** Maxillary line.

Dolan & Jacoby describe three lines for evaluating the occipitomental projections which can be used as an adjunct[10] (Fig. 5.17). These are known collectively as Dolan's lines.

- The 'orbital line' extends along the inner margins of the lateral, inferior and medial walls of the orbit, passing over the nasal arch to follow the same structures on the opposite side.
- The 'zygomatic line' extends along the superior margin of the arch and body of the zygoma, passing along the lateral margin of the frontal process of the zygoma to the zygomaticofrontal suture.
- The 'maxillary line' extends along the inferior margin of the zygomatic arch, the inferior margin of the body and buttress of the zygoma and the lateral wall of the maxillary sinus.

These authors also describe evaluation lines for the modified Caldwell projection. The first extends along the outer margin of the orbital process of the frontal and zygomatic bones. The second is the innominate line or oblique orbital line. The third extends along the inner margin of the orbit down to break into two roughly parallel lines meeting at the inferior orbital foramen: the medial of these two lines is the posterior lacrimal crest, the lateral is the lamina papyracea. The line then continues along the orbital margin inferiorly, laterally and superiorly (Fig. 5.18).

The 'four S's' described by Delbalso et al are a good reminder of what to look for on radiographs.[11] They stand for Symmetry, Sharpness, Sinus and Soft tissue.

Symmetry

With the exception of the frontal sinuses, the face is reasonably symmetrical in most people. Occasionally a hypoplastic maxillary antrum or previous old trauma can cause confusion,

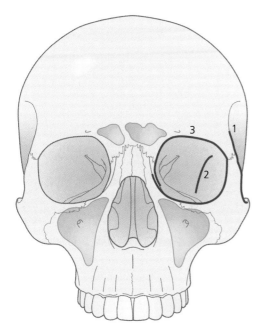

Fig. 5.18: Dolan's lines for the modified Caldwell projection.

but any asymmetry noticed should draw the examiner's attention to that area for further evaluation (Figs 5.1, 5.2, 5.6, 5.10).

Sharpness

This refers to the accentuated sharpness brought about by fracture fragments being rotated or displaced into tangent with the X-ray beam and thus appearing accentuated on the image (Fig. 5.10). A number of radiographic signs have been described based on this principle, such as the 'bright sign', 'railroad track' and 'trapdoor sign', some of which are discussed below. The converse of this principle is loss of normal sharp outline when a fragment is rotated out of tangent.

Sinus

Nearly all the midface fractures involve one or more of the paranasal sinuses (Figs 5.1, 5.2). Indeed, Valvassori & Hord have used this to provide a classification scheme for such midface injuries.[12] A number of abnormalities discussed below may be apparent in the sinuses.

Soft tissues

Swelling, foreign bodies and emphysema may all be apparent (Fig. 5.2) and help in the evaluation of the patient.

'Hot' sites and fracture patterns

Three fractures following Le Fort's three great lines of weakness[13] have come to be known as the three great transfacial fractures, namely the Le Fort I, II and III (although these are in reverse order to Le Fort's original assignation). These, together with the zygomatic fractures, orbital blow-out fractures and localized nasoethmoidal complex fractures, form the basis of most midface fracture classifications.

Two points should be noted. If these fracture lines/lines of weakness are mapped onto the image of an occipitomental 10° or modified Caldwell projection in those areas where fractures are easily manifested to the observer (namely, where bone is either thick or is seen in tangent), then a pattern emerges and certain sites provide likely hunting grounds for recognizing injury ('hot' sites). Second, these sites (Fig. 5.19) are not precise because the lines of weakness are not precise and vary slightly from individual to individual. Hence they are indicated on the diagram as zones where fractures are most likely to be seen and particular attention should therefore be given to these areas. This approach speeds up and enhances the discovery process. It does not, however, obviate the need for a complete study of the radiograph.

Allied to this notion is the idea of fracture patterns, inherent in the classifications of midface fractures. Using these allows the examiner, having identified a fracture, to direct his or her attention to other likely sites. Thus, for example, having identified a fracture of an inferior orbital rim and knowing that this may not be localized but be part of a tripod, Le Fort II or nasomaxillary fracture, the examiner can proceed to double-check the zygomatic arch, frontozygomatic suture, nasal arch, lateral antral wall on the same side and the inferior orbital rim and lateral antral wall on the other side. Similarly, an arch fracture may be isolated, part of a tripod or Le Fort III fracture. Likewise, a lateral antral wall fracture may be part of a tripod, Le Fort II or Le Fort I fracture, or may be localized or dentoalveolar in origin or indeed may be a combination of these, as it may with the other examples.

That a fracture at a single site may occur as part of several different fracture types or patterns is important. Failure to appreciate this can lead to error (clinically as well as radiologically). Malar fractures, for example, are common but not every inferior orbital rim fracture is due to a malar injury. One of the most frequently misinterpreted fractures

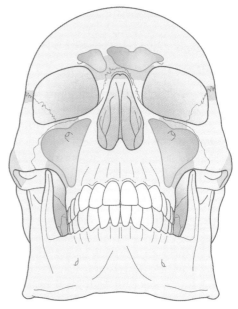

Fig. 5.19: 'Hot sites' for identifying fractures on the occipitomental projection.

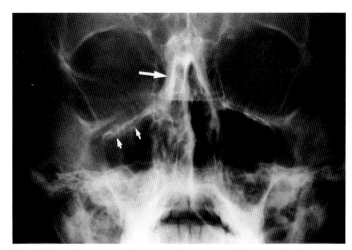

Fig. 5.20: Fracture of the frontal process of the maxilla. Seen on an occipitomental projection with only 40° angulation. Note the narrowing of the right nasal arch (long arrow) when compared with the opposite side, and the depressed medial portion of the inferior orbital rim (short arrows).

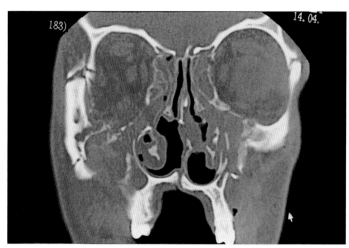

Fig. 5.21: Coronal CT showing extensive fracturing at all the Le Fort levels with severe comminution and palatal splitting.

involving the inferior orbital rim is a fracture of the frontal process of the maxilla (Fig. 5.20).

One should not, however, be too rigid about such patterns or classifications, because hybrid and mixed forms, particularly in the Le Fort type of injuries, are more common than pure forms. Indeed, in severe high-impact injuries, particularly of the panfacial type, the facial skeleton may 'egg-shell' into dozens of fragments, making any attempt at ordered classification fruitless (Fig. 5.21). Concomitant injury patterns also occur and identification of one should alert the examiner to check whether the other is present. Examples include the association of depressed zygomatic arch fracture with coronoid process of mandible fracture; the association of Le Fort I and palatal fractures with mandibular injury; and that between a parasymphysis fracture and a fracture of the opposite condylar neck or body.

The concept of completeness and incompleteness

Not all fractures will be apparent on clinical examination. Similarly, for a variety of reasons, not all will be discovered by either plain radiograph (Fig. 5.1) or CT scanning. What is important is whether the bone fragment is loose or displaced.

Some bone injury is only visible microscopically. Hair line fractures may only become visible radiologically after about 7–10 days when decalcification at the fracture edges occurs. Greenstick fracturing – where there is a fracture through one side of the cortex with buckling on the other – and pure buckle fractures are common in children, particularly in the condylar neck. In these circumstances only angular displacement may be seen and the fragment is usually stable, albeit in an incorrect position. In the skull vault fractures are commonly seen to 'peter out', without ending at a bone edge. In addition to this, separation and movement may occur at sutures and be indiscernible radiologically. At certain suture sites this can be

a most difficult problem for the radiologist. The fronto-zygomatic suture is a case in point. This may be visible as a lucent line in some normal individuals and in a few normal people may be so only on one side. The radiologist may therefore be unable to confirm a fracture or separation there, even though at surgery it is obviously loose and unstable.

Direct radiographic signs of fracture

All the signs of injury may be considered as being abnormal densities – either more lucent or more opaque than normal – or as being abnormalities of position, either incorrectly oriented or incorrectly located.

Separation sign

This is sometimes called the cortical defect or 'crack' (Figs 5.1–5, 5.9, 5.11, 5.22). Fry et al[14] have pointed out that the radiographic appearance of fracture lines may vary in width, according to:

- the amount of destruction
- the amount of displacement
- the angle of projection of the X-rays
- the stage of repair.

Such a break in the continuity of bone allows X-rays to pass unimpeded and results in a lucent line on the image, but only provided part of the fracture plane is oriented in tangent to the X-ray beam *and* there is sufficient depth (thickness) of bone. Many of the bones of the face are extremely thin plates. In the absence of other signs the visibility of a fracture in such a thin plate depends to a large degree on its orientation. Thus continuous fracture lines are rarely seen on radiographs of the midface. In a Le Fort I or II fracture, for example, the fracture line may be seen at the lateral antral wall on a frontal projection but not seen as it passes across the front and back walls of the antrum, where the bone is not only thin but oriented 'en face' to the X-ray beam. When its plane of cleavage rotates or curls or suddenly alters direction,

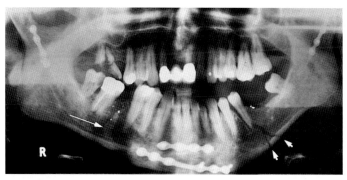

Fig. 5.22: Bilateral mandibular body fractures. The fracture on the left shows true comminution (short arrows) and there is widening of the periodontal membrane on the mesial aspect of the premolar. The fracture on the right is only evident on this view as an overlap sign of increased density (long arrow). A fractured right upper molar is also present. There are plates for previous fractures in this patient who has epilepsy.

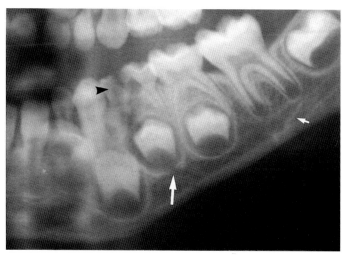

Fig. 5.23: Fracture of the mandible, seen on part of a panoramic tomograph. There is a separation sign across the condensed bone of the lamina dura of a tooth bud (large arrow). A vertical fracture of the deciduous tooth above is present (arrowhead). The dense band distally (small arrow) is a pseudo-overlap sign due to superimposition of the hyoid bone.

a fracture line may seem to disappear even though it continues further in the bone in question. This accounts both for some fractures which appear to be incomplete and, to a lesser extent, for the pseudocomminution which is often seen in the mandible. In this latter situation the fracture is visible as a lucent line on both the lingual and buccal cortex (Fig. 5.3) and if these lines do not coincide geometrically, it can appear as if two fractures are present. Close examination will usually reveal that they approximate at a bone margin. Such changes in orientation also account for fractures in the frontal bone which appear to 'end' at the orbital margin. These almost always continue into the orbital roof.

The margin of fracture lines should be inspected. In fresh fractures the margins are well defined and sharp: rounding off indicates either that it is not a fracture or that infection or non-union is occurring. The width of a fracture line may increase slightly due to decalcification in the healing process, prior to ossification of the fracture callus. More extensive widening can be due to displacement, intervening bone loss (e.g. ballistic injuries) or infection. However, this latter is a delayed feature and in any event takes at least 10 days to become apparent, as time is needed for removal of calcium salts. Where displacement is the cause, the width of a fracture provides additional information: wide gaps indicate periosteal tearing and, in the calvarium, dural tearing. Cortical or condensed bone does not only exist at the perimeter of bone: the condensed bone of the mental foramen and the margins of the dental canal may demonstrate a separation sign. The lamina dura of tooth sockets and developing tooth buds should also be inspected for the presence of fracture lines. In children a fracture may only be visible as a lucency crossing the wall (lamina dura) of a developing tooth bud (Fig. 5.23).

A number of pitfalls exist for the unwary. Neurovascular channels produce lucent lines, as do sutures. Such channels and sutures can also cause confusion on CT scanning. Knowledge of anatomy is important here, but there are clues on the film: the margins of such anatomical lucent structures tend to be sclerotic (dense), unlike fresh fractures. A thin line of air between the tongue and palate (palatoglossal gap)

can simulate a fracture on plain films, as indeed can streaks of soft tissue emphysema. A clue to these, as to many other imitators, is the bone margin; if the lucency goes beyond the bone margin it is not a fracture of that particular bone and is therefore probably spurious. Some care is needed, however: a lucent line projecting beyond a bone does not exclude a fracture, only a fracture of the bone in question. This problem occurs especially in the midface, where there is much superimposition of bone.

Sutural diastasis

Separation of a fragment of bone from the rest of the facial skeleton may, in part or in whole, occur along a suture line. There are well-recognized sites in the face where such separation may be seen, such as the frontozygomatic suture (Figs 5.1, 5.11), the frontonasal suture, the nasomaxillary suture and, in young children, the internasal suture. Recognition of such suture separation is easy where the gap is well marked but since such sutures in the normal may be seen as thin lucent lines, mild degrees of separation may be impossible to appreciate.

Overlap sign

This occurs where there is a displacement at the fracture site such that two fragments overlap, either wholly or in part. The thickness of bone here will be greater and show as a band of increased opacity (Figs 5.22, 5.24). It may be the only sign of fracture. It is sometimes called the 'double density' sign or 'cortical duplication', but these are misnomers because, if the fracture plane is oblique and overriding is incomplete, the increase in thickness may be less than double. The margins of this band of increased opacity may be sharp or blurred, depending on the obliquity of the fracture line with respect to the

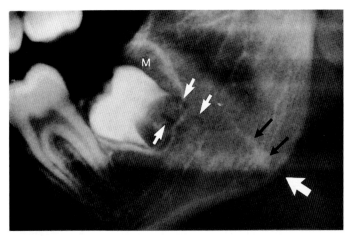

Fig. 5.24: Left angular fracture of the mandible (part of a panoramic projection). The fracture is difficult to see but note the presence of several signs. There is widening of the periodontal ligament (m). Faint fracture lines cross the lamina dura and region of the dental canal (small white arrows). There is a linear density due to overlap of fracture fragments (black arrows) and a tiny step deformity of the cortical margin (large white arrow).

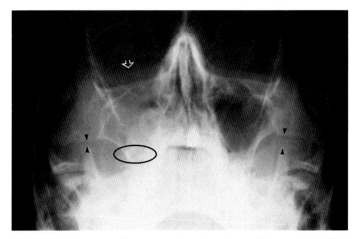

Fig. 5.25: Abnormal linear density sign. An occipitomental 10° projection showing a subtle minimally displaced malar fracture. The antrum is opaque, the soft tissues are slightly swollen (open arrow) and there is a 'bright sign' (abnormal linear density) projected over the inferior lateral antral wall (circled). Note also the reduced gap (arrowheads) between the tip of the coronoid process and the inferior margin of the buttress on the same side due to the displacement of the malar bone.

X-ray beam. Care must be exercised with this sign, as normal structures such as the soft palate can produce a similar appearance. In addition, foreign bodies or displaced bone fragments from another site can project over the bone being examined.

Abnormal linear density

This is seen when a fracture fragment is displaced and/or rotated so that it is seen 'end on' in an abnormal position. This gives rise to a non-anatomical linear opacity. A common example occurs when a fragment of the antral wall rotates to produce a linear opacity projected over the antrum: the so-called 'bright sign' (Fig. 5.25). Other examples include the 'trapdoor sign' of an orbital floor fracture and the 'railroad' or 'parallel line' sign which occurs when the lateral orbital wall is rotated to parallel the innominate (or oblique orbital) line. It is occasionally seen in high condylar neck fractures, when bone fragments may be seen projected over the sigmoid notch on panoramic, oblique or lateral views. A further and important example is the increased density seen in the anterior fragment of a depressed zygomatic arch fracture on frontal projections (Fig. 5.11). As with the 'overlap' sign, foreign bodies such as glass shards may mimic this sign, as may normal antral septa and other superimposed anatomical structures.

Disappearing fragment sign

The absence of bone from an expected position is the 'opposite' of the abnormal linear density (Fig. 5.10). A bone structure which normally produces an image, e.g. the orbital floor or lateral antral wall, is displaced or rotated out of tangent to the beam, resulting in a gap appearing. This sign is most commonly seen where there are thin bone plates. It too has its counterpart on CT images and in CT there is a special example: the empty glenoid fossa, implying mandibular condylar neck fracture or dislocation.

Abnormal angulation/curvature

This may be seen in children with greenstick or buckle fractures of the condylar neck, in the antral walls and in the zygomatic arches (especially the outward bowing from frontal impact to the malar bone). It may be the only clue to injury or an obvious feature of an otherwise readily recognizable injury (Fig. 5.26).

Step deformity

This is due to displacement of bone in the plane at right angles to the X-ray beam, giving rise to a sharp step in the contour of the outer margins of the bone cortex (Figs 5.2, 5.24). It is seen notably in the mandible, but can be seen elsewhere in the face and is recognizable on CT and plain film images.

Displaced bone

A large fragment or an entire osseous structure may change its location (Figs 5.4, 5.12). Examples are depression of the orbital floor and margin in tripod injuries or of the midface with respect to the skull base and mandible in Le Fort fractures. This displacement may be the most immediate or obvious feature but is always seen in conjunction with other signs.

Widening of the periodontal ligament

This sign is an important but often overlooked clue to fracture (Figs 5.3, 5.22, 5.24). In any individual socket the periodontal ligament has a uniform thickness all round the tooth and is equivalent in thickness to that around adjacent teeth. The ligament may appear wider/thicker in some disease processes and in local injury, such as partial extrusion. However, in the absence of such extrusion, a periodontal liga-

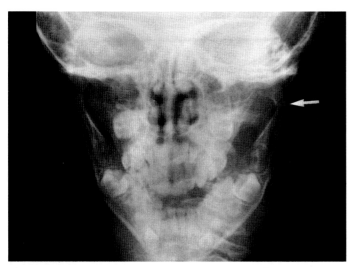

Fig. 5.26: Greenstick injury. Note the angular deformity of the left condylar neck (arrow) on this PA projection of a child's mandible.

ment appearing wider on one side than the other (e.g. wider mesially than distally) should raise the possibility that a mandibular fracture passes into it.

The indirect radiographic signs of fracture

Soft tissue swelling

This is a common and fairly non-specific sign (Fig. 5.2) and is often present with no underlying fracture. Occasionally, if localized, it may direct the attention to a particular area of the face on the radiograph. For example, soft tissue swelling over one cheek will direct attention to that side; swelling over the nasal arch will direct attention to the nasomaxillary structures. Swelling may also affect the airway and this should always be inspected on any lateral views and on CT images, bearing in mind that free blood may give a similar opacification.

Paranasal sinus opacification

Complete opacification, mucosal thickening (localized or general) and fluid levels in the sinuses may all be seen following trauma (Figs 5.1, 5.2, 5.5, 5.25). These signs may be due to pre-existing disease (Fig. 5.10) or just a severe nose bleed but should nevertheless be regarded with suspicion. Recognition of a fluid level requires the X-ray beam to be horizontal (or nearly so: up to about 10° tilt does not usually matter). A fluid level in the sphenoid sinus on a horizontal beam lateral view of a severely injured patient should always be taken as indicating a skull base fracture (Fig. 5.5) and further studies undertaken to prove or disprove the supposition. Opacification of the frontal sinus can be problematic if there is much overlying soft tissue swelling and if the AP dimension of the frontal sinus is small, it can be impossible to determine from the PA films whether the sinus is fully aerated or full of blood or CSF, unless a fluid level is seen. Opacification in the frontal or ethmoidal air cells may also be due to herniation of brain tissue.

Air in the soft tissues

Soft tissue gas has several causes, including infection, penetrating injury, sinus fracture and also rupture of the trachea, larynx or esophagus, with dissection up to the face. Emphysema from facial fracture is fairly common, particularly if there has not been much delay between the time of the trauma and the acquisition of images. Abnormally located air is usefully divided into three groups: soft tissue, orbital and intracranial. Very rarely, air may also occur in the intravascular space (e.g. cavernous sinus) or in the spine (pneumorachis).

Soft tissue emphysema

Apart from superior dissection of air due to laryngeal, tracheal or esophageal laceration, air in the soft tissue of the face is usually stated to be due to communication via a fracture with a paranasal sinus (Fig. 5.2). This can be misleading: although uncommon, it is encountered from time to time in patients whose only injury is a fracture of the mandible, particularly fractures around the angle. As with other signs, there are pitfalls: air lateral to the maxillary antrum may be mimicked by lateral extensions of the sphenoid sinus and by pacchionian granulations in the skull vault. Rarely air may be localized and under tension within the soft tissues, i.e. soft tissue pneumatocele. Occasionally air is seen in other sites, such as the temporomandibular joint. Soft tissue emphysema is always more extensive and widespread on CT images than one would expect from the plain radiographs.

Patients with facial fractures should be discouraged from nose blowing, sneezing, etc., as increased air pressure can force large amounts into the soft tissues, increasing the risk of infection. This can also result in extension of emphysema down the neck, over the chest and into the mediastinum. However, whenever air is seen in the soft tissues below the mandible (i.e. in the neck or below), every effort should be made to exclude other causes, such as laryngeal, tracheal or esophageal laceration.

Intraorbital air (Figs 5.1, 5.2, 5.10)

Intraorbital air, as seen on the plain film, must be differentiated from the deep sulcus of the upper lid in the elderly or enophthalmic patient. Air is usually seen superiorly in the orbit but can occur anywhere, even within the globe. Large amounts can collect in the preseptal space and, on occasion, behind the globe. There are even a few cases of 'tension pneumo-orbitism' presenting much like retrobulbar hemorrhage, with chemosis and threatened vision. Most cases of intraorbital air are said to be due to medial orbital wall fractures but air here can result from orbital floor injury. It can also occur as a delayed manifestation of an orbitoantral fistula, particularly in patients who have had 'blow-out' floor fractures repaired; these patients experience swelling and crepitus following nose blowing when they get colds.

Pneumocephalus/intracranial air

Air may collect in any of the spaces where blood collects, namely extradural (epidural), subdural, subarachnoid (cortical,

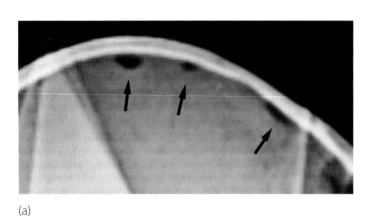

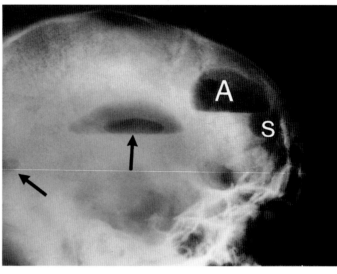

(a) (b)

Fig. 5.27: Examples of pneumocephalus. **(a)** CT (part of the lateral scanogram) following an orbitoethmoidal injury showing bubbles of subarachnoid air (arrows) beneath the calvarium. **(b)** Lateral skull X-ray in a patient with delayed pneumocephalus following repair of frontoethmoidal injury. Note aerocele (A), air in the body and occipital horns of the lateral ventricles (arrows) and in the subdural space (S).

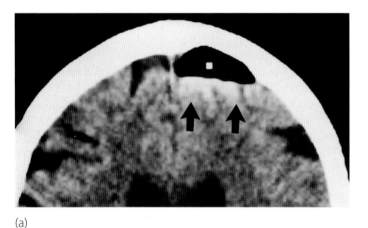

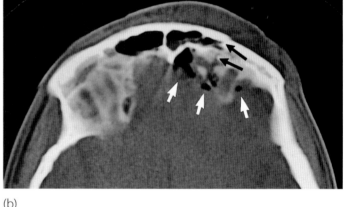

(a) (b)

Fig. 5.28: Examples of pneumocephalus. **(a)** Axial CT following an orbitoethmoidal injury showing air in the subarachnoid space (white cursor mark) limited medially by the falx (unlike epidural air). The increase in density of the brain tissue immediately behind this air (arrows) is a beam hardening artefact and should not be mistaken for brain contusion. **(b)** Axial CT following an injury to the frontal sinus. Note the thickened soft tissues in front of the sinus, fracturing of both anterior and posterior sinus walls (black arrows) and small collections of intracranial air (white arrows) due to dural tearing.

basal cistern and intraventricular) and in the brain substance (aerocele) (Figs 5.5, 5.27, 5.28). All sites except extradural imply tearing of the dura. Only occasionally seen on plain films, and then usually in only small amounts, pneumocephalus should nevertheless be looked for, particularly behind the frontal sinuses on the brow-up cross-table lateral projection obtained in the casualty/emergency room. The amount of air seen is very variable, but on CT images extremely small volumes (0.5 ml or less) can be recognized and so it is not uncommonly encountered on CT images of patients with severe injury. Intracranial air may arise from the air cavities of the petrous bones but more commonly from breaches around the ethmoid roof, sphenoid sinus and especially the frontal

sinus. When very tiny amounts of air are seen immediately adjacent to bone, it may be impossible to determine whether it is extradural or subdural.

The rate of disappearance of intracranial air depends on the amount originally present and whether there is an ongoing leak. Small amounts disappear in a few days; large amounts may take a week or more. If very large amounts are present then the air may be under pressure, forming a tension pneumocephalus or aerocele. This is an emergency, as it acts much like large intracranial blood collections. The appearance of pneumocephalus may be delayed – not just by a few days, but in some cases years or decades after injury; this is often associated with unexpected CSF rhinorrhea, which may be profuse.

Investigation of recurrent or delayed pneumocephalus is similar to that for recurrent or delayed CSF leak (see below).

Changes to the occlusal plane

Changes in the occlusion are always best assessed clinically, but gross changes are visible radiologically (Fig. 5.12) and can aid the radiologist (who may have limited information on the request form). Thus premature occlusion on one side may suggest a unilateral Le Fort I or dentoalveolar injury. An open anterior bite might suggest one of the Le Fort or condylar neck fractures.

Dental injury

Missing teeth and fractured teeth draw attention to areas of impact. Abnormal alignment of several adjacent teeth in the upper jaw may suggest the rotation of a dentoalveolar fragment.

CT evaluation approaches

CT imaging provides a series of slices through the facial skeleton. Assessing these requires analysis of each image, with its soft tissue and bony abnormalities, together with an ability to stack up these images to provide a 3D image in the mind. Gentry et al have developed the concept of a series of horizontal, coronal and sagittal struts or buttresses.[15] These can be used to evaluate the CT images of patients with facial trauma (Box 5.1). Such an approach allows for a more thorough assessment of the CT images. With a few exceptions, these struts are best evaluated when the plane of the image slice is perpendicular to the strut plane.

Specific signs on CT

Many of the changes described in relation to plain radiographs are applicable to CT imaging (Figs 5.6, 5.13, 5.14, 5.21). However, CT is very sensitive to soft tissue changes, many of which are not readily visible on plain films. It may demonstrate changes in position of the globe, the relationship of extraocular muscles to bone shards and blow-out fractures, accurately locate foreign bodies and demonstrate lens rupture or dislocation. CT can demonstrate hemorrhage at various intracranial sites, in the orbit and in the globe (Fig. 5.29). It can identify fractures which would otherwise be difficult to see on plain radiographs and it more accurately displays and localizes displaced bone fragments (Figs. 5.6, 5.13, 5.14, 5.30, 5.31). On the other hand, very thin walls located between structures of lower opacity may, because of partial voluming, disappear on CT images.

Specific Problems

Dental and dentoalveolar injury

Injury may involve the relationship of the tooth to its socket, the substance of the tooth itself or the surrounding bone.

Box 5.1 Facial struts[15]

Horizontal plane struts

Superior:	Orbital roof
	Fovea ethmoidalis
	Cribriform plates
Middle:	Orbital floor
	Zygomatic arch
Inferior:	Hard palate
	Alveolar ridge

Sagittal plane struts

Midline:	Perpendicular plate of ethmoid
	Vomer
	Nasal septal cartilage
Parasagittal:	Medial orbital walls
	Medial walls of maxillary antra
	Pterygoid plates
Lateral:	Lateral orbital walls
	Lateral walls of maxillary antra

Coronal plane struts

Anterior:	Anterior wall of frontal sinus
	Anterior walls of maxillary antra
	Nasoethmoidal complex
	Frontozygomatic buttress
	Anterior maxillary alveolus
Posterior:	Posterior walls of maxillary antra
	Pterygoid plates

There is, of course, a lot of overlap – an injury to a tooth may result in changes in all three of these and in major trauma frequently does.

Purpose of radiography in the acute phase of dental injury

- To assess the physiological development of the root apex. If the root formation is incomplete – that is, a wide open and funnel-shaped canal with a developmental sac still evident – the young tooth has marked healing potential. With advanced root development the canal is narrow and there is a greater likelihood of vascular damage and pulp necrosis.
- To assess the size of the pulp and its relationship to the fracture – but beware: a fracture here may appear to involve the pulp when it does not.
- To identify the presence of a root fracture.
- To identify the presence of foreign bodies such as tooth fragments in the soft tissues.
- To identify the presence of alveolar bone fracture.
- To assess any other abnormalities in the area and the condition of adjacent teeth.
- As a baseline for prognosis.

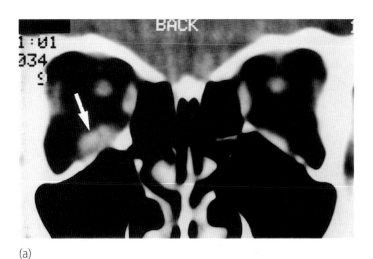

(a)

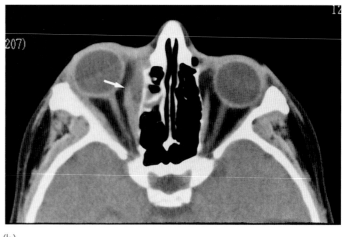

(b)

Fig. 5.29: Orbital injuries. **(a)** Coronal CT scan demonstrating hemorrhage in and around the right inferior rectus muscle sheath (arrow) due to penetrating injury. A large wooden twig was removed but was not separately identifiable on the CT studies. **(b)** Axial CT of the orbits. A posttraumatic subperiosteal orbital hematoma is displacing the medial rectus muscle (arrow) and causing proptosis.

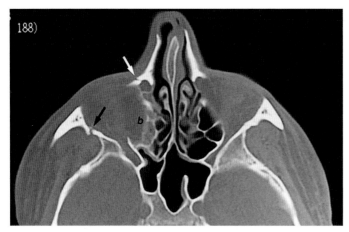

Fig. 5.30: Axial CT in a patient with malar and maxillary trauma. Part of a more extensive injury showing a fracture of the lacrimal duct (white arrow) and sphenomalar suture diastasis (black arrow). An inferomedial blow-out fracture is also evident (b).

Foreign bodies and missing teeth

General

Every effort must be made to locate missing teeth (Figs 5.32, 5.33) and dentures, and all lacerations and penetrating injuries must be suspected of harboring foreign bodies. In facial trauma the most common foreign bodies are windscreen glass and road grit. Teeth and foreign bodies may be ingested, inhaled or implanted into soft tissues; foreign bodies may also impale the patient.

Foreign bodies may implant anywhere and may be a great distance from the mucosal or skin breach. A very high index of suspicion must be maintained with any laceration in or around the eye, including the lids, and particularly in children, who are often poor historians. Orbital roof penetration is a well-recognized injury and is all too often overlooked, with such disastrous delayed results as CSF leak, orbital meningocele, meningitis, brain abscess and death. CT should be considered

in all suspicious cases, especially in children. Wooden objects are notorious for harboring organisms and producing abscesses and can be very difficult to detect (Fig. 5.29a). If the history is appropriate and CT negative, with no evidence of metallic foreign body, then MRI should be undertaken.

Avulsed teeth have been found implanted in the frontal sinus and as far away as the patient's forearm. The most common site for teeth or tooth fragments to become implanted is the oral soft tissues – the gingiva, the floor of mouth and the lips and tongue – but they may propel into the nasal cavity, palate or maxillary sinus. If careful examination of routine plain radiographs of the face does not reveal their whereabouts, and there are oral or lip lacerations, a soft tissue lateral radiograph should be obtained. If still unlocated, a chest radiograph (PA and lateral) should be obtained (Fig. 5.33). Inhaled teeth are distinctly uncommon but the results can be grievous, with lung collapse, pneumonia, lung abscess or even death occurring. Delayed removal beyond 24 hours is associated with increased morbidity and hospital stay: imaging should be expeditious. Ingested teeth are rarely a problem once they have entered the esophagus and are usually passed without problem. Large ingested foreign bodies and dentures may, however, be a problem and if stuck in the esophagus, may perforate into the mediastinum. Some foreign bodies and many dentures are not radiopaque and a contrast swallow examination with fluoroscopy may be needed to confirm their presence and locate them. This should be done as soon as possible otherwise edema around the impacted foreign body can make removal difficult and increases the likelihood of esophageal perforation.

Long impaled foreign bodies in the esophagus should be left in place until CT and, if appropriate, angiography have demonstrated their exact anatomical relationships and any underlying vascular damage. Sharp, elongated or pointed objects greater than 10 cm in length (6 cm in children) in the stomach should be considered for removal, as should blunt round objects greater than 2.5 cm, as they may fail to pass the pylorus.

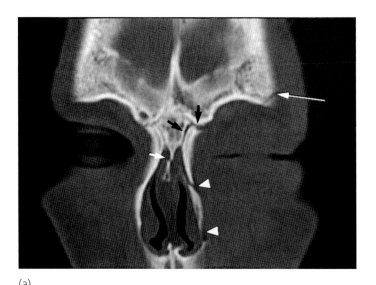

(a)

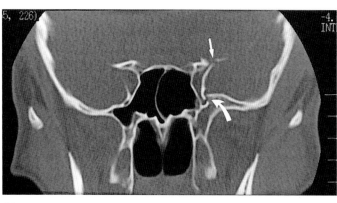

(b)

Fig. 5.31: Coronal CT in a patient with a central middle third injury. **(a)** Separation of the nasofrontal and nasomaxillary sutures (black arrows). Fractures of the nasal septum (short white arrow), the nasal plate of the frontal process of the maxilla (arrowheads) and of the superior orbital rim (long white arrow). **(b)** Same patient showing a sphenoid fracture involving the inferior part of the superior orbital fissure, floor of the middle cranial fossa (curved arrow) and the root of the anterior clinoid process (straight arrow).

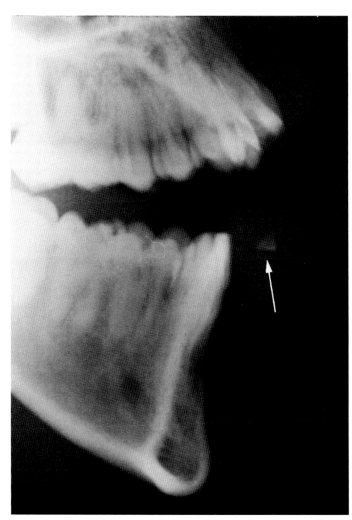

Fig. 5.32: Missing dental fragment seen in the lower lip on a soft tissue lateral projection (arrow).

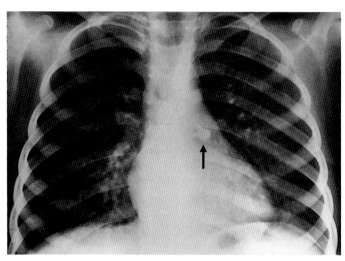

Fig. 5.33: Inhaled tooth. The chest X-ray in a young child demonstrating a molar tooth (arrow) in the left main bronchus.

Orbital foreign bodies

Foreign bodies in the orbit may be isolated or part of more widespread facial injury. They may be intra- or extraocular. Most extraocular intraorbital foreign bodies do not need removal except in special circumstances, e.g. organic material and those impinging on the optic nerve. Projecting foreign bodies, whether intra- or extraocular, need removing. Intraocular foreign bodies need removal as they may cause sympathetic ophthalmitis or premature cataract. Most intraocular foreign bodies that are clearly identifiable on ophthalmoscopy or slit-lamp examination do not require radiological assistance.

The purpose of imaging is twofold: first, to confirm a foreign body is present and second, to locate it. Methods used for confirmation that a foreign body is present and to demonstrate its approximate site include plain radiography, special techniques (bone-free radiographs, limbal ring and allied procedures), ultrasound and CT. MRI should not be used in any patient who may have a metallic fragment in the orbit, as the magnetic field may displace the fragment and endanger sight, but it has an important place in detecting wood, if it has not been identified on CT. When the patient is having CT examination to assess facial or cranial fractures, this alone may provide all the information required, both identifying the presence of a foreign body in the orbit and determining its position (whether intra- or extraocular, and its exact location within these compartments). CT is particularly useful when there are multiple foreign bodies, but is less accurate than ultrasound in demonstrating intraocular damage.

If CT imaging is not otherwise being performed the initial radiograph is a plain lateral view centered to the outer canthus, with the patient looking straight ahead. If no opaque foreign body is seen, then either no foreign body is present or it is a non-radiopaque foreign body requiring other imaging modalities to identify and locate it. If an opaque foreign body is seen, two views are taken, a PA projection with 35° elevation of the orbitomeatal line, and a lateral view with a double exposure, one exposure in upward gaze and one in downward gaze. Those tiny fragments that lie in a very anterior position may be demonstrable on bone-free radiographs: this technique involves a dental film being placed in the inner canthus, with a central ray directed just behind the outer canthus to include as much of the globe (and lids) as possible.

Such simple views may provide all the information required. If further detail regarding the exact location of an intraocular foreign body is needed then some special localizing technique is required. In these circumstances the most appropriate is ultrasound; the limbal ring radiographic technique can be used, but requires the assistance of an ophthalmologist for its attachment. Extremely tiny (less than 0.3 mm) foreign bodies may not be visible using standard radiographic methods and ultrasound is better here, although CT is preferred for extraocular intraorbital foreign bodies.

Projectile extraocular metallic or glass foreign bodies posterior to the equator are associated with a higher likelihood of ocular injury, but most do not need removal unless they are compromising the optic nerve or unless it is incidental to some other necessary surgical proceedure. Anterior extraocular metallic or glass foreign bodies do not require imaging if they are clinically palpable, the history is reliable and the eye examination is normal. CT should be considered if a ruptured globe is suspected, the foreign body is not palpable, there are significant ocular findings, the patient is a poor historian or if there is a possibility of multiple foreign bodies.

Organic matter such as wood and cotton incites an inflammatory reaction and can lead to a fungal cellulitis. In children especially, there may be no history of injury and little in the way of any physical evidence. The most common site is the superior orbit and foreign body material here may lead to abnormal extraocular motility, proptosis, ptosis, acute cellulitis and even osteomyelitis. Again, especially in children,

there is the risk that the injury is orbitocranial and this has a high mortality if unrecognized. Ultrasound is helpful in assessing the globe but not elsewhere in the orbit. CT is probably the best modality. However, the appearance of organic matter on CT varies considerably: wood may have densities between +110 and −446 Hounsfield units, dry wood looking like air and green wood being isodense to orbital fat or even muscle. CT cannot be used to exclude organic material, as it correctly identifies the foreign body in only about half of all cases. It does show well such secondary effects as abscess, osteomyelitis, periosteal thickening, optic nerve changes and any fractures or intracranial damage. Success with MRI is also variable. Dry wood is hypointense to fat on T1 and T2 weighting, mimicking bone fragments and air. Green wood, with a higher water content, is hypo- or isointense to fat on T1 and T2 weighting. The surroundings of the foreign body may enhance following contrast administration and also some surrounding hyperintensity may be seen on T2 weighting.

Nevertheless, reliable MRI identification of the foreign body is not much better than with CT and the added advantage CT has in assessing bone and its ability to exclude metal (contraindicated with MRI) makes it the first choice. History and a high degree of suspicion are most important and even if imaging is unhelpful, exploration may be necessary. Exploration without adequate imaging, however, is courting disaster as additional foreign body fragments and even intracranial foreign body and damage may be missed.

Pathological fractures

A pathological fracture is one that occurs in bone that has been weakened by disease. This disease process may be local, widespread or generalized. When such a process is present, the fracture may occur with less force than would normally be expected. Indeed, it often occurs with normal physiological loading such as mastication and sometimes spontaneously. Fracturing may occur during extirpation of teeth or surgery for cysts (Fig. 5.34). The list of potential causes is as long as

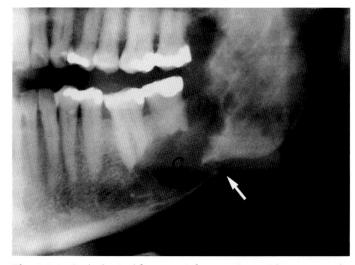

Fig. 5.34: Pathological fracture. A fracture (arrow) has occurred following surgery for a dentigerous cyst (c).

the list of diseases which weaken bone but includes cysts, malignant tumors (primary or secondary), osteomyelitis and osteoradionecrosis. Allied situations can also weaken bone, e.g. osseous implants. Developmental conditions such as ectopic teeth can also predispose to fracture. The patient may well be aware of the traumatic incident, but occasionally will present with no more than deranged occlusion. Clinically there may be less – or no – crepitus on movement and less pain than expected.

Recognition that the fracture is pathological is usually easy, there being a cyst or destructive lesion involving the bone or a clinical history of irradiation with irradiation bone changes adjacent to the fracture. Occasionally the problem may not be so obvious, particularly if the disease is generalized, e.g. myeloma. In the face the mandible is by far the most common bone to be involved. As the site of the fracture is determined by the disease, the pattern and location are often atypical: fractures of the body and ramus are more common. Once a pathological fracture is recognized further head and neck imaging is unlikely to be helpful, other than to stage malignancy and assess its operability.

Injury to secretory glands and their ducts

Significant injury to the parotid gland is usually the result of penetrating injury and of itself does not usually require imaging. Stenson's duct and the major duct tributaries are most at risk. Sialography can be of some help in suspected cases by identifying and locating any disruption of the duct (Fig. 5.35). Injury to the other salivary ducts rarely if ever requires imaging, except in late cases with stenosis.

Injury to the lacrimal drainage pathways is a fairly common sequel to severe fractures in the naso-orbitoethmoidal region. Injury may be direct from laceration/penetration or the result of shearing fractures in the bony canal. Imaging has a part to play in recognizing fractures of the bony canal and later in assessment of the lumen of the drainage apparatus. Fractures involving the bony canal are best identified on CT imaging using bony windows (Fig. 5.30). Fractures of the nasolacrimal fossa are usually avulsions of an intact fossa, comminution of the fossa itself being less frequent, although extensive comminution can occur in the surrounding bone. In contrast, most fractures involving the canal are comminuted and

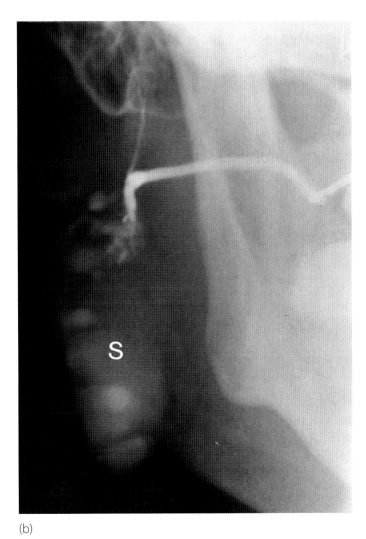

(a)

(b)

Fig. 5.35: Parotid sialogram showing duct trauma. **(a)** Lateral oblique projection. **(b)** PA projection. The patient fell through a plate glass door and developed swelling, having been sutured elsewhere. There is a laceration of a primary duct tributary (long arrow) with spurting of contrast medium (short arrows) into a large traumatic sialocele. Note the contrast puddling in the sialocele (s).

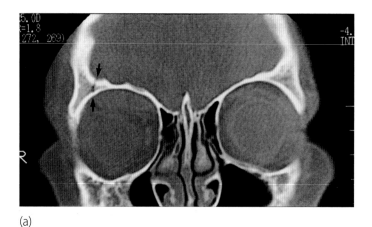

(a)

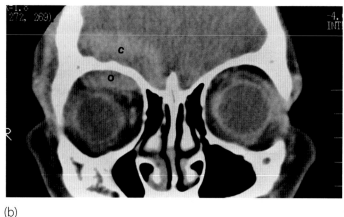

(b)

Fig. 5.36: Coronal CT in a child with an isolated orbital roof fracture. Clinically thought to have an orbital floor fracture because there was limitation of upward gaze with diplopia. **(a)** Bone window setting showing an isolated fracture of the orbital roof (arrows). **(b)** Soft tissue window setting at the same level showing intracranial hemorrhage (c) and subperiosteal hemorrhage at the orbital roof (o). The orbital floor and the superior orbital rim were intact.

especially so in the inferior canal. An important point to note on CT images of the nasolacrimal duct is that they are opaque in most normal people, but can be aerated, and that no significance can be attached to this even if one side is aerated and the other opaque.

Dacryocystography is used to assess the lumen of the naso-lacrimal canaliculi, sac and duct and involves introduction of contrast media via the lower canaliculus, although the upper – or, rarely, both – canaliculi may be used. Such dacryocystography is recorded by either plain radiography or from fluoroscopy, but CT has been used by some workers. Unless repeated attacks of dacryocystitis have occurred, the majority of lesions will be found either at the bony ring or in the canal, rather than the sac, which usually escapes injury.

Upper third facial injuries

Injury here has more scope for disaster than anywhere else in the face. The upper third of the face comprises the frontal bone, which contains the frontal sinuses. These sinuses are undeveloped in early childhood and may remain so in a few adults. They are extremely variable, may show marked asymmetry and may have extensions right out to the external angular process and right back along the orbital roof into the lesser wing of the sphenoid bone. These structures have an intimate relationship to the orbital contents and the brain. The lateral part of the frontal bone is exceptionally strong, but fracturing of the external angular process may occur, sometimes in association with a malar injury. Experiments with holographic interferometry show that supraorbital ridge loading causes stress in the form of surface perturbations in the orbital roof, some 5–8 mm in front of the optic foramen.[16] Blows to this part of the frontal bone are particularly associated with the onset of blindness (a fact noted by Hippocrates). Often, little will be found on imaging – not even a local fracture – but isolated orbital roof fractures may be seen (Fig. 5.36) and in the very young are more common than orbital floor fractures. Occasionally, ill-defined hemor-

rhage or a subperiosteal hematoma may be identified close to the orbital apex.

Most orbital roof fractures extend to the orbital rim. The dura over the roof is thin and firmly attached, so dural tearing is common. However, as the frontal sinus may extend along the roof, not all roof fractures will involve dura. When dura is torn the usual problems arise: CSF may leak into the orbit and large defects (greater than 1–1.5 cm) may allow dural herniation and pulsating exophthalmos. In addition, intra-orbital hemorrhage or bone spicules may affect extraocular muscle action, including the levator apparatus.

Fractures of the frontal sinus may involve the anterior wall, posterior wall and/or the nasofrontal duct. Undisplaced fractures of the anterior wall only require stabilization if there are other adjacent fragments. Displaced fractures of the anterior wall are more common (Fig. 5.37). These require treatment, both for cosmetic reasons and because bone fragments or mucosal tears may block the nasofrontal duct and lead to mucocele or pyocele formation. Clear visualization of the nasofrontal duct is not always possible on imaging, but any injury in this area should be regarded as compromising the frontal sinus drainage. Also, combined anterior and posterior wall fractures nearly always involve the duct, unless the fracture is laterally placed. If the posterior

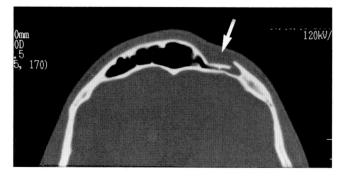

Fig. 5.37: Frontal sinus injury seen on an axial CT. There is a depressed fracture of the anterior wall of the frontal sinus (arrow).

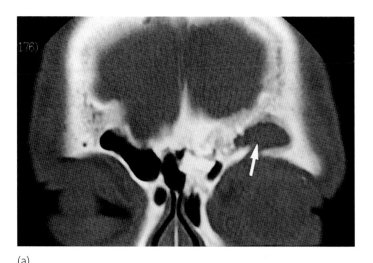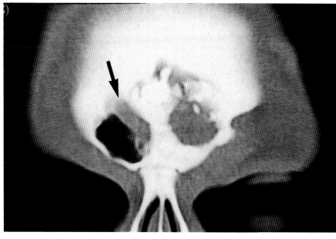

(a)   (b)

Fig. 5.38: Coronal CT of a patient with a frontal sinus mucopyocele. Previous fracture with incomplete obliteration with bone chips. **(a)** A far left loculus (white arrow) was left uncleared and unfilled. **(b)** As was a right-sided loculus which drained to the left (black arrow). 18 months later CT shows that these loculi have filled with pus, bone erosion is taking place and the bone chips are being resorbed.

wall is intact but the nasofrontal duct is involved or at risk, the sinus will need to be obliterated. It is essential here to recognize and report the extent of pneumatization of the frontal sinus: if locules in the orbital roof or far laterally are not obliterated mucocele and pyocele are likely to result (Fig. 5.38). Fractures of the posterior wall may involve the dura, leading to CSF leak. This is most likely if the fracture is displaced or comminuted. Undisplaced fractures with no evidence of CSF leak may be treated as above, but otherwise the sinus needs to be cranialized. Good imaging and accurate assessment are therefore essential.

Plain films (modified Caldwell and lateral), although useful as initial scout imaging, are notoriously unreliable and difficult to interpret. Some significant and severe injuries can be almost impossible to see. This is, in part, due to the curvature of the anterior and posterior walls of the frontal sinus which results in only small portions of these walls being in tangent to the X-ray beam. Additionally, apart from recognizing pneumocephalus, plain radiographs will not allow assessment of underlying soft tissues such as brain, meninges and orbital contents. For this reason CT is virtually mandatory.

Dural tearing and CSF leak

Severe blunt trauma as well as penetrating injury may breach the dura. Cerebrospinal fluid leak and pneumocephalus are the potential consequences, leading in turn to infection such as meningitis or, if brain tissue is involved, abscess formation. Pneumocephalus has already been described (see above), but the two conditions commonly coexist, although they may not be apparent at the same time. Fractures of the ethmoid and sphenoid sinuses with dural tearing and CSF leak commonly occur with Le Fort II, III and naso-orbitoethmoidal fractures, but the CSF leak in these cases is usually short-lived and ceases with fracture reduction and fixation. Only a few

persist, and it is only those that persist for more than 2 weeks or are recurrent or delayed, or exhibit expanding pneumocephalus or develop meningitis, that require detailed investigation. Recurrence can be delayed for decades.

The most common site of persistent CSF leaks is the frontal sinus and with acute trauma to this sinus, CT is virtually mandatory because plain films are notoriously unreliable in demonstrating fractures of the posterior table, let alone the commonly occurring coexistent intracranial damage. Wide fracture separation or displacement of fragments greater than the thickness of the posterior table implies dural tearing and therefore these signs should be sought on the CT images of patients with acute trauma. Rarely CSF may enter the orbit, forming a cyst, or, even more rarely, leak into the conjunctiva (orbitorrhea) to present like epiphora.

Considerable ingenuity has been expended in developing tests not only to prove that leaking fluid is CSF but especially to locate the dural breach. Most of the location methods used in the past were superseded by the introduction of iodinated contrast media in the intrathecal space during CT (CT cisternography). This method is now rarely used, as there are inherent risks in introducing such material into the CSF and, as with nearly all the other methods, it is only reliable if the patient is actively leaking at the time of the study. More recently, Lloyd and co-workers[17] have shown that with improvements in CT technology, high-definition CT is all that is required to demonstrate accurately the site of the leak (Fig. 5.39) and that this does not depend on active CSF leak at the time of the investigation. In their series persistent bone defects were identified and these were nearly always accompanied by some soft tissue opacification in the adjacent sinus and in about a quarter of cases by pneumocephalus.

However, the use of CT with or without intrathecal contrast media still exposes the patient to ionizing radiation. MRI avoids both this and the injection with contrast medium. In 1994, el Gammal and Brooks,[18] as well as

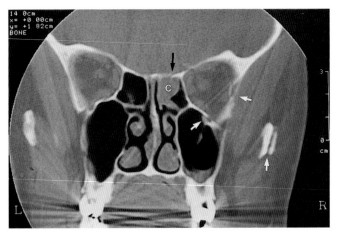

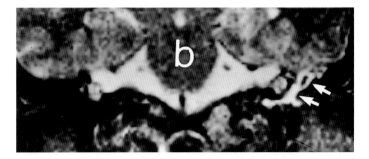

(a)

(b)

Fig. 5.39: Coronal CT showing CSF fluid leak into the sinuses (c). The floor of the anterior cranial fossa is fractured (black arrow). Note also fractures of the orbital floor, lateral orbital wall and malar arch (white arrows). There is a fluid level in the antrum.

Fig. 5.40: MRI showing a CSF leak. T2-weighted coronal **(a)** and axial **(b)** reconstructions. **(a)** High signal (white) CSF is seen leaking through a dural tear in the tegmen on the coronal study. The CSF fills the middle ear cavity (white arrows), surrounding the ossicles (black signal void). **(b)** CSF is seen in the mastoid air cells (long arrow), middle ear cavity (large short arrow) and escaping through the tympanic membrane to pool in the scaphoid fossa of the pinna and drip off the helix margin (small short arrows). (b = brain stem, c = cerebellum)

El Jamel and co-workers,[19] demonstrated that magnetic resonance cisternography provided an important alternative. CSF gives a high signal on T2-weighted images and as such, provides its own contrast (Fig. 5.40). MRI can also display intracranial anatomy and trauma pathology in great detail and images can readily be obtained in any plane.

The choice between modalities remains controversial. Hegarty, in 1997, looked at a control group having MRI for temporal lobe epilepsy and found that 42% fulfilled the criteria for diagnosis of CSF fistula.[20] However, the year before, Stafford-Johnson [21] had published the findings in 24 patients with CSF leaks and found the technique 100% reliable in identifying the site of leak; all were confirmed at surgery. High-resolution CT has a high incidence of false positives, especially in the region of the cribriform plate. Both modalities may be helpful, but CT is likely to be used in most centers, because it is faster and more widely available. Nevertheless, MRI should be considered if CT is equivocal or unhelpful. Furthermore, MRI is the procedure of choice in evaluating those rarer consequences of dural tearing, namely meningocele and encephalocele: these may present clinically with pulsating exophthalmos or hypoglobus (if through the orbital roof), as a soft tissue mass in the nasal cavity or as soft tissue opacification of the frontal and ethmoid sinuses on plain radiographs.

Compartment syndromes

Acute compartment syndromes

These comprise acute retrobulbar hemorrhage and tension pneumo-orbitism. Some degree of retrobulbar hemorrhage is common in orbital trauma and is recognizable on CT imaging as patchy areas of increased attenuation (Fig. 5.41). Most cases probably decompress, either due to the increased orbital capacity that occurs with coexistent blow-out injury or via breaches into the sinuses. In other cases hemorrhage is too small to be of significance to vision. Cadaver experiments

in the young show that the orbital septum can withstand pressures between 70–100 mmHg (rarely as high as 120 mmHg) before rupture. In the elderly the septum is weaker and as little as 10–15 mmHg pressure may be enough to cause rupture.[22] Nose blowing can cause intranasal pressures as high as 114 mmHg. If there is a wall defect in the orbit air can be transmitted into the orbit at these high pressures and with a valve mechanism, the air can remain trapped there. Similarly, bleeding into the orbit can achieve high pressures. Unfortunately retinal vessels and the optic nerve cannot withstand pressures of 65–70 mmHg for long and blindness may ensue. Higher pressures still will also cause central retinal artery occlusion, with irreversible damage.

The hemorrhage or air in such circumstances may be retrobulbar and within the fat or may be subperiosteal. Subperiosteal hemorrhage is more common in the young and is most often situated at the orbital roof. It is usually less of a problem because the subperiosteal space is continuous with the presep-

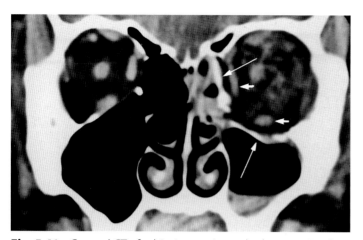

Fig. 5.41: Coronal CT of orbits in a patient who has sustained blow-out fractures and intraorbital hemorrhage (left/right orientation reversed). Note the fluid level in the maxillary antrum, opacification of the ethmoidal air cells on the affected side and medial wall and orbital floor blow-out fractures (long arrows). There is patchy increase in density within the orbital fat due to widespread hemorrhage and edema. Comparison with the normal side shows that on the affected side the inferior and medial rectus muscles are displaced downwards (short arrows) and there is apparent elongation of the cross-sectional image of the medial rectus, these changes being due to septal tethering.

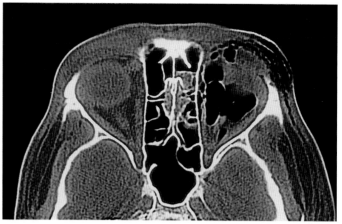

Fig. 5.42: Axial CT in a patient with tension pneumo-orbitism. There is extensive air in the postseptal as well as the preseptal space (courtesy P Ayliffe).

tal space and it only becomes a problem if the collection is very large or it is directly compressing the optic nerve.

The cardinal clinical signs of acute retrobulbar hemorrhage causing a compartment syndrome are pain, progression of increasing proptosis and decreasing visual acuity (leading to blindness). Signs indicating that active treatment is required are decreasing visual acuity and loss or impairment of the afferent pupillary reflex.

Tension pneumo-orbitism is exceedingly rare, but presents with clinical findings that are very similar to acute retrobulbar hemorrhage (Fig. 5.42). Preseptal air is never vision threatening. Air behind the globe is nearly always innocuous and self-limiting, most of the intraorbital air resorbing within a few days to a week. There are, however, enough cases in the literature to warrant a more cautious attitude.

Hunts and co-workers suggest classifying orbital emphysema into four groups.[23]

- Stage I: No proptosis/dystopia, no loss of vision, no increase in intraocular pressure, no central retinal artery occlusion
- Stage II: As in Stage I, except proptosis/dystopia is present
- Stage III: Proptosis/dystopia present, loss of vision; possible rise in intraocular pressure. No central retinal artery occlusion
- Stage IV: All above positive, including central retinal artery occlusion

They suggest imaging as follows.

Stage I patients are common and no special imaging is required. It is recognized radiologically. Stage II patients

require CT to rule out other intraorbital lesions. Stage III patients require emergency CT if available, to localize air to allow needle aspiration. Stage IV patients (suggested by no light perception) require rapid orbital decompression and this should not be delayed by acquiring further imaging. Under their regime, the use of CT in Stage III patients with loss of vision is, however, debatable.

The onset of blindness in acute compartment syndromes can be extremely rapid and although these conditions are identifiable on CT, as a general rule no imaging should take place as this merely prolongs the time to treatment and risks the blindness becoming permanent. Such cases require either immediate needle aspiration (if air) or a lateral cantholysis and canthotomy under local anesthesia in the emergency room. Only if this is unhelpful should CT be considered (to identify and locate the blood or air).

Chronic compartment syndromes

These occur very slowly and manifestation may be delayed. They include hematocysts, posttraumatic cholesterol cysts, chronic abscess formation around foreign bodies, CSF cysts, meningoceles, encephaloceles and posttraumatic frontal sinus mucoceles. Most are distinctly rare. They almost invariably cause dystopia, usually proptosis, sometimes hypoglobus and occasionally other or mixed forms. They may also cause diplopia. When associated with a breach in the orbital roof there may be a pulsating exophthalmos, which needs to be differentiated from the pulsating exophthalmos of posttraumatic carotocavernous fistula. CT is the usual method of investigation and is satisfactory, although if not otherwise precluded, MRI is probably now the imaging modality of choice.

Enophthalmos

That posttraumatic enophthalmos (Fig. 5.43) is due to orbital volume expansion has been repeatedly confirmed using CT imaging. Whitehouse et al have attempted to predict the final degree of enophthalmos using CT to measure orbital volume.[24] In 11 patients scanned more than 20 days post

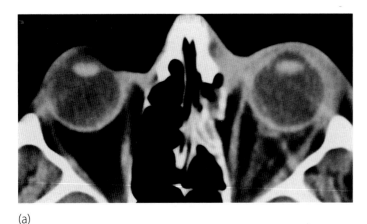

(a)

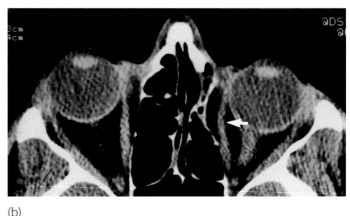

(b)

Fig. 5.43: Orbital enlargement leading to enophthalmos (patient in Fig. 5.41). **(a)** Axial CT with medial wall blow-out fracture. Patchy hemorrhage in the orbital fat is not as obvious as on the coronal image (Fig. 5.41). There is preseptal swelling and very slight proptosis. **(b)** Axial CT obtained as part of a 3D volumetric study 9 months after injury. Note again the medial wall displacement. The edema and hemorrhage have resolved and the patient has become slightly enophthalmic. The medial rectus muscle on the affected side appears slack (arrow) when compared with the opposite side.

injury and 25 scanned within 20 days of injury, they concluded that enophthalmos was less marked than would be predicted from orbital volume expansion when enophthalmus was measured within 20 days (due, no doubt, to hemorrhage and edema), but that after this time resolution of edema and hemorrhage permitted a good correlation between orbital volume expansion and the degree of enophthalmos, each 1 cc of increase in orbital volume corresponding to 0.8 mm enophthalmos. They suggest that CT-measured orbital volume can be done early and that it will allow prediction of the expected final degree of enophthalmos, allowing appropriate early surgery.

In some patients detailed imaging may not be required, other than that demanded by additional problems such as diplopia and to provide information about the integrity of the medial wall. Many patients will, however, require volume-increasing surgery. Detailed preoperative assessment of such cases is best provided by 3D CT volumetric analysis, ideally using a spiral (helical) technique. Volume changes can then be measured and their location identified; models can be generated using computerized milling, so allowing more accurate placement and volume of implant material.

Blow-out and blow-in fractures

Blow-out fractures (Figs 5.10, 5.14, 5.41, 5.43, 5.44)

In patients with suspected blow-out fractures three main questions have to be addressed by imaging.

1. Is a fracture present?
2. What is its effect?
3. If present, how extensive (how far posteriorly) is it?

Imaging in the initial stages has little part to play in the direct investigation of these disorders. In an article on the role of plain radiography in the management of suspected orbital blow-out fractures, 100 consecutive patients were reviewed.[25] The plain films made no difference to patient

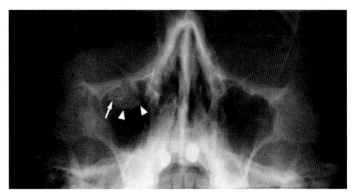

Fig. 5.44: Blow-out fracture of the right orbital floor seen on an occipitomental projection. Note the soft tissue herniation (arrowheads) and displaced bone fragments (arrow). Soft tissue swelling of the cheek is also present.

management, the decision to operate being guided exclusively by clinical criteria. It was recommended that patients in whom a competent clinician finds no direct evidence of an orbital fracture (orbital emphysema, enophthalmos, decreased infraorbital sensation, deformity, pseudoptosis or certain types of eye movement disturbance) should not undergo plain radiography; that patients with minor degrees of the above signs and symptoms should be given a follow-up clinical appointment or a request form for CT, which they are instructed to present for CT imaging after a given interval, or a delayed appointment for CT – in either of the latter cases cancelling the appointment or tearing up the form if these symptoms improve over a period to be determined by the clinician; and finally, that patients found to have 3 mm or more of enophthalmos and/or diplopia strongly suggestive of orbital tissue entrapment or prolapse, or with signs of a major or symptomatic fracture, should be directly referred for CT. The authors made the point that all patients with diplopia should have formal orthoptic assessment.

In the adult most small orbital floor blow-out fractures are rather posteriorly situated, in the thinnest portion of the orbital floor, medial to the infraorbital groove and anterior to the inferior orbital fissure, and an important aspect of imaging is the delineation of the posterior extent of the fracture. In one series, 95% of patients with diplopia persisting 6 months postoperatively had fractures extending more than 2 cm posterior to the orbital rim. Indeed, the risk of such postoperative diplopia was even greater in such cases than that associated with combined medial and floor injury.[26]

However, large blow-outs (hammock type), whether of the pure or the impure (orbital rim involved) type, are less likely to cause problems with orbital tissue tethering than the smaller ones (Fig. 5.45). In children and young adults smaller fractures, particularly of the trapdoor type, are more common and, because of the greater elasticity of bone, despite being small, can be of greater clinical importance. This is because incarceration and strangulation of even small amounts of prolapsed orbital tissue (not necessarily muscle) cause severe limitation in eye movement.

de Man and co-workers therefore recommend surgery as soon as possible in such cases.[27] In their paper they describe 15 patients under 15 years of age almost all of whom had linear closed trapdoor fractures, different from the open trapdoor or hammock type seen in older patients. These children had unequivocal forced duction tests, did not improve conservatively and required early surgery. Anderson, discussing two patients less than 8 years old, emphasized the immature morphology of the antrum and orbit, but pointed out that this did not prevent escape of orbital contents.[28] Using logistic regression, Koltai demonstrated that the age at which the probability of lower orbital fracture exceeds orbital roof fracture was 7.1 (+/−1) years, noting that the very young were more likely to have a roof fracture.[29] In 1999 Cope[30] reported on 45 cases and commented that such cases of floor fracture were especially rare under the age of 8 years, but that up to the age of 9 years children were more likely to have small defects in the anterior orbital floor, which were of a linear trapdoor type: more than half of these patients had persistent diplopia. From the age of 13 to 15 years the fracture was more likely to be of an open door type and less than one-third had persistent diplopia.

In 1998, Jordan et al pointed out that young patients may not exhibit all the usual signs.[31] They described 20 cases with no ecchymosis or edema, but who had marked motility restriction in up and down gaze. They termed the condition the 'white-eyed' blow-out fracture. In these patients there was very minimal evidence of floor disruption on imaging, CT showing a small crack in the floor or a small trapdoor defect with little bone displacement: some had a very small degree of tissue hematoma (tear drop sign). In this group, those having a 2–3 week wait for surgery had slower and in some cases incomplete resolution of gaze restriction. They, therefore, also recommended surgery was done early, within 2–4 days of injury.

Although plain films should not be requested to assess blow-out fractures it is of course reasonable to obtain plain radiographs in patients with clinically suspected orbital rim fractures and this may reveal a blow-out fracture (Figs 5.10, 5.24). Despite some authors claiming a high degree of accuracy in diagnosing orbital floor blow-out fractures using plain radiographs,[32] reports vary considerably. Furthermore, in most patients diplopia will resolve without intervention, being due to causes other than tethering. Selection for imaging, therefore, is based on clinical criteria and, in adults, on the evolution of signs and symptoms. In any event, few surgeons would be happy operating without the additional information available from CT.

Both CT and MRI may be used to address the questions posed at the beginning of this section. CT has the advantage of delineating the skeletal tissues more effectively than MRI and, in any event, is frequently indicated for other concomitant facial injury outside the orbit. MRI, on the other hand, is more sensitive in assessing the soft tissue components, such as the orbital fat and its displacement; also alternative imaging planes are easier to achieve with MRI.

CT imaging (Figs 5.13, 5.41, 5.45, 5.46) is best done in the coronal position, as this displays the floor (where most injuries occur) better than the axial position and displays the medial wall as well as the axial position. Coronal imaging can be done prone with neck extended, supine with hyperflexion of the neck or supine with extension of neck into the 'hanging head' position or by reconstruction from axial imaging. The

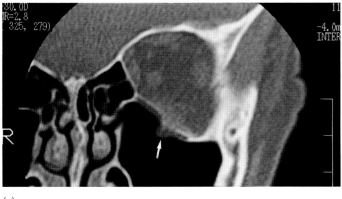

(a)

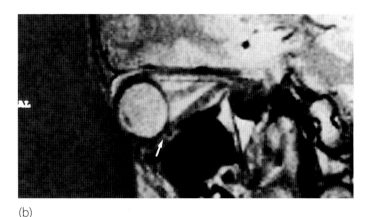

(b)

Fig. 5.45: Tiny blow-out fracture in a child. **(a)** Coronal CT showing a tiny amount of soft tissue below the orbital floor (arrow). No fracture can be reliably identified. **(b)** Sagittal MRI (STIR setting) showing high signal crossing the orbital floor (arrow). At surgery a minute (5 mm) undisplaced linear fracture was identified tethering the orbital septal apparatus.

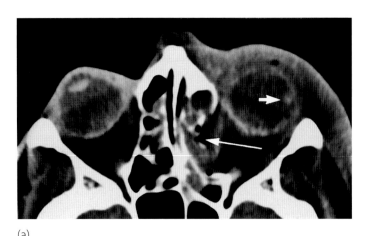

(a)

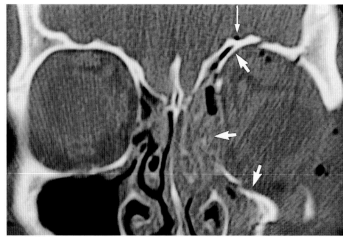

(b)

Fig. 5.46: Orbital blow-out fractures. **(a)** Axial CT image showing preseptal soft tissue swelling, vitreal hemorrhage (short arrow) and a medial orbital wall blow-out fracture (long arrow). **(b)** Coronal CT image of the same patient. There are further blow-out fractures of the orbital roof and floor. Note the opaque maxillary antrum and ethmoidal air cells and the air in the cranium (long arrow), orbit and soft tissues. There are fractures of the medial orbital wall and the orbital floor with depression of these walls (short arrows). The base of the external angular process of the frontal bone and the roof of the orbit are fractured with cranial displacement of the medial segment of the roof. The orbital volume increase is obvious.

former two methods are preferable as they place antral blood/fluid inferiorly, allowing more accurate assessment of soft tissue changes in the upper antrum.

All the signs seen on plain radiographs may be evident and in addition, further important information is acquired regarding the position of the extraocular muscles relative to the fracture and the presence of hemorrhage and bone spicules. The coronal scans alone may provide adequate information, but direct sagittal or sagittal reconstructions, in selected cases, may display the posterior extent of an orbital floor fracture and its relationship to the inferior rectus in a more readily appreciated way. On CT images muscle can be difficult to see if there is much surrounding edema and hemorrhage, but displacement can sometimes be inferred by the absence of a muscle from its usual position.

Blow-in fractures

These are common at the orbital roof. A high index of suspicion should be entertained especially in children and/or if there is ptosis, evidence of restriction to the superior rectus muscle or hematoma confined to the upper lid. Bone fragments may not only involve the superior rectus and levator muscles, but also the superior division of the oculomotor nerve. CSF may leak; meningoceles and encephaloceles may cause proptosis – sometimes pulsating. Blow-in fractures also occur at the orbital floor due to buckling, again especially in children, and also at the medial wall in association with severe naso-orbitoethmoidal fractures (Fig. 5.47). If roof and floor blow-in fractures are suspected coronal CT is the best projection; with medial wall fractures axial or coronal CT is satisfactory.

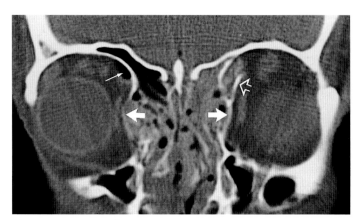

Fig. 5.47: Blow-in fractures seen on a CT image of a patient who has sustained a severe naso-orbitoethmoidal fracture. Both medial orbital walls have become displaced laterally, bulging into the orbital cavities (large arrows) as a result of the severe concertina effect of the primary injury. Note air in the right orbit (small arrow). There is a bone fragment in the left orbit which has displaced below the superior oblique muscle (open arrow).

References

1 Johnson DH 1984 CT of maxillo-facial trauma. Radiologic Clinics of North America 22: 131–44

2 Masters SJ, McClean PM, Arcarese JS et al 1987 Skull x-ray examinations after head trauma: recommendations by a multidisciplinary panel and validation study. New England Journal of Medicine 316: 84–91

3 Jennett B 1978 If my son had a head injury. British Medical Journal 1: 1601–1603

4 Heiskanen O, Marttila I, Valtonen S 1973 Prognosis of depressed skull fracture. Acta Chirurgica Scandinavica 139: 605–608

5 McAuley CE, Sherman HF, Jones LM, Carter DM, D'Amico F 1992 The 'missed injury': a prospective evaluation of delayed diagnosis in blunt multisystem trauma. Journal of Trauma 22: 948

6 Velmahos GC, Theodorou D, Tatevossian R et al 1996 Radiographic cervical spine evaluation in the alert asymptomatic blunt trauma victim: much ado about nothing? Journal of Trauma 40: 768–774

7 Beirne JC, Butler PE, Brady FA 1995 Cervical spine injuries in patients with facial fractures: a 1 year prospective study. International Journal of Oral and Maxillofacial Surgery 24: 26–29

8 McGrigor DB, Campbell W 1950 The radiology of war injuries. Part VI, wounds of the face and jaw. British Journal of Radiology 23: 685–696

9 Trapnell DH 1985 Diagnostic radiography. In: Rowe NL, Williams JLI (eds) Maxillofacial injuries. Churchill Livingstone, Edinburgh

10 Dolan KD, Jacoby CG 1978 Facial fractures. Seminars in Roentgenology 13: 37–51

11 DelBalso AM, Hall RE, Margarone JE 1990 Radiographic evaluation of maxillofacial trauma. In: DelBalso AM (ed) Maxillofacial imaging. WB Saunders, Philadelphia

12 Valvassori GE, Hord GE 1968 Traumatic sinus disease. Seminars in Roentgenology 3: 160–171

13 Le Fort R 1901 Étude experimentale sur les fractures de la machoire supérieure. Revue de Chirurgie 23: 208–227, 360–379 and 479–507

14 Fry WK, Shepherd PR, McLeod AC, Parfitt GJ 1942 The dental treatment of maxillofacial injuries. Blackwell Scientific, Oxford

15 Gentry LR, Manor WF, Turski PA, Strother C 1983 High resolution computed tomographic analysis of facial struts in trauma: 1. Normal anatomy. American Journal of Roentgenology 140: 523–532

16 Anderson RL, Panje WR, Gross CE 1982 Optic nerve blindness following blunt forehead trauma. Ophthalmology 89: 445–455

17 Lloyd MNH, Kimber PM, Burrows EH 1994 Post-traumatic cerebrospinal fluid rhinorrhoea: modern high-definition computed tomography is all that is required for the effective demonstration of the site of leakage. Clinical Radiology 49: 100–103

18 el Gammal T, Brooks BS 1994 MR cisternography: initial experience in 41 cases. American Journal of Neuroradiology 15: 1647–1656

19 El Jamel MS, Pidgeon CN, Toland J, Phillips JB, O'Dwyer AJ 1994 MRI cisternography, and the localization of CSF fistulae. British Journal of Neurosurgery 8: 433–437

20 Hegarty SE, Millar JS 1997 MRI in the localization of CSF fistulae: is it of any value? Clinical Radiology 52: 768–770

21 Stafford Johnson DB, Brennan P, Toland J, O'Dwyer AJ 1996 Magnetic resonance imaging in the evaluation of cerebrospinal fluid fistulae. Clinical Radiology 51: 837–841

22 Muhammad JK, Simpson MT 1996 Orbital emphysema and the medial orbital wall: a review of the literature with particular reference to that associated with indirect trauma and possible blindness. Journal of Cranio-maxillofacial Surgery 24: 245–250

23 Hunts JH, Patrinley JR, Holds JB, Anderson RL 1994 Orbital emphysema: staging and acute management. Ophthalmology 101: 960–966

24 Whitehouse RW, Batterbury M, Jackson A, Noble JL 1994 Prediction of enophthalmos by computed tomography after 'blow-out' orbital fracture. British Journal of Ophthalmology 78: 618–620

25 Bhattacharya J, Moseley IF, Fells P 1997 The role of plain radiography in the management of suspected orbital blow-out fractures. British Journal of Radiology 70: 29–33

26 Biesman BS, Hornblass A, Lisman R, Kazlas M 1996 Diplopia after surgical repair of orbital floor fractures. Ophthalmic Plastic and Reconstructive Surgery 12: 9–16

27 de Man K, Wijngaarde R, Hes T, de Jong PT 1991 Influence of age on the management of blow-out fractures of the orbital floor. International Journal of Oral Maxillofacial Surgery 20: 330–336

28 Anderson PJ, Poole MD 1995 Orbital floor fractures in young children. Journal of Cranio-maxillofacial Surgery 23: 151–154

29 Koltai PJ, Amjad I, Meyer D, Feustel PJ 1995 Orbital fractures in children. Archives of Otolaryngology and Head and Neck Surgery 121: 1375–1379

30 Cope MR, Moos KF, Speculand B 1999 Does diplopia persist after blow-out fractures of the orbital floor in children? British Journal of Oral Maxillofacial Surgery 37: 46–51

31 Jordan DR, Allen LH, White J, Harvey J, Pashby R, Esmaeli B 1998 Intervention within days for some orbital floor fractures: the white-eyed blowout. Ophthalmic Plastic and Reconstructive Surgery 14: 379–390

32 Kim SH, Ahn KJ, Lea JM, Choi KH, Han SH 2000 The usefulness of orbital lines in detecting blow-out fracture on plain radiography. British Journal of Radiology 73: 1265–1269

Appendix: Radiography of Facial Injuries

Definitions

Orbitomeatal baseline

Syn: Radiographic baseline, tragocanthal line, canthomeatal line. This line passes from the outer canthus of the eye to the middle of the external auditory meatus. The line projected forward passes through the nasion (helpful to note when the canthus reference point is uncertain). It is this line that is most often used in facial radiography.

Anthropological baseline

Syn: Anatomical baseline, Reid's baseline, line of Frankfurter. This line passes from the infraorbital point to the superior border of the external auditory meatus. The orbitomeatal and the anthropological baselines are approximately 10–12° to each other.

Glabellomeatal line

This line passes from the center of external auditory meatus to the center of the glabella and makes an angle of about 15° to the orbitomeatal line.

Sagittal plane

Any plane parallel to the median sagittal plane. The median sagittal plane is a vertical plane that divides the skull into left and right halves.

Coronal plane

Any plane parallel to the meatal (or auricular) plane. The meatal plane is perpendicular to the anthropological baseline and passes through the external auditory meati.

Tube angulation vs orbitomeatal line elevation

Neck extension may be impossible, because of either concurrent spinal injury or pre-existing disease such as osteoarthrosis or ankylosis, or because of a severe upper dorsal kyphosis or gibbus deformity. In such patients the inability to elevate the orbitomeatal baseline can be compensated by an equivalent caudal tilt of the central ray. Severe degrees of tube tilt produce greater distortion, but this is usually acceptable for most cases.

Posteroanterior (PA) vs anteroposterior (AP)

This terminology refers to the direction of the path taken by the X-ray beam. PA means the tube is posterior to the patient and hence the beam passes from back to front; AP means the reverse. In facial trauma patients frontal films should *always* be done in the PA projection, *never* the AP. In the AP projection, on both Caldwell or other occipitofrontal views, the lateral orbital margins can be superimposed over (and are therefore obscured by) the parietal and temporal bones,

where these latter are seen in tangent. Similarly on the AP Waters/occipitomental group of views, including the occipitomental 30° view, both the lateral orbital margins and the zygomatic arches can be superimposed over the margins of the calvarium. Furthermore, there is a significantly higher radiation dose to the lens of the eye with AP than with PA projections. Finally, geometric sharpness is greatest in those anatomical parts closest to the film, namely the face in a PA projection. Imaging should always be delayed until the patient can co-operate with the radiographer to provide PA views.

Projections for the middle and upper thirds of the face

The occipitofrontal 15–20° (Caldwell) projection

Caldwell's view is equivalent to 15–20° elevation (standard 17°) of the orbitomeatal baseline, the glabellomeatal line used by Caldwell and the orbitomeatal line being about 8° to one another. This view projects the petrous bones over the lower one-quarter to one-third of the orbit. It should be remembered that this view was designed for sinus imaging rather than trauma. For this reason a modification is recommended – the occipitofrontal 25° projection or modified Caldwell view.

The occipitofrontal 25° (modified Caldwell) projection

With the orbitomeatal baseline horizontal (perpendicular to the film plane) the central ray is angled 25° caudad, with a possible variation in some individuals of 26° or 27°. The advantage of this view is that it provides good visualization of the orbital floor (projecting the petrous bones just below the orbit).

Waters projection

This was described by Waters and Waldron as a modification of the occipitofrontal positions, in order to obtain a better view of the maxillary antra whilst retaining a view of the frontal and ethmoidal sinuses. The orbitomeatal baseline elevation (or tube depression) should be 37°. This tilt of tube or orbitomeatal baseline will usually project the petrous bone over the inferior portion of the antra, obscuring it. Occasionally, the same problem occurs with the true occipitomental position (45° elevation) and for this reason a modification is preferred – the occipitomental 10° projection.

The occipitomental 10° projection

The orbitomeatal baseline is elevated 45° and the central ray angled 10° caudad and centered to the lower orbital margin. This projection provides a margin of safety, ensuring the petrous bones are projected below the maxillary antra so that the whole of the lateral sinus wall is clear.

The occipitomental 30° projection

The orbitomeatal baseline is elevated 45° and the tube angled 30° caudad, centering to the lower orbital margins. This projection provides a superior view of the malar arches and the anterior aspect of the inferior orbital margins, allowing assessment of displacement of these structures. It is used in preference to the submentovertical projection for assessing the arches.

In both the occipitomental 10° and 30° projections it is very important not to allow any rotation of the patient from the sagittal plane. In some individuals the arches can project very close to the image of the inner table of the lateral calvarium. Where the latter is seen in tangent, slight rotation will superimpose one arch over the calvarium, diminishing the clarity with which the arch is seen.

The occipitomental projection view with only 40° elevation of the orbitomeatal baseline

This is the best view to diagnose orbital blow-out fracture on a plain film. Centering is to the inferior orbital margin. However, with CT scanning available this projection should rarely be necessary.

The lateral projection

In this projection the median sagittal plane is parallel to the film plane and the central ray is perpendicular to the film plane. By convention it is obtained as a left lateral (i.e. left side of patient closest to film) but this is not essential in acute trauma work. Centering should be to the body of the zygoma, about 2.5 cm below the outer canthus of the eye.

The lateral soft tissue projection

This view provides useful information about foreign bodies, e.g. windscreen glass. It also gives a good view of the nasal bones, the nasal plates of the frontal processes of the maxilla and the nasal spine of the maxilla. It is not required, however, for assessing isolated simple nasal trauma which is better investigated clinically.

The upper occlusal projection

An occlusal film is placed in the mouth as far back as possible. Positioning is more likely to be successful and gagging overcome if the equipment and patient position are set up beforehand, the patient is asked to swallow hard just before inserting the film and the film is placed gently, trying to avoid contact with the tongue and oral mucosa until the last moment. The central ray is directed down 45° to the film plane, centering to the anterior nasal spine. This view is occasionally useful to assess the palate, although palatal fractures are usually either clinically obvious or best demonstrated by CT scanning.

Projections for the lower third of the face

Posteroanterior projection of the mandible (PA mandible)

This is a standard projection and part of most mandibular trauma series, whether it be two views (PA mandible and OPG), three views (PA mandible and two lateral obliques) or five views (PA mandible, two rotated PA views and two lateral obliques). For this projection the patient faces the film cassette. The median sagittal plane and the orbitomeatal plane are perpendicular to the film plane. Centering is to the midpoint of the rami with central beam perpendicular to the cassette.

Lateral oblique group

The standard projection here is the 30° lateral oblique. For this the patient has the sagittal plane parallel to the film plane and the central ray is angled 30° cranially, centered to the mandibular angle closest to the film. The head should be extended to throw the image of the mandible off the cervical spine. If more of the body of the mandible needs to be seen the patient can be rotated face towards the film cassette to bring the body of the mandible parallel to the cassette. Some workers use a slightly higher angle, 35–40°, for the central ray where the ramus is the main area of interest. An alternative to tube tilt is to use an angle board.

Rotated PA mandible projection

Rarely used except where panoramic tomography is not available. The patient is turned from the PA position away from the parasymphyseal region of interest by 8–10°, dropping the chin towards the cassette and centering 1 inch behind the opposite angle at the level of the midpoint of the rami with the central beam perpendicular to the film plane.

Lower occlusal projection

An occlusal film is placed in the mouth and a dental X-ray unit used to expose the film from below the mandible. This is occasionally useful in the symphysis region where both panoramic and PA mandible projections may be suboptimal.

Extraoral submental projection (superoinferior symphysis projection)

This can be helpful in patients who will not tolerate an occlusal film in the mouth. The film is placed underneath the chin and exposed from above with a dental X-ray unit.

Reverse Towne's projection (Haas position, nuchofrontal position)

This is a reverse of the half axial or Towne's projection. The patient faces the cassette with both the median sagittal plane and the orbitomeatal line perpendicular to the film plane. The central ray is then directed at an angle of 30° upwards, centering to about 4 cm above the superior orbital margins. It is seldom that an injury is seen on this view that cannot be seen with careful inspection on the PA mandible view.

Frontal open mouth projection

The PA mandible projection taken with the mouth open undoubtedly gives a good view of the condyle. Unfortunately, most patients with significant trauma here have trismus and are reluctant to open the mouth far enough for this view to be useful. The central ray is angled up 12°, centering to the nasion with the mouth open. Like the reverse Towne's view, and for the same reasons, this view should rarely be needed.

Panoramic radiography

There are two forms of this type of radiography: an intraoral and an extraoral technique. The intraoral technique where the tube and film are static is seldom used for trauma and is not widely available. In the extraoral form the tube and the film move relative to the patient to provide an image of a curved plane, usually the mandible. The extraoral panoramic systems thus provide a modified tomographic technique that takes into account the curvature of the mandible. The image layer is made to conform with the shape of the mandible and objects outside the image layer are blurred. Great care is needed in positioning as the image plane is thin and even slight errors in positioning can result in parts of the mandible being outside the image plane and thus blurred. This may be unavoidable with grossly displaced fracture fragments.

Panoramic zonography

Based on the well-established methods of panoramic radiography used for examination of the mandible, the panoramic principle has been extended to a variety of other image layer tracks to enable examination of the middle third of the face, temporal bone and upper cervical spine and to provide additional imaging of the temporomandibular joints. A further advantage of this equipment is the ability to perform the examinations, including standard panoramic views of the mandible, on a supine patient.

6 Principles of Facial Soft Tissue Injury Repair

Barry L Eppley, Amardip Bhuller

Introduction

Injuries to the face commonly result in a significant psychological response that is unparalleled by the response to injury elsewhere on the body, especially if it is the result of interpersonal violence. The importance of facial appearance in modern society and its implication in both vocational and social status makes changes to facial features, particularly by injury, an emotionally charged occurrence. Patients fear facial disfigurement and scars and risk loss of their self-esteem. Surgical repair of facial injuries is understandably associated with high expectations of a complete return to a normal facial appearance. Often the final result, fairly or unfairly, is judged to be a reflection of the surgeon's skill and ability.

Accepting the obvious skin/mucosal involvement, facial trauma frequently includes injury to the deeper anatomical structures, both hard and soft tissue, and an understanding of the mechanism of injury and a complete understanding of the anatomy of the region are essential for satisfactory management of both the patient in general and the injury in particular.

Wound Assessment

History/examination

Apart from general aspects of the history that are common to all patient contacts, a complete history of the incident leading to the injury should be taken and if not available from the patient, the details should be obtained from anyone present at the time of the incident/injury and/or those in immediate attendance after. Understanding the mechanism of injury will alert the surgeon to the possibility of associated injury and/or contamination (bacterial/viral or foreign body) and sequelae that might not otherwise be apparent. For example, when dealing with a penetrating knife wound it is necessary to know the type of weapon, the degree of force used and the postures of the patient and the assailant when the injury was caused in order to usefully assess the degree of tissue damage and possible contamination and the depth and direction of penetration and hence the possibility of involvement of deeper structures. Similarly, when the injury results from a road traffic accident the type of accident (motorcycle, motor car, etc.), the position of the patient in the accident (pedestrian, driver, passenger/pillion, etc.) and the circumstances and relative speeds of the vehicles involved all alert the surgeon to the possibility of associated injury either underlying the presenting facial trauma or involving other systems.

The specialized nature of the structures of the face demand that special attention be paid to injuries of specific facial regions. Lacerations to the brow, eyelid, nose, lip and ear require careful assessment and treatment to avoid deformity and potential interference with function. Lacerations to the lateral face, temple and naso-orbital regions risk injury to branches of the facial nerve and parotid and lacrimal ducts. Injuries to the eyelid and orbit almost always require ophthalmological evaluation to establish visual status and the presence or absence of corneal damage.

A history of the tetanus status is essential as part of the general medical history. Whilst facial wounds often appear quite clean, they are still at risk and require tetanus prophylaxis. For clean minor wounds, no treatment is necessary if the immunization status is current. If more than 10 years has elapsed since the last booster injection, tetanus toxoid should be given. In contaminated wounds, all patients should receive tetanus toxoid unless they have been immunized within the last 5 years.

Biomechanics

An appreciation of the concept of relaxed skin tension lines (RSTLs) of the face is relevant to treatment and outcome. In a cadaver model exposed to blunt facial trauma, the induced soft tissue lacerations have been shown to parallel the cleavage lines of the face (RSTLs) and were more severe on the forehead than on the zygoma or maxilla.[1] Furthermore, it was shown that these injuries were inherent in the biomechanical and structural property of the dermis of the skin and independent of muscle or bony attachments. It has been postulated that the direction of skin lacerations in blunt trauma occurs as a protective mechanism to minimize injury to the underlying blood supply as both vessels and collagen bundles parallel the RSTLs (Fig. 6.1). In addition, the esthetic outcome of skin injuries is partially related to their relationship to the RSTLs, scars having a better prognosis if they parallel the RSTL or are in natural skin creases. Thus with immediate repair, if the laceration is irregular but parallels the RSTL, it can be excised and closed as a straight line. If it runs perpendicular or oblique to the RSTL, it should be closed as it presents since the irregularities may offer better camouflage of the resultant scar.

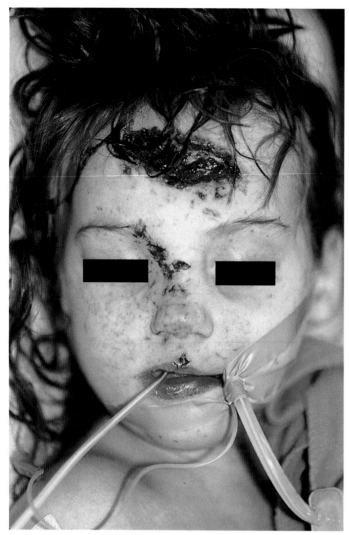

Fig. 6.1: Impact of forehead on windshield in motor vehicle accident of a 5-year-old female. Glass injuries have occurred to the nose and note the forehead skin separation that parallels the RSTLs.

Need To Exclude Fractures

Classification

Soft tissue trauma of the face may be classified according to the tissue insult (contusions, abrasions, lacerations, avulsions and burns (chemical or thermal)) or the mechanism of injury (dogbite, etc.) which often involve a combination of the former elements dependent upon the mechanism.

Contusion

Blunt trauma to the face will always result in some degree of swelling and bruising, which occurs variably dependent upon the area involved. Eyelids or lips, for example, will develop a relatively greater amount of swelling than forehead or cheek tissues. If subcutaneous vessels are ruptured, a hematoma may occur which may or may not require primary or secondary management. In general, there is no specific treatment for most facial contusions with the exception of ear or septal hematomas, which require immediate evacuation.

Many facial lacerations have contusions at their skin edges, requiring sharp debridement to minimize the long-term risks of adverse scarring, pigmented changes and underlying soft tissue atrophy. Red dermal bleeding is the hallmark of viable skin and such tissues should not usually be debrided.

Abrasion

Most abrasions that occur on the face are superficial and involve loss of the epithelium with exposed papillary dermis. These injuries will heal quite rapidly with topical agents (Fig. 6.2). Impact of the face against particulate surfaces (e.g.

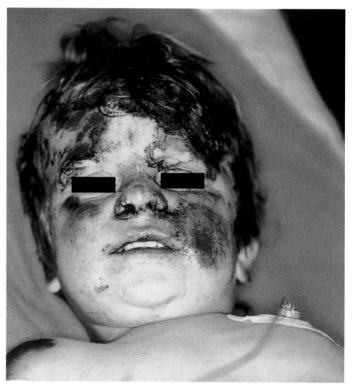

(a)

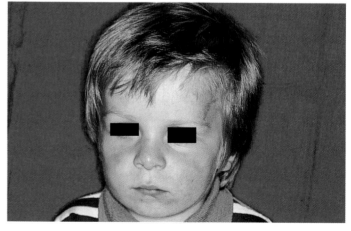

(b)

Fig. 6.2: (a) Four-year-old male child who sustained multiple facial abrasions while falling from a moving car. **(b)** The superficial wounds went on to heal completely by topical therapy without scarring as evident 3 months after the injury.

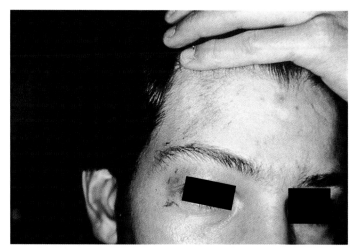

Fig. 6.3: Traumatic tattooing that occurred from a close-range discharge of a firearm that was not primarily treated.

asphalt, gravel) or exposure to explosive charges (e.g. powder burns from gunshots) usually results in the implantation of foreign material. The frictional contact between otherwise benign particulate matter results in dermal exposure and injury that may mimic a second- or third-degree burn depending upon the depth. If allowed to heal, the growth of new epithelium over the contamination results in the phenomenon known as 'traumatic tattooing', leading to permanent discoloration (Fig. 6.3). Prevention requires meticulous debridement and may occasionally necessitate the use of a dermabrader. Petroleum-based liquids, such as grease and oil, can be removed with organic solvents such as acetone or ether. After adequate cleansing, the partially denuded dermis may be covered with either antibiotic ointment alone or medicated non-adherent gauze dressing (e.g. Xeroform). Complete healing via re-epithelization occurs within 7–10 days and erythema resolves within several months thereafter.

Lacerations

Facial lacerations occur as a variety of specific types, which affect the risks of scarring and eventual need for scar revision. Recognition of these permits modifications in the surgical repair techniques.

Sharp objects generally create wounds with clean straight edges, which are easy to repair and produce fine scars. Minimal or no debridement is necessary and the apposition of tissues is done with a layered closure. As sharp objects often penetrate deeper than initially perceived, careful exploration of the wound should be carried out in areas where vital structures lie underneath. Revision of linear scars is often not needed (Fig. 6.4) unless they violate the RSTL where they may be improved by geometric rearrangement.

Stellate lacerations usually result from blunt injury, explosions or crushing forces, which strike with enough force in a single area to 'fracture' the surrounding tissue in non-cleavage planes. Multiple flaps of skin are created, often with contused edges, around a more central area of tissue damage or loss (Fig. 6.5). The elastic recoil of the skin often gives the false

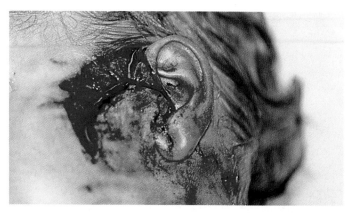

(a)

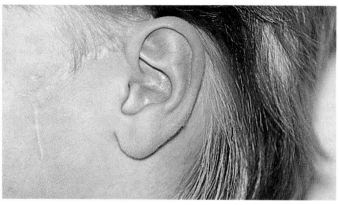

(b)

Fig. 6.4: (a) Laceration and pre-auricular skin avulsion from a dogbite in a 4-year-old male. **(b)** Scar revision will not improve the resultant scar after primary closure as it appears one year later after maturity as it parallels the RSTL and is quite narrow.

perception of significant tissue loss. This type of laceration should be repaired as it presents and only grossly non-viable tissue should be debrided. Despite the best initial repair, these lacerations often heal poorly, with a large number requiring secondary revision.

Tangential lacerations which undermine and lift up skin edges or those lacerations which have a curvilinear or semicircular shape result in the 'trapdoor' deformity. The laceration heals with a heaping up of tissue on its concave side due to contracture from unopposed fibrosis as well as lymphatic and venous obstruction (Fig. 6.6). By creating a sharp vertical edge on the flap side, undermining the undersurface of the side opposite to the flap and advancing it at the same level and placing the initial suture support deep to the dermis between the flap and the surrounding tissue (Fig. 6.6), the deformity may be averted or at least reduced.

Avulsions

Facial defects due to traumatic avulsion are relatively uncommon, occurring almost exclusively from gunshot or large sharp-edged weapon injuries. For small defects, the surrounding tissue can be mobilized and the defect closed. In general, the use of local random or pedicled flaps should be discouraged during the initial repair, as the viability of

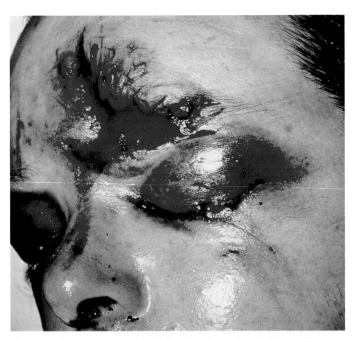

Fig. 6.5: Direct impact of the forehead on the dashboard in an unrestrained passenger involved in a motor vehicle accident. The significant blunt force has 'fractured' the forehead and eyebrow tissues.

surrounding tissues can be difficult to evaluate in the primary setting. In larger defects that are not amenable to primary closure, wet-to-dry dressings can be placed until the appropriate time for reconstruction. Such dressings can be used for long periods as the zone of viability demarcates and granulation tissue develops. In more uncommon circumstances, the avulsion defect can initially be covered with a split-thickness skin graft. This allows the facial wound to heal before more complex methods of facial reconstruction with better esthetic outcome are carried out at a later date (e.g. tissue expansion, serial graft excision, local flaps) (Fig. 6.7).

Bites

Bite wounds, even on the well-vascularized face, have a significant risk of infection due to their high rate of contamination. Not only do they introduce highly infective bacterial flora but also the bite wound is often a combination of multiple types of injury, including penetrating, contusing and avulsing. Bites come from either animals or humans and each has its own distinctive bacterial content. Animal bites, particularly from dogs, are polymicrobial and include *Staphylococcus aureus*, β-hemolytic streptococcus and the anaerobes bacteroides and fusobacterium.[2] *Pasteurella multo-*

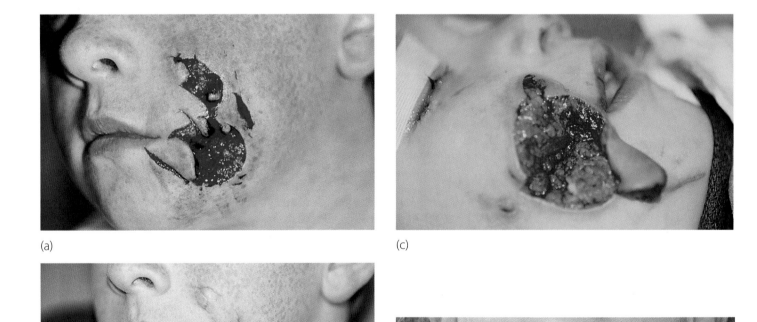

(a)

(b)

(c)

(d)

Fig. 6.6: (a,b) Semicircular-type lacerations frequently result in the classic trapdoor scar deformity. **(c,d)** Several surgical manuevers at the time of primary repair, such as deep suture support, same-level undermining on the side opposite the semicircular flap and the creation of sharp vertical edges on the flap, may be helpful in its postoperative prevention. (**a** = dogbite in a 12-year-old male; **b** = 6 months postoperative repair with a trapdoor scar deformity; **c** = dogbite flap avulsion in a 6-year-old female; **d** = 6 months postoperative repair without a trapdoor scar deformity)

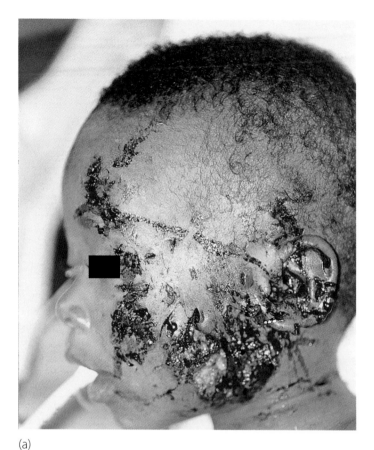

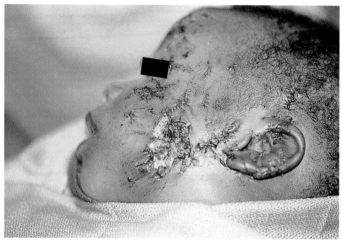

(a)

(b)

Fig. 6.7: Facial lacerations and avulsion injury with pre-auricular tissue loss in a 4-year-old male child who was unrestrained in a motor vehicle accident. **(a)** Immediately after injury. **(b)** After closure of lacerations, the area of tissue loss is evident. The tissue was impossible to close primarily due to wound tension and would have resulted in significant distortion of the surrounding tissues. **(c)** A split-thickness skin graft was placed for primary repair. Even though it is hyperpigmented, it allowed time for the wound to heal and will be removed later by secondary tissue expansion.

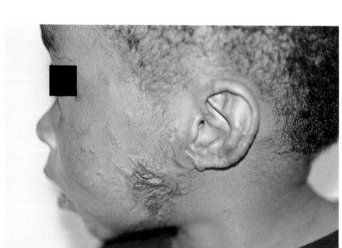

(c)

cida may also be found, especially in cat bites. Human flora usually has a higher concentration of anaerobes such as bacteroides but also commonly contains staphylococcus and α-hemolytic streptococcus. Differences also exist in bite wound locations, with human bites being far more prevalent on the lips, nose and ear while most animal bites are more random, involve more surface area and are more avulsive due to the innate 'pull-back' response of the victim.

For most wounds that are seen within 24 hours primary treatment includes operative irrigation, limited debridement and primary closure. With this approach, the infection risk is fairly low and the resultant scars are better[3] (Fig. 6.8). Only small puncture wounds would be left to heal secondarily. For wounds that occurred more than 24 hours earlier or large avulsion injuries, closure is controversial. The author prefers primary closure, accepting that the infection risk is higher, in the hope of obtaining both a more expeditious treatment and a better scar. Some surgeons prefer delaying closure of such wounds for up to 1 week although whether this truly decreases the risk of infection is not clear. Adjunctive pharmacological treatment is essential, usually consisting of broad-spectrum (combined aerobe-anaerobic coverage) antibiotics, such as amoxicillin with clavulanic acid, tetanus immunization and rabies prophylaxis as necessary.

Documentation

The recording of facial injuries is important for two main reasons: patients may benefit and cope better with the outcome if they are able to compare the present with the original injury; the injury may at some point be the subject of a medicolegal action and accurate recording, preferably with photographs, will facilitate the process.

Recording of the injuries on a handwritten facial cartoon is the most primitive method. One novel method of recording facial information is the MCFONTZL system,[4] which represents a simplified method of recording blunt facial soft tissue injuries. The system divides the face into 12 different esthetic units using the mnemonic M-C-F-O-N-T-Z-L. The soft tissue laceration is recorded using an asterisk mnemonic which records the information along the rays of the asterisk in a clockwise direction under the

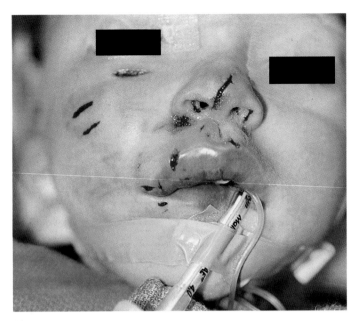

(a)

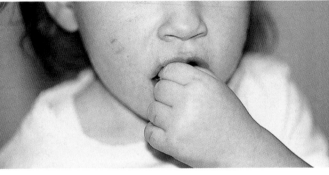

(b)

Fig. 6.8: Almost all dogbite injuries can be primarily repaired in the face without a significant risk of postoperative infection. **(a)** Multiple small lacerations and puncture wounds from a dogbite in a 2-year-old female child. **(b)** Uncomplicated wound healing seen after 6 postoperative months.

following headings: location, depth of penetration, branching, direction, size and the presence/absence of soft tissue defects. However, conventional color slides or prints document the injuries in such a graphic and detailed manner that where possible they should be the method of choice. Digital photography may gradually replace conventional light photography though arguably it could be more prone to exploitation.

Soft Tissue Handling

Operative setting

The patient with facial lacerations should always be treated promptly, in an ideal world as soon as an assessment has been made to eliminate other injuries. The majority of facial injuries requiring soft tissue repair are not extensive and may be treated in the outpatient setting under local anesthesia. Whilst this usually is the quickest way, it has some disadvantages. The local anesthetic solution distorts the tissues and

may be painful. There is a risk that incomplete anesthesia is achieved which may prevent careful cleaning and suturing. More extensive injuries or complex repairs involving the eyelids, nose, lips or ears should be managed in the operating theater under either local anesthesia with sedation or general anesthesia. As a general rule, if the procedure is to take longer than an hour, complex facial structures are involved or there is any question of involvement of deeper structures, the procedure should be carried out in the operating theater.

Children more frequently require management in the operating theater because of their greater anxiety and the level of their co-operation and understanding is more limited. As a general rule, if the repair is to take more than 15 minutes and is more than a simple laceration, it should be carried out in the operating theater.[5]

Anesthesia

The administration of local anesthesia for the repair of facial wounds serves three purposes: to anesthetize the wound during an awake procedure; to provide postoperative analgesia at the repair site; and to facilitate hemostasis, irrespective of the surgical setting. A number of technical points should be considered.

First, the local infiltration should be injected through the existing wound edges where there may already be reduced sensation resulting from the injury. Second, the volume of the syringe should be matched to the needle size. It is least painful to use a small 30 G needle with either a 1 cc or 3 cc syringe. The small needle combined with the low pressure of infiltration from the low-volume reservoir is the most comfortable (Fig. 6.9**a**). Whilst a larger 25 G needle with a 10 cc syringe is appropriate for intraoral and facial blocks (due to the need for longer needle length), it will cause more discomfort during direct local infiltration. Third, buffering the pH of the local anesthetic will reduce the discomfort during infiltration.[3] As all local anesthetics containing epinephrine are acidic (pH less than 4), they cause a burning sensation on contact with the subcutaneous tissues. For large-volume infiltrations, adding a small amount of bicarbonate eliminates this source of immediate tissue pain (Fig. 6.9**b**).[6] Fourth, the use of regional nerve blocks can be invaluable when there is extensive injury. They not only expedite the onset and distribution of the anesthetic but also lessen the total volume of solution required. The supraorbital, infraorbital and mental nerves are the most commonly blocked. Finally, consideration should be given to the use of long-acting local anesthetics for postoperative pain relief. The infiltration of bupivacaine (Marcain) in and around the wound site gives up to 24 hours of pain relief, which is particularly useful in children.

A full understanding of the pharmacology and pharmokinetics of the drugs used is essential. The safe limits of local anesthetic volumes should be well known and include 7 mg/kg for lidocaine with epinephrine, 4 mg/kg for lidocaine without epinephrine and 1 mg/kg for bupivacaine.

Recently, a number of topical anesthetics have become available that provide for skin anesthesia in cream formulations.[7] The two best known are EMLA (eutectic mixture of two local

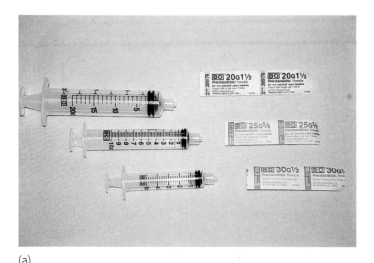

(a)

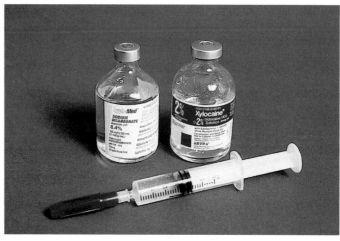

(b)

Fig. 6.9: (a) To lessen injection pain in the face in the awake patient, the smallest needle (30 gauge) in a small syringe (1 or 3 ml) is the most effective. It creates a small puncture wound and causes little pain by fluid pressure and tissue distension. Large syringes require larger needles and are best used for the administration of regional blocks. **(b)** Buffering local anesthesia that contains epinephrine with bicarbonate will neutralize the acidic pH and contribute to less injection pain.

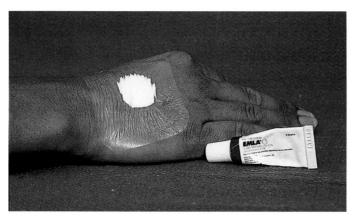

Fig. 6.10: Topical anesthetics, such as EMLA, are commonly used to prevent pain from the insertion of venous catheters. Their effectiveness and practicality of use in the closure of facial lacerations are more questionable.

anesthetics, 2.5% prilocaine and 2.5% lidocaine) and TAC (a mixture of 0.5% tetracaine, epinephrine at a concentration of 1:2000 and cocaine 11.8%). Both preparations need to be applied to the skin a significant length of time prior to injection or manipulation in order to achieve dermal penetrations of 3–4 mm (Fig. 6.10). They should not be applied to open wounds or around mucous membranes or the eyes. Whilst both achieve some degree of skin anesthesia and are often promulgated for use in small lacerations in children, they have some practical limitations that severely limit their use in facial wound repair. The time lapse before onset of anesthesia, difficulty in keeping the topical creams to the desired area and lack of anesthesia of the deeper tissues make their use, whilst theoretically appealing, often less than practical.

Wound preparation/debridement

Fortunately the majority of facial wounds will be seen early, usually within hours after their occurrence, but even those seen much later, even after 24 hours, can usually be closed after thorough irrigation and debridement.

Initial cleansing of the wound should be carried out using either a gentle soap (e.g. Ivory soap) or a dilute Betadine (5% ophthalmic) solution. Use of either agent causes little if any cellular damage to open wounds yet reduces bacterial counts. Most other cutaneous preparatory agents, including alcohol, hydrogen peroxide, benzylkonium chloride or hexachlorophene, are quite toxic to live cells. A general rule is never to use any solution that is not well tolerated by the conjunctival lining of the eye.

Removal of hair is usually not necessary and its presence can be a guide to good anatomical reconstruction. Eyebrow and eyelash hair should never be removed as their regrowth cannot be assured. Scalp and associated hair removal should be limited to facilitate tissue repositioning only. Facial hair (beards, moustache, goatee) can freely be removed as it impedes a good skin repair and always regrows. The wound(s) should be meticulously examined for the presence of foreign bodies, especially if the history of the injury suggests that foreign bodies may be present. The facial wounds of road traffic accident victims commonly contain embedded glass. In many instances the glass is better identified by listening for the 'chink' of a metallic instrument against the glass rather than trying to visualize it. In wounds that are contaminated with dirt and other debris, pressure irrigation with an 18 G needle and 20 cc syringe generates sufficient pressure to dislodge implanted particles and reduce the bacterial count. Given that there is no convincing evidence that antibiotic irrigations in the facial region are advantageous and that there is a risk of toxicity to the cornea, saline irrigation should be sufficient in most cases.

An abrasion may contain particulate material, which could result in a 'traumatic tattoo' if not removed. Light scrubbing of the wounds can be carried out using a surgical scrub brush or a toothbrush. A dermabrader with a very fine diamond wheel, however, is usually much more effective as some

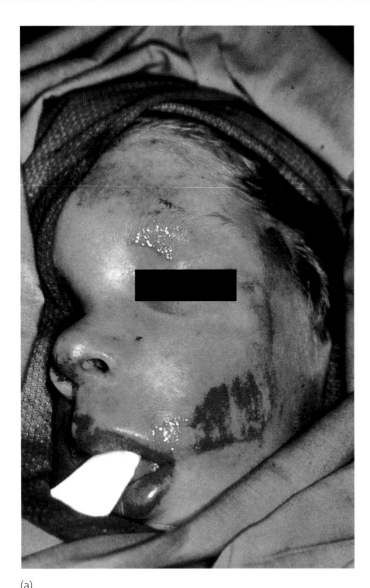

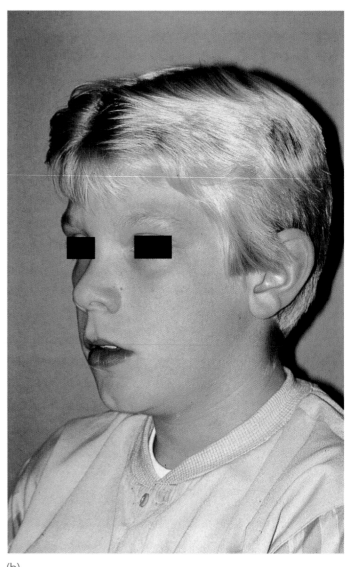

(a)

(b)

Fig. 6.11: Dermabrasion into the papillary dermis is a reliable method for removing impregnated material and preventing traumatic tattooing. **(a)** Dermabrasion removal of asphalt debris. **(b)** Scarless healing at 9 months after surgery.

removal of the papillary dermis is necessary to remove or expose many of the embedded particles (Fig. 6.11).[8] Those particles not removed with the dermabrader can be systematically removed with a number 11 blade. It is important not to dermabrade too deep into the reticular dermis or expose the underlying fat as this will likely result in hypertrophic scarring. It is better to have to do a secondary laser or dermabrasion procedure than manage hypertrophic scarring. Furthermore, a light dermabrasion heals quite rapidly within 5–7 days, particularly in the adult male due to the epithelial contributions from the beard skin.

Excision of the wound edges is generally not advised unless the tissues are obviously crushed and non-viable. As the blood flow to the facial skin is extensive and receives contributions from both the dermis and underlying perforators, it is often remarkable how little soft tissue attachment may be needed for survival (Fig. 6.12). Furthermore, it is always easier secondarily to remove excess scar and tissue than it is to recruit replacement.

Wound closure techniques

It should be remembered that the face is unique amongst all other tissues in the body and merits a 'different' approach from many aspects of traditional wound care.

Tissue handling principles

The following guidelines should be followed.

1. Reduce operative tissue damage

The tissues should be handled gently with fine instruments and if necessary, loupes should be used.

2. Minimize sharp debridement

Most facial wounds require minimal excision but, when needed, it should be carried out with the scalpel held at right angles to the skin surface. In hair-bearing areas, the incision should parallel the hair follicles to reduce the possibility of damage.

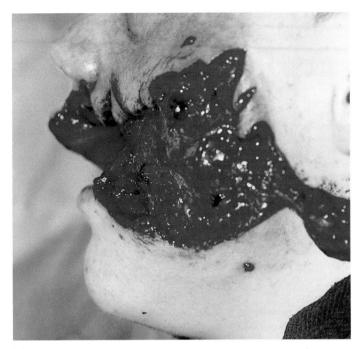

(a)

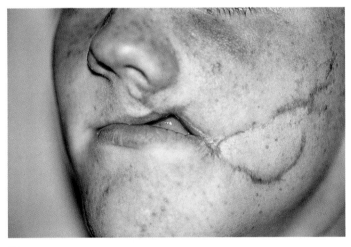

(b)

Fig. 6.12: Gunshot wound to the face with lateral facial flap avulsion. **(a)** Lateral facial skin flap hanging on by a small skin pedicle. **(b)** Complete survival of the hanging skin flap after primary repair.

3. Repair wounds as they present

The classic teaching is to close wounds along tension lines and the natural folds (RSTLs) of the facial skin. In reality, facial wounds tend to be random and adherence to this concept is frequently impractical. Important facial landmarks should be aligned and the wounds repaired as they present. Allow for natural healing and would maturation to make the first attempt at optimizing scars.

4. Closure in layers

Good dermal support is one of the primary keys to flat narrow scars. As skin sutures are removed early to prevent track marks, a lack of dermal support may allow scars to widen, particularly if they cross the RSTLs. If necessary,

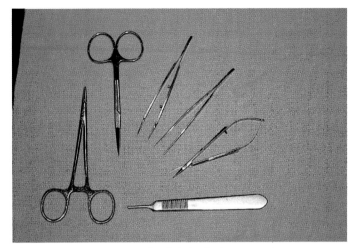

Fig. 6.13: Instrument set for facial soft tissue repair.

undermine the wound margins to create a deeper layer for suturing and eversion of the wound edges. Tension across the wound should be reduced to a minimum.

5. Use fine sutures and remove early

With good dermal support and the rapid epithelialization of facial tissues, the sutures should be removed between 5 and 7 days after insertion. Alternate sutures may be removed after 3 days.

Instrumentation

The finest and most precise instruments should be used. A large number of instruments are not necessary (Fig. 6.13).

Suture types

Fundamentally there are two types, absorbable and permanent.[9] Whilst used by surgeons of all specialties, their composition and technical details are frequently either not known or misunderstood.

Absorbable sutures

Sutures that absorb include gut (plain or chromic), Dexon, Vicryl, Maxon and PDS.

A plain gut suture is composed of twisted collagenous strands of sheep or beef intestinal wall. As the result of its animal origins it is being withdrawn from use in Europe. This suture is rapidly absorbed by phagocytosis, maintaining strength for up to 10 days with complete absorption within 70 days. When heat treated, a fast-absorbing gut suture is created with accelerated tensile strength loss and absorption. Wound support is provided for only 5–7 days and it is used primarily for epidermal suturing. When gut is coated with a chromium salt solution, chromic gut suture is created which is more resistant to body enzymes, resulting in slower absorption and maintenance of strength for up to 14 days. It also has advantages of better tensile strength and knotting capability. A mild chromic gut suture is also made that is absorbed more rapidly, between 3 and 5 days. The remainder of absorbable sutures are synthetically derived and have much longer retention.

Dexon is a braided suture composed of a glycolic acid polymer, which breaks down by hydrolysis and maintains strength for up to 30 days. Vicryl, similarly, is a polymer but incorporates lactide and calcium stearate (lubricant) with the glycolic acids. Because of the lactide, which is hydrophobic, hydrolysis is slowed and complete absorption takes up to 70 days to occur. Significant strength is maintained at 21 days after placement. Maxon is also of glycolic acid composition but has the addition of trimethylene carbonate in a monofilament form, the tensile strength is prolonged and complete absorption can take up to 180 days. PDS is also a synthetic monofilament but is made from the polyester derivative polydioxanone. It glides easily through tissue, has significant memory, takes about 180 days to absorb and has extended wound strength up to 6 weeks. These features account for its frequent use as an absorbable subcuticular suture. Monocryl (poliglecaprone) is a monofilament suture that is also used for subcuticular closure and which maintains its strength for several weeks, with complete absorption at 120 days.

Practically, the types of absorbable sutures used in the face are limited to the gut and Vicryl/Dexon sutures. Closure of the skin when suture removal is not desired, as can be the case in young children, should be performed with 5-0 or 6-0 plain gut. Any of the other absorbable sutures cause too much inflammation and take too long to dissolve. Plain or fast-absorbing gut sutures are also suitable for closure of the mucous membranes of the eye, nose and mouth.

Dermal closure should be carried with 5-0 gut or 5-0 Dexon and Vicryl. While some postoperative suture extrusion will occur with the longer lasting absorbables, it does not seem to be as significant as in other areas of the body. This is probably due to the smaller-sized sutures used in the facial region. Deeper structure apposition, including fascia and muscle, can be performed using the larger 3-0 and 4-0 longer absorbing sutures and benefits from their increased strength retention.

Non-absorbable sutures

Monofilaments have replaced the traditional braided silk suture materials. They offer smooth tissue passage, minimal tissue reactivity and easy handling by virtue of their elasticity. Such features make them well suited for retention and skin closure. Nylon, derived from the synthesis of polyamide polymers, and polypropylene (Prolene), a linear hydrocarbon polymer, are both commonly used in the facial region. They are extremely inert and can hold tensile strength for years. The flexibility of the polypropylene is superior to nylon and accounts for its popularity in the pull-out subcuticular technique of skin closure.

Either of these sutures, ranging in sizes from 5-0 to 7-0, can be used for facial skin closure depending upon the specific site. In the scalp, the blue coloring of prolene makes it easier to remove.

Suturing techniques

Whilst all techniques, including simple, continuous, subcuticular, horizontal and vertical mattress (Fig. 6.14), will, on

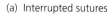
(a) Interrupted sutures

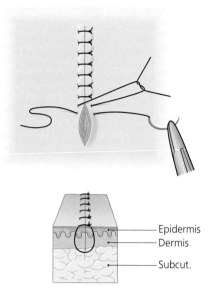

Epidermis
Dermis
Subcut.

(b) Continuous sutures

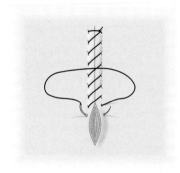

(c) Intracuticular sutures

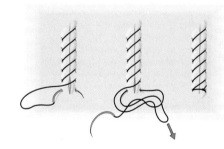

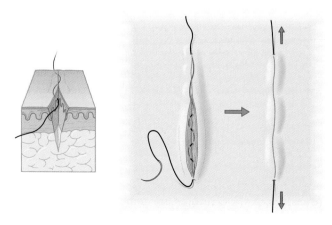

Fig. 6.14: Commonly used facial suturing techniques.

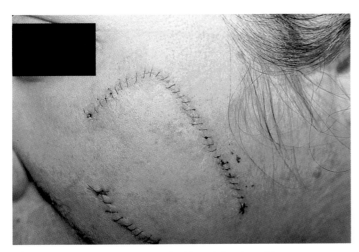

Fig. 6.15: Running, non-interlocking 6-0 nylon skin suture repair.

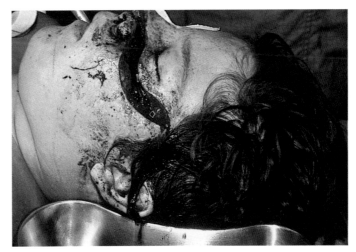

(a)

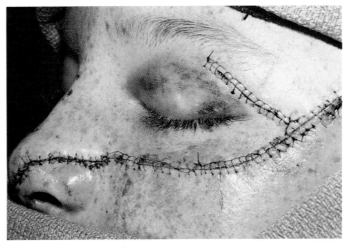

(b)

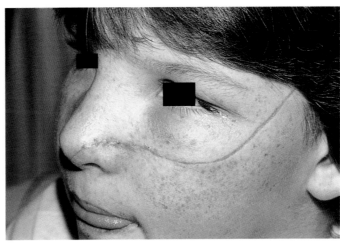

(c)

Fig. 6.16: Knife laceration to face. **(a)** Preoperative. **(b)** Multilayer wound repair with running, interlocking 6-0 nylon for skin repair. **(c)** One year postoperative.

occasion be used, the simple and continuous should be the ones most exclusively used. The vascularity of the wound edges, already compromised as a result of the injury, should not be further jeopardized by the suturing technique. The simple interrupted or the continuous non-interlocking suture techniques provide the least strangulation of tissue (Fig. 6.15). There is no real advantage to a running interlocking suture but if used, the suture loops should not be too tight (Fig. 6.16). Occasionally, an interrupted vertical mattress suture may be of value to evert the skin edges but good dermal support usually makes the use of this suture technique unnecessary.

Skin sutures of 6-0 or 7-0 size should be used. Sutures should be placed close enough to the wound margin (1–2 mm) to optimally relieve wound tension. The suture should be tied with an allowance for postoperative edema and without blanching of the wound margins. Suture track marks are usually due either to the suture being tied too tightly, causing tissue necrosis, or delayed removal, resulting in epithelialization of the suture track.

On the scalp a larger suture, usually a 3-0 or 4-0, is used with the sutures placed further from the wound margins. Due to the structure and vascularity of the scalp the tissues can tolerate a tighter closure if required for hemostasis. Dermal sutures should not be used as they may injure hair follicles. Deep support comes from closure of the galea. Metallic staples can also be used and are probably the least compromising to the vascularity, as they do not completely encircle the apposed tissues. Their use, however, is usually retained for rapid closure and ease of removal in the hair-bearing scalp where track marks are less relevant.

The importance of layered closure in facial wounds cannot be overemphasized.

Skin adhesives

The use of a glue for skin (epidermal) repair has long appealed. Previously attempts at developing a skin adhesive have been fraught with handling problems and histoxicity but a recent cyanoacrylate derivative, octyl-2-cyanoacrylate (Dermabond, Ethicon, New Jersey), has had significant success without the previous problems (Fig. 6.17). The adhesive is quite durable but flexes with the skin. Multiple studies have demonstrated its equivalency to 5-0 and 6-0 skin

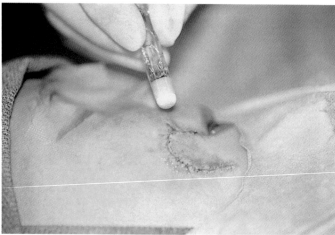

Fig. 6.17: Cyanoacrylate adhesive (Dermabond) for skin closure comes in a bullet-ampoule dispenser.

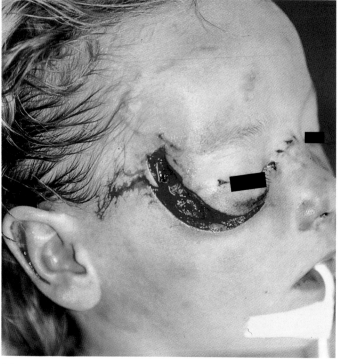

(a)

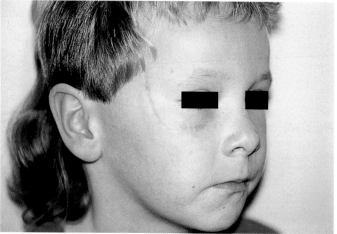

(c)

sutures in facial surgery.[10,11] It is still important to provide dermal suture support (Fig. 6.18) and care must be taken to seal the epithelium without allowing the liquid to flow between the wound margins where it will harden and block epithelial/dermal healing. It is particularly useful after suture removal instead of taping as it secures the wound edges better and does so in a near-invisible fashion.

Postoperative Care

Dressings other than a line of an ointment to prevent drying of the tissues are usually not required. Some surgeons use antibiotic creams but the use of cloromycetin has some theoretical risks of producing aplastic anemia and is best avoided. In reality it is still used very widely. Extensive taping obscures the wound margins and does not allow the wound exudate to

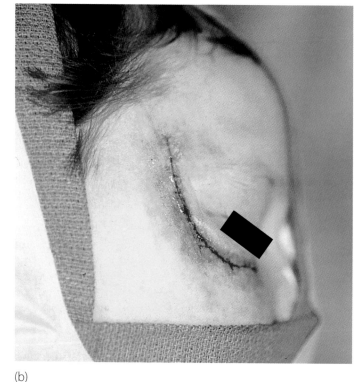

(b)

Fig. 6.18: Closure of facial dogbite wound with topical skin adhesive. **(a)** Preoperative. **(b)** Skin closure with good dermal support. **(c)** One year postoperative.

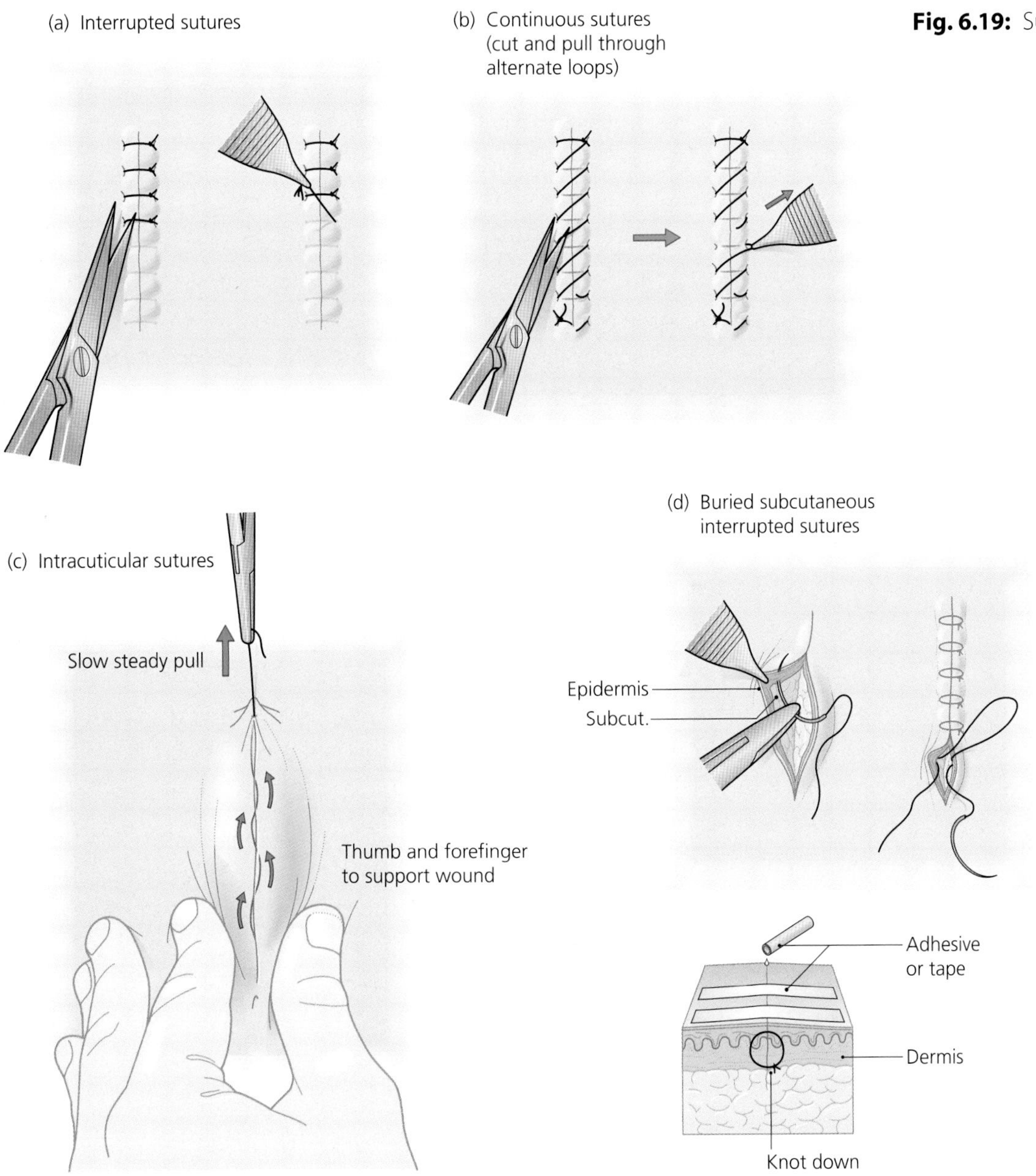

(a) Interrupted sutures

(b) Continuous sutures (cut and pull through alternate loops)

Fig. 6.19: Suture removal techniques.

(c) Intracuticular sutures

Slow steady pull

Thumb and forefinger to support wound

(d) Buried subcutaneous interrupted sutures

Epidermis

Subcut.

Adhesive or tape

Dermis

Knot down

be cleaned from the edges. Crusting is removed with dilute hydrogen peroxide and antibiotic ointment is reapplied 2–3 times per day. Face and hair washing can be performed within 48 hours as it has been shown that the wetting of sutures with soap and water, particularly on the face, does not increase the incidence of wound infection. Keeping the suture line clean and soft without crusting makes it easier to remove the sutures.

There is good evidence that more rapid healing can be achieved by applying negative pressure dressing over the wound. This removes inflammatory exudates and speeds up healing. It has little place in routine closure, but in difficult areas with abrasions or tissue loss it may have a place.

Facial sutures are usually removed 5–7 days after placement while those in the scalp remain longer, being removed from 2 to 3 weeks later. Removal of sutures, although rarely discussed, can be both uncomfortable and cause anxiety for the patient. Fine instruments, a delicate touch and several simple maneuvers can make the experience more tolerable for the patient (Fig. 6.19).

Following suture removal, the wound can be supported using either Steri-strips/brown tape or a recent introduction, cyanoacrylate adhesive.

References

1 Lee RH, Gamble WB, Robertson B, Manson P 1997 Patterns of facial lacerations from blunt trauma. Plastic and Reconstructive Surgery 99: 1544–1554

2 Wolff KD 1998 Management of animal bites to the face. Experience in 94 cases. Journal of Oral and Maxillofacial Surgery 56: 838–843

3 Donkor P 1997 A study of primary closure of human bite injuries to the face. Journal of Oral and Maxillofacial Surgery 55: 479–481

4 Lee RH, Gamble WB, Robertson B, Manson P 1999 The MCFONTZL classification system for soft tissue injuries to the face. Plastic and Reconstructive Surgery 103: 1150–1157

5 Kolta PJ 1996 Management of facial trauma in children. Pediatric Clinics of North America 43: 1253–1275

6 Eppley BL, Sadove AM 1989 Reduction in injection pain by buffering of local anesthetic solutions. Journal of Oral and Maxillofacial Surgery 47: 762–763

7 Hirko MK, Lin PH, Greisler HP, Chu CC 1996 Biologic properties of suture materials. In: Chu C, von Fraunhofer J, Greisler H (eds) Wound closure biomaterials and devices. CRC Press, New York pp 237–288

8 Cronin ED 1996 A new technique of dermabrasion for traumatic tattoos. Annals of Plastic Surgery 36: 401–402

9 Ratner D 1994 Basic Suture materials and suturing techniques. Seminars in Dermatology 13: 20–26

10 Spotnitz WD 1997 The role of sutures and fibrin sealants in wound healing. Surgical Clinics of North America 77: 651–659

11 Toriumi DM, O'Grady K, Desai D, Bagal A 1998 Use of octyl-2-cyanoacrylate for skin closure in facial plastic surgery. Plastic and Reconstructive Surgery 102: 2209–2215

Principles of Reduction of Fractures and Methods of Fixation

Malcolm Cameron, Peter Ward Booth

Introduction

This chapter will give an overview of the principles of facial fracture reduction and fixation rather than detailed surgical techniques, which are found elsewhere in this book.

Poorly treated facial injuries are hopefully rarely seen nowadays in the developed world. Poor outcome is not just in terms of gross disfigurement. Thought must also be given to poor function, the morbidity of the procedures, pain and chronic infection, although the latter is rare. Severe functional problems such as diplopia, anesthesia and enophthalmos are not infrequent yet less significant problems like nasal obstruction and malocclusion are more common but equally annoying to patients (Fig. 7.1). Ankylosis is a severe complication but fortunately rarely seen. Any one of these complications, however rare, is of course extremely disabling to a patient. It is all too easy for surgeons who work in the facial region every day to become complacent, yet nothing is so important to patients as their face, mouth and jaws, in terms of both appearance and function.

Minimizing the risk of suboptimal outcome relies on accurate diagnosis, careful surgical planning, careful surgery and attentive follow-up and audit (Fig. 7.2). Poor outcome occurs for many reasons and in the majority of cases will be multifactoral.

- Coexisting surgical and medical problems may delay treatment and provision of optimal treatment.
- Poor preoperative preparation, notably poor diagnostic imaging and scans which may not show the full extent of the injuries (Figs 7.3–7.6).
- Inadequate surgical access.
- Inexperience of the operating surgeon should no longer be a factor as subspecialization continues. However, surgeons

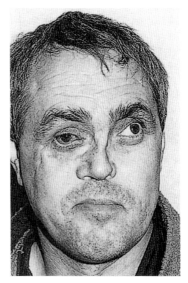

Fig. 7.2: This patient, who had multiple assaults, rarely attended for treatment. It shows the functional and cosmetic disaster of failure to treat facial trauma.

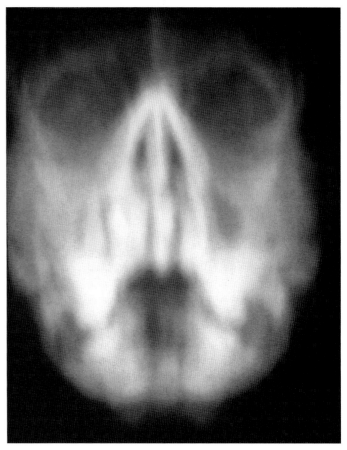

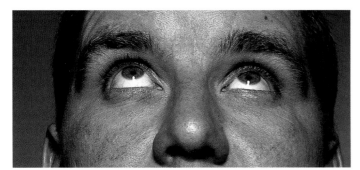

Fig. 7.1: Established enophthalmos and restricted upward eye movements have left this patient with persistent diplopia. In his case it affected his ability to undertake his work.

Fig. 7.3: A useless X-ray, caused by an unco-operative patient who has moved during imaging.

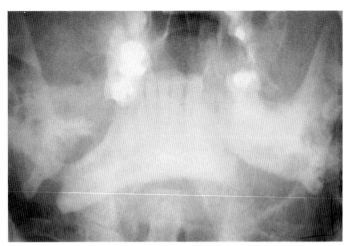

Fig. 7.4: A useless film because of poor exposure which ideally will require a lower occlusal film to check the obliquity of the fractures.

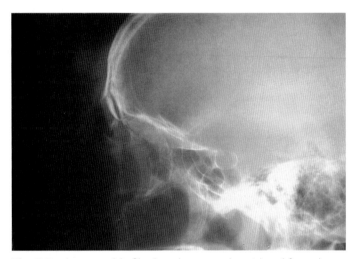

Fig. 7.5: A reasonable film but the nasoethmoid and frontal areas are not well shown by these standard views.

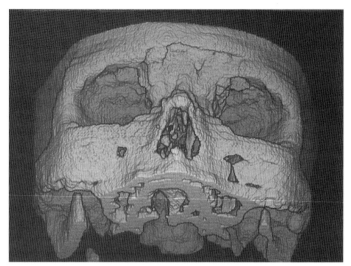

Fig. 7.6: The CT (normally 3-D films offer little extra information over standard CT) gives much more information relevant to planning the surgery.

do still use old techniques, like inappropriate use of compression plating, and frequently do not adequately audit their results.

- Motivation and social factors may prevent patients seeking treatment or attending for follow-up. This is important even in modern industrialized societies.
- Controversy still exists in certain areas of facial traumatology. These debates usually reflect the lack of a 'most effective' treatment. Often there is not a 'wrong' or a 'right' method, both methods having disadvantages. It is therefore a balance based on using the method in which the 'disadvantages' are least for a given patient. Management of the condylar neck fracture is a classic example; open approaches have 'mechanical' advantages, yet may have higher morbidity from the surgical approaches necessary.
- Finally there are still some accident and emergency departments who fail to refer the patients promptly or to a specialist in maxillofacial traumatology.

Methods of Reduction and Stabilization

Introduction

The maxillofacial region is in many ways unique. In the past, failure to appreciate its differences from the rest of the bony skeleton has led to poor outcomes and unnecessary morbidity. Whilst it is acknowledged that maxillofacial surgeons have used experience and research from general orthopedics to great effect and benefit, the mindless transfer of orthopedic techniques and principles is sometimes unhelpful. We must recognize that as surgeons we are vulnerable to 'market forces' from the manufacturers of fixation devices. The same companies, of course, have helped to introduce highly effective innovations! In the past fixation devices used in general orthopedics were offered to maxillofacial surgeons but without proper evaluation of their outcomes with regard to facial injuries. Proper evaluation takes many years and it thus took a long time before the shortcomings of these devices became apparent. We must, therefore, be careful not to be seduced by innovations and always look critically at new devices and ideas. If available, relevant supporting publications should also be scrutinized.

In recent years we have been exposed to two such new innovations from general orthopedics: osteogenic distraction and bioresorbable fixation devices. Both these ideas have a lot to offer the maxillofacial traumatologist and are strongly promoted by the supply industry. They may not, however, be the ultimate answer to our surgical requirements in the way that the sales teams would have us believe. Whilst innovation is the precursor of progress, many new techniques, instruments and materials may in reality not stand the test of time.

The facial stigma of unreduced unstabilized fractures is fortunately rarely seen, but when it happens it may be severe. Minor cosmetic changes after facial injuries are common and in modern societies 'good' results are often not enough – 'perfection' is demanded. Indeed, for the surgeon a less than perfect outcome is always unsatisfactory. The common causes of poor cosmetics are:

- bad choice of surgical access. All skin incisions may, we stress *may*, form bad scars so 'hidden' or mucosal incisions should be used wherever possible (Figs 7.7–7.10)
- inability to operate early. This prevents the normal skin draping if early healing has begun
- operating too early. Excessive swelling makes the precise placement of incisions difficult (Fig. 7.11)
- poor reduction of bone fractures. An open procedure greatly reduces this risk
- poor understanding of the fracture sites, leading to poor reduction and/or stabilization, usually because of inadequate clinical and radiological examinations.

Posttraumatic functional problems may well be more significant than any esthetic considerations and taken together, such patients often feel markedly disabled.

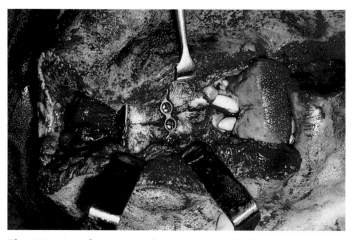

Fig. 7.7: Use of an existing laceration is desirable.

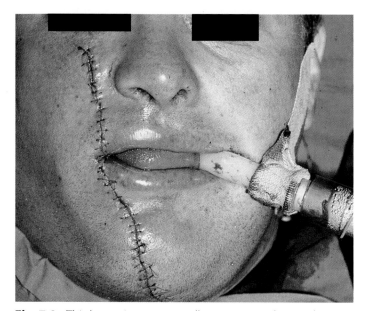

Fig. 7.8: This laceration gave excellent access and a good scar can be expected due to its site and careful closure.

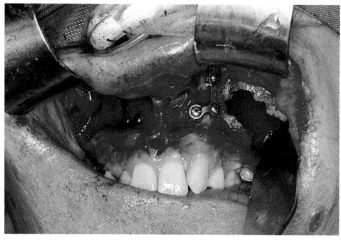

Fig. 7.9: Intraoral mucosal incisions give ideal results, but limited access to the periorbital region.

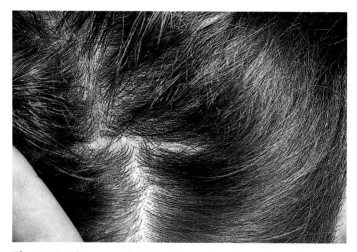

Fig. 7.10: The coronal incision is excellent, but it has to be placed carefully, especially in men. It must be raised and closed carefully to avoid hair loss or a broad scar. This scar is successful.

- Poor primary care, in particular meticulous wound cleaning and suturing.
- Visual problems, such as loss of vision, diplopia, with or without enophthalmos, are totally disabling.
- Loss of masticatory efficiency, from iatrogenic malocclusion, is possibly the most common functional problem encountered following facial trauma.
- Impairment of speech and swallowing is very rarely seen.
- Persistent epiphora and anosmia are troublesome but rare.
- Neurological damage, either motor or sensory, is very common early after trauma and can persist, leaving very significant problems.

Inadequate reduction and/or stabilization even in less severe cases is associated with poor esthetics and poor function. In addition, there may be associated pain and/or chronic infection, but this is less than might be seen in general orthopedic practice. Unfortunately, inadequate reduction and stabilization is probably not as rare as we would like it to be, but only by careful follow-up and audit can this be truly established.

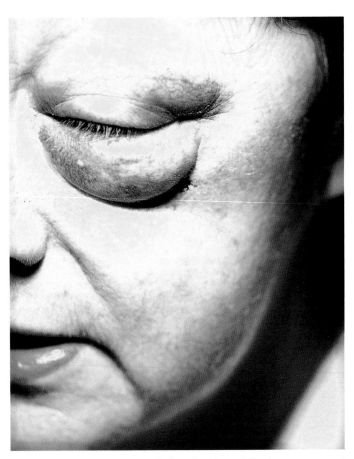

Fig. 7.11: The excessive swelling will make it difficult to get a good result with any periorbital scar and delay may be the best course.

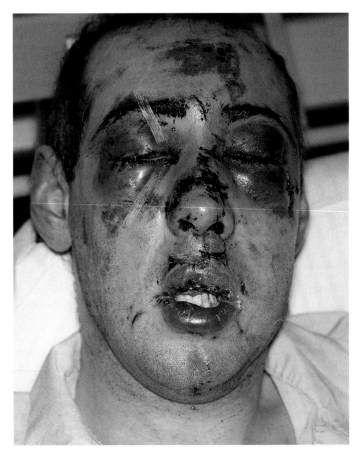

Fig. 7.12: Although this patient had no intracranial bleeding and his GCS score did not deteriorate, drowsiness delayed surgery by 10 days.

Whilst it is easy to record a very poor outcome from Figure 7.2, which was a result of the patient not seeking treatment, it is sometimes less easy to decide what is a 'perfect' result. The aim of reduction and stabilization is to return the patient to the preinjury status. It is self-evident that we must ensure the morbidity of the surgery does not exceed the traumatic injury itself; for example, the inappropriate and overzealous open reduction of an uncomplicated, minimally displaced orbital rim fracture. It is important to recall that bone, as a living structure, will remodel, especially in young patients.

More difficult decisions have to be made in Third World countries where resources and manpower are limited. Is it reasonable to undertake a 1-hour open reduction of a fractured malar or accept the less than perfect reduction by a closed 'lift' procedure? Similarly, should we spend a long time reducing a nasal fracture in a pugilist, who will probably reappear with a fractured nose again in 3 months time? Such decisions will be determined by the attending doctor, on an individual basis. It is, however, important to have targets of excellence, which may be modified in the light of individual patients and circumstances.

Suboptimal outcomes unrelated to socioeconomic factors (like failing to attend after a fracture) are not as uncommon as we would like them to be and only by careful follow-up and audit can the extent be fully established.[1] Poor outcomes may occur for a variety of other reasons.

- Coexisting medical problems, particularly head injuries (Fig. 7.12), may delay definitive surgery, making it difficult to achieve good reduction. Secondary correction of primary problems is rarely as good as primary surgery.
- Inadequate preoperative investigations, particularly appropriate imaging, may fail to reveal the true extent of the bony injuries. It is quite acceptable to delay surgery until adequate plain films and scans are available.
- Inadequate surgical planning, notably failing to plan the surgical access or the need for bone for grafting. Adequate patient consent requires that these important eventualities are considered and discussed before embarking on any procedure. Informed consent, of course, is becoming an ever more important issue in these increasingly litigious times.
- Very severe fractures, particularly grossly comminuted fractures, can be extremely difficult to reduce and stabilize. Only by concentrating trauma in the hands of surgeons with a special interest can these technical difficulties be overcome.
- Less commonly, surgeons (often from anatomically related specialties) with limited experience in facial trauma may not appreciate the structure and function of the oral and maxillofacial region fully and may therefore gain less than ideal results.

■ Occasionally patients, often from poor social backgrounds or who abuse alcohol or drugs, refuse or fail to attend for treatment. These patients then require secondary procedures.

State of the art

Reduction

There are many controversies related to both reduction and fixation and these will be discussed later in this chapter. The 'gold standard' of reduction, based on our current level of knowledge, is an 'open' approach for most fractures. This is based on the principle that only by an 'open' approach can access be gained to the fracture to precisely reduce and stabilize the fragments. Only by this aggressive approach can full form and function be most reliably achieved. An 'open' approach demands great ingenuity to provide, as far as possible, access utilizing pre-existing lacerations, transmucosal incisions or carefully placed skin incisions in the hair line. Presently, transmucosal incisions, via oral and conjunctival mucosae, should be seen as the 'ideal', although the latter may have complications in 25% of cases, particularly excessive scleral show (Fig. 7.13).

Skin incisions should be placed with esthetics in mind and should, if possible, avoid the visible facial skin. Even the best-placed incision, in the most skilled hands, can form a bad scar. Typically these non-facial skin incisions are the Gilles temporal approach and coronal flaps. Both these approaches should confine the incisions to the hair-bearing area. To be successful, these incisions must be placed at right angles to the hair follicles to prevent hair loss and, in the case of coronal incisions, high and posteriorly in male patients to avoid exposure in the event of male-pattern hair loss. Only on rare occasions should it be necessary to either extend on to or place the incision on the exposed skin. Periorbital fractures are the most common reason for visible skin incisions. There is accumulating evidence that the transconjunctival approach,[1] with or without lateral canthotomy, gives excellent access to all parts of the periorbita. The lateral canthotomy extension provides excellent exposure of the frontozygomatic suture when extended from a transconjunctival incision. Only superior wall or medial superior rim fractures cannot be accessed by this approach. The short skin extension into the so-called 'crowsfoot' area appears not to have any significant morbidity and is rarely visible. Another option is to combine a transconjunctival approach with a superior blepharoplasty incision. The latter has very few complications and is of course hidden when the eyes are open (Fig. 7.14).

The notable exception to these is the relatively invisible retromandibular incision used to approach the mandible's condylar neck. Whilst a pre-auricular incision provides an excellent approach in terms of morbidity and visibility of the fracture, it frequently fails to give good access to fix the fracture. The submandibular or Risdon approach rarely gives easy access to the high fracture line and is associated with a significant risk of damage to the facial nerve, notably the mandibular branch, a fact which is often noted in the literature but rarely documented. Surgical access is the basis of another chapter, but the most acceptable approach for condylar neck reduction and fixation is the retromandibular approach. In this approach most of the access is gained by a blunt dissection through the parotid, which appears to have a low risk of facial nerve damage.[2] Although the scar is well positioned behind the mandible there is unfortunately a risk of an unsightly scar in those patients who are prone to hypertrophic or keloid scar formation.

Although most facial fractures are best treated by an 'open' approach it should by no means be used for all fractures. Minimally displaced or undisplaced fractures may clearly require no active surgical intervention. Many pediatric facial fractures can usually be treated without surgical intervention. Like adults, however, childhood fractures may be so displaced that intervention is indicated, but the ability of the facial skeleton to remodel means a perfect reduction may not be essential. The risk of damage to developing dentition may indeed make intervention undesirable. The exception to the rule is in children with orbital wall injuries in whom there should be a low threshold for surgical intervention, especially when the risk of persistent diplopia is higher in younger children.

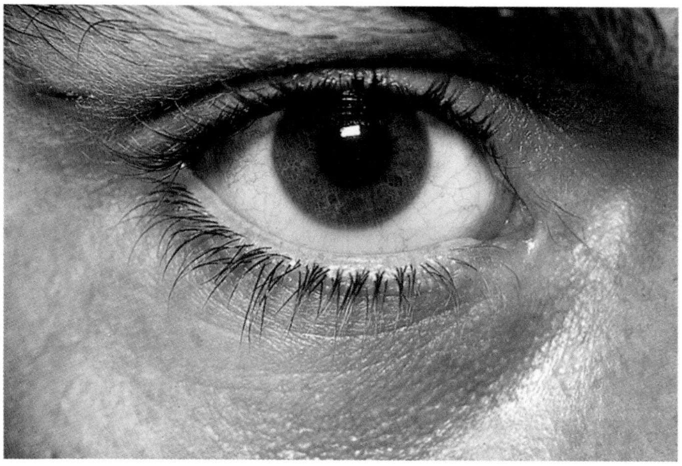

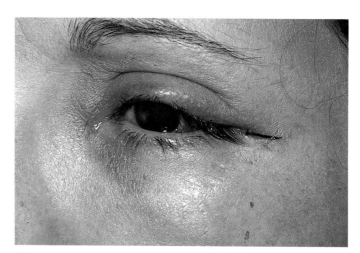

Fig. 7.13: A very nice blepharoplasty incision is marred by excessive scleral show.

Fig. 7.14: This superior blepharoplasty is an excellent approach but provides limited access.

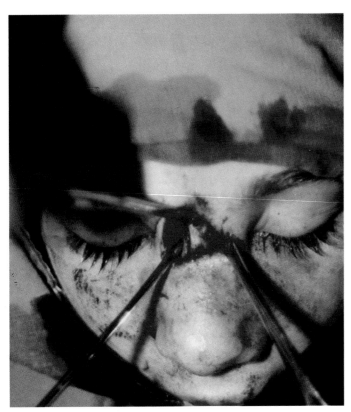

Fig. 7.15: A small laceration allowed excellent access to place a plate and provide a stable reduction, far superior to that possible with nasal packs and plaster of Paris splints.

Nasal fractures traditionally have been treated 'closed', but the poor outcomes may suggest that this philosophy is in need of review (Fig. 7.15).

Loss of bone or gross comminution requires immediate bone grafting, if proper reduction and stabilization is to be achieved. This is important at certain sites, for example in the orbital walls or in nasoethmoid fractures. In the past there has been a reluctance to undertake immediate grafting. Gruss has shown the importance of such an approach. Certainly the hope that a secondary procedure will achieve the same results is too optimistic.

In summary, therefore, the majority of facial fractures in adults with any significant displacement will require reduction under direct vision to ensure a precise position. Access is equally as important as good reduction and can be gained in most cases via transmucosal or cutaneous incisions within the hair line.

Fixation

As new ideas and philosophies develop, the controversies move on to new areas. In the past heated debates raged over which type of intermaxillary fixation (IMF) gave the best results. Once osteosynthesis became the 'gold standard', the site and size of the implants entered the arena. Nowadays it is accepted by the mainstream of maxillofacial surgery that 'small is good'. The use of 'biological' semirigid miniplate or microplate fixation gives excellent outcomes in terms of both good bone healing and reduced surgical morbidity. The use of

orthopedic heavy compression plates has no role in routine facial trauma. This means that mini- and microplates are used and the emphasis is on carefully placing the plates to maximize their biomechanical potential. Heavy reconstruction, non-compression plates only have a role in mandibular continuity defects or in gross fragmentation of the mandible.

The new 'debate' is now between resorbable plates of different materials versus non-resorbable plates (see later in this chapter). The previous debate revolved around how best to achieve fixation. Whilst a debate is taking place over the benefits of resorbable fixation devices, most of the true controversy over fixation devices is historical.

There is now a clear recognition that after good exposure of the fracture is achieved, stabilization is by the smallest appropriate fixation device. The fixation or osteosynthesis device is a plate and it is the accepted 'gold standard' that the plates for the vast majority of facial fractures are 'miniplates' or 'microplates'. 'Miniplates' are of varying dimensions, but the word is used to distinguish them from heavy plates used to provide 'compression' osteosynthesis, which of course requires bicortical screws, preventing the correct biomechanical placement of the plate. The latter does not have a place in modern maxillofacial surgery, except in very rare exceptional cases. Osteosynthesis with plates having two screws, usually on either side of the fracture, is able to provide three-dimensional stability of the fracture, unlike wire osteosynthesis which provides no more than monoplane traction, with no useful two- or three-dimensional stability, except in a few sites like a frontozygomatic suture fracture. The smallest device is used to minimize periosteal stripping around the fracture, which is helpful for fast healing, and of course the smaller devices are less likely to be felt by the patient.

There is a certain latitude in the size of the device used and for example, a grossly comminuted fracture may require a heavy (but non-compression) plate long enough to span the comminution. These plates can be retained by bi- or monocortical screws. A mandibular fracture in a young adult/child may only require a microplate. In certain sites, particularly the mandible, the muscular vectors demand that more than one plate is needed to provide stability, for example in the parasymphyseal area.

As previously mentioned, the materials used for the plates are the source of much debate. Currently titanium alloys are the materials most widely used. The decision to remove plates once their function has ceased, after say 3 months, is still controversial. The Strasbourg Osteosynthesis Research Group (SORG) has produced guidelines, which seem to be logical. These advocate removal of non-functional devices when healing has been completed. However, removal is undertaken only if the perceived risk is insignificant compared with the risk of retention of the plate. So, for example, if there is chronic infection around a plate then clearly the morbidity of removing the plate is less than leaving a focus of chronic infection. In contrast, the complications of raising a coronal flap to remove a titanium plate on the zygomatic arch, which is not palpable and is not infected in an adult, are greater than leaving it in situ. For most patients removal of asymptomatic plates often requires a general anesthetic and this to many represents an unnecessary risk and morbidity compared with leaving the plate. So for most surgeons in the UK and USA elective plate removal is not undertaken. In Germany, however, demand from patients to remove the non-functional device pushes the 'equation' towards elective plate removal.

Outcomes

Outcome measurement of reduction and fixation is not perfect and concentrates on 'measurable' benefits. There are studies recording complications of different surgical access approaches. In the past outcomes of miniplate osteosynthesis have been reported.[3,4] Most of these relate to the mandible, as it is easier to 'measure' occlusion rather than cosmetic outcomes of, say, zygoma fractures. These studies have also looked at complications like plate infection, screw loosening and wound infection. Many animal studies have looked at the biomechanics of miniplate fixation and the reaction of the tissues to the devices and material toxicity. Little evidence exists of the quality of the reduction with 'open' versus 'closed' reduction. Randomized studies of osteosynthesis are exceptionally rare.

Controversies

Reduction

This has been the source of much controversy, although the need for reduction per se is not in doubt. The controversy surrounds the 'balance' between maintaining perfect reduction during the healing process and inadequate reduction which may lead to either non-union (including fibrous union) or malunion. 'Perfect' reduction may be biologically impossible in microscopic terms, except in the first few days of reduction. Even then, the 'price' of perfect reduction may be harmful, as very heavy rigid and large implant devices are needed. This in its own right may have adverse effects.

- It creates such rigidity that there is stress shielding not only at the fracture site but on the adjacent normal bone. If bone is not under normal stresses and strains of function it will become osteoporotic.
- The heavy devices will deprive the periosteum of its blood supply.
- Even if initially there is perfect reduction, the pressure between the bone ends, and around the implant retaining screws, will quickly lead to bone resorption and the stability and reduction will be lost.
- Perfect reduction using heavy implants is technically difficult.

Much of the controversy has arisen as the result of the greater 'choice' offered by open reduction and the plethora of fixation devices. Prior to open reduction, closed techniques had only limited opportunities to perfectly reduce and perfectly stabilize the fracture. In the preantibiotic era and before better access surgery was available, closed reduction was effective at least at obtaining union of bone ends. As open techniques became safely available, the impetus was on avoiding the problems of closed treatment, importantly malunion and non–union. Early on in the 'open era', the approach was to produce perfect reduction maintained by heavy compression plates. In the maxillofacial region this technique had a high morbidity. This ranged from the surgical access (the technique usually uses an extraoral approach) producing scarring and nerve damage through to the fixation devices producing poor reduction, nerve damage, multioperations and infections. That said, some European centers continue to advocate the use of the AO system for mandibular fractures, pointing out that 'thoroughly experienced' operators have a low complication rate in a compliant population. But even in such groups the overall complication rate was 7% using the AO system.[5] Few studies can compare with those of Ellis and his co-workers, who clearly show the success of miniplating in mandibular fractures, and similar less controlled but larger studies confirm this miniplating non-compression technique, which really has ended the debate on routine osteosynthesis for facial fractures.[1,5]

In an attempt to reduce these failings of heavy compression plates, different less rigid techniques were developed, in some respects intuitively rather than by any careful science. The work was pioneered by Michelet,[6] popularized and investigated by Champy and the clinical outcomes evaluated by Pape and Ellis.[1,2] The success of these modifications was confirmed by biomechanical studies. The subsequent development of osteogenic distraction and better understanding of the role of callus formation has enhanced the move towards 'biological' reduction and stability. 'Biological' reduction and stability means creating an environment which maximizes healing without allowing malunion, non-union or fibrous union to occur. This is in marked contrast to the earlier pronouncements of study groups like the Arbeitsgemeischaft fur Osteosynthesefragen (AO) who proposed heavy rigid fixation and compression reduction. Whilst its work was innovative, it is not a principle normally used in maxillofacial surgery today.

Open or closed?

Terminology can be confusing; the terms 'closed' or 'open' treatment are to be preferred to 'conservative' or operative. 'Open' means a deliberate surgical intervention to open and explore the fracture site, normally by a surgical incision or using a laceration. Of course, fractures involving the teeth-bearing areas are biologically 'open' but this does not normally afford surgical access. Some surgeons refer to intermaxillary wiring as 'conservative' treatment, yet others refer to a 'soft diet' alone as 'conservative'. The use of IMF (or mandibular maxillary fixation – MMF) has a well-documented morbidity and even mortality which certainly does not fit with the concept of 'conservative'!

Open therefore means the intention to expose the fracture and normally reduce and fix it under direct vision. Closed, on the other hand, means no direct visualization of the fracture site and blind fixation, normally indirectly or by relying on non-surgical stabilization. In contrast, the vague term 'conservative' may mean no treatment at all, no surgical treatment or, for some surgeons, the use of IMF (MMF).

Not all displaced fractures need reducing. However, only severe medical problems, preventing general anesthesia, should prevent open reduction if otherwise indicated. Many fractures can be treated by sedation and local anesthetic even using open reduction. Open reduction involves exposure of the fracture, either through the skin or mucosa. Once opened, the fracture can then be reduced and directly fixed through the incision. Closed reduction is 'blind' reduction, relying on the fragments 'locking' together. This is more likely if the periosteum is intact. Examples of closed reduction include fixing the teeth in occlusion (IMF/MMF), elevation of a fractured zygoma or using an arch bar to stabilize dentoalveolar fractures. In these circumstances reduction normally occurs without direct visualization of the fragments in their final position.

In maxillofacial surgery the most common method of closed treatment is IMF (MMF) which relies on the correct positioning of the teeth to control the reduction (see Fig. 7.3). For mandibular fractures, open reduction and internal fixation has traditionally been performed using intraoperative IMF (MMF) to secure the occlusion prior to plate placement. Although the IMF (MMF) is released at the end of the operation it may be reapplied if necessary. This 'belt and braces' approach could be questioned for a number of reasons.[7]

■ Not using IMF (MMF) reduces operating time.
■ It is safer for the surgeon[8] but is it more comfortable for the patient? There is ample evidence of the short- and long-term risk to the patient of using IMF (MMF). There is good evidence of reducing airflow and weight loss and long-term TMJ function is adversely affected.[9]

Thirty years ago facial fractures were typically managed by closed methods. Open reduction was reserved for cutaneously compound fractures or certain unstable mandibular fractures. This evolution towards open reduction has improved the precision of the reduction, since the fragments can be carefully examined and manipulated. What has led to this change in philosophy?

In the preantibiotic era and prior to modern aseptic techniques, surgeons were extremely cautious about open reduction. Experience, particularly from general orthopedics, suggested that open reduction almost invariably led to local infection, severe osteomyelitis and frequently death of the patient. Little enthusiasm for open reduction existed and this was further fueled by the lack of a suitable implant material, necessary to stabilize the fracture. This problem continued beyond the introduction of modern sterile techniques and antibiotics. Although more suitable implants became available, the biomechanics of the systems often lacked a scientific base. Bad experiences created a climate of antipathy towards routine open reduction.

Historically, the avoidance of open reduction by our predecessors was based on sound surgical principles that were valid for the day but, in fact, difficult to achieve then for a variety of reasons. In contrast, these principles are relatively easy to achieve nowadays.

■ Open reduction should only be used if the procedure itself does not have a significant or unacceptable morbidity.
■ It should also be followed by direct fixation of the fracture, to ensure the full benefits of the procedure are gained.

Closed reduction

Disadvantages of closed reduction

Closed reduction can be problematic. 'Closed' means that only the position of the teeth, palpation or postoperative X-rays are used as a guide to the accuracy of reduction. The most common problem with closed reduction therefore is poor fracture alignment. In many cases closed reduction relies on positioning the teeth correctly, on the assumption that this will produce correct orientation of the bony fragments. Whilst it is necessary for the occlusion to be correctly restored, the teeth per se have only a limited 'control' over the final position of the bones. This significantly diminishes as fractures extend away from the dental arches (e.g. in the zygomatic complex, which is not related to the teeth at all). Even in mandibular fractures, muscle tone and activity may displace bone fragments despite firm location of the teeth.

This problem becomes compounded in cases of pre-existing malocclusion, a frequent predisposition to mandibular fractures. In cases of a depleted dentition or injury to the teeth themselves, then reduction of the occlusion becomes less reliable in reducing the bony fractures. Errors of reduction are tolerated much less in facial fractures than in general orthopedics. Inadequate reduction, even in the presence of a normal occlusion, may still be associated with poor esthetics and functional problems. Facial fractures are most common in the young and it is unacceptable to leave these patients with long-standing facial deformity or dysfunction.

Closed reduction for maxillary and mandibular fractures demands IMF (MMF). This is a technically simple procedure which may not require a general anesthetic. It has a number of disadvantages which are discussed later in the chapter. In passing, patients dislike IMF (MMF) and it can be dangerous.

Advantages of closed reduction

Perhaps the greatest advantage of closed reduction has been demonstrated in war zones, when treating maxillary or mandibular fractures. In the UK, particularly in the Second World War, this technique was of great importance. Custom-made cast silver splints were constructed and sectioned at the fracture site. IMF was slowly applied via the splints and a slow reduction and then fixation of the fractures was achieved. This was predominantly carried out away from the front line, often without the need for anesthetics. Closed reduction also worked well in missile injuries, stabilizing continuity defects. At that time, with the available technology and limited facilities, it proved to be a perfectly adequate method.

Today in many Third World countries, with limitations imposed by too many patients, too few maxillofacial surgeons and inadequate resources, these simple basic techniques still have a place. Cast silver splints have been replaced by simple arch bars, which are a lot easier and cheaper to manufacture. It should, however, be stressed that in some developing countries local manufacturers can economically produce locally made plating systems for internal fixation, although not necessarily out of exotic materials. Costs of the plating system should not prevent their use. There are in fact significant 'hidden' costs to closed reductions using IMF (MMF). These include the costs of extra patient supervision, often involving intensive care, increased morbidity, for example poor ventilation and persistent trismus. There may also be delays in returning to work.

Closed treatment may be an acceptable compromise, for instance in a patient with medical problems which preclude a general anesthetic or sedation. IMF (MMF) may be used to treat simple minimally displaced fractures very effectively. However, those very conditions which preclude a general anesthetic may also contraindicate IMF (MMF) (e.g. uncontrolled epilepsy, chronic respiratory disease). In addition, patients dislike having their teeth wired together and may not comply with prolonged treatment. Alternatively, simple open reduction is now possible under local anesthetic with supplementary 'awake' sedation.

The choice between 'open' and 'closed' reduction may be clear in some cases, but there are many in which both are equally acceptable. Nowadays with good outcomes from surgery and anesthesia, open reduction offers the chance of better reduction and direct osteosynthesis. This is very important as this means a safer postoperative recovery and earlier return to normal function and discharge in the majority of cases.

The debate over 'open' or 'closed' treatment of facial fractures is no more sharply focused than in condylar fractures. Those in favor of closed reduction point to the good results of IMF (MMF). Union always occurs and surgical complications are rare. Those in favor of open reduction underline that modern techniques and, most importantly, surgical experience allow for safe reduction and quicker discharge from hospital and quicker return to work. They also underline that closed reduction is frequently associated with poor long-term function. This includes reduced mouth opening, malocclusions and deviation on opening. Pain and clicking of the TMJ are also cited as problems, but this is such a common symptom to make it a very unreliable indicator of outcome. At a recent symposium[10] the controversies and disagreements were highlighted. However, certain areas of agreement could be reached (Fig. 7.16).

Terminology can add to the confusion and the following may be more appropriate.

■ It is best to refer to closed or open treatment, not 'conservative', since that has different meanings for different surgeons. The use of IMF should also be qualified as 'rigid fixed IMF' and training elastics, which allow guided opening of the jaws.

■ The terms 'displaced' and 'dislocated' (from the fossa) are best used to describe the position of the condylar head. These are less confusing than terms like 'subluxed'.
■ Description of the level of the fracture can be limited to 'Intracapsular', 'neck' and 'low'. Fractures may extend to more than one site.

There is a need for prospective studies to evaluate the best methods of treatment. Closed treatment is not always associated with good results while open reduction in experienced hands has a low morbidity. Closed treatment seems to be an effective method of treating children with condylar fractures.

At the present time pure intracapsular fractures can be treated by closed methods. Research suggests that the open treatment may be indicated but further work is needed.

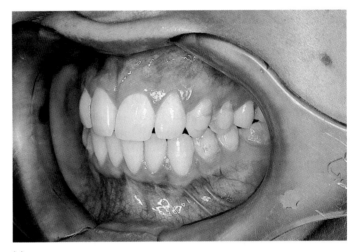

(a)

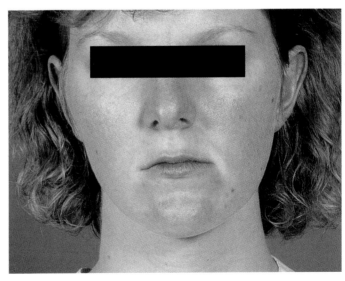

(b)

Fig. 7.16: Two examples of teenagers who had similar displaced fractures of the condylar neck. **(a)** has perfect symmetrical opening and a normal occlusion, **(b)** has a mandibular asymmetry and deviates on opening. Both were treated 'closed' without IMF; these two cases reflect the confusion in the literature.

Immobilization by *rigid* IMF (MMF) is not ideal. The use of *function*-guided elastics as a method of closed treatment has a more therapeutic role.

Clinical and radiological evaluation may not define those who will get a poor result from closed treatment (except where there is no or minimal displacement).

There are increasing numbers of publications showing that open reduction may produce excellent outcomes, with low morbidity. At present there is inadequate evidence to identify which surgical approach or type of fixator is the best. However, it does seem that single microplate fixation is inadequate and associated with plate fracture. In contrast, Marker with a large series obtained excellent results with a closed treatment regime.[11]

This important topic is further discussed in the appropriate chapter.

There is little doubt that the innovation of open reduction and miniplate fixation has improved outcomes and patient safety and comfort. Innovation however never ceases, and recently the use of locking screws attached to small plates is becoming popular. The principle is to function like an intra oral external fixator, since contact between the bone and the plate is not important. It is hoped this will make the fixation easier to use and equally rigid. These plates are larger and obviously much more expensive. Whilst there have been good studies to show that the system works,[12] a randomized study against existing systems is not yet available. Caution must be exercised to ensure the innovation is treating the existing problems, and not just a manufacturers marketing 'gimmick'.

Timing of reduction

The best time to reduce fractures is not clearly defined in the literature. With regard to open injuries, it is generally assumed that the longer the delay, the more the wound becomes contaminated and so the greater the risk of poor outcome due to infection. This seems logical, but what is not clear is the time frame over which this applies. There is clearly a difference between 5 hours and 5 days but is there a significant difference between, say, 2 hours and 24 hours after fracture? Few studies have been able to quantify these variations although some studies[13] have failed to show any differences in complications between those treated under 24 hours and after 24 hours post injury.

More worrying are the assumptions based on the orthopedic literature which, if applied too inflexibly to maxillofacial injuries without due thought for function and form, result in unsatisfactory outcome. The rich blood supply and rapid mucosal healing make comparison of outcomes between long bone and mandible fractures unrealistic.

There is little doubt that after long delays (around 14 days), initial healing is well established and this makes mobilization and reduction difficult. Soft tissues become adherent to the displaced bones, making reduction even harder to achieve. This is particularly important in the canthal region of the eye. Once displacement is established the canthal ligament is unlikely to ever settle into its correct position.

Delays inevitably occur as life-threatening conditions clearly need to take precedence. Here the greatest problem relates to patients with associated head injuries, in whom fears over long maxillofacial reconstruction lead to delay in definitive surgery. Some units have shown that early intervention is possible without any significant morbidity. For this to be possible close working relations with anesthetists and neurosugeons are essential.

Fixation

The debate about stabilization and its effect on bone healing has been a constant source of controversy. At times such dogmatic views have been expressed that readers may have felt the matter has reached the level of religious or political debate. It is perhaps reassuring to know that a similar debate rages in orthopedics, with equal vigor.

The debate is relatively new, since it is only in modern times that biomechanical products have become available to stabilize fractures. In addition, it is also only recently that the anesthetic skills and the reliable control of infection have become available to allow these developments to be carried out with low morbidity. Until the 19th century, only crude external devices were applied, if at all, to stabilize fractures and achieve some kind of union. Limited function was considered successful treatment. In the 20th century a few isolated reports of stabilizing facial fractures began to appear. Fixation mostly relied on use of the dentition with crude forms of IMF (MMF). This use of the dentition persisted with only the odd exception until the 1950s.

In orthopedics in the 19th century it was well recognized that any attempt to open a fracture was accompanied by a significant rise in mortality. Death was due mainly to the use of unsterile instruments and no understanding of aseptic techniques. Once the fundamentals of sterility were applied and safe anesthesia became possible, the desire to develop improved methods of fixation increased. Centuries of caution meant for many that the idea of open reduction and placement of foreign bodies (plates) was totally unacceptable. This was the general view despite early reports of internal plate fixation as far back as 1886. It was therefore left to enthusiastic individuals to develop the modern concept of osteosynthesis. Roberts and Battersby[14] in the UK and Speissl in Basle all made significant contributions to this development. General acceptance of open osteosynthesis did not appear in the maxillofacial literature until the organized research of the AO group in the 1950s. Even then this work was only accepted in the German-speaking countries. It is now hard to believe that the first osteosynthesis courses in maxillofacial surgery run in English only occurred in the 1970s.

Although many surgeons continued to avoid open approaches they became frustrated by the shortcomings of poorly reduced and unstable fractures. Current debate about poor results frequently becomes blurred by confusion between poor *reduction* and poor *stabilization*. Even if the 'best' fixation is used, it will be of little value if reduction is inadequate. Similarly, an anatomically reduced fracture will displace if it is inadequately stabilized. This is particularly important in the maxillofacial region where a well-healed but displaced fracture may carry significant morbidity (e.g. malocclusion, diplopia and a 'flat face'). Such outcomes are clearly unacceptable. Maxillofacial surgery has significantly benefited from the research carried out in orthopedics but again, the transfer of orthopedic concepts and techniques to the maxillofacial region still carries problems.

Anatomical peculiarities of the facial skeleton can make the application of some orthopedic concepts and techniques very difficult. The excellent blood supply to the bones, overlying skin and mucosa provides favorable conditions for healing and enables the placement of plates with low morbidity. This is at variance with general orthopedics where blood supply may be poor, especially to the distal extremities in elderly patients. Degloving injuries of the fractured mandible often heal uneventfully, a situation rarely seen in the lower limb after a comparable soft tissue insult. Yet many parts of the facial skeleton are only paper-thin and this precludes *rigid* fixation. That said, the mechanical loads, i.e. displacing forces created by the muscles of mastication, do not compare with those in the limbs.

In maxillofacial surgery there are several advantages to be gained from rigid fixation.

- To maintain reduction.
- To restore early function at the fracture site, surrounding muscles and joints. In the case of the jaws this means restoration of normal mastication, deglutition and speech.
- To minimize healing time.
- To prevent infection by movement at untreated fracture sites.

What is the effect of no fixation? Although rarely seen nowadays, there are still plenty of examples of non-treated fractures (predominantly in specimen jars in medical museums!). The study of non-treated fractures is, however, an unhelpful view of the 'end' stages rarely seen nowadays and therefore inapplicable to modern practice. Animal studies have yielded much more information. The work of the AO group provided much of the earlier data. These studies plotted the progress of untreated radius fractures in dogs, through to a displaced fibrous union. Although it is reasonable to question the relationship between young animals and humans, particularly when considering, for example, an elderly osteoporotic patient with mandibular fracture, animal models do provide some useful data.

From this animal work a better understanding of fracture healing emerged. The AO group divided the bone-healing process into direct and indirect.

Direct healing was seen to occur in, for example, a 1 mm hole cut into bone. Because there was complete stability, there was immediate growth of bone into the hematoma. This was then replaced and remodeled into trabecular bone. No intermediate cartilage formation occurred nor was there proliferative callus formation.

Indirect healing classically occurred across a mobile long bone fracture. Here a quite different process developed. Initial hematoma formation preceded ingrowth of fibrous

tissue and blood vessels. This underwent remodeling accompanied by proliferative osteoid growth at the periosteum – callus formation (Fig. 7.17). Callus provided early stability for osteoid formation to occur across the fracture. Once united, remodeling of the callus and the osteoid then occurred to produce trabecular bone. However, in both humans and animals, where mobility was excessive there was proliferative but incomplete formation of callus, which was unable to stablize the fracture. That is, it failed to bridge the fracture site. At best a malunion was the final result but frequently other complications intervened, including osteomyelitis. Indirect healing therefore became associated with the traditional problems of fracture management:

- infection
- malunion
- non-union
- excess callus formation

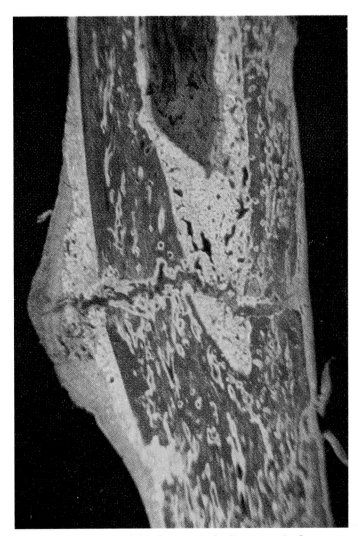

Fig. 7.17: The normal development of callus around a fracture. Whilst excessive callus formation occurs with excessive motion, it is not per se a sign of abnormal healing. Futile attempts to prevent any callus formation produced more and more rigid fixation systems. Champy's work with miniplates demonstrated that complete rigidity was in fact a disadvantage.

and in practical terms:

- prolonged hospitalization
- prolonged immobilization
- prolonged antibiotic regimes
- joint dysfunction
- secondary surgery to encourage union or eliminate infection
- opening of a second donor site for bone grafting.

Researchers and clinicians contrasted these problems with animal models of direct healing, in which perfect reduction led to production of osteoid and trabecular bone without callus formation and ultimately to early healing and restoration of normal function. With hindsight it is easy to see this was comparing unlike starting points; that is, the results of inadequate versus adequate stability and not recognizing there are many degrees of rigidity in the fixation between 'adequate' and 'inadequate' stability. Whilst the argument at first sight may appear to be one between direct and indirect healing, it is in fact a question of stability during the healing period. Indirect healing does not necessarily lead to instability and failure. The problems listed above were the result of *inadequate stability*.

That said, research workers of 30 years ago decided that direct healing had to be the goal and this led to the artificial situation of absolute stability. The engineers set about providing methods of fixation, which produced sufficient stability for direct healing to take place. Even the early enthusiasts recognized that in a biological system in which bone itself had some flexibility, absolute rigidity was not possible. In order to distinguish between the inadequate stability of some systems, like wire ligatures used alone, the AO workers referred to the need for absolute stability. Only this would achieve direct healing, they stated. Again, in hindsight, the thinking was muddled since to get stability in a mandible required (by their 'rules') compression plates. For these to work bicortical screws were needed. To use bicortical screws in a dentate patient required the plate to be moved to the lower border of the mandible, biomechanically the wrong site!

There is no doubt that the philosophies of dynamic compression osteosynthesis had an enormous impact on orthopedic trauma services as it became established practice in most trauma units. This was not the case in maxillofacial surgery. Certainly a number of large maxillofacial units in the German-speaking countries whole-heartedly accepted this philosophy but the technique did not become widely accepted around the world as it was in orthopedics. There are a number of reasons for this.

- Even the strongest advocates of the system did not apply heavy compression plates to all facial fractures. Only mandibular fractures were treated in this way.
- The complex curvature of the mandible creates difficulties for a system designed to provide straight-line compression.
- The presence of teeth and the inferior alveolar nerve forced the placement of the compression plates in zones already exposed to compression by muscle activity and not in tension.

- Too much compression (especially in comminuted fractures), inadequate compression at the upper border and straightening of the natural curvature of the mandible may all produce malocclusions.
- The precision of reduction in maxillofacial surgery is far in excess of anything demanded in orthopedic surgery.
- Skin incisions are required in most cases, with scarring and a small risk of damage to the mandibular branch of the facial nerve. IMF (MMF) may be unpleasant but it is only temporary with no risk of scarring and permanent nerve damage. Interestingly, these aspects are not discussed in the AO/ASIF manual.
- Dynamic compression plating (DCP) is an unforgiving and difficult technique. This is not a reason for not using it but, as will be discussed later, the advantages of this technique can in most cases be achieved by a simpler and less morbid procedure.
- Although scientifically unproven, fears existed that the plates were so rigid that stress shielding delayed healing strength.
- Contact from these long wide plates reduced the periosteal blood supply. This might be important in the elderly atrophic mandible with already impaired blood supply.
- There is normally a need for a second, often extraoral operation to remove these thick bulky plates.

Overall, there was a significant complication rate when using the AO system for mandibular fractures. In one series this was as high as 13%.[5]

Even with many modifications the use of heavy compression systems failed to be universally acceptable and is now becoming a historical footnote. It has, however, provided valuable research data and nowadays its influence lies in the limited use of lag screws, particularly useful in condylar neck fractures popularized by Ecklet and his co-workers. More recently, even in units where the AO system was accepted, there has been a move away from compression to monocortical non-compression miniplates.

Miniplates

Miniplates were, however, to find almost universal acceptance, because they provided a well-engineered system which achieved good stable bone union, but without the technical difficulties and, most important, with lower morbidity.

In maxillofacial surgery two separate events have been responsible more or less for the cessation of dynamic compression. Michelet[6] and then Lodde developed an osteosynthesis system comprising smaller plates, which were inserted along the lines of tension. Fortunately Lodde was working with Maxine Champy who was aware of the need to publish and disseminate this information. Dieter Pape who, having being schooled in the traditional heavy compression plates, provided thorough audit of these new systems, took up this concept in Germany. Together with his background, this undoubtedly gave the system much credibility and long term reviews were published.[1]

Secondly, studies in animal models showed that micro-movement, using semirigid or biological fixation, produced earlier healing, as measured by strength at the fracture site.

Non-compression and smaller sized plates ('miniplates') have now become the standard method of internal fixation in many units. This has effectively shown that indirect healing, if combined with adequate fixation leading to good stability, can still produce excellent bone healing comparable to those systems aiming to produce direct healing. More importantly, miniplates were placed transorally using monocortical screws and thus had much less morbidity than the compression systems.

Michelet's work was essentially intuitive, but it was developed and evaluated by Champy. Champy[15] undertook animal studies and made measurements in human volunteers, to support the concept. This work was initially confined to the mandible.

The principle of the miniplate technique is to identify the line of tension within the mandible at the site of the fracture. The plate is then applied across the fracture along this line, without compression. In a way analogous to suspension bridges, huge loads can be controlled by relatively small structures, relying on the tensile strength of the materials. Miniplates can control relatively large loads. More importantly, since compression is unnecessary, the plate can be anchored to the bone using only monocortical screws. As a result the plate can be placed where it is biomechanically desirable and not only where there is room to place a bicortical screw. Monocortical screws can be safely placed in the outer cortex over dental roots and the inferior alveolar nerve, so long as care is taken whilst drilling.

Champy's studies examined the loads at different parts of the mandible, in particular the forces in play anteriorly. These are complicated in part due to the curve of the bone and partly by the attachment of the muscles, each pulling in different directions. These displacing forces need to be controlled, if a small plating system is to work. Posterior to the canine the mylohyoid muscle pulls medially, whilst anterior to the canine the genial muscles and digastric tend to pull posteroinferiorly, resulting in additional rotational forces. In this region a single miniplate would provide inadequate fixation and two plates are necessary to prevent displacement.

In comminuted or sagittal fractures miniplating needs to be modified. In both circumstances whilst the plate may be correctly placed along the lines of tension, because the fractures do not have solid contact in the area of compression the fragments will 'slip' past each other and tension will not be generated. The plate is then left functioning as the only means of fixation in all directions. These plates are not designed to take these kinds of loads. Scenarios like this can occur if there is a sagittal split of the mandible or in cases where there is gross comminution, particularly at the lower border. In the former example, a position or lag screw placed at the lower border can control the rotatory element and generate the appropriate forces. In comminuted fractures careful repositioning and fixation of all the fragments are needed, although smaller fragments may become devitalized.

The simplicity of miniplate application has reduced the risks of malocclusions, compared with the very rigid and unforgiving heavy compression plates. Champy and his colleague Pape have audited hundreds of cases and demonstrated an exceptionally low complication rate. The technique is carried out entirely via the transoral route with no need for skin incisions or trocar punctures. The plates are small and can be left in situ if desired. In addition, light elastics can be used to 'fine tune' the occlusion if necessary. The technique, although originally not recommended by Champy, has been extended into treating all facial skeleton fractures. With better understanding of the biomechanics, smaller plates are now recommended for the upper face and cranium.

As is often the case, full scientific explanation follows clinical success and to some extent this is true of the small plate tension systems. Although Lodde and Champy undertook biomechanical studies, later complemented by Champy and Pape's audit, recent studies have added further to our understanding. Kroon[16] demonstrated that at the angle there are circumstances when tension and compression are reversed. Bos, in a recent paper[15] using finite element analysis, has accurately documented the forces and directions within the functioning mandible. However the forces generated in a non-injured jaw are significantly different to the smaller loads generated in the fractured mandible. More recent scientific mathematical models have not confirmed Kroon's work[16] but have suggested greater torsional movements in body fractures.

Extensive audits of miniplates have confirmed their effectiveness. In addition, miniplate fixation utilizing and ignoring Champy's principles has been compared to transosseous wiring. Miniplates are associated with fewer complications, especially when Champy's principles are adhered to.

Despite the trend in the orthopedic literature towards biological or 'semirigid' fixation, it must not be forgotten that *excessive* movements are associated with excessive callus formation, less strength and ultimately delayed union. Most important of all are the excellent predictable results that are obtained from miniplates.

At the present time, the literature suggests that an optimal number of micromovements at the fracture site are ideal for healing. 10 000 cycles per day will produce non-union, whereas 10 cycles per day encourage good union. However, the optimal number of cycles is unclear even in animal models and translation into humans with fractures is extremely difficult. For an overview of the mechanobiology of bony healing the reader is directed to a recent review by Carter et al.[17] Huge variations in the site and nature of the fractures, let alone unrelated variables like age, nutritional, muscle bulk and hormonal status, may all have significant effects on the healing process. The precise degree of stability still eludes researchers. What is clear is that the miniplating concept, which has minimal morbidity, now has sound biological principles to account for its effectiveness. Being semirigid imparts some advantages to the bone-healing process and this degree of fracture mobility should not be seen as a disadvantage.

Intermaxillary fixation (IMF/MMF)

Plate fixation is favored now by many maxillofacial units in the developed world. However, by far the greatest number of facial fractures worldwide do not occur within industrialized societies. It is from emerging nations, who see the greatest volume and range of facial injuries, that many of the future developments will come. At the present time, however, many of these countries do not have the resources to pay for expensive plating systems. They are therefore obliged to use more traditional methods of fixation, particularly IMF (MMF), despite the previously discussed hidden costs. By contrast, in developed countries it was recognized a decade ago that using miniplates was actually cheaper than IMF (MMF) when the 'hidden costs' of, for example, intensive care were considered.[18]

Intermaxillary fixation was first reported in the 17th century and is most commonly used for fractures of the mandible. Its principle is simple: the teeth arise from the bone fragments to which they are firmly attached. By securing them in occlusion with the upper, intact arch not only will the fracture be stabilized, but it will also be reduced to the correct position.

Unfortunately IMF (MMF) cannot be applied to all fractures.

- Fractured jaws are often associated with pre-existing malocclusions, which may be difficult to define accurately.
- There may be an inadequate number of teeth to provide stability.
- Although the teeth may appear to be in the correct position, muscle attachments may still displace the bony fragments.
- This approach is unsuitable for fractures which do not involve the teeth-bearing structures such as malar and nasoethmoid fractures.
- In combined lower and upper face fractures neither jaw is capable of stabilizing nor allowing accurate reduction of the fractures.
- IMF (MMF) is not without risk, especially in the early postoperative period, where the patient may vomit and intraoral swelling may not be detected. As a result, patients who have had a general anesthetic frequently require the first postoperative night in an intensive care ward. In the UK this costs about £1000 per night and certainly offsets any savings made from not using expensive plating systems.
- Patients may lose weight and those with respiratory disorders, like asthma, have been shown to have deterioration in the respiratory function.
- Patients dislike it.

Disadvantages of osteosynthesis are of a technical nature and to abandon it in favor of a less satisfactory method because of technical errors is not in the best interest of the patients. The fundamental problem of IMF (MMF) is the unpleasant nature of the procedure and its poor results, especially in midface trauma. Many feel that it is inappropriate even in simple fractures.

Other methods of fixation

Extraoral pin fixation was, prior to plating, an important method of fixation. It was used in two main ways. In midface fractures it can be used to indirectly secure upper and/or lower arch bars to another fixed point, usually the cranium. Alternatively it can be used as a direct fixator across a fracture, commonly the mandible or malar. Unfortunately patients dislike the bulky apparatus and care is required not to injure themselves with it. Even modern miniature devices are still very intrusive. Placement normally involves skin punctures and these can leave unsightly scars. The external fixator has had a new lease of life as a means of callus distraction but although it is a very successful technique, the cutaneous scarring and awkwardness of the fixator are still important problems.

As a means of securing the dental arches to a fixed point, external fixators have been quite successful. Fixation involves the use of a halo frame around the skull. The halo frame is mechanically very stable and was initially developed for traction of unstable cervical injuries. However, the system of rods and joints to link the halo to the jaws is less rigid. Previously, cast silver cap splints were used to secure the apparatus to the dental arches. The main advantage of this system is that it can provide anterior traction to a fractured maxilla. It also acts as a guide to establishing the correct vertical height in patients with multiple facial fractures, particularly those with bilateral condylar neck fractures. The cranial attachment may be modified to attach posteriorly if a craniotomy is necessary. Levant developed a very compact, efficient modification by creating a bar attached to two supraorbital pins.

Fixators placed across fractures, usually in the mandible, have several attractions. They can be quickly applied, there is minimal exposure and stripping of the periosteum around the fracture. The degree of rigidity can be modified during healing (dynamization), thereby reducing the potential effects of stress shielding. The position of the fractures can also be adjusted if postoperative radiology shows inadequate reduction. These fixators can also be used to provide callus distraction in appropriate cases.

In modern times, the main role of this type of treatment is to provide rapid 'first aid' stabilization in the multiply injured patient or where there are limited facilities prior to transfer to a definitive care center. In those areas where gunshot wounds are common, this method of fixation provides good 'long-term' temporary fixation, until the contaminated wounds have healed. The external fixator is also particularly useful in maintaining space and orientation in continuity defects.

The obvious problems around the face are the unacceptable inconvenience of these devices in the short term and cosmetics in the long term. Pin sites frequently become infected and leave unsightly scars. After 6–8 weeks loosening of the pins in the bone occurs. In order to obtain effective stability, two pins are required each side of the fracture.

Special Considerations

Children and the atrophic mandible

Both these groups respond differently to treatment modalities.

Children

Childhood facial fractures are marked by rapid healing and rapid remodeling. In many ways, therefore, these are easy fractures to treat and have minimal complications. These factors are, of course, a function of growth and excellent blood supply. In most fractures reduction and fixation is not necessary. However, there is a risk of ankylosis in intracapsular mandibular joint fractures and early mobilization is desirable. If fixation is required microplating systems are normally adequate. The problem of plate removal is heightened in this group, with fear of impairing further growth.

Atrophic edentulous mandibular fractures <10 mm

In the atrophic mandible the picture is the complete opposite. The severely atrophic edentulous mandible often has a poor outcome, especially in those in whom the radiographic height of the mandible is 10 mm or less (Fig. 7.18). It is characterized by a poor blood supply and slow reparative efforts. In addition, the older population may be in poor general health which sometimes precludes prolonged general anesthesia. Patients are commonly female with osteoporotic bones, making screw fixation difficult and unreliable. The thin atrophic mandible has very little separation between the compressive and tension zones and this often demands greater strength in the osteosynthesis, which has to control both. Interfragmentary contact is poor, brittle and unstable. The poor blood supply within the central cancellous bone places greater demands on having an intact periosteal blood supply, making use of heavy large plates less desirable. It is therefore not surprising that these fractures are some of the most demanding to treat.

Management of the edentulous mandible is discussed in detail in Chapter 15. It is, however, important to note the absence of good studies reporting outcomes of treatments. The current literature would appear to suggest that equally good results could be obtained by very different methods. Two retrospective studies[19,20] show that most problems arise in those patients with mandibles less than 10 mm in height at the fracture site. These are fortunately rare, both units

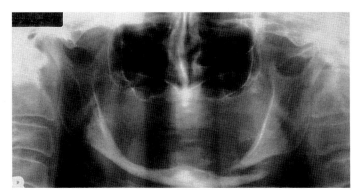

Fig. 7.18: A typical severely atrophic mandible. This was successfully treated with small plate fixation.

reporting only about 15 patients in 10 years. Both papers draw attention to anecdotal poor results from traditional methods, particularly the use of Gunning splints. It appears from these studies that equally good results were achieved by heavy rigid fixation and minimal stabilization. In the latter case fresh rib bone grafts were used not only to provide the stabilization, but presumably also bone morphogenic protein, to hasten healing. This is clearly a finding that warrants further investigation.

Edentulous jaws, not atrophic (greater than 10 mm)

This is an area of special interest as traditional methods of fixation are severely compromised by the lack of teeth. Gunning splints are useful here. This essentially consists of using modified dentures secured to the upper and lower jaws as a method of IMF (MMF) and stabilization. Splints are wired to the jaws, in the maxilla passing through the alveolus and in the mandible around the lower border. However, in the maxilla the wires frequently cut through the atrophic edentulous alveolus and are therefore modified by using wires passed higher up the facial skeleton. These are passed through the pyriform rim and/or around the zygomatic arch. In midface fractures the direction of 'pull' of the wire tends to be posteriorly. This is highly undesirable in patients in whom the fracture has been displaced posteriorly. In the mandible the solid bone makes the fixation much more rigid. Problems also arise with oblique fractures where it may be difficult to have a good distribution of the wires around the jaws.

This system is inherently unstable because of the stretching of the wires, which then become loose. The use of screws to locate the Gunning splints has helped somewhat, especially in the lower jaw. The use of open reduction with appropriate sized plates has greatly improved the management of these fractures.

Condylar neck fractures

Controversy abounds in this area of traumatology. Is it better to treat 'closed', relying on the musculature activity and dental occlusion to allow return to normal function, or should we be opening, reducing and fixing these injuries? The closed approach has been shown in some studies to have poor outcomes, yet other studies show good results.[15] Open reduction and fixation ensures the correct posterior facial height is restored but has complications[16] from the surgical access, long operative time and in some cases avascular necrosis of the condylar head. There presently appears to be a trend towards surgical therapy, notably in cases where the condylar head is displaced from the fossa.[21]

Until there is clear evidence for and against these two methods, controversy must remain but there are areas where agreement exists.

- In children conservative, non-operative approaches are the norm.
- In combination with displaced midface fractures, there is a need to establish the posterior vertical height of the

face. This requires that at least one of the condylar necks must be intact, so open surgery is needed if there is a bilateral fracture.

- If IMF (MMF) is used it should allow opening of the jaws and therefore guiding elastics should be used.
- Opening of intracapsular fractures has a high risk of leading to avascular necrosis of the condylar head.
- Low 'subcondylar' neck fractures are least likely to need open reduction.
- Grossly displaced neck fractures are most likely to need open reduction.

Classification of condylar fractures

There are many classifications but the simple one shown below seems to provide good comparisons with outcomes:

- intracapsular
- extracapsular:
  — neck
  — low
- isolated or in association with other mandibular fractures
- adult/child.

Open treatment

Whilst open treatment allows direct visualization of the fracture, consequent improved reduction and, it is presumed, better fixation, this must be balanced against the potential risk to the facial nerve and maxillary artery. Even via an optimally placed access incision, the approach to the condyle is often difficult and of course leaves a facial scar. That said, several approaches have been suggested which are cosmetically acceptable, for example the widely used retromandibular approach.[2]

Open reduction and fixation ideally leads to an improved outcome in terms of function and preservation of posterior facial height as well as minimizing the risk of malocclusion. With this, however, the surgeon must consider the risk of postoperative infection, fixation device failure or fracture and avascular necrosis of the condylar head. One of the advantages of closed treatment of condylar head fractures is that it is simple! In some surgeon's hands very effective.[11] But if the outcome is suboptimal the patient may be left with a poor occlusion or even an anterior open bite if a bilateral condylar injury has been sustained. Deviation on mouth opening is another unwanted consequence of inadequately treated condylar fractures. At the present time there are not enough sound data to help decide protocol so clinical decisions should be made on an individual patient basis.

Plate removal

Plates are foreign bodies and as such should ideally be removed once they have assisted fracture healing. Normally plates are made of titanium, which is 'inert' but of course is bioactive, especially where the plates contact bone and/or screws.

Plate removal is commonly undertaken in orthopedics and many maxillofacial units in Europe. However, in the UK and the US plates are not routinely removed. Removal is undertaken in the event of symptoms, which occur in 5–20% of all cases. Fewer plates need removal in the midface and those patients having elective orthognathic surgery.[13] Removal often requires the added risks of another general anesthetic or further surgery which are on balance considered too great to justify routine removal.

Debate has become more vigorous with the introduction of new materials. Titanium, for example, is said to be more 'biocompatible' than many traditional materials, such as vitallium and stainless steel which corrode. The concept that plates are completely 'bioinert' is not true and studies on dental and other implants have demonstrated titanium in the lymphatics.[22]

As a result there has been a move towards developing 'biodegradable' materials. These materials do not currently have the range of properties to substitute all desirable characteristics of the metallic plating systems. Further understanding about how these materials are actively degraded is required. The process seems to involve either active phagocytosis and/or enzymatic degradation. Neither process is truly 'inert'. This is a rapidly developing field[17] and whilst some animal studies suggest that complete degradation occurs, great caution is needed. Of course, the degree of degradation is also dependent on how carefully the local tissues are examined for degradation products, for example using electron microscope studies or simple light microscopy. EM studies suggest these products remain, but what is not certain is the relevance of these fragments. We have all, however, been warned by the successful litigation regarding certain types of breast implant, yet with the flimsiest of scientific evidence to support the litigation. Will EM deposits of 'resorbable' plates be similarly implicated in a variety of apparently unrelated conditions?

Ideal properties of biodegradable materials

There are several features which resorbable or biodegradable plates and screws must exhibit before they become an accepted alternative to the various metal miniplates and screws currently available. Clearly they must be non-toxic but this cannot be measured just in terms of local tissue reaction. They must be non-allergenic and, in the long term, non-carcinogenic and non-teratogenic. Data on these latter two features are not available for humans. Equally importantly, the degradation products must also be non-toxic.

The physical properties will be most closely scrutinized by surgeons. Good strength and ease of handling are of paramount importance. These devices must provide adequate stability, enabling some movement yet permitting reliable bone healing. They should have limited 'memory' to allow correct adaptation and bending. The plates and screws should degrade completely within an acceptable time scale. One notable advantage of biodegradable materials over their metal counterparts will be their non-interference with imaging.

Several biodegradable materials have been trialed over the past few years.

- Polylactic acid (PLA) – four types depending on the L and D configuration (PLLA, PDLA)
- Polyglycolic acid (PGA)
- Polydioxanone (PDS)
- Co-polymers of PLA and PGA and self-reinforcing polymers of PLLA and PDLLA

It is known that pure PGA and PLLA cause adverse reactions and so they are no longer used. At present there is much interest in the self-reinforced co-polymer of PLLA and PDLLA. These plates can be sterilized by gamma radiation which actually improves the resorption characteristics, enabling them to resorb faster. This carries the benefit of avoiding ethylene oxide remnants found on metallic fixation devices. These devices can easily be manipulated into the desired shape, typically using hot water baths at 70°C. Above all, of course, these devices do not require a second operation for removal.

Conclusion

It is clear that maxillofacial surgeons have, through research and experience, advanced the management of facial fractures over the past two decades. It is important that the specialty keeps abreast of developments in the management of fractures from other disciplines but equally, we should remain critical and ensure that we appraise and audit new techniques and materials.

It is essential that management of our patients continues to be based on the sound principles of care used throughout surgery. Accurate diagnosis, by careful history, thorough examination and carefully chosen special tests, should lead to evidence-based treatment plans. The treatment plan should take account of the patient's general medical condition as well as the type of injury. It is entirely reasonable to delay treatment until all the required information is available, especially adequate imaging.

In our ever more litigious society experienced surgeons should discuss the treatment choices with the patient so that truly informed consent can be obtained. Equally, experienced surgeons should actually perform or direct any operation so the benefit of that experience is appreciated by the patient or passed on to a trainee. The public rightly expects good outcomes and the only way to ensure this is to audit our activity carefully.

Open reduction now carries low morbidity, for example in terms of cosmesis and risk of infection, and should be considered the technique of choice for facial fractures unless there is an overriding reason for using the closed method. Equally, internal fixation with miniplates has become established as the gold standard although this standard may change over the next few years as the use of biodegradable plates becomes more commonplace.

It is important to keep in mind the problem areas of facial fracture management, notably childhood bony injuries and the edentulous lower jaw. The threshold for open reduction and internal fixation is higher in children than adults as immature facial bones have greater capacity to heal without intervention and the use of plating systems, although they may initially assist healing, may impair later growth. Treatment of edentulous jaws has been improved by the use of miniplates but it is important to be aware of the severely atrophic mandible which requires extra care in management.

The management of condylar fractures is likely to remain controversial for some time; the very fact that these injuries are treated in so many ways is testament to this. Ideally, prospective research is required to establish the optimum choices for condylar fractures in any given circumstance.

References

1 Sneddon KJ 2003 Audit of 40 cosequective subconjunctival approaches to the orbital floor. In press.
2 Cheynet F, Aldegheri A, Chossegros C, Bourezak Z, Blanc JL 1997 The retromandibular approach in fractures of the mandibular condyle. Revue de Stomatologie et de Chirurgie Maxillofaciale (Paris) 98(5): 288–294
3 Pape H-D 1997 Microplate osteosynthesis – 5 years of clinical use of a new technique. International Journal of Oral and Maxillofacial Surgery 26(1): 65
4 Ellis E 3rd. Treatment methods for fractures of the mandibular angle. International Journal of Oral and Maxillofacial Surgery 1999 Aug; 28(4): 243–52
5 Zachariades N, Papademetriou I 1995 Complications of treatment of mandibular fractures with compression plates. Oral Surgery, Oral Medicine, Oral Pathology, Oral Radiology and Endodontics 79(2): 150–153
6 Michelet FX, Deymes J, Dessus B 1973 Osteosynthesis with miniature screwed plates in maxillofacial surgery. Journal of Maxillofacial Surgery 1: 79–84
7 Fordyce AM, Lalani Z, Songra AK, Hildreth AJ, Carton AT, Hawkesford JE 1999 Intermaxillary fixation is not usually necessary to reduce mandibular fractures. British Journal of Oral & Maxillofacial Surgery 37(1): 52–57
8 Avery C, Johnson P 1992 Surgical glove perforation and maxillofacial trauma: to plate or wire? British Journal of Oral and Maxillofacial Surgery 30: 31–35
9 Hayter JP, Cawood JI 1993 The functional case for miniplates in maxillofacial surgery. International Journal of Oral and Maxillofacial Surgery 22(2): 91–96
10 Bos RR, Ward Booth RP, de Bont LG 1999 Mandibular condyle fractures: a consensus. British Journal of Oral and Maxillofacial Surgery 37(2): 87–89
11 Marker P, Nielsen A, Bastian HL 2000 Fractures of the mandibular condyle. Part 2: results of treatment of 348 patients. British Journal of Oral and Maxillofacial Surgery 38(5): 422–426
12 Ellis E, Graham J 2002 Use of a 2.0 mm locking plate/screw system for mandibular fracture surgery. Journal of Oral and Maxillofacial Surgery 60(6): 642–645
13 Brown JC, Trotter M, Cliffe J, Ward Booth RP, Williams ED 1989 The fate of miniplates in facial trauma and orthognathic surgery. British Journal of Oral and Maxillofacial Surgery 27: 306–315
14 Battersby TG 1974 The plating of mandibular fractures. British Journal of Surgery 1: 79
15 Lodde JP, Champy M 1976 Justification biomecanique d'un nouveau materiel d'osteosynthese en chirurgie faciale. Annales de Chirurgie Plastique 21: 115–121
16 Kroon FH, Mathisson M, Cordey JR, Rahn BA 1991 The use of miniplates in mandibular fractures. An in vitro study. Journal of Craniomaxillofacial Surgery 19(5): 199–204
17 Carter DR, Blenman PR, Beaupre GS 1988 Correlations between mechanical stress history and tissue differentiation in initial fracture healing. Journal of Orthopaedic Research 6(5): 736–748
18 Brown JS, Grew N, Taylor C, Millar BG 1991 Intermaxillary fixation compared to miniplate osteosynthesis in the management of the

fractured mandible: an audit. British Journal of Oral and Maxillofacial Surgery 29(5): 308–311

19 Newman L 1995 The role of autologous primary rib grafts in the treatment of fractures of the atrophic mandible. British Journal of Oral and Maxillofacial Surgery 33: 386–387

20 Luhr HG, Reidick T, Merten HA 1996 Results of treatment of fractures of the atrophic mandible by compression plating: evaluation of 84 cases. Journal of Oral and Maxillofacial Surgery 54: 250–254

21 Rasse M 2000 Recent developments in therapy of condylar fractures of the mandible. Mund Kiefer Gesichtschir 4(2): 69–87

22 Kim YK, Yeo HH, Lim SC 1997 Tissue response to titanium plates: a transmitted electron microscopic study. Journal of Oral and Maxillofacial Surgery 55(4): 322–326

23 Jorgenson DS, Mayer MH, Ellenbogen RG, Centeno JA, Johnson FB, Mullick FG, Manson PN 1997 Detection of titanium in human tissues after craniofacial surgery. Plastic Reconstructive Surgery 97: 976–979

8 Alloplastic Biomaterials for Facial Reconstruction

Barry L Eppley

Introduction

The use of implantable biomaterials and devices plays a critical role in reconstruction of most traumatic facial injuries, particularly that of the underlying bony skeleton. Significant advances in materials science and engineering during the latter half of last century have made the internal use of alloplastic implants an integral part of many primary and secondary facial procedures. Their frequency of modern surgical use can also be traced to the simultaneous development of broad-spectrum antibiotics, an improved understanding of the healing of bone and soft tissues and the remarkable tolerance of well-vascularized facial tissues to alloplastic materials.

As these alloplastic implants are made from a wide array of biomaterials and have diverse physical structures and properties, the facial surgeon may have difficulty interpreting the merits of the particular biomaterial and its appropriateness for the specific facial site. As the immediate future will bring not only new types of biomaterials but also promises to merge pharmacologic technology (e.g. antibiotics, growth factors) with existing biomaterials, completely new types of surgical implants will be forthcoming in the near future. It is therefore imperative that the facial surgeon develop a fundamental knowledge base upon which informed decisions concerning the selection of a synthetic implant can be made, based upon their chemical composition, physical structure and the proposed site of tissue implantation.

Alloplastic Materials, Biocompatibility and Wound Healing

The concept of an alloplastic material is synonymous with the term 'synthetic'. This indicates that they are manufactured from non-human, non-animal and hence non-organic sources. Therefore, they should not be confused with allografts, heterografts or xenogeneic materials which are derived from organic sources and represent a completely different type of surgical implant which carries different risk considerations from alloplastic materials (e.g. immunologic rejection, transmission of viral diseases). Alloplastic implants provide an array of reconstructive materials that offer solutions to many facial needs and often simplify the operative procedure in terms of time and complexity of technique.

For the alloplastic material to be clinically successful, it must be *biocompatible*, implying an acceptable interaction between the host and the implanted material. The level of

material biocompatibility is influenced by several major factors, including the host reaction to the physical characteristics of the implant material, the tissue site of implantation and the surgical technique of placement.[1] The difficulty in developing consistent and long-term biomaterial success after implantation underscores the complex interactions between an implant and the body and explains why so few safe and effective biomaterials exist despite the tremendous advances that have been made in biomaterial development and engineering over the past 50 years.

The end-stage healing response to most biomaterials is the formation of an enveloping fibroconnective tissue scar or fibrous encapsulation. This is initiated with the surgical implantation procedure which generates an acute inflammatory response due to the induced tissue damage and is subsequently followed by a cascade of events including chronic inflammation, granulation tissue development, foreign body reaction and ultimately an enveloping fibrosis. This fibrous capsule represents the body's reparative response, which is to separate the body from the foreign material, and is, in essence, a biologic barrier between self and non-self. Almost all biomaterials implanted in the face will develop a surrounding fibrous scar with the one exception of metallic plates used for bone fixation which can develop bone attachment directly to the implant.

Principles of Facial Alloplastic Material Selection and Surgical Placement

While the composition of the alloplastic material implanted has an impact on biocompatibility, the anatomic location of placement and the surgical technique used to put it there carry an equal, and often greater, impact on long-term clinical success. Ensuring that the biomaterial is appropriately matched to the tissue plane within which it will be implanted is ultimately the responsibility of the treating surgeon.

The tissue quality of the recipient site must be initially assessed and emphasis is placed on *vascularity* and *adequacy of soft tissue coverage*. Decreased vascularity due to scar or prior surgeries or irradiation compromises the establishment of a normal fibrovascular tissue encapsulation and significantly limits a proper inflammatory response should the surface of the biomaterial become inoculated or infected secondarily. Soft tissue coverage over an implant should be as thick as possible. As a general rule, the thinner the overlying tissue coverage, the greater the likelihood over time that implant exposure or extrusion may occur. Alloplastic implants that are more deeply placed (e.g. subperiosteal, submuscular) rarely develop exposure. Implants placed immediately under the skin or with thin overlying subcutaneous fat may develop eventual thinning of the skin, particularly if the material lacks sufficient *flexibility* or if it is placed in an area of significant *tissue mobility*. In either case, the overlying dermis of the skin thins due to pressure of the underlying avascular implant. Placement of an implant into or through a tissue plane of existing or recent *contamination* significantly increases the risk of subsequent infection. As most alloplastic implants never establish an intramaterial vascular supply and have an affinity for bacterial adhesion, alloplastic tolerance is very low for contaminated wounds or in direct proximity to facial sinuses. Fortunately, implant placement in the face is fairly forgiving.

The *size of the implant* should be considered in relation to that of the tissue pocket or wound cavity. An implant that places the surrounding soft tissue under tension is more likely to extrude or develop exposure, particularly if there are other simultaneous adverse tissue or implant characteristics. In certain clinical situations, the overlying soft tissue can safely stretch and expand to accommodate large biomaterial placements. However, this is most safely done when the implant has a thick overlying soft tissue layer or is placed in the submuscular plane.

Lastly, implant mobility should be minimized by *fixation* to the most stable adjacent structure whenever practical or be placed in a well-contained, healthy tissue pocket. This not only ensures the desired postoperative implant position but prevents migration or exposure of the implant to other less desired tissue planes.

Patients undergoing alloplastic facial implants should receive an intravenous antibiotic infusion during placement followed by a postoperative oral course. Other than coverage for staphylococcus or streptococcus, dependent upon the path of insertion (intraoral, transcutaneous, transconjunctival), no specific antibiotic or duration of administration has yet been shown to be of superior clinical advantage. The rationale for antibiotic coverage is to prevent or eliminate any bacterial inoculation that may have occurred on the implant surface. No large clinical trials have been conducted to confirm that this is true but it appears to have no compelling disadvantage. Additional antibiotic coverage in certain types of facial implants is often sought by washing or soaking of the implant prior to intraoperative insertion. The value of this technique is best determined by the hydrophilicity or wetting ability of the implant material. An increased hydrophilic nature of a biomaterial allows increased amounts of antibiotic solution to be drawn into the implant. Whether this antibiotic impregnation actually lowers the postoperative infection rate is unknown but this intraoperative technique is widely used, particularly in non-metal implants. In less hydrophilic or overtly hydrophobic biomaterials, antibiotic soaking only mechanically removes any bacteria or contamination that has inadvertently become attached to the implant surface during the placement process. Therefore, it is likely no more effective than washing with any non-antibiotic solution.

Intraoperative handling of the implant is another method of decreasing the risk of postoperative infection. Extensive handling or exposure of the implant prior to insertion should be avoided. The implant should not be removed from its sterile packaging until the pocket or recipient site has been fully dissected and irrigated. Once removed from its sterile package or container, the implant should be handled by instruments with minimal contact with the contaminated gloved hand. Ideally, new gloves should be used if the implant is to be manually handled. Lastly, implant contact with the surrounding skin or oral cavity should be minimized to prevent a final source of bacterial transmission onto the implant surface. Whether these intraoperative techniques actually decrease the risk of postoperative infection is difficult to prove but they appear to be reasonable and prudent precautions to decrease potential postoperative complications.

Alloplastic Implant Types

While many types of implants have been used over the past 25 years, only some classifications of biomaterials have a significant clinical history of successful use for either soft or hard tissue replacement and repair. The following biomaterials are currently commercially available for surgical implantation: the polymers dimethysiloxane, polytetrafluoroethylene, polyethylene, polyesters, polyamides and acrylic, titanium and gold metals, calcium phosphate-based biomaterials and cyanoacrylate adhesives.

Dimethylsiloxane (silicone)

The use of silicone is widespread throughout many areas of medicine and surgery with a remarkable paucity of significant adverse tissue reactivity. Its use in the face is primarily as onlay implants for reconstruction of zygomatic, maxillary, nasal and mandibular contours (Fig. 8.1). Silicone is a polymer created from interlinking silicon and oxygen (positions 14 and 8 respectively on the Periodic Table of Elements) with methyl side groups (only *non-carbon* chain polymer used in all medical implantation devices). As a result, the backbone of this polymer has alternating monomers of dimethylsiloxane ($SiO(CH_3)_2$) which is extremely resistant to degradation in the body due to the very strong and stable silicon–oxygen bonds. When the monomers of dimethylsiloxane are linked together, polydimethylsiloxane is formed and the amount of crosslinking between different strands of polydimethylsiloxane results in variable physical forms. With minimal crosslinking, a gel is formed which was commonly used as the filler material for breast implants. When combined with silica particles and other chemical reagents, a silicone gel can be converted (i.e. vulcanized) into a solid rubber. Varying the elasticity of silicone rubber allows it to have great clinical versatility for its use as various facial implants. The excellent biocompatibility of silicone materials in the body may have some relation to its close proximity to carbon (position number 6) on the Periodic Table of Elements.[2]

Implants composed of solid silicone represent one of the earliest alloplastic materials used with extensive applications

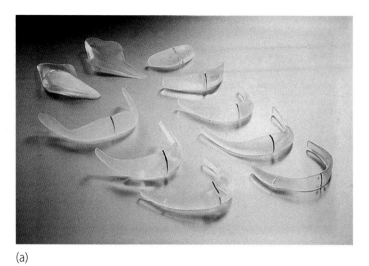
(a)

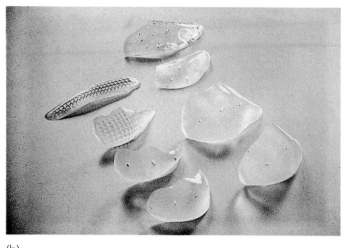
(b)

Fig. 8.1: Silicone (silastic) implants available for a wide variety of onlay facial contouring procedures. **(a)** Mandibular chin implants. **(b)** Midfacial malar implants.

for facial skeletal augmentation procedures.[3] While initially developed for use in the chin, an extensive array of implants are now available for every conceivable facial site including the chin, parasymphysis, inferior border and mandibular ramus (angle), paranasal, infraorbital, maxillary, malar, orbital floor and globe, nasal dorsum and columella, as well as the ear (Fig. 8.1). Solid silicone offers the advantages of easy sterilization by steam autoclaving or irradiation without degradation of the implant, is easily modified intraoperatively by scalpel or scissors, retains its flexibility through a wide temperature range, can be stabilized by suture or screw fixation through the implant and is very economical in cost.

Solid silicone has a high degree of chemical inertness, is hydrophobic, extremely resistant to degradation and no significant clinical toxicity or allergic reactions appear to exist. Tissue ingrowth or attachment to the implant does not occur and it acts as a relatively inert filler with a predictable surrounding fibrous encapsulation which may change very little, if at all, over a long period of implantation. When the implant is exposed to mechanical loading, fragmentation of the material and a synovitis may occur due to its poor mechanical properties. Therefore, it should not be used in the temporomandibular joint as an arthroplastic or interface material.

Polytetrafluoroethylene

The perfluorocarbons represent a very biocompatible group of carbon-based biomaterials with use in almost every specialty of surgery, as well as dentistry. They have a carbon ethylene backbone to which is attached four fluorine molecules (PTFE).

The bonding of highly reactive fluorine to carbon creates an extremely stable biomaterial which is not biodegradable in the body due to the lack of any known human enzyme to disrupt the fluorine–carbon bonds.[2,3] In addition to its chemical stability, its surface is very non-adherent with significant antifrictional properties. Due to the lack of crosslinking in its

molecular structure, it is very flexible with a low tensile strength.

PTFE was originally introduced in facial surgery in the 1980s as a skeletal augmentation material known as Proplast, in which it was combined with either graphite (Proplast I), alumina (Proplast II) or hydroxyapatite (Proplast-HA) as either preformed or block facial implants. It is now no longer available in the United States due to its withdrawal, from the misconceived approach of using it in the temporomandibular joint as either a meniscal replacement or as part of a glenoid fossa or condylar joint prosthesis where it was exposed to mechanical loads resulting in delamination, material fragmentation, particulation and subsequent foreign body reactions.

PTFE has now been 'reborn' as a subcutaneous augmentation material (SAM, WL Gore, Flagstaff, AZ). Based on the manufacturer's extensive experience with other surgical implants composed of PTFE (vascular prostheses, soft tissue patches, sutures), a variety of blocks, preformed implants, strips and strands are available for facial augmentation from subperiosteal to subdermal placement (Fig. 8.2). Essentially, the material is composed of fine expanded PTFE fibrils which are oriented and held together by solid pieces of the same material. The fibrillar composition results in non-interconnected surface openings with pore sizes of 10–30 μm. This allows for some soft tissue ingrowth, less fibrous encapsulation and little tendency for migration. The material is easily shaped with scalpel and scissors, may be resterilized if not used (stable at temperatures up to 325°F), threads easily through subcutaneous tissue and into tissue pockets and can be anchored to adjacent tissues by sutures or screws.

With its long history of use as a vascular prosthesis since 1975 and in other abdominal and thoracic surgery applications, its clinical safety is well established and extensive histologic evaluations of its tissue response have been done. It has been approved as an implant material for facial applications since 1994 and has been widely employed for subdermal implantation in the lip, nasolabial folds, glabella, nasal dorsum and other subcutaneous facial defects, as slings for

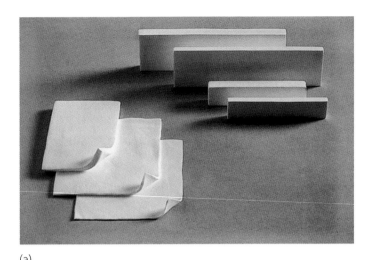

(a)

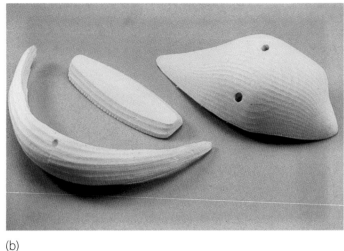

(b)

Fig. 8.2: Gore-Tex SAM (subcutaneous augmentation material) implants available as strands and cords for subdermal implantation and blocks **(a)** preformed implants **(b)** for subperiosteal onlay implantation.

ptotic tissues of the eyelid and face and for bony augmentation of the midface, malar and mandibular areas.[4,5] In block form, its compressive deformability by handling has been improved by the addition of reinforcement layers. Its ease of removal in subcutaneous sites due to the lack of significant ingrowth offers an advantage in the event of infection or if additional augmentation or modification of the material is required secondarily. In areas of thin skin with little subcutaneous substance (e.g. nasal dorsum), PTFE like all other inorganic materials should be used cautiously due to the higher potential for secondary complications.[6]

Polyethylene

This biomaterial has a simple carbon chain structure that differentiates it from PTFE by the lack of fluorination of the ethylene monomer. It is currently available commercially in three major grades: low and high density and ultrahigh molecular weight polyethylene (PE). Ultrahigh molecular weight PE is used for load-bearing orthopedic implant fabrications due to its superior mechanical properties with little propensity for creep. High-density PE (HDPE) is used in facial surgery due to its higher tensile strength over low-density grades. Like PTFE, it is non-resorbable and highly biocompatible with no tendency for chronic inflammatory reactions. While HDPE and PTFE are chemically similar, HDPE has a much more firm consistency that resists material compression but permits a degree of flexibility. In addition, it has an intramaterial porosity with a pore size between 125 and 250 μm which permits extensive fibrovascular ingrowth throughout the implant. Limited bone ingrowth may occur in select clinical circumstances but the material should not be considered osteoconductive.

While it can be produced in a variety of physical forms, it initially experienced significant use as a mesh for abdominal and chest wall reconstruction (Marlex) and is still favored by some surgeons due to its superior tensile strength. More recently, high-density polyethylene (HDPE) has been used successfully as a facial augmentation material with a variety

of preformed facial, ear, orbital and cranial implants available[7,8] (Medpor, Porex Medical, Fairburn, GA) (Fig. 8.3). The fibrous ingrowth into HDPE has several important clinical manifestations: eventual stabilization of the implant to the recipient site, more difficulty with secondary removal and minimal settling (underlying bone resorption) of the implant in areas of overlying soft tissue tension (e.g. chin). HDPE can be shaped intraoperatively with some difficulty compared to other softer biomaterials, can be loaded with antibiotics by syringe vacuum impregnation (displaces the air within the material, the material itself is hydrophobic) and accepts drilling and fixation techniques without fracturing the implant. Care should be taken when placing the material immediately underneath a thin soft tissue cover as it can be exposed by trauma or develop subsequent infection.

Polyesters

The polyester compounds are one of the most widely used families of biomaterials in surgery. They comprise a diverse

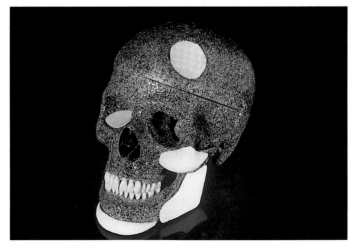

Fig. 8.3: Polyethylene craniofacial implants which demonstrate the porous surface of the material and a variety of onlay facial applications.

group of surgical devices that have a wide range of shapes (e.g. suture, mesh, vascular conduits, plates and screws) and sites of tissue implantation, with physical properties that extend from resorbable to permanent implants. They are composed of either large linear aromatic (permanent) or aliphatic (resorbable) thermoplastic polymers by the establishment of ester linkages between the carbon bonds.

Polyethylene terephthalate

Besides suture materials, the most widely recognized surgical implants of this group are the synthetic meshes such as Dacron (DuPont Chemical, Philadelphia, PA) and Mersilene (Ethicon, Somerville, NJ), also known as polyethylene terephthalate (PET). This material has a long history as knitted and woven prostheses for arterial vessel replacement. Like Marlex, PET mesh is also used for abdominal and chest wall replacement. The knitted multifilament mesh material is essentially non-reactive, becomes encased in an interwoven fibrous tissue matrix and should be non-resorbable. It has found limited applications in facial surgery but has some proponents as an onlay facial and nasal augmentation material. It is now primarily used in genioplasty procedures where it is rolled onto itself, sutured, shaped and inserted as an onlay to the symphyseal region.[9] Due to the fibrous ingrowth and its soft flexible nature, fixation to the implantation site without palpable edges is usually assured. Secondary removal may be difficult, however, and it is often necessary to remove a cuff of surrounding tissue. For this reason, use of PET mesh in areas of thin overlying skin (e.g. nose) should be avoided.

A special use of PET mesh was its application as a craniofacial reconstructive material where it was reinforced with polyurethane (Xomed, Jacksonville, FLA). Available in either a mandibular reconstructive tray or as a sheet for cranial coverage, it offered the capability of providing a porous material for either bone graft containment or defect coverage. Due to the development of metallic mesh and other more stable metal reconstructive systems, Dacron-polyurethane implants are rarely used today.

Resorbable polymers

The aliphatic polyesters are the most widely utilized class of resorbable polymers in surgery today and the poly(α-hydroxy) acids, consisting of six-membered lactone rings known as lactide and glycolide, comprise most resorbable implantable devices commercially sold. Through ring opening polymerization of lactide and glycolide, the homopolymers of polylactic (PLA) and polyglycolic (PGA) acids are created. With over 20 years of human use, these resorbable polymers have a very safe history and this accounts for the wide array of surgical devices available.

While the clinical applications for these polymers extend from tissue repair and regeneration to drug delivery in a wide range of medical and dental specialties, they initially achieved awareness in surgery as braided resorbable suture material. Beginning with the introduction of Dexon suture (pure PGA,

Davis & Geck, Wayne, NJ) in 1971, a co-polymer of PGA/PLA suture (Vicryl, 90% PGA/10% PLA, Ethicon, Somerville, NJ) soon followed. More recently, improvements in handling properties have been obtained by the development of smooth resorbable monofilament sutures composed of new poly(α-hydroxy) acids including Maxon (polyglyconate = glycolide/trimethylene carbonate co-polymer, Davis & Geck) and Monocryl (polyglecaprone 25 = glycolide/e-caprolactone co-polymer, Ethicon).

From a non-suture implant standpoint, the most common current application in facial surgery is as bone fixation devices. Introduced in 1996, plates and screws composed of 82% PLA and 18% PGA (LactoSorb, Walter Lorenz Surgical, Jacksonville, FLA) became available for craniomaxillofacial applications. This co-polymer combination captures the more hydrophilic and rapidly resorbing PGA with the more hydrophobic and very slowly resorbing PLA to produce workable fixation devices that maintain strength long enough (6–8 weeks) for craniofacial bone healing while assuring eventual complete resorption (approximately 1 year depending upon polymer mass and site of implantation) without inflammatory reactions.

Like suture material, the resorption of these devices is a two-phase process beginning with a physicochemical process of absorption of water (hydrolysis), which separates the ester linkages, followed by a metabolic cellular response through fibrovascular ingrowth which permits macrophages to clear the monomeric debris.[10] As a general rule, molecular weight reduction via hydrolysis precedes strength loss which precedes mass loss. Thus, a resorbable implant will have lost its mechanical strength long before the polymer material is resorbed. The use of essentially amorphous (very little to no crystallinity, low molecular weight) polymeric materials appears to be the primary reason why previous negative experiences in orthopedic and maxillofacial surgery with inflammation and lack of device resorption have not occurred with these contemporary resorbable implants. While achieving initial success in immature bone in pediatric craniofacial surgery, their use has now been successfully extended to midfacial fracture sites[11,12] (Fig. 8.4). Further work is needed to determine their potential effectiveness in more load-bearing applications for the mandible.

Given the large number of resorbable implants currently in use in orthopedic surgery (suture anchors, bone pins, meniscal staples, bone plates, bone screws) and the diverse number of new poly (α) esters and manufacturing methods available, different polymeric varieties of resorbable implants for craniomaxillofacial surgery from various manufacturers are assured in the immediate future.

Polyamide

Polyamides are organopolymer derivatives of nylon, chemically related to the polyester family of materials, and are best known clinically as a mesh material (Supramid).[3] They are very hydroscopic, structurally unstable in vivo and undergo hydrolytic degradation. Histologically, the material is degraded with a mild foreign body reaction. While once used

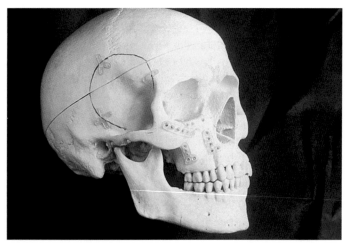

(a)

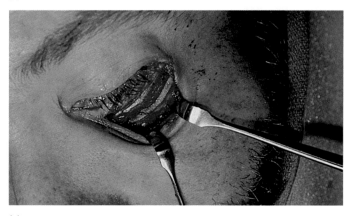

(c)

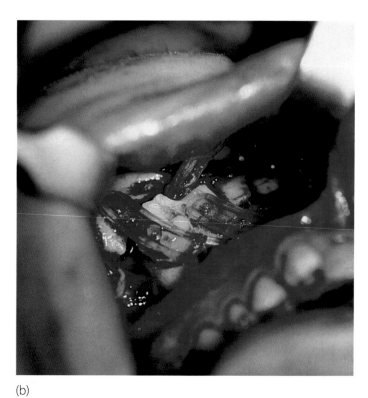

(b)

Fig. 8.4: (a) Resorbable polymer (LactoSorb) craniomaxillofacial bone plate and screw fixation devices used in the fixation of facial fractures. **(b)** Zygomatic fracture fixation with cranial bone grafts across the face of the maxilla. **(c)** Infraorbital rim fracture fixation.

for nasal contouring and augmentation genioplasty, clinical experience demonstrated that fibrosis and resorption of the material occur over time. While still used by some surgeons for orbital floor reconstruction, this material is now largely of historical interest.

Acrylic

Acrylic biomaterials are derived from polymerized esters of either acrylic or methylacrylic acids. With a long history of use in orthopedic surgery as a bone cement for joint prostheses, polymethyl methacrylate resin (PMMA) is fabricated intraoperatively (cold curing) by mixing a liquid monomer with a powdered polymer. An exothermic reaction results (temperatures can be as high as 80°C) as the two polymers cure (8–10 minutes), creating a rigid, nearly translucent plastic. While the monomer is extremely allergenic and cytotoxic, the mixing and initial polymerization process occurs outside the body and very little free monomer ever comes into tissue contact. Once formed, PMMA is impervious, non-biodegradable and is tolerated in the body by the development of a relatively avascular fibrous capsule. While having a long history of use in orthopedic surgery as a bone cement for fixation of joint replacements, it has achieved its greatest use in plastic surgery for cranioplasty procedures for filling full-thickness cranial defects or in secondary forehead contouring[13] (Fig. 8.5).

Specifically, it is a powdered mixture of methyl methacrylate polymer and methyl methacrylate-styrene copolymer and a benzyl peroxide monomer, being essentially identical to the acrylic materials used in dentistry (Cranioplastic, Codman and Shurleff, Randolph, MA). This mixture offers numerous advantages for these procedures including a very low cost, intraoperative fabrication and adaptation (contourable with a handpiece and burr after curing), can be loaded with antibiotics by mixing antibiotic powder in the acrylic resin, is very durable and can be heated or autoclaved without change in its physical form. While PMMA is rigid, the adjunctive use of metal mesh reinforcement decreases the risk of fracture on impact and more closely approximates the strength of cranial bone. Due to the capability of antibiotic impregnation and its documented postoperative release, PMMA beads have been used in the treatment of infected craniofacial fractures and reconstructions.

There are, however, several unique disadvantages with PMMA. It has a very profound and offensive odor when mixed which has caused allergic reactions through its fumes in operative personnel in the same room (female support staff who are pregnant or are trying to become pregnant should be asked to leave the operating room), the high cure temperatures require cool irrigation after placement until set to prevent thermal damage to adjacent tissues, and the material has a very high bacterial adhesion property which makes it poorly tolerated in the body once infected or in close prox-

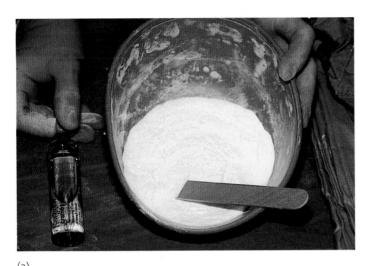

(a)

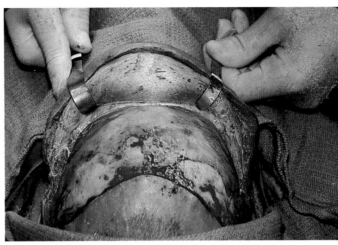

(b)

Fig. 8.5: Liquid monomer and powdered PMMA polymer which is mixed and cured intraoperatively for a frontal cranioplasty. **(a)** Liquid and powder components. **(b)** Cured in situ for frontal cranioplasty.

imity to the oral cavity, air-filled sinuses or in tissues with recent infection.[14] Furthermore, thinning of the overlying skin, implant exposure and infection can occur with long-term implantation in pediatric cranioplasties.

A distinct variation of PMMA with some different physical properties is HTR, an acronym for hard tissue replacement. It is a composite of polymethylmethacrylate (PMMA) and polyhydroxyethylmethacrylate (pHEMA) and has significant strength, interconnected porosity, marked hydrophilicity and a calcium hydroxide coating that imparts a negative surface charge. While it has a long clinical history of use in dentistry and jaw implantation as a granular bone replacement material, it is also available as a preformed (heat-cured) craniofacial implant that is custom manufactured to the patient's defect from a CT scan (HTR-PMI, Walter Lorenz Surgical, Jacksonville, FLA). It is useful as a replacement for large full-thickness defects involving the cranial, frontal and orbital regions where sufficient autologous material may not be available or there is significant morbidity with the size of the donor defect (Fig. 8.6). This typically occurs when craniotomy bone flaps are lost due to postoperative infection or when significant cranial bone is lost due to trauma. Unlike traditional PMMA, the interconnected porosity of the material allows extensive fibrovascular ingrowth throughout the implant and may allow for some limited bony ingrowth at the implant–tissue interface.[15] The custom designing of the implant allows for a reconstructive procedure that produces an optimal cranial contour in a short period of operative time. The precise interlocking of the implant to the defect allows for good stabilization or the material may be drilled and fixation hardware applied. Cost of this reconstructive approach is significantly higher than pure PMMA due to the CT scan and preoperative implant fabrication time.

Metals

Metals have been used in facial surgery for the past 30 years for skull reconstruction, repair and reconstruction of cranio-

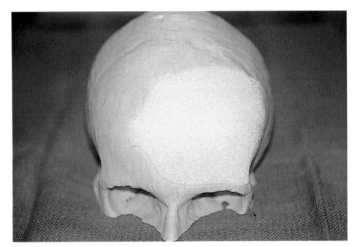

Fig. 8.6: Computer-generated cranial implant, composed of sintered HTR granules creating an anatomic prosthesis with interconnected porosity, for reconstruction of a large frontal-orbital defect.

facial and upper extremity skeletal injuries, and most recently as an adjunct to oral and craniofacial prosthetic rehabilitation. The biocompatibility of metal implants is primarily determined by their surface properties and corrosion (electrochemical conversion of a metal to its base compounds) resistance. After implantation, an oxide layer quickly forms on the metal's surface which determines its resistance to corrosion and the amount of leaching of metals or oxides to the adjacent tissues.[16] The combination of corrosion and metal ion release may cause pain and localized tissue reactions around the implant, necessitating its removal. Migration of metal ions to distant tissue and organ sites has been reported but their long-term implications are presently unknown.

Essentially, stainless steel, vitallium and titanium have been used successfully in human implantation. Stainless steel implants (alloy of iron, nickel and molybdenum with a surface layer of chromium oxide), however, have a higher corrosion potential, greater amount of metal ion release and are more likely to require secondary removal. The nickel content also contributes to an increased incidence of allergic reactions. As a result, the use of stainless steel for craniofacial implants has dramatically decreased. Vitallium was introduced in the 1930s to help overcome the corrosion problem with stainless steel. It is a cobalt-chromium alloy that has comparable strength to stainless steel and its development as a bone-plating system in the 1980s helped revolutionize facial skeletal surgery.[17] While it also forms a chromium oxide surface layer, it is much more highly resistant to corrosion than stainless steel due to its higher concentration of chromium in the alloy. Due to radiographic imaging and artefact scatter concerns, vitallium has subsequently lost favor for most craniofacial indications due to the increased popularity of titanium where these issues are not a concern.

Unlike other metals manufactured for medical devices, titanium is a pure material (element 22 on the Periodic Table) and, perhaps for this reason, there have been no reports of titanium allergy, toxicity or tumorigenesis. It is most commonly manufactured and available clinically as either pure titanium or as an alloy with small amounts of other metals (e.g. Ti-6A1-4V, 6% aluminum and 4% vanadium) which improve the strength of the material considerably. Titanium

forms a titanium oxide surface layer which is very adherent and highly resistant to corrosion and even if the oxide layer is damaged, it reforms in milliseconds. This superior corrosion resistance makes titanium highly biocompatible. In addition, the low density of the metal allows it to have minimal X-ray attenuation and hence a lack of artefact on CT or MR images. These properties, combined with its strength, make titanium the best metal currently available for the requirements of craniomaxillofacial bone stabilization [18] (Fig. 8.7).

Titanium has developed a unique role due to its association with the concept of osseo-integration. Osseo-integration is defined as a direct contact between metal and bone, without a fibrous interface, at the light microscopic level. This healing response provides the needed stability for long-term retention of bone-anchored dental prostheses. While the biocompatibility of titanium for this purpose is important, other parameters also contribute, including surgical technique (keeping the thermal insult to the bone during drilling to less than 44° C), osseous quality of the implant bed, implant design and exposure to amount and duration of postoperative loading conditions.[19] The scientific principle of osseo-integration of titanium implants has revolutionized prosthetic reconstruction of the edentulous mandible and maxilla as well as single tooth replacement. Its success in the demanding intra-

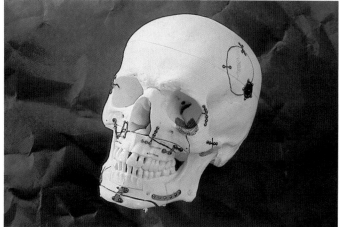
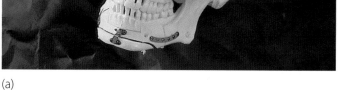

(a)

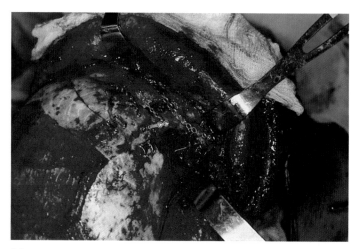

(b)

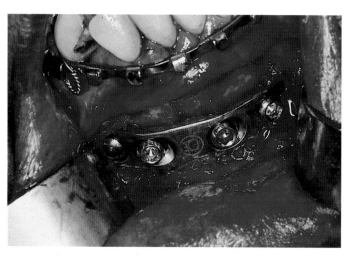

(c)

Fig. 8.7: (a) Titanium plates and screws are the standard method of metal fixation of all facial fractures. **(b)** Complex fronto-orbital zygomatic fracture fixation. **(c)** Mandibular symphyseal fracture fixation.

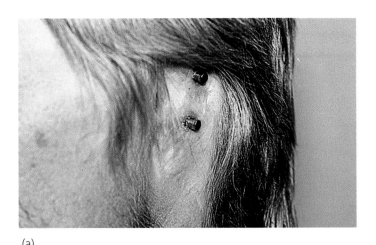

(a)

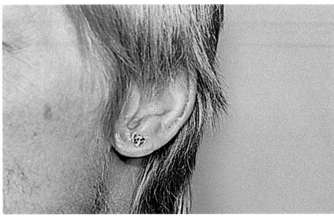

(b)

Fig. 8.8: Titanium endosseous implants placed into the mastoid for retention of an ear prosthesis after traumatic ear loss. **(a)** Preoperative ear loss. **(b)** Postoperative prosthetic ear in place.

oral environment has led to numerous craniofacial applications for extraoral retention of facial prostheses and hearing aids which have a reasonable retention rate even in irradiated bone (Fig. 8.8).

The newest application of titanium is in the form of bone-anchored suturing devices. Used as either a titanium anchor screw or a self-deploying barbed anchor, they are designed to be implanted into bone onto which resorbable or permanent sutures are placed. The suture anchor is composed of a titanium body with internal wire arcs (which spring apart after anchor insertion) composed of a titanium-nickel alloy (Nitonol). This provides a secure method for attaching soft tissue to a bone site. While utilized mainly in orthopedic surgery, their continued refinement and miniaturization have led to certain facial surgery applications such as orbital canthal repositioning and facial soft tissue re-attachment and suspensions.[20]

Lastly, we come to gold. While it was one of the first surgical implants, gold is only commonly used today in dentistry. Unlike other pure metals, gold is a noble element (number 79 on the Periodic Table) that does not develop a layer of oxide on its surface after implantation. As a result, it is exceptionally well tolerated in the body but is generally not used as a conventional metal implant due to its lack of strength (i.e. softness) and expense. It has one surgical use as an upper eyelid implant for the treatment of acquired ptosis in facial nerve palsies.[21] It is produced from 99.99% pure gold and is available in different spherically shaped sizes with weights between 0.6 and 1.6 grams (MedDev, Palo Alto, CA). The gold weights are placed in a subcutaneous plane above the tarsus and have a low rate of postoperative exposure or extrusion (Fig. 8.9).

Calcium phosphate

Implants composed of calcium phosphate have been commercially available for nearly 20 years as bone replacement/augmentation materials. Unlike most other alloplasts that are inert, these materials are bioactive (capable of osteoconduction) and have the potential to develop actual tissue ingrowth

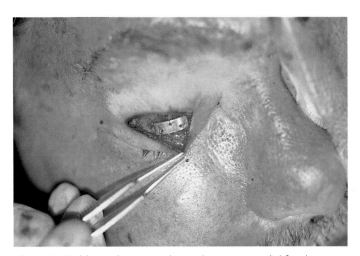

Fig. 8.9: Gold weight inserted into the upper eyelid for the treatment of lagophthalmos in traumatic facial nerve palsy.

and integration into the recipient site after placement. As a result, they are very well tolerated with essentially no inflammatory response, minimal fibrous encapsulation and no negative effects on local bone mineralization. Calcium phosphate materials are not osteo-inductive by themselves but they do provide a physical substrate onto which new bone from adjacent surfaces may be deposited and potentially guided into areas occupied by the material.

Almost all currently available calcium phosphate materials are manufactured as hydroxyapatite (HA)$(Ca_{10}(PO_4)_6(OH)_2)$, which is the principal inorganic component of bone accounting for up to 70% of the calcified skeleton. It can be manufactured as either ceramic or non-ceramic apatites and can be formed into a wide variety of physical configurations.

Ceramic hydroxyapatite is made from crystals which are sintered at high temperatures into a hard non-resorbable solid. Appearing initially as either dense granules or blocks, they became available in the early 1980s and were used in maxillofacial reconstruction, particularly alveolar ridge augmentation. The dense form of the granules was prone to migration prior to significant fibro-osseous ingrowth and the

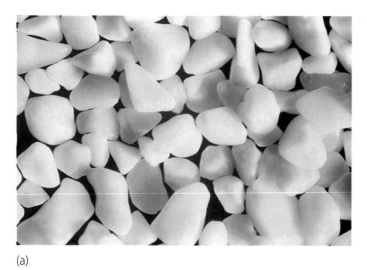

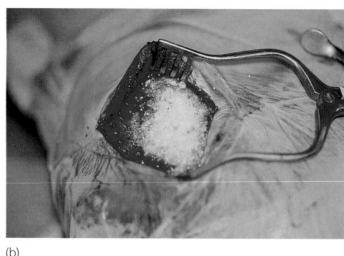

(a)   (b)

Fig. 8.10: (a) Porous hydroxyapatite granules used to fill in a small outer table defect in the frontal calvarium. Granules, 10×.
(b) Granules used to cover a small partial-thickness cranial defect which are held in place by a resorbable mesh cover to prevent migration.

dense blocks were difficult to shape and prone to extrusion. Therefore, dense HA was replaced by a different physical structure. Porous forms of HA are based on the structure of marine corals (calcium carbonate skeleton) which has interconnecting porosity of a size (50–200 μm) that permits fibrovascular and osseous ingrowth as well as the potential for cell-mediated resorption and osseous replacement. Of the available porous HA forms, the granules have achieved the greatest current use as an augmentation material for the craniofacial skeleton[22] (Fig. 8.10). The block forms have been primarily used as an interpositional graft material in facial skeletal osteotomies, are shaped and contoured with some difficulty due to potential fracturing and should not be used in load-bearing facial areas. After tissue ingrowth is complete, nearly half of the block implant remains as residual HA which does appear to resorb, albeit very slowly at approximately 1% per year. While very biocompatible and well tolerated after placement, preformed hydroxyapatite has been of less value than initially perceived due to con-

tinued handling and recipient site containment issues, inability to tolerate any significant load bearing and incomplete to no bony replacement.

Non-ceramic (i.e. not sintered to make a stable physical structure) forms of hydroxyapatite come as powder and liquid mixtures that are mixed intraoperatively, filled or contoured into the bony defect and subsequently convert in vivo by direct crystallization without heat formation to pure hydroxyapatite.[23] Multiple varieties of these mixtures currently exist which form a dense cement that sets in 5–30 minutes, dependent upon the types of calcium phosphate powders and liquid solvents used. After intraoperative setting, the material converts to hydroxyapatite within hours to days. Due to its limited shear resistance, its use is restricted to non-stress bearing craniofacial regions as an onlay contouring material[24] (Fig. 8.11). Experimental animal work indicates that initial fibrovascular ingrowth is followed by slow material resorption, without change in shape, and bone replacement. In humans, however, significant bony

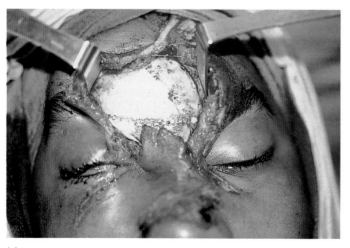

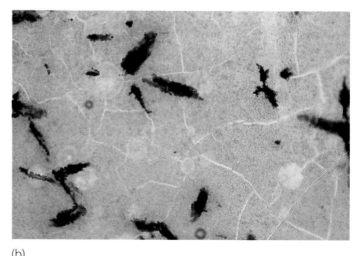

(a)   (b)

Fig. 8.11: (a) Hydroxyapatite liquid and powder composite used to reconstruct a traumatic impaction of the frontal bone after surrounding bone stabilization. **(b)** Histology demonstrating non-porous nature of the set material, undecalcified, Goldner's stain, 10×.

ingrowth and replacement has yet to be confirmed. Whether this biologic behavior changes with a longer period of implantation (e.g. 5–10 years) is not yet known given its short clinical history. The lack of shape changes postoperatively makes it ideal as an onlay reconstructive material.

Cyanoacrylate

The use of tissue adhesives in surgery has been studied for nearly three decades for diverse applications including tissue adhesion and wound closure, vascular embolization, hemostasis, closure of cerebrospinal fluid leaks and application of skin grafts. Historically, the autologous and homologous fibrin tissue adhesives have achieved the most use for these applications due to their safety and reliability. Synthetic cyanoacrylate derivatives first described in 1949, despite tremendous success for non-medical uses, have not been as successful for surgical purposes due to their handling problems and associated histoxicity. The adverse tissue reactions are due to the by products of cyanoacrylate polymer degradation, cyanoacetate and formaldehyde. This degradation is affected by the length of the alkyl (R) group of the cyanoacrylate derivative. Shorter chain derivatives such as methyl- and ethylcyanoacrylates degrade quickly but have more tissue toxicity than longer chain derivatives such as butyl-2-cyanoacrylate (Histoacryl, TriHawk International, Montreal, Canada). Histoacryl has sufficient strength and reliability for skin closure and is approved for use in Europe and Canada but not the United States.

A more recent cyanoacrylate derivative, octyl-2-cyanoacrylate (Dermabond, Ethicon, Somerville, NJ), has now been approved for skin closure in the United States. It has an eight carbon alkyl constituent off the carboxyl group which slows degradation and by product release into the surrounding tissues. Additionally, plasticizers have been added which make the adhesive bone both stronger (three times stronger than butyl-2-cyanoacrylate) and more durable but allowing flexion with the skin. Multiple studies have demonstrated its equivalence to 5–0 and 6–0 skin sutures in esthetic facial surgery and repair of traumatic facial wounds[25] (Fig. 8.12). It is important to remember, however, that dermal suture support is still needed (in wounds that traverse the full thickness of the dermis) and the superficial skin must be held together as the adhesive is applied to prevent deposition of the cyanoacrylate polymer into the wound, potentially delaying or preventing wound healing. The cost of a single ampoule of the material (generally enough to cover 15–20 cm of wound closure) is roughly twice that of conventional nylon suture for the same size wound.

Management of Alloplastic Infection

While a number of different complications can occur with any implant-related procedure (e.g. migration, extrusion, palpability),[26] the one common factor that is shared by all biomaterials is the risk of infection. Adhesion of bacteria to an implanted biomaterial surface is an essential step in the pathogenesis of infection and has been described as a two-phase process. There is an initial reversible physical phase (physicochemical interaction between bacteria and material surface) and an irreversible cellular phase (cellular interactions between bacteria and material surface). The initial attachment of bacteria to the material surface is the beginning of adhesion and occurs through actual contact between the two initiated by a variety of physical forces and may be reversed by mechanical washing or irrigation. In the second phase, a firmer adhesion of the bacteria to the surface occurs through a variety of bacterial surface polymeric structures including capsules, pili or slime. Once strongly adherent, this biofilm results in colonization, protection against phagocytosis, interference with the cellular immune response and reduction of antimicrobial agent effectiveness. It is likely that the reversible phase usually occurs intraoperatively during implantation and the second phase occurs in the early postoperative period which coincides with the timing of a large number of implant infections, typically appearing within weeks to months after the initial surgery.[27] Alloplast infections that occur years after implantation must be

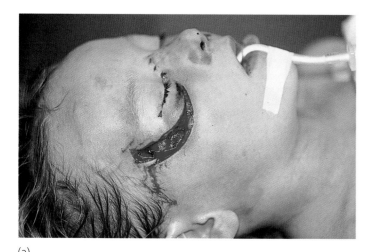
(a)

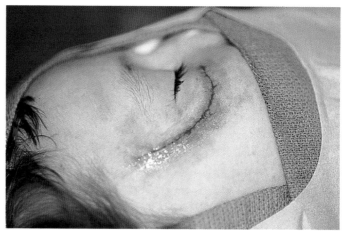
(b)

Fig. 8.12: Dermabond skin adhesive used on a large facial laceration from glass from a motor vehicle accident. **(a)** Open laceration. **(b)** Epidermis closed with adhesive after placement of dermal sutures.

initiated by hematogenous spread or by direct violation of the surrounding capsule (e.g. needle injection, secondary surgery).

When a purulent infection occurs, antibiotics and drainage alone will usually not provide a permanent solution. Once established, the bacterial biofilm is essentially impenetrable by antibiotics. At this point, drainage and removal of the material is advised. Reimplantation should not be done for at least 3–6 months to allow complete resolution of infection and inflammation in the adjacent tissues. Salvage of the alloplastic implant can be considered by its removal, extensive irrigation of the anatomic site, mechanical scrubbing and/or sterilizing the implant to remove the biofilm, reinsertion and a prolonged postoperative antibiotic course, providing the patient understands the inherent risk of recurrent infection with this approach.

Numerous biomaterial characteristics have been shown to influence bacterial adhesion, including chemical composition of the material (e.g. *S. epidermidis* often causes polymer implant infection, *S. aureus* is usually found in metal implant infections), surface roughness (irregular surfaces typically promote bacterial adhesion), surface configuration (bacteria colonize porous material surfaces preferentially) and surface hydrophobicity (hydrophilic materials are more resistant to bacterial adhesion than hydrophobic materials).[27] This would suggest that smooth, non-porous, non-resorbable biomaterials have lower rates of infection. However, alloplastic implant infections are multifactorial and the host–material interactions are far more complex than this simplistic explanation. It remains unclear at present whether any real infectious risk differences exist amongst the different alloplastic materials available and the varying clinical problems that they are designed to treat.

References

1 Rubin JP, Yaremchuk MJ 1997 Complications and toxicities of implantable biomaterials used in facial reconstructive and aesthetic surgery: a comprehensive review of the literature. Plastic and Reconstructive Surgery 100: 1336

2 Constantino PD 1994 Synthetic biomaterials for soft-tissue augmentation and replacement in the head and Neck. Otolaryngology Clinics of North America 27: 223

3 Eppley BL 1999 Alloplastic implantation. Plastic and Reconstructive Surgery 104: 1761

4 Lassus C 1991 Expanded PTFE in the treatment of facial wrinkles. Aesthetic Plastic Surgery 15: 167

5 Maas CS, Gnepp DR, Bumpous J 1993 Expanded polytetrafluoroethylene (Gore-Tex soft tissue patch) in facial augmentation. Archives of Otolaryngology and Head and Neck Surgery 119: 1008

6 Daniel RK 1994 The use of Gore-Tex for nasal augmentation: a retrospective analysis of 106 patients. Plastic and Reconstructive Surgery 94: 228

7 Bikhazi HB, van Antwerp R 1990 The use of Medpor in cosmetic and reconstructive surgery: experimental and clinical evidence. In: Stucker, F (Ed) Plastic and reconstructive surgery of the head and neck. Mosby, St Louis, p 271

8 Wellisz T 1993 Clinical experience with the Medpor porous polyethylene implant. Aesthetic Plastic Surgery 17: 339

9 McCullough EG, Hom DH, Weigel MT, Anderson JR 1990 Augmentation mentoplasty using Mersilene mesh. Otolaryngology and Head and Neck Surgery 116: 1154

10 Pietrzak WS, Sarver DS, Verstynen ML 1997 Bioabsorbable polymer science for the practicing surgeon. Journal of Craniofacial Surgery 8: 87

11 Eppley BL, Prevel CD, Sadove AM, Sarver D 1996 Resorbable bone fixation: its potential role in cranio-maxillofacial trauma. Journal of Craniomaxillofacial Trauma 2: 56

12 Eppley BL 2000 Zygomaticomaxillary fracture repair with resorbable plates and screws. Journal of Craniofacial Surgery 11: 377

13 Prolo D 1985 Cranial defects and cranioplasty. In: Wilkins RH, Rengachary SS (Eds) Neurosurgery, vol. 2. McGraw-Hill, New York, p 1647

14 Manson PN, Crawley WA, Hoopes JE 1986 Frontal cranioplasty: risk factors and choice of cranial vault reconstructive material. Plastic and Reconstructive Surgery 77: 888

15 Eppley BL, Sadove AM, German RB 1990 Evaluation of HTR polymer as a craniomaxillofacial graft material. Plastic and Reconstructive Surgery 86: 1085

16 Altobelli DE 1992 Implant materials in rigid fixation: physical, mechanical, corrosion, and biocompatibility considerations. In: Yaremchuk AJ, Gruss JS, Manson PN (Eds) Rigid fixation of the craniomaxillofacial skeleton. Butterworth-Heinemann, Boston

17 Munro IR 1989 The Luhr fixation system for the craniofacial skeleton. Clinics in Plastic Surgery 16: 41

18 Mercuri MR 1995 Titanium implants in maxillofacial reconstruction. Otolaryngology Clinics of North America 28: 351

19 Holt GR 1994 Osseointegrated implants in oro-dental and facial prosthetic rehabilitation. Otolaryngology Clinics of North America 27: 1001

20 Antonyshon OM, Weinberg MJ, Dagum AB 1996 Use of a new anchoring device for tendon reinsertion in medial canthopexy. Plastic and Reconstructive Surgery 98: 520

21 Kelly SA, Sharpe DT 1992 Gold eyelid weights in patients with facial palsy: a review. Plastic and Reconstructive Surgery 89: 436

22 Byrd HS, Hobar PC, Shewmake K 1993 Augmentation of the craniofacial skeleton with porous hydroxyapatite granules. Plastic and Reconstructive Surgery 91: 15

23 Costantino PD, Friedman CD, Jones K 1991 Hydroxyapatite cement. I.Basic chemistry and histologic properties. Arch Otolaryngol Head Neck Surgery 117: 379

24 Costantino PD, Friedman CD, Chow LC, Sisson GA 1992 Experimental hydroxyapatite cement cranioplasty. Plastic and Reconstructive Surgery 90: 174

25 Toriumi DM, O'Grady K, Desai D, Bagal A 1998 Use of octyl-2-cyanoacrylate for skin closure in facial plastic surgery. Plastic and Reconstructive Surgery 102: 2209

26 Rubin JP, Yaremchuk MJ 1997 Complications and toxicities of implantable biomaterials used in facial reconstructive and aesthetic surgery: a comprehensive review of the literature. Plastic and Reconstructive Surgery 100: 1336

27 An YH, Friedman RJ 1998 Concise review of mechanisms of bacterial adhesion to biomaterial surfaces. Journal of Biomedical Materials Research 43: 338

Section 2
Definitive Management

9 Surgical Access

Barry L Eppley

Introduction

Despite the importance of understanding the technical details of a specific facial surgical procedure, little can be accomplished without proper access through the skin or mucosa. Such access provides critical exposure to the defect site. With this exposure, the contemporary techniques of rigid fixation, placement of bone grafts or biomaterials or alteration of regional bony or soft tissue anatomy can be done. It can be argued, therefore, that a thorough understanding of the different methods of contemporary surgical access has permitted many of these more well-known advances in facial reconstructive surgery to be realized.

In traumatic injuries, a laceration often provides the access to complete the necessary repair of underlying facial structures. More commonly, however, additional facial or intraoral incisions are needed. In secondary reconstructions, use of old lacerations or completely new incisions are required. Either approach adds scar burden and potential associated morbidity which in the facial area may be as potentially deforming or visually noticeable as the original injury. Therefore, it is important that the surgical approach and its anatomical and technical aspects be understood and well executed. Often in facial reconstruction, getting there is far more difficult than what one does once there.

Many areas of the facial skeleton can be accessed by an intraoral approach and this should be the first choice. Those areas not accessed via the mouth can usually be reached via a coronal incision, made within the hair. Both these approaches minimize the risk of visible scars.

Periorbital fractures, in isolation, can be accessed by a transconjunctival approach and with a lateral canthoplexy, virtually all the common zygomatic fracture sites can be visualized.

Principles

The face is full of many intricate, delicate and vital structures from the scalp down to the neck. Rearranging and repairing many of these facial components is often not unduly difficult but exposing and finding them without additional morbidity can be. Unlike most surgical disciplines where a direct cutdown to the defect site is usually done, facial surgery often requires remote incisions with great emphasis on their healed esthetic result. The appearance of the incisional scar or revised laceration can add or detract from the facial result as much as the original traumatic problem.

Three factors separate facial access from the remainder of the body. First, the prominent location and social importance of the face mandates that incisions be placed in locations that are as inconspicuous as possible. Second, the presence of peripheral nerves makes both the location of the incisions and the dissection around them of critical importance. Loss of sensory input and, more importantly, weakness or loss of facial movement can be devastating for many patients and very difficult to correct secondarily. Third, the compact nature of facial structures exposes structures in the path of dissection to injury, particularly the more remote the incision is from the defect site. Complete knowledge of facial muscle, nerve, tendon, bone as well as dental anatomy is important to avoid such injuries. Naturally the intraoral approach should be used whenever possible to avoid skin incisions.

Incision Placement

Relaxed skin tension lines (RSTL)

The old concept of the lines of minimal tension (RSTL) is obvious in the older face and these lines are good choices for incision placement as they heal with less chance of scar hypertrophy and may be less noticeable due to decreased skin shadowing. In the younger face and in most cases of surgical access, however, this concept has less utility than is often perceived. RSTLs are of most value in scar revision and reconstruction of local defects due to resection of skin cancer. In most cases of facial access, no one would think of using any conspicuous skin area for incision placement. The first principle is to use a remote incision that lies in the nearest 'hidden' skin crease. Essentially, this creates a list of 14 basic facial incisions including the coronal, four periorbital (upper eyelid crease, supraorbital, lower eyelid subciliary, lower eyelid transconjunctival), five cervicofacial (high cervical, submental, retromandibular, rhytidectomy, pre-auricular), two transoral (maxillary and mandibular vestibular) and two nasal (endonasal, external open) incisions.

Short versus long incisions

In theory, a shorter incision results in less of a scar burden. Therefore, many surgeons limit their incisional length, often at the expense of adequate exposure. As the skin can stretch and slide over the surface of deeper structures, a short incision may be capable of moving over a considerable distance and permitting the necessary manipulation of the underlying structures. In a very limited number of facial procedures (e.g. repair of zygomatic arch fractures, endoscopic brow lift or subcondylar mandibular fracture repair), the short incision can serve as a remote portal for endoscope or instrument insertion.

On a practical basis, however, the use of remote skin creases permits their full length to be used without excessive scar as the crease is already hidden. Therefore, a longer incision is permitted as there is no disadvantage to using the full crease as long as one does not extend the incision beyond the anatomic boundary of the skin crease. For example, the full length of the pre-auricular incision can be used from the temporal hair line to the bottom of the earlobe or the subciliary incision can be used from the medial punctum to the lateral canthal crease as long as it does not extend beyond the lateral orbital rim.

Cold versus hot cutting

The use of 'cold steel' (scalpel) undoubtedly causes the least skin injury with only sharp cutting of the epidermal and dermal surfaces. Bleeding of the dermal edges may promote one to cauterize some of the edges, inducing the potential for increased scar formation. This temptation can be avoided by the use of preincisional infiltration with local anesthesia containing epinephrine. High concentrations work best and 1:100 000 epinephrine solutions work very well provided that one waits the obligatory 7–10 minutes for maximal vasoconstrictive effect. In addition, not all skin edges need to be immediately cauterized as most bleeding will stop with some pressure and time.

Despite these basic steps, it remains appealing to use a thermal instrument to do the skin and subcutaneous cutting for the immediate hemostatic effect. Traditionally, the use of cautery was associated with significant burning of the skin edges due to the width of the blade and the energies used. Today, fine-tip needle cautery composed of better metals and low energies makes it possible to significantly reduce the zone of the thermal injury on the skin edges (e.g. Colorado needle, Colorado Biomedical). It is particularly useful for periorbital and pre-auricular incisions without any increase in adverse scarring. It should not be used, however, in hair-bearing areas due to follicular injury and hair loss immediately adjacent to the incision. Hot cutting should never be used in the scalp and this inevitably results in a wider, more noticeable scar due to traumatic alopecia along the incision line.

Coronal Access

An incision in the hair line between the temporal regions provides unparalleled exposure to the upper craniofacial skeleton as well as to much of the orbitozygomatic regions. Fractures of the frontal bone and sinus, naso-orbital ethmoid region and Le Fort II and III patterns provide the main reason for its use in trauma. In exceptional cases, complex fractures of the zygomatic arch may justify its use. Its major advantages include the relative simplicity of its execution, negligible rate of complications and the hidden location of the scar within the hair line.

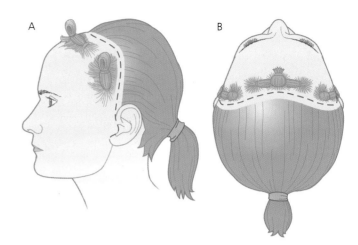

Fig. 9.1: Location of coronal incision 3–4 cm behind the frontal hairline.

Technical points

- The location of the incision in females and non-alopecic males in 3–4 cm behind the frontal and temporal hair line. In balding males, more of a W-pattern is chosen across the frontal component in anticipation of further recession. In the completely bald male, make the incision as if there were hair. It is remarkable how well bald scalp skin heals with minimal scarring (Fig. 9.1).
- The ability to turn the scalp flap and attain the desired skeletal exposure is dependent upon the inferior extent of the incisions in the temporal and auricular areas. The inferior extent of the incision can run in either the pre-auricular or postauricular areas without compromising anterior exposure. When placing the incision in the pre-auricular area, go retrotragal to further hide the scar (Fig. 9.1).
- Shaving the incision site is optional. Shaving the hair offers no significant improvement on postoperative wound infections. It does help the speed of closure and is more comfortable for the patient during suture removal.
- A large running W-plasty or zigzag pattern hides the scar better by intermingling the hair pattern around the scar (Figs 9.2, 9.3).
- Cut the incision with a scalpel down to the galea below the hair follicles. A thermal cautery can be used thereafter without increasing postoperative alopecia around the scar. Injectable vasoconstriction, clamps or running sutures are all preferable hemostatic measures to electrocautery for the skin edges.
- Raise the scalp flap forward in the subgaleal level. Only incise the periosteum directly above the bone area to be treated. This limits the amount of bleeding bone surface (Fig. 9.4).
- To avoid injury to the frontal branch of the facial nerve, stay at the deep temporal fascial level. The nerve lies lateral to the superficial layer of the temporalis fascia (Fig. 9.5). Incise the periosteum on the superior surface of the zygoma and zygomatic arch which will then reflect the superficial fascia outward, protecting the nerve (Figs 9.5, 9.6).

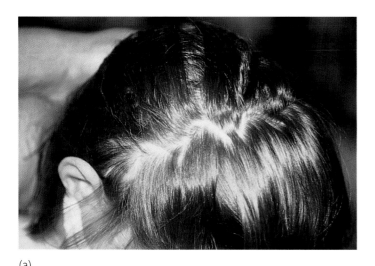

(a)

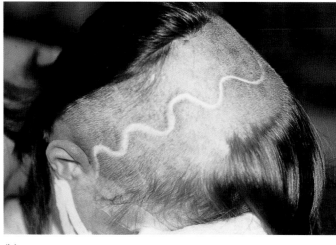

(b)

Fig. 9.2: Wavy coronal incision used in pediatric cranial vault surgery. **(a)** Preoperative view of secondary surgery showing the intermingling of the hair and hiding of the scar. **(b)** Scalp is shaved showing the width and pattern of the scar which hides itself fairly well despite being wider than desired.

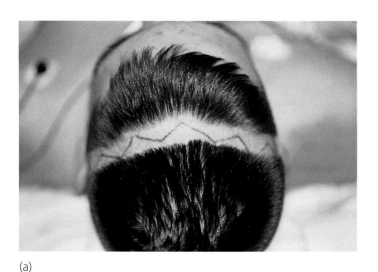

(a)

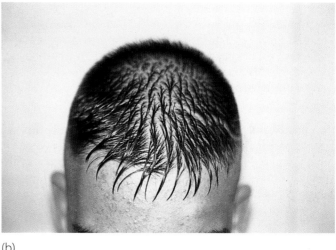

(b)

Fig. 9.3: Broken line, irregular coronal incision makes hair intermingle with improved camouflage of the scar. **(a)** Preoperative incision marking for frontal access. **(b)** Six month postoperative view through short hair.

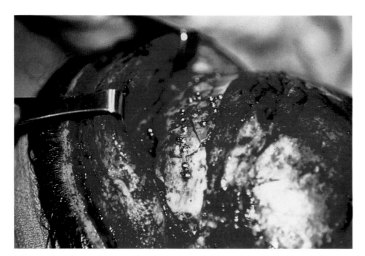

Fig. 9.4: Frontal sinus fracture repair. The periosteum is only incised and raised directly above the operative site which limits bone bleeding to the repair site.

- Across the supraorbital rim, dissect out the neurovascular bundle from the notch. When it is a foramen, do an ostectomy to release the bundle. Dissection can be carried onto the nasal bones and medial orbits easily. Look for the lacrimal sac and medial canthal tendons (Fig. 9.7).
- Prior to closure, resuspend all soft tissues if necessary, including the lateral canthal tendon and the temporalis muscle.
- The scalp skin closure should be done in two layers with non-strangulating sutures (non-interlocking) or staples.

From a coronal incision perspective, mention should be made of endoscopic scalp access. Although this is of very limited value in facial trauma and is used almost exclusively in endoscopic brow lifting, this approach may achieve wider application in the future as endoscopic techniques and instrumentation improve. At least two incisions are required for the placement of the endoscope through one (non-

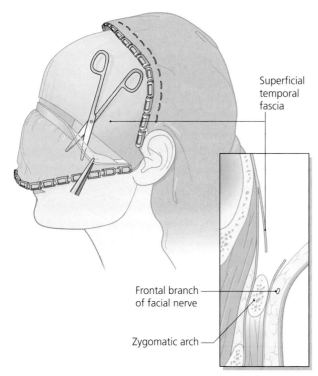

Fig. 9.5: Location of the frontal branch of the facial nerve in the temporal area. Incising the deep temporal fascia 1–2 cm above the zygomatic arch with dissection directly onto the arch will protect the nerve branch superiorly.

dominant hand) and instruments (dominant hand) through the second incision. These incisions are small (1–2 cm in length) and are placed immediately behind and perpendicular to the frontal or temporal hair line (Fig. 9.8). Two or four incisions may be used depending upon the extent of dissection needed across the supraorbital and frontal areas.

Temporal Access

Special mention should be made of the smallest incision used for facial fracture repair, that of the transtemporal or classic Gilles approach. Its use is limited strictly to repair of zygomatic fractures, most commonly the zygomatic arch. Traditionally, its very small size was used for blind manual instrumentation of the arch or zygomatic body. Now with the advent of endoscopic techniques, it can also serve as a portal for either instrument or endoscope insertion.

Technical points

■ The incision is placed several centimeters behind the frontotemporal hair line.
■ Dissection proceeds directly down to and through the deep temporal fascia. This permits instruments to be directed along the temporal bone inferiorly (Fig. 9.9).

Periorbital Access

Surgical access to the entire orbit is not possible through any one single incision. A series of standard incisions (two upper

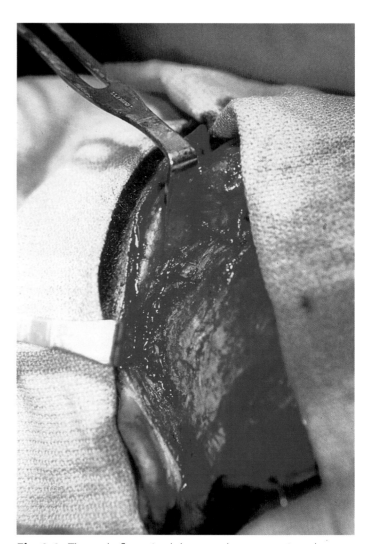

Fig. 9.6: The scalp flap raised down to the zygomatic arch, protecting the frontal branch of the facial nerve by incising the deep temporal fascia above the arch and then continuing toward the bone.

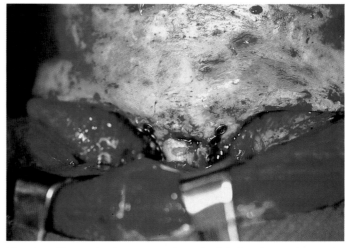

Fig. 9.7: The scalp flap can easily and safely be elevated over the bony nose and medial orbits for access as in this Le Fort III fracture repair.

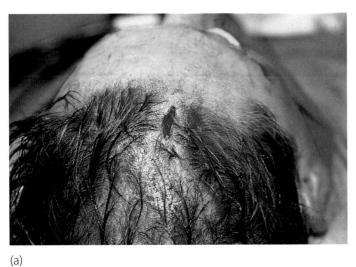
(a)

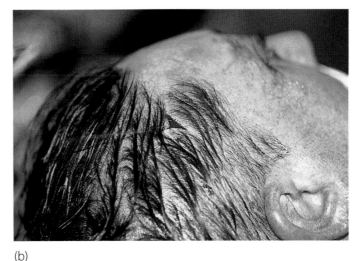
(b)

Fig. 9.8: Frontal and temporal incisions for endoscopic brow lifting. **(a)** Parasagittal frontal incisions. **(b)** Temporal incision for lateral brow access.

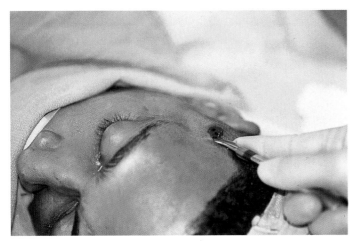

Fig. 9.9: Small temporal incision for instrument manipulation of the zygomatic arch.

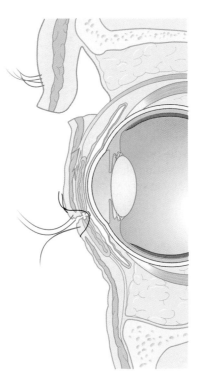

Fig. 9.10: Sagittal section through orbit with the plane of dissection between the orbicularis muscle and the levator in the upper eyelid incision.

and two lower) must be used and even these do not always provide complete access to medial orbital structures. Because of the thin and delicate structures of the eye and its relative intolerance to poor surgical technique, these incisions must be well placed and superb attention to small detail is necessary to avoid postoperative scar problems. In addition, intraoperative globe protection is important and corneal protectors and an ophthalmic lubricating ointment should always be used.

Upper eyelid

The upper eyelid usually offers a well-defined supratarsal crease which permits access to the superolateral orbital bone, lacrimal gland and lateral canthal tendon. This is a natural location for an incision which is known to heal inconspicuously as is demonstrated in the commonly performed blepharoplasty procedure. In addition to skin and the orbicularis muscle which overlies the tarsus and conjunctiva, the upper eyelid contains the levator superioris

aponeurosis which must not be cut or postoperative ptosis will develop.

Technical points

- The incision should be made either in the well-defined supratarsal crease or at least 10 mm above the upper lid margin. An extension can be carried out laterally in a skin crease but should not extend beyond the lateral orbital rim.
- A skin-muscle (orbicularis) muscle flap is raised superiorly and laterally without violation of the underlying levator aponeurosis or orbital septum (Fig. 9.10).
- Use of the full length of the supratarsal crease incision extends exposure from the medial supraorbital rim to the lateral canthus (Fig. 9.11).

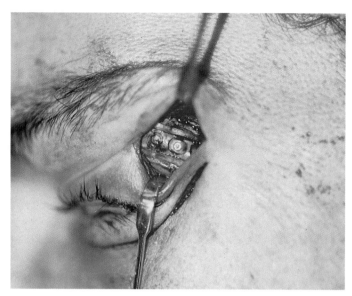

Fig. 9.11: Lateral portion of upper eyelid crease incision used for access to frontozygomatic fixation.

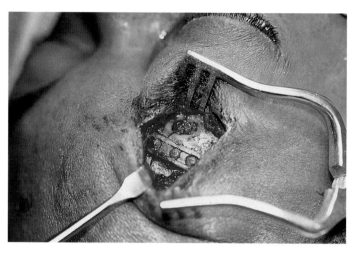

(a)

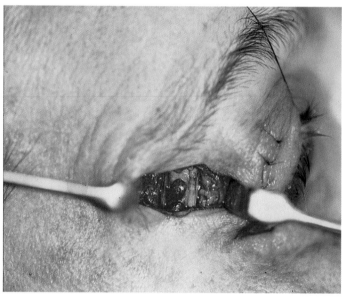

(b)

Fig. 9.12: Supraorbital rim incisions produce more noticeable scars but provide direct access to the supraorbital portions of the lateral orbital rim. **(a)** Medial supraorbital rim incision for frontal sinus fracture repair. **(b)** Lateral supraorbital rim incision for frontozygomatic fixation.

Supraorbital eyebrow

This very limited incision offers simplicity by direct access to the supraorbital rim, portions of the frontal sinus and the frontozygomatic region. When made laterally, there is no potential involvement of branches of the supraorbital nerve. When made more centrally, the branches of the supraorbital nerve are often in the way, limiting access. Care should be taken to dissect and preserve them when possible.

Technical points

- The incision can be made at the junction of the eyebrow and skin or within the eyebrow itself. Unfortunately, when made in the brow itself, hair loss is not uncommon. An incision in this area should not extend beyond the medial or lateral tail of the brow unless the patient is aware of the postoperative presence of the scar (Fig. 9.12).
- When undermined, either above or below the periosteum, the skin can slide along the brow, improving the amount of access.

External lower eyelid

The lower eyelid offers numerous incisional opportunities for exposure to the lower orbit extending from the medial orbital rim and wall, orbital floor and the lateral orbit. All of these incisions are based on skin creases which are present in the lower eyelid, some of which are most obvious in the older patient. From superior to inferior, these include the subciliary, lower lid or subtarsal and infraorbital incisions. Short of the infraorbital incision which lies at the orbital-cheek groove and always leaves a conspicuous scar, advocates exist for the remaining two. Because of the very thin skin of the eyelids and the usual presence of some skin laxity, healing is superb with virtually no chance of hypertrophic scar formation with any of these choices. As the lower eyelid is essen-

tially a static structure and is suspended by the medial and lateral canthal tendons, a preoperative appreciation of lower lid laxity is essential. In addition, an understanding of lid tightening and canthal manipulation procedures is necessary not only to postoperatively treat but more importantly to intraoperatively prevent subsequent ectropion.

Technical points

- The location of the external skin incision may be placed at two levels: subciliary or lower blepharoplasty (subtarsal) (Fig. 9.13). For incision selection, considerations are given to the presence of a prominent skin crease to guide incision placement, the risk of postoperative ectropion (with increased risk factors the incision should be placed

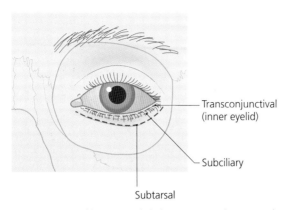

Fig. 9.13: Location of lower eyelid skin incisional approaches.

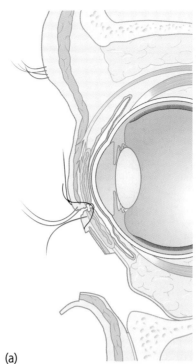

Fig. 9.14: Subciliary and subtarsal incisional approaches. **(a)** Sagittal plane through orbit demonstrating a lower eyelid skin-muscle flap raised anterior to the orbital septum. **(b)** Subciliary incision with lateral canthal extension used for infraorbital rim and floor access in zygomatic-orbital fracture repair.

(a)

further from the lashline) and the age of the patient. Extended access can be gained by lengthening the incision beyond the lid margin in a skin crease, which is almost always done.

- Regardless of the incision used, a skin-muscle flap should be raised. This is technically easier to perform and leaves a good blood supply to the skin. Some limited subcutaneous dissection can be done inferiorly (3–5 mm) and the muscle then transected if desired (stepped incision). Whether this contributes to a lessened risk of ectropion is controversial.
- When possible, stay in the preseptal plane down to the rim which avoids the nuisance of orbital fat herniation into the wound (Fig. 19.14a).
- Once at the infraorbital rim level, make the periosteal incision on its anterior surface. This allows the periosteum to be raised without directly cutting through the orbital septum.
- Wide subperiosteal undermining throughout the orbit can then be done. In this process, the inferior oblique muscle, which is the only orbital muscle which does not originate from the apex, will be stripped from its anterior attachment. The fact that you do not see it means the periosteal incision was adequately anteriorly placed (Fig. 9.14b).
- With extended periosteal elevation on the lateral orbital wall, the lateral canthus may be inadvertently/intentionally stripped for exposure. Do not forget to reattach it prior to closure.
- Closure consists of closing the dermis and skin. Suturing the periosteum, muscle or septum is likely to encourage ectropion. Suture suspension to the forehead is helpful for several days after surgery to prevent vertical lid shortening. A suture is placed below the lower eyelashes and taped to the forehead.

Transconjunctival approach

The transconjunctival approach to the inferior orbit is performed through the inner lower eyelid at the inferior fornix level. It has become popular due to the lack of any external skin scar and the belief that ectropion risk is significantly reduced with its use. In addition, the technique is fairly rapid to perform and does not involve any skin or muscle dissec-

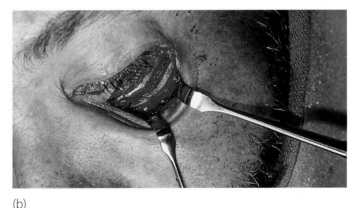

(b)

tion. Its main disadvantage is that exposure to the medial orbit is limited due to the presence of the lacrimal drainage system. If extended by a lateral canthotomy, it provides access to all the fracture sites in zygomatic complex injuries.

Technical points

- The incision is made midway between the lower margin of the tarsal plate and inferior conjunctival fornix.
- Two paths of dissection down to the orbit exist, the preseptal and the retroseptal. The retroseptal approach is more direct and easier to perform but orbital fat will be encountered (Fig. 9.15a).
- A lateral canthotomy is frequently needed with a lateral canthal skin incision for maximal exposure (Figs 9.15b,c).
- Periosteal incision and elevation is done which is aided by a traction suture through the cut end of the conjunctiva.
- Closure consists of a lateral canthopexy suture and dermal and skin closure of the lateral canthal skin incision. Reattachment of the lateral portion of the tarsal plate to the superior portion of the lateral canthal tendon is a

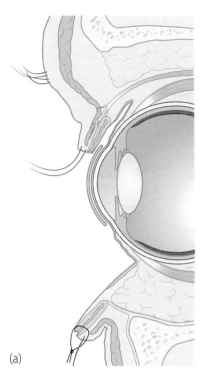

Fig. 9.15:
Transconjunctival incisional approach.
(a) Sagittal plane through orbit demonstrating transconjunctival approach.
(b) Transconjunctival approach to orbital floor repair.
(c) Transconjunctival approach with lateral canthal extension for wider access to the orbital floor.

(a)

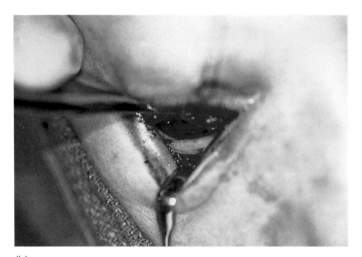

(b)

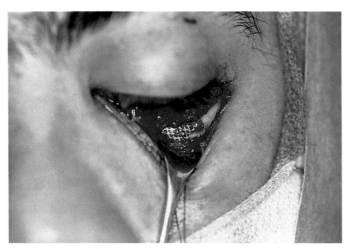

(c)

critical element in the closure of this approach. It is not necessary to close the conjunctiva and the cornea may be abraded if any sutures are placed.

Transoral Approaches

Intraoral incisions through the mucosa provide excellent exposure to the midface and mandibular structures. These approaches are very easy to perform and have minimal morbidity, other than some risk of trigeminal nerve damage and postoperative loss of sensation of facial skin, mucosa and the anterior dentition. Essentially they are 'scarless' approaches for wide degloving of the lower two-thirds of the facial skeleton.

Maxillary vestibular

This intraoral approach is probably the simplest of all facial approaches to perform, with the least morbidity. It allows complete exposure from the anterior zygomatic arches, infraorbital rim, pyriform aperture, down to the alveolus. The only nerve structure exposed is the infraorbital which is easy to find, always present in the same location below the infraorbital rim, and has a quick sensory recovery. As long as one is in the subperiosteal plane, dissection can proceed safely and rapidly.

The other potential problem with midfacial degloving is the detachment and superolateral retraction of the nasolabial musculature. In some patients, adverse facial effects may occur which include widening of the alar bases, rolling inward of the upper lip and slight loss of tip projection. Proper closure technique will avoid these problems in those patients at risk.

Technical points

■ The incision is made at least 5–6 mm above the mucogingival junction. It is important to leave an inferior cuff of mucosa and muscle to facilitate closure. The incision does not need to extend posterior to the maxillary first molar. The stretch of the mucosa allows adequate exposure without risk of injury to the parotid duct with long posterior incisional extensions.
■ Wide subperiosteal dissection can be done to provide extensive midfacial exposure (Fig. 9.16).
■ Closure should incorporate a muscle layer with medial advancement of the superior tissues and a V-Y mucosal closure. In some patients (those with normal to wide preoperative alar base width), an alar cinch suture technique can be used.

Mandibular vestibular

The mandibular vestibular approach, like the maxillary vestibular, is relatively easy to perform with little morbidity. It differs, however, in the amount of exposure to the anterior surfaces of the bone. Due to the mental nerve and the curvilinear structure of the mandible, access is more limited to the anterior body and the lower border of the ramus of the mandible. The issue of muscle detachment and retraction also impacts this approach at the anterior mandible where

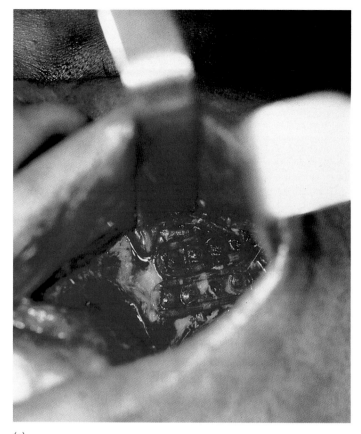

(a)

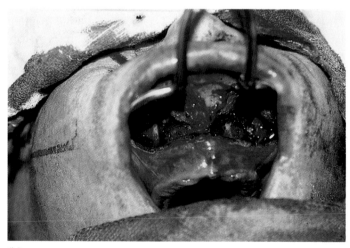

(b)

Fig. 9.16: Maxillary vestibular incision and wide degloving of the midface. **(a)** Unilateral maxillary vestibular incision for access to zygomatic fracture repair. **(b)** Complete maxillary vestibular incision for extensive intraoral exposure in Le Fort I fracture repair.

detachment of the mentalis, without proper reattachment, may result in postoperative ptosis of the chin tissues.

Technical points

- The incision anteriorly runs between the canines and is placed slightly up on the lip side of the vestibule to leave a good cuff of mucosa and muscle for closure.

- Wide subperiosteal dissection is done with attention to the exit of the mental nerve from its foramen which is situated between the first and second premolars. The mental nerve and its branches can be dissected for greater exposure without significantly increasing the risk of permanent nerve injury (Fig. 9.17).
- The incision can be extended posteriorly or a separate incision made along the ascending ramus of the mandible where the entire lateral body and ramus can be widely dissected in the subperiosteal plane (Fig. 9.18).
- Anterior closure requires good mentalis muscle reapproximation to prevent postoperative chin ptosis. Posteriorly, a single layer closure over the body and ramus is adequate.

Transfacial Approaches

Seven basic transfacial incisions can be used, of which five access the mandible and two the nose. Incisional access to the mandible and soft tissues of the lateral face and upper neck are complicated primarily by the presence of branches of the facial nerve. If it were not for these structures, other than the importance of the esthetics of the visible scar, access and closure would almost be as easy as the intraoral vestibular approaches. Due to cross-innervation of the buccal branches of the facial nerve and their increased size, the real risks are to the marginal mandibular and frontal branches which are small and have little chance of recovery if significantly stretched or cut.

Pre-auricular approach

The use of this incision is primarily for access to the temporomandibular joint (TMJ). Its limited length and exposure mean that it is less useful for more anterior structures. In the pathway to the joint are the parotid gland, superficial temporal vessels, auriculotemporal nerve and branches of the facial nerve. Although it would be ideal to save all of these structures during the dissection, the most important preservation is of the frontal or temporal branch of the facial nerve. One or two temporal branches cross the lateral sur-face of the zygomatic arch at the level of the superficial temporal fascia. The crossing point, however, is highly variable and can be anywhere from 10 to 30 mm in front of the external auditory canal. Therefore, a safe plane of dissection to the TMJ is to stay on the cartilaginous anterior surface of the canal and retract all soft tissue forward which will also protect the temporal vessels and the auriculotemporal nerve.

Technical points

- The incision follows the junction of the skin and ear from the temporal area down to the earlobe, with the exception of the tragus. Extending the incision retrotragal hides the scar better and has no risk of tragal deformity as this is not a skin excisional procedure (Fig. 9.19).
- Dissection above the zygomatic arch is down to the superficial temporal fascia. Below the arch, the dissection proceeds along the external auditory canal.

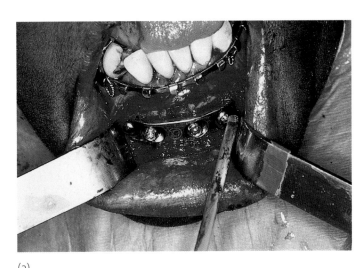

(a)

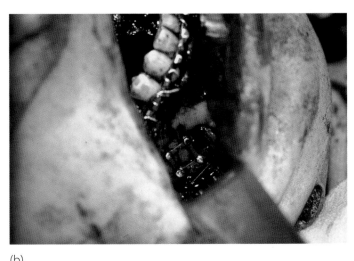

(b)

Fig. 9.17: Mandibular vestibular incision for exposure to the mandible. **(a)** Anterior vestibular incision between the mental nerves for symphyseal fracture repair. **(b)** Anterolateral vestibular incision with mental nerve dissected out in parasymphyseal fracture repair.

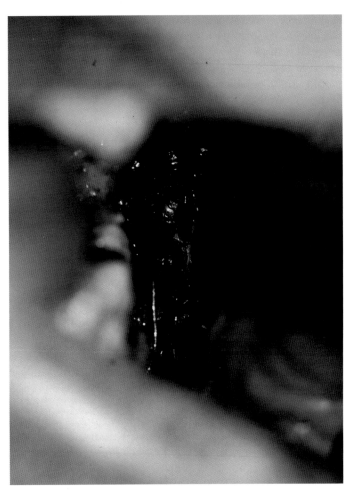

Fig. 9.18: Posterior mucosal incision along the ascending ramus for access to superior border plate fixation.

■ The joint is entered by incising the temporal fascia and developing a subperiosteal plane down into the superior joint space with retraction of the tissues in front of the canal (Fig. 9.20).

■ Closure of the joint capsule is controversial as this may contribute to postoperative adhesions. Closure of the temporal fascia should be done before skin closure.

Rhytidectomy

The facelift approach is an extension of the pre-auricular approach and inferiorly incorporates the retromandibular approach. Calling it a facelift denotes only the location of the skin incision and has nothing to do with dissection or manipulation of the superficial facial fascial planes. It primarily places the great auricular nerve, which is the most commonly injured structure in a facelift, and the marginal mandibular branch of the facial nerve at risk. The elevation of the skin flap may injure the greater auricular nerve inferiorly as it emerges from the deep fascia at the middle of the posterior border of the neck to cross over the sternocleidomastoid muscle at a 45° angle toward the posterior border of the mandible. The deeper dissection to approach the mandible places the facial nerve branch at risk.

Technical points

■ As in the pre-auricular incision with a retrotragal extension, the incision is identical until one reaches the earlobe. At this point, the posterior extension can take one of two routes. A traditional rhytidectomy incision is carried onto the back of the ear and cut into the hair line at the level of the tragus (Fig. 9.21**a**). An alternative and preferable approach is to curve the incision back and downward from the earlobe into a high cervical crease (Fig. 9.21**b**). While this makes a slightly more visible scar, the anterior exposure obtained by the neck extension is greatly improved.

■ The skin flap is quickly raised and is best done with blunt scissors pointed upwards with a spread and pushing maneuver.

■ Access to the mandible is done as for the retromandibular approach.

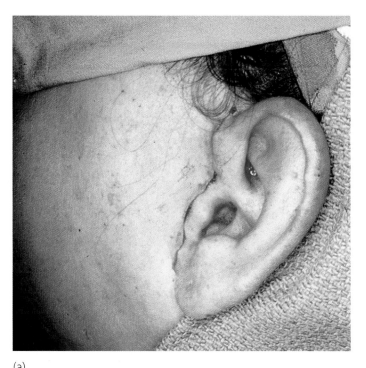

(a)

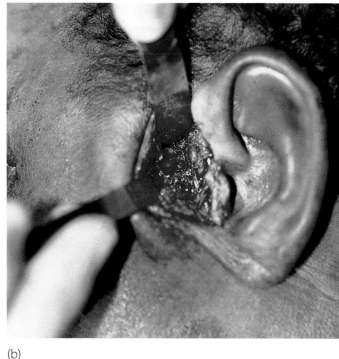

(b)

Fig. 9.19: Pre-auricular incisional approach. **(a)** Pre-auricular incision; the incision should go retrotragal and not pretragal as in this patient. **(b)** Retrotragal pre-auricular incision hides the scar better with no increased morbidity.

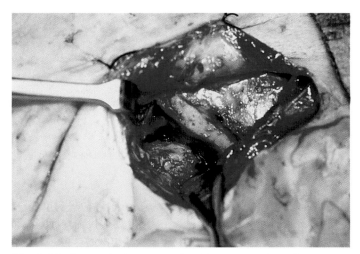

Fig. 9.20: Pre-auricular approach with exposure into the superior joint space of the TMJ.

■ Skin closure should be performed over a drain which exits posteriorly.

Retromandibular approach

This commonly used approach is useful for exposing the posterior ramus of the mandible and the low subcondylar region. It is the shortest distance from the skin to this area but requires identification of the marginal mandibular branch of the facial nerve. Essentially, the path of dissection to the posterior mandible is done between the superior and inferior divisions of the facial nerve. Short of the angular region, access to the superior and anterior ramus is somewhat limited by the mass of overlying parotid gland and soft tissue.

Technical points

■ The incision is placed in a vertical orientation directly beneath the earlobe, paralleling the posterior border of the ramus. The incision may be placed more posteriorly in a skin crease but access becomes further away.
■ Dissection cuts through the parotid gland with exposure of the facial nerve. A more posterior incision avoids the inferior branch of the facial nerve and the parotid gland but exposure is more limited.
■ Division of the pterygomasseteric sling is necessary to approach the bone.
■ Once in the subperiosteal plane of the mandible, retractors placed in the sigmoid notch and/or the anterior ramus aid greatly in exposure.
■ Closure of the pterygomasseteric sling, parotid capsule and platysma layer should be done before skin closure.

Submandibular approach

Approach from a high cervical incision, historically referred to as a Risdon incision, is a standard method for procedures on the posterior body and ramus of the mandible. The exact location of the incision varies but all place it below the inferior border of the mandible. The single greatest obstacle in the dissection is the marginal mandibular branch of the facial nerve. While its course is somewhat variable, this branch is below the inferior border of the mandible in many cases when it is posterior to the crossing of the facial artery. Anterior to the facial artery, it is almost always above the inferior border. It is rarely lower than 1–1.5 cm below the inferior border and, for this reason, the incision is often placed two finger-breadths or 2 cm below the inferior border.

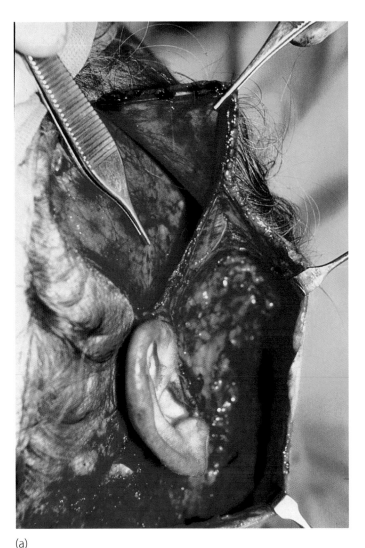

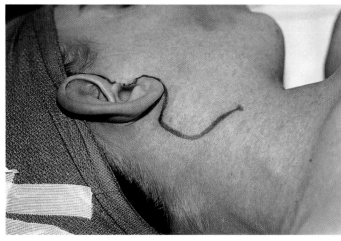

(a)

(b)

(c)

Fig. 9.21: Facelift-type approaches. **(a)** Traditional full facelift with temporal fascial plane (forceps) separated from the submusculoaponeurotic plane inferiorly. **(b, c)** Traditional superior facelift approach combined with an anterior neck incision for improved access to facial vessels necessary in this free gracilis facial reanimation procedure.

Technical points

- A skin crease that is 1.5–2.0 cm below the inferior border is chosen for the incision. It may be horizontally more posterior or anterior dependent upon what part of the mandible is to be treated. Turning the head away from the side to be treated helps move the nerve more superiorly.
- Once through the platysma, the underlying cervical fascia, the facial artery and vein and the marginal mandibular nerve are to be found. Often the facial vessels need to be ligated in more anterior approaches (Fig. 9.22). The nerve should be stimulated for location, but it should lie superiorly.
- Division of the pterygomasseteric sling, subperiosteal dissection and exposure of the mandible are then performed (Fig. 9.23). Closure proceeds as in the retromandibular approach.

Submental approach

The most anterior inferior border approach to the mandible and midline neck structures is an extension of the submandibu-

lar approach. It is used for access to the anterior mandible for symphyseal manipulation. It differs from all other cervicofacial approaches by having no significant anatomic structures between the skin and the bone. Dissection may be sharp, with impunity.

Technical points

- The submental skin crease is chosen for the incision. In young patients, a skin crease may not be present and incision placement should be behind the inferior border as the neck will be on some extension.
- Access is direct to the bone where good exposure can be achieved for fracture repair or implant placement (Fig. 9.24).

Nasal Approaches

The nasal bones and cartilages are approached through two basic approaches: endonasal, where all the incisions are within the nasal cavity, or an external open method which incorporates a columellar skin incision. Either approach can

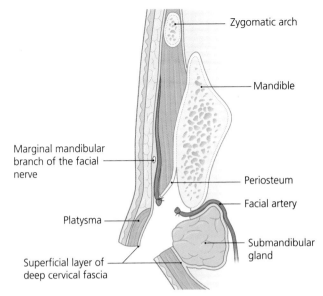

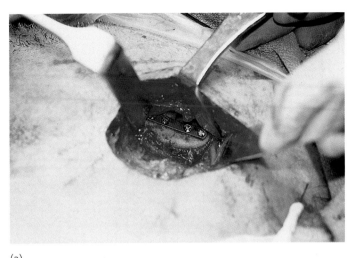

(a)

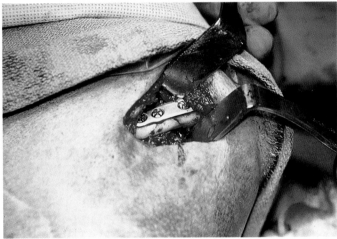

(b)

Fig. 9.22: Coronal illustration of the path of dissection in the submandibular approach. The initial dissection goes through the platysma muscle to the superficial layer of the deep cervical fascia. It then moves above the submandibular gland to the periosteum of the mandible.

be effective in experienced hands, but they differ primarily by the amount of exposure and visualization of the nasal structures. They are unique facial incisions as they provide access to a structure composed of both bone and cartilage.

Endonasal approach

A variety of mucosal incisions exist for intranasal access for treatment of dorsal, tip and septal deformities. These include the marginal, intercartilaginous and transfixion incisions (Fig. 9.25) which represent standard closed approaches to nasal surgery. An intercartilaginous incision permits approach to the nasal dorsum. A unilateral transfixion incision alone (hemitransfixion) allows access to the septum. The combination of the marginal, intercartilaginous and transfixion incisions allows the complete delivery of the lower lateral cartilages. There is little use for the isolated marginal incision except in secondary cases for graft placement for the treatment of alar retraction.

Technical points

- A marginal incision follows the caudal margin of the lower lateral cartilage as opposed to the margin of the nostril. It is important to appreciate the relationship of these two structures as the caudal cartilaginous margin and the rim are closer together medially than laterally (Fig. 9.25). Thus, the incision diverges from the rim as it goes laterally. It is important to avoid traversing the soft triangle, a medial alar rim zone formed by two juxtaposed layers of skin unsupported by cartilage, to avoid postoperative alar rim notching.

Fig. 9.23: Surgical procedures with submandibular approach. **(a)** More posterior approach for access to an angle fracture. **(b)** More anterior approach for access to a body fracture.

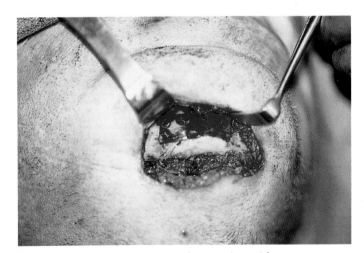

Fig. 9.24: Submental approach for symphyseal fracture repair.

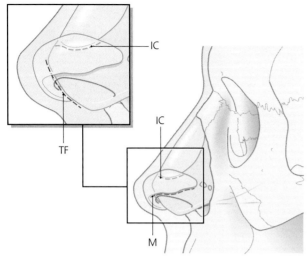

Fig. 9.25: Sagittal view of intranasal incisions.
IC = intercartilaginous incision, M = marginal incision,
TF = transfixion incision which follows the caudal border of the septum, inset.

- The intercartilaginous incision is placed at the junction of the upper and lower lateral cartilages. With the lower lateral cartilage everted, the inferior edge of the upper lateral cartilage is visible protruding into the vestibule. The incision is made parallel to the cephalic margin of the lower lateral cartilage, avoiding the nasal valve area (Fig. 9.25).
- A transfixion incision is made at the caudal end of the septum. A hemitransfixion incision is made only through one nostril, leaving the membranous septum intact on the opposite side. A full transfixion incision traverses both sides, extends inferiorly to sever the columella and lip from the septal cartilage and anterior nasal spine and connects superiorly to the intercartilaginous incision for complete separation of the soft tissues overlying the dorsum and columella from the septum. This allows complete exposure of the septum and delivery of the lower lateral cartilages (Fig. 9.26). These incisions and dissection create a bipedicled flap of lower lateral cartilages lined with vestibular skin based medially and laterally for its vascularity.
- Isolated septal exposure is done through a transfixion incision. For septal manipulation, the incision is placed at the caudal end of the septum. For cartilage graft harvest, the incision may be placed more posteriorly

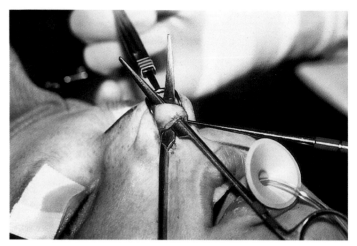

Fig. 9.26: Lower lateral cartilage delivery technique through intranasal incisions.

directly over the septum. In either case, wide subperichondrial dissection is done.
- Closure of the septum and intranasal incisions is done with small resorbable sutures with external taping and/or splints. Quilting resorbable sutures are used through the septum to close dead space. No intranasal packing is used.

External (open) approaches

The recent popularity of the external rhinoplasty approach has been primarily due to the amount of exposure obtained and the resultant increased ease and reliability of nasal tip and dorsal manipulation. It caused considerable debate during its early introduction and quickly became the most controversial 6 mm of skin incision in the entire face. However, its ability to guide surgeons in rhinoplasty and improve the postoperative results, particularly in the tip and dome area, have rightly confirmed its place as a recognized method of nasal access. With some experience and careful dissection technique, the resultant columellar scar is of little consequence.

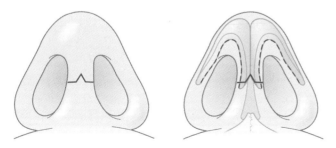

Fig. 9.27: Transcolumellar incisional designs.

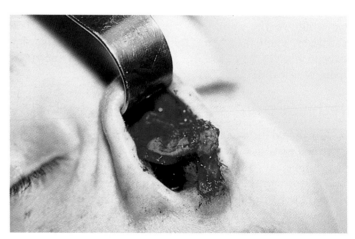

Fig. 9.28: Complete exposure of the lower two-thirds of the nose through the open approach.

Technical points

- The external approach consists of bilateral marginal incisions connected by a mid-columellar incision. The marginal incision follows the caudal margin of the lower lateral cartilage rather than the margin of the nostril. The columellar incision is made at the narrowest portion of the columella between the columella-lobule junction and the flare of the feet of the medial crura. Multiple types of skin incisions can be used but most commonly, an invert V and stair-step pattern is employed (Fig. 9.27).

- The two incisions are connected with care taken not to transect the medial crura which are quite superficial, particularly in the transition from the columella to the dome.

- The skin is dissected off the dome and lower lateral cartilages and up onto the upper lateral cartilages to the dorsum, providing wide exposure of the lower two-thirds of the nasal framework (Fig. 9.28).

- Closure is done with small permanent sutures on the columellar skin (no dermal suturing) and small resorbable sutures for the nasal mucosa. External taping or splinting is done to adapt the skin to the underlying skeleton.

10 A Logical Approach to the Controversies Around Orbital Trauma

Leo F A Stassen, Gordon N Dutton, Nils–Claudius Gellrich

The management of orbital injuries is one of the most interesting and difficult areas in facial trauma. The consequences of an orbital injury are dramatic. They vary from a loss of vision, diplopia, loss of an eye, epiphora, a disturbing loss of facial sensation to an unsightly and unacceptable appearance of the eye and the hard and soft tissues around it (Fig. 10.1). These injuries demand a careful attention to detail but they are often underestimated and undertreated.

Introduction

When we look at each other, all areas of the face are important but there is no doubt that the eyes and how they appear play a very important part in how we initially perceive each other. The eyes are the outward expression of our minds (Fig. 10.2).

Persistent enophthalmos (sunken eye), hypo- or hyperglobus (dropped/raised level of the globe), strabismus (squint), diplopia (double vision), deteriorated visual acuity/blindness, a false eye, ectropion (eyelid turned out), entropion (eyelid turned in), scarring, fat atrophy, zygomatic malalignment and canthal dystopia are significant debilitating problems (Fig. 10.3). They are unfortunately common complications of orbital/zygomatic surgery. All lead to a major grief reaction to a loss of function (vision) or esthetics or both. Psychological support and counseling are required.[1]

It is essential to take both the soft and hard tissues into consideration. If we ignore either, our patient care will be compromised. Treatment must avoid exacerbating the problem by the positioning of our facial access incisions (Figs 10.4–10.6).[2,3] It is possible to expose most of the face and orbit with esthetic incisions – bicoronal, transconjunctival, transcaruncular, lower lid and intraoral.[2-5] Endoscopic assessment of injuries and orbital fracture repair is becoming more common.[6-8]

How do we ensure that we get the best results for our patients? The controversies surrounding orbital injuries include the following.

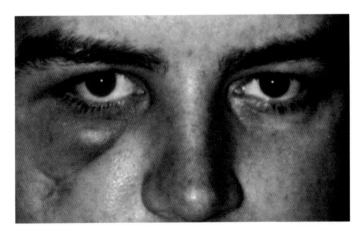

(a)

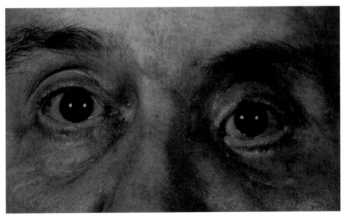

(b)

Fig. 10.1: Long-term consequences of an orbital injury.
(a) Severe right orbital injury, soft and hard tissues. **(b)** Severe left orbital injury: soft and hard tissues, diplopia, loss of vision, enophthalmos, hypoglobus, canthal dystopia.

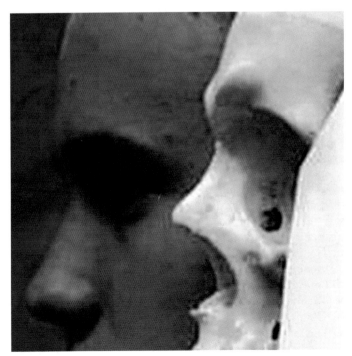

Fig. 10.2: Soft and hard tissue relationship.

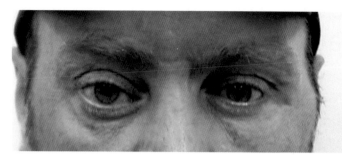

Fig. 10.3: Canthal dystopia.

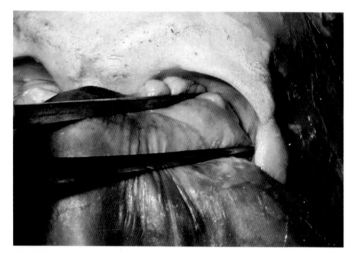

Fig. 10.4: Coronal exposure.

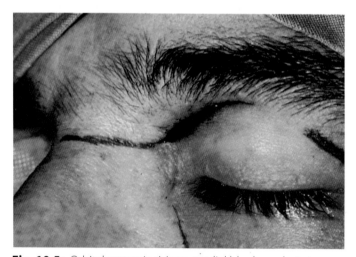

Fig. 10.5: Orbital access incisions: medial blepharoplasty to explore medial wall.

- The type, detail and extent of preoperative clinical examination and investigations that are required.
- The timing of primary surgery (early or late).
- Incisions for fracture exposure.
- The type of fixation at primary and secondary surgery (none, multiple, resorbable plates, non-resorbable plates).
- Bone grafting vs alloplastic materials.
- The management and prevention of diplopia.
- The prevention of enophthalmos.
- The management of infraorbital nerve numbness/dysesthesia.

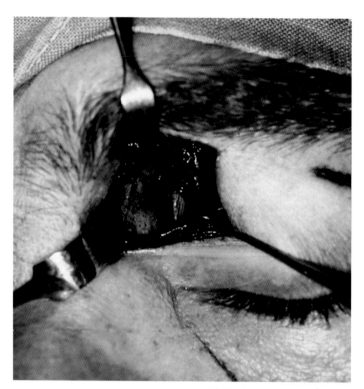

Fig. 10.6: Medial wall exposure via upper blepharoplasty with extensive subperiosteal dissection and preservation of nerves and vessels.

- The management of a patient with decreasing visual acuity or the acutely blind eye.
- The management of ocular injuries.
- Length of follow-up.

Assessment, preoperative investigations, collaboration with others, timing of surgery and methods of treatment, follow-up and secondary management all demand consideration.

Orbital injuries can occur alone but are most often associated with other injuries, such as zygomatic (malar), frontal sinus, naso-orbitoethmoidal, Le Fort II / III fractures and skull fractures. They are a mixture of low-force (zygomatic fracture, orbital floor, naso-orbitoethmoidal) and high-force injuries (supraorbital rim, orbital roof and frontal sinus) (Fig. 10.7). Orbital injuries are complicated by their proximity to the brain, eye, nasolacrimal apparatus, facial nerve and sinuses.

The etiology of orbital injuries depends on which country one works in. In the UK, orbital injuries are most often caused by assaults usually in association with alcohol but they also occur following road traffic accidents, horse riding accidents, falls, sport and industrial accidents. Gunshot injuries are rare but are becoming more common. The greater the force, not surprisingly, the more comminuted and displaced the fracture and the greater the association with other serious injuries. High-force injuries (orbital roof, supraorbital rim) have a mortality of 12% from associated injuries (head, neck, chest). Zygomatic and orbital injuries involving the floor and medial wall are low-impact (force) injuries. Injuries involving the medial canthal area (naso-orbitoethmoidal) are intermediate-impact (force) injuries.

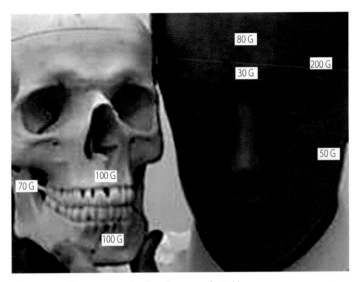

Fig. 10.7: Forces required to fracture facial bones.

The principles of acute trauma life support for maxillofacial surgery must not be forgotten and are similar to those for any injury (Fig. 10.8).

Airway
Breathing
Circulation/cervical spine
Disability, drainage (intracranial hematoma, retrobulbar hemorrhage), drugs (for cerebrospinal leak, fractures)
Expose and examine eyes, ears and the back of the head
Facial nerve
Go over it all again
Help

Facial injuries are sometimes considered as 'less important' in the severely injured patient. They should be treated after the life-threatening injuries have been dealt with and in conjunction with any other procedures (orthopedic/surgical) rather than be left unattended. If a CT scan is requested to rule out an intracranial injury, it is sensible to use the opportunity, if injury is suspected, to assess the orbit and nasoorbital area. Facial lacerations demand attention to detail and a maxillofacial surgeon should be part of the acute trauma

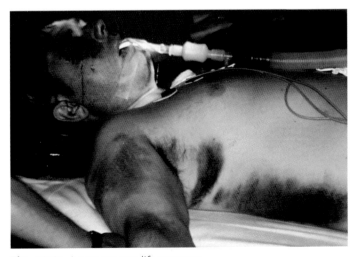

Fig. 10.8: Acute trauma life support.

team. Once the patient is stable, lacerations should be explored and sutured within the first few hours.

Blindness is a serious complication following an orbital injury. In a prospective study undertaken by al-Qurainy et al (1991), the incidence of severe ocular injury in 438 zygomatic fractures was 12%, with 2.5% having a significant traumatic optic neuropathy.[9] The incidence of diplopia was 20% and even with early surgery, long-term diplopia occurred in 1%.[10] These prospective studies led to the development of a scoring system for eye injuries and highlighted the acronym BAD ACT (blowout fracure, acuity, diplopia, amnesia, comminuted trauma) (see Appendix 1). If a serious eye injury is suspected or identified, urgent collaboration with ophthalmology is required and consideration of urgent exploration is essential.[11]

Visual acuity must be assessed and recorded. If the patient is conscious but swollen around the eyes, the assessment can be made easier by explaining to the patient that you need to examine his eyes, that you will be helping him to open his eyes and then ask him to open his eyes whilst gently elevating the upper lid and depressing the lower lid. If an attempt is made to prise open the eyes, the orbicularis oculi spontaneously contracts and resists the attempt.

Edema of the retina (Berlin's edema) is the most common cause of decreased visual acuity but an intraocular injury or a retrobulbar hemorrhage or an optic nerve lesion must be ruled out. In head and neck trauma, an optic nerve injury is the third most common major cranial nerve injury following olfactory and facial nerve injuries. With severe facial injuries, these potentially serious problems must be identified during the secondary survey. Traumatic optic nerve lesions (TONL) often occur acutely and are missed or ignored because of the other potentially more serious injuries. Two percent (0.7–5.0%) of all closed head injuries and 20% of all frontobasal injuries show some kind of visual pathway damage. In these injuries, it is usually the intracanalicular part (Figs 10.9, 10.10) of the optic nerve that is affected and not surprisingly, TONL most commonly are found with frontal (72%) or frontotemporal (12%) injuries.

The first orbital surgery should give the best outcome and it needs to be thorough. The main aim of orbital surgery is the restoration of the anatomy to its normal and esthetic form with preservation of vision, movement, globe position, esthetics and lacrimation. It is essential to address the 'whole' problem. It is wise to remember the morbidity of surgery as well as its advantages but also to consider the problems of neglected treatment. A patient who survives is likely to do better from all aspects if he is not left with severe deformities. It is often not possible, for patients with significant soft tissue injuries, to return the face to its preinjury state.

Assessment and investigations should be thorough, including access to plain radiographs, CT, MRI, US and spiral 3D reconstruction.[12–18] Usually more than one type of investigation is required to get a clear picture. A provisional surgical plan is made but the final assessment can only be made after surgical exposure and exploration of the injuries.[19]

Orbital surgery requires a multidisciplinary team involving a maxillofacial surgeon, facial plastic surgical experience, an ophthalmic surgeon with access to orthoptists, a neurosurgeon

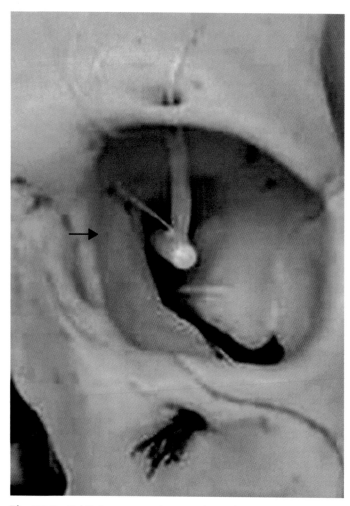

Fig. 10.9: Orbital apex – optic nerve (arrow).

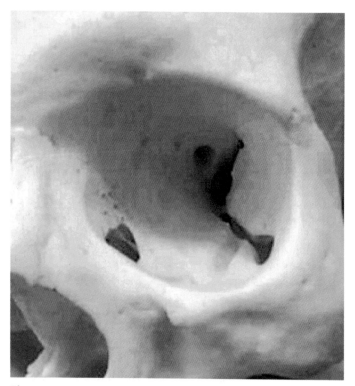

Fig. 10.10: Orbital apex to show optic foramen.

and a radiologist. Intraoperative fluoroscopy, cameras and CT screening are becoming more common and are likely to influence the direction of future treatment in this area.[20–22] Radiological screening will help assess the position of the zygoma and its arch, the correction of enophthalmos, orbital wall/optic canal exploration and extensive orbital reconstruction. The zygomatic arch, infraorbital rim and buttress positions are of paramount importance in supporting the zygoma and ensuring optimal orbital reconstruction.[19,23,24] Endoscopic assessment of the arch, rim and orbital floor at the time of surgery is relatively straightforward and is likely to influence future treatment.[6,7,8,17]

Secondary problems are usually related to one or more of the following:

- the complexity of the initial soft and hard tissue injury
- delayed treatment
- excessive scarring
- failure of adequate support of soft tissues
- fat atrophy
- inadequately treated zygomatic fractures
- comminuted zygomatic fractures (Fig. 10.11), missed medial and floor injuries
- bone loss
- a failure of adequate fixation or fixation methods.[23–29]

Clinical Assessment of Orbital Injury

A thorough history and clinical examination are undertaken (see Appendix 2) to determine the possibility of a penetrating, chemical or blunt injury or any such combination to the eye and soft tissues. Evidence of a head injury (amnesia), a neck injury (10%), loss of smell (anosmia), deterioration or loss of vision, development of double vision (diplopia – vertical, horizontal or rotatory), eye movements (painful or not) and the eye position in the three planes (proptosis or enophthalmos, hypoglobus or hyperglobus or an orbital dystopia) should be recorded.

Orbital trauma can result in displacement of the globe in any direction. Proptosis occurs in the acute phase due to hematoma and/or swelling of orbital tissues. As the swelling subsides, proptosis resolves and may become enophthalmos. Persistent proptosis may be due to subperiosteal hematoma or intraorbital bone fragments. Enophthalmos is a common late sequel, which may result from a combination of expansion of the orbit, prolapse of soft tissue through a blow-out

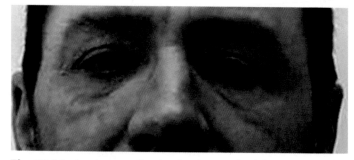

Fig. 10.11: Inadequate fixation leading to flat left zygoma with lateral canthal drift.

fracture, necrosis of soft tissue (rare) and intraorbital fibrosis. There is often an associated impairment of ocular motility. Vertical displacement of the globe is common. Upward displacement may result from hematoma/edema in the acute phase or orbital floor impaction causing a reduction in orbital volume. Downward displacement (hypoglobus) is far more common, particularly in patients with comminuted orbital floor/lateral wall or roof fractures. Horizontal lateral displacement of the globe can result particularly from naso-orbito-ethmoidal fractures and when the medial canthal ligament is severed. Traumatic herniation of the globe into the maxillary sinus can occur. Good recovery of visual function and esthetics is achievable after effective repair.

Eye position can be measured using an exophthalometer but is best assessed from the CT or MRI scans. The exophthalometer is of little benefit for patients with lateral orbital disruption, the most common orbital injury. Surgeons have developed exophthalometers based on the ear canals and supraorbital positions but these are less accurate than CT scan assessment, which also allows an assessment of orbital fat volume and helps determine the need for surgery.[12,13,16,22,30–32]

Facial sensation is tested. Altered facial sensation around the orbit may be the only initial clinical sign of a blow-out fracture. The alar of the nose should be gently touched and the patient asked if he can feel one side and then the other and if they feel the same.

Facial nerve injury compounds any orbital injury and should be actively sought. If the nerve is severed through a laceration, the laceration should be explored and the nerve primarily repaired with the aid of the microscope.

Intercanthal (medial and lateral) and interpupillary measurements are taken (see Appendix 2). The use of local anesthetic to enable a full clinical assessment for medial canthal disruption is advised.

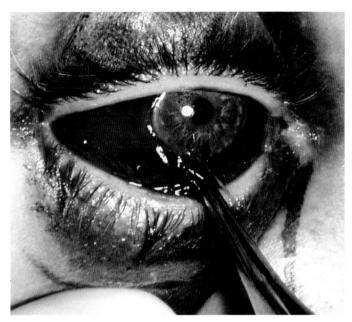

Fig. 10.13: Forced duction test, picking up attached conjunctiva at margin of cornea.

Mouth opening should be assessed as any displacement of the zygomatic complex can impinge on the temporalis muscle or coronoid process and interfere with jaw movement. Trismus is not an uncommon complication of a zygoma/orbital fracture.

It is an advantage to have a diagram or photograph in the notes to demonstrate grazes, bruises, the presence of periorbital or lid lacerations and to record any loss of soft or hard tissue.

Forced duction tests under local anesthetic can be helpful but are not necessary in the conscious patient (Figs 10.12–10.14). The clinical sign of pain on looking up or laterally

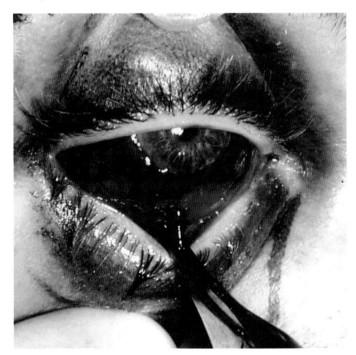

Fig. 10.12: Forced duction test, picking up adventitial tissue around inferior rectus muscle.

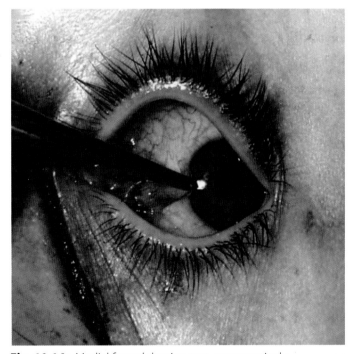

Fig. 10.14: Medial forced duction test, peroperatively.

with diplopia is evidence of entrapment. The pain is thought to be due to the entrapped tissue disturbing the periosteum. A Hess test will help display any restriction but it is important to look for the clinical sign of pain (slight grimace) and retraction of the globe on eye movement.

Applied Surgical Anatomy

The orbit (Figs 10.15–10.17) has several important anatomical features. If we know and appreciate the anatomy, this enables us to understand the injuries and to postulate how to reconstruct them. The orbital skeleton should be returned to its norm with enough strength to resist disrupting forces. There is argument about simple elevation, single, two-point and three-point fixation.[23,24] It is recognized that even with frontozygomatic and infraorbital rim fixation, posterolateral orbital rim rotation can be missed. It is advisable with unstable zygoma fractures to view the frontozygomatic fracture and either the buttress (intraoral) or the zygoma/sphenoidal fracture line to prevent the development of enophthalmos.[33]

The orbit can be anatomically classified in many ways. It has been described in relation to its bony components; it is made up of seven bones. It has been divided into anterior, middle and posterior thirds to help differentiate the sites for the

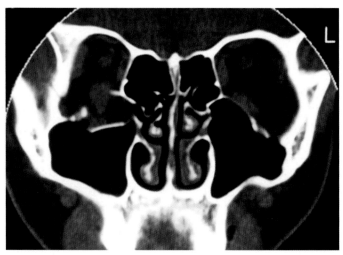

Fig. 10.16: CT scan showing orbital floor fracture.

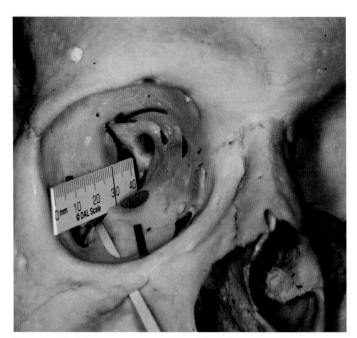

Fig. 10.17: Measurements to aid orbital dissection. Orange arrow = superior fissure. Red arrow = inferior fissure. Green ring = posterior floor, retrobulbar bulge. Red line = anterior floor (concave). Yellow line = infraorbital nerve in groove and exiting from canal through infraorbital foramen. Red triangles = anterior and posterior ethmoidal arteries.

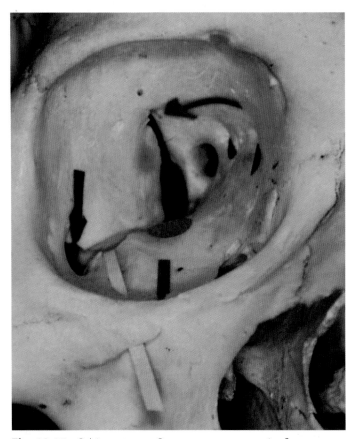

Fig. 10.15: Orbit anatomy. Orange arrow = superior fissure. Red arrow = inferior fissure. Green ring = posterior floor, retrobulbar bulge. Red line = anterior floor (concave). Yellow line = infraorbital nerve in groove and exiting from canal through infraorbital foramen. Red triangles = anterior and posterior ethmoidal arteries.

causes of hypoglobus (anterior orbital floor), enophthalmos (middle) and visual/neurological problems (posterior) (see Fig. 10.9). It is important to recognize that the correction of hypoglobus requires the globe to be lifted and the repair +/– bone grafting to the anterior half of the orbit. The prevention and correction of enophthalmos require the globe to be pushed forwards with repair of the lateral and medial walls and reconstruction of the retrobulbar bulge.[34] The orbit has been described according to its anatomical walls; it has a floor, a medial wall, a roof, a lateral wall, an apex and an orbital rim. The latter method is the easiest to comprehend and combining it with the other classifications allows for a logical anatomical assessment and for a logical treatment of orbital injuries.

The orbit is a quadrangular pyramid with its base on the facial surface. Its apex is the optic foramen and the medial end of the superior orbital fissure.

The orbital rim is composed of cortical bone. Its strength arises from its circumorbital continuity. If the rim is broken, the strength, particularly of the inferior, medial and lateral walls of the orbit, is significantly decreased. The dissipation of the forces required to fracture the rim is often transmitted to the floor and medial wall, leading to concomitant damage in both.[35] An isolated orbital rim fracture may have initially few symptoms, presenting with only infraorbital anesthesia but presenting later with enophthalmos or dysesthesia, epiphora (secondary to nasolacrimal obstruction) or dacrocystorhinitis. These patients should be followed up for at least 6 weeks before discharge (Fig. 10.16). Symptomatic infraorbital nerve problems warrant treatment.[36,37]

The floor is very thin and S shaped. It is concave anteriorly and convex posteriorly (see Figs 10.15, 10.17). It is traversed anteriorly by the infraorbital groove and canal (lateral to medial). The infraorbital canal is suspended from the floor. This groove and canal carry the infraorbital nerve from the pterygopalatine fissure below the inferior orbital fissure to the infraorbital foramen and further weaken the floor. This anatomical relationship accounts for the clinical sign of facial numbness, paresthesia or dysesthesia affecting the alar of nose, cheek, upper lip and anterior teeth, following an orbital floor or zygomatic fracture. The floor is fractured either by buckling (dissipation of orbital rim forces) or by rapid expansion of the orbital contents, leading to a fracture of the floor or the medial orbital wall.[35] Floor fractures are usually medial to the nerve. If a fracture involves the whole floor, the infraorbital nerve supports the floor like a piece of string camouflaging the initial clinical signs of hypoglobus and enophthalmos.

The anatomy of the postbulbar bulge (maxillary sinus expansion posterior to the globe) is important in maintaining the eye's anterior–posterior position and must be reconstructed to prevent enophthalmos. Volume changes on CT examination illustrate clearly the importance of this area in the development of enophthalmos. This area is often not explored due to a reluctance to dissect far enough into the orbit. It is essential to dissect the inferior fissure free from the orbital contents at least to behind the infraorbital nerve (see Fig. 10.16). The inferior orbital fissure is traversed by only minor vessels, lymphatic channels and fibro-fatty tissue. The infraorbital nerve passes below the fissure to enter the infraorbital groove. These tissues are carefully dissected under magnification by a combination of bipolar diathermy and knife dissection. The floor must be fully explored, which in the adult usually means a dissection along the floor and lateral wall for at least 35 mm (Fig. 10.17).

The majority of failed explorations are due to a reluctance to adequately free up this area and get completely around any floor fracture/defect. The difficult areas are the junction of the infraorbital groove and the inferior fissure and the identification of the posterior aspect of the retrobulbar bulge as it passes posteriorly and medially to the inferior fissure. The periosteum needs to be incised on either side of the fissure and elevated gently. Care needs to be taken at the junction of the infraorbital groove and fissure to dissect the infraorbital nerve free of the orbital tissues. This subperiosteal dissection, particularly with careful eye retraction, magnification and a light source (head light), enables a full exploration of the orbital floor and its lateral and medial walls. The transconjunctival or lower eyelid skin incision does not need to be extended, if the orbital periosteum is well mobilized. The inferior rectus and inferior oblique muscles are protected by remaining in a subperiosteal plane. The anatomy of the nasolacrimal sac and canal should be kept in mind.

It has been suggested that an inferior orbitotomy may help in exploring the large blow-out fractures. In our experience an inferior orbitotomy is used occasionally in secondary procedures but is usually not necessary in the acute situation. An inferior orbitotomy may be useful to decompress the infraorbital nerve in patients with an infraorbital nerve dysesthesia or persistent numbness (Figs 10.18–10.22). Resolution and protection of cheek/lip sensation is best achieved, even with

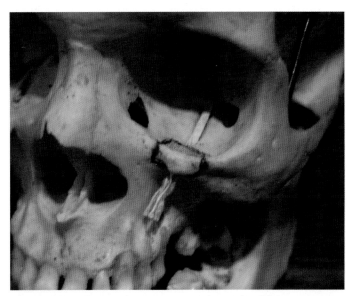

Fig. 10.18: Inferior orbitotomy to explore orbital floor or decompress infraorbital nerve.

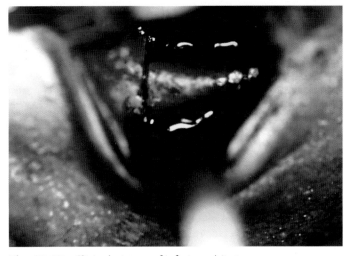

Fig. 10.19: Clinical picture of inferior orbitotomy.

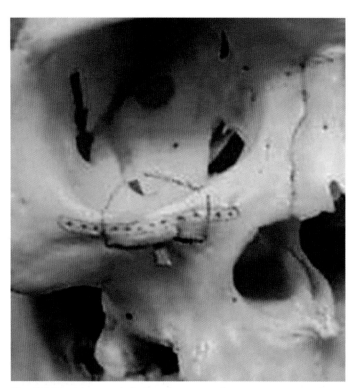

Fig. 10.20: Plate on inferior orbitotomy for reconstruction of orbital rim.

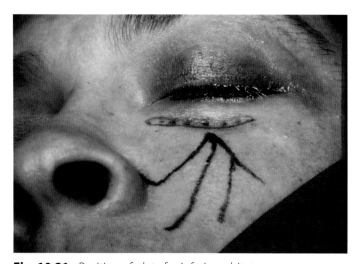

Fig. 10.21: Position of plate for inferior orbitotomy.

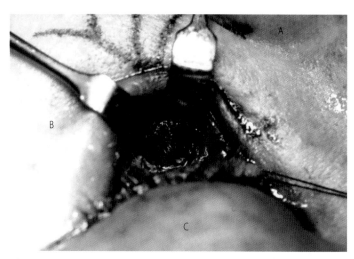

Fig. 10.22: Infraorbital nerve exposed. A = nose, B = cheek, C = eyelid.

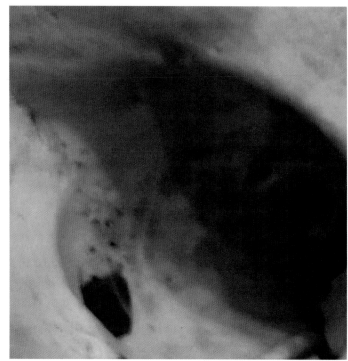

Fig. 10.23: Thinness of medial wall.

minimal infraorbital rim disruption, with reduction and fixation of the fractured zygoma/infraorbital rim at the frontozygomatic and/or infraorbital rim.[36,37]

The anterior floor supporting the globe is reconstructed to prevent hypoglobus (usually with bone graft). It is our preference to use autogenous bone either from the cranium, mandible or opposite lateral maxillary sinus wall, although nasal septum, ear cartilage and fascia lata have been used with success.[38,39] Alloplastic material (silastic) has a tendency to extrude but despite this silastic remains the most frequently used material in the UK.[40,41] Resorbable material, although useful in small defects, resorbs and potentially leaves the patient with late enophthalmos. Very large defects are well restored with a combination of metal (titanium or vitallium)

and autogenous bone. The posterior floor (bulbar bulge) is reconstructed with layers of bone to correct and prevent enophthalmos. There is still a reluctance to undertake bone grafting in the acute management of these injuries. Primary bone grafting in facial injuries has been shown to give good long-term results.[27,38,39,41,42]

The medial wall is paper thin (Fig. 10.23). It obtains its strength from the continuity of the ethmoidal air cells and from their multiple septa. If fractured, the forces of injury are rapidly dissipated and thus protect the brain and eye. Nasal fractures frequently involve the medial wall and the inferior orbital rim.

Although nasal radiographs are not usually taken, there should be a high index of suspicion of medial wall injuries in the anterior collapsed nasal fracture. If there is any clinical indication of nasal or cheek numbness, radiographs should be taken. Medial wall defects tend to be small, minimally displaced and are easily missed. There is a high incidence (30–50%) of medial wall fractures associated with floor fractures.[13,28] Medial wall injuries contribute to enophthalmos and can cause horizontal diplopia. The medial wall is traversed by the anterior and posterior ethmoidal arteries at about 24 and 34 mm from the anterior lacrimal crest (orbital rim). If the medial wall is being explored, they should be identified and coagulated. Bleeding can easily be arrested by bipolar diathermy. Although these are relatively low-pressure vessels, they do contribute to the problem of visual impairment, ophthalmoplegia and proptosis secondary to a retrobulbar hemorrhage (Fig. 10.24).

The nasolacrimal sac is sited anteriorly between the orbital rim and the posterior lacrimal crest. It is protected by the anterior and posterior bands of the medial canthal ligament (Figs 10.25, 10.26) and drains through the nasolacrimal duct to the inferior meatus of the nose. It is important when treating orbital injuries to protect the canaliculi, the sac and the duct when placing incisons and osteosynthesis. Obstruction in the duct or damage to the sac can cause epiphora (tearing) and recurrent dacrocystorhinitis.

Telecanthus, medial canthal dystopia, nasal deformity, epiphora (tearing) and dacrocystitis are also complications of medial orbital wall/nasal injuries and can only be addressed by considering them in the acute phase and by reconstructing the areas anatomically.

The lateral orbital wall is fairly strong, supported by the temporalis muscle but weakened inferiorly by the inferior orbital fissure and posterosuperiorly by the superior orbital fissure. It is sensible to understand the relationship between these two fissures (see Figs 10.9, 10.15). Fractures in the lateral wall and displacement are usually associated with zygomatic fractures. Inferior displacement of the zygoma

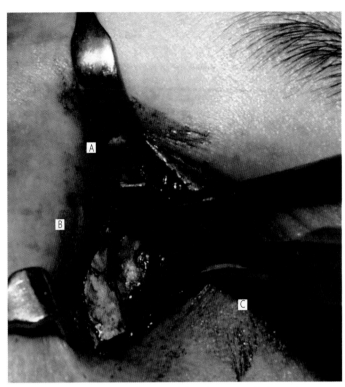

Fig. 10.25: Dissection of lacrimal fossa. A = medial canthus, B = fossa, C = nasolacrimal sac retracted.

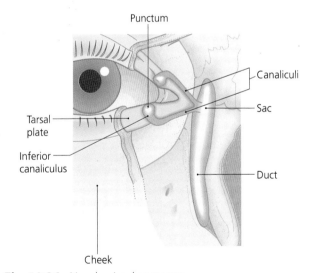

Fig. 10.26: Nasolacrimal anatomy.

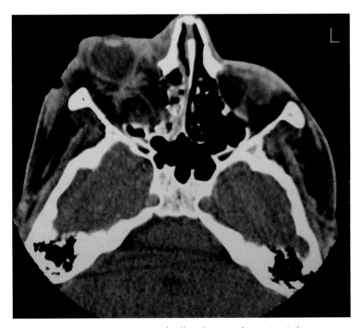

Fig. 10.24: CT showing retrobulbar hemorrhage in right eye.

leads to displacement of the lateral canthus and to a unilateral mongoloid slant to the palpebral fissure (see Fig. 10.11). Undercorrected or overcorrected lateral displacement (lateral wall) is the most common cause of enophthalmos and hypoglobus (low placement of eye). This is compounded, if zygomatic fixation at the frontozygomatic suture is not secure, because of the masseteric and temporalis muscles pulling the zygoma inferiorly leading to an osteodistraction force at the frontozygomatic suture with elongation of the lateral wall. This is a very important concept in secondary reconstruction and explains the need to resect a measured piece (usually 5 mm) of the lateral orbital rim in a malar (zygomatic) osteotomy (Fig. 10.27)

Adequate reduction of the zygoma is difficult to determine on the table and it is probable that ultrasound, fluoroscopy, CT navigation or endoscopy will become more popular.[6,7,8,20,21] Postoperative radiographs or some accurate analysis are an integral part of assessing the postoperative zygoma/orbit position. Reoperation should be undertaken earlier rather than later to avoid the long-term sequelae. In some countries (USA, Australia) postoperative spiral CT scans are taken for the moderate-to-complex orbital reconstructions to assess orbital volume, zygoma and bone graft position and orbital wall reconstruction. This is the gold standard and enables clinicians to improve future treatment of these patients.

The orbital roof is protected by the very strong supra-orbital rim but fractures are common in association with frontal sinus and naso-orbitoethmoidal fractures (Figs 10.28, 10.29). These can be both blow-out but more commonly blow-in fractures, leading to hypoglobus and proptosis.[32] This injury is also associated with diplopia due to displacement of the trochlea, which transmits the tendon of the superior oblique muscle of the eye.[43] Consideration of the orbital roof is essential in any craniofacial injury. The orbit's relationship with the frontal sinus is a natural defense mechanism against injury to the brain or eye with dissipation of the forces through fracturing of the walls of the air-filled sinus. If injured, this area warrants reconstruction because of damage to the frontonasal duct leading to mucoceles, sinusitis and possible meningitis. An isolated blow-in fracture with proptosis is relatively easily treated and is best done in collaboration with a neurosurgeon via a subcranial or transcranial approach.

The orbital apex is not well understood (see Figs 10.9, 10.10, 10.15, 10.17). It transmits the optic nerve with its retinal artery, which is an end-artery. Injury or constriction of this vessel may lead to acute or insidious blindness following an orbital injury (traumatic optic nerve lesion – TONL) and development of traumatic optic atrophy (Fig. 10.30). There is an increasing tendency, although unproven need, to explore this area to decompress the optic nerve and this will be discussed later under ocular injuries.

Other important anatomical factors in the apical area include the posterior aspects of the inferior and superior orbital fissures, the tendinous ring origin of the ocular muscles, the oculomotor, the trochlear, the abducens and ophthalmic (branches) nerves. Injury to this area leads to a number of well-recognized syndromes. The orbital apex syndrome is blindness (optic nerve injury). The clinical signs of superior orbital fissure syndrome are gross and persistent periorbital edema, proptosis (due to loss of tone of muscles of the eye), ophthalmoplegia and ptosis (third, fourth and sixth cranial nerves), subconjunctival hemorrhage, pupil

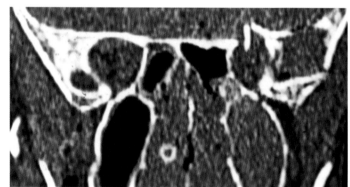

Fig. 10.28: Orbital blow-in fracture.

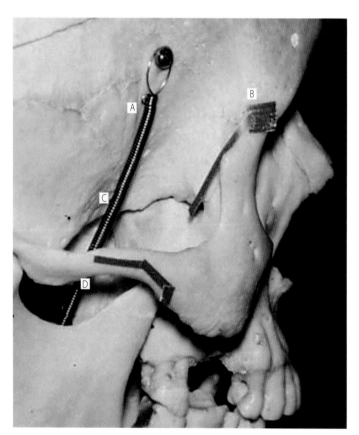

Fig. 10.27: Malar osteotomy cuts. A = Calvarial bone graft to augment floor, retrobulbar area and any bone defects, B = Resect (5mm), C = Osteotomy into inferior fissure, D = Arch osteotomy.

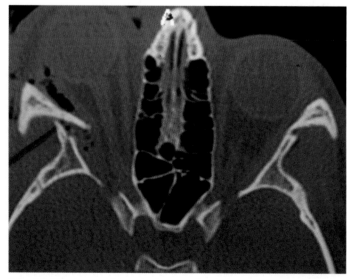

Fig. 10.29: Lateral blow-in fracture leading to proptosis and impingement on lateral rectus and indirectly on optic nerve.

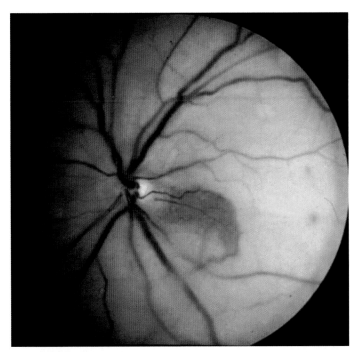

Fig. 10.30: Traumatic optic atrophy with preservation of a small retinal artery (normal color in that area).

dilatation, an absent direct light reflex but a persistent indirect light reflex (second nerve is normal), loss of accommodation, corneal reflex and sensation to the forehead (frontal nerve). Treatment for these has been conservative in the past. It is now advisable to consider orbital apex exploration, if a patient has an acute visual loss with no intraocular cause, in an effort to save vision.

It is necessary when operating to understand the dimensions of the orbit and how far it is safe to dissect down any individual wall.[34,44] It is for this reason that the availability of a dried or plastic skull in theater is advocated to facilitate an understanding of orbital dissection. It is possible through orbital incisions to mobilize the orbital contents so that they are free except for the superior fissure, the tendinous muscle origin/optic nerve and the nasolacrimal/medial canthal area.[2,3] This allows for a thorough exploration of all the orbital walls, floor and roof.

In the case of avulsive orbital defects, the remaining orbit should be reconstructed. The bony +/− soft tissue defect should be reconstructed with primary autogenous bone grafting, supported with rigid fixation (low-profile plates) and covered with soft tissue through local rotation flaps or free vascular tissue, rather than waiting for the scarring process to proceed. Scarring will further compromise the orbital outcome.

Assessment

Orbital injuries require a thorough investigation including an ophthalmic assessment,[9–11] an orthoptic assessment, photographs (preinjury, prior to repair and postoperatively), plain radiographs, CT assessment +/− MRI, occasionally 3D reconstruction and possibly stereolithic models. Ultrasound

has been shown to be useful in the A&E department and in theater for assessing zygomatic/orbital fractures and in particular medial and floor blow-out fractures.

Radiology is covered in Chapter 5. Briefly, plain radiographs are very useful and if carefully assessed can give good information. Comparison in a non-injured patient between the left and right zygoma, orbit and maxillary sinus usually indicates symmetry. Comparison in the injured can therefore give an accurate assessment of the displacement, accepting that there may have been a previous injury.

Occipitomental views at 10° and 30°, a submentovertex (if no neck injury) and a lateral face give the most information. It is advisable to look at the zygomatic arch (particularly posteriorly), the orbital rim (buckling/separate fragment), the frontozygomatic junction (F–Z distraction/diasthesis), the lateral maxillary buttress (displacement), the body of the zygoma (comminution) and the distance between the coronoid tip and the buttress to assess the amount of displacement (Figs 10.31, 10.32). A comparison and estimate of the size and shape of the quadrangular orbit and the maxillary sinus (black triangle) can help in both the acute and secondary assessment. The lateral face X-ray is mainly for looking at the nasal projection, frontal sinus and for height changes in those patients with associated maxillary fractures.

Tomography is rarely used but can be helpful to identify the position of metallic foreign bodies. This assessment should be done with some external metallic marker.

CT assessment is the investigation of choice for any patient with a blow-out fracture, diplopia, a comminuted orbital fracture and prior to secondary reconstruction (Figs 10.16, 10.24, 10.28, 10.29, 10.33, 10.34). Coronal and transverse images (1–2 mm) are required to be able to see the floor and the medial wall. CT allows the clinician to look at the bony orbit, the air sinuses around the orbit (frontal, ethmoidal and maxillary), the soft tissues for evidence of edema and hema-

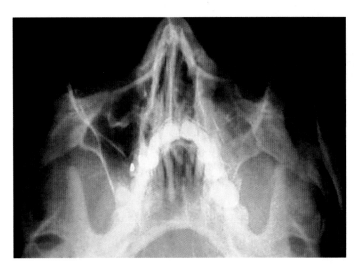

Fig. 10.31: Occipitomental view of a fractured left zygoma, not suitable for simple elevation. Note radiopaque and decreased size of triangle (maxillary sinus); decreased distance between the coronoid tip and zygoma body of the left as compared to the right side; left zygomatic arch (two fractures with distal disruption); multiple fractures along infraorbital rim with naso-orbital disruption.

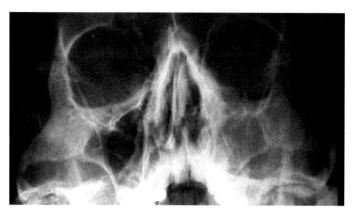

Fig. 10.32: Occipitomental view of a fractured left zygoma, not suitable for simple elevation. Note altered axis of orbital quadrangle horizontal to vertical; radiopaque and decreased size of triangle (maxillary sinus); left zygomatic arch (two fractures with distal disruption); loss of gentle curve of lateral maxillary sinus wall on the left; decreased distance between the coronoid tip and zygoma body on the left (overlap) as compared to the right side.

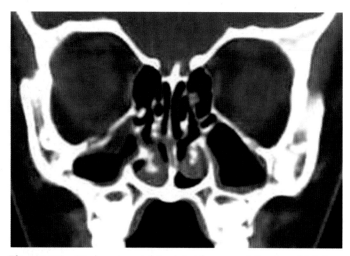

Fig. 10.33: CT showing right orbital floor crack fracture (child).

toma and the muscles for edema and fibrosis. Conventional 3D CT scans can be misleading (Fig. 10.35). Spiral 3D CT scans are much more accurate but still lack definition because of the very thin bones that make up the orbit. Stereolithic models have been used and are helpful but they are expensive and have not been accurate enough to allow for planning plate positioning and bending.[18]

CT is very useful for orbital volume assessment in orbital blow-out in the acute situation and once the swelling has settled, gives an idea of the amount of augmentation required and whether surgery is indicated (Fig. 10.34). It is advisable in all cases of enophthalmos to determine any bony defects, lateral displacement and the amount of bone required to restore the orbit to normal. CT navigation devices have been shown to be very useful in helping reconstruct orbital fractures and determining the position and amount of bone grafting required.[15,20,29,61] Orbital bone grafting should be combined with some assessment of intraocular pressure.[39]

MRI scans can be very helpful particularly for looking at soft tissues and have been shown to be just as accurate as CT scans in identifying blow-out fractures of the medial wall.[13,14,34] An MRI and CT scan can improve the information gained particularly for assessment prior to secondary correction.[30,31] Spiral CT scan remains the gold standard. Ultrasound is particularly useful in the acute situation in A&E or in a severely injured patient on intensive care to assess for an orbital injury.[17] It is particularly good at picking up buttress wall, medial wall and zygomatic arch fractures.

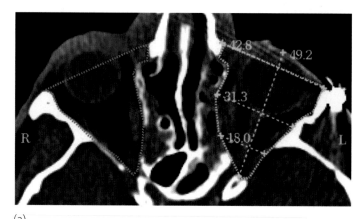

(a)

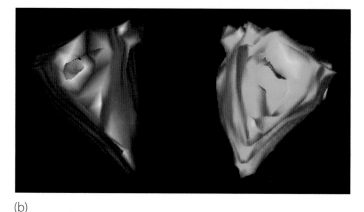

(b)

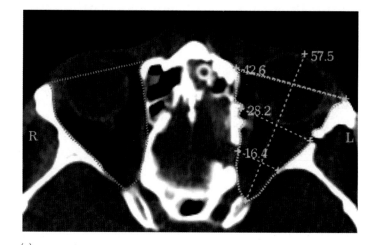

(c)

Fig. 10.34: CT of left orbital injury. **(a)** Computer measurements. **(b)** Computer-generated volume 3D assessments. **(c)** Postoperative measurements.

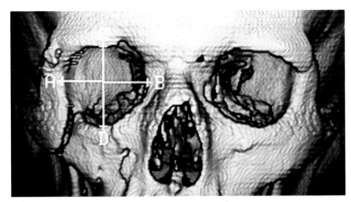

Fig. 10.35: 3D CT scan showing difficulty in interpretation because of thinness and computer reconstruction of floor and medial wall, although showing displacement of body of right zygoma.

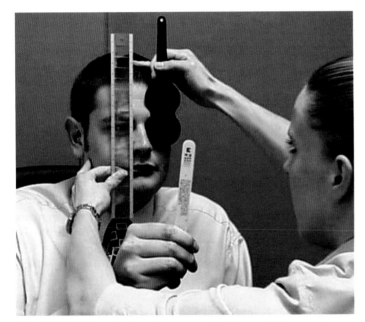

Fig. 10.36: Cover test and assessment of hypoglobus.

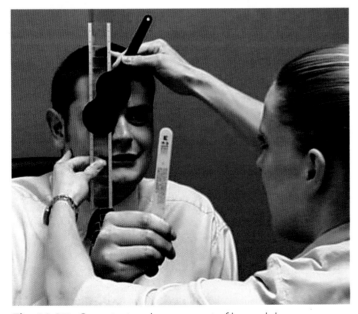

Fig. 10.37: Cover test and assessment of hypoglobus.

Fluoroscopy can be used to assess the bony positions and the vascular supply.[21]

Orthoptic tests (Figs 10.36–10.41) include the cover test, diplopia test, Hess test, binocular fixation tests and field tests. Ocular pressure is also assessed.

The Hess test is very useful for assessing and reviewing patients with diplopia. It allows clinicians to distinguish between edema, entrapment, neurological impairments and a previous strabismus. It is important to recognize that with entrapment the non-injured eye will overreact, because of the muscle straining in both eyes, in an attempt to get the injured eye to move (Fig. 10.38). This makes the discrepancy in eye movements appear greater than it really is.

The diplopia test should be increased from the nine cardinal positions to 25 to allow the testing of central gaze, peripheral gaze (<25°) and extreme peripheral gaze (>25°). The type of separation, vertical or horizontal, should be indicated on the form (Fig. 10.41).

It is essential to work closely with an ophthalmology department to enable assessment of these patients for ocular injury, to have access to orthoptists and to an ophthalmologist with a particular interest in managing diplopia.[9,10,11,29,45,46]

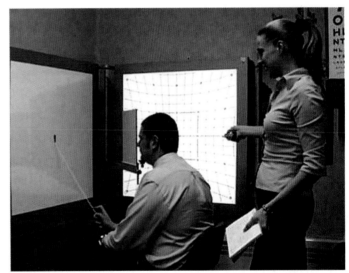

(a)

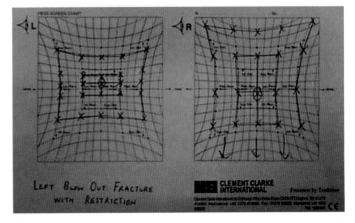

(b)

Fig. 10.38: Hess test. **(a)** Test in progress. **(b)** Print-out showing decreased movement of the left eye and overaction of the right.

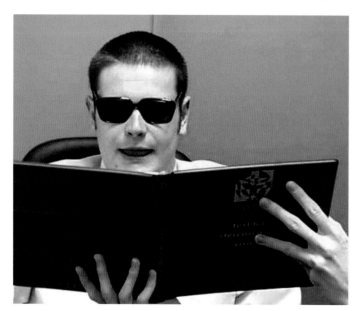

Fig. 10.39: Test for stereotactic vision.

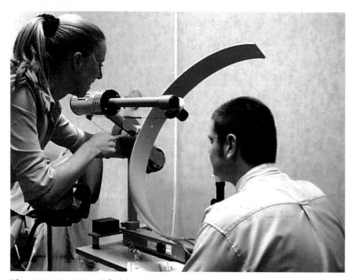

Fig. 10.40: Visual field testing.

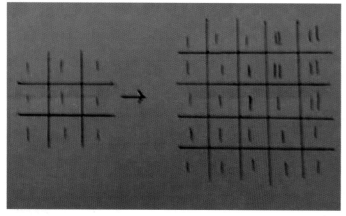

Fig. 10.41: Diplopia test showing double vision on looking up and to the left at extreme vision.

The Timing of Surgery

The timing of surgery is controversial for a number of reasons. Are the facilities available for accurate assessment, stabilization, intensive care and treatment? Is the surgical team available (surgeons, anesthetists, nurses)? Will the patient survive the severity of the head injury and/or other injuries? Are CT and neurosurgical support available for an accurate assessment? Many of these problems have been resolved with the universal availability of CT and the development of telemedicine. This enables neurosurgical, ophthalmological and other consultations to proceed. If the patient has a Glasgow Coma Scale score of >6, no evidence of an intracranial hemorrhage or midline shift and intracranial pressure monitoring is <15 mmHg lying down, facial surgery can proceed early and at the same time as other surgical procedures, e.g. orthopedic fixation.[47–49] It is probably best for the definitive surgery to proceed as soon as investigations are complete and the team can be brought together. This should be early or within 5–14 days at the latest. Soft tissue results appear to be better with early surgery.[26] The results for severe orbital and craniofacial fracture reconstruction have also been shown to be better from an esthetic and functional point of view if the surgery (full reconstruction) can be undertaken early. If there is a considerable threat to life from chest injury, abdominal bleed or severe head injury, facial surgery should be delayed for a few days. It is inappropriate to keep patients waiting 2–3 weeks before providing definitive treatment as the surgery becomes more difficult and the eventual outcome is less good. An advantage of early surgery appears to be the ability to limit the amount of fibrosis by limiting the ingrowth of fibroblasts and avoiding two insults – the injury and the delayed repair. Surgery is usually performed under steroid and antibiotic cover.[50]

Swelling of the soft tissues can make assessment more difficult but the development of CT scanning and the acceptance of the need to explore these injuries more thoroughly through coronal, facial and oral incisions have led to a better understanding of the extent of the facial injuries. Surgical correction has been further improved by the acceptance of primary bone grafting with rigid low-profile fixation for bony defects, orbital wall fractures and naso-orbital injuries. It is important to control any mobilized facial soft tissue by reattaching the periosteum supporting the facial soft tissue envelope to the facial bones. This prevents the unsightly facial soft tissue ptosis often associated with panfacial fractures.[26] The periosteum is supported with non-resorbable monofilament sutures to the orbital rim and temporalis muscle fascia. Careful attention to a layered closure of any soft tissue lacerations or incisions and to facial suturing is essential.[25] All facial sutures should be removed by 5 days at the latest.

There is a view that more simple orbital injuries (blow-out fractures) should be allowed to settle before deciding on surgery (<10 days) to enable ophthalmological, orthoptic and radiographic investigations to be completed. A few days allows for the diplopia secondary to edema or a hematoma to settle. Early surgery (<10 days) has been shown to give better results than delayed surgery (>3 months), particularly in children.[10,45,51,52,54] Orbital (lower lid) incisions are easier in the less swollen patient and enable the identification of a crease line. The latter problem can be avoided by the use of a transconjunctival or transcaruncular incision with adequate subperiosteal dissection to enable satisfactory access.

Prevention and Management of Enophthalmos

Prevention is much easier than cure. The etiology of enophthalmos is usually that the bony socket is too big following a zygomatic fracture, with inadequate reduction of the orbital rim, arch and buttress.[30,31] Enophthalmos may also occur if the orbital content is decreased by loss of orbital contents (fat) through the floor or medial wall or both or by loss of the globe or its rupture. Fat atrophy was considered to be a major cause of enophthalmos and was thought to be secondary to a vascular insult due to the trauma or the surgery. This is no longer considered to be a significant cause although cicatricial enophthalmos is well described.

It is not uncommon for an orbital blow-out fracture to be missed. The signs may be subtle because of orbital swelling and the only sign may be some numbness of the cheek/nose. Radiographs are difficult for the non-maxillofacial surgeon to interpret but the late signs are very obvious: enophthalmos,

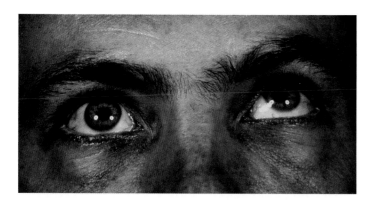

(a)

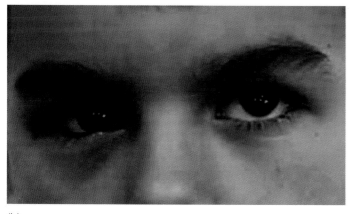

(b)

Fig. 10.42: Limitation of movement of right eye. **(a)** Movement. **(b)** Hypoglobus. Both patients complained of pain on looking up. Difference in level of light reflex allows for a clinical measurement and an assessment in time.

hypoglobus, supratarsal hollowing, supratarsal hooding, diplopia, numbness of the cheek and an altered palpebral fissure (Fig. 10.1). The palpebral aperture (opening and width) should be measured. The altered palpebral fissure presents as an asymmetry and is classically described as almond shaped but can have different shapes – rounded, widened, narrowed.

An accurate assessment of the extent of the orbital injury with plain radiographs and CT, adequate exposure, anatomical reconstruction and primary bone grafting should prevent the development of enophthalmos (see Chapter 12). The extent of surgery and the exposure required are proportional to the severity of the injury. The common problems relate to comminution of the zygomatic arch or infraorbital rim, failure to augment the orbital floor posteriorly or to explore the medial wall and inadequate stabilization.[23,24] It is advisable to follow patients for at least 6 months following an orbital injury to rule out the possibility of late enophthalmos and for at least 12 months to assess the outcome of infraorbital nerve anesthesia.[36,37]

Disorders of Ocular Motility

Acute disturbance in eye movement following trauma (Fig. 10.42) may be due to orbital edema, hematoma, direct orbital injury with associated extraocular muscle injury, periorbital fat entrapment, injuries to the third, fourth and sixth cranial nerves or disorders of the central control of eye movement.[10,11,16,28,29,43,45,46,51,53,54] Persistent diplopia is usually due to entrapment of the periorbital fat or fibrosis around the extraocular muscles.

Diplopia

Double vision (diplopia) is a common and debilitating sequel to orbital injury. Diplopia is usually associated with a blowout fracture of the floor or medial wall but can occur following roof or lateral wall injuries.[10] Hematoma, edema of extraocular muscles or their surrounding fascia or entrapment of the orbital fat septa are the principal causes (Figs 10.33, 10.43). Entrapment of extraocular muscles is now not considered the cause of diplopia in the acute phase but ischemic injury leading to fibrosis is considered important in secondary surgery. This ischemia may be secondary to the initial trauma or surgery. Cranial nerve palsies must be distinguished from the above causes which is relatively easily done with the advantage of orthoptic tests (Fig. 10.44). Trauma can lead to a previous latent squint breaking down and becoming manifest which is easily detected by orthoptic testing.

It is necessary to test visual acuity in each eye before testing for diplopia. Double vision usually does not occur in patients with poor vision in one eye or those who have received successful patching for amblyopia in the past and who effectively only use one eye at a time. Testing for diplopia should be done with the patient's reading glasses in place. If visual acuity is so bad that diplopia is not a problem, surgical repair may not be required unless the limited eye movement is esthetically unacceptable. Although monocular diplopia can occur, it is rare and warrants ophthalmological

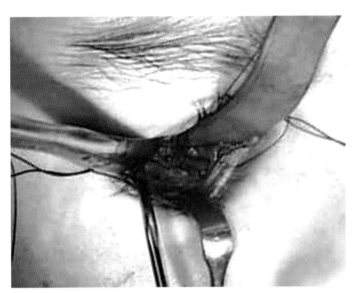

Fig. 10.43: Orbital floor crack fracture with fascial entrapment (CT in Fig. 10.33).

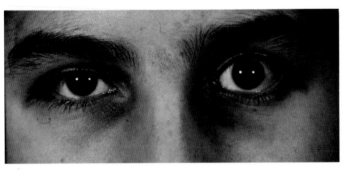

(a)

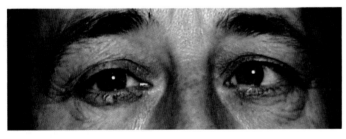

(b)

Fig. 10.44: Cranial nerve palsy. **(a)** Right oculomotor (third) nerve palsy. **(b)** Left abducens palsy secondary to carotico-cavernous sinus fistula.

assessment. It is usually due to corneal scarring, lens dislocation, cataract formation or retinal detachment.

Orbital floor blow-out fracture

Diplopia (double vision) may be vertical, horizontal or both. There may be restriction of upward and downward gaze with a sudden onset of pain, engendered by eye movement. The clinician should look for a slight retraction of the globe on attempts at upward gaze. A positive forced duction test may be elicited. Orbital emphysema may be present for 24 hours following injury. Enophthalmos may occur but is often camouflaged for 24–48 hours. It is associated with an asymmetric palpebral fissure, when compared to the normal eye. Ptosis of the upper eyelid due to enophthalmos may occur. When the patient attempts to lift that eyelid the other lid is also elevated, causing pseudo lid retraction on the contralateral side. Fast up-and-down eye movements (saccades) help to differentiate between muscle bruising and entrapment. In muscle bruising a slower eye movement occurs and with entrapment a rapid movement occurs but of incomplete amplitude. Increased intraocular pressure occurs on attempts at upward gaze due to tethering of the globe. Infraorbital nerve anesthesia may occur and may be accompanied by persistent pain and dysesthesia. Patients with an orbital injury and altered infraorbital sensation should be presumed to have a blow-out until proven otherwise by a review a few days later.

In the literature, there is an apparent difference in the way these patients are treated depending on whether they are seen by ophthalmology or oral and maxillofacial surgery.[10,53,54] Working co-operatively in a joint clinic has helped resolve some of the gray areas.[10,45] All patients have a thorough maxillofacial and ophthalmic assessment. Surgery depends on the severity of the problem. If the injury is severe, there is little controversy. If there is clinical entrapment (diplopia), enophthalmos, hypoglobus, infraorbital nerve anesthesia, both specialties, following investigations, advise surgery. If there is entrapment but no enophthalmos, no hypoglobus or infraorbital anesthesia, ophthalmologists prefer to wait and if diplopia persists, to correct it with muscle surgery.[53] In our practice, we have found the best results for persistent diplopia (>3 days with orthoptic evidence of entrapment) are achieved with early surgery.[10,45,54]

There are many surgical approaches to the orbital floor, all with advantages and disadvantages (Fig. 10.45). These are the infraorbital, lower lid, blepharoplasty, transconjunctival, medial canthal, transcaruncular, transmaxillary sinus and coronal approaches. All approaches have their place.[34] It is important to be comfortable with all incisions to give the patient the best available treatment.

Correction of enophthalmos alone is a decision that the team will make with patient involvement. Enophthalmos of >2 mm is noticeable and >4 mm is clinically obvious. Patients must be aware of the risks of surgery, with an incidence of 3/1000 of blindness in the acute repair and 1/1800 of blindness following delayed corrective surgery.[42]

There is an indication for immediate infraorbital nerve decompression for acute or persistent dysesthesia. This is achieved more easily through a lower eyelid incision or a transconjunctival incision and an inferior orbital rim orbitotomy than an intraoral incision and attempting to decompress the nerve with a burr from below (see Figs 10.18–10.22). Access is better and it is easier to free the whole nerve. Incisions in eyelid skin or transconjunctivally heal very well and are imperceptible at 1 month.

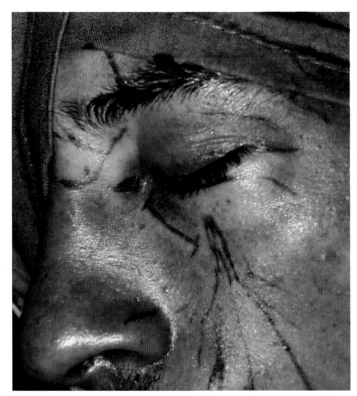

Fig. 10.45: Multiple access incisions. Medial blepharoplasty (dissecting supraorbital nerve), lateral blepharoplasty, medial canthal, lower blepharoplasty, lower lid and lateral orbital.

Medial wall blow-out fracture

Medial wall blow-out fractures accompany orbital floor blow-out fractures in about 50% of cases. Entrapment of the orbital fat septa medially results in horizontal diplopia and restriction of abduction with retraction of the globe. Early surgical repair is indicated in these cases. These are usually small defects and easily repaired with a thin piece of bone (maxillary sinus) or some alloplastic material. Access to the medial wall is through the transcaruncular, medial canthotomy (see Fig. 10.25), medial upper blepharoplasty and coronal approach.

Blow-in fracture

Fractures of the orbital roof may be undisplaced or the bone may blow in or blow out.[32] Symptoms following blow-in fractures of the orbital roof, floor and medial wall vary. These injuries can interfere with eye position, motility and optic nerve function. If symptoms persist, treatment is by open reduction and fixation. Perforating injuries of the orbital roof can lead to bone fragments being displaced into brain tissue. Damage to levator palpebrae superioris and the superior rectus muscle leads to ptosis and impaired upward gaze respectively. Fracture at the posterior aspect of the orbital roof where it is weakest and in the region of the optic canal and superior orbital fissure can result in profound damage to

the optic and oculomotor nerves. Prolapse of orbital tissue into the frontal sinus has been described.

Trauma to the trochlea

The superior oblique muscle passes through the trochlea, which is close to the medial superior orbital margin. Injury in this area can lead to entrapment of the superior oblique tendon, which causes restriction of elevation of the eye in adduction.[43] Simple stripping of the periosteum and repair of the bony skeleton in the area seems to resolve the problem. Detachment of the trochlea at the time of coronal dissection does not carry any long-term problems.[3]

Cranial nerve injury

In severe head injury, damage to the third, fourth and sixth cranial nerves is commonly seen. Postmortem studies have shown that the nerves may even be avulsed from the brain stem.

Oculomotor (third cranial) nerve injury results in ptosis, dilatation of the pupil and abduction with slight depression of the globe due to the unopposed actions of the remaining lateral rectus and superior oblique muscle function (see Fig. 10.44) There may be no recovery, normal recovery or recovery with aberrant regeneration. This injury will lead to paradoxical eye movement. Eyelid elevation occurs on adduction or looking down. Spontaneous recovery may take 4–6 months.

Trochlear (fourth cranial) nerve palsy may result from a contre-coup injury against the tentorium cerebelli. The superior oblique muscle causes depression of the globe in adduction, therefore vertical double vision occurs. There may be a torsional element in which the two images appear to be rotated with respect to each other. Torsional diplopia is usually following bilateral fourth nerve injuries. Spontaneous recovery may take 4–6 months. Surgery of the squint is deferred to allow spontaneous recovery to take place.

Abducens (sixth cranial) nerve injury causes loss of abduction. The sixth cranial nerve passes very close to the lateral orbital wall and the lateral rectus muscle. It is prone to injury following zygomatic or orbital injuries or orbital reconstruction. It usually recovers spontaneously. The sixth cranial nerve passes through the cavernous sinus and may thus also be injured following the development of a traumatic carotico-cavernous sinus fistula (see Fig. 10.44). Surgery is deferred to allow spontaneous recovery to take place following treatment of the fistula.

Surgery for persistent diplopia following entrapment or nerve injury depends on what is possible. Surgery may be undertaken on the healthy eye to weaken a muscle pull and is best performed using an adjustable suture technique. The major surgery is one with the patient under general anesthetic and the final adjustment (tightening or relaxation) completed with the patient sitting up awake under local anesthetic and a little sedation to enable fine adjustments to be made.

Disorders of Central Control of Eye Movements

Impairment of convergence

Impaired convergence may result from a closed head injury. The presumed cause is an upper midbrain injury. Treatment is with prisms on glasses.

Loss of fusion

Fusion of the images provided by the two eyes is required for single vision. Patients who have required orthoptic treatment for squint during childhood may have a reduced fusional capacity and a head injury can result in double vision when fusion is lost. Spontaneous recovery may occur. The subjective nature of double vision due to fusion can make it difficult to analyse objectively when compensation is involved. Treatment is with prisms on glasses.

Skew deviation

Skew deviation is characterized by vertical deviation of the eyes on lateral gaze. This can result from closed head injury and results in double vision on lateral gaze. Spontaneous recovery usually occurs.

Parinaud's syndrome

Injury to the region of the superior rectal plate can lead to dilated pupils, impairment of accommodation and convergence and impaired upwards gaze.

Posttraumatic nystagmus

Posttraumatic nystagmus may result from damage to the labyrinthine system or from brain stem trauma. This can be very difficult to treat and is outwith the remit of this chapter.

Eye Injuries

Decreasing visual acuity or blindness demands urgent assessment. The differential diagnosis includes traumatic optic nerve lesions, retrobulbar hemorrhage and vitreal hemorrhage.

Retrobulbar hemorrhage

This is an eye-saving diagnosis but is underdiagnosed in serious orbital injuries.[59] The patient presents with an orbital injury, proptosis, pain, developing ophthalmoplegia, decreasing visual acuity, dilating pupil and on ophthalmoscopy has pallor (arterial compression) or venous dilatation (venous compression) of the disc. If time allows, with the support of medical treatment an ultrasound or preferably a CT scan should be obtained, to determine the site of the hemorrhage to facilitate an urgent decompression (see Fig. 10.24). Medical treatment involves:

- mannitol 20%, 2 g/kg IV over 5 minutes
- dexamethasone 8 mg IV
- acetazolamide 500 mg IV and then 1000 mg orally over 24 hours
- surgical decompression remains the most certain option.

If visual acuity is deteriorating rapidly, a four-wall decompression under local anesthetic is required to prevent a permanent loss of vision. It is probably easier in the non-operated patient to decompress initially through a medial blepharoplasty rather than the usually recommended lateral canthotomy (see Fig. 10.5).

Traumatic optic nerve lesions

The optic nerve may be damaged at the junction of the eye, within the orbit or within the optic canal. This is a common long-term cause of decreased visual acuity following an orbital injury.[60] A significant percentage (2%) of patients with an orbital injury have an ocular injury severe enough to render them blind in that eye.[9,11] The incidence of blindness in those patients with more severe orbital fractures (fronto-orbital) is significantly higher.

Partial tearing of the optic nerve from the eye leads to the tearing of nerve fiber bundles with a corresponding visual field defect. Hemorrhage at the optic nerve head can initially be seen which evolves into optic nerve pallor (see Fig. 10.30). As the pigment epithelium of the retina heals a crescent of pigmented change may be seen in the late stages. The distribution of the nerve fiber loss dictates whether central vision is lost or not. The mechanism of damage probably results from torsion of the globe with respect to the optic nerve.

Traumatic optic nerve lesions (TONL) generally occur acutely. Two percent (0.7–5.0%) of all closed head injuries and 20% of all frontobasal injuries show some kind of visual pathway damage, in which the intracanalicular part of the optic nerve is affected (see Figs 10.28, 10.29).

TONL most commonly are secondary to frontal (72%) or frontotemporal (12%) injuries. These patients often have associated complex general injuries. In about 60% of patients with severe midface or skull base fractures a routine neuro-ophthalmologic investigation with evaluation of optic nerve function is not possible because of the patient's conscious level or swelling. Some means of testing is required to distinguish permanent from temporary TONL. Electrophysiological testing of the visual pathways with flash ERG/VEP is a known method in the non-acute situation but is not frequently used in the acute situation to assess TONL. This test allows a diagnostic assessment of vision and facilitates the decision on whether to operate (decompress) or not (Fig. 10.46). Total avulsion of the optic nerve is very rare but occurs with severe orbital injuries and results in immediate blindness (Fig. 10.47). Decompressive surgery is not indicated in avulsion injuries.

The first clinical step is the assessment of vision, followed by gross visual field testing and if necessary the swinging flash light test. If the patient is unconscious and a decision on visual pathway function or a diagnosis of visual pathway damage cannot be made, electrophysiological testing with flash ERG/-VEP is undertaken. Visual pathway function is classified as *normal*, *pathological* or *absent* and treatment

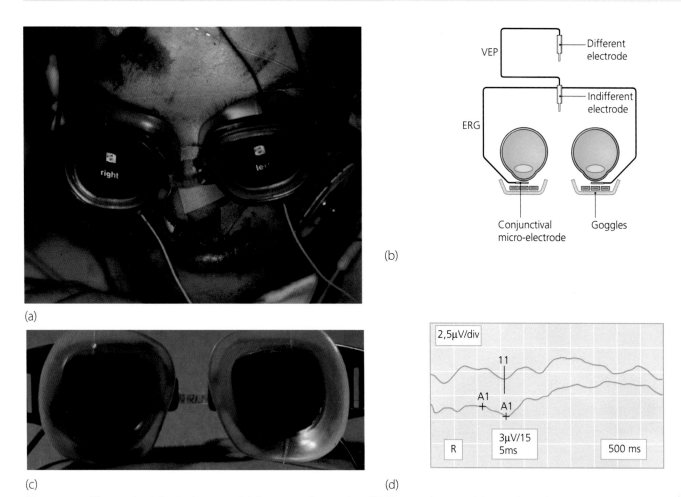

Fig. 10.46: Electrophysiological testing. **(a)** Patient with goggles. **(b)** Electrical set-up. **(c)** Goggles. **(d)** Print-out.

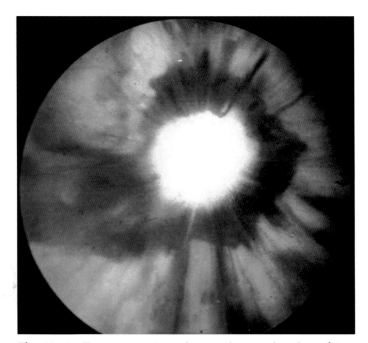

Fig. 10.47: Traumatic optic avulsion with immediate loss of vision and decreased intraocular pressure.

decisions are made on the basis of this. The checkerboard VEP investigation would be superior for the detection of TONL but is unfortunately not applicable in the unconscious or unco-operative patient.

If decreased visual acuity is detected, an axial spiral CT scan of the midface and the frontal skull base with reconstructed coronal planes is performed. This enables visualization of the orbit, optic canal, optic chiasma and displaced bones in order to identify where the origin for the TONL might be. This helps indicate whether to treat or not to treat a patient surgically. It is important to recognize that a compressive TONL does not necessarily require a displaced fracture in the optic canal. A whiplash type injury with no displacement, an occult fracture or simply edema can result in compression and may need decompression (Fig. 10.48). Most patients with a confirmed posttraumatic afferent disorder of the visual pathway (TONL) have a fracture in the bony optic canal or the posterior third of the orbit or a space-occupying intraorbital lesion (retrobulbar hemorrhage).

Three-dimensional CT reconstructions are of no additional diagnostic value and might be misleading because of the window threshold normally used and the thinness of the bony structures in the area. MRI is better than CT scanning at showing optic nerve edema or hematoma but CT is still preferred to assess for bony injuries. High-resolution axial

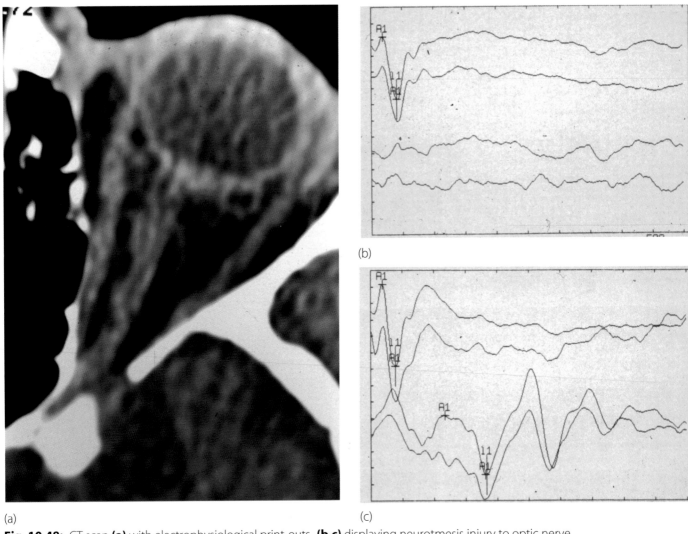

(a)

(b)

(c)

Fig. 10.48: CT scan **(a)** with electrophysiological print-outs **(b,c)** displaying neurotmesis injury to optic nerve.

spiral CT scan with coronal reconstruction is the gold standard to detect midface and skull base fractures. Plain radiographs are usually of little value in detecting the bony lesions responsible for visual pathway damage. Ultrasound is a valid method, especially for detection of retrobulbar hematoma, but is of limited value for optic nerve injuries.

Therapy of TONL

There are basically four options and research can support all of them:

■ wait and see
■ conservative treatment
■ surgical treatment
■ combined conservative and surgical treatment.

The diagnosis of TONL is important. Patients with orbital injuries in association with severe midface or skull base fractures should be investigated on a routine basis. If there is no evidence of a TONL in the unconscious patient, a wait-and-see policy is acceptable. It is the delay to the onset of treatment that limits the prognosis for a successful visual pathway treatment.

Glucocorticoids dominate the conservative treatment. Their therapeutic effect is related to their antiedematous, anti-inflammatory and antioxidative effects. They prevent vasospasm, which in turn helps prevent neuron death. They inhibit the gliofibrillary scarring of the traumatized optic nerve.

There has been one study advocating high-dose steroids, undertaken in the US in 1994. Treatment with methylprednisolone must be started not later than 8 hours following the trauma with an initial IV bolus of 30 mg/kg bodyweight, followed by 5.4 mg/kg bodyweight over the following 48 hours. This protocol originates from a spinal cord injury study (NASCIS). The rationale for the methylprednisolone megadose is the reduction it produces in free radicals, the decrease in secondary posttraumatic lesions due to impaired lipid peroxidation and the improved perfusion of the CNS. With this dose of steroid, blood glucose level needs to be monitored and antacid therapy commenced prophylactically. Treatment with acetazolamide and mannitol infusion has been described, although there is still no evidence for their value.

Joseph's team correlated the severity of the external trauma, the location and extent of the fracture and TONL with the amount of brain contusion, swelling, hematoma and intracranial bleeding.[55] In combination with neuro-ophthalmologic findings, they undertook a prospective study but despite early promise, they were unable to define the need for early optic nerve decompression. They believe optic nerve decompression must be a case-orientated decision, based on the clinical and CT findings.

Clinical findings have been correlated with individual fractures and show that the prognosis for the afferent disorder of the visual pathway depends on whether or not the optic canal is involved.

A retrobulbar hematoma needs to be differentiated from a bone-related TONL. If there is a posttraumatic globe protrusion present together with an ipsilateral afferent disorder of the visual pathway, the intraorbital pressure within the orbital compartment has to be released by opening the orbital septum. This should be done in conjunction with medical treatment and an urgent CT scan. If there is any delay in obtaining a CT, treatment should be started. Decompression depends on the site of the bleed. In the first author's experience this is usually medially and a medial blepharoplasty approach is preferred. This is easily performed under local anesthetic and sedation in the A&E department. The only contraindication for this emergency operation is a pulsating exophthalmos, which may be due to a carotico-cavernous sinus fistula. In this rare case pretherapeutic imaging is performed including angiographic investigations.

The controversy with regard to surgical treatment of TONL relates to the extent of surgery, the surgical approach and its timing. The aim of surgical therapy of TONL is to mechanically release the nerve along the optic tract but especially in the optic canal area, where bone fragments might impinge on the nerve or where relative narrowing of the canal (hematoma, edema) might be present. If there is evidence of TONL, an urgent decompression procedure is considered to relieve the optic nerve in its canal. The dura over the optic nerve or chiasma is not incised.

Surgical approaches are variable and all have some advantages. Besides the transethmoidal, it is now possible with transcranial, sublabial, transsphenoidal and endonasal microsurgical approaches to reach the area of interest. The method chosen depends on previous surgical experience.

TONL in craniofacial reconstruction

There is a danger of visual loss with any orbital procedure, both in primary and secondary orbital reconstruction, and patients should be warned about it. The risk can be reduced by using computer-assisted surgery (Fig. 10.49). Modern navigation systems allow for a precise preoperative planning and intraoperative control of any contour changes, i.e. all changes close to the optic canal can be directly controlled. This is important in defining the most posterior position of bone transplants or alloplastic grafts to augment the orbit.[20,22,39,58] During the operation three infrared cameras are used to detect the position of preset markers via integrated LEDs and changes in the patient's position monitored via LEDs attached to a Mayfield clamp.

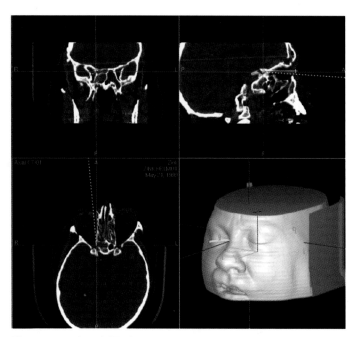

Fig. 10.49: Spiral CT 3D peroperative reconstruction with probe identifying surgical area under investigation (review with Fig. 10.34).

Changes in pupillary diameter or shape are not uncommon during complex orbital reconstructions. Obviously optic nerve injury needs to be ruled out. As the patient is under general anesthetic, the function of the visual pathway cannot be judged clinically and therefore flash ERG and VEP can be used intraoperatively to assess vision and to confirm lack of compression of the optic nerve by the grafting procedure.

Eyelid injury

The most common injury is a bruise. The pattern of bruising depends on whether the leakage of blood is superficial or deep. Superficial bruising extends down onto the face. Deep bruising gives rise to a demarcation line resembling the eye of a panda, with blood constrained behind the septum, and this type of bruising usually follows an orbital fracture. A subconjunctival hemorrhage with a posterior limit is usually due to a direct ocular injury, whilst a subconjunctival hemorrhage with no posterior limit is a common sequel to an orbital fracture (Fig. 10.50). Swelling of the eyelids is very common and is exacerbated if a patient with an orbital fracture blows his nose, leading to the clinical sign of crepitus. Massive swelling can be a sign of a retrobulbar hemorrhage or orbital vein obstruction.

Lacerations need special care, particularly those affecting the medial eyelids with the potential for injury to the nasolacrimal apparatus and canthal area (Fig. 10.51). These lacerations should be examined under magnification and with good lighting. The canthal area should be assessed. Lid margins must be accurately realigned. The layers of the eyelid should be identified and repaired with 5.0 or 6.0 resorbable sutures to the deep layers, ensuring proper apposition of the orbicularis oculi, and fine monofilament sutures to the skin of the eyelid. Tears of the medial canthus should be identified

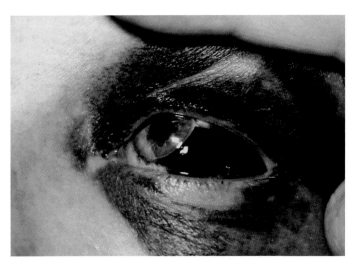

Fig. 10.50: Bruising/subconjunctival hemorrhage.

and primarily repaired with non-resorbable sutures. The nasolacrimal apparatus, if injured, should be repaired over appropriate stents.

Corneal abrasion

Corneal injury causes severe pain, blurring of vision, photophobia and lacrimation. Damage to the corneal epithelium may be due to direct injury or may result from inadequate eyelid closure due to facial palsy or loss of eyelid tissue. Alcohol-based skin preparations must never be used on the eyelids prior to surgery as these can cause corneal epithelial loss. Incomplete eyelid closure during surgery is another hazard to be avoided. Fluorescein staining of the cornea identifies the pathology (green). Antibiotic ointment is instilled as a prophylaxis against secondary infection.

Corneal foreign body

Superficial corneal foreign bodies can be lifted off with the pointed end of a hypodermic needle, preferably using binocular magnification, using one drop of topical local anesthetic. A short-acting cycloplegic agent such as cyclopentolate 1% (which diminishes pain due to ciliary spasm) and a topical antibiotic are instilled. Topical diclofenac has recently been shown to afford good pain relief.

Blunt eye injuries

Closed injury causes damage due to both distortion and concussion of the globe (during the brief duration of the injury) and concussion. Both types of injury can be seen. A high-speed blow to the eye causes marked globe distortion. The eye is compressed, resulting in anteroposterior shortening and coronal distension. The cornea and sclera are unable to distend. Therefore the iris, ciliary body, zonule of the lens and peripheral retina may be torn from their insertions. In severe cases, rupture of the sclera has been described. Distortional injury can also cause tearing of the choroid, which is associated with subretinal hemorrhage, and in very severe cases avulsion of the optic nerve.

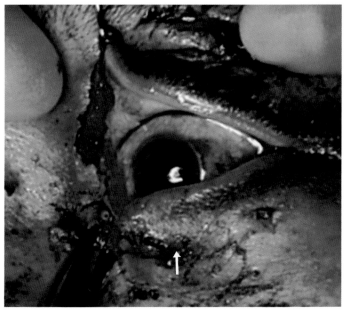

(a)

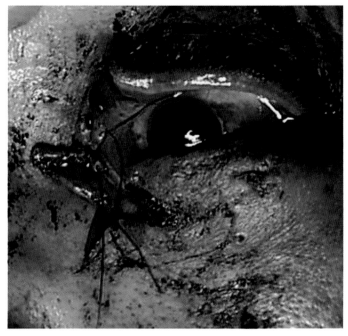

(b)

Fig. 10.51: Nasolacrimal laceration. **(a)** Laceration with probable nasolacrimal injury (arrow = punctum). **(b)** Exploration of canalicular system with fine nylon sutures.

The concussional component of the injury can damage the cornea, the lens, the retina, the choroid and the optic nerve, all of which are susceptible to transient or permanent damage. These injuries are best assessed by an ophthalmologist.

Conjunctiva

Swelling of the conjunctiva is commonly associated with subconjunctival hemorrhage and resolves spontaneously.

Cornea

The cornea is made up of five layers: the epithelium and its basement membrane, the stroma and the endothelium with its basement membrane. Damage to the epithelium results in an erosion, which requires the topical application of anesthetic (long acting) and a topical antibiotic.

Stromal and endothelial damage causes corneal edema. This is because the pumping action of the endothelium, which retains the cornea's transparency, ceases to function following the injury. In the majority of cases, corneal edema clears spontaneously.

Anterior chamber, iris and anterior chamber angle

Ripping of the iris from its root is a common sequel to blunt injury. Tearing of fine vessels in the iridocorneal angle results in bleeding in the anterior chamber and hyphema (Fig. 10.52). The hyphema is managed conservatively in the majority of cases. Spontaneous rebleeding into the eye is rare but is more likely to occur in those patients who are given aspirin, which is contraindicated in ocular hemorrhage. Severe hemorrhage can impair the drainage of aqueous humor, which will lead to a raised intraocular pressure. A

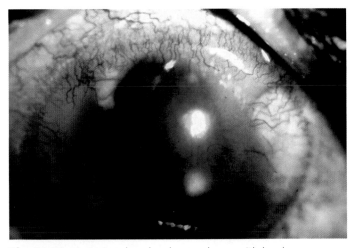

Fig. 10.52: Anterior chamber hemorrhage with hyphema.

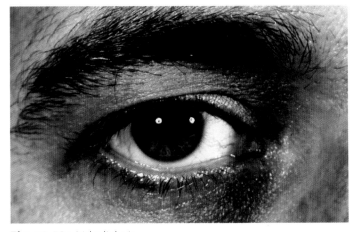

Fig. 10.53: Iridodialysis.

hemorrhage in the anterior chamber may be complicated by blood staining of the cornea.

Traumatic iritis is common. An injury to the iris causes the release of protein and inflammatory cells into the anterior chamber. These are seen on slit-lamp microscopy. Treatment is with topical steroids to diminish the inflammation and with pupil dilatation (cyclopentolate), to decrease the probability of the iris sticking to the lens (posterior synechiae). Deepening of the anterior chamber suggests that the lens may have been subluxated or even become dislocated.

Iridodialysis (tear in the iris) results from the iris being ripped from its root (Fig. 10.53). Traumatic mydriasis is common. The dilated pupil does not react directly or consensually. In severe cases, pupil sphincter ruptures can be seen on the slit lamp and this results in a permanent widely dilated pupil. More commonly, a mid-dilated pupil can result from such injury and spontaneous recovery can take place.

Angle recession occurs when the iris is partially stripped from its root without being torn completely. Rarely, severe injuries can lead to 360° recession. The iridocorneal angle contains Schlemm's canal. The healing response can give rise to fibrosis and scarring in this area, which diminishes the outflow of aqueous and can cause raised intraocular pressure, either acutely or many years later. Angle recession takes place at the time of injury and can be visualized by gonioscopy (slit-lamp examination using a mirror or prism system to see into the angle). This pathology can easily be missed if detailed slit-lamp eye examination is not carried out and can lead to glaucoma in the long term.

Lens

The lens can be damaged in a number of different ways. Subluxation of the lens is a common sequel to a severe blunt injury. Macroscopically the principal clinical sign comprises wobbling of the iris or iridodonesis. Dislocation of the lens into the vitreous is less common. Occasionally the lens can be dislocated into the anterior chamber. This is an acute ophthalmic emergency and is more common in people with underlying spontaneous lens subluxation, such as those with Marfan's syndrome. Such lens injuries cause changes in refraction both because the lens is moved and because it does not accommodate for near vision so well. Traumatic cataract can be the result of severe concussional injury. In cases of severe injury the pupil margin impacts upon the anterior surface of the lens, leaving a permanent pigmented ring.

Rarely, rupture of the lens capsule can take place. Aqueous fluid then enters the lens and this in turn causes opacification or cataract formation for which the only effective treatment strategy is cataract surgery, when the acute effects of the injury (e.g. traumatic iritis) have resolved.

Ciliary body

The ciliary body performs two principal functions: the production of aqueous humor and accommodation of the lens. Damage to the ciliary body can therefore lead to reduction in aqueous humor formation and a reduced intraocular pressure.

Impaired accommodation is common after blunt eye injury. Patients complain of blurring of vision and eye strain, particularly when reading. Reading matter held in front of the affected eye cannot be seen in focus as close as the unaffected eye and in some cases reading glasses which give balance to the focusing system are required.

Tearing of the ciliary body from its root is rare and is called traumatic cyclodialysis. A persistent very low intraocular pressure results which may necessitate surgical repair of the injury.

Retina

The distortional effects of blunt injury can lead to tearing of the peripheral retina (known as retinal dialysis) or peripheral retinal hole formation. The vitreous gel adheres firmly to the peripheral retina. The acute coronal distension of the injury distorts the vitreous, which can pull and tear the peripheral retina. The majority of cases of retinal dialysis are secondary to trauma. Tears of the peripheral retina can lead to water from within the vitreous passing through the tear and lifting off the retina. Progressive retinal detachment results (Fig. 10.54). Patients who are short-sighted or who have conditions predisposing to retinal detachment such as myopia, Stickler's syndrome or Marfan's syndrome are at a significant risk. Approximately 10% of traumatic retinal detachments occur at the time of the injury, 70% within 2 years and 20% more than 2 years after injury. If the tear passes through a retinal vessel then bleeding into the vitreous can take place. This gives rise to the sensation of seeing floaters in the visual field. Blunt injury to the globe can also cause damage to the vitreous humor which can collapse, leading to the formation of strands in the vitreous, which can also give rise to floaters.

Treatment of retinal detachment is complex and not always successful. It is therefore important to prevent retinal detachment by identifying and treating dialysis and retinal holes by photocoagulation and/or cryotherapy. Exudative retinal detachment can occur as a rare sequel to blunt eye trauma. In such causes, spontaneous flattening of the retina takes place but the prognosis for recovery of vision is poor.

Traumatic retinal edema is also known as commotio retinae or Berlin's edema (Fig. 10.55). Whitening of the retina is seen. If the edema takes place at the posterior pole, blurring of vision occurs. Peripheral edema, which causes peripheral visual field impairment, may not be symptomatic and may be missed. The majority of patients report rapid improvement in vision during the first 40 minutes after injury. In some cases of severe injury, improvement does not take place and fluorescein angiography reveals breakdown in function of the pigment epithelium in the retina. Permanent visual impairment can ensue and such pathology may be accompanied by the development of a traumatic retinal hole or pigmentary changes in the retina known as traumatic pigmentary retinopathy. This clinical pattern is very similar to retinitis pigmentosa.

Choroidal tears

Choroidal tears due to blunt injury characteristically occur circumferential to the optic disc (Fig. 10.56). Initially extensive subretinal hemorrhage is seen but as the hemorrhage

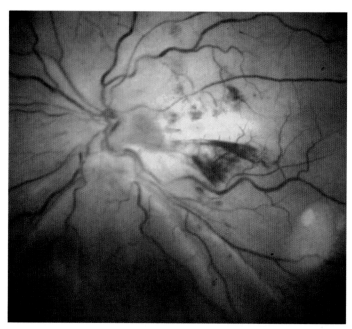

Fig. 10.54: Retinal detachment.

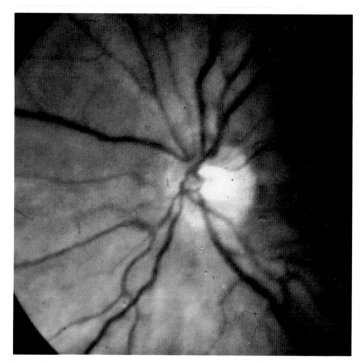

Fig. 10.55: Traumatic retinal edema or commotio retinae (Berlin's edema).

resolves, the tear becomes apparent. If the tear passes through the fovea, central vision is lost but in tears which do not affect the fovea, the prognosis is much better. Occasionally, the healing response can include the growth of new blood vessels, which can grow under the macula and cause secondary visual loss.

Choroidal effusion looks very similar to retinal detachment. However, there are no holes in the retina and the appearance is more ballooned in nature. Severe hypotonia (which may be due to cyclodialysis) is the principal underlying cause.

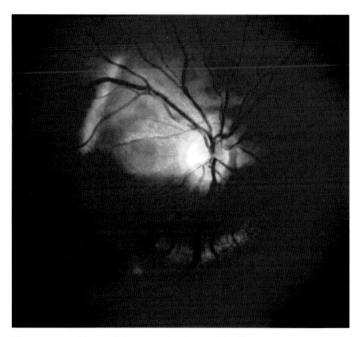

Fig. 10.56: Choroidal tear with choroidal effusion.

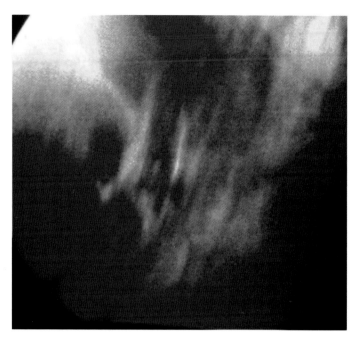

Fig. 10.57: Vitreal hemorrhage secondary to a perforating eye injury.

Injury to the sclera

Injury to the sclera is most common in the superonasal quadrant and is in 18% of scleral tears associated with an orbital fracture. If an eye has a very low intraocular pressure, rupture of the sclera posteriorly may be present and requires imaging studies to diagnose this.

If a scleral rupture is not repaired, persistent hypotonia or the ingrowth of fibrous tissue can develop. Surgical exploration is indicated in the majority of cases of persistent hypotonia for which there is no clear explanation as repair of the scleral rupture is usually accompanied by restoration of intraocular pressure and prevents the complication of fibrous ingrowth. In addition, sympathetic ophthalmia in which inflammation of the other eye occurs can rarely complicate scleral rupture.

Perforating eye injuries

Orbital and facial fractures may rarely be accompanied by perforating eye injury, particularly following road traffic accidents. The presence of multiple facial lacerations increases the index of suspicion that there may be an underlying perforating eye injury.

Visual function is determined if possible. The eyes are examined by gentle retraction of the eyelids, without direct pressure on the bottom of the eye. There may be an obvious perforation or some irregularity of the pupil, opacification of the anterior chamber due to intraocular hemorrhage or a shallow anterior chamber. Prolapse of iris, ciliary body or vitreous may be observed. Loss of vision secondary to a vitreal hemorrhage may be the only clinical sign of the injury (Fig. 10.57).

Perforation of the globe by a small, fast, flying missile necessitates appropriate radiological examination. Immediate transfer to the care of an ophthalmologist is indicated. A pad is applied to the eye and pressure to the globe is avoided. Primary surgical repair is carried out within 24 hours. If surgical treatment is delayed, prophylactic intravenous broad-spectrum antibiotic treatment is indicated.

Indirect ophthalmic sequelae to injury

Traumatic retinal angiopathy (Purtscher's retinopathy)

Multiple cotton wool spots at the posterior pole of the eye are observed (Fig. 10.58). A sudden increase in intravenous pressure due to severe head or chest injury is thought to give rise to a reactive precapillary arteriolar spasm in the retina which in turn causes multiple small retinal infarcts. A similar appearance is observed in patients who sustain long bone

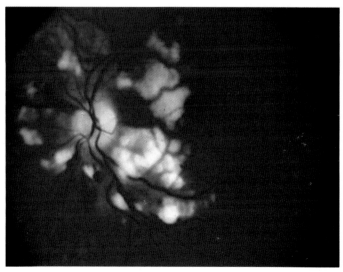

Fig. 10.58: Traumatic retinal angiopathy.

fractures with secondary fat emboli. Impairment of loss of central vision ensues in one or both eyes. There is no specific treatment but fortunately spontaneous resolution with return of normal visual function takes place in the majority of cases.[58]

Carotico-cavernous sinus fistula and arteriovenous anastomosis

The formation of a fistula between the arterial and venous systems may occur a few days following severe skull injury (see Fig. 10.44). The ophthalmic features include pulsating exophthalmos, ophthalmoplegia, chemosis and markedly dilated blood vessels on the conjunctiva and eyelids. The intraocular pressure is raised. Loss of vision may ensue without treatment.

Papilledema

Swelling of the optic nerve head due to raised intracranial pressure may be observed. In the acute phase, swelling does not take place but the absence of spontaneous venous pulsation and failure of the retinal veins to collapse when pressing the upper eyelid during ophthalmoscopy is a useful clinical sign.

Facial palsy

Incomplete eyelid closure as a sequel to traumatic facial palsy can give rise to corneal ulceration and infection. Patients who do not manifest a Bell's phenomenon (in which the eye rolls up when the eyelids are closed) are particularly at risk. Eye ointment is required to prevent drying of the cornea. Tarsorrhaphy or injection of levator palpebrae superioris with botulinum toxin to produce eyelid closure may be required if ulceration has developed.

Conclusion

The management of orbital injuries is a challenging area. It requires an ability to collaborate with others and to understand the surgical anatomy, physiology and potential complications. A thorough assessment, full investigations, satisfactory exposure, anatomical reconstruction with appropriate material and audit of our results will improve the lot of our patients.

References

1 Errington J 1999 Facing the future (editorial). British Journal of Oral and Maxillofacial Surgery 37: 161–163
2 Ellis E III, Zide MF 1995 Surgical approaches to the facial skeleton. Williams and Wilkins, Baltimore, pp 7–65
3 Kerawala CJ, Grime RJ, Stassen LFA, Perry M 2000 The bicoronal flap (craniofacial access): an audit of morbidity and a proposed surgical modification in male pattern baldness. British Journal of Oral and Maxillofacial Surgery 38(5): 441–444
4 Baumann A, Ewers R 2000 Transcaruncular approach for reconstruction of medial orbital wall fracture. International Journal of Oral and Maxillofacial Surgery 29(4): 264–267
5 Ilankovan V 1991 Transconjunctival approach to the orbital region: a cadaveric and clinical study. British Journal of Oral and Maxillofacial Surgery 129(3): 169–172
6 Jin HR, Shin SO, Choo MJ, Choi YS 2000 Endonasal endoscopic reduction of blowout fractures of the medial orbital wall. Journal of Oral and Maxillofacial Surgery 58(8): 847–851
7 Chen CT, Lai JP, Chen YR et al 2000 Application of endoscope in zygomatic fracture repair. British Journal of Plastic Surgery 53(2): 100–105
8 Lee CH, Lee C, Trabulsy PP, Alexander JT, Lee K 1998 A cadaveric and clinical evaluation of endoscopically assisted zygomatic fracture repair. Plastic and Reconstructive Surgery 101(2): 333–345; discussion 346–347
9 al-Qurainy IA, Stassen LF, Dutton GN, Moos KF, el-Attar A 1991 The characteristics of midfacial fractures and the association with ocular injury: a prospective study. British Journal of Oral and Maxillofacial Surgery 29(5): 291–301
10 al-Qurainy IA, Stassen LF, Dutton GN, Moos KF, el-Attar A 1991 Diplopia following midfacial fractures. British Journal of Oral and Maxillofacial Surgery 29(5): 302–307
11 al-Qurainy IA, Titterington DM, Dutton GN et al 1991 Midfacial fractures and the eye: the development of a system for detecting patients at risk of eye injury. British Journal of Oral and Maxillofacial Surgery 29(6): 363–367
12 Fox LA, Vannier MW, West OC, Wilson AJ, Baran GA, Pilgram TK 1995 Diagnostic performance of CT, MPR and 3DCT imaging in maxillofacial trauma. Computerized Medical Imaging and Graphics 19(5): 385–395
13 Ilankovan V, Hadley D, Moos K, el-Attar A 1991 A comparison of imaging techniques with surgical experience in orbital injuries. A prospective study. Journal of Craniomaxillofacial Surgery 19(8): 348–352
14 Maya MM, Heier LA 1998 Orbital CT. Current use in the MR era. Neuroimaging Clinics of North America 8(3): 651–683
15 Mauriello JA Jr, Lee HJ, Nguyen L 1999 CT of soft tissue injury and orbital fractures. Radiologic Clinics of North America 37(1): 241–252, xii
16 Cahan MA, Fischer B, Iliff NT, Clark NL, Manson PN 1996 Less common orbital fracture patterns: the role of computed tomography in the management of depression of the inferior oblique origin and lateral rectus involvement in blow-in fractures. Journal of Craniofacial Surgery 7(6): 449–459
17 McCann PJ, Brocklebank LM, Ayoub AF 2000 Assessment of zygomaticoorbital complex fractures using ultrasonography. British Journal of Oral and Maxillofacial Surgery 38(5): 525–529
18 Holck DE, Boyd EM Jr, Ng J, Mauffray RO 1999 Benefits of stereolithography in orbital reconstruction. Ophthalmology 106(6): 1214–1218
19 Gruss JS, Van Wyck L, Phillips JH, Antonyshyn O 1990 The importance of the zygomatic arch in complex midfacial fracture repair and correction of posttraumatic orbitozygomatic deformities. Plastic and Reconstructive Surgery 85(6): 878–890
20 Stanley RB Jr 1999 Use of intraoperative computed tomography during repair of orbitozygomatic fractures. Archives of Facial Plastic Surgery 1(1): 19–24
21 Kobienia BJ, Sultz JR, Migliori MR, Schubert W 1998 Portable fluoroscopy in the management of zygomatic arch fractures. Annals of Plastic Surgery 40(3): 260–264
22 Watzinger F, Wanschitz F, Wagner A et al 1997 Computer-aided navigation in secondary reconstruction of post-traumatic deformities of the zygoma. Journal of Craniomaxillofacial Surgery 25(4): 198–202
23 Kasrai L, Hearn T, Gur E, Forrest CR, Manson P 1999 A biomechanical analysis of the orbital zygomatic complex in human cadavers: examination of load sharing and failure patterns after fixation with titanium and bioresorbable systems. Journal of Craniomaxillofacial Surgery 10(5): 400–403
24 Kasrai L, Hearn T, Gur E, Forrest CR 1999 A biomechanical analysis of the orbitozygomatic complex in human cadavers: examination of load sharing and failure patterns following fixation with titanium and bioresorbable plating systems. Journal of Craniomaxillofacial Surgery 10(3): 237–243

25 Key SJ, Thomas DW, Shepherd JP 1995 The management of soft tissue facial wounds. British Journal of Oral and Maxillofacial Surgery 33: 76–85

26 Phillips JH, Gruss JS, Wells MD, Chollet A 1991 Periosteal suspension of the lower eyelid and cheek following subciliary exposure of facial fractures. Plastic and Reconstructive Surgery 88(1): 145–148

27 Dufresne CR 1992 The use of immediate grafting in facial fracture management. Indications and clinical considerations. Clinics in Plastic Surgery 19(71): 207–217

28 Burm JS, Chung CH, Oh SJ 1999 Pure orbital blowout fracture: new concepts and importance of medial orbital blowout fracture. Plastic and Reconstructive Surgery 103(7): 1839–1849

29 Harris GJ, Garcia GH, Logani SC, Murphy ML, Sheth BP, Seth AK 1998 Orbital blowout fractures: correlation of preoperative computed tomography and postoperative ocular motility. Transactions of the American Ophthalmological Society 96: 329–347; discussion 347–353

30 Ramieri G, Spada MC, Bianchi SD, Berrone S 2000 Dimensions and volumes of the orbit and orbital fat in posttraumatic enophthalmos. Dentomaxillofacial Radiology 29(5): 302–311

31 Raskin EM, Millman AL, Lubkin V, della Rocca RC, Lisman RD, Maher EA 1998 Prediction of late enophthalmos by volumetric analysis of orbital fractures. Ophthalmic Plastic and Reconstructive Surgery 14(1): 19–26

32 Penfold CN, Lang D, Evans BT 1992 The management of orbital roof fractures. British Journal of Oral and Maxillofacial Surgery 30(2): 97–103

33 Burns JA, Park SS 1997 The zygomatic-sphenoid fracture line in malar reduction. A cadaver study. Archives of Otolaryngology and Head and Neck Surgery 123(12): 1308–1311

34 Stassen LFA, Kerawala C 1999 Peri- and intraorbital trauma and orbital reconstruction. In: Ward-Booth P, Schendel SA, Hausamen J (eds) Maxillofacial surgery, vol 1. Churchill Livingstone, Edinburgh

35 Bullock JD, Warwar RE, Ballal DR, Ballal RD 1999 Mechanisms of orbital floor fractures: a clinical, experimental, and theoretical study. Transactions of the American Ophthalmological Society 97: 87–110; discussion 110–113

36 Vriens JP, Van Der Glas HW, Moos KF, Koole R 1998 Infraorbital nerve function following treatment of orbitozygomatic complex fractures. A multitest approach. International Journal of Oral and Maxillofacial Surgery 27(1): 27–32

37 Tengtrisorn S, McNab AA, Elder JE 1998 Persistent infra-orbital nerve hyperaesthesia after blunt orbital trauma. Australian and New Zealand Journal of Ophthalmology 26(3): 259–260

38 Lee HH, Alcaraz N, Reino A, Lawson W 1998 Reconstruction of orbital floor fractures with maxillary bone. Archives of Otolaryngology and Head and Neck Surgery 124(1): 56–59

39 Forrest CR, Khairallah E, Kuzon WM 1999 Intraocular and intraorbital compartment pressure changes following orbital bone grafting: a clinical and laboratory study. Journal of Plastic and Reconstructive Surgery 104(1): 48–54

40 Morrison AD, Sanderson RC, Moos KF 1995 The use of silastic as an orbital implant for reconstruction of orbital wall defects: review of 311 cases treated over 20 years. Journal of Oral and Maxillofacial Surgery 53(4): 412–417

41 Courtney DJ, Thomas S, Whitfield PH 2000 Isolated orbital blowout fractures: survey and review. British Journal of Oral and Maxillofacial Surgery 38: 496–503

42 McGurk M 1998 Blow-out fractures of the orbit and enophthalmos. In: Langdon JD, Patel MF (eds) Operative maxillofacial surgery, part 7. Chapman and Hall Medical, London

43 Haug RH 2000 Management of the trochlea of the superior oblique muscle in the repair of orbital roof trauma. Journal of Oral and Maxillofacial Surgery 58(6): 602–606

44 Karampatakis V, Natsis K, Gigis P, Stangos NT 1998 Orbital depth measurements of human skulls in relation to retrobulbar anesthesia. European Journal of Ophthalmology 8(2): 118–120

45 Cope MR, Moos KF, Speculand B 1999 Does diplopia persist after blowout fractures of the orbital floor in children? British Journal of Oral and Maxillofacial Surgery 37(1): 46–51

46 Iliff N, Manson PN, Katz J, Rever L, Yaremchuk M 1999 Mechanisms of extraocular muscle injury in orbital fractures. Plastic and Reconstructive Surgery 103(3): 787–799

47 Derdyn C, Persing JA, Broaddus WC et al 1990 Craniofacial trauma: an assessment of risk related to timing of surgery. Plastic and Reconstructive Surgery 86: 238–245

48 Jordan DR, Allen LH, White J, Harvey J, Pashby R, Esmaeli B 1998 Intervention within days for some orbital floor fractures: the white-eyed blowout. Ophthalmological Plastic and Reconstructive Surgery 14(6): 379–390

49 Verhoeff K, Grootendorst RJ, Wijngaarde R, de Man K 1998 Surgical repair of orbital fractures: how soon after trauma? Strabismus 6(2): 77–80

50 Flood TR, McManners J, el-Attar A, Moos KF 1999 Randomised prospective study of the influence of steroids on postoperative eye-opening after exploration of the orbital floor. British Journal of Oral and Maxillofacial Surgery 37(4): 312–315

51 Egbert JE, May K, Kersten RC, Kulwin DR 2000 Pediatric orbital floor fracture, direct extraocular muscle involvement. Ophthalmology 107(10): 1875–1879

52 Bansagi ZC, Meyer DR 2000 Internal orbital fractures in the paediatric age group: characterisation and management. Ophthalmology 107(5): 829–836

53 Putterman AM 1991 Management of blowout fractures of the orbital floor. III The conservative approach. Survey of Ophthalmology 35: 292–298

54 Manson PN, Iliff N 1991 Management of blowout fractures of the orbital floor. II Early repair of selected injuries. Survey of Ophthalmology 35: 280–292

55 Levin LA, Beck RW, Joseph MP, Seiff S, Kraher R 1999 The treatment of traumatic optic neuropathy: the International Optic Nerve Trauma Study. Ophthalmology 106(7): 1268–1277

56 Steinsapir KD, Goldberg RA 1994 Traumatic optic neuropathy. Survey of Ophthalmology 38(6): 487–518

57 Girotto JA, Gamble WB, Robertson B et al 1998 Blindness after reduction of facial fractures. Plastic and Reconstructive Surgery 102(6): 1821–1834

58 Stassen LFA, Goel R, Moos KF 1989 Purtscher's retinopathy: an unusual association with a complicated malar fracture. British Journal of Oral and Maxillofacial Surgery 27: 296–300

59 Gellrich N-C, Schramm A, Rustmeyer J, Neubacher U, Eysel UT 2002 Quantification of the neurodegenerative impact on the visual system following sudden retrobulbar expanding lesions – an experimental model. Journal of Cranioxmaxillofacial Surgery 30: 230–236

60 Gellrich N-C, Schimming R, Zerfowski M, Eysel UT 2002 Quantification of histomorphological changes after calibrated crush of the intraorbital optic nerve in rats. British Journal of Opthalmology 86(2): 233–237

61 Gellrich N-C, Schramm A, Hammer B, Rojas S, Cufi D, Lagrèze W, Schmelzeisen R 2002 Computer-assisted reconstruction of unilateral posttraumatic orbital deformities. Plastic and Reconstructive Surgery 110(6): 1417–1429

Appendix 1

Eye Scoring System and Referral to Ophthalmologist

Total score

0	4	Do not refer
5	11	Routine referral
11	14	URGENT referral

Visual acuity

6/12	4
6/24	8
6/36	12
NPL	16

NPL = no light perception

Fracture type

Comminuted	3
Blowout	3
Other	0

Diplopia

Yes	3
No	0

Amnesia

Yes	5	(retrograde or antegrade)
No	0	

Female

Yes	1
No	0

Age

>35	1

RTA

Yes	1
No	0

Total _____

BAD ACT: B = blow-out, A = acuity, D = diplopia, A = amnesia, CT = comminuted trauma

Appendix 2: Clinical History and Examination

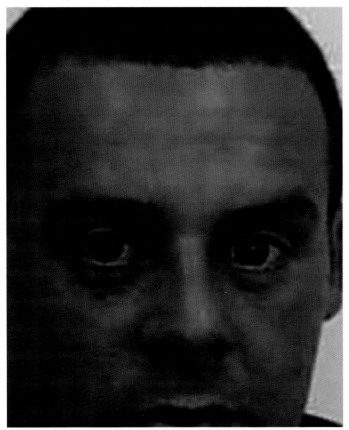

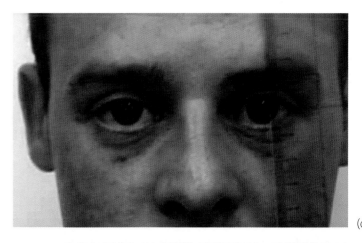

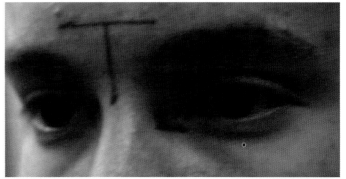

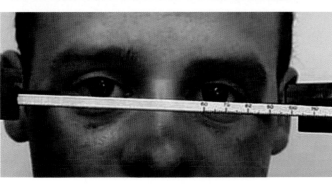

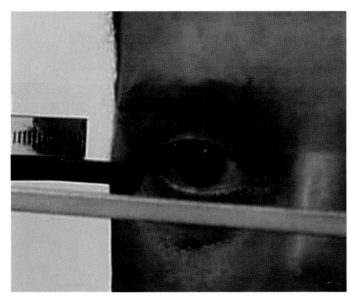

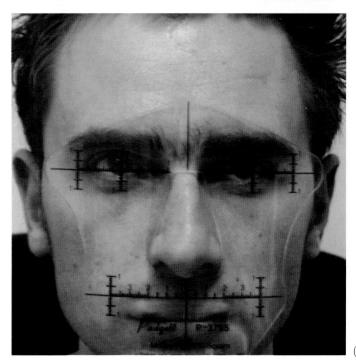

Fig. 10.59: Measurements. **(a)** Left orbital injury, enophthalmos, hypoglobus. **(b)** Hertel exophthalometer, unsuitable to use because of lateral wall dystopia. **(c)** Assessing enophthalmos. **(d)** Pseudo correction of orbital dystopia by rotating head allows measurement of the hypoglobus (see Figs 10.36, 10.37). **(e)** Measurement of canthal area. **(f)** Facial measurements using the McCoy Facial Square.

Name: DOB: Age: Sex: M/F

Injury: Date: Time: Location:

Drugs: alcohol / other

How: assault / road traffic accident / fall / sport / industrial / firearm / other

Others involved:

Amnesia Retrograde / Antegrade / Both

Visual acuity:		Right eye 6/6, 6/12, 6/36, NPL	Left eye 6/6, 6/12, 6/36, NPL
Pupil size:		Symmetrical / asymmetrical, Size:	
			right pinpoint, 3 mm, 5 mm, >8 mm
			left pinpoint, 3 mm, 5 mm, >8 mm
		Reaction to light:	right direct / indirect
			left direct / indirect

Eye movements: Right eye: normal / limited / globe retraction
                                  Left eye: normal / limited / globe retraction
                                  Diplopia yes / no
                                  Specify:

Right eye:		Normal	proptosis / enophthalmos hypoglobus / hyperglobus lateral dystopia / medial dystopia
Left eye:		Normal	proptosis / enophthalmos hypoglobus / hyperglobus lateral dystopia/medial dystopia

Canthal area:		Intercanthal distance:	medial____mm	Right____Left____
		Intercanthal level:	medial Right = Left	asymmetric____mm
		Intercanthal distance:	lateral____mm	Right____Left____
		Intercanthal level:	lateral Right = Left level / mongoloid / anti-mongoloid	asymmetric____mm

Palpebral fissure:		Width:	Right:____ Left:____	Height:	Right:____ Left:____
Facial nerve function:		Right Left	normal normal	weak weak	Specify____ Specify____
Eye closure:		Right Left	complete, incomplete, Bell's phenomenon Y / N complete, incomplete, Bell's phenomenon Y / N		
Jaw movement:		Mouth opening mm R (lateral) L (lateral)	____ ____ ____		

Fig. 10.59: (g) Orbitofacial evaluation form.

11 Frontal Sinus Fractures

Nicholas J Baker, Barry T Evans, G Neil Dwyer, Dorothy A Lang

Introduction

The treatment of fractures of the frontal sinus has become less contentious as the contemporary principles of modern maxillofacial trauma management have become more widely adopted. The rationale to treat fractures of the frontal sinus has always been to produce a 'safe' sinus and reduce the long-term risks of complications. Early treatment was based on experience from the management of infective frontal sinus disease extrapolated to equate with the frontal sinus involved in trauma. The difficulty has been in predicting exactly which patients are at risk of developing complications. Progress has been hampered by small numbers of patients in retrospective reviews. Complications may develop many years after the initial trauma, often presenting to teams not involved in the initial management.

The aim of this chapter is to provide an overview of currently accepted principles of management of frontal sinus fractures based on the experience of others and our own experience of over 100 consecutive cases of craniofacial trauma managed between 1988 and 2000.

Historical Perspectives

Traditionally, in view of the perceived risk of infection and neurological deterioration, craniofacial injuries have been managed in at least two separate stages. These injuries were treated as separate entities by neurosurgeons and maxillofacial surgeons working in isolation. Understanding of the aims of other specialties was limited and the overall management of these patients suffered as a result of the fragmented nature of the treatment. Initial treatment usually consisted of urgent craniotomy for the evacuation of intracranial clots, elevation of depressed bone fragments and the repair of the dura over the convexity of the brain. Wounds were debrided and loose bone fragments were discarded. Facial fracture repair was carried out 7–14 days or longer after the initial neurosurgical management. Formal anterior fossa exploration and reconstruction was seldom carried out, basal repair being limited to those cases of persistent cerebrospinal fluid (CSF) rhinorrhea. Fixation of facial fractures was usually achieved with closed techniques by means of bone pins, halo frames and internal suspension wires normally attached to the teeth with the patient placed into intermaxillary fixation. Direct visualization of fracture sites by elevation of the periosteum was kept to a minimum for fear of devitalizing bone fragments. Primary bone grafting was rarely, if ever, performed. Contour defects of the forehead were treated secondarily, often by

means of alloplastic material such as methyl methacrylate. The limitations of traditional frontobasal repair, combined with the lack of co-ordination of treatment, resulted in inadequate functional and cosmetic results, particularly in the critical frontal nasoethmoid, and orbital regions. Satisfactory secondary correction of these posttraumatic sequelae was difficult and often produced unsatisfactory results.

Management of the frontal sinus was based upon historical experience in the treatment of acute and chronic frontal sinusitis. Initial techniques were based on the Reidel procedure of sinus ablation with excision of the bony walls. This produced severe frontal deformity and was subsequently replaced by several modifications to exenterate the sinus mucosa yet preserve the bony anatomy of the sinus. All of these techniques carried a significant failure rate and were replaced by techniques to obliterate the sinus by excising the sinus mucosa, plugging the nasofrontal ducts and obliterating the sinus with autogenous or alloplastic materials.

Fractures of the frontal sinus form an integral part of craniofacial fracture management and cannot be considered in isolation. This chapter examines the contemporary principles of craniofacial fracture management with particular reference to management of the frontal sinus.

Classification of Craniofacial Fractures

Fractures of the nasofronto-orbital region account for approximately 5% of facial fractures.[1] Fractures involving the anterior or posterior wall of the frontal sinus occur in 2–12% of cranial fractures.[2] Combined frontobasilar and facial injuries may be isolated to the cranio-orbital area or be part of more extensive injuries involving the upper, middle and lower facial regions. Craniofacial fractures may be divided into central and lateral groups.

Central injuries

Central injuries are those that involve the skull base adjacent to the paranasal sinuses – the frontal, ethmoid and sphenoid sinuses. Central injuries are subdivided into two types depending on the location of the fracture.

Type I Cribriform fracture

This is a linear fracture through the cribriform plate without involvement of the ethmoid or frontal sinuses.

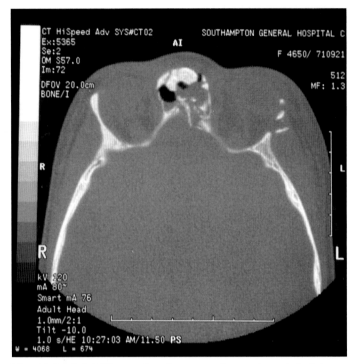

Fig. 11.1: Axial CT scan showing a type I central craniofacial injury with disruption at the level of the cribriform plate.

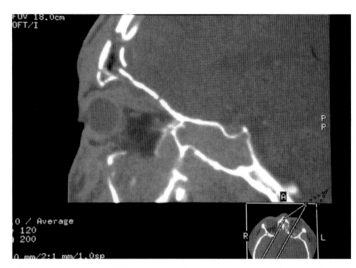

Fig. 11.2: Sagittal CT scan showing a type II central craniofacial injury with fractures involving the anterior and posterior walls of the frontal sinus.

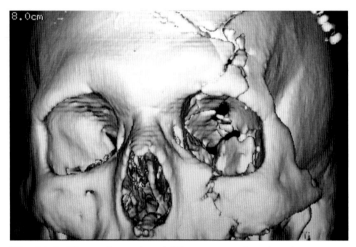

Fig. 11.3: Three-dimensional CT reconstruction showing a lateral craniofacial injury with fractures of the frontal bone, orbital roof and zygomatic complex.

These fractures may result from relatively low-energy injuries, which would not cause fractures in stronger areas of the anterior skull base. The dura covers this area with the arachnoid layer and both form tubular sheaths around the branches of the olfactory nerves, with the dura being continued into the periosteum of the nose and the arachnoid into the neurolemma of the nerve. The cribriform plate is thin, easily fractured and may be difficult to repair, resulting in a high propensity for the development of CSF fistulae (Fig. 11.1).

Type II Frontoethmoidal fracture

These fractures involve the medial portion of the anterior cranial fossa with direct involvement of the frontal and/or ethmoid sinuses. In common with type I fractures, CSF pools towards the midline and this may prevent brain herniation and seal by brain or adjacent tissues[3] (Fig. 11.2).

Lateral injuries

Lateral injuries involve the frontal bone and orbital roof. These fractures may lie lateral to the frontal sinus or involve the superior or inferior walls of the lateral frontal sinus. In this area the brain is completely invested in dura and, in contrast to central injuries, the brain lies superior to the fracture site. CSF fistulae are therefore more likely to subside spontaneously as a result of gravity and brain herniation through the dural laceration (Fig. 11.3).

Complex injuries can occur where a combination of central and lateral fracture patterns occurs (Fig. 11.4).

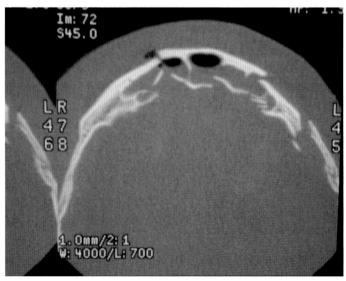

Fig. 11.4: Axial CT scan showing a combination of central and lateral craniofacial fractures.

Clinical Features

Up to one-third of patients with a head injury and a Glasgow Coma Score (GCS) of 8 or less can expect to have a major injury elsewhere in the body.[4] These patients must have all life-threatening conditions treated and stabilized before a full assessment of all other injuries is undertaken. In addition, patients who are unconscious, particularly if they have sustained facial injuries, are unable to protect their own airway and should be intubated. The nature and severity of the craniofacial injuries are assessed once the patient has been stabilized following emergency treatment.

The risk of cervical spine injury in the unconscious patient with craniofacial injuries must be assumed until it can be cleared radiologically. The cervical spine should be stabilized with a hard cervical collar as part of the management of the airway and the collar must be left in position until the cervical spine has been imaged. Radiographs should be taken to visualize the cervical spine from a lateral and anteroposterior direction and a further film to visualize the odontoid peg. All seven cervical vertebrae must be visualized, including the cervicothoracic junction. If there is any doubt on the plain radiographs or a soft tissue injury is suspected, a computed tomogram (CT) and/or magnetic resonance imaging (MRI) of the cervical spine must be obtained in the unconscious patient.

Clinical examination

An initial assessment of the level of consciousness can be made using the acronym AVPU – Awake, responds to Vocal commands, responds to Pain or Unresponsive. This provides a baseline against which more detailed assessment of the level of consciousness may subsequently be made.[5]

Once the patient has been stabilized a more detailed assessment of the level of consciousness is made and a thorough examination of the head and neck performed. A full neurological assessment should also be included for focal or general neurological signs. The assessment of the level of consciousness should be repeated and recorded at regular intervals to detect any deterioration in the patient's condition. The GCS allows a rapid and repetitive means of assessing the level of consciousness by individual or multiple clinicians and allows direct comparison of clinical findings. Any deterioration in the level of consciousness as evidenced by the GCS is an indication for an urgent CT scan. The GCS has three components: eye opening, best verbal response and best motor response. The score in each group is totaled to give a final score of between 3 and 15. A score of 8 or less indicates the patient is unconscious.[6]

Following assessment of level of consciousness, examination of the head and neck should be undertaken, including the cervical spine if the patient is conscious. This should be performed in a systematic manner starting with inspection of the scalp and working downwards, noting any physical signs and palpating all bony margins. The eyes should be examined, recording the visual acuity, pupillary responses, range of eye movement and the presence of diplopia or restricted eye movements. Visual fields should be tested to confrontation. The intercanthal distance should be noted, particularly if nasoethmoidal injury is suspected. Sensation to light touch and pinprick should be tested in all three divisions of the trigeminal nerve. Facial nerve function should be assessed, particularly if a base-of-skull fracture is suspected or in the presence of facial lacerations which may involve the peripheral branches of the nerve. If the patient is conscious it is important to inquire about loss of smell or hearing and if necessary, these should be formally tested. Initial assessment may be difficult in the acute situation due to the presence of blood in the nasal airway or external meatus.

Inspection of the external auditory meatus should be performed to examine for the presence of hemotympanum, lacerations, damage to the tympanic membrane and the presence of otorrhea.

Anterior rhinoscopy should be undertaken to examine for the presence of CSF rhinorrhea and nasal septal hematoma. This area may be difficult to visualize in the presence of blood. Clear secretions from the nose can be tested for glucose by the glucose oxidase test. This should only be used to confirm that the secretion is *not* CSF, as both nasal and lacrimal secretions may contain glucose.[7] This test is unreliable and has been replaced by immunoelectrophoresis of the secretions for β_2 transferrin as this will identify CSF and will not produce false positives in the presence of nasal or lacrimal secretions or blood.[8] β_2 transferrin is present in CSF but absent in tears, saliva, nasal secretions and serum except perhaps in neonates and individuals with deranged liver function.

Intraoral examination should be performed to examine for bruising, swelling and mobility of the tooth-bearing segments. The patient's occlusion should be checked for evidence of derangement.

Clinical findings

Skull vault fractures may present with localized scalp swelling and bruising with varying levels of consciousness. A range of neurological signs may also be present. The presence of an underlying intracranial hemorrhage correlates with the presence of a skull fracture and the patient's level of consciousness.[9]

Fractures involving the anterior fossa may show bilateral circumorbital ecchymoses, nasal epistaxis and CSF rhinorrhea. A variety of eye signs may be demonstrated, including visual loss, and the patient may complain of loss of smell. Middle fossa fractures may demonstrate Battle's sign (bruising around the mastoid process), blood in the external auditory meatus and CSF otorrhea. There may be evidence of hearing loss or facial nerve weakness.

In craniofacial fractures, bruising around the eyes is common and there may be evidence of subconjunctival hemorrhage. Subconjunctival hemorrhage as a physical sign merely demonstrates that bleeding has occurred below the orbital periosteum. Visual loss may occur as a result of the intracerebral insult or trauma directly to the optic nerve itself, usually within the optic canal. Fractures extending into the orbital apex are fortunately rare, as this area is the strongest part of the orbital skeleton. Fractures of the optic canal may occur, particularly in severe high-energy injuries.[10] Orbital fractures involving the superior orbital fissure may also occur and give rise to a range of physical signs depending upon the individual nerves involved (the superior orbital fissure syndrome).[11] The oculomotor, trochlear and ophthalmic divisions of the trigeminal and abducens nerves all pass through the superior orbital fissure and may produce limitation of eye movement, pupillary dilatation (mydriasis) and sensory disturbances in the frontal region (the supraorbital and supratrochlear branches of the ophthalmic division of the trigeminal nerve). The superior orbital fissure syndrome secondary to trauma is also fortunately a rare occurrence.

Pupillary mydriasis may be an indication of rising intracranial pressure as a result of its effect on the oculomotor nerve as it passes forwards from the posterior aspect of the brain stem on its intracranial course. This occurs as a result of transtentorial herniation and is always secondary to a fall in the GCS.[12] The oculomotor nerve contains parasympathetic fibers to the iris of the eye and is responsible for pupillary constriction (miosis). Direct damage to the oculomotor nerve may also occur either intra- or extracranially to produce an isolated third nerve palsy. The eye takes up an abducted and depressed position with an associated mydriasis and upper eyelid ptosis. The direct pupillary reflex will be absent, but the consensual pupillary reflex will be present if the ipsilateral optic nerve and the contralateral oculomotor nerve are both functioning normally. This is in contrast to an isolated optic nerve lesion when the ipsilateral direct and contralateral consensual pupillary reflexes will both be absent.

Damage to the abducens and trochlear cranial nerves occurs less frequently. An isolated abducens nerve palsy will produce an inability to abduct the eye and an isolated trochlear nerve palsy will produce an inability to abduct the eye in downwards gaze. In all cases of damage to the third, fourth and sixth cranial nerves there will be diplopia when assessing the range of eye movements. With any suspected orbital or globe injury an ophthalmic opinion must be sought. If eye signs are present, particularly restricted eye movements or diplopia, an orthoptic assessment should be performed, including a Hess chart.

The eyes should be assessed for the presence of enophthalmos. Assessment of enophthalmos in the acute situation may be difficult as swelling of the periorbital tissues can mask its presence. Enophthalmos may occur with either orbital floor or medial wall blow-out fractures, if there is also rupture of the periorbita. Disruption to the medial orbital walls is invariably present in severe nasoethmoidal injuries and is therefore often present in craniofacial injuries. Disruption to the attachments of the medial canthal tendons may also occur with nasoethmoidal injuries. The medial canthal tendon has an anterior limb that attaches to the anterior lacrimal crest and a posterior limb lying posterior to the lacrimal sac. Disruption to the anterior limb of the tendon alone does not produce telecanthus (increase in the intercanthal distance). Telecanthus is a sign of disruption to both anterior and posterior limbs of the tendon and necessitates reattachment of the anterior limb to prevent persistence of the deformity postop-

eratively. The intercanthal distance should be checked in suspected nasoethmoidal and craniofacial injuries. The normal intercanthal distance is 25.5–37.5 mm in women and 26.5–38.7 mm in men. Injuries to the medial canthal tendon may also occur with lacerations to the area in the absence of underlying fracture.

A fracture involving the frontal sinus may be suggested by the presence of a laceration in the region of the supraorbital ridge, glabella or lower forehead.[13]

Traumatic hypertelorism may also occur in severe fronto-orbito-nasoethmoidal injuries with a true increase in the interorbital distance. Failure to appreciate the distinction between traumatic telecanthus and hypertelorism will lead to inadequate treatment with a poor functional and cosmetic result.

Radiological Assessment

CT scanning has revolutionized the management of craniofacial trauma by allowing precise delineation of injuries prior to surgery. This allows for exact preoperative planning prior to intervention. Assessment of both skeletal and soft tissue elements is possible utilizing appropriate bone and soft tissue windows. Scanning is performed in both the axial and coronal planes to allow visualization of all anatomical structures. The coronal views are essential for assessment of the orbital and frontal sinus roofs and floors as well as a detailed assessment of the cribriform plate, the jugum sphenoidale (roofs of the ethmoid sinuses) and optic canals (Fig. 11.5). All other fractures are usually demonstrated on the axial views. Two to three millimeter slices are required to allow evaluation of the skull base and orbits. Three-dimensional CT reconstruction often adds little in the way of practical information in assessing patients with craniofacial trauma but may be of benefit in selected complex cases[14] (Fig. 11.6).

Indications for CT scanning

CT scanning should be performed in all patients with suspected craniofacial injuries. In addition a CT must also be obtained under any of the following circumstances.

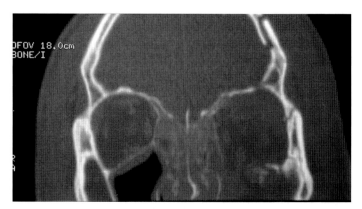

Fig. 11.5: Coronal CT scan demonstrating an increase in left orbital volume secondary to disruption of the orbital roof and floor and zygomatic complex.

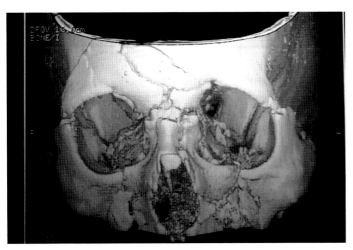

Fig. 11.6: Three-dimensional CT reconstruction demonstrating complex frontal, nasoethmoidal, orbital floor and midface injuries.

1. Basal skull fracture
2. GCS less than 8
3. Confusion persisting after resuscitation
4. Deteriorating level of consciousness or progressive focal neurological deficit
5. Seizure
6. Neurological symptoms or signs including headache or vomiting
7. CSF rhinorrhea or otorrhea

CT scanning is particularly useful in precisely delineating the site and extent of injury associated with the frontal sinus. Axial views will demonstrate disruption to the anterior and posterior walls of the sinus. CT scanning may be used to assess injury to the ostia or ducts of the sinus. The level of fracture and degree of disruption of the base of the sinus are predictive of the probability of ductal obstruction.[13]

Plain skull radiographs do not add to the information gained from CT scan and are unnecessary in patients who are to be scanned.

Plain radiographs of the midface may give an extra overall dimension to information gained from the CT scan. It may be difficult to obtain satisfactory views in the unconscious patient, but plain films are of particular benefit in assessing facial symmetry following internal fixation of fractures.

If mandibular injury is suspected, the mandible should be imaged using plain films or as part of the overall CT scan.

Rationale for the Treatment of Craniofacial Fractures

Current management of craniofacial trauma is based upon the principles of pediatric craniofacial surgery outlined by Paul Tessier in 1967 and adopted to the application of craniofacial trauma by Merville in 1978. This was the first time that combined injuries were addressed in a definitive single-stage repair. A frontal bone flap was raised to allow inspection of the dura and its repair. The frontal sinus was cranialized and

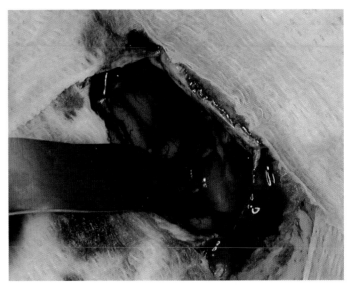

Fig. 11.7: Intradural exploration reveals the brain plugging a dural tear. Failure to repair this type of injury despite the absence of a CSF leak places the patient at a lifelong risk of infection.

the fronto-orbital and facial injuries treated during the same anesthetic.[15]

The aims of treatment in craniofacial injuries have been refined to address the problems arising if treatment is not undertaken. These aims are the prevention of early and late complications, and in particular infective sequelae, and to achieve restoration of satisfactory form and function.

Prevention of late infective sequelae

Dural tears in communication with the nasal cavity and paranasal sinuses are common in craniofacial fractures and if untreated, may leave the patient at significant risk of developing meningitis. The absence of an overt CSF leak does not indicate the absence of a dural tear. In the presence of a dural tear the brain may act to plug the hole in the dura and prevent the CSF leak (Fig. 11.7).

In 1954 Lewin showed the risk of meningitis to be at least 25% in patients with CSF rhinorrhea and cranial base fractures communicating with the paranasal sinuses in the absence of dural repair.[16] Eljamel & Foy (1990) looked at a series of patients with acute traumatic CSF fistulae and found an overall incidence of meningitis of 30.6% before dural repair with a 10-year cumulative risk in excess of 85%.[17] Surgical repair of the dura reduced the overall risk of meningitis from 30.6% before surgery to 4% following surgery with a reduction in the cumulative risk at 10 years from 85% before dural repair to 7% after dural repair.[18]

In 1989 Poole & Briggs published their approach to the management of craniofacial trauma based on their experience of 48 patients over a 7-year period. Their indications for combined craniofacial repair were:

1. radiological evidence of displaced fractures involving the posterior wall of the frontal sinus, the cribriform plates or orbital roofs with or without the presence of CSF rhinorrhea

2. displaced fractures of the frontal bone or upper orbital skeleton
3. extensive bone loss as a result of the injury or initial debridement procedure.[19]

Sakas et al (1998) outlined the need for surgical intervention in patients with or without CSF rhinorrhea based on the results of detailed neuroimaging. They identified certain factors which were linked to a high long-term risk of developing posttraumatic meningitis:

- proximity to the midline – particularly central type cribriform fractures (Type I)
- large fracture displacement (>1 cm)
- prolonged rhinorrhea (>8 days).

The effects were shown to be cumulative, with fracture patterns showing a combination of these factors at particular risk.[3]

Our group has refined these criteria to determine the indications for combined craniofacial repair.[20]

1. Central injuries that show clinical or radiological evidence of displaced fractures of the posterior wall of the frontal sinus, cribriform plate and roof of the ethmoid sinuses with or without a CSF leak.
2. Lateral injuries with displaced fractures producing contour deformity, globe displacement or ocular motility disturbance.
3. Extensive bone loss in the supraorbital rim or orbital roof resulting from either the injury or debridement procedure.
4. Growing skull fractures in association with the orbital roof or frontal sinuses. This is a rare complication, which may occur in 0.6% of linear skull fractures in pediatric patients. The fracture is associated with a dural laceration with arachnoid herniating into the dural tear, preventing primary dural healing and resulting in progressive enlargement and eversion of the fracture line. 90% of these fractures occur before the age of 3 years. These fractures may result in significant functional and cosmetic disturbances.

Based on these criteria, we have reviewed 100 consecutive cases of craniofacial trauma managed jointly in Southampton. This has demonstrated a dural tear in direct communication with the nasal cavity or paranasal sinuses irrespective of the presence of a CSF leak in 86% of patients.[21] Based on the findings of Eljamel & Foy,[17] if these dural tears had been left untreated we may have expected a potential meningitis risk of 69% over a 10-year period. In contrast, in our series there have been no cases of early or late postoperative meningitis or cerebral abscess and no postoperative deaths.[21] This study confirms the validity of our original criteria for combined craniofacial repair.

The frontal, ethmoid and sphenoid sinuses must be effectively isolated from the intracranial contents. This is achieved by watertight dural repair, appropriate management of the frontal sinus, bone grafts to cover the ethmoid sinus roofs if required and vascularized soft tissue flaps (pericranial/galeal frontalis) inserted between the dural repair and the underlying bone grafts.

Prevention of posttraumatic cranio-orbital deformity

Accurate three-dimensional reconstruction of the frontal bandeau and orbital roofs is a prerequisite to satisfactory orbitofacial reconstruction. This may be achieved by aiming to reproduce the precise premorbid projection and convex curvature of the supraorbital rims. Laterally the temporal buttresses of the frontal bone determine the projection and width of the upper midface. The position of the glabella in the midline determines the projection of the nasoethmoidal complex and may require primary bone grafting in comminuted injuries or when bone is lost (Fig. 11.8).

The convexity of the orbital roof in the anteroposterior and lateral planes must be reproduced to prevent globe displacement and disturbed ocular motility. Inaccurate reconstruction of the superior orbital rim and orbital roof resulting in inferior globe displacement is one of the most difficult posttraumatic deformities to correct satisfactorily. The premorbid ocular position can be re-established by wide exposure and accurate reduction of the zygomatic arch and lateral orbital rim. The inner orbital skeleton can be reconstructed secondarily to the lateral position.[20, 26]

Timing of Surgery

Early combined repair of craniofacial injuries has been demonstrated to be effective in improving functional and cosmetic results with acceptable morbidity and mortality and no adverse effect on neurosurgical outcome in selected patients.[22] The advocates of early intervention cite a better outcome in terms of functional and cosmetic results. This must be balanced against unacceptable morbidity as a result of the surgical procedure itself. Benzil et al looked at a series of patients with craniofacial trauma who were operated on within 24 hours in a single-stage combined surgical repair and

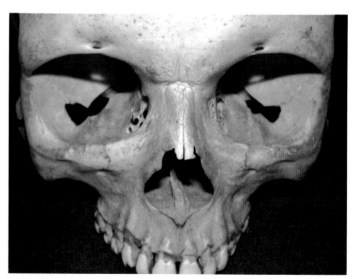

Fig. 11.8: Precise appreciation of premorbid anatomy is essential in craniofacial trauma management to allow accurate reconstruction and prevention of posttraumatic deformity.

demonstrated a 15% rate of postoperative CSF fistula and 8% meningitis.[23]

Other series report a mortality rate as high as 11.8% in patients undergoing early surgical intervention but apparently balanced by a good neurosurgical, functional and cosmetic outcome in 79.2% of patients.[24] If patients are excluded for early intervention as a result of certain clinical criteria – elevated intracranial pressure (ICP), severe associated injury or medical condition or a poor prognosis for survival due to cerebral injury – there is no significant difference in survival in patients who undergo early, middle or late surgical repair.[22]

Our criteria for case selection for early surgery are based on:

- GCS above 13 following resuscitation
- a stable ICP less than or equal to 15 mmHg in a cardiovascularly stable patient
- no CT evidence of midline shift or effacement of the basal cisterns and/or third ventricle.

A retrospective review of over 100 consecutive patients treated jointly at Southampton since 1988 has shown a good recovery according to the Glasgow Outcome Score of 87%. The rate for revisional facial surgery in this group was 14% with no postoperative cases of CSF fistula or meningitis and no postoperative deaths. Emergency neurosurgical procedures within the first 24 hours were required in 15% of patients and 27% required preliminary procedures for orthopedic and abdominal injuries. The mean time to surgery from injury to combined craniofacial repair was 10 days in the group of patients fitting our criteria and 20 days in the group of patients failing to meet the criteria for early surgical repair. This demonstrates that there is no detriment to neurological, functional or cosmetic outcome in patients undergoing early combined craniofacial repair that fit the criteria. In addition, there appears to be no significant disadvantage in delaying surgery for up to 3 weeks in patients not fitting the criteria.[25]

Principles of Surgical Management[20,26]

Order of treatment

The reduction and fixation of the cranial vault and anterior fossa should usually precede the treatment of the facial fractures, i.e. the treatment proceeds from above downwards. With severe comminution or bone loss in the frontobasal region, the reconstruction may have to commence with the facial fractures. The full extent of any bone loss in the cranial vault and anterior skull base may then be determined and any missing bone replaced with primary autogenous bone grafts.

Adequate exposure

Management of craniofacial fractures requires complete subperiosteal exposure of all fracture sites and complete exposure of the basal dura in relation to the fractures. The standard approach is to combine a coronal flap with a low

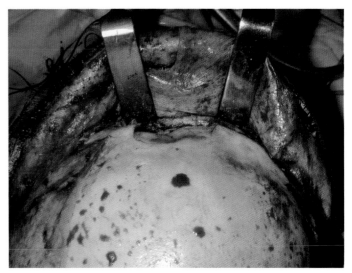

Fig. 11.9: A coronal flap allows wide access to a fracture involving the anterior wall of the frontal sinus.

bifrontal craniotomy (Fig. 11.9). Raveh et al published a series of 395 patients advocating an extracranial-subcranial approach to repair craniofacial fractures and associated dural tears.[27] This is achieved by incisions confined to the hair borders of the eyebrows with no nasal extension. Dural repair is performed microsurgically along the ethmoid, sellar and temporal planes via an extracranial approach. The nasofronto-orbital injuries, including the management of the frontal sinus, are also treated via this approach. In this series the surgery was performed within 48 hours of the injury and with the aim of avoiding frontal lobe retraction and anosmia. Despite a low incidence of postoperative CSF fistula and no cases of meningitis, there were five postoperative deaths in this series. Endoscopic repair of CSF fistulae has been reported with the aim of reducing the morbidity of standard approaches.[28] Given the nature of dural tears and their unpredictable pattern, the risk of missing tears by this approach must place the patient at long-term risk of infective sequelae.

The standard approach combining a coronal incision with a low bifrontal craniotomy allows wide access to the entire craniofacial skeleton. Fracture patterns may be directly assessed and repaired (Fig. 11.10). Dural repair can be performed under direct vision with easy access and dural tears not easily appreciable can be addressed via intradural exploration and repair (Fig. 11.11). This has been our approach in over 100 patients, with no deaths or infective sequelae and excellent outcome.[21]

Access to the entire craniofacial skeleton can be achieved with a combination of esthetically acceptable incisions. A coronal incision extended into the pre- or postauricular region on each side to the level of the tragus allows access to the frontal and temporal bones and upper facial skeleton, particularly the zygoma, lateral orbit, orbital roof and nasoethmoidal regions. The supraorbital neurovascular bundles should be identified and freed from their bony canals in the supraorbital rim as they provide sensation to the skin of the forehead up to the vertex and provide the vascular pedicle for

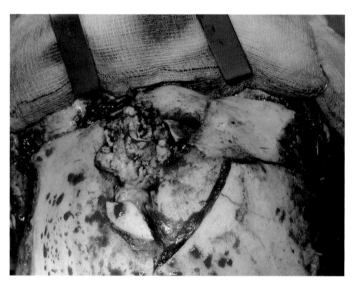

Fig. 11.10: A comminuted fracture of the frontal bone is widely exposed to assess fracture pattern prior to craniotomy.

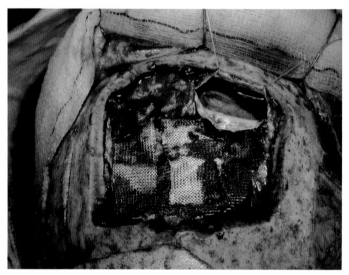

Fig. 11.11: Intradural dural exploration allows direct inspection of the basal dura and detection of dural tears that may otherwise have been missed.

any subsequent pericranial or galeal frontalis flap used for anterior cranial fossa repair. The temporalis fascia should be split above the root of the zygomatic process of the temporal bone. When splitting the fascia, an incision orientated superiorly at 45° to the base of the zygomatic arch is necessary to preserve the frontal branch of the facial nerve, which runs in the plane between the two layers of the temporalis fascia. Dissection may then continue deep to the nerve.[29] The coronal flap may be combined with a lower eyelid incision (transconjunctival – with or without lateral extension, subtarsal or subciliary) to gain access to the inferior orbital rim and floor and the medial and lateral orbital walls. The suborbital incisions should be made before raising the coronal flap to prevent edema. An alternative to suborbital incision is to do a lateral orbitotomy via the coronal flap, which gives excellent access to the orbital floor and medial wall by retracting the globe laterally.

The projection and width of the upper midface are determined by the accurate restoration of the position of the body of the zygoma in three-dimensions in relation to the cranial base. The key to this task is the accurate restoration of the length of the zygomatic arches. The accurate positioning of the body of the zygoma in three dimensions is also the most critical factor in restoring the correct orbital volume and hence the correct position of the ocular globe. If there is disruption to the medial canthus but there is still attachment to bone, this can be reduced and plated back into position. If there is no bony attachment, the ligament can be picked up with a permanent suture. This can be passed transnasally and fixed to the contralateral posterior lacrimal crest. Following extensive lateral orbital subperiosteal dissection, the lateral canthus should be reattached to a fixed reference point just below the frontozygomatic suture.

An intraoral vestibular incision allows access to the lower midface. All of these incisions may be linked subperiosteally and no attempt should be made to retain the periosteal attachment of small pieces of bone fragments. Occasionally large facial lacerations may be utilized to gain access to fracture sites but often the access is inadequate without unacceptable extension of the laceration.

A low bifrontal craniotomy will allow access to the anterior cranial fossa and basal dura as far posteriorly as the lesser wing of the sphenoid and jugum sphenoidale. Exposure of the basal dura does not necessitate sectioning intact olfactory nerve filaments. Intradural exploration allows identification and preservation of the olfactory tracts.

Definitive reduction and fixation of fractures should be undertaken only after the entire fracture pattern has been assessed by direct inspection. This is of particular importance when attempting to mobilize fractures of the orbital roof as this may be potentially dangerous if the optic canal is involved.

Minimal brain retraction

A low subfrontal exposure will minimize frontal lobe retraction. This may be achieved either by removing the supraorbital fracture fragments or by performing an osteotomy of the superior orbital margin. Retraction will then be at the expense of the orbital contents rather than the frontal lobe. Spinal drainage may be used in selected cases to reduce further frontal lobe retraction.

Rigid fixation of fractures

Rigid fixation systems have been specifically designed which allow accurate and stable three-dimensional reconstruction of the craniofacial skeleton (Fig. 11.12). Stable reconstruction of hard tissues following fracture resists later distortion as a result of muscle pull and scar contracture.

The number of plates and screws used should be kept to a minimum and placed at sites where they may easily be removed if necessary without significant morbidity. Plates should be placed on the convexity of the outer table of the skull and never intracranially.[30]

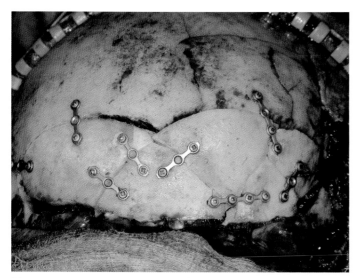

Fig. 11.12: Accurate reduction of a comminuted frontal bone fracture and internal fixation with multiple monocortical plates and screws.

Primary bone grafting

Primary autogenous bone grafting may be necessary to replace severely comminuted or missing bone segments. It has been suggested that bone gaps in excess of 5 mm should be replaced with bone grafts.[30] The need for a bone graft is dependent on the site of the defect and the extent to which it is subject to the forces of muscle pull and soft tissue contracture. Bone grafting is most commonly required for fractures involving the anterior cranial fossa, the orbital roofs, the frontal bandeau, the anterior wall of the frontal sinus, the orbital floor and medial and lateral orbital walls, the nasal skeleton and the anterior aspect of the maxilla (Figs 11.13a,b).

In the management of craniofacial fractures, the usual donor sites when considering bone grafting are the calvaria, ribs and iliac crest. Calvarial bone is a particularly attractive option for craniofacial fractures as there is no additional donor wound and if the inner table is harvested, there is no visible donor site defect. Full-thickness calvarial grafts may be harvested from children under the age of 1 without the need to reconstruct the donor site as bone regeneration can be expected to occur. Inner table calvarial bone may be used to provide a satisfactory volume of bone to reconstruct craniofacial fractures in the majority of patients. The outer table is split from the inner table of calvarium to provide the graft material and the outer table can then be repositioned to avoid a defect at the site of the craniotomy (Fig. 11.14). Calvarial bone can be difficult to contour satisfactorily and in complex defects such as the orbital floor and walls, split rib may be the graft material of choice.

Rigid fixation of primary autogenous bone grafts reduces subsequent resorption and volume depletion (Figs 11.15a,b). The combination of bone grafting and rigid fixation allows the complete and stable reconstruction of the craniofacial skeleton following trauma.

Management of the Frontal Sinus
Surgical anatomy

The frontal sinuses are derived from the frontal recess portion of the middle meatus or occasionally from an air cell of the ethmoid infundibulum. The sinuses are radiologically

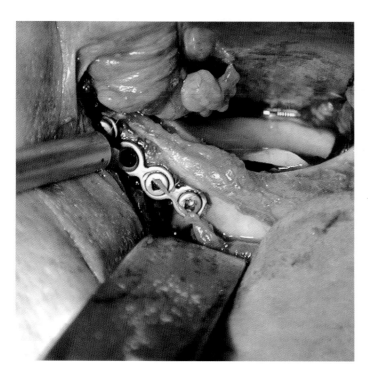

(a)

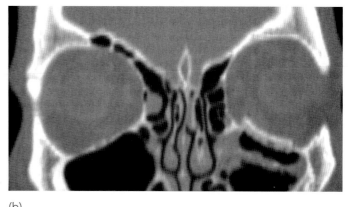

(b)

Fig. 11.13: (a) Split inner table calvarial bone graft has been harvested for reconstruction of large orbital floor defect.
(b) Postoperative coronal CT showing satisfactory graft position lying passively across orbital floor defect.

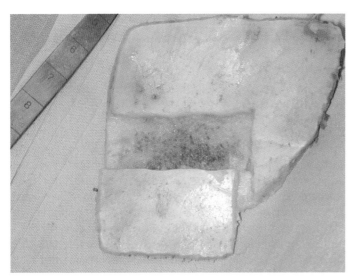

Fig. 11.14: Split calvarial inner table taken from the craniotomy bone flap can yield a large volume of autologous bone for primary grafting. The bone flap can be repositioned without contour deformity.

evident at 5–6 years of age and become adult sized by 10–12 years of age.[13]

The frontal sinus is a pyramidal, air-filled cavity lying within the lamina of the frontal bone, creating an anterior and posterior wall to the sinus. The size and shape of the sinus vary between individuals and sides. The anterior wall of the sinus is the stronger of the walls but itself is a bone of low resistance to both low-and high-energy impact. The brows and buttress of the supraorbital rims demarcate the lower anterior border of the frontal sinus and offer some protection to the anterior wall of the sinus. The posterior wall of the sinus is thinner and weaker and separates the sinus from the dural covering of the brain in the anterior cranial fossa. The sinus floor consists of membranous bone,

which is the thinnest of the sinus boundaries. It forms up to two-thirds of the medial orbital roof and is the most susceptible area to trauma. A thin septum usually arises from the midline of the sinus floor, partially or completely separating the two sides of the sinus. The inferior aspect of the sinus is intimately related to the orbits, ethmoids and nasal cavity (Fig. 11.16).

Drainage of the frontal sinus is variable. A true nasofrontal duct exists in only 15% of the population, varying from a few millimeters to 1 cm in length.[31] In the remaining 85% the frontal sinus drains directly into the anterosuperior portion of the middle meatus via an ostium without a true duct or occasionally by a communication through the ethmoids via the ethmoidal infundibulum.[13] The proximal opening is a more constant feature, lying in the posteromedial aspect of the frontal sinus floor.[32]

Rationale for management of the frontal sinus

Injury to the frontal sinus is an integral part of most central craniofacial injuries and some lateral craniofacial injuries. The principles involved in the management of the frontal sinus are essentially no different from the overall management of the craniofacial fracture, i.e. to avoid late infective sequelae and the satisfactory restoration of form and function. However, its unique anatomical position and physiological function means the frontal sinus must be assessed and managed as a separate entity within the overall fracture pattern. Adverse outcomes of acute and chronic sinusitis, mucocele, mucopyocele, osteomyelitis, meningitis and cerebral abscess have all been reported following treated and untreated frontal sinus fractures.[2]

The rationale for management of the injured frontal sinus has been aimed at attempting to eliminate the risk of infection and mucocele development. The risk of infection is

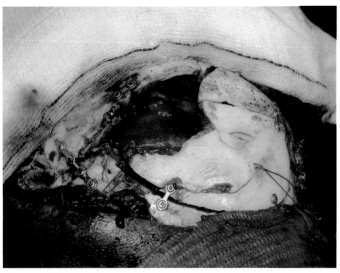

(a)

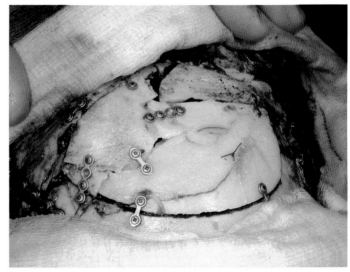

(b)

Fig. 11.15: (a) Large residual defect in the frontal region following removal of multiple comminuted bone fragments and replacement of the craniotomy bone flap. **(b)** Reconstruction of the defect with split inner table calvarial bone taken from the craniotomy bone flap.

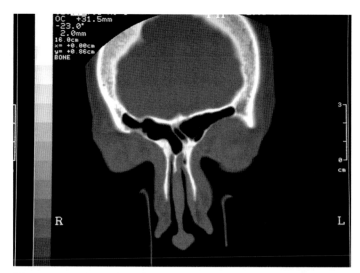

Fig. 11.16: Coronal CT showing the position of the frontal sinus and its immediate relations. Note the septum dividing the sinus in the midline.

linked to communication between the nasal cavity and dural tears via the frontal sinus. A mucocele is a collection of mucus within the sinus with gradual enlargement and destruction of the bony walls. The etiology appears to be related to obstruction of the nasofrontal duct in a diseased or injured frontal sinus.[33] This may become infected to form a mucopyocele. It may also be complicated by localized osteomyelitis or intracranial complications of an epidural or subdural abscess. Unfortunately these complications may occur many years after the initial injury and hence the actual risk of complications is unclear. Historically management of frontal sinus injury has been extrapolated from experience gained in treating patients with acute and chronic frontal sinusitis. This has led to confusion and controversy over the management of frontal sinus injuries, which still exists today.

Our experience and that of other contemporary units treating large numbers of craniofacial injuries suggest that the frontal sinus can be managed reliably and effectively with minimal long-term risk of morbidity. This is based upon clinical and radiological evaluation of each case combined with planned surgical intervention based on these findings.

Classification of frontal sinus fractures

Luce classified frontal sinus fractures into anterior, anterobasilar and frontal skull fractures with extension into the sinus. The fractures were further classified as closed or open, depending upon the presence of an overlying laceration, and whether there was an associated CSF leak.[13]

Gonty et al classified frontal sinus fractures into four groups based on the fracture pattern[2] (Box 11.1). Each of these has its merits, particularly in descriptive terms, but is not particularly helpful in terms of management.

We believe that frontal sinus fractures can be categorized into one of three groups related to management.

1. Fracture of the anterior wall
2. Fracture of the sinus with disruption of the posterior wall
3. Fracture involving the floor of the frontal sinus

Surgical management of the frontal sinus

Safe surgical management of the frontal sinus is based on thorough clinical and radiological evaluation of the nature of the injury, allowing precise preoperative surgical planning. This allows patients to be fully assessed in terms of the risks of developing late complications, which in turn determine management of the frontal sinus.

Fractures of the anterior wall of the frontal sinus

In a series of 72 frontal sinus fractures, isolated fractures of the anterior wall of the frontal sinus occurred in 18% of patients.[34] These fractures may occur with relatively minimal trauma and few clinical signs. Bruising and tenderness over the region of the sinus and the presence of a laceration may all be indicative of an underlying fracture. A CT scan should supplement plain radiographs if there is any doubt.

Undisplaced fractures of the anterior wall require no surgical intervention. Minimally displaced fractures with no evidence of clinical deformity when any edema has subsided may also be managed conservatively. Displaced fractures should be explored via a coronal incision. An overlying laceration is not ideal for surgical exploration and is best avoided. The anterior wall should be reduced and fixed in the anatomical position to restore normal forehead contour (Figs 11.17a–c). Occasionally in severely comminuted fractures primary bone grafting will be required. If a concomitant craniotomy has been performed a split inner table calvarial bone graft is ideal. Otherwise, outer table calvarial or iliac crest bone may be harvested.

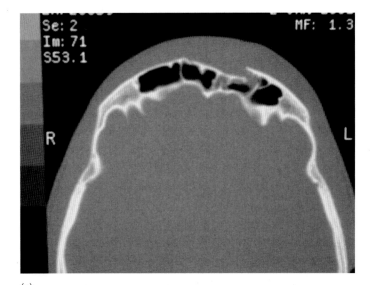

(a)

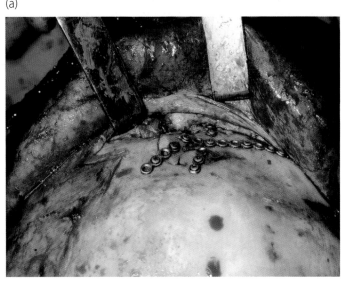

(b)

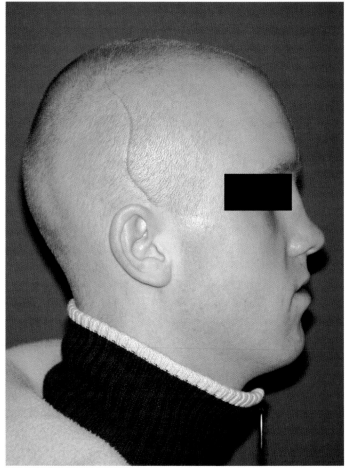

(c)

Fig. 11.17: (a) Axial CT scan showing a displaced fracture involving the anterior wall of the frontal sinus. **(b)** Reduction and fixation of anterior wall of frontal sinus fracture seen in Fig. 11.8. **(c)** Early postoperative view showing satisfactory restoration of forehead contour.

Fractures of the frontal sinus with disruption of the posterior wall

When there is a fracture involving the frontal sinus, involvement of the posterior wall is relatively common. In a series of 72 fractures of the frontal sinus, the posterior wall was involved in almost 80% of cases.[34] If the frontal sinus is large it may absorb much of the force, leaving the posterior wall intact, even if there is gross comminution of the anterior wall. If the sinus is small, there is a greater likelihood of posterior wall involvement.[35] Occasionally a high-energy injury to the nasoethmoidal area can produce relatively minimal primary deformity at the site of impact, with the energy being transmitted to the weaker posterior wall of the frontal sinus with disruption at this site (Fig. 11.18). This 'burst' phenomenon may also occur with skull fractures. The etiology is analogous to orbital floor fractures where the energy of the force is transmitted through the infraorbital margin to the relatively weaker area of the orbital floor, producing a fracture remote from the point of impact. These injuries

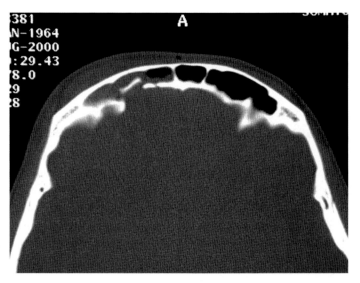

Fig. 11.18: Axial CT scan showing isolated displaced fracture involving the posterior wall of the frontal sinus with no disruption of the anterior wall.

can be easily missed without appropriate imaging, thus placing the patient at lifelong risk of developing infective complications.

Disruption of the posterior wall of the frontal sinus with or without a CSF leak has been reliably demonstrated to be associated with a high incidence of dural tear.[21] Undisplaced fractures of the posterior wall may be treated conservatively. We consider a fracture of the posterior wall to be displaced if the displacement is greater than the width of the posterior wall itself. When there is displacement or other radiological findings on CT scan suggestive of a dural tear, e.g. aerocele, surgical exploration is warranted because of the inherent risks of long-term infective sequelae.

Fractures involving the posterior wall of the frontal sinus are approached via a coronal flap. A low bifrontal craniotomy allows access to the frontal sinus and inspection of the basal dura. Dural tears are not necessarily confined to the convexity dura immediately behind the fracture but may frequently be basal, making direct dural repair technically difficult and potentially hazardous if the repair is performed inadequately. Under these circumstances it is both safer and easier to perform an intradural dural repair owing to the superior access and visibility afforded by this approach. Dural tears can be closed primarily or, when complex, a pericranial patch can be sutured across the defect and sealed with fibrin glue.

The posterior wall of the frontal sinus is removed in its entirety (cranialization of the frontal sinus) and the mucosa lining the sinus is meticulously removed (Fig. 11.19). The nasofrontal duct on each side is plugged with autogenous bone chips and the nasal cavity is effectively sealed from the cranial cavity with a vascularized pericranial or galeal/frontalis flap raised with the coronal flap (Fig. 11.20). The flap is inlaid over the sinus floor via the inferior aspect of the craniotomy and care should be taken when repositioning the bone flap at the end of the procedure not to damage or inhibit the vascularity of the flap (Fig. 11.21).

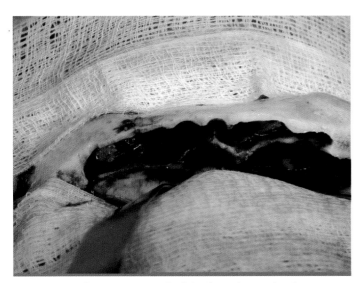

Fig. 11.19: The posterior wall of the frontal sinus has been removed to the level of the floor of the anterior cranial fossa and all mucosa removed.

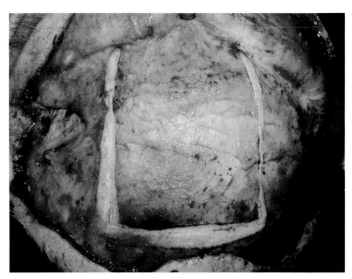

Fig. 11.20: A pericranial flap has been raised with the coronal flap for later use following cranialization of the frontal sinus. Note the split in the temporalis fascia to preserve the frontal branch of the facial nerve.

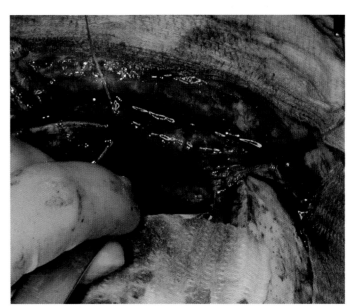

Fig. 11.21: A pericranial flap is being inlaid to separate the repaired dura from the cranialized frontal sinus.

Fracture involving the floor of the frontal sinus

Isolated frontal sinus fractures without concomitant involvement of the anterior or posterior walls of the sinus is uncommon. In a series of 72 fractures of the frontal sinus only two patients (1.44%) had isolated fractures involving the floor of the frontal sinus.[34] When isolated fractures of the sinus floor occur they are almost inevitably associated with a fracture of the nasoethmoidal complex. The rationale to treat these injuries from the view point of the frontal sinus has been to prevent the later development of a frontal sinus mucocele and its inherent complications. Schenck et al have postulated two types of mucocele: a pressure mucocele in an obstructed sinus and a trauma mucocele after infection or blunt trauma to the sinus mucosa.[33] There is little evidence to suggest the late development of a mucocele in an adequately treated frontal sinus. In two series of frontal sinus mucocele, only 4% and 6% of patients respectively gave a previous history of trauma and in all cases the frontal sinus had not been primarily explored.[13]

Disruption to the drainage of the frontal sinus is more likely to occur in nasoethmoidal fractures. Historically these fractures have been treated by closed reduction and therefore we would anticipate reports of frontal mucocele as a long-term complication of inadequately treated nasoethmoidal fractures. This is not reflected in the literature. It is tempting to suggest that isolated fractures of the floor of the frontal sinus may be treated conservatively and, if drainage of the sinus appears satisfactory, this is acceptable. Contemporary management of nasoethmoidal fractures is aimed at open anatomical reduction of fractures, internal fixation and, if necessary, primary bone grafting. Under these circumstances, if disruption to the drainage of the frontal sinus is suspected on imaging, direct inspection of the frontal sinus is recommended. If there is concomitant posterior wall fracture the sinus should be managed as outlined above.

A number of series have been published where the sinus cavity is maintained with the expectation that the nasofrontal duct would continue to function. When fractures are reduced and rigidly fixed with or without primary bone grafting and the dura is repaired and isolated from the contents of the nasal cavity with a vascularized flap, the long-term risk of mucocele is minimal. It appears that under these circumstances function of the nasofrontal duct will resume. It is the presence of inadequately treated fractures, comminuted sequestra, foreign bodies and torn mucosal shreds which leaves the patient at long-term risk of mucocele.[35]

Controversies

Obliteration or cranialization of the frontal sinus?

We have advocated cranialization of the frontal sinus for fractures with disruption of the posterior wall of the sinus. In our series of over 100 patients, reconstruction of the basal dura and base of skull was carried out using peri-cranial flaps in 71 cases, pericranial and fascial grafts in 23 cases and cranialization of the frontal sinuses in 59 cases where there was disruption of the posterior wall of the frontal sinus. There have been no cases of postoperative meningitis or cerebral abscess and no postoperative deaths.[21] Significant complications of intracranial sepsis have been demonstrated in cases where posterior sinus wall fractures have been treated conservatively.[36] This is not surprising in light of the incidence of dural tears associated with disruption of the posterior wall of the frontal sinus and the long-term risk associated with leaving a dural tear in communication with the nasal cavity via the frontal sinus.[21] Management of acute and chronic infections of the frontal sinus has evolved from ablation of the sinus by excision of the bony walls to exen-

terate the sinus of diseased mucosa but preserving the bony confines. These techniques carried a significant failure rate and were replaced by procedures to obliterate the sinus by excising the mucosa, plugging the nasofrontal duct and allowing the sinus to fill by osteoneogenesis.[13]

Obliteration of the frontal sinus has been described using autogenous materials such as fat, muscle or bone or the use of synthetic materials such as hydroxyapatite or lyophilized cartilage. Obliteration of the sinus with fat appears to be the most popular choice but failure rates of up to 25% have been reported.[37] In a series of 46 fractures of the frontal sinus treated by obliteration with fat, only 28% of patients developed no postoperative complications. Two patients in this series developed meningitis and one patient developed a cerebral abscess after treatment.[38] Other series have demonstrated variable complication and success rates with sinus obliteration. Free fat grafts can be expected to undergo a significant rate of necrosis when used to obliterate the frontal sinus, as any non-vascularized graft is dependent upon the vascularity of the recipient site to survive. It is therefore illogical to consider obliteration of the sinus where there is disruption of the posterior wall and an associated dural tear. Cranialization of the sinus with separation of the sinus from the nasal cavity with a vascularized flap is the procedure of choice under these circumstances.

Management of the nasofrontal duct

Patency of the nasofrontal duct has been considered to be important in preventing infection of the frontal sinus and the development of a mucocele. This is certainly the case when considering acute and chronic frontal sinusitis. However, the role of the nasofrontal duct in trauma may have been overstated because of previous experience with sinus diseases. It has already been demonstrated that infection is an extremely rare sequelae of an adequately treated fracture of the frontal sinus. In addition, a mucocele is a rare complication of trauma to the frontal sinus and those cases that arise tend to do so in inadequately managed fractures. This is supported by the paucity of reports of mucocele complicating isolated fractures of the nasoethmoidal complex where disruption to sinus drainage may be greater than when the frontal sinus itself is involved in trauma.

In fractures of the frontal sinus where there is radiological evidence of disruption to sinus drainage the fracture should be explored and treated on its merits according to the criteria outlined above. There is no place for attempts to re-establish drainage of the sinus. Attempts to surgically re-establish the function of an incompetent nasofrontal duct have a failure rate of nearly 30% due to subsequent scar formation and stenosis.[38]

The key to nasofrontal duct function lies with the inherent principles of contemporary maxillofacial trauma management. When fractures are anatomically reduced and rigidly fixed, with or without primary bone grafting, and comminuted bone and torn denuded mucosa are removed, the long-term risk of mucocele formation is minimal.

Key points

- Craniofacial fractures are classified as central, lateral or complex injuries depending upon the site of the fracture.

- Preoperative CT imaging in axial and coronal planes allows precise delineation of fractures and accurate planning for management.

- The rationale for the management of craniofacial injuries is to prevent late infective sequelae and cranio-orbital deformity.

- Untreated dural tears have an unacceptably high risk of the long-term development of meningitis.

- Early combined repair of craniofacial injuries is effective in improving functional and cosmetic results with acceptable morbidity and mortality with no adverse effect on neuro-surgical outcome in selected patients.

- The principles of the surgical management of craniofacial fractures are based upon adequate exposure, minimal brain retraction, rigid fixation of fractures and primary bone grafting where necessary.

- Fractures involving the anterior wall of the frontal sinus are treated on the basis of cosmesis.

- Displaced fractures of the posterior wall of the frontal sinus have a high risk of dural tear and are treated by cranialization of the sinus and isolation of the sinus contents from the nasal cavity with a vascularized pericranial flap.

- The risk of mucocele development is minimal in adequately treated fractures of the frontal sinus.

- There is no place for obliteration of the frontal sinus or attempts to re-establish drainage of the nasofrontal duct in contemporary management of frontal sinus fractures.

Use of prophylactic antibiotics

The question of prophylactic antibiotics remains. Retrospective analyses of the use of antibiotics in patients with traumatic CSF leaks have given conflicting results in attempting to demonstrate a benefit. There is no strong evidence for prophylactic antibiotic therapy in these patients.[39,40] Patients who have suffered one episode of meningitis are liable to experience further instances of infection. This group may benefit from the provision of prophylactic antibiotics.

Outcomes

The rationale for the treatment of craniofacial fractures has been stated as the prevention of late infective complications and late cranio-orbital deformity. We have followed the criteria outlined above for over 10 years in treating over 100 patients in Southampton. Of these patients 87% have made a good recovery according to the Glasgow Outcome Score with a revisional facial surgery rate of 14%. There have been no cases of postoperative CSF leakage, postoperative meningitis or late intracranial abscess. There have been no cases of mucocele to date and the postoperative mortality for the series is zero. The only major postoperative complication has been the loss of the frontal bone flap due to postoperative infection in one case.

References

1 Ionnides CH, Freihofer HP, Friens J 1993 Fractures of the frontal sinus: a rationale of treatment. British Journal of Plastic Surgery 46: 208–214

2 Gonty AA, Marciani RD, Adornato DC 1999 Management of frontal sinus fractures: a review of 33 cases. Journal of Oral and Maxillofacial Surgery 57: 372–379

3 Sakas DE, Beale DJ, Ameen AA et al 1998 Compound anterior cranial base fractures: classification using computerized tomography scanning as a basis for selection of patients for dural repair. Journal of Neurosurgery 88: 471–477

4 Jones N 1997 Craniofacial trauma. Oxford University Press, New York

5 American College of Surgeons 1993 Advanced trauma life support course manual. American College of Surgeons, Chicago

6 Teasdale G, Jennet B 1974 Assessment of coma and impaired consciousness: a practical scale. Lancet 2: 81–84

7 Kirsch AP Diagnosis of cerebrospinal fluid rhinorrhoea: lack of specificity of the glucose-oxidase test tape. Journal of Pediatrics 71: 718–719

8 Meurman OH, Irjala K, Suonpaa J, Laurent B 1979 A new method for the identification of cerebrospinal fluid leakage. Acta Otolaryngologica 87: 366–369

9 Teasdale GM, Murray G, Anderson E et al 1990 Risks of acute traumatic intracranial haematoma in children and adults: implications for managing head injuries. British Medical Journal 300: 363–367

10 Zacharides N, Vairaktaris E, Papavassilou D, Triantafyllou D, Mezitis M 1987 Orbital apex syndrome. International Journal of Oral and Maxillofacial Surgery 16: 352–354

11 Bowerman JE 1969 The superior orbital fissure syndrome complicating fractures of the facial skeleton. British Journal of Oral Surgery 7: 1–6

12 Palmer JD 1996 Neurosurgery. Churchill Livingstone, New York

13 Luce EA 1987 Frontal sinus fractures: guidelines to management. Plastic and Reconstructive Surgery 80: 500–508

14 Broumand SR, Labs JD, Novelline RA, Markowitz BL, Yaremchuk MJ 1993 The role of three dimensional computed tomography in the evaluation of acute craniofacial trauma. Annals of Plastic Surgery 31: 488–494

15 Merville LC, Derome P 1978 Concomittant dislocations of the face and skull. Journal of Maxillofacial Surgery 6: 2–14

16 Lewin W 1954 Cerebrospinal fluid rhinorrhoea in closed head injuries. British Journal of Surgery 42: 1–18

17 Eljamel MS, Foy PM 1990 Acute traumatic CSF fistulae: the risk of intracranial infection. British Journal of Neurosurgery 4: 381–385

18 Eljamel MSM, Foy PM 1990 Post-traumatic CSF fistulae, the case for surgical repair. British Journal of Neurosurgery 4: 479–483

19 Poole MD, Briggs M 1989 Cranio-orbital trauma: a team approach to management. Annals of the Royal College of Surgeons 71: 187–194

20 Evans BT, Lang D, Neil-Dwyer G 1996 Current management of craniofacial trauma. In: Palmer JD (ed) Neurosurgery. Churchill Livingstone, Edinburgh

21 Evans BT, Webb AAC, Baker NJ, Neil-Dwyer G, Lang DA 2001 The indications for combined surgical management of craniofacial trauma. (In press)

22 Derdyn C, Persing JA, Broaddus WC et al 1990 Craniofacial trauma: an assessment of risk related to timing of surgery. Plastic and Reconstructive Surgery 86: 238–245

23 Benzil DL, Robotti E, Dagi TF, Sullivan P, Belvivino JR, Knuckey NW 1992 Early single-stage repair of complex craniofacial trauma. Neurosurgery 30: 166–171

24 Piotowski WP, Beck-Mannagetta J 1995 Surgical techniques in orbital roof fractures: early treatment and results. Journal of Craniomaxillofacial Surgery 23: 6–11

25 Webb AAC, Evans BT, Baker NJ, Lang DA, Neil-Dwyer G 2001 Case selection and timing of surgery in craniofacial trauma. (In press)

26 Baker NJ, Evans BT, Neil-Dwyer G, Lang DA 1999 The surgical management of craniofacial trauma. In: Ward-Booth P, Schendel SA, Hausamen J (eds) Maxillofacial surgery. Harcourt Brace, London

27 Raveh J, Vuillemin T, Sutter F 1988 Subcranial management of 395 combined frontobasal-midface fractures. Archives of Otolaryngology Head and Neck Surgery 114: 1114–1122

28 Jones NS, Becker DG 2001 Advances in the management of CSF leaks. British Medical Journal 322: 122–123

29 Al-Kayat A, Bramley P 1978 A modified pre-auricular approach to the temporomandibular joint and malar arch. British Journal of Oral Surgery 17: 91–103

30 Yaremchuk MJ, Gruss JS, Manson PN 1992 Rigid fixation of the craniomaxillofacial skeleton. Butterworth-Heinemann, Boston

31 Gross CL 1984 Pathophysiology and evaluation of frontoethmoid fractures. In: Mathog RH (ed) Maxillofacial trauma. Williams and Wilkins, Baltimore

32 Heller EM, Jacobs JB, Holliday RA 1989 Evaluation of the frontonasal duct in frontal sinus fractures. Head and Neck 11: 46–50

33 Schenk NL, Rauchbach E, Ogura J 1974 Frontal sinus disease. II. Development of the frontal sinus model: occlusion of the nasofrontal duct. Laryngoscope 84: 1233–1247

34 Wallis A, Donald PJ 1988 Frontal sinus fractures: a review of 72 cases. Laryngoscope 98: 593–598

35 Gruss JS, Pollock RA, Phillips JH, Antonyshyn O 1989 Combined injuries of the cranium and face. British Journal of Plastic Surgery 42: 385–398

36 Newman MH, Travis LW 1973 Frontal sinus fractures. Laryngoscope 83: 1281–1292

37 Sailer HF, Grätz KW, Kalavrezos ND 1998 Frontal sinus fractures: principles of treatment and long term results after sinus obliteration with the use of lyophilized cartilage. Journal of Cranio-maxillofacial Surgery 26: 235–242

38 Wilson BC, Davidson B, Corey JP, Haydon RC 1988 Comparison of complications following frontal sinus fractures managed with exploration with or without obliteration over 10 years. Laryngoscope 98: 516–520

39 Klastersky J, Sadeghi M, Brihaye N 1976 Antimicrobial prophylaxis in patients with rhinorrhea or otorrhea: a double-blind study. Surgical Neurology 6: 111–114

40 MacGee EE, Cauthen JC, Bracken CE 1970 Meningitis following acute traumatic cerebrospinal fistula. Journal of Neurosurgery 33: 312–316

12 Nasoethmoid Fractures

Peter Ayliffe, Peter Ward Booth

Introduction

The nasoethmoid region is an important area of the face not only for cosmesis but also in determining facial projection and width. The region relies for form and strength on a complex interrelationship between uniquely specialized soft tissues and bones formed into buttresses and thin plates.

Nasoethmoid fractures represent a spectrum of injury from simple nasal fractures with minimal ethmoid involvement through to grossly comminuted fractures with displacement. The complex anatomy and direction of the force together with the degree of development of the paranasal sinuses and related structures often mean that the fracture patterns extend posteriorly into the orbit, the skull base and the frontal sinus. Indeed, fractures of the frontonasal duct as it traverses the anterior part of the labyrinth of the ethmoid should be considered in all nasoethmoid fractures. In more than 50% of individuals the frontonasal duct is continuous with the anterior ethmoidal sinus through the infundibulum which means that all nasoethmoid fractures should be considered to be compound fractures. Nasoethmoid injuries should also be considered as fractures of the orbit, with all the recognized and associated problems.

State of the Art

Management of these injuries requires a clear understanding of the anatomy. Since the standard texts do not emphasize certain important aspects of surgical anatomy, it is a controversial area. We would therefore refer the reader to the extensive review of the surgical anatomy under the heading 'Controversies' at the end of this chapter.

The 'gold standard' of care of patients with nasoethmoid injuries begins with:

- careful clinical evaluation
- detailed radiological examination
- careful ophthalmic examination
- rarely, secondary special examinations, particularly to verify the function of the lacrimal apparatus.

This protocol should establish a precise diagnosis. With this information, normally using an open approach, precise reduction and stabilization should be possible, leading to a good outcome.

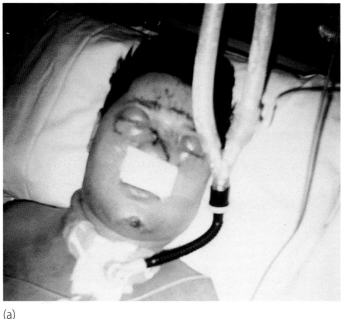

(a)

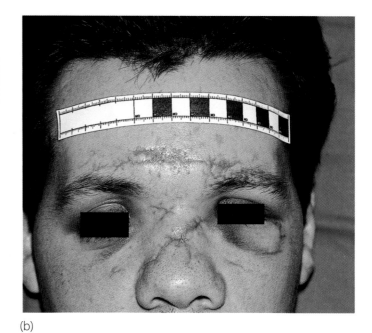

(b)

Fig. 12.1: **(a)** Severe injuries and the problems of immediate care may allow a traumatic telecanthus from a nasoethmoid fracture to be overlooked. **(b)** Once the swelling has settled the fracture and displacement of the canthi are obvious. Hopefully delay in diagnosis will not happen if there is a careful initial examination; this patient was seen at first in a non-specialist environment.

Clinical Examination

The clinical findings will obviously be related to the time of examination of the patient post injury. Soft tissue injuries are usually readily evaluated by clinical examination. However, gross edema or emphysema initially may mask the full nature of the injuries. If the patient is examined soon after the injury gross swelling may mask canthal detachment, for instance (Fig. 12.1).

Clinically nasoethmoid fractures may present with traumatic telecanthus and impaction of the bridge of the nose, producing a characteristic appearance (Fig. 12.2). Telescoping of the nasal dorsum into the ethmoid region (Fig. 12.3) and the lack of distal support leads to nasal tip elevation. Depression of the nasal bridge with lack of normal form in the frontonasal angle projects the nostrils almost horizontally, giving a 'pig snout' appearance when the swelling has subsided (Fig. 12.4).

Some workers[23] have attempted to classify these bony fractures. These classifications have not proved useful in clinical practice to date and they do not correlate well with outcome; thus they are infrequently used. It is, however, important to distinguish the severity of the fracture. Clearly greater problems occur with compound comminuted fractures with gross displacement than with simple fractures.[40]

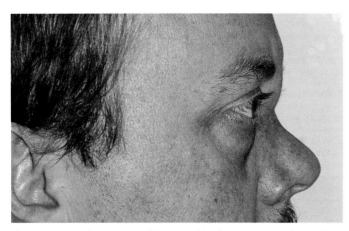

Fig. 12.2: Displacement of the nasal bridge into the ethmoids causes this characteristic 'pig snout' appearance, caused by the relative upturning of the nasal tip.

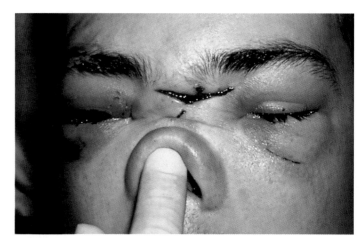

Fig. 12.3: Comminution of nasal bones further adds to the problem with no support and the soft tissue is easily depressed.

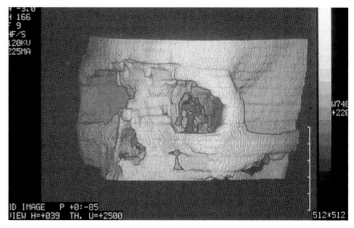

Fig. 12.4: The CT of the patient in Fig. 12.2 demonstrates the cause of the soft tissue appearance by displacement of the nasal bridge.

In nasoethmoid trauma, comminution and actual detachment from bone of the canthus represent important and poor prognostic criteria for a satisfactory outcome.

In trauma to this region the bones most commonly fracture in such a way as to leave a fragment with the medial canthal lig-

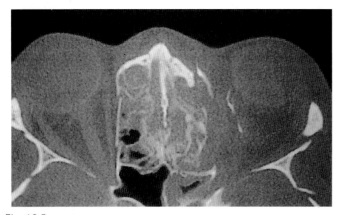

Fig. 12.5

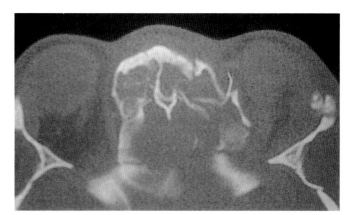

Fig. 12.6

Fig. 12.5, 12.6: Overriding of the bony fragments can cause sectioning of the canthal ligament.

ament attached. However, the oblique slope of the nasal bones and their concavoconvexity from above down and their concavity anteroposteriorly mean that anterior forces can cause overriding of bony fragments. The fragments can be pushed posteriorly and disrupt the lacrimal sac (Fig. 12.5) or guillotine the canthal ligament. This can be seen on CT scans (Fig. 12.6) and clinically, when careful exploration of lacerations in this area will reveal the extent of the damage to either the canthal attachment (Fig. 12.7) or the lacrimal system or both.

The eyelids should be held and distracted laterally. This maneuver is particularly directed at pulling the canthus to ensure it is still attached to stable bone. If the canthus is detached or if the canthal-bearing bone fragment is small then the canthal apex will move laterally and the canthal angle will be blunted (Fig. 12.8). In situations where the nasoethmoid bone fragments are severely impacted, the canthal-bearing fragment can become wedged in an incorrect position and the distraction test will be falsely negative.

More severe forces may extend the fractures into the base of skull (Fig. 12.9) through the cribriform plate of the ethmoid; frequently this is associated with a leak of cerebrospinal fluid. Tears in the dura may occur if a fragment

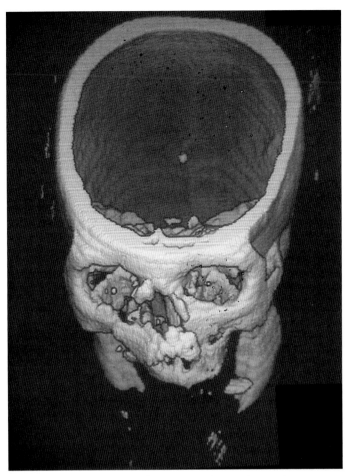

Fig. 12.9: A 3D CT scans shows severe impaction and comminution involving the cribiform plate.

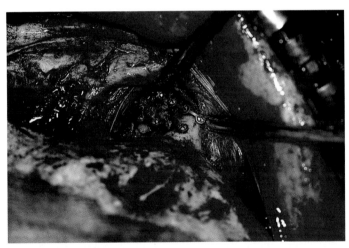

Fig. 12.7: In this case the ligament is still attached to a piece of bone which has been plated.

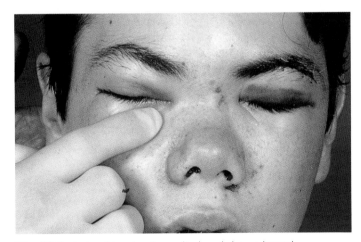

Fig. 12.8: Lateral tension is applied and shows lateral movement caused by damage to the medical canthal attachment.

of misplaced bone punctures the membrane. Shearing forces may tear the dura, particularly if the crista galli is fractured as is often seen with severe displaced nasoethmoid fractures. The energy of impact may also be dissipated through the frontal sinus and fractures of the posterior wall of the frontal sinus are a common finding in association with high-energy trauma causing severely displaced nasoethmoid fractures that extend into the skull base and anterior cranial fossa.

An appreciation of the midline of the patient's face is important and also determination of any asymmetry in the canthi. The intercanthal and interpupillary distances should be measured. Although a gross increase in the intercanthal distance (normal range 24–39 mm in Caucasians) is diagnostic, borderline cases can be difficult. A better guide in clinical practice is to relate the intercanthal distance to the interpupillary distance provided there is no globe displacement due to gross orbital disruption. Normally the intercanthal distance is twice the interpupillary distance. If the bone attachment has itself been fractured and displaced laterally with the canthus then this needs to be explored more formally at the time of surgery in order to fix the medial canthus to prevent late complications of canthal drift.

A full ophthalmic examination is obviously essential but this may be compromised by the neurological status of the patient. It is important to examine the function of the optic nerve and the ocular reflexes. In a posteriorly impacted nasoethmoid fracture the optic nerve can be compressed due to collapse of the bony complex into the sphenoid sinus and direct compression of the nerve in the canal. In the unconscious patient the swinging flashlight test is particularly important and the fundus should be examined thoroughly for signs of optic nerve compression. In patients who have sustained sufficient trauma to cause compression of the optic nerve, there is a high incidence of injuries to the globe itself.

The lacrimal apparatus is damaged infrequently, usually as a result of direct penetrating trauma or due to overriding fragments of sharp bone. Thus lacerations in this area must be carefully explored. Dye can be introduced into either of the lacrimal puncta and backflow will usually demonstrate the leak. If doubt remains radiological confirmation may be needed.

Bony injuries are frequently difficult to examine well enough to give a precise diagnosis. Even in the most swollen patients, however, it is normally possible to gauge the extent of the fractures by careful clinical examination. This is important in order to obtain X-ray examinations which are well 'targeted' to gain maximum information.

Radiological Examination

Good-quality X-rays are normally required but in patients with marked swelling the fine bones of the nasoethmoid region may be effaced by the soft tissue shadows. Again, careful orbital and other facial bone examination is required. Occipitomental views (10° and 45°) are most helpful as an initial screening examination. Lateral face or skull radiographs are usually disappointing in nasoethmoid trauma; occasionally an occlusal film will show the ethmoid disruption.

Good-quality cut CT scans are extremely valuable, if not essential, particularly in high-energy trauma where the frontal sinus and base of skull may be disrupted (Fig. 12.10). Since reconstructed and 3D images contain artefacts, it is helpful if the patient is fit enough to allow axial and coronal cuts to be made. These images must of course be used to

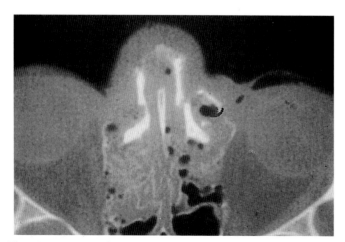

Fig. 12.10: A good-quality CT gives unrivalled detail, essential for nasoethmoid fractures, in this case even showing damage to the lacrimal sac.

exclude any related fractures or injuries, particularly orbital wall fractures.

Special radiology, such as a dacrocystogram, is not normally used for primary surgery, as direct examination is usually possible at the time of surgery.

Timing of Treatment

This is a difficult problem for all facial surgery, but especially in nasoethmoid trauma. Delays in treatment can lead to difficulty in repositioning the soft tissues, particularly the canthal ligaments, and identifying any damage to the lacrimal duct system. Early treatment may, however, be impossible because of other injuries, commonly head injuries. Edema presents significant problems when operating in this region and delay can allow this to settle. Many patients with these injuries will be treated at about 7–10 days, but the earlier surgery can be undertaken, allowing for other injuries and swelling, the more satisfactory.

Anatomy

If a satisfactory treatment is to be achieved a good understanding of the normal anatomy is essential. There are certain anatomical structures that are disproportionately important. This section will discuss these structures in turn.

The bony anatomy

The nose is the most conspicuous feature of the bony skeleton in this region. The two nasal bones and the vertical midline bony septum form its major structural components. The nasal bones superiorly articulate through a serrated joint with the nasal part of the frontal bone. Laterally they articulate with the frontal process of the maxilla. Superiorly the bones are thick; they gradually thin to the notched inferior borders that are continuous with the lateral nasal cartilages. The medial borders are thicker above than below and the two nasal bones articulate with each other around the midline of the nose. The pair of nasal bones have a vertical crest on their posterior surface which forms part of the midline septum of the nose. They articulate with the nasal spine of the frontal bone, the perpendicular plate of the ethmoid bone and the cartilage of the nasal septum from above downwards.

The structural arrangement of the nasal skeleton in a pyramidal form along with the frontal process of each maxilla together form the major buttresses of the anterior midface. They provide strength and act to protect the relatively thin sheets of the lacrimal bone, the cribriform, perpendicular and orbital plates of the ethmoid bone more posteriorly. The frontonasal buttresses provide considerable strength to resist the energy transmitted from a direct anterior blow, but there is relatively little strength to resist a lateral blow. Once the thick nasal bridge collapses, the forces are dissipated into the air cells. Whilst this mechanically protects the base of the skull as a natural 'crumple zone', relatively small forces in patients with large pneumatized air cells can cause collapse of the whole complex.

The bones of this region are important in providing the area of insertion to that part of the medial canthal ligament which attaches anterior to the lacrimal sac. The medial canthal ligament provides the primary functional support of the eyelids medially by connecting the orbicularis muscle to the medial orbit, lateral nose and lacrimal diaphragm.

The eyelids

The skin of the eyelids, at less than 1 mm thick, is the thinnest in the body[1,2] and almost transparent. The skin over the medial canthal ligament is smooth and shiny, unlike the skin of the temporal eyelids. It is firmly attached to the underlying structures in this region and has very few hairs. The few that are present are fine and have only rudimentary sebaceous glands. In the medial part of the lower lid bundles of muscle fibers fan out from the underlying preseptal muscle and insert directly into the skin and are responsible for the vertical wrinkles seen in this area (muscles of Merkel).[3] There are no such muscle fibers in the upper lid.

The axis of the palpebral fissure is not horizontal; the lateral angle is about 2 mm above and behind the medial angle. An increase in the obliquity of the palpebral fissure is characteristic of Mongolian races as is a fold of skin passing from the medial end of the upper lid to the lower, obscuring the caruncle, a feature known as epicanthus. Epicanthus occurs in the human fetus but disappears with nasal development in Caucasians. It persists in some cases of congenital ptosis.

The palpebral fissure at the lateral canthus is acute, measuring 30–40°, and is placed directly against the globe. At the medial canthus it is more rounded; the lower margin is horizontal and the upper passes downwards and medially (Fig. 12.11). It is separated from the globe by a little recess, the lacus lacrimalis. Within this is a yellowish elevation, the lacrimal caruncle, an area of skin containing modified sweat and sebaceous glands. Lateral to the caruncle is the plica semilunaris, a reddish narrow crescentic fold of conjunctiva

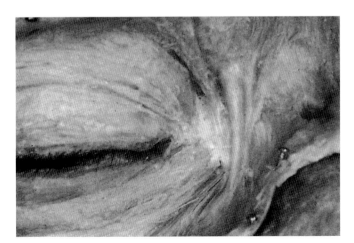

Fig. 12.11: Superficial dissection of the ligament. The angular artery and fat have been removed to demonstrate the muscles and the extent of attachment of the ligament over the frontonasal buttress.

lying vertically with its concavity facing laterally. It lies partly under cover of the caruncle and its lower horn reaches to the middle of the lower fornix; the upper does not extend quite so far. This fold represents the third eyelid or membrana nicitans of lower animals. The connective tissue stroma of the plica contains numerous vessels, a lobule of fat and some muscle. Similar structures are found within the caruncle and arise from the medial capsulopalpebral muscle of Hesser while some arise from the medial rectus.[1]

The lacrimal drainage system

The lacrimal papilla are elevations at the medial end of the lid margins just lateral to the plica semilunaris; they are pierced by the small round or transversely oval apertures of the lacrimal puncta. The puncta are situated in line with the openings of the tarsal gland ducts and lie about 1 mm medial to the nearest opening, dividing the lids into ciliary and lacrimal parts. The superior punctum is slightly nearer to the nasal side, being 6 mm from the medial canthus, and the lower is 6.5 mm from the canthus. Each punctum is surrounded by dense fibrous tissue continuous with the tarsus. This keeps the punctum patent and is surrounded by fibers of the orbicularis, which pass on to and attach to the medial canthal ligament.

Each lacrimal canaliculus is lined by stratified squamous epithelium upon an extensive corium of elastic tissue. Macroscopically they consist of a vertical and a horizontal part; the vertical components are about 2 mm long and then bend medially almost at right angles to become the horizontal portions. At the junction of the two is a dilatation or ampulla. Both horizontal components of the canaliculi slope towards the common medial canthal ligament within the substance of the pretarsal components of the upper and lower eyelids. They take a convergent course, the lower in a slight upward inclination for 8 mm and the lower in a downward inclination for 7.5 mm within the lid margins. They have pretarsal fibers of the orbicularis in superficial and deep relationship over the medial third of their course. The tarsal glands lie below the canaliculi and the ciliary glands of Moll and the ciliary glands of Zeiss lie superficially. The canaliculi pierce the lacrimal fascia either separately or in common. They enter the lacrimal sac through the valve of Rosemüller at a small diverticulum called the sinus of Maier. This lies behind the middle of the lateral surface of the lacrimal sac about 2.5 mm from its apex.

The membranous lacrimal sac lies in the lacrimal fossa formed by the frontal process of the maxilla and lacrimal bone. The sac is open and continuous below with the nasolacrimal duct; a constriction marks the junction between the two. The sac is enclosed by a splitting of the orbital fascia called the lacrimal fascia or lacrimal diaphragm; it is the action of the attached muscles that is in part responsible for the normal aspiration of tear fluid.[4] The lacrimal fascia is adherent to the sac around the fundus but otherwise it is separated by a thin layer of areolar tissue. The medial canthal ligament is attached to the lacrimal fascia in front and behind the sac. The lacrimal sac extends for about 3–5 mm above the horizontal component of the ligament. A thin layer of orbicularis covers the sac below the medial canthal ligament and it is therefore in this region that herniations, abscesses and fistulae tend to come to the surface.

The medial canthal ligament

The medial canthal ligament when viewed from the anterior aspect is a diamond-shaped fibrous band, longer in its horizontal dimension. It has a superficial anterior limb that averages 11.7 mm in length, with an average width of 4.9 mm.[5,6] It is attached to the frontal process of the maxilla just lateral to its suture with the nasal bone behind the angular vein and the angular artery more medially. This anterior attachment extends laterally to the anterior lacrimal crest (Figs 12.12, 12.13). The area of this insertion averages 25.3 sq mm. This forms an extensive attachment to the frontonasal buttress. The angular vein lies 8 mm from the medial canthal apex.

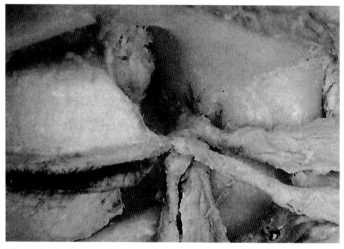

Fig. 12.12: The major muscle components of the ligament are displayed. Riolan's muscle can be seen. The strong attachment to the posterior lacrimal crest and medial orbital periosteum can also be seen.

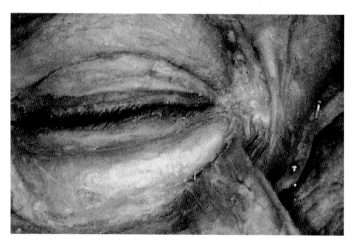

Fig. 12.13: The vertical component of the ligament can be seen lateral to the angular vein. The inferior orbicularis muscle has been retracted medially to show the orbital septum. The orbital fat can be seen bulging forward from below.

The extent of medial aspect of the ligament beyond the anterior lacrimal crest is demonstrated by the fact that the crest is only 2–3 mm from the medial commissure of the eyelids and just lateral to the canthal apex.

The medial canthal ligament may require reconstruction or replacement following nasoethmoid trauma, resection for neoplastic disease, congenital deformity or detachment during craniofacial surgery. The anatomical arrangement of the individual components is important to both the functional role of the ligament and the cosmetic appearance of the face. An understanding of the three-dimensional arrangement is essential for the satisfactory management of this region.

Historically, the eponym 'Horner's muscle' has been applied to the muscularis orbicularis oculi pars lacrimalis or tensor tarsi, as described by William Edmonds Horner (1793–1853) in 1822.[7] Reiffler[8] has shown that the muscle was actually first discovered by Jacques Francois-Marie Duvernay approximately a century earlier. The first published description appeared in 1730 in a manuscript by Johan Caspar Schobinger, one of Duvernay's pupils,[9,10] who clearly credited Duvernay with the discovery. The first published illustration of the muscularis orbicularis oculi pars lacrimalis was in the second plate of the first atlas published by Duvernay in collaboration with the engraver Jacques-Fabian Gautier d'Agoty in 1745,[11] in which Duvernay described the structure as 'le petit muscle des paupières'.

Reconstruction of the medial canthal ligament remains a challenging clinical problem and is associated with a significant failure rate.[12] Debate continues over the best surgical method and techniques for its reconstruction.[5,13–24] Much of this is probably related historically to a poor understanding of the anatomy and physiological function of this area, demonstrated by the confusion over the nomenclature that has been employed in the past. The structure has been referred to as the medial canthal tendon, medial canthal ligament, tensor tarsi, medial palpebral tendon and medial palpebral ligament, to name the most commonly used labels in the published literature. Dagum et al,[24] in their experimental work, clearly show that the structure behaves biomechanically as a ligament, demonstrating the extensibility and strain behavior that is typical of a ligament rather than of a tendon. Furthermore, from the histological point of view the structure is composed of fibrous tissue more characteristic of a ligament than a tendon. Thus it would seem more appropriate to call the structure the medial canthal ligament.

Several contributions have been made in modern times to our understanding of the medial canthal ligament, many of them based on anatomical studies. Duke Elder published comprehensive descriptions of the anatomy and histology of the orbital region in 1931 and 1961.[25,26] For many years these remained the standard authoritative texts and much of his work remains relevant today. Wolfe's textbook in 1954[3] contributed to our three-dimensional understanding of the ligament, but the meticulous dissections and precise descriptions of the anatomy by Jones remain outstanding references.[27–31] In 1961 he published a paper that included photographs of his dissections, displaying the muscular origins of the medial canthal ligament.[32] In this paper he described a deep head of the preseptal orbicularis muscle, which has subsequently been referred to as Jones' muscle by Edelstein[22] and other authors.

Edelstein also postulated that the deep attachments of the orbicularis muscle provide the major positional support for the eyelid medially and activate the lacrimal pump by generating negative pressure in the lacrimal sac during blinking. Edelstein's statement that 'The primary functional support for the medial eyelid is from the deep attachments of the orbicularis muscle to the posterior lacrimal crest and lacrimal diaphragm' is in contradiction to many earlier observations that the posterior component of the ligament is thin and insignificant.

Robinson & Stranc dissected the medial canthal ligament in six cadavers and found it to be a band of fibrous tissue, which acts as an insertion for the orbicularis oculi muscle to the medial orbit, into the lacrimal bone and the frontal process of the maxilla.[5] The most lateral parts of the medial canthal ligament act through the upper and lower palpebral extensions and they attach to the margins of the tarsal plates lateral to the caruncle. Medial to the caruncle the ligament bifurcates into superficial anterior and deep posterior limbs. They found the posterior limb difficult to define and suggested it consisted of lacrimal fascia, Horner's muscle and areolar tissue. They concluded that the posterior limb lacked strength because of its weak fibers and that the underlying bone is thin and incapable of providing solid anchorage.

In 1976 Warwick provided one of the most comprehensive descriptions of the medial canthal region.[1] In this he uses many of Wolff's dissections and histological preparations and discusses in detail the relationship of the ligament to the lacrimal system.

Anderson in 1977[33] demonstrated in a cadaveric study a superior branch of the medial canthal ligament that attaches to the periosteum of the frontal bone. He postulated that by attaching to the frontal bone, it gave additional support to the ligament in cases where the anterior limb was accidentally or surgically detached, e.g. dacrocystorhinostomy. This vertical component had been demonstrated before and labeled as the corrugator superciliaris muscle[34] and can be seen in the anatomical preparations by Jones[4] where it is labeled as the superficial and deep origins of the upper part of the orbital muscle. It is clear that it attaches to the anterior aspect of the ligament and lacrimal fascia just posterior to the angular vein and lateral to the procerus muscle. From these illustrations it can be seen that this muscle would lose its attachment to the medial canthal ligament when the anterior portion is resected and is therefore unlikely to be the sole reason for stability of the canthal ligament following disruption of the anterior limb.

Zide & McCarthy in 1983[19] dissected 12 medial canthi in fresh human cadavers under magnification. They found that the medial canthus attaches to the medial bony orbit in a tripartite manner. The vertical and horizontal components comprise two parts and the deep heads of the pretarsal and preseptal muscles arise from the posterior lacrimal crest as described by previous authors.[3,22,32] However, they empha-

size that the medial canthal ligament attaches far beyond the anterior lacrimal crest as depicted in most anatomical texts. This gives support to the empirical observation by Converse & Smith,[14,16] made before this tripartite arrangement was widely known, that the optimal position for surgical replacement of the medial canthal ligament was posterior and superior to the insertion.

Manson et al published an anatomical study of the region in 1986.[35] They substantiated the gross anatomical findings of the anterior limb described by previous authors. They further described the association of the posterior ligamentous attachments to the medial check ligament, the medial horn of the levator aponeurosis as described by Koorneef[36,37] and to Lockwood's ligament[38,39] as they insert with the orbital septum into the lacrimal bone.

Ayliffe discussed the importance of the three-dimensional arrangement of the muscles that attach to the medial canthal ligament.[6] He demonstrated the relative complexity of the posterior components of the structure, particularly the posterior insertion of the superior orbital part of the orbicularis oculi, a previously undescribed arrangement. Furthermore, he demonstrated the thickening of the periosteum of the medial orbital wall which acts to reinforce the triangular nature of the ligament in the third dimension. By broadening the base of the triangle in the horizontal plane, it serves not only to make the posterior attachment of the ligament strong but it also strengthens the whole structure. This observation emphasizes the importance of reconstructing the posterior attachment.

Our current understanding of the anatomy and relations of the medial canthal ligament is therefore one of a complex three-dimensional association between highly specialized structures.

Laterally the ligament is attached to the tarsus through a small strip or bands of fibrous tissue. The pretarsal orbicularis runs superficial and deep to the canaliculi at the lid margin and is referred to as Riolan's muscle.[34] The superficial fibers form the anterior crus of the medial canthal ligament and insert into the frontal process of the maxilla and anterior lacrimal crest. The posterior crus or deeper limb of the pretarsal orbicularis arises from the posterior lacrimal crest and lacrimal bone behind the lacrimal sac.

The preseptal muscle forms the horizontal raphe; it decussates to insert into both the anterior and posterior limbs of the medial canthal ligament, sometimes referred to as Jones' muscle and Horner's muscle respectively. The inferior part of the orbital orbicularis attaches medially to the lower border of the medial canthal ligament, the nasal part of the frontal bone and the medial orbital margin inferiorly.[34] The superior orbital orbicularis attaches to the medial canthal ligament, into the posterior lacrimal fascia[6] and into the upper half of the posterior lacrimal crest.[3] A discrete vertical muscular component is inserted into the cephalic aspect of the medial canthal ligament and anterior aspect of the lacrimal fascia; it attaches superiorly to the frontal bone.[19,33] This vertical stabilizing muscular element measures 1–2 mm thick and 5–7 mm long and lies just lateral to the angular vein. It is separated from the orbital part of the orbicularis by adipose tissue.

In the past the deeper reflected part of the ligament has been described as a thin fascial expansion[5,40] but it is now known to be a more substantial part of the ligament,[6,22,32] having a thickness of 1–3.3 mm.[5] It extends more posteriorly over the medial orbital wall as a thickening of the orbital periosteum.[6] It is important for maintaining the medial aspect of the palpebral fissure in proximity to the globe and thus its position is significant to lacrimal drainage.[22] The deep crus is a strong component of the ligament and the reason why a posterior and superior position has been advocated when reattaching or reconstructing the ligament.[14,16] Behind the sac the ligament attaches to the lacrimal fascia and the posterior lacrimal crest. The superior orbicularis muscle makes part of its insertion into the ligament and also the posterior lacrimal fascia at this point. It runs posterosuperiorly behind the sac and behind the posterior aspect of the medial third of the superior canaliculus.

Behind the orbicularis lies the orbital septum and the check ligament of the medial rectus. The inferior oblique arises from the floor of the orbit just lateral to the lacrimal fossa. A few fibers often take origin from the lacrimal fascia and the posterior lacrimal crest. Lockwood's ligament is a fascial sling and an important component of the global support mechanism; it extends from the zygomatic bone in around the lateral canthus and the lateral check ligament. It inserts into the inferior border of the medial canthal ligament with the medial check ligament[35] and also inserts into the lacrimal bone at the posterior lacrimal crest.

The medial canthal ligament is a complex and strong, interlocking three-dimensional arrangement of many individual components and structures. The skin over the lateral nose and eyelids is unique to this site, both in its structure and in the relationship it has to the underlying structures. The lacrimal drainage apparatus is intimately related to the ligament. The insertions of the many individual muscular components into the frontal process of the maxilla, the lacrimal bone and their attachments and relationships to the ligament are extremely complex. Lockwood's suspensory ligament and the orbital and capsulopalpebral fascia are important structures for support of the globe and are intimately related to the medial canthal ligament. All the individual structures affect the overall integrity of the ligament. The complex three-dimensional interlocking triangular arrangement of the muscular and ligamentous components described by Ayliffe[6] gives the structure its strength. It is therefore not appropriate to dismiss any individual component as unimportant. Each individual component should be considered when dealing with the pathology and reconstruction of this region.

Treatment

This should only begin when the surgeon has a clear understanding of the injuries and has a clear plan and objective. This plan must of course involve integrating surgery for the nasoethmoid fracture with any other facial injuries. A clear plan and objective can only follow a careful clinical and radiological examination. Since these fractures are often part of panfacial fractures, the more peripheral facial injuries will be treated first.

A classification of nasoethmoid injuries can be helpful in executing a coherent plan. A useful practical classification has been published by Ayliffe.

- *Type I*: en bloc minimal displaced fracture of the entire nasoethmoid complex (Fig. 12.14)
- *Type II*: en bloc displaced fracture, usually associated with large pneumatized sinus and minimal fragmentation (Fig. 12.15)
- *Type III*: comminuted fracture but canthal ligaments firmly attached with bone fragments which are big enough to plate (Fig. 12.16)
- *Type IV*: comminuted fracture with free canthal ligaments not large enough to capture by bone plating (Fig. 12.17)

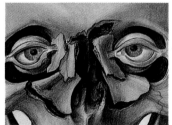
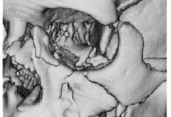

Fig. 12.14: Bone plating, Type I fracture.

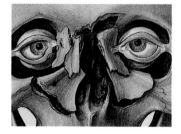
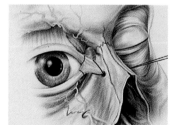

Fig. 12.16: Canthopexy, Type III fracture.

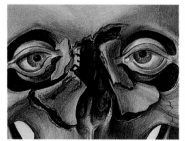
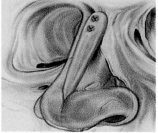

Fig. 12.15: Bone grafting, Type II fracture.

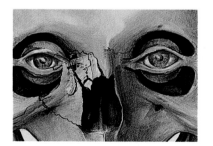
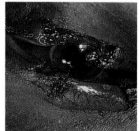

Fig. 12.17: Lacrimal repair, Type IV fracture.

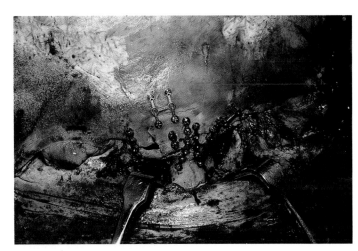

Fig. 12.18: Microplates placed via a coronal incision provide good reduction and stability.

- *Type V*: gross comminution needing bone grafting (Fig. 12.18)

The introduction of mini and micro bone plates has revolutionized the treatment of these injuries. The principal benefit is the ability of the bone plate to provide 3D stability to the fractures and maintain the projection of the nose.

The aims of treatment should be to restore normal anatomy and physiological function, particularly with respect to a patent functioning lacrimal system, and prevention of complications due to involvement of the frontal sinus and nasolacrimal duct. Symmetrical fixation of the bones, restoration of orbital volume, globe position, frontonasal angle and nasal projection are essential for a satisfactory cosmetic outcome. Stable symmetrical fixation of the canthus in three dimensions with good apposition of the eyelids against the ocular globe and a nice cosmetic curve to the medial canthal angle are all essential for a satisfactory esthetic and functional result.

Sequencing surgical treatment

1. Access and exposure.
2. Reconstruction of the cranial base, frontal bandau, outer orbital frame and management of the frontal sinus and decompression of the optic canal if necessary.
3. Frontonasal buttress and orbital rim. Usually these fragments are easy to locate and reduce.
4. The nasal dorsum should be reconstructed and nasal projection restored either, ideally, by plating the bone fragments or using grafts that can be cantilevered from the glabella with miniplates. It is important to contour the frontonasal angle.
5. Medial orbits. When the nasoethmoid complex is disrupted in a patient with panfacial trauma, the projection of the face will be correct if surgical treatment is sequenced correctly. Following reconstruction of the mandible, zygomas, frontonasal buttress and maxilla and location of the correct occlusion, the outer orbital frame will be correct and it is

only at this stage that the true nature and size of the medial orbital defect can be accurately assessed and reconstructed.
6. Medial canthal ligament.
7. Lacrimal system.
8. Closure and drain.
9. Consider secondary external support of the medial canthal ligament.
10. Nasal plaster.
11. Dressings and antibiotic eyedrops.

Hard tissues

The principle is simple: reduce and stabilize the fractured fragments to stable normal bone.[41] In practice, there is a significant difference between achieving this in a simple non-comminuted, minimally displaced fracture compared to a grossly compound comminuted 'bag of bones' fracture.

There is, however, little doubt that the best results are achieved with any fracture using the following principles.

1. Prompt treatment aids good reduction and reduces complications.
2. Good surgical exposure, either through existing lacerations or via a coronal flap or both.
3. Reduce and stabilize bone fragments using small, low-profile osteosynthesis plates.
4. Bone grafting immediately may be indicated if there is gross comminution of key bone buttresses or the orbital walls.

Surgical exposure and access

The aims of the surgical exposure should be to explore the injuries in order to diagnose the nature of the injuries, expose all fracture sites, preserve all bone fragments, give access to reconstruct the area and not compromise function or esthetics. Excessive subperiosteal dissection, especially in children, may lead to subperiosteal new bone formation in the postoperative period. In the canthal area this can cause blunting of the canthal angle and the appearance of pseudo-telecanthus. No individual approach fulfills all these criteria. The use of an existing laceration is obvious, but as this may cause contamination it is not without its complications. Under these circumstances surgery should be carried out as soon as the patient is fit for anesthesia.

There are few skin incisions around the nose and forehead that are satisfactory. This is in marked contrast to the excellent cosmetic results and wide access produced by the coronal flap.[42] The coronal approach has the advantage of providing access to harvest outer calvarial bone for primary reconstruction of bony deformities. Even with this flap care must be taken to place it well into the hair line or as posteriorly as possible in male patients to avoid exposure of the scar should recession of the hair line occur incisions at the hair line leave unsatisfactory scars, particularly as the hair thins. A simple strip shave or no shave is required to make this incision. A full head shave is not indicated or justified.

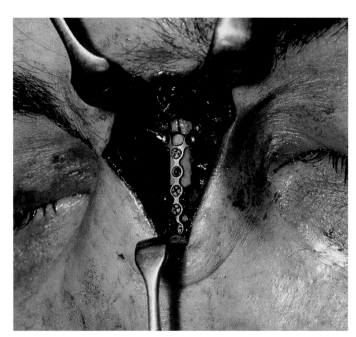

Fig. 12.19: Bone grafting and microplate stabilization of a bone graft needed as there was gross comminution. The access is through an existing laceration.

Reduction and stabilization

Microplates will stabilize very small fragments and provide good three-dimensional stability. Particular care must be taken to identify and stabilize any bone fragments which have the canthi attached without stripping the medial canthal ligament from them. In cases of gross comminution or in patients who have a midline split of the nose it may be helpful to place a plate over the bridge of the nose horizontally, to pull the fragments into a good sharp narrow arch (Fig. 12.19).

Bone grafting

This is infrequently required but in cases of gross comminution, particularly of structurally important bones, an immediate bone graft is indicated. It is critically important to make sure that both onlay grafts and any plates that are used to correct comminution of the nasal dorsum are contoured to reconstruct the frontonasal angle (Fig. 12.20, 12.21).

If bone grafting is to be delayed the soft tissues may contract down, making later secondary grafting difficult and possibly leading to erosion through the tight skin. Unfortunately these grossly comminuted fractures are often compound, making a less than ideal environment for immediate grafting.

Soft tissues

As with any soft tissue injury, treatment consists of:

- examination
- debridement
- management of specialized structures
- closure, drainage and dressings
- postoperative care.

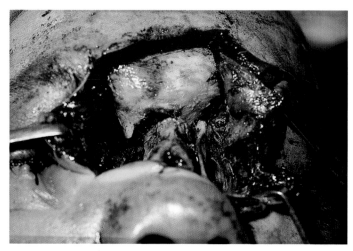

(a)

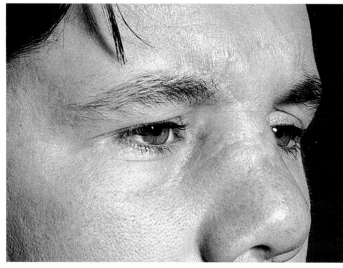

(b)

Fig. 12.20: (a) Late treatment was undertaken with a bone graft. **(b)** The final result is poor and scarring can be seen on the dorsum of the nose caused by some skin breakdown over the bone graft. This case illustrates the problems of late secondary treatment.

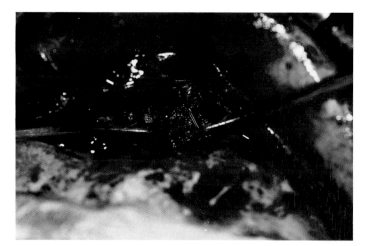

Fig. 12.21: The canthal ligament is attached to a small fragment of bone. The modern microplates allow even these small fragments to be reduced and stabilized, avoiding much less successful treatments, like wire canthopexy.

The lacrimal drainage system

Pure soft tissue damage to the lids may result in lacrimal system damage, particularly shearing injuries to the eyelids medial to the lacrimal puncta that may transect the canaliculi. Undoubtedly lacrimal damage is underdiagnosed in nasoethmoid trauma with between 3% and 18% of patients subsequently requiring dacrocystorhinostomies. Careful exploration and suture is required at the time of initial repair. The vulnerable parts in lid lacerations are the canaliculi, particularly the short medial segment lying between the medial canthi before it enters the sac, as the lid margin is particularly vulnerable in this site. Careful approximation of the severed ends of the canaliculi should be performed and then the duct should be cannulated with fine-bore polyethylene or silicone tubes through the puncta along the length of the canaliculus into the lacrimal sac to prevent stenosis. Careful identification of both ends of the canaliculus is obviously essential for this. The use of pigtail probes should be avoided in unicanalicular injuries as this can damage the normal canaliculus. Repair of the canaliculus may be carried out secondarily together with a dacrocystorhinostomy if necessary but scar tissue and technical difficulties make this a difficult endeavor. The evidence suggests that primary repair leads to better results.

The whole lacrimal system including the intra-bony lacrimal sac and duct are at risk in displaced nasoethmoid fractures. In patients with bicanalicular lesions and gross disruption of the region, intubation of both puncta can be carried out and the soft silicone tubes should be left in situ for at least 6 months.

The detached medial canthus

In trauma to the nasoethmoid area, care must be taken to diagnose any damage to the canthi and lacrimal system as mentioned above.

The nature of the reconstructive problem depends on the type of lesion. If the canthus is attached to a small fragment of bone this should be identified. With modern microplates it is possible to fix the bone fragment in its normal anatomical position and this usually gives excellent and stable results provided the fixation is solid enough.

The ligament is usually attached to a fragment of bone (see Fig. 12.21). The canthi can on rare occasions be detached or avulsed from the bone and this presents a difficult problem. Complete detachment is unusual in the absence of damage to the underlying bone or in the absence of penetrating injuries. One cause of complete detachment is careless surgical exploration and this should be guarded against as subsequent identification and reattachment may be difficult and lead to disappointing results.

When the ligament is detached from the bone it can be located lateral to the lacrimal sac by passing a needle through the canthal angle and identifying the needle on the deep surface posterior to the lacrimal sac. Once located, a fine wire suture is passed through the surface of the canthal ligament deep to the lacrimal canaliculi and sac. This wire is either passed transnasally[12] to the opposing canthus if this is attached, or through a bony point on the other side of the nose. The wire is directed so as to pull the ligament medially and posteriorly. The use of tendon anchor screws can be considered provided there is a large enough fragment of bone of sufficient strength in the appropriate position to fix the screw. In the author's experience this leads to a rather sharp medial canthal angle; however, this technique does have the advantage of making a posterior attachment easy to attain and good positioning of the lid margin against the globe of the eye can be achieved. It also has the advantage of minimum subperiosteal dissection. The technique of transnasal canthopexy is easily described but those experienced in the procedure recognize its shortcomings.

Following 'capture' of the canthus it may be possible to reduce and fix it directly to plates placed on the anterior and posterior lacrimal crests. Direct canthopexy does give stable results but it is important to position the attachment posteriorly enough to maintain the medial eyelid in close approximation to the globe and to restore a normal lacus. Failure to do this may lead to problems with lacrimal drainage and recurrent inflammation. Direct canthopexy may involve extensive subperiosteal stripping in order to attach the canthopexy plates.

In true detachment it is difficult to 'hold' the canthus. The fine wire very easily cuts through the delicate ligament, especially if edema puts any significant pressure on the repair or if the treatment is delayed and undue strain is applied when tightening the wire. For this reason it may be helpful to support the canthal reattachment from the cutaneous surface. This can be carried out using a preformed clear acrylic button (Fig. 12.22). The risk of this procedure is skin necrosis, but with clear acrylic the status of the skin can be monitored.

Pediatric Considerations

In children the paranasal air sinuses may not be fully developed and therefore direct blows to the nasoethmoid region tend to concentrate the energy in the area of the primary force. This tends to cause gross comminution and collapse of the nasoethmoid region.

Before the frontal sinus has developed the dissemination of energy through the cranial base will differ and the consequent fracture pattern does not follow that of adults. Often the nasoethmoid fragment may be disrupted in continuity with the frontal bone, either in its entirety (Fig. 12.23) or on a fragment that extends superiorly. In these cases the nasoethmoid component will be rotated in the direction of the frontal bone. The whole complex needs to be fully exposed via a coronal approach when the nature of the distortion can be accurately diagnosed. It is often not possible to relocate the fragment in its correct anatomical position as a small discrepancy in the frontal bone will be magnified in the nasoethmoid region and distal nose. There is a risk of leaving the nasoethmoid fragment angled incorrectly. A better approach in these cases may be to formally osteotomize the nasoethmoid fragment from the frontal bone at the frontonasal suture and relocate and fix it formally following relocation of the frontal bandau, taking care to maintain the frontonasal angle, nasal projection and symmetry.

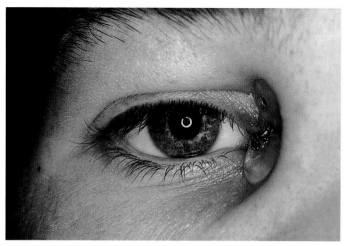

(a)

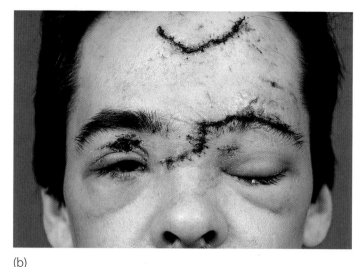

(b)

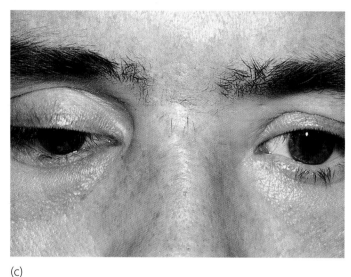

(c)

Fig. 12.22: (a) The clear acrylic button 'supports' the wire canthopexy and is not a substitute for wiring if there is no bone to plate. Without these buttons the wires will frequently cut through the canthus. **(b)** Preoperative appearance, again a late presentation. **(c)** Postoperative appearance showing a satisfactory result is possible even in late presentations. The enophthalmus is due to a prosthetic globe.

During direct canthopexy extensive subperiosteal stripping, in children particularly, may cause to the deposition of subperiosteal new bone, leading to blunting of the canthal angle. It is useful in children to give secondary external support to the reconstruction not only to prevent canthal drift but also the acrylic buttons approximate the soft tissues and help to prevent subperiosteal new bone deposition.

Outcomes

There are few good reviews comparing different methods of repair.

Anosmia is a severely debilitating sequela of nasoethmoid trauma and can be a result of fractures where there is gross comminution of the cranial base or severe posterior displacement of the nasoethmoid complex causing shearing of the olfactory system. Inappropriate removal of bone fragments or aggressive dissection in order to repair dural tears at the time of reconstruction can cause postoperative anosmia.

Late drift of the canthus can occur if the canthal-bearing bone fragment is not fixed properly or if the ligament is not captured or attached to the bone adequately in cases of complete detachment. Subperiosteal new bone formation is a problem in cases where it is necessary to strip the periosteum widely in order to fix the bony fragments; it is a particular problem in younger patients.

Lacerations that occur as a result of the initial trauma will cause scarring. Sometimes these lacerations can be used to give access to the fractures but they rarely provide access to the whole complex and rarely allow for the complete management of the injury. The use of lacerations in isolation usually leads to compromises in the surgical treatment of nasoethmoid fractures and to disappointing results. There are few surgical incisions in the local area that give direct access to the more usual nasoethmoid fractures and they usually lead to conspicuous scars. Delayed surgery allows scarring to develop, impeding reduction of the fractures.

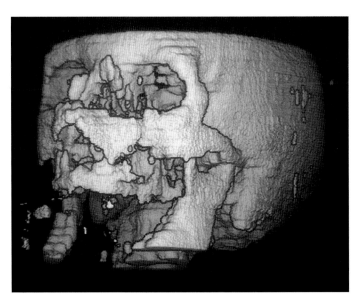

Fig. 12.23: The CT scan shows extensive involvement of the frontal sinus.

Controversies

Two main areas exist: timing and reduction.

Timing

There is no doubt that operation on an established, partly healed fracture rarely produces a good result. The main problem is difficulty in mobilizing the soft tissue and identifying soft tissue structures like the canthal ligament and lacrimal drainage system. Against this argument is the case for delay to allow the swelling to settle. This is an entirely valid argument since open reduction or, more relevant, the placement of incisions is less satisfactory in the presence of gross edema. Nerves may not be seen and incisions on the skin may turn out to be poorly placed once the swelling resolves.

Other systemic factors, in particular head injuries, may preclude early surgery. A frontal injury is much more likely to be associated with a head injury than a mandibular injury. Unfortunately there is not a uniform international approach by neurosurgeons to early intervention for non head injuries. In some units early intervention has been successfully undertaken, but in the majority of cases, neurosurgeons believe early intervention for non-life threatening conditions poses a greater risk than benefit for the patient. Each case is of course handled on its merits. In any event resolution of edema and systemic stability often follow the same timescale.

In effect, 'timing' is largely driven by events and not negotiable. However, this does not justify the long delays which can occur, often due to poor communications between surgical teams. These long delays push the patient into the poor outcome group outlined in the opening paragraph. Delays of up to 10 days will in most cases not significantly damage the final result.

Reduction

This is the argument for and against open reduction. Closed reduction is quick, avoids skin incisions and is thus superficially attractive. The argument against closed reduction, and this applies to the whole facial skeleton, is of course inadequate reduction and fixation, producing a poor functional and esthetic outcome.

Nowhere in the facial skeleton is this latter argument more true than in the nasoethmoid and orbital regions. These are both complex, three dimensional structures, made of fine bones. In the nasoethmoid region, closed reduction means the use of large lead plates placed over the complex to squeeze the bones into the 'correct' shape. The position can sometimes be improved by pulling the complex forward by running wires through the lead plates to pull them forward to an external fixator, like a halo. In the rare case of an intact nasoethmoid complex which has been displaced en bloc, results might be satisfactory. This is, however, a rare scenario and most leave a poor esthetic and functional outcome.

The argument about needing incisions on the face for proper open reduction is true. However, if well-placed coronal incisions are used most nasoethmoid incisions can be easily reduced and fixed with no other incisions. This does mean that the raising of this flap must be executed with care and thought. It must be placed high, especially in males, are minimum damage must be done to hair follicles. Most importantly, sensory and motor nerves must be seen, isolated and not damaged.

In summary, avoiding long delays of over 10 days and open reduction and fixation are well-established approaches, which should be adopted.

References

1 Warwick R 1976 Chapter 2. In: Eugene Wolff's anatomy of the eye and orbit, 7th edn. WB Saunders, Philadelphia, pp 182–237

2 Jakobiec FA 1982 Ocular anatomy and teratology. Harper & Row, Philadelphia, pp 677–731

3 Wolff E 1954 The anatomy of the eye and orbit, 4th edn. Blakiston, Philadelphia

4 Jones LT 1961 An anatomical approach to problems of the eyelids and lacrimal apparatus. Archives of Ophthalmology 66: 111–124

5 Robinson MD, Stranc MF 1970 The anatomy of the medial canthal ligament. British Journal of Plastic Surgery 23: 1–7

6 Ayliffe PR 2002 The anatomy of the medial canthal ligament. British Journal of Oral and Maxillofacial Surgery (in press)

7 Horner WE 1822 A description of a muscle connected with the eye lately discovered by W. E. Horner, M.D., one of the Professors of Anatomy in Philadelphia. London Medical Report and Review 18: 32–33

8 Reifler DM 1996 Early descriptions of Horner's muscle and the lacrimal pump. Survey of Ophthalmology Vol 41(2): 127–134

9 Schobinger JC 1756 Dissertatio medico-chirurgica de fistula lacrimali. Quam pro doctoratu consenquendo defendet. In: Haller A (ed) Disputiones physico-medico anatomico-chiurgicae selectae, vol 1, pp 195–212

10 Schobinger JC 1757 Sur la fistule lachrymale (abridged translation by Macquart HJ). In: Haller A (ed) Collection de theses medico-chirurgicales, sur les points les plus importans de la chirurgie theorique et pratique, vol 4. Vincent, Paris, pp 240–262

11 Duvernay JFM, Gautier d'Agoty J-F 1745 Essai d'anatomie, en tableaux imprimes, qui representent au naturel tous les muscles de la face, de col, de la tete, de la langue, it du larinx. Chez Gautier, Paris

12 Freihofer HPM 1980 Experience with transnasal canthopexy. Journal of Maxillofacial Surgery 8: 119–124

13 Callahan A 1962 Secondary reattachment of the medial canthal ligament. In: Scheie HG (ed) Surgical techniques. University of Pennsylvania Hospital, Philadelphia, pp 240–241

14 Converse JM, Smith B 1966 Naso-orbital fractures and traumatic deformities of the medial canthal region. Plastic and Reconstructive Surgery 38: 147–162

15 Bostwick J, Jurkiewicz MJ 1976 Functional anatomy of the eyelids as related to reconstruction. American Surgeon 42: 696–700

16 Converse JM, Smith B, Wood-Smith D 1977 Malunited fractures of the orbit. In: Converse JM (ed) Reconstructive plastic surgery. WB Saunders, Philadelphia , p 1016

17 Munro IR, Das JK 1979 Improving results in orbital hypertelorism correction. Annals of Plastic Surgery 2: 499–507

18 Bass CB 1979 Medial canthal ligament reconstruction. Annals of Plastic Surgery 3(2): 182–185

19 Zide BM, McCarthy JG 1983 The medial canthus Revisited – an anatomical basis for canthopexy. Annals of Plastic Surgery 11(1): 1–9

20 Callahan A, Callahan MA 1983 Fixation of the medial canthal structures: evolution of the best method. Annals of Plastic Surgery 11: 242–245

21 Rodriguez RL, Zide BM 1988 Reconstruction of the medial canthus. Clinics in Plastic Surgery 15(2): 255–262

22 Edelstein JP, Dryden RM 1990 Medial palpebral tendon repair for medial ectropion of the lower eyelid. Ophthalmic Plastic and Reconstructive Surgery 6(1): 28–37

23 Markowitz BL, Manson PN, Sargent L CA et al WA 1991 Management of the medial canthal tendon in nasoethmoid-orbital fractures: the importance of the central fragment in classification and treatment. Plastic and Reconstructive Surgery 87: 843–853

24 Dagum BD, Antonyshyn O, Hearn T 1995 Medial canthopexy: an experimental and biomechanical study. Annals of Plastic Surgery 35(3): 262–265

25 Duke-Elder WS 1938 Textbook of ophthalmology, vol 1. Mosby, St Louis

26 Duke-Elder WS, Wybar KC 1961 The anatomy of the visual system. In: Duke-Elder WS (ed) System of ophthalmology, vol 2. Mosby, St Louis

27 Jones LT 1956 Epiphora: its relation to the anatomic structures and surgery of the medial canthal region. Transactions of the Pacific Coast Ophthalmology Society 37: 31

28 Jones LT 1963 The anatomy and physiology of the ocular appendages. In: Reeh MJ (ed) Treatment of lid and epibulbar tumors. Charles C Thomas, Springfield, pp 16–21

29 Jones LT 1964 The anatomy of the upper eyelid and its relation to ptosis surgery. American Journal of Ophthalmology 57: 943– 959

30 Jones LT 1970 New anatomical concepts of the ocular adnexa. In: Mustardé JC, Jones LT, Callahan A (eds) Ophthalmic plastic surgery up-to-date. Birmingham, Ala, Aesculapius Publishing, Birmingham, Alabama, pp 3–6

31 Jones LT, Reeh MJ, Wirttschafter JD 1970 Ophthalmic anatomy. American Academy of Ophthalmology and Otolaryngology, Rochester, pp 39–48

32 Jones LT 1976 New concepts of orbital anatomy. In: Tessier P, Callahan A, Mustardé JC et al (eds) Symposium on plastic surgery in the orbital region. Mosby, St Louis p 11

33 Anderson RL 1977 Medial canthal tendon branches out. Archives of Ophthalmology 95: 2051–2052

34 Bergin DJ 1987 Anatomy of the eyelids, lacrimal system and orbit. In: McCord C, Tanenbaum M (eds) Oculoplastic surgery, 2nd edn. Raven Press, New York, p 41–71

35 Manson PN, Clifford CM, Su CT, Illiff NT, Morga R 1986 Mechanisms of global support and posttraumatic enophthalmos: I. The anatomy of the ligament sling and its relation to intramuscular cone orbital fat. Plastic and Reconstructive Surgery 77(2): 193–202

36 Koorneef L 1981 Sectional anatomy of the orbit. Aeolus Press, Amsterdam, pp 1–29

37 Koorneef L 1987 Spatial aspects of the orbital musculo-fibrous tissue in man. Swets and Zeitlinger, Amsterdam

38 Lockwood CB 1886 The anatomy of the muscles, ligaments, and fascia of the orbit, including an account of the capsule of Tenon, the check ligaments of the recti, and of the suspensory ligament of the eye. Journal of Anatomy and Physiology 20: 1

39 Whitnall SE 1932 Anatomy of the human orbit and accessory organs of vision, 2nd edn. Oxford University Press, London, p 152

40 Leipziger LS, Manson PN 1992 Nasoethmoid orbital fractures. Clinics in Plastic Surgery 19(1): 167–193

41 Champy M, Lodde AW, Wilk A, Grasset D 1978 Plate osteosynthesis in midface fractures and osteotomies. Deutsche Zeitschrift fur Mund, Kiefer und Gesichtschirurgie 8(2): 26–36

42 Sheperd DE, Ward Booth P, Moos KF 1985 The morbidity of bicoronal flaps in maxillofacial surgery. British Journal of Oral and Maxillofacial Surgery 23(1): 1–8

13 Nasal Fractures

Barry L Eppley

Introduction

The nose is the most prominent feature of the face and has little protection or support. It is the most easily fractured of the facial bones[1] and not surprisingly, the most commonly fractured.[2] Fractures occur twice as often in men as in women and are often the result of automotive accidents, interpersonal violence or sporting injuries. One report indicates that over one-third of all nasal fractures are associated with alcohol use.[2]

Despite a relatively low incidence of facial fractures in children, it is estimated that 25% of all nasal fractures occur in patients less than 12 years old.[3] Fractures can occur in newborns due to malposition in utero and during birth, in infants and toddlers as a result of bumps and falls as they begin to crawl and then walk, and in children and teenagers as they participate in competitive sports. Because the child's nose is more cartilaginous than bony, fractures can be difficult to diagnose and frequently the fractures go undiagnosed until a deformity subsequently develops.

Repair of nasal fractures is considered to be a relatively simple procedure[4] but it is associated with relatively high revision rates.[5,6] Results of inappropriate treatment include cosmetic external deformity, internal nasal airway obstruction with resultant snoring and sinusitis. In children, delayed or abnormal growth of the nose and midface can occur and, more rarely, disturbance of the dentition.

Classification

The type of nasal injury sustained is dependent upon the age of the patient and the direction and intensity of the forces applied. Most nasal fractures in adults result from a lateral blunt force. Typically, both the nasal bone and the frontal process of the maxilla are involved unilaterally (Fig. 13.1a). With greater force, bilateral displacement of the nasal bones is seen. As the nasal bones increase in thickness from their inferior aspect upwards towards the junction with the frontal process, most nasal fractures occur in the midsection below the thicker portion, with the base of the nasal pyramid remaining in situ. Frontal rather than lateral blows result in posterior displacement or impaction of the nasal bones. The fracture line is again located along the midsection (Fig. 13.1b). More severe force causes disruption at the frontonasal suture and as the impact force increases nasal, orbital and ethmoidal fractures occur in combination. In children, the relatively large amount of cartilage and open suture lines predispose to an open book-type fracture which results in a

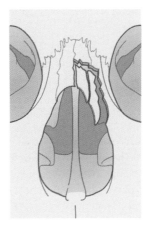
(a)

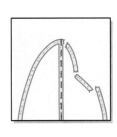

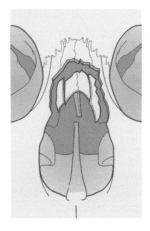
(b)

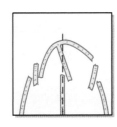

Fig. 13.1: Nasal bone fracture patterns. **(a)** Simple unilateral (type I). **(b)** Comminuted bilateral (type III).

flattened appearance to the nose (Fig. 13.1c). The bony component of these fractures is classified as type I (simple unilateral), type II (simple bilateral) and type III (comminuted, unilateral, bilateral or frontal).[5]

The septal component, the most important but often undiagnosed feature, requires accurate reduction and alignment if secondary deformities are to be avoided.[7] The septum tends to follow the displacement of the nasal bone fractures and, conversely, the nasal bones tend to unite in the direction of the deviated septum. The extent of the septal injury determines the appropriate technique for septal correction.[5] Lateral force results in displacement of the septal

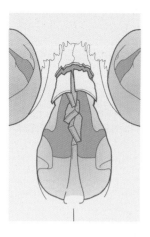
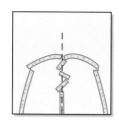

(c)

Fig. 13.1: (c) Open book (children).

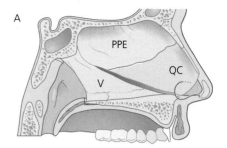
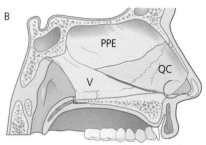

Fig. 13.2: Sagittal views of nasal septal fracture patterns. **(a)** Fracture and dislocation of the septum from the maxillary crest typically caused by low impact forces. **(b)** Vertical fractures through the quadrangular plate typically caused by higher impact, particularly frontal, forces. V = vomer, PPE = perpendicular plate of ethmoid, QC = quadrangular cartilage.

cartilage from the maxillary crest, producing a partial or complete obstruction on one side of the nasal cavity. The fracture dislocation usually occurs along the vomerine groove (Fig. 13.2a). Greater force, particularly associated with frontal impact, may extensively fracture the septum in a more vertical direction through the thin central region of the quadrangular cartilage, which extends between the perpendicular plate of the ethmoid above and the upper edge of the vomer below[5] (Figs 13.2b,c). Almost all septal fractures result in some telescoping of the cartilages, loss of vertical central support and widening of the base of the septum. The septal component of these fractures is classified as type IV (nasal bone and septal dislocation), which is subdivided into type IVa (associated with a septal hematoma) and type IVb (associated with an open nasal laceration).[5]

Assessment

Understanding the mechanism and direction of the forces involved should provide an accurate three-dimensional mental image of the disrupted nasal anatomy.

Examination includes a visual assessment of the nasal deviation, location of any lacerations, degree of swelling and bruising present. Palpation may reveal specific areas of tenderness, crepitus or a bony step. It is necessary to distinguish between simple nasal fractures and more complex facial fractures. Complex nasal fractures predominantly relate to the fracture extending into the nasoethmoid complex. Such fractures may be associated with much more serious complications, more difficult to treat and often accompanied by other injuries like head injuries. For example, once the nasoethmoid complex is fractured there may be detachment of the medial canthal ligament or fractures extending into the frontal sinus and/or cribriform plate. These more complex fractures require CT scanning and an open reduction. The intercanthal distance may be increased in severe injuries, indicating a more complex nasoethmoid injury.

An intranasal examination, to determine the status of the septum, should always be carried out under adequate lighting and using a nasal speculum. A septal hematoma requires

immediate evacuation. Decongesting the nose with a topical decongestive agent can be beneficial. A full endoscopic examination is advised for a complete assessment of the septum (particularly at the posteroinferior junction with the perpendicular plate of the ethmoid), turbinates and inferior meatuses. This may have to be delayed until the operating room. Airway patency is in part self-determined by the patient's own assessment of their breathing before and after injury.

Radiographic examination, although routinely performed, is often of questionable value.[8] Plain films are of little benefit (other than for medicolegal reasons) as they are rarely helpful in determining the need for surgery or the type of surgical intervention required (Fig. 13.3a). A CT scan provides better information, particularly of the position of the septum and patency of the airway, but is more costly and does not replace a good history and physical examination, particularly if an endoscopic assessment is performed (Fig. 13.3c).

Management

Not all nasal fractures require surgical manipulation. The main criteria for surgery are the obvious presence of a cosmetic deformity or a functional (breathing) impairment that is not due primarily to intranasal swelling (mucosal edema/bruising) or retained blood. If either exists, then surgery is justified and should be carried out as soon as the precise deformity is evident. The extent of the bony/cartilaginous deformity determines the appropriate treatment. Murray et al[9] have shown poor outcomes for the treatment of 'simple' nasal fractures and suggested a more aggressive treatment is indicated. In many cases with

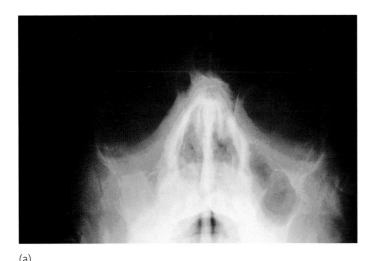

(a)

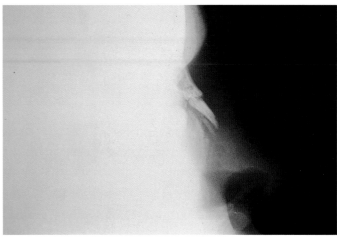

(b)

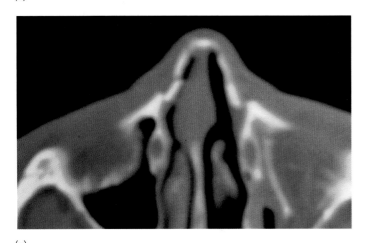

(c)

Fig. 13.3: Radiographic assessment of nasal fractures. **(a,b)** Plain radiographs are not only often misleading as to whether a nasal fracture exists but do not provide an assessment of the cartilaginous septum. **(c)** CT scans offer a much better view of nasal anatomy as can be seen in this depressed bilateral nasal bone fracture with a vertical septal fracture, dislocation and telescoping of the segments (axial view).

significant deviation of the septum (more than half the nostril width) small fractures occur in the septum close to the rigid support of the palatal groove. They have suggested a mini septoplasty be carried out acutely, to prevent late deformation of the septum at the fracture site.

Closed reduction

A general anesthetic greatly facilitates a successful closed reduction. Whilst local anesthesia alone is often used, to do so seems unduly punitive to the patient and probably limits the thoroughness of the technique.[10] The authors prefer to carry out the reduction under general anesthesia supplemented by 4% topical cocaine.

The nasal bones can usually be manually manipulated back into a midline position. If required, depressed nasal fragments can be elevated using the Boies (straight) elevator internally with digital manipulation externally (Fig. 13.4). Minor dislocations of the septum along the vomerine groove can be reduced with the same instrument. Walsham forceps may be required for severe impactions as a method of grasping the septum and lifting. When using Walshams to reposition the nasal bones compression or crushing of the skin should be avoided. Support for the nasal bones and septum is

usually provided by gel foam packing, which also aids hemostasis.

Following reduction, the nose is taped and splinted for one week. A small piece of Telfa is placed in the nasal vestibule overnight to absorb any drainage. Because of the well-documented reports of recurrent deviation following closed reduction, patients are followed closely for one year (Figs 13.5, 13.6).

Open reduction

Open reduction is reserved for those patients who have an unstable intraoperative result following closed reduction, have failed previous attempts at closed reduction or who have presented more than 4 weeks from the time of injury. The key to successful open reduction is management of the septum.[7] Persistent deviation of the septum is the most common cause of misalignment of the nasal bones.

The septum is approached through a hemitransfixion incision. A mucoperichondrial flap is usually elevated on one side of the septum only but both sides can be raised if necessary. The cartilage segments are repositioned, with resection only if it aids the repositioning of the remaining fragments. When the quadrangular cartilage is dislocated from the maxillary

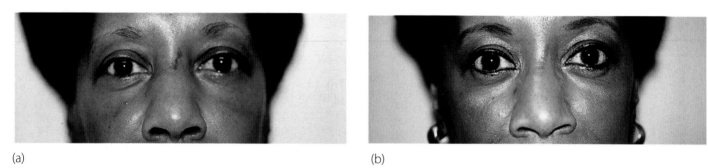

(a) (b)

Fig. 13.4: Technique of bimanual closed reduction of nasal fractures. **(a)** The straight elevator is used internally to push out or over the displaced nasal bone while the external fingers mold it into the proper position. **(b)** Septal relocation is done by pushing the septum over and evaluating with a speculum immediately thereafter.

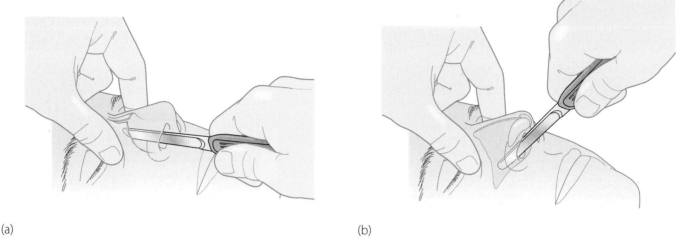

(a) (b)

Fig. 13.5: 52-year-old female who sustained a high frontal impact with a type II nasal fracture. **(a)** 1 week after injury. **(b)** 1 month after closed reduction.

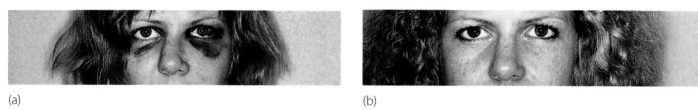

(a) (b)

Fig. 13.6: 30-year-old female with type III nasal fracture secondary to domestic violence. **(a)** 1 week after injury. **(b)** 3 months after closed reduction.

crest, removal of an inferior strip of cartilage may be necessary to permit reduction (Fig. 13.7a). In common with the traditional septoplasty, at least 1 cm of cartilage must be preserved along the caudal border and dorsum for adequate support (Fig. 13.7b). Bent cartilage may be crosshatched on the concave side to aid straightening. Caudal septal dislocations are fixed to the anterior nasal spine with a permanent figure-of-eight suture. In cases where the septum is fractured and unstable, an internal straight splint composed of resorbable polymers may be placed submucosally on one side of the septum and the overlying mucosa repositioned and adapted by sewing through it.[11] More commonly, the carti-

lage is secured into position and the mucosal flaps adapted with through-and-through sutures of 4/0 plain gut on a straight needle. If the mucosa is significantly torn, silastic splints are placed on each side and sewn into place for support (Fig. 13.8).

Open reduction of the nasal bones is usually carried out after the septal support is re-established through an intercartilaginous incision. Lateral and if necessary medial osteotomies are performed to facilitate the reduction of the fracture. Appropriate reduction of the bones usually corrects any deformities of the tip or supratip cartilages. The dressings and follow-up are as for closed reductions (Fig. 13.9).

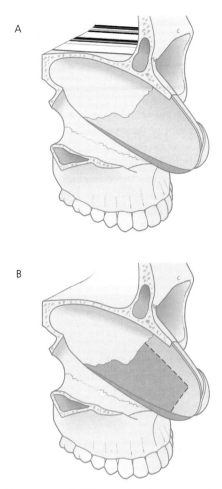

Fig. 13.7: Management of the septum in open reduction.
(a) Resection of inferior end of cartilaginous septum permits repositioning in the midline. **(b)** More extensive cartilage resection can be done if necessary (although not preferred) but 1 cm of dorsal and caudal support must be maintained.

The treatment of nasal fractures in children differs from that of adults. Unrecognized injuries can result in nasal and midface deformities later in life so accurate diagnosis and treatment remain important. Care must be taken to avoid damage to the growth centers. Since these fractures are often of the greenstick type, the use of closed reduction techniques

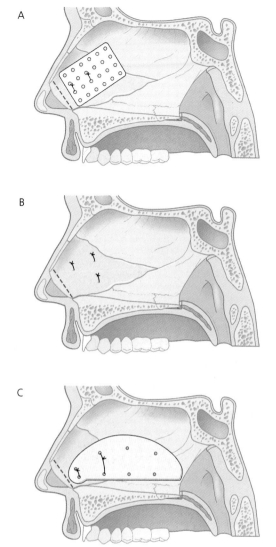

Fig. 13.8: Septal support techniques in open reductions.
a) An internal rigid splint composed of resorbable polymers can be placed directly against the cartilage and secured into position with external transmucosal sutures. **(b)** Through-and-through sutures coapt the mucosa to the septum as well as providing structural support. **(c)** When the external mucosa is severely torn, extramucosal internal silastic splints can be bilaterally placed and sutured into position.

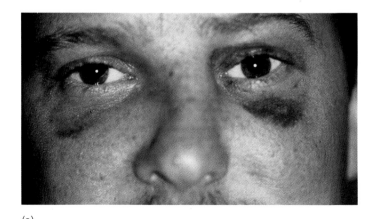

(a)

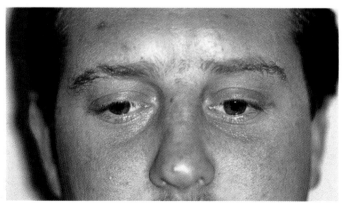

(b)

Fig. 13.9: 30-year-old male with nasal fracture treated with open reduction. **(a)** Preoperative. **(b)** 6 months postoperative result.

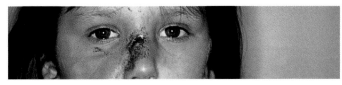

(a)

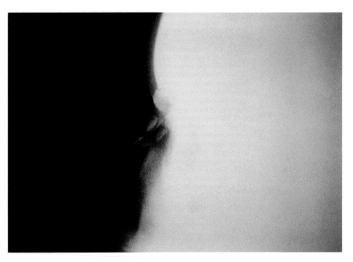

(b)

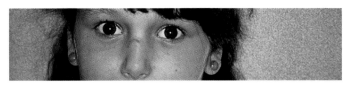

(c)

Fig. 13.10: 5-year-old female with nasal fracture secondary to bicycle accident. **(a)** Preoperative. **(b)** Preoperative plain radiographs. **(c)** 3 months postoperative result.

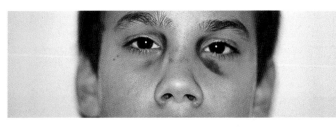

(a)

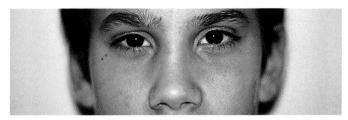

(b)

Fig. 13.11: 10-year-old male with nasal fracture secondary to sporting accident. **(a)** Preoperative. **(b)** 6 weeks postoperative after open reduction with no cartilage resection.

is effective in the majority of cases (Fig. 13.10). When required, open reduction is performed but without removal of bone or cartilage (Fig. 13.11).

Outcome

The treatment of the relatively 'simple' nasal fracture is perceived to be highly successful but close examination of postoperative results is often disappointing. The need for revision is historically high, ranging from 10% to 50% in reported series. Using the approaches described above, the need for revision in the more severe type III fractures should not exceed 10–20%. Results obtained for treatment of type I and II fractures should include no more than a 10% revision rate.[2,5]

Complications

Both closed and open reductions of nasal fractures are associated with few complications.

Epistaxis

Epistaxis can occur but is usually controlled with conservative measures including upright positioning, mild sedation and topical vasoconstrictive agents. Packing can dislocate the reduction and should only be used as a last resort.

Septal hematoma

Septal hematomas can occur at the time of injury or following reduction. Unrecognized septal hematomas can lead to necrosis of the cartilage and on occasion saddling of the middle third of the nose in severe cases. Immediate evacuation is always indicated as described above.

Infection

Infection is uncommon. Prophylactic antibiotics are routinely given although their benefit is often debated. A septal abscess requires drainage and further antibiotics. Osteitis of the nasal bones, which is very rare, requires bony debridement and intravenous antibiotics.

Synechiae

Synechiae can occur secondary to lacerations of the nasal mucosa. This problem can most often be treated under local anesthesia by incising the scar band and placing packing between the septum and the lateral nasal wall.

Conclusion

Nasal fractures are the most common facial bone injury. Despite perceptions that they are relatively easy to treat, revision due to secondary deformity is not uncommon. Careful assessment of the injury, an understanding of the underlying bony/cartilaginous deformity (including the important role of the septum), followed by appropriate treatment will lead to the best cosmetic and functional outcome.

References

1 Swearington JJ 1965 Tolerance of human face to crash impact. Federal Aviation Agency, Oklahoma City

2 Wang TD, Facer GW, Kern EB 1990 Nasal fractures. In: Gates GA (ed) Current therapy in otolaryngology: head and neck surgery, vol 4. BC Decker, Philadelphia, pp. 105–109

3 Goode RL, Spooner TR 1972 Management of nasal fractures in children. Clinical Pediatrics 11: 526

4 Verwoerd CDA 1992 Present day treatment of nasal fractures: closed versus open reduction. Facial Plastic Surgery 8: 220

5 Rohrich RJ, Adams Jr WP 2000 Nasal fracture management: minimizing secondary nasal deformities. Plastic and Reconstructive Surgery 106: 266

6 Murray JAM, Maran AGD 1980 The treatment of nasal injuries by manipulation. Journal of Laryngology and Otology 94: 1405

7 Gunter JP, Rohrich RJ 1988 Management of the deviated nose: the importance of septal reconstruction. Clinics in Plastic Surgery 15: 43

8 Logan M, O'Driscoll K, Masterson J 1994 The utility of nasal bone radiographs in nasal trauma. Clinical Radiology 49: 192

9 Murray JA, Maran AG, Busuttil A, Vaughan G 1986 A pathological classification of nasal fractures. Injury 17(5): 338–344

10 Cook JA, McRae DR, Irving RM, Dowie LN 1990 A randomized comparison of manipulation of the fractured nose under local anesthesia and general anesthesia. Clinical Otolaryngology 15: 343

11 Eppley BL 2000 The use of resorbable spacers for nasal spreader grafts (discussion). Plastic and Reconstructive Surgery 106: 922

14 Maxillary and Panfacial Fractures

Jeremy D McMahon, David A Koppel, M Devlin, Khursheed F Moos

Introduction

In 1968, Rowe & Killey,[1] in their second edition of a text on facial fractures, distilled the experience of a half century in the management of facial trauma. The lessons came primarily from an unforgiving teacher – the theater of war. Europe had been convulsed by two conflicts in which the warring sides employed weaponry of previously unimagined destructive power. The first of these wars was characterized by a conflict of attrition which laid waste much of a generation of the young men of Europe and her former colonies. Many sustained facial avulsive and ballistic injuries. In the Second World War civilian populations, as well as combatants, were subject to attack with high explosives and projectiles. What evolved out of this experience was a management protocol that was safe and provided resource-efficient treatment. The largely closed treatment techniques allowed a return to satisfactory function for most patients. Persistent deformity in many was accepted.

The last three decades, of relative peace and prosperity for much of the developed world, have seen major developments with advances in resuscitation techniques, imaging and other diagnostic tools, anesthesia and instrumentation. Concomitantly there has occurred an increase in the available resources to manage the, usually sporadic, trauma that occurs in peacetime. Patient expectations of outcome have also steadily risen. Innovative surgeons have exploited these changes in an attempt to achieve much improved results in facial form. A paradigm shift has occurred with the emphasis on wide exposure with precise reduction and fixation of fractured segments, the direct antecedent of this change being experience gained in the management of craniofacial deformity by wide exposure and osteotomy, with direct osteosynthesis of mobilized fragments.[2]

We believe there has been a steady improvement in outcome; however, validation of this belief with objective data has not been achieved. What has emerged is a treatment protocol, which aims to deliver excellent results but is resource expensive. As such, this treatment paradigm may not readily translate to the battlefield where mass casualties stretch resources to the point where only life-saving treatment can be given immediately. The techniques learnt in the preceding era must not be lost. It is regrettable but probable that they will be required again, in some form, by today's or tomorrow's generation of surgeons.

What follows in this chapter is largely a management protocol applicable to civilian peacetime practice, where considerable resources are available, and brought to bear on the management of relatively small numbers of individuals at any one time.

Classifaction of Midface Fractures and Outcomes

Le Fort's 1901 classic treatise, describing experimentally induced midfacial fracture patterns, has remained in use for a century and continues to have utility (Fig. 14.1). However, a

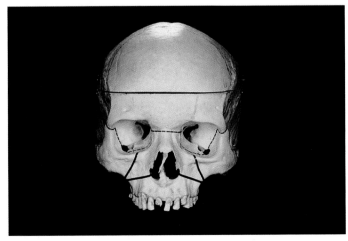

(a)

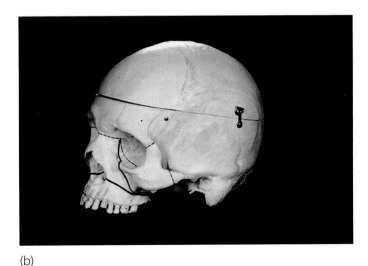

(b)

Fig. 14.1: (a,b) Le Fort's 1901 description of experimentally induced midfacial fractures. Le Fort I – black line, Le Fort II – red line, Le Fort III – green dashes.

satisfactory classification schema should accurately describe the major clinical features present and allow the stratification of patients presenting according to severity, for the purposes of measuring outcome. Le Fort's simple classification has important deficiencies in both respects. It fails to adequately account for fractures at multiple levels, asymmetric fracture patterns, separation of major fragments, comminution of vulnerable areas, as well as concurrent anterior cranial fossa and mandibular fractures.[3] All of these features have a bearing on management protocols and outcome.

A number of workers have made useful contributions in an attempt to provide more comprehensive classification systems for the mid and upper face. Developments in the 1980s incorporated, and recognized the significance of, sagittal palatal fractures,[4] naso-orbitoethmoid comminution[5] and involvement of the anterior cranial fossa.[6] In addition, varying degrees of zygomatic complex involvement have been classified, as have frontal injuries. These descriptions have the virtue of being clinically significant with classification of fractures of each of the major midfacial subunits facilitating communication between clinicians and the planning of surgical intervention. However, where several subunits are involved, it is descriptively cumbersome. For example, a patient with a frontal sinus fracture, naso-orbital ethmoid fracture with traumatic telecanthus, pyramidal maxillary fracture and displaced zygomatic complex would have a number of different classification labels applied. Applying distinct, perhaps overlapping, scoring systems to the various components of a complex facial injury has not, to our knowledge, been validated in the stratification of injury severity.

More recently, comprehensive scoring systems applicable to facial trauma have been described. Guerrissi devised a maxillofacial trauma scoring system which aims to identify patients with potentially life-threatening maxillofacial injuries, allowing appropriate triage as well as quantifying the severity of facial injuries for the purpose of stratification, according to functional and esthetic impact.[7] This scoring system has the disadvantage of being descriptive of both bony injuries and soft tissue injuries and is therefore subject to potential difficulties with interpretation. Furthermore, it has not, to our knowledge, been validated in a prospective study.

An alphanumeric scoring system has been devised by Cooter & David[3] and a prospective evaluation of this method has recently been reported. This instrument expresses the degree of facial disruption as a percentage. The authors claim it offers a detailed analysis of fracture pattern and accurately represents the severity of bony injuries. That contention is supported by the authors' published data. In 100 patients studied prospectively, both the maxillary fracture and total facial fracture scores demonstrated a strong correlation with complications/adverse sequelae. Whilst it is hardly surprising that greater degrees of facial disruption are associated with a greater likelihood of less favorable outcomes, the strong correlation coefficient suggests a useful objective stratification instrument. Accurate stratification of the severity of injury allows comparison of outcomes between centers and where variations exist in treatment methodology. Moreover, the pattern of adverse results observed in this study is revealing.

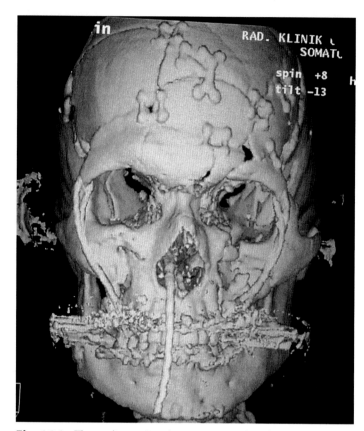

Fig. 14.2: Three-dimensional reconstructed CT following anterior cranial fossa repair and fixation of the midface with internal suspension wires and intermaxillary fixation as an interim measure. Note the substantial residual malposition of major midface fragments (courtesy R Schmelzeisen).

The majority of posttreatment problems were seen in the orbital region (20% of patients) and principally comprised enophthalmos, orbital dystopia and canthal deformities. Eight percent had occlusal abnormalities post treatment, 8% had nasal problems, while wound and implant-related problems occurred in 9%. The overall adverse sequelae rate was 36% in this group of patients who, in the majority, had sustained high-energy injuries. These data, from a major craniofacial surgical center, emphasize that residual deformity following treatment of midfacial trauma of more than moderate severity is commonplace.

A recent publication from two major North American centers also found worse outcomes with respect to physical problems, and also psychosocial well-being, in patients with severe midface injuries. Patients with severe midface disruption were compared to patients with less severe facial disruption and a second control group of patients, who had sustained injuries other than to the facial region.[8] Specifically excluded from all three groups were those with a severe brain injury, spinal cord injury, major burns or an extremity requiring amputation. Only 55% of those with more severe Le Fort type fractures returned to work compared with 70% of those with less severe midface fractures and the age- and sex-matched general injuries group. This study found a 23% incidence of persistent diplopia (minimum follow-up 18 months) following Le Fort type fractures. This figure is similar to the 20% incidence of diplopia after midface fracture in a sample of 363 patients managed in the West of Scotland.[9] In the former study 35% of patients reported epiphora and the prevalence of this problem increased with severity of facial injury. Difficulty with mastication was reported in 31% (trismus, malocclusion, pain, residual nerve injury). Subjectively reported altered smell and taste occurred in 35% and a third of patients reported persistent areas of facial numbness. This work emphasizes that the functional and psychosocial costs of midfacial injuries are high. Minimizing long-term disability requires early intervention of the highest standard and subsequent follow-up care which seeks to rectify remediable problems and provides appropriate referrals to other healthcare professionals when necessary.

Haug et al[10] also found that more superior levels of midfacial fracture resulted in a higher incidence of adverse sequelae. This study sought, retrospectively, to compare largely closed management of maxillary fractures with open reduction and internal fixation using complications/adverse sequelae rates as the outcome measure. No difference was observed and the authors concluded that '. . . given the advantage of airway protection, enhanced nutrition, and a more rapid return to pretraumatic functioning, open reduction with rigid internal fixation may be the preferred modality of treatment'. The lack of a demonstrable benefit from

techniques which employ wide exposure and direct fixation is disappointing and surprising. It is clear that less invasive management strategies leave substantial fragments malpositioned (Fig. 14.2) and it has been assumed that more precise reduction and fixation would lead to improved outcomes. There are two possible explanations. Either the method of outcome measurement was insufficiently sensitive to detect a difference or the extended exposure required to effect precise reduction and fixation of all fragments was associated with adverse effects, nullifying a potential benefit. These explanations are not mutually exclusive but it is our belief that the former is the most significant factor.

What we currently lack are objective methods which assess both functional and esthetic outcomes. Measuring complication rates and requirement for revisional surgery provides only limited information. Adverse outcomes vary from the trivial and transitory to the functionally and/or esthetically disabling. Thresholds for revision procedures vary widely between both patients and surgeons. Our lack of progress in developing good outcome measures can be explained. The diverse functions performed by the facial region (special senses, mastication, verbal and non-verbal communication, humidification) imply a diverse range of potential problems. Nevertheless, just as fracture configurations tend to follow certain patterns, so do adverse outcomes. Advances in measuring esthetically adverse results may emerge with the

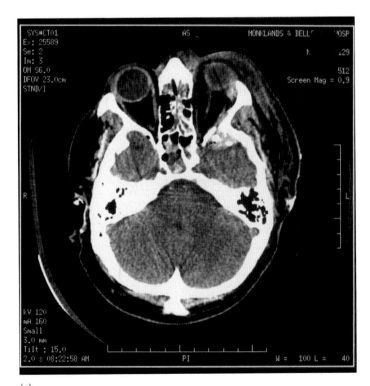

(a)

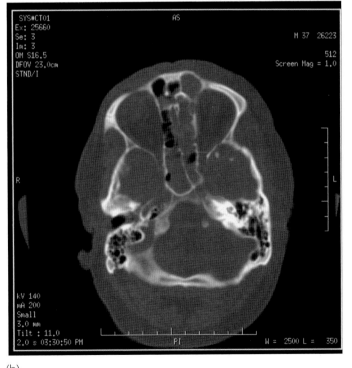

(b)

Fig. 14.3: (a,b) CT axial scans demonstrating craniofacial fractures involving the right lateral orbit extending to the orbital apex. There is a small associated extradural hemorrhage and a traumatic optic neuropathy was present. Neurosurgical intervention was not required. The traumatic optic neuropathy was managed with high-dose corticosteroids with subsequent improvement in visual acuity. Associated mandibular fractures were managed operatively. In this circumstance the displaced zygomatico-orbital complex was not treated as part of the primary management. Because of the risks associated with mobilization of the zygomatico-orbital complex this is one of the few circumstances where secondary delayed management with osteotomy and bone grafting is advocated. This case illustrates the importance of CT imaging in delineating the relationships of facial injuries to those which may be present in the skull base.

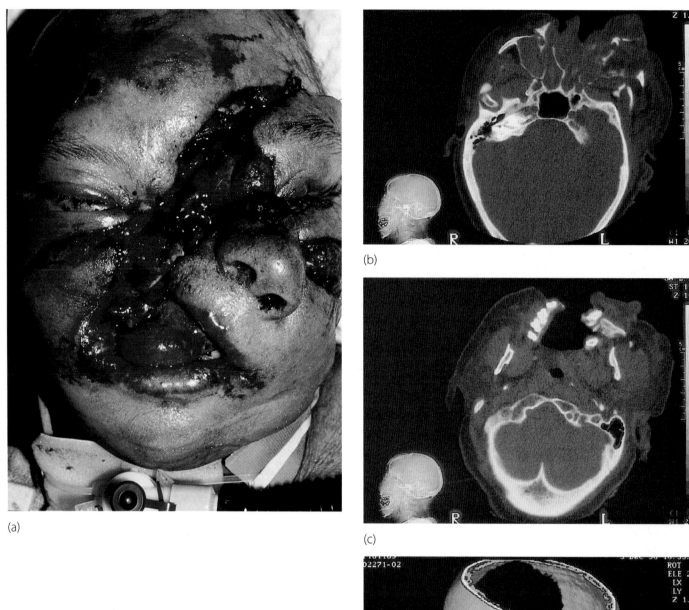

(a)

(b)

(c)

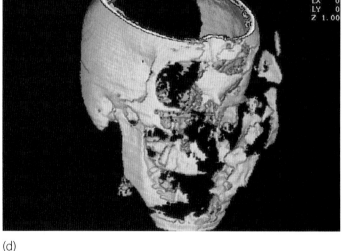

(d)

Fig. 14.4: (a) Severe panfacial injury. **(b,c)** Careful clinical examination and scrutiny of axial (and coronal where possible) CT images provides as much information as 3D reformatted images in most circumstances **(d)**.

advent of three-dimensional facial imaging modalities. Much of the perceived disfigurement following facial injury is a consequence of asymmetry, which should be quantifiable with digitization of facial form and the use of software algorithms. There are of course significant obstacles to the development of such a tool. All individuals have some degree of facial asymmetry and this cannot be controlled for. It seems probable that asymmetry in some facial subunits will have a disproportionate effect in producing perceived disfigurement.

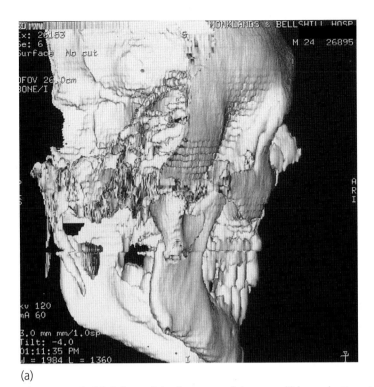 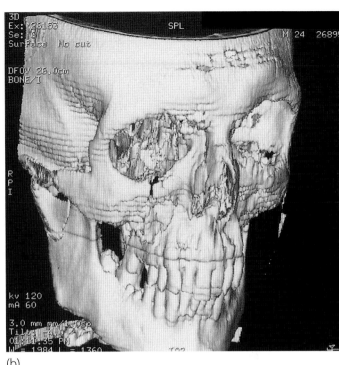

(a)   (b)

Fig. 14.5: (a,b) Subcondylar fractures of the mandible are better visualized in 3D reformatted images compared with axial scans.

Whether or not three-dimensional imaging generated data can be validated against professional and non-professional observer ratings of disfigurement/deformity only active research will tell. However, refinements in technique to produce improved outcomes demand that we look critically and carefully at results and further develop objective outcome measures despite the very substantial obstacles that exist.

Diagnosis

The diagnostic objectives in the patient presenting with panfacial and maxillary fractures are no different from those which apply to other injuries localized to the craniomaxillofacial region. However, the greater energy imparted in producing panfacial trauma implies a higher probability of associated injury, particular to the brain and cervical spine.

Diagnostic questions include the following.

1. Is there an actual or potential airway problem?
2. Is there ongoing hemorrhage?
3. What is the nature and likely outcome of any accompanying head injury?
4. Has a cervical spine injury been diagnosed or definitively excluded?
5. Is there an occult life-threatening injury not detected on primary and secondary survey, i.e. is further investigation and/or consultation required? A further comprehensive top-to-toe evaluation is a prudent measure in the 48-hour period following admission and prior to any subsequent major intervention.
6. What is the precise extent, location and nature of all injuries to the craniomaxillofacial region?

7. Are there non-life threatening injuries present which require management by other specialties?
8. Is there co-morbidity which will impact upon treatment and subsequent rehabilitation?

What follows is primarily a discussion of question 6, that is, the extent, location and nature of injuries to the facial region, but all the above issues require an answer in the planning of definitive management. Not only the necessity but also the urgency of liaison with additional specialties such as neurosurgery, ophthalmology, vascular surgery, interventional radiology and orthopedics requires careful consideration based on timely, detailed and repeated assessment. Early involvement of the required team(s) and good communication will minimize delays and optimize treatment.

The full assessment begins with a detailed history of the injury. This should be taken from the patient when possible and or eye witnesses, ambulance and other emergency team staff. The object of the detailed history taking is to clearly define the mechanism of injury and to gain an appreciation of the energy involved. This serves two main functions: first, to indicate the probable extent of the facial injuries and second, to highlight probable associated injuries. A past medical history is important with regard to any intervention but in the multiply injured patient it is often necessary to obtain this from relatives. In addition to this it may be helpful to obtain preinjury photographs and dental records of the patient to assist in the planning of surgery.

A detailed craniofacial examination should take place as soon as practicable following admission. All findings must be detailed and diagrams are very useful. Detailed inspection should identify lacerations, incised wounds, abrasions and contusions. These should all be inspected carefully with con-

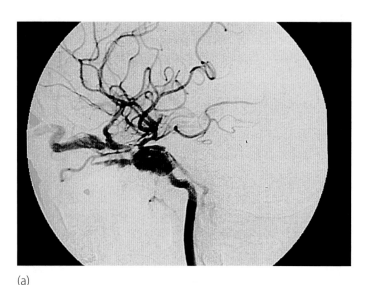

(a)

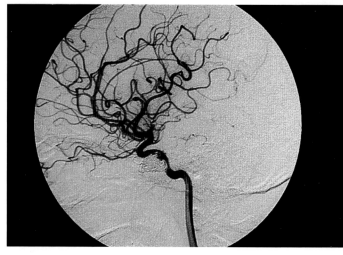

(b)

Fig. 14.6: (a,b) A traumatic carotico-cavernous fistula managed with embolization.

sideration given to underlying structures that may be damaged, particularly the seventh cranial nerve. During inspection consideration should be given to the possibility of a CSF leak. The bony structures should be palpated for contour, steps and mobility. The eyes should be examined in detail, including fundoscopy. However, dilatation of the pupils should only be carried out following discussion with the neurological service. The ears should be examined and blood behind the tympanic membrane, tympanic perforations and external auditory canal tears noted.

The history and clinical examination guide the use of further investigations. Plain radiographs taken under less than ideal circumstances are usually non-contributory. Furthermore, plain film images frequently fail to give sufficiently detailed information as to the nature and extent of skull base fractures, orbital wall injuries, pterygoid plate fractures and sagittal fractures of the maxilla and condylar process of the mandible. CT scanning is the major diagnostic investigation and both axial and coronal scans have a significant role. In the absence of coronal scans reconstructed scans are of use. We advocate the use of the computer workstation to view the images, particularly the multiplanar reconstructions, which allow a greater appreciation of the three-dimensional nature of the injuries than hard copies.

Interpretation of CT scans is first directed towards determining the presence, extent and location of skull base involvement as well as underlying brain parenchymal injury and intracranial hemorrhage. The axial images will reveal posterior wall of frontal sinus fractures. The cribriform plate region is often more clearly seen on the coronal images with the orbital roof region well visualized in both axial and coronal planes. Fractures detected in the anterior cranial fossa are often associated with dural tears that communicate with the upper airway. Subsequent meningitis is a short and longer term subsequent risk, although this is not well quantified. Anterior cranial fossa repair is frequently indicated with varying thresholds across neurosurgical units. Consultation is, however, always indicated in the presence of such injuries. The middle

cranial fossa scans are next scrutinized. Here we pay particular attention to the greater wing of sphenoid in the lateral orbit. Where fractures extend into the middle cranial fossa, mobilization/reduction of anterior zygomatico-orbital segments risks exacerbating/producing intracranial hemorrhage, dural tears and direct brain injury (Fig. 14.3). Fractures involving the orbital apex with potential involvement of the optic foramen are occasionally seen. In the presence of a traumatic optic neuropathy accompanying such injuries, high-dose steroids are recommended. Other workers perform optic nerve decompression procedures in addition.

Three-dimensional CT reconstructions do not currently have a large role to play in the assessment of facial injuries. The interpolation of data between images means that the true extent of injury is frequently underestimated. There is little information that cannot be obtained from a careful scrutiny of the axial and coronal images (Fig. 14.4). The only exception to this we have found is the particular case of the mandibular condyle where 3D images give a clearer indication of the level of fracture of the condylar process, and its orientation, than is readily appreciable from the planar images (Fig. 14.5).

Angiography is not often necessary but can be utilized both diagnostically and therapeutically. In cases of penetrating neck wounds injury to important vessels can occur and angiography should be considered. Interventional techniques are utilized when other measures to arrest hemorrhage have not been, or are not likely to be, successful (Fig. 14.6).

The utilization of evoked responses, particularly to assess the optic pathway, has been advocated but at present this type of investigation is a research tool. In the future it may have a more major role in assessing the optic pathway in the unconscious patient.

A full dental assessment, both clinically and with the use of dental casts, is important. The use of dental models allows the occlusion to be planned and for the construction of custom-made arch bars and an acrylic interocclusal wafer. It is often necessary to section the models mimicking the fractures to allow for an accurate reduction. The inspection of wear facets, the use of preinjury photographs and, if available, preinjury orthodontic casts aid the correct re-establishment of the dental occlusion.

Once the full assessment and targeted investigations have been performed the following key questions can be answered and, particularly for more complex injuries, a planning meeting for the surgical team convened to formulate an individualized operative strategy. These can be prolonged procedures and planning optimizes efficiency with respect to both intraoperative decision making and allocation of resources.

- Skeletal assessment:
    Is the anterior cranial fossa involved?
    Is the frontal sinus involved?
    Extent of naso-orbital ethmoidal injuries
    Extent of malar-orbital injuries, particularly the medial orbital wall
    Extent and type of maxillary injuries
    Extent and type of mandibular injuries (particularly condylar)
    Is there any bone loss (either absolute or effective)?
- Soft tissue assessment:
    Extent and type of lacerations
    Is there any tissue loss?
    Injury to cranial nerves
    Globe/optic tract injury
- Is there any potential for vascular injury?
- Is there potential for exacerbation of a coexisting head injury?
- Is there a spinal cord injury (particularly cervical spine) that might be exacerbated?

The main aspects of the formulated management plan should be:

- timing of intervention(s)
- airway management
- surgical access
- sequencing of repair
- bone graft donor sites
- soft tissue repair/reconstruction.

These aspects must be considered in relation to the general state of the patient with particular reference to the current and anticipated respiratory status, cardiovascular status, nutritional state, co-existing injury and co-morbid disease.

Operative Strategy: State-of-the-Art Management

Management principles

Restoring the preinjury form and function to the facial region requires the precise anatomic reconstitution of the craniofacial skeleton and overlying soft tissue drape. The cranial cavity must be sealed off from the upper aerodigestive tract, preventing subsequent infection. Orbital volume and configuration must be restored, providing support and projection to the globes and supporting structures. The form of the

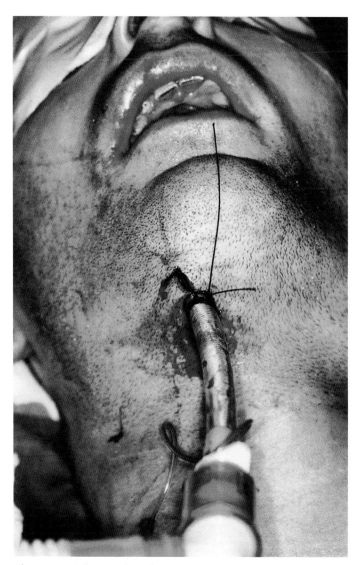

Fig. 14.7: Submental intubation is a simple technique which gives unimpeded access to the facial region and is a useful alternative to tracheostomy where it is envisaged that airway support will be required for a short duration.

external nose is restored and an unimpeded nasal airway re-established. Correct jaw relationships are re-established and maintained with a precise restoration of the pre-existing dental occlusion. The form of the face is restored in three-dimensional space, i.e. width, anteroposterior projection and vertical height. The soft tissue drape of the face must be supported in its preinjury location before scar development and maturation lead to soft tissue shrinkage. It is the secondary alteration in the character of soft tissues that so often frustrates secondary attempts to correct posttraumatic deformity. Primary repair represents the best opportunity to restore form and function.

Achieving these goals requires appropriate surgical access to, and exposure of, the craniofacial skeleton. All fractures are exposed directly, allowing accurate assessment of the degree of bony comminution and displacement. Failure to achieve a direct visualization of all fractures and bone segments is a common reason for persistent deformity.[11] This

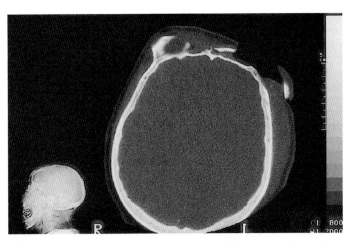

Fig. 14.8: Despite extensive disruption of the anterior frontal sinus wall the force transferred in this injury has been dissipated in disrupting this well-pneumatized frontal sinus, leaving the posterior wall intact.

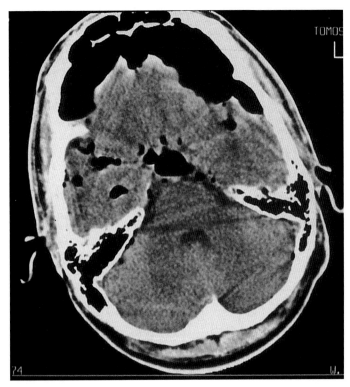

Fig. 14.9: Extensive disruption of the anterior cranial fossa including the posterior wall of the frontal sinus. Air is entrapped within the anterior and middle cranial fossae.

problem particularly applies in the orbital and nasoethmoidal regions where procedures are performed through small incisions in patients who have a comminuted fracture pattern. Comminuted fractures in this region are an indication for the wider exposure afforded by a coronal flap, usually in combination with a lower eyelid access incision. Having visualized the fracture anatomy, reduction and internal fixation are performed, linking unstable segments to adjacent stable areas of the craniofacial skeleton. Severely damaged areas, with comminution, represent areas of effective bone loss and are replaced with primary bone grafting, restoring support and

contour. Only in the presence of a heavily contaminated or infected wound is primary bone grafting omitted and recourse made to delayed grafting techniques. The results will not be as favorable when delay in grafting is necessitated because of the effects of fibrosis and tissue shrinkage.

Where elements of the bony skeleton and soft tissue are absent, primary bone grafting and on occasions flap repair indicated, no attempt should be made to reduce the size of defects by accepting a less than anatomical reduction. Advancement of local tissues across areas of loss creates secondary deformity which may be irreversible. Where there is skin or mucosal loss, this should, in general, be managed with grafting or occasionally free tissue transfer, in the primary treatment phase.[12] Absolute or effective bone loss is similarly managed with bone-grafting techniques. In the case of composite tissue loss, a composite free flap primary repair may be indicated. The overriding principle is to restore and maintain spatial relationships.

An inevitable consequence of the surgical exposure required to effect precise reduction and stabilization of the facial skeleton is that the overlying soft tissue drape is detached. Often, whilst producing good restoration of skeletal form, results are compromised because of failure to restore the correct relationship of the soft tissues to the underlying facial skeleton.[13] This applies particularly to the orbital region. The medial canthal tendon is an obvious problem area. However, wide exposure means that the lateral canthus is also on occasions inferiorly displaced and requires reattachment at its normal location 2 mm cephalad and posterior to its medial counterpart. An important superficial muscular aponeurotic system supporting adhesion exists around the orbital rim. In addition, a series of the muscles of facial expression (zygomaticus major, zygomaticus minor, levator labii superiorius, levator labii alaeque nasi) arise from the periosteum in the infraorbital region. Detachment of periosteum in this area allows its descent along with the origin of these muscles of facial expression. Unless reattached, thinning in the infraorbital region is seen with a corresponding fullness of the nasolabial fold. This may also contribute to the lower eyelid retraction and scleral show sometimes seen following the fixation of fractures of the infraorbital rim via a lower eyelid approach.

In the temporal region, a further system of adhesions exists supporting the superficial musculo-aponeurotic system (SMAS). Loss of support and descent of the SMAS may contribute to, and accentuate, the temporal hollowing seen following coronal flap access to the upper and midface skeleton. It is probable, however, that much of this hollowing is a consequence of ischemic atrophy of the fat pad lying between the leaves of deep temporal fascia above the zygomatic arch. This fat is perfused by the middle temporal artery, a branch of the superficial temporal artery, which is susceptible to injury during dissection to expose the zygomatic arch.

Management of the soft tissue drape following treatment of facial fractures has received insufficient attention in the literature, with some notable exceptions.[13] The authors do not pretend to have clear answers to all of these soft tissue drape problems but seek here to give them their deserved

Key points

- Restore and maintain spatial relationships
- Replace missing and severely damaged (comminuted) bone segments
- Replace missing soft tissue cover
- Restore the correct relationship of the soft tissue drape to the underlying facial skeleton

attention and describe some practical solutions we have adopted in attempting to restore proper facial soft tissue support.

Timing

Procedures performed at admission are confined to those which are life saving. The maxillofacial surgeon may be called upon to provide a surgical airway or arrest hemorrhage. Thereafter, early procedures are limited to debridement of wounds with excision of necrotic tissue and closure of wounds where there has been no tissue loss. The opportunity is taken to perform a thorough examination under anesthesia. Impressions for dental models are obtained. These procedures should only be performed on a warm and stable patient. Second- and third-look procedures and appropriate debridement are indicated where there has been massive tissue injury with necrosis and where marginally viable tissue is present.

Our aim is to perform a definitive repair within 5–7 days of admission. This can be delayed for up to 2 weeks without substantially compromising outcome, depending upon the age of the patient, but these delayed procedures present greater technical difficulty in achieving adequate reduction and fixation. Beyond 2 weeks, progressive difficulty is encountered, at least in part, because of the accelerated callus formation seen in head-injured patients. Furthermore, beyond 7 days, internal healing and fibrosis, in the setting of malpositioned skeletal support, will prevent a natural redraping of the mimetic soft tissues of the face. In our practice, the most common reason for a longer delay is an accompanying brain injury.

Airway management

In panfacial fractures, where unrestricted access is required to the mid and lower face, a surgical airway is our usual practice. Submental intubation provides an alternative route to tracheostomy where it is envisaged that the period of ventilatory support is likely to be short (48 hours)[14] (Fig. 14.7). Where an anterior cranial fossa repair is to be performed, a surgical airway is usually indicated. This reduces the potential for the development of a cranial aerocele associated with coughing in the early postoperative period.

In maxillary fractures where there is no skull base involvement, we have found that nasotracheal intubation allows adequate access. However, where the upper midface is involved

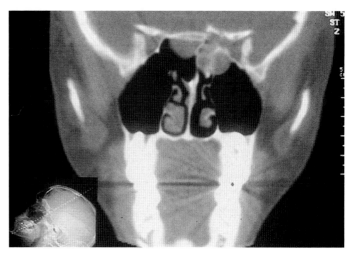

Fig. 14.10: Fracture extending across sphenoid ridge. Such fractures jeopardize the optic nerve and internal carotid artery.

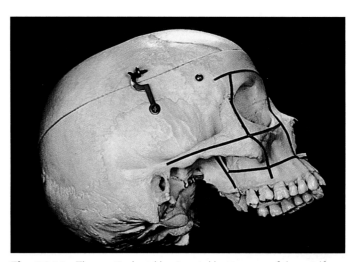

Fig. 14.11: The vertical and horizontal buttresses of the midface define the lines of elective osteosynthesis. Note the absence of a sagittal buttress between the palate and the frontal bar in the central midface.

and a coronal flap indicated, either submental intubation or tracheostomy is recommended to ensure a safe and unencumbered procedure.

Access

Manson et al[13] divide the facial skeleton into anterior and posterior areas from the viewpoint of access requirements. Low-level midfacial fractures, pyramidal fractures and fractures of the horizontal body of the mandible may be approached via buccal sulcus and small cutaneous incisions, provided there are no more than one or two large fragments. The presence of multiple fractures at a higher level, comminution of facial subunits or fractures of the condylar process of the mandible necessitates posterior access incisions – a coronal flap in the case of upper and midface injuries. The essential point is that not only must the location of the injury be considered in planning access, but also severity of the

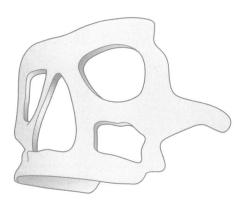

Fig. 14.12: Model depicting the horizontal and vertical lines of elective osteosynthesis for the midface, since the bone is thicker at these sites (courtesy R Schmelzeisen).

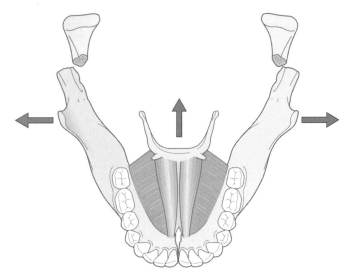

Fig. 14.13: Fractures involving the symphysis and condylar regions of the mandible frequently result in an increase in facial width with decreased anterior projection. This position is maintained by the pull of the suprahyoid musculature.

injury. Greater fragmentation implies greater difficulty in achieving adequate stability, necessitating better fixation, with or without bone grafting, and therefore wider exposure.

However, detachment of the soft tissue drape, and in particular periosteum, from the facial skeleton has secondary consequences as outlined above. Exposure commensurate with visualization and accurate reduction and fixation is required but no more than that. Where periosteum can be left attached it should be, maintaining the correct spatial relationship between the facial skeleton and overlying mimetic soft tissues in at least a few points. This is likely to greatly facilitate accurate and secure repositioning of intervening areas of detachment. Our preferred adjective to describe access and exposure is 'appropriate' rather than 'wide'.

Key points

- Consider degree of comminution as well as site of fractures in planning access

- Leave soft tissue drape attached to craniofacial skeleton where possible

---

Surgical anatomy of the facial skeleton

The face may conceptually be divided into three zones or subunits, each subserving different purposes. The upper subunit is composed of the frontal bone whose principal purpose is protection of the frontal lobes of the brain but also forms the roof of the orbit and encloses the cribriform plate of the ethmoid, subserving the special sense of olfaction. It contains the frontal sinus whose extent varies from individual to individual, with a trend towards increasing pneumatization with age.

Sufficient force directed over the frontonasal region produces a central fracture with fracture lines that may involve the frontomaxillary and weak frontoethmoid vomerine buttress. If the frontal sinus is large, it absorbs a large proportion of the force and the posterior wall may

remain intact without dural exposure or injury (Fig. 14.8). With small linear cracks in the posterior wall of the frontal sinus, the dura may be intact but with greater disruption dural tears occur, leading to CSF rhinorrhea. If the frontal sinus is rudimentary and/or the fracture extends beyond the sinus, large segmental fractures are seen involving the orbital roof/floor of the anterior cranial fossa (Fig. 14.9). These may extend across the sphenoid ridge and in so doing, jeopardize the internal carotid arteries and optic nerve as the latter lie within the confined space of the optic canal (Fig. 14.10). It is safer to expose the anterior fossa prior to disimpacting the maxilla under such circumstances. Laterally, extensive fractures involving the frontal bone, greater wing of sphenoid, temporal and parietal bones present the potential for injury to the middle meningeal artery. Displacement of bony segments in this region must involve neurosurgical colleagues. Mobilization of depressed fractures of the zygomatic complex under such circumstances should also be performed with direct visualization through a coronal flap and in an institution with neurosurgeons present and forewarned.

The middle subunit of the face has a very different structure, characterized by areas of lower structural integrity and enclosed within a bony framework of supportive pillars or struts. Gruss & McKinnon[15] made an important conceptual advance in the mid 1980s in describing the vertical 'supportive pillars' of the midface: the paired frontonasal maxillary pillars anteromedially, zygomatico-maxillary pillars laterally and the pterygoid processes posteriorly. In individuals with fully developed sinuses, these pillars are relatively weak in the midface superior to the alveolar process of the maxillae. It is unfortunate for the surgeon undertaking repair of midfacial fractures that the most robust of these supportive pillars, the pterygoid plates (in fact muscular processes), are inaccessible for direct operative repair. Added to this schema, subsequent authors have described horizontal facial buttresses. Superiorly the

Key points and pitfalls

- Principle of subunit reconstruction

- Horizontal and vertical buttresses mark sites of elective osteosynthesis in the midface

- Bone grafting is frequently required in the relatively weak midface

- Lack of central midface sagittal buttress explains the frequent midface collapse following severe injury

- Excessive width and corresponding lack of anteroposterior projection are common errors in the repair of midface fractures

frontal bar of the upper facial subunit is included. Inferiorly, the horizontal buttress is described as comprising the maxillary alveolus and palatal processes, with a contribution from the horizontal process of the palatine bone. The middle horizontal buttress is composed of the zygomatic arches, body of the zygomatic bones and the infraorbital rim. These transversely orientated supportive elements link the zygomaticomaxillary processes and nasomaxillary processes[13,16] (Fig. 14.11). This conceptual model has utility because it marks important horizontal and vertical lines of elective osteosynthesis in repair of the facial skeleton (Fig. 14.12). In reality, surgeons could naturally use these thicker bony struts for osteosynthesis, since outside these areas, the bone is too thin for adequate fixation of the plates.

Manson makes the point that what is notably absent is a robust sagittal supportive pillar in the central part of the face which extends from posterior to anterior.[13] The septovomerine complex is weak. The lateral wall of the nose between the perpendicular processes of the palatine bone and the nasomaxillary processes has very little structural integrity. Central midface collapse is therefore a common consequence of severe midfacial injury and requires specific attention if successful repair is to be achieved.

The mandible forms the skeletal structure of the lower face. Its surgical anatomy is described elsewhere in this text. It has good structural integrity as a consequence of its functional role and well-developed associated musculature. The specific problem presented by mandibular fractures in association with midfacial injuries lies with its importance in re-establishing correct facial width. The fracture pattern where difficulties commonly arise are those occurring in the symphysis and parasymphyseal region and particularly when associated with fractures of the condylar process(es). Force delivered from an anterior direction produces retrodisplacement of the mandible as it fractures, with widening at the mandibular angles. Displacement is maintained by the insertion of the suprahyoid musculature into the symphyseal region of the mandible, which also places torsional forces on the fracture segments[11] (Fig. 14.13).

When there is a corresponding sagittal fracture of the maxilla or an absence of teeth, guides to the re-establishment

of facial width are lost and an operative strategy designed to overcome this difficulty must be planned.

Sequence of operative repair in panfacial injuries (Fig. 14.14)

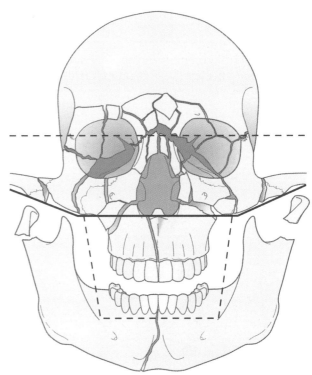

Fig. 14.14: (a) Descriptively panfacial fractures may be divided into two facial halves separated by a fracture at the Le Fort I level. The upper facial half is subdivided into an upper unit comprising the frontal bone and a midfacial unit. The lower facial half is subdivided into an occlusal unit and a lower basal unit.[11]

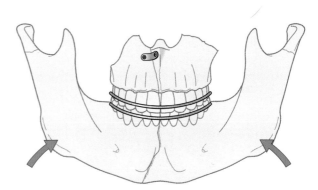

Fig. 14.14: (b) Establish facial width at the occlusal level. Sagittal fractures of the maxilla and mandibular fractures with splaying of the vertical rami lead to errors with excessive width and deficient anterior projection. Pressure should be applied to the gonial angles to close any lingual gap in the anterior mandible. A useful guide to the correct reduction is the point at which the anterior fracture just starts to open on its labial or buccal surface. At this point the lingual cortex is acting as a fulcrum.

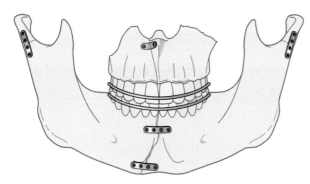

Fig. 14.14: (c) Fixation of the mandibular condyles where feasible helps prevent excessive width as well as restoring posterior facial height.

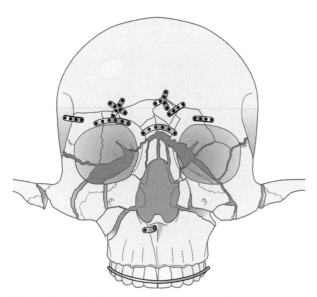

Fig. 14.14: (d) Reassembly of the upper facial subunit precedes midface repair.

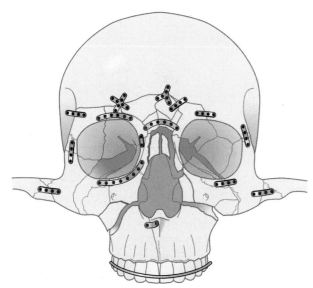

Fig. 14.14: (e) Start midface repair at the least injured part of the orbits and use all visual clues to establish the correct anterior projection.

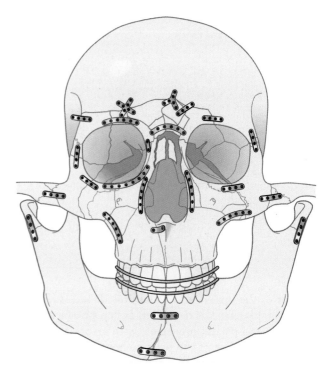

Fig. 14.14: (f) Buttress reconstruction is completed by miniplating the nasomaxillary and zygomatico-maxillary vertical buttresses.

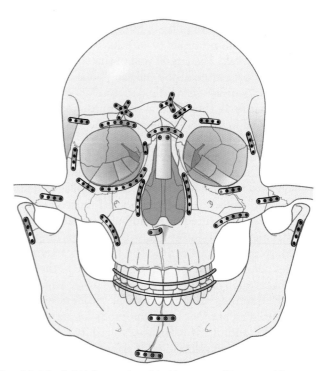

Fig. 14.14: (g) Volumetric orbital bone grafting, nasal bone grafting and medial canthopexy are performed where necessary and prior to inset of any pericranial or galeofrontalis flap and soft tissue redraping.

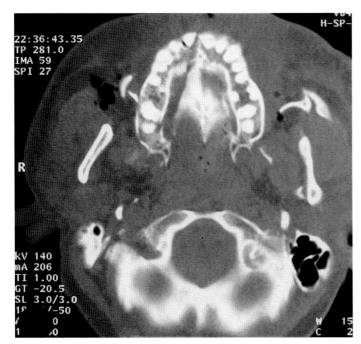

Fig. 14.15: Axial CT image of a parasagittal fracture of the palate in a patient with panfacial trauma.

Manson describes panfacial fractures as comprising two facial halves separated by a fracture at the Le Fort I level. The lower facial half is further divided into an upper occlusal level, comprising the maxillary and mandibular alveolar processes with their associated teeth as well as the palate, and a lower unit comprising the vertical ramus and horizontal basal mandible. The upper facial half is divided into an upper unit, comprising the frontal bone with its supraorbital ridges and roof of orbits, and a midfacial unit[13] (Fig. 14.14a). This model has descriptive utility and is employed here.

Our preferred operative sequence is to commence with management of the lower facial half. The occlusal subunit is first reconstituted. This is an important determinant of lower facial width. Sagittal fractures of the maxilla, in association with mandibular fractures, result in loss of all reference points for re-establishing the correct width, and therefore anterior projection, in the lower face (Fig. 14.15). Standard techniques relying on establishment of a seemingly correct dental occlusion, followed by fixation of mandibular fractures, and then relating upper facial repair to this will not infrequently result in decreased anterior projection and increased lower facial width. Manson and co-workers found split palate fractures accompanying 8% of mid-face fractures.[17] However, where midface fractures are a consequence of motor vehicle accidents, the incidence of sagittal fractures rises and has been reported in as many as 20–25% of such patients.

Rowe & Killey[1] pointed out that gross separation of the maxilla must result in associated fractures of the zygomatico-orbital complex, an observation subsequently demonstrated to be generally correct.[18] Denny & Celik studied the distribution of sagittal fractures of the maxilla in a series of patients and found about 15% comprised dentoalveolar fractures with the remainder involving the palatal vault.[19] These were equally distributed between true sagittal and parasagittal fractures. Manson stated that while sagittal fractures occur in younger individuals, parasagittal fractures are preponderant in adults.[20] The palatal suture is structurally akin to the cranial sutures. Pearsson & Thilender[21] found synostosis of the palatal suture to occur between 15 and 19 years of age, firmly uniting the lateral palatal segments, thus making parasagittal fracture, in the thinner bone at this site, more probable with advancing years. A lip laceration extending into the gingivobuccal sulcus, accompanied by tooth loss, is strongly suggestive of sagittal fracture of the maxilla. A mucosa tear in the palate is sometimes seen. However, sagittal fractures may be present in the absence of any of these signs. Careful palpation for such injury and scrutiny of axial and coronal CTs is therefore required since this is an important diagnosis to make in correctly re-establishing facial width.[17] Displacement of the dentoalveolar fragments occurs in a superior and lateral direction.

Manson and others have advocated direct exposure of the palatal fracture via a longitudinal incision and limited subperiosteal exposure of the palatal shelves.[17,20] Reduction by the application of lateral arch pressure followed by plate and screw fixation in the palate re-establishes facial width, but does not necessarily prevent incorrect angulation of segments. Further plate fixation across the fracture at the anterior alveolus decreases the likelihood of improper angulation or malrotation of segments.

Dentoalveolar segment fractures can greatly complicate treatment and require precise methods of fixation. In this circumstance, it is our opinion that best results are achieved with the use of an acrylic occlusal splint which has sufficient palatal coverage to control angulation of the dentoalveolar segments and yet allows buccal inspection of occlusal relationships. Whilst acrylic splints should be constructed in patients with panfacial trauma, other than in the specific circumstance of dentoalveolar fractures, we prefer to avoid any intervening wafer and establish dental intercuspation by direct examination. This allows the identification of small but important occlusal discrepancies indicating imperfect fracture reduction.

The use of wire intermaxillary fixation using Erich or custom-made arch bars is our standard practice. Prior to placement in intermaxillary fixation, mobilization of the maxilla should be achieved. However, where there exists a skull base fracture and an anterior cranial fossa repair is indicated, mobilization of the maxilla should be deferred until this can be performed with the anterior fossa floor under direct vision. Adequate maxillary mobilization is important. Failure to obtain adequate mobilization, and correction of the posterior maxillary lengthening, prior to fixation invites relapse into an anterior open bite on release of intermaxillary fixation.

Having established arch width, and therefore anterior projection at the occlusal level, fractures of the mandible are then fixed. The management of mandibular fractures is discussed elsewhere in this text and here we confine our comments to the particular problem of low face width and posterior facial height in patients with panfacial trauma.

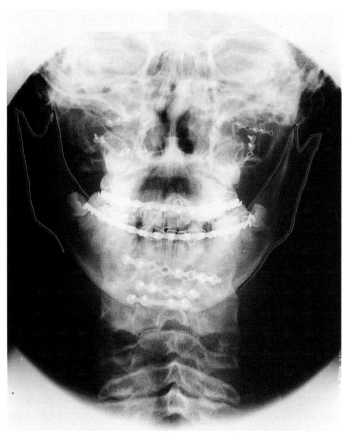

Fig. 14.16: This patient sustained a parasymphyseal fracture as well as high condylar fractures of the mandible, in association with midfacial injuries. Open reduction and fixation of the mandibular symphysis without due consideration to the condylar injuries has resulted in a mandible with excessive width posteriorly, inadequate projection in an anteroposterior plane, as well as a reduction in height in the posterior face. This is a common error in fractures of this pattern.

After considering the fracture pattern and examining the mandibular arch form, it should be possible to predict any tendency to arch widening. In this regard a lateral crossbite should be viewed with the greatest scepticism. As stated above, the fracture pattern most commonly resulting in increased width is that which involves the symphyseal or parasymphyseal region and especially in conjunction with fractures of the condylar process[22] (Fig. 14.16). Under such circumstances all fractures should be exposed prior to the reduction and fixation of any one of them. It is advisable where there is clear widening of the arch to expose the lingual cortex of the mandible via an upper cervical skin incision. Pressure should be applied at the gonial angles to close any lingual fracture gap occurring in the body of the mandible (Fig. 14.14b). A small lingual gap in the symphyseal region is magnified at the gonial angles and must be closed if the lower facial width is to be reestablished and the correct anterior projection achieved.

Before fixation of body fractures, it is prudent to examine any condylar fracture to ensure fragment alignment; indeed, fixation of fractures in the vertical ramus prior to those in the anterior part of the mandible has been advocated.

However, treatment of condylar fractures is not always feasible. As the energy imparted in fracturing the mandible increases, the location of fractures has a tendency to move from a predominance of subcondylar fractures to more superior locations in the neck and intra-articulator region[23] so that, in panfacial injuries, intracapsular fractures are not uncommon. Fortunately the loss of height that occurs with such injuries is usually less than that which occurs with fracture dislocations occurring in the condylar neck, an injury pattern which also occurs in higher energy trauma but which can and should be treated by open reduction and internal fixation. Where a coronal flap is indicated for treatment of fractures of the mid and upper face, detachment of the masseter insertion along the zygomatic arch provides good access to the condylar process of the mandible. In the absence of a coronal flap, our currently preferred approach to the condyle is a retromandibular incision and transparotid dissection.

Fixation of condylar process fractures is important in re-establishing posterior facial height and preventing subsequent anterior open bite deformity. It indirectly helps establish midfacial height by correctly orientating the occlusal and thus maxillary plane angle, in relation to the skull base (Fig. 14.14c). In the case of intracapsular condylar fractures, with collapse, less precise clues to the correct maxillary and mandibular plane angle must be relied upon. The reassembly of midfacial fragments that provides the basis for correct orientation under such circumstances is prone to error in angulation even where there has been no loss of bone segments.

Management of the upper facial unit

Injuries to the frontal bone, the frontal sinus and the anterior cranial fossa often require, and benefit from, neurosurgical and craniofacial surgeons co-operating in a multidisciplinary team. The balance between the neurosurgical concerns of the patient with a brain injury and the need to treat facial injuries often seems to lead to conflict. This can be resolved with close co-operation and communication between the neurosurgical and craniofacial teams. The neurosurgical needs of the patient have to take priority, as minimizing injury to the brain outweighs the importance of an improved outcome following on from the early repair of craniofacial fractures. The neurological outcome may be adversely affected by brain retraction in the early stages of an evolving head injury. It is primarily for this reason that we prefer a delayed approach (day 5–7) to the repair of craniofacial injuries.

Anterior fossa fractures are often complex and they do not follow stereotypical patterns. The anterior fossa floor may be significantly disrupted with no other fractures more superficial to the area. Imaging should be in two planes (axial and coronal). It is also useful to utilize multiplanar reconstructions on the CT workstation to view, and fully appreciate, the three-dimensional nature of the fractures. It should also be remembered that, even with the most advanced scanners, all the fractures may not be apparent due to the overlapping of thin bone fragments and data interpolation.

Where an anterior cranial fossa repair is indicated, access to the anterior cranial fossa through a frontal craniotomy is followed by dural repair. Fractures involving the orbital roof may be impacted and should be reduced under direct vision. Where fractures of the anterior cranial fossa extend to the sphenoid ridge, it may be safer to perform an osteotomy and advance the frontal bar into the correct position, leaving posterior fractures unreduced and grafting resulting defects in the orbital roof with split calvarial bone.

The anterior skull vault is not subjected to muscular forces and stable fixation is readily achieved with osteosynthesis wires and small (1 mm) plating systems. The latter have the advantage of more readily providing the correct contour when comminution has occurred. Fixation plates should, wherever possible, be placed in a transverse plane. This orientation facilitates their removal, should it become necessary, via a local incision parallel to the relaxed skin tension lines.

The management of frontal sinus injuries is an important issue and remains the subject of some controversy. The frontal sinus drains via the short frontonasal duct into the anterior end of the hiatus semilunaris of the middle meatus, in the lateral wall of the nose. Frontonasal duct obstruction leads to entrapment of mucus with chronic infection. The frontal sinus mucosa may then develop mucus retention cysts. By an unknown mechanism, mucoceles erode adjacent bone and may extend intracranially or into the orbit. If the mucoid contents of the cyst become infected, a mucopyocele results. Mucopyocele formation may lead to orbital or cranial abscess formation, orbital cellulitis, meningitis or osteomyelitis of the frontal bone. These complications can occur many years after the initial repair and it is this long-term risk that makes obtaining satisfactory data so difficult.

Reports to date have described this complication in small numbers of trauma cases and none of these reports have been comparative trials. In an attempt to avoid such adverse consequences, a number of authors have recommended frontonasal duct and frontal sinus obliteration where fractures involve the frontal sinus. Abdominal fat, temporalis muscle and bone graft have been recommended for this purpose. The danger of using fat in the presence of comminuted or missing sinus walls has been emphasized in an animal experimental model[24] and there is no reason to believe non-viable muscle would pose any less risk. Furthermore, prior to obliteration, all sinus mucosa must be removed by thorough curettage and burr obliteration. This represents a considerable undertaking in a well-pneumatized frontal bone where the sinus may extend posteriorly almost to the lesser wing of sphenoid and laterally to the zygomatic processes of the frontal bone. The posterior wall is thin and dural injury a risk. Filling the resultant defect with bone graft requires a large amount of what is a valuable commodity in panfacial trauma.

Our experience is in accordance with that of Gruss et al.[25] Where anterior cranial fossa repair is required, 'cranialization' of the frontal sinus should be performed. The posterior or cranial wall of the frontal sinus is burred away in its entirety and the sinus mucosa curetted and burred, ensuring thorough removal. The frontonasal ducts are identified inferomedially and obliterated with bone graft with subsequent placement

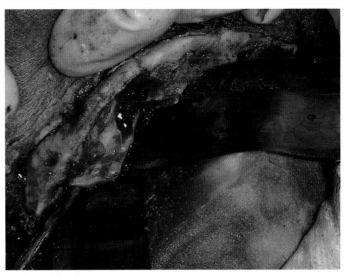

Fig. 14.17: Where an anterior cranial fossa repair is planned due consideration must be given to the requirement for a pericranial or galeofrontalis flap inset to seal the floor of the anterior fossa. Such thin flaps are readily introduced through the craniotome cut at the inferior edge of the frontal bone flap. This slide shows removal of the posterior wall (courtesy Robert Bentley, Kings College Hospital, London).

of a pericranial or galeofrontalis flap inset to seal the anterior cranial fossa from the nasal cavity below (Fig. 14.17). Where injury is limited to the anterior wall of the frontal sinus without dural involvement, no attempt is made at sinus obliteration, Gruss et al state that:

... when bone is securely reduced and grafts rigidly applied ... when non delayed debridement is accomplished, the chance of mucocoele formation is minimal. The premise that the naso-frontal duct will resume function in a majority of patients appears legitimate. Early intervention and reconstruction are hallmarks of this approach. The presence of improperly reduced bone segments, comminuted sequestra, foreign bodies, and torn mucosal shreds leave the patient susceptible to the development of mucopyocoele ...

Where the anterior wall of the sinus and nasoethmoidal region are comminuted, stenting of the nasofrontal ducts for 4 weeks with silastic tubing (a portion of nasogastric tube is suitable) seems prudent. These can be inserted through the anterior wall defect prior to reconstitution and brought out through the external nares to which they are secured.

After debridement the anterior wall is reconstructed by reassembly of bone fragments with bone grafting where necessary (Fig. 14.14d). It is often necessary to map and mark the fragments to allow reassembly (Fig. 14.18). If a map is not used it is surprisingly difficult, and time consuming, to piece the jigsaw back together correctly, even with only a few pieces. On occasions bone deformation prior to fracture occurs and under such circumstances a perfect reduction cannot be achieved.

Inadequate reduction in the supraorbital ridge is a potential problem and leads to flattening with inadequate anterior projection (Fig. 14.19). The senior author has performed secondary correction of this deformity regularly over a practic-

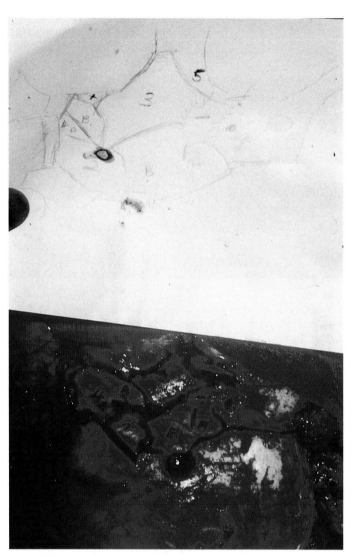

Fig. 14.18: Prior to removing frontal bone fragments a map is constructed of the constituent pieces. This greatly facilitates reassembly.

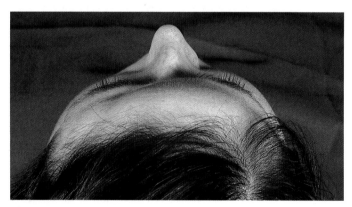

Fig. 14.19: Posttraumatic recession or 'flattening' of the supraorbital region.

ing career at Canniesburn Hospital. Comminution of the supraorbital ridge may require primary bone grafting to prevent this occurrence and this particularly applies when major segments are displaced and anterior cranial fossa repair is not

judged to be indicated. Onlay bone grafting is indicated with split rib being a good donor material, allowing the restoration of an even contour with a symmetric anterior projection.

Reconstruction of the orbital rim and roof can also be problematic when comminuted. Exophthalmos and downward displacement of the globe, which is very difficult to safely correct secondarily, may occur. Care must be exercised in contouring the orbital rim and ensuring the reconstructed roof of the orbit is approximately 3 mm cephalad to the rim where it lies above the globe. This can only satisfactorily be achieved from above with exposure of the anterior cranial fossa. Failure to reconstruct the orbital roof where there is a large bony dehiscence risks the development of a pulsating exophthalmos.

Where anterior cranial fossa repair is required, insetting of the pericranial or galeofrontalis flap and fixation of the frontal bone flap is deferred until midface repair is complete. This maintains unimpeded access.

Midface fractures

In the midface zygomatico-orbital and nasoethmoid reconstruction, re-establishing the correct width and anterior projection in relation to a stable frontal bar, follow on from fixation of the upper face (Fig. 14.14e). Finally, with a stable upper midface, the occlusal unit is fixed in the anterior vertical buttress regions at the appropriate height (Fig. 14.14f).

The midface presents several major reconstructive difficulties following severe facial trauma. Comminution of this delicate structure is the rule rather than the exception in panfacial injury. The greater the comminution, the more difficult it becomes to achieve adequate stability, even in the presence of precise reduction and fixation of individual fragments. Furthermore, errors of a few millimeters in restoring orbital volume and configuration, canthal reattachment and occlusal relationships are noticeable and often difficult to correct with secondary procedures. A wide midface, with collapse in an anteroposterior plane, enophthalmos and traumatic telecanthus were common sequelae of management with closed techniques in a former era and continue to frustrate contemporary efforts. As elsewhere in the facial skeleton, a complete diagnosis and the planning of an operative strategy, bearing in mind common errors, maximize the likelihood of a satisfactory outcome.

On the basis of preoperative imaging and intraoperative findings, the least injured part of the orbital region is identified and repair of the midfacial skeleton commences at that point. A successful approach has been to identify an intact greater wing of sphenoid in the lateral orbit. If not fractured, this robust structure gives a good indication of the correct angulation and therefore width and anterior projection of the lateral midface. Gruss[11] prefers to rely on the zygomatic arches and commence reconstruction at this point. Our experience, however, has been more in accordance with Manson et al,[13] who have found few clues to the correct lateral projection of the zygomatic arch. A common error is to overreduce laterally, the result of which is an increased facial width and inadequate anterior projection. If the greater wing of sphenoid is fractured and the zygomatic arch used as the key to the lateral facial reconstruction, it is important to recall that the zygomatic arch has a straight sagittal orientation between the zygomatic process of the temporal bone and the zygomatic prominence. A temporary wire placed at the frontozygomatic suture establishes vertical height in this region and allows manipulation in the transverse and anteroposterior planes. The zygomatic arch is a muscular process giving origin to the masseter muscle. It is therefore subject to significant functional stress and is not of itself robust. Subsequent displacement with loss of anterior projection, following initial good reduction of fixation, has been described. We routinely fix this region with a 1.5 mm plate and screw system in adults, believing that lighter fixation provides insufficient stability.

Fixation of the medial orbital region takes as its reference the nasal process of the frontal bone, reconstituted or uninjured. The frontal process of the maxilla is the key structure in this region since this forms a substantial part of the important frontonaso-maxillary vertical buttress. Establishing the correct transnasal width of this structure, and therefore restoring anterior projection to the nasal pyramid, is problematic. Common errors in the naso-orbitoethmoid region are increased width and collapse in an anteroposterior plane and malposition of medial canthal tendons. Whilst height of the fractured frontal process of the maxilla can generally be readily established if it is not comminuted, the orientation of this structure in all other planes is difficult as a consequence of the frequent fragmentation of nasal bones and inferior orbital rim which occurs. Reduction of the frontal process of the maxilla where it meets the frontal bone is therefore frequently associated with significant angular errors. All visual clues must be utilized to achieve its correct orientation. Fixation of the frontal process of the maxilla at the glabella is followed by reassembly of the inferior orbital rim which is frequently fragmented. Every effort should be made to retrieve fragments displaced posteroinferiorly into the maxillary sinus and ensure the jigsaw of fragments is reassembled with plate fixation. Visual assessment of the width at the medial canthal level is important at this stage (Fig. 14.14f).

Having re-established the horizontal and vertical buttresses of the upper midface, fixation of the occlusal unit at the correct vertical height is performed with fixation at the zygomatico-maxillary and nasomaxillary vertical buttresses. It is important to consciously seat the mandibular condyles into the glenoid fossae if an anterior open bite dental relationship is to be avoided. To prevent persistent posterior maxillary lengthening, it may be necessary to remove displaced bone fragments in the posterolateral maxilla at the Le Fort I level. Primary bone grafting is indicated anteriorly where there has been comminution. At this point the vertical and horizontal midfacial buttress reconstruction should be complete (Fig. 14.20).

Bone grafting of the medial, lateral and inferior walls of the orbits is next accomplished with the emphasis on precise volumetric reconstruction. In most cases, the canthus remains attached to a fragment of bone, and thus can be reduced using a small plate via a coronal incision.

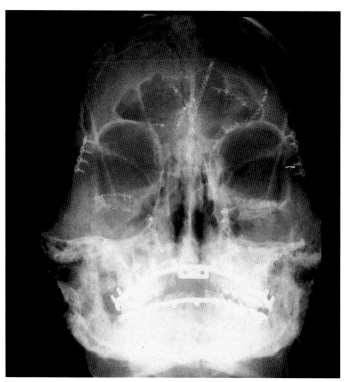

Fig. 14.20: Plain radiograph of patient with upper and midfacial fractures. Fixation devices are placed along the midfacial vertical and horizontal buttresses.

Medial canthal tendon reattachment is performed after orbital wall reconstruction. This key soft tissue structure inserts into the anterior lacrimal crest of the frontal process of the maxilla and the posterior lacrimal crest on the lacrimal bone. Treatment is aimed at restoring attachment at the anterior lacrimal crest. Exposure and identification of the medial canthus are required for a successful repair of traumatic telecanthus. Attempts to identify and reposition a totally detached medial canthus via a coronal flap have been unsuccessful in correcting telecanthus in our experience and that of others.[13] The medial canthus is readily exposed via a short 4–5 mm horizontal incision commencing 2–3 mm medial to the medial commissure of the palpebral fissure. Dissection through this small wound brings the 2–3 mm white band of fibrous tissue that forms the medial canthal tendon into clear relief. Its attachment to the frontal process of the maxilla where this is a substantial fragment should not be disturbed. Where comminution exists, however, transnasal canthopexy is indicated.

Common errors in canthal repositioning are twofold. First, undercorrection in width is overcome by direct canthal ligament exposure and wire capture. The other common error is fixation of the canthus too far anteriorly, creating an unnatural appearance of the medial canthus. It is essential to locate the canthus behind the most anterior part of the globe within the orbital rim. This can be achieved by passage of the transnasal canthopexy wire through a cantilevered microplate fixed in the glabellar region. This plate terminates at the desired location for canthal attachment and the transnasal wire is passed through the vacant screw hole at the end of this plate.

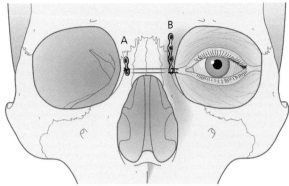

Fig. 14.21: (a) Medial canthopexy. The medial canthus is directly exposed and captured with wire. The wire is passed through the distal hole of a miniplate on the ipsilateral side (positioning plate), passed transnasally and tied over a 'toggle' plate on the contralateral side of the nasoethmoid complex. A toggle plate; B positioning plate.

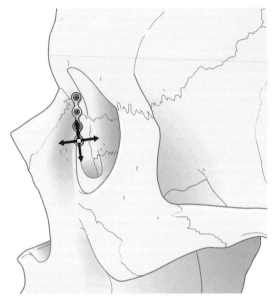

Fig. 14.21: (b) Medial canthopexy. Once the medial canthus has been captured and the transnasal wire has been placed, the positioning plate is moved into the desired location and then fixed with screws in the accessible glabella region. Final tightening over the 'toggle' plate is then performed.

The wire then passes across the nasal pyramid and is tied over a 'toggle' (short length of plate) on the contralateral side at the desired canthal width (Fig. 14.21). Subsequent canthal drift is to be anticipated and overcorrection is desirable. It is probable that this drift is, at least in part, a consequence of delayed bone resorption in the glabellar region. Each canthus is managed independently of its counterpart.

Collapse of the glabellar region is a consequence of two factors. As elsewhere in the face, excessive width leads to inadequate anterior projection; therefore reducing the width of the bony radix to approximately 20 mm in Caucasians is an important treatment objective. Effective bone loss due to comminution, with subsequent small fragment resorption, explains both early and delayed inadequate projection of the

Key points and pitfalls

- Establish the facial width at the occlusal level

- Repair of fractured mandibular condyles is important in preventing excessive lower facial width as well as restoring posterior facial height

- If the anterior cranial fossa is fractured defer maxillary mobilization until the anterior fossa is exposed

- Cranialize the frontal sinus if anterior fossa repair is performed, otherwise repair anterior wall and stent frontonasal duct

- Commence midface repair at the least injured part of the orbits

- The greater wing of sphenoid provides a good guide to zygomatic width and anterior projection when uninjured

- Excessive width and inadequate anterior projection are common errors in naso-orbitoethmoid repair

- Where there is comminution of the midface primary bone grafting and intermaxillary fixation enhance stability

nasal pyramid where the intercanthal width is satisfactory. Primary bone grafting with split calvarium is indicated where comminution of the nasal bones has occurred. The bone graft is cantilevered with plate or screw fixation to the glabella. Common errors in primary nasal bone grafting are obliteration of the radix, giving a Greco-Roman nose. Over-extension of the bone graft into the nasal tip gives an unnatural appearance in this region and may result in graft exposure due to ulceration through the skin.

There are difficulties in establishing adequate stability of fixation in the midface. The delicate bone architecture, its fragmentation and the necessity of using relatively light fixation devices all contribute. Manson points out that the lever principle means that relatively small forces at the occlusal level result in significant deforming influences where the first point of good fixation is the frontal bar.[13] Where significant fragmentation of the midface has occurred, postoperative intermaxillary fixation is therefore a prudent measure during the initial healing phase. Primary bone grafting seems to enhance both the initial and subsequent development of midfacial stability following operative repair and is also recommended.

Closure and soft tissue drape

Surgical anatomy

Moss et al[26] have recently made the point that true ligaments exist in the medial midface (zygomatic and masseteric ligaments) as well as in the lower face (mandibular ligament). These connective tissue condensations comprise a discrete cylindrical attachment of fibrous tissue that arises from either deep fascia or periosteum. They then cross the sub-SMAS

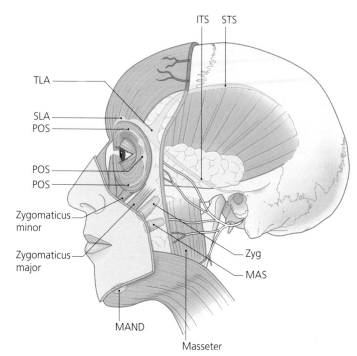

Fig. 14.22: Schematic diagram of the ligamentous and septal retaining apparatus for the superficial musculoaponeurotic system and overlying integument.[24] Supraorbital ligamentous adhesion (SLA), temporal ligamentous adhesion (TLA), superior temporal septum (STS), inferior temporal septum (ITS), periorbital septum (POS), zygomaticus major, zygomaticus minor, zygomatic ligament (Zyg), masseteric ligament (MAS), mandibular ligament (MAND). Note that the important attachments around the orbit and temporal region retain the SMAS only, whereas the ligamentous structures of the cheek region and mandible run from deep structures, traverse SMAS and insert into dermis.

plane to the undersurface of SMAS, where they divide into numerous branches and then attach to the dermis through a subcutaneous fascial system. More superior attachments around the orbit and temporal region differ in that they retain the SMAS plane only, allowing considerable mobility to occur at a cutaneous level (Fig. 14.22). Rather than true ligaments, these attachments take the form of fibrous tissue septa and adhesions. An adhesion (temporal ligamentous adhesion) supports the region immediately superior to the eyebrow at the junction of the middle and lateral thirds. Located at the intersection of the temporal, frontal and periorbital region, this fibrous adhesion is a well-defined structure from which three further zones of fixation radiate. The temporal ligamentous adhesion inserts onto the deep surface of frontalis muscle where it meets temporoparietal fascia laterally. It is a broad adhesion lying about 1 cm above the superolateral orbital rim. From this adhesion, the superior temporal septum radiates posterosuperiorly, arising from the pericranium along the superior temporal line and inserting into the line of junction between the temporoparietal fascia and galea. The inferior temporal septum takes an oblique course along a line extending from the lateral corner of the temporal ligamentous adhesion toward the root of the zygomatic

process. It comprises crisscross fibers that pass from the deep temporal fascia to their insertion into the deepest layer of the temporoparietal fascia.

The division of deep temporal fascia into its deep and superficial leaves, with an intervening fat pad, is above the level of the inferior temporal septum. The most cephalad temporal branches of the facial nerve lie on the deep surface of the temporoparietal fascia, just caudal to this inferior temporal septum. Thus, in developing a coronal flap, incising the outer layer of the deep temporal fascia cephalad to the inferior temporal septum will preserve this supporting structure and facilitate repositioning of the SMAS layer at the time of closure. It also ensures that the temporal branches of the facial nerves are protected.

A periorbital septal adhesion gains origin from three-quarters of the circumference of the orbital rim extending from the corrugator origin around to the inferomedial bony origin of the orbicularis oculi. The septum has two or more broader adhesions named the lateral brow and lateral orbital ligamentous thickenings. The lateral orbital thickening is located superolaterally to the lateral canthal tendon insertion, whereas the lateral brow thickening arises from a bony crest on the lateral supraorbital rim. Both of these ligaments insert into and retain the deep surface of orbicularis occuli.[26] Esthetic surgeons recognize the importance of these supporting structures in facial rejuvenation procedures, aiming to release and reposition them superiorly and posteriorly.

Zygomaticus major, zygomaticus minor, levator labii superioris and levator labii superioris alaeque nasi originate in a line across the malar eminence and along the infraorbital region to the frontal process of the maxilla. All originate from periosteum and are important in supporting the soft tissue of the cheek and upper lip. In the lower face the mandibular ligament is found in the anterolateral region of the mandible adjacent to the origin of depressor angulioris.[27] Furthermore, the importance of the mentalis muscle in preventing lip and chin ptosis has been emphasized in the esthetic facial literature. In accessing the facial skeleton, utilizing wide-exposure subperiosteal dissection, release of many of these, particularly periorbital, supporting structures will occur. Recognizing that these attachments of the mimetic soft tissues have important esthetic consequences, it is apparent that accurate periosteal repositioning is an important part of treatment. Where this is not feasible, additional measures should be taken to re-establish support for the SMAS layer.

Operative details

Closure commences with the re-establishment of periosteal continuity across the inferior orbital rim. Where periosteal continuity cannot be re-established suspension of the periosteum and thus the mimetic soft tissue drape must be provided for. The zygomatic ligament as it lies medial to zygomatic minor directly supports the skin of the midface. Often the cheek prominence is not directly fractured and, where possible, periosteum should be left undisturbed at this location to prevent detachment of the zygomatic ligament. If

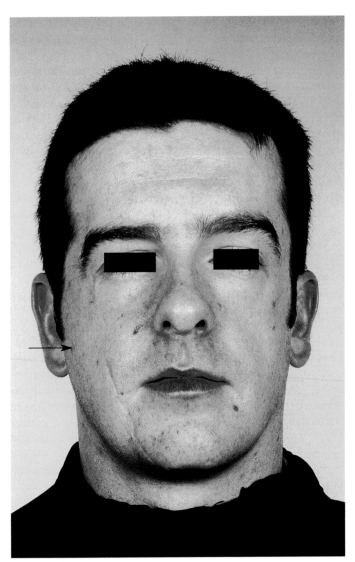

Fig. 14.23: Lateral canthal descent and a mildly 'skeletonized' lateral orbit with hollowing in the temporal fossa and fullness below (arrow). This patient sustained a right-sided orbital injury. There has been SMAS descent on the right. Note the comparative vertical positions of the most anterior part of the hair line.

with a non-resorbable suture and secured to the lateral orbital rim 2 mm cephalad and posterior to the medial canthus. It is prudent to overcorrect.

Closure of the incision in the deep temporal fascia created in raising the coronal flap is important in our opinion. Detachment at the zygomatic arch of the lateral SMAS will often have been necessary and any gap in closure of the deep temporal fascia above implies lateral SMAS descent, since an adhesion exists between the two layers, with consequent fullness below and hollowing above. A 'skeletonized' lateral orbit is a not uncommon consequence of severe orbital injury and its repair; SMAS descent may be an important contributor (Fig. 14.23).

When an anterior cranial fossa repair has not been necessary closure of periosteum in the supraorbital region is usually performed continuously with that of deep temporal fascia. Every effort is made to restore height of periosteal redraping. Where an anterior cranial fossa repair has been performed, suspension sutures may be employed in the frontal region from supraorbital periosteum to superior bone anchoring points. The highest point of the eyebrow is at the junction of the middle and lateral thirds in the youthful face and this should be borne in mind when applying suspension sutures. Closure of the galeal layer at the coronal incision provides further support for the SMAS, as well as being important in preventing subsequent scar widening.

In creating exposure to the anterior mandible the mentalis muscle is an important structure. Maintenance of an adequate cuff of muscle attached to the labial surface of the mandible to allow layered closure may be helpful in preventing subsequent lower lip and chin ptosis. Where muscle re-approximation is not possible the use of bone anchoring devices is advisable. Chin supportive strapping is recommended while substantial postoperative soft tissue edema is present. Periosteal layer closure in buccal sulcus incisions is achievable if exposure is created with this goal in mind. Wherever feasible, an effort should be made to achieve closure of periosteum and muscle origins followed by mucosal closure in a double-layered wound approximation.

Management of Ballistic and Avulsive Injuries of the Face

Gunshot wounds to the face have recently been reported to be associated with a mortality of 14.5% all due to injuries other than the facial wound. This relatively high mortality, despite modern trauma resuscitation protocols, emphasizes the need for particular care in the early management of individuals injured in this way.[29]

Low-energy ballistic injuries do not differ significantly from blunt trauma in their effects on the damaged parts and management is the same. In marked contradistinction, high-energy avulsive and ballistic injuries have a different pathophysiology. The zone of tissue injury sustaining direct impact is typically avulsed, pulverized, destroyed by the impact. This

detachment is necessary non-resorbable sutures should be used to resuspend the cheek tissue. We use two 2-0 nylon sutures from the periosteum of the cheek and infraorbital region to the deep temporal fascia above and lateral to the frontozygomatic suture.

Lateral canthal descent is commonly seen after treatment of orbital trauma requiring extensive periosteal detachment. Where a lateral canthotomy has been performed for access, the lower tarsal plate should be directly reattached to the lateral orbital rim. We have observed relatively frequent abnormalities of contour of the palpebral fissure where lateral canthotomy and cantholysis have been performed for access. Other workers have reported a similar experience.[28] After a period of enthusiasm our current practice is to avoid lateral canthotomy in accessing the orbit. Where a canthotomy is not performed the lateral canthal orbital septum is grasped

zone typically widens from the surface point of impact as the energy imparted dissipates through the affected tissues and secondary projectiles (bones and teeth) are recruited. Surrounding the resulting zone of tissue necrosis exists a zone of relative tissue injury, the extent of which varies with the degree of energy transferred. Within this zone of relative injury an evolving pattern of tissue loss develops over ensuing days. Previously marginally viable tissues may become necrotic as the massive swelling associated with an acute inflammatory response and bacterial insult combine to adversely affect areas of marginal perfusion. Ultimately, the inflammatory response subsides, macrophage infiltration is seen at tissue level and the contused soft tissue components heal with a variable degree of internal fibrosis, depending upon the magnitude of the injury sustained. The effects of fibrosis are to render affected areas variably hypovascular, rigid and contracted.

What previous generations of surgeons have learnt is the primacy of an adequate blood supply. At each stage the surgical team seeks to exert a favorable influence by minimizing the potential for further bacterial insult and avoiding any intervention which may add surgical trauma in the wound evolution stage or otherwise adversely impact upon tissue perfusion. The essential difference between what is proposed here and more traditional management protocols is one of timing. High-energy ballistic and avulsive wounds have largely been managed with a regimen of debridement, sequential dressings, external skeletal fixation and delayed secondary reconstruction following scar maturation. The problem with this strategy is that fibrosis with contracture fixes soft tissues and displaced bone segments in rigid, hypovascular, collagen-rich scar. Deformity occurring as a consequence is often impossible to correct secondarily. Collapse of the central facial region is frequently seen. The use of external fixators to maintain the spatial relationship of major bony fragments, and thus associated soft tissue relationships, is all too frequently frustrated by fibrosis, shrinkage and collapse inwards of intervening bone and soft tissue. Thus, while tissue perfusion has been maximized by minimal interference, the ultimate functional and esthetic outcome is frequently compromised.

It is for these reasons that treatment protocols which seek to optimize functional and esthetic outcome, without compromising safety, utilizing serial debridement and a delayed primary reconstruction are gaining increasing acceptance in civilian practice.[30] These are complex injuries with potential loss of mucosal lining, bone and overlying soft tissue, which will have serious consequences for the affected functional and esthetic subunits of the face. Management of these injuries challenges the resourcefulness of the resuscitation team, the maxillofacial trauma surgical team and rehabilitation specialties. These patients, managed according to the described protocol, will also challenge the resources of all but large hospitals.

Having secured the airway, active external bleeding is controlled. Truncal, head and limb injuries take precedence over facial injuries in the early (day 1) management. It is, however, frequently possible to perform an initial debride-

ment concurrently with the management of trunk or limb emergency treatment. In managing bleeding in the head and neck region, care is taken to preserve vascular pedicles which may be used later in definitive reconstruction. However, expanding hematomata should be investigated with angiography and embolization performed where indicated. After resuscitation and treatment of life-threatening problems a tracheostomy is performed, replacing the orotracheal tube. Even if the airway is patent, massive swelling is to be anticipated over the ensuing 48 hours. Necrotic soft tissue is excised, fragments of teeth and devitalized detached bone fragments are removed. Significant bone fragments attached to viable soft tissue should be left undisturbed. Severed branches of the facial nerve are repaired or tagged for later identification. The wound is copiously lavaged with a warmed normal saline solution and broad-spectrum antimicrobials are administered.

Following this initial procedure an intermediate phase of wound management ensues the purpose of which is wound stabilization. This phase is necessitated by the evolving pattern of tissue loss seen where high levels of energy are imparted to the tissues. The treatment strategy is to minimize loss of marginally viable tissue by doing nothing which further impairs tissue perfusion and to control all variables that lead to bacterial growth. Hematomata, persistent dead space, retained foreign bodies and necrotic tissue are the principal culprits favoring infection. To stabilize the wound, planned serial re-exploration is performed every 24–36 hours. Any necrotic tissue is debrided, hematoma evacuated, the wound lavaged and an antibiotic-impregnated non-adherent dressing applied.

Robertson & Manson[30] advocate reduction and fixation of fractures within the first day or so after admission, with primary closure of wounds or advancement of mucosa to skin where tissue loss has occurred. The authors cite optimal support for soft tissue healing as their reason for early skeletal fixation by wide exposure and direct fixation, and minimization of bacterial colonization as the reason for early wound closure. Until further evidence emerges demonstrating the safety of such an approach, we do not advocate the use of such aggressive intervention during the wound stabilization period. Attempts to advance tissues and achieve closure early in the wound evolution may lead to tension, and thus ischemia, of already vulnerable wound margins as progressive and gross tissue edema develop. As swelling starts to resolve and the wound stabilizes, generally after 72 hours, primary closure of wounds becomes safe. Serial evaluation in the operating theater is repeated until no further debridement is required and the wound is stable and viable.

By day 5–10 definitive management is possible. The principles of definitive management are the same as that for blunt trauma and low-velocity ballistic injuries. Precise skeletal fixation is achieved by appropriate exposure and internal fixation of bone segments, with primary bone grafting of midfacial defects. Restoration and maintenance of correct spatial relationships to support the soft tissue drape is emphasized. The survival of bone grafts, and that of major fragments converted to free grafts by wide exposure, is dependent upon a well-vascularized and complete soft tissue cover. This often presents a considerable challenge in the management of high-energy avulsive and ballistic injuries.

Rotation and advancement of tissue within the zone of relative injury requires careful judgment and can be hazardous. Where there has been loss of mucosal lining, as well as bone and other soft tissues, composite free flap transfer is usually indicated. Where there has been considerable soft tissue loss in the absence of a skeletal defect we would also give serious consideration to the import of a soft tissue

---

Key points

- Initial debridement is followed by an evolving pattern of tissue loss

- Serial debridement is performed during the evolution phase to stabilize the wound

- Wound stabilization is followed by primary reconstruction

---

flap. Where free tissue transfer is employed recipient vessels outside the zone of relative injury should be utilized. Once the definitive reconstruction has stabilized, secondary revision of bulky or color-mismatched tissue can be performed. Serial excision of skin flaps is frequently possible with rotation or advancement of local skin without disturbing now well-established spatial relationships.

Management of Fractures of the Edentulous Maxilla

Trauma in the elderly is an increasing phenomenon due to increased longevity. It is reckoned that in the USA the geriatric population will have expanded by 50% in 2050. Around 6% of maxillary fractures occur in the edentulous.[31] As in the dentate, fractures of the edentulous maxilla are less common than mandibular fractures until the age of 65 years, when the incidence of maxillary fractures equals that of mandibular injuries.[32] The probable explanations are the increasing maxillary pneumatization that occurs with age, the declining bone resilience, and atrophy of the relatively strong alveolar process. Maxillary fractures in the elderly population tend therefore to be more comminuted.

Triage of the elderly patient who has sustained a facial injury is crucial at the outset of treatment. The in-hospital mortality rate for elderly patients with a craniomaxillofacial injury in one review was 11.1%. This reflected the likelihood of a coexistent head injury and the fact that this age group may have significant coexisting disease. The Glasgow Coma Scale and trauma scores have a direct relation to eventual outcome. In the group of patients above, the significant mortality rate occurred predominantly in those with a lower GCS and a higher trauma score.

Non-union is extremely rare in the maxilla and for undisplaced or minimally displaced fractures, where there is no obvious comminution, simple management with a soft diet and appropriate analgesics will allow adequate healing.

Where definitive surgical management of the fractured edentulous maxilla is indicated the goals are the same as in the dentate population. Facial height, width and anterior projection must be restored with anatomical reduction of the facial buttresses. Primary bone grafting and augmentation of the anterior and middle facial buttresses should form an integral part of the definitive management.[31]

In our own practice we have observed a high incidence of malposition of the Le Fort I segment in the open reduction and internal fixation of edentulous fractures. We believe this to be a consequence of the lack of intraoperative visual clues to guide the correct positioning of this alveolus-palatal fragment. An overreliance on the correct reassembly of comminuted buttresses is the operative strategy we believe to be directly responsible. Errors have occurred in all three dimensions with the maxilla rotated, canted and retro-

---

Key points and pitfalls

- Comminution is likely to be present

- Buttress reconstruction augmented with bone graft is often required

- Overreliance on reassembly of comminuted fragments will frequently result in malposition of the Le Fort I segment

- Use of dentures or splints and intraoperative intermaxillary fixation is recommended

---

positioned. Whilst some of these errors can be compensated for in denture construction this is by no means universally the case. Dentures and acrylic splints can provide useful aids to the repositioning of the maxilla where the mandible is intact and therefore reduction of mandibular fractures, when present, is essential. We advocate the use of some form of prosthesis which allows for intraoperative intermaxillary fixation in all cases where open reduction and internal fixation are undertaken.

References

1 Rowe NL, Killey HC 1968 Fractures of the facial skeleton, 2nd edn. Churchill Livingstone, Edinburgh

2 Wolfe SA 1997 The influence of Paul Tessier on our current treatment of facial trauma, both in primary care and in the management of late sequelae. Clinics in Plastic Surgery 24: 515– 518

3 O'Sullivan ST, Snyder BJ, Moore MH, David DJ 1999 Outcome measurement of the treatment of maxillary fractures: a prospective analysis of 100 consecutive cases. British Journal of Plastic Surgery 52: 519–523

4 Manson PN, Glassman D, Vanderkolk C, Petty P, Crawley WA 1990 Rigid stabilization of sagittal fractures of the maxilla and palate. Plastic and Reconstructive Surgery 85: 711–717

5 Gruss JS 1986 Complex nasoethmoid-orbital and midfacial fractures: role of craniofacial surgical techniques and immediate bone grafting. Annals of Plastic Surgery 17: 377–390

6 Jackson IT 1986 Classification and treatment of orbitozygomatic and orbitoethmoid fractures. The place of bone grafting and plate fixation. Annals of Plastic Surgery 16: 77–81

7 Guerrissi JO 1996 Maxillofacial injuries scale. Journal of Craniofacial Surgery 7: 130–132

8 Girotto JA, McKenzie E, Fowler C, Redett R, Robertson B, Manson PN 2001 Long-term physical impairment and functional outcomes after complex facial fractures. Plastic and Reconstructive Surgery 108: 312–327

9 Al-Quiranny JA, Stassen LF, Dutton GN, Moos KF, EI-Attar A 1991 Diplopia following midfacial fractures. British Journal of Oral and Maxillofacial Surgery 29: 302–309

10 Haug RH, Adams JM, Jordan RB 1995 Comparison of the morbidity associated with maxillary fractures treated by maxillomandibular and rigid internal fixation. Oral Surgery, Oral Medicine, Oral Pathology, Oral Radiology and Endodontics 80: 629–637

11 Gruss JS 1995 Advances in craniofacial fracture repair. Scandinavian Journal of Plastic and Reconstructive Hand Surgery 27 (suppl): 67–81

12 Foster RD, Anthony JP, Singer MI, Kaplan MJ, Pogrel MA, Mathes SJ 1997 Reconstruction of complex midfacial defects. Plastic and Reconstructive Surgery 99: 1555–1565

13 Manson PN, Clark N, Robertson B et al 1999 Subunit principles in midfacial fractures: the importance of sagittal buttresses, soft tissue reductions, and sequencing treatment of segmental fractures. Plastic and Reconstructive Surgery 103: 1287–1306

14 Caron G, Paquin R, Lessard MR, Trepanier CA, Landry P-E 2000 Submental endotracheal intubation: an alternative to tracheotomy in patients with midfacial and panfacial fractures. Journal of Trauma 48: 235–240

15 Gruss JS, Mackinnon SE 1986 Complex maxillary fractures: role of buttress reconstruction and immediate bone grafts. Plastic and Reconstructive Surgery 78: 9–22

16 Stanley RB 1990 Rigid fixation of fractures of the maxillary complex. Facial Plastic Surgery 7: 176–184

17 Hendrickson M, Clark N, Manson PN et al 1998 Palatal fractures: classification, patterns, treatment with rigid internal fixation. Plastic and Reconstructive Surgery 101: 319–332

18 Rimmell F, Marenette LJ 1993 Injuries of the hard palate and the horizontal buttress of the midface. Otolaryngology Head and Neck Surgery 109: 499–505

19 Denny AD, Celik N 1999 A management strategy for palatal fractures: a 12 year review. Journal of Craniofacial Surgery 10: 49–57

20 Manson PN, Glassman D, Vanderkolk C, Petty P, Crawley WA 1990 Rigid stabilization of sagittal fractures of the maxilla and palate. Plastic and Reconstructive Surgery 85: 711–717

21 Persson M, Thilender B 1977 Palatal suture closure in man from 15 to 35 years of age. American Journal of Orthodontics 72: 42–51

22 Ellis E, Tharanon W 1992 Facial width problems associated with rigid fixation of mandibular fractures. Journal of Oral and Maxillofacial Surgery 50: 87–94

23 Marker P, Nielsen A, Bastian HL 2000 Fractures of the mandibular condyle. Part 1: Patterns of distribution and causes of fracture in 348 patients. British Journal of Oral and Maxillofacial Surgery 38: 417–421

24 Donald PJ, Ettin M 1986 The safety of frontal sinus fat obliteration when sinus walls are missing. Laryngoscope 92: 190–193

25 Gruss JS, Pollock RA, Phillips JH, Antonyshyn O 1989 Combined injuries to the cranium and the face. British Journal of Plastic Surgery 42: 385–398

26 Moss CJ, Mendelson BC, Taylor GI 2000 Surgical anatomy of the ligamentous adhesions in the temple and periorbital regions. Plastic and Reconstructive Surgery 105: 1475–1490

27 Furnas DW 1989 The retaining ligaments of the cheek. Plastic and Reconstructive Surgery 83: 11–16

28 Yaremchuk MJ 1999 Orbital deformity after craniofacial fracture repair: avoidance and treatment. Journal of Craniomaxillofacial Trauma 5: 7–12

29 Demetriades D, Chahwan S, Gomez H, Falabella A, Velmahos G, Yamashita D 1998 Initial evaluation and management of gunshot wounds to the face. Journal of Trauma 45: 39–41

30 Robertson B, Manson PN 1999 High energy ballistic and avulsive injuries. Surgical Clinics of North America 79: 1489–1502

31 Crawley WA, Azman P, Clark N et al 1997 The edentulous Le Fort fracture. Journal of Craniofacial Surgery 8: 298–306

32 Farmand M, Bauman A 1992 The treatment of the fractured edentulous maxilla. Journal of Craniomaxillofacial Surgery 20: 341–344

15 Mandible Fractures: Principles of Treatment

Bernard J Costello, Ramon L Ruiz

Introduction

Over the past three decades, there has been a rapid development of techniques used in the management of craniomaxillofacial trauma. The most significant advancements related to the management of fractures of the mandible are based on specific technical refinements in the rigid internal fixation methods now routinely utilized. Contemporary mandible fracture management techniques have allowed for decreased infection rates and biological stable fixation of bone segments. This philosophy produces bony union and restoration of preinjury occlusion and normally eliminates the need for wire maxillomandibular immobilization. All this adds up to a faster, safer, more comfortable return to function.[1] The aim of this chapter is to present an overview of general treatment principles and outline major advances in the management of mandibular fractures.

Historical perspectives

Historical references to mandible fracture diagnosis and treatment date back to 1650 BC as evidenced by the Edwin Smith Surgical Papyrus.[2,3] The patient described ultimately succumbed, likely from infection secondary to the mandibular fracture. Hippocrates also described the treatment of mandible fractures with circumferential dental wiring in some of his initial writings.[4] However, it was Salicetti, in 1275, who first presented maxillomandibular fixation as a treatment for fractures of the mandible.[5,6] Much later, Gilmer was the first to apply the technique clinically and describe its utility in more detail.[7,8]

Despite a few early attempts at rigid internal fixation, for most of the 20th century[9,10] the management of mandibular and maxillary fractures was limited to the application of maxillomandibular fixation or Gunning-type splints for the edentulous. Later external frames were used in combination with pin fixation. Fracture treatment by open approach and direct transosseous wiring was avoided in the preantibiotic era since it almost inevitably produced infection and osteomyelitis. It was reserved for use in select cases involving the posterior mandible (i.e. ramus/angle) or in edentulous patients.[11] In the German-speaking countries, surgeons like Luhr and Spiessl reintroduced the idea of utilizing miniature bone plates in the repair of mandibular fractures in 1968 and 1972.[12]

In 1976, Spiessl and others continued to advance techniques of open reduction and internal fixation (ORIF) and developed the principles now advocated by the Arbeitsgemeinschaft fur Osteosynthesefragen (Association for Osteosynthesis/Association for the Study of Internal Fixation (AO/ASIF).[13] This concept was unfortunately based on trying to 'fit' orthopedic principles and, worse, orthopedic materials to the complex and very different structures of the facial skeleton. The belief was that callus formation represented a failure of the healing process, because of excessive and undesirable movements across the fracture. Thus more heavy and complex methods were devised to increase the stability across the fracture. These plates were bulky, difficult to use and always required large skin incisions. This philosophy failed to see that perfectly good reduction and healing could be achieved by very unstable fixation methods like wiring of the teeth together. Whilst mandibular maxillary wire fixation was potentially dangerous and unpleasant, it was very effective in healing bones. These crude, heavy plating systems did, however, demonstrate the benefits of avoiding wire maxillomandibular fixation, including comfort, return to normal mastication and normal oral function.

It is interesting how local cultures and traditions fashioned these developments. It was normal practice in some centers for patients with their teeth wired together to remain in hospital for the 6 weeks of fixation. It is hardly surprising therefore that the complications of these compression plating systems seemed like a step forward compared with 6 weeks in hospital. In reality, these heavy compression plates had a high morbidity. The neck scars were undesirable, nerve damage to both the facial and inferior alveolar nerves was common and infection of the plates frequent, and a second operation to remove the plates always necessary. Despite the compression and bicortical screws, it is likely that resorption around the screws meant the system was not very stable during the 6–8 weeks of bone healing. Biomechanically, the bicortical screws forced the plates into the wrong position, at the lower border of the mandible. The principles of heavy compression plating could not be applied to the thin bones of the upper facial skeleton.

One useful technique to arise from this principle of applying orthopedic material to the facial skeleton was the use of lag screws, which is a simple technique of producing interfragmentary stability by compression. These have a large screw hole bored on the outer fragment and allow the tightening of the screw to compress the fragments together. In a few sites in the mandible it can be a simple effective treatment via the intraoral approach but since the screw must cross the fracture at right angles it has limited use.

The AO group must be congratulated on its excellent educational record, excellent research history and advancing the better care of patients.

In 1973, Michelet introduced techniques for mandible fixation utilizing smaller 'miniplates', placed via the transoral approach. The principle was rather like a suspension bridge, to define lines of tension in a fracture. This meant smaller, thinner, lighter plates could be used. Importantly, however, because of the smaller 'miniplates', monocortical screws were used, allowing the plate to be placed in lines of tension, not in places where bicortical screws could be used.[14] Champy further refined and researched these techniques. From his work these techniques have become standard clinical practice.[15] The use of small miniplates was successfully extended into the rest of the facial skeleton, being refined and miniaturized for the periorbital and cranial non-load bearing areas.

Most recently, bone-plating systems made from resorbable polymer have been introduced. Although these materials show significant promise, they have been utilized most often in the non-load bearing cranial and orbital regions. Published reports examining the use of resorbable hardware in the maxillofacial skeleton are limited and, to date, many manufacturers have not approved their plating systems for use in the mandible.[16] Despite some encouraging clinical reports and growing enthusiasm among surgeons, a careful analysis of outcome measures using these materials and critical evaluation of their potential advantages must be completed before widespread use is advocated. The resorbable materials themselves and the techniques used in their application continue to be redefined at a rapid pace in this early phase of development.[17,18]

Epidemiology

The circumstances and pattern of injury to the mandible are variable based upon the population studied as well as the environment in which they live. Etiologies of mandible fractures include assault, motor vehicle crashes, work-related injury, falls, sport-related injury, pathologic fractures and projectile missiles. The Canniesburn trauma database, which has been running for nearly three decades, uses the following categories:

- assault
- road traffic accidents
- sports injuries
- industrial or workplace accidents
- 'falls', which may be a trip or a medical syncope. Some patients state this as a cause when they are punched to the ground, which is a weakness of this section.

Several authors examining the incidence of mandibular fracture have reported differences between their respective clinical settings. In urban populations, the most frequent cause of mandibular fractures was interpersonal violence, while surgeons in more rural areas found motor vehicle crashes to be the most common etiology.

Haug completed a 5-year review of facial trauma in a mostly urban setting and found assault to be the most common cause of isolated mandibular fractures.[19] Ellis et al reviewed 2137 facial trauma cases over a 10-year period and found that mandible fractures were present in 45% of cases.[20] In this series in urban Scotland, motor vehicle crashes comprised only 15% of the fracture cases. Olson et al's review of cases in more rural Iowa had 48% of fractures caused by motor vehicle crashes.[21] Adekey reviewed the facial trauma in Nigeria and found that approximately 76% of the cases were caused during motor vehicle crashes.[22]

State-of-the-Art Management

Diagnosis

The diagnosis of mandibular fractures must begin with a careful history and clinical examination. Immediate attention must always be given to problems associated with airway compromise and bleeding which may endanger the patient's life. The immediate care of the traumatized patient is covered in other chapters. In outline, however, once the airway, breathing and circulation have been adequately assessed, a quick neurologic function evaluation should be performed. If the patient requires intubation, it is helpful to assess neurologic function prior to placement of the endotracheal tube. Standard trauma protocols such as those described in the Advanced Trauma Life Support guidelines from the American College of Surgeons should be utilized for a comprehensive evaluation.

In eliciting a history, information about the mechanism of injury will often suggest a specific fracture pattern and may provide the surgeon with valuable insight regarding the potential for concomitant injuries. Patients who sustain fractures involving the mandible will often report a paresthesia or change in their occlusion noted immediately after the traumatic event. In addition to focused questions about the traumatic event, the surgeon must carefully review the patient's past medical and surgical history, medication use and known drug allergies. Temporomandibular joint dysfunction and any previous non-surgical or surgical treatment should be carefully documented.

When a mandibular fracture is suspected, meticulous clinical examination of the maxillofacial region is critical and should be carried out prior to the ordering of radiographic imaging studies. A number of symptoms and clinical findings are highly suggestive of mandibular fracture and are listed in Box 15.1. Without question, a change in occlusion is the most common physical finding in patients with fractures of the mandible. When examining the occlusion, it is important to consider that the patient may have had an abnormal dental or skeletal occlusal relationship (Class II or Class III) prior to the injury. Changes in occlusion will likely accompany fractures of the mandible, but may also be present in soft tissue trauma of the TMJ, fractures of the alveolus, dental fractures or fractures of the maxilla. When the fracture traverses a region of the mandible that includes the inferior alveolar nerve, some level of neurosensory disturbance involving this nerve will result. Abnormalities in the mandibular range of motion or deviation of the mandible are also indicative of fracture, as can

Box 15.1   Signs and symptoms of mandible fractures

- Change in occlusion
- Paresthesia anesthesia or dysesthesia
- Localized pain
- Altered range of motion/deviation of the mandible
- Changes in facial contour, symmetry and dental arch form
- Lacerations, hematoma, ecchymosis
- Mobility of teeth
- Crepitus or mobility of bone segments
- Palpable bony steps

be an inability to close completely. These restrictions may also be the result of internal TMJ injury or hematoma. Sublingual ecchymosis is highly suggestive of a fracture involving the mandibular arch form. Another indication of fracture is a bony step which is most easily recognized by careful palpation along the inferior border of the mandible.

Radiographic studies

In clinical situations where the mechanism of injury or physical findings are suggestive of a fracture of the mandible, radiographic studies are necessary to confirm the diagnosis and plan subsequent treatment. In principle, these should be at least two films taken at right angles to each other. There is a tendency in accident and emergency departments to keep taking films until a fracture is seen. It is important therefore for these departments to be given protocols by the maxillofacial department on which films should be taken and when to progress to special investigations like CT scans.

When isolated mandibular fracture is suspected, the standard radiographic assessment consists of a panoramic radiograph and one additional posteroanterior view of the mandible (usually an open mouth Towne's) (Fig. 15.1). A diagnostic-quality panoramic radiograph is the most comprehensive view possible with a single film and allows satisfactory visualization of all regions of the mandible (condyle, ramus, body and symphysis).[23] It is also useful in examining the existing dentition, presence of impacted teeth with respect to the fracture, alveolar process and position of the mandibular canal. The panoramic tomogram also includes the maxilla and some of the midfacial structures, but not at the same level of quality as the mandible. The Towne's view adds another anatomic dimension and is especially useful in ruling out displaced condylar fractures. Some machines will produce selective tomograms of the temporomandibular regions as well (Fig. 15.2). Dedicated tomograms or transcranial views of the TMJ can be obtained as separate studies to further delineate the displacement of fractured segments. In situations where a panoramic view of the mandible is not

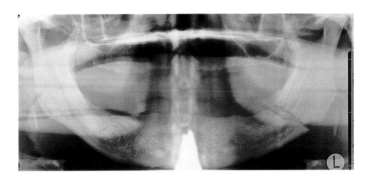

(a)

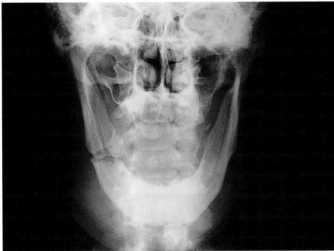

(b)

Fig. 15.1: (a) Panoramic tomogram of left mandibular angle fracture in an edentulous patient. **(b)** Reverse Towne's view of right mandibular angle fracture.

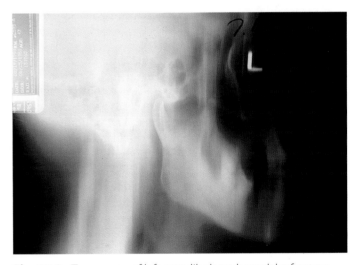

Fig. 15.2: Tomogram of left mandibular subcondylar fracture.

available, a series of different views of the mandible is required to adequately view all the anatomic regions of interest. This is more labor intensive and costly and subjects the patient to a higher dose of radiation. Despite the good visualization of the dentoalveolar structures obtained by a panoramic radiograph, additional periapical or occlusal radiographs are often helpful in viewing specific areas of

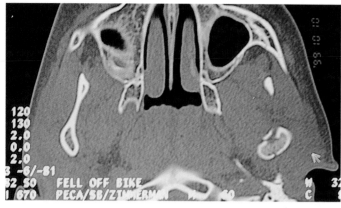

(a)

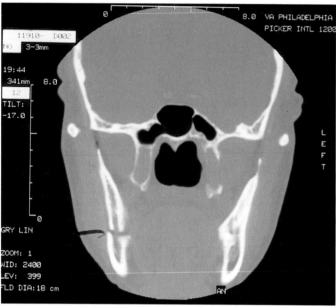

(b)

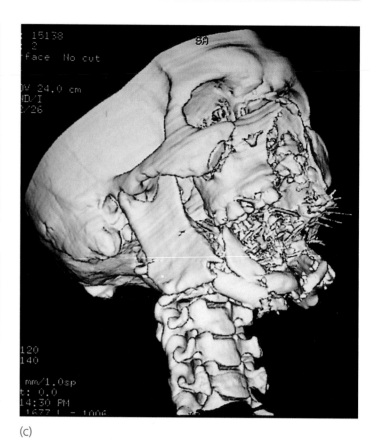

(c)

Fig. 15.3: (a) Axial CT scan of pediatric left condylar head fracture (intracapsular). **(b)** Coronal CT scan of right mandibular ramus fracture. **(c)** Three-dimensional reconstruction CT of a massive comminution injury to both the mandible and maxilla from a self-inflicted gunshot.

concern with more detail, especially when tooth or alveolar fractures are suspected. Parasymphysis fractures often benefit from occlusal films to display any obliquity of the fracture, which will certainly change the fixation methods.

One of the most compelling reasons for utilizing a panoramic radiograph as part of the initial evaluation of isolated mandibular fractures is its subsequent use during the postoperative period. Even in cases where more extensive radiographic studies are ordered at the time of the initial assessment, it is the panoramic view that is subsequently obtained and utilized to follow the patient's long-term progress. This likely has to do with the excellent visualization, availability and cost effectiveness of the radiographic study.

Computed tomography (CT) currently offers the most detailed and comprehensive view of the facial skeleton. Current protocols allow for axial, coronal and reconstructed three-dimensional images to be formulated (Fig. 15.3). Despite this superior three-dimensional visualization, the use of CT scans for the diagnosis of isolated mandibular fractures is uncommon and may be cost-prohibitive. In the authors'

experience, the use of CT scans is reserved for cases involving complex (comminuted, avulsive, etc.) mandibular injuries or concomitant midfacial or orbital injuries. In some cases where a condylar fracture is suspected, the CT will allow for detailed three-dimensional imaging. Another useful application of the CT scan is in clinical situations (cervical spine injury, head injury) where the patient is not able to submit to routine radiographic positioning and techniques. Very young patients with limited co-operation may also be candidates for CT scan evaluation, but will often require sedation during the study. When the CT scan is utilized, 2 mm incremental axial and coronal cuts usually allow for detailed imaging of the facial skeleton.

Other studies can be helpful in very specific circumstances, but are rarely required. Magnetic resonance imaging (MRI) is of very limited value in evaluating bony injuries. It may be helpful to delineate injuries to the intracapsular structures of the TMJ, associated soft tissues or in cases of condylar displacement into the middle cranial fossa. Ultrasound has occasionally been used to determine condylar position after fractures. Angiography in conjunction with interventional

Box 15.2 Classification of mandible fractures

Relationship of fracture segments
Simple: No external contamination
Compound: Communication with the external environment
Comminuted: Multiple segments of bone that have been splintered or crushed
Greenstick: One cortex is compromised, but the other is intact
Pathologic: Pre-existing disease or lesion associated with a fracture site
Multiple: Two or more lines of fracture on the same bone, but not communicating with one another
Impacted: One fragment is telescoped within the adjacent fragment
Atrophic: Decreased bony mass of the fractured bone in question
Indirect: Fracture is present at a site distant from the point of impact
Complex: Associated soft tissue injury

Anatomic
Symphysis
Body
Angle
Ramus
Coronoid
Condylar process
Dentulous
Partially edentulous
Edentulous
Primary or mixed dentition

Biomechanical
Favorable: Muscle pull will tend to keep the fracture reduced
Unfavorable: Muscle pull will tend to distract the segments

radiology techniques can be utilized in situations where significant bleeding is associated with facial fractures.[24–29]

Classification of mandible fractures

The classification scheme for fractures involving the mandible is based on previous orthopedic experience. Despite some similarities, a number of important differences exist between long bones and the mandible. These include differences in the developmental pattern, presence of the dentition, complex muscle attachments and simultaneously active bilateral articulations. Fractures of the mandible are often described using terms that refer to the relationship of the fractured segments, anatomic region, associated muscular anatomy and/or the involvement of the dentition. Box 15.2 outlines the different terms utilized. The influence of the pterygomasseteric muscle sling with respect to displacement of the fractured bone ends must be taken into account especially when consideration is given to closed management of the fracture (Fig. 15.4). Most fractures are most accurately described utilizing a combination of terms.

Treatment

Surgical access

Closed techniques

There is a subgroup of patients who present with mandibular fractures and may require essentially no treatment. These are cases in which the mandible appears stable, the fracture pattern is favorable, there is no displacement of the bone segments or change in occlusion and the patient is motivated to be compliant. Management in these rare instances consists of careful observation, liquid diet and limited physical activity. The patient must be kept under relatively close clinical surveillance and the surgeon must remain prepared to change the treatment plan should any change in the clinical situation arise. If occlusal discrepancies or other signs of fracture displacement develop, then either closed or open reduction techniques should be implemented early.

When mandibular fractures are treated with closed reduction, the clinician depends on some type of external stabilization method. Currently, the most common form of external stabilization consists of Erich arch bars, which are applied to the maxilla and mandible using circumdental wire ligatures and wire loops used to achieve maxillomandibular fixation (Fig. 15.5). Other jaw-wiring methods include Ivy loops, Stout wiring, Ernst and Gilmer ligatures. Some commercially available products have attempted to make the process of applying maxillomandibular fixation faster. Bonded arch bar systems tend to be cumbersome to place due to the need for an absolutely dry field during the bonding procedure and require that the patient's dentition be in good condition. Another system for achieving maxillomandibular fixation involves the use of bone screws, which are modified to allow for passage of a wire ligature. One of the potential complications of such a system is that the surgeon may unintentionally distract the condyles out of their glenoid fossae when the fixation wires are overtightened. Edentulous and partially edentulous patients with severe fractures may benefit from the use of occlusal splints (Gunning-type) to maintain interocclusal dimension and re-establish arch relationships. At times massive comminution of the mandible with significant soft tissue loss may benefit from a period of external pin fixation (Fig. 15.6**a**). When soft tissue loss compromises the quality of coverage, then this technique should be considered. Acrylic bars can be easily fabricated with the aid of an endotracheal tube and acrylic resin. The reaction is exothermic, so great care should be taken to avoid burning the patient's skin during the bar's fabrication (Fig. 15.6**b**).

Despite the tremendous advances in maxillofacial plating system technology, there remain a number of good indications for the implementation of closed reduction and external fixation techniques in the management of mandibular fractures. Certainly non-displaced, stable fractures of the mandible, as described above, may lend themselves to closed management. One of the most appropriate indications for closed reduction is a grossly comminuted fracture where there may be a number of small bony fragments within the injured segment. In comminuted fractures, the periosteal stripping required for an open approach may result in a loss of

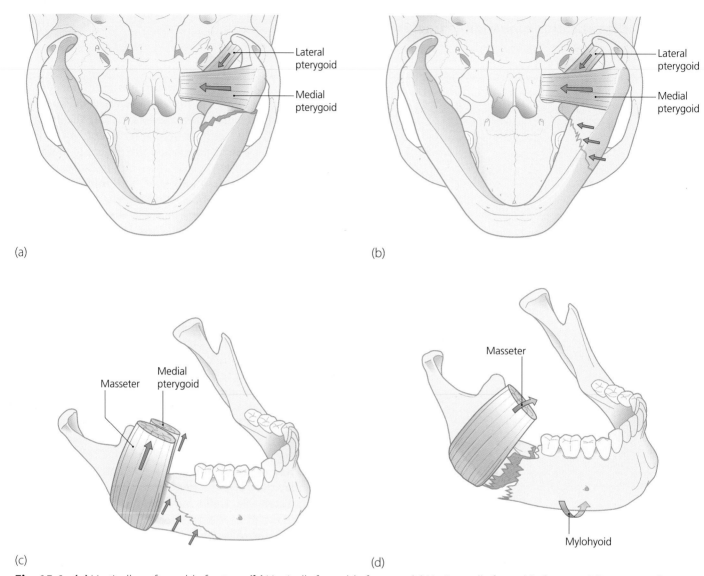

Fig. 15.4: **(a)** Vertically unfavorable fracture. **(b)** Vertically favorable fracture. **(c)** Horizontally favorable fracture. **(d)** Horizontally unfavorable fracture.

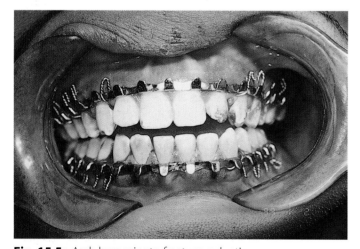

Fig. 15.5: Arch bars prior to fracture reduction.

vascular supply and necrosis of the smaller bone fragments. This is especially relevant in mandibular fractures associated with gunshot wounds where additional hard and soft tissue necrosis is anticipated for several weeks following the initial

injury. Another relative indication for closed reduction of a mandibular fracture is when a compromised soft tissue matrix is present. This may be the result of a pre-existing condition (e.g. radiation therapy) or related to the traumatic injury which caused the fracture itself (e.g. avulsive loss of tissue).

Perhaps the most commonly utilized and valuable role for closed reduction of a mandibular fracture is in the treatment of pediatric patients. Stabilization of pediatric mandibular fractures should be accomplished using the least invasive modality possible. Surgeons treating a child with a mandibular fracture must be aware of developing tooth buds that can be damaged when applying bone plates and screw fixation.[30] In addition, closed reduction and external stabilization obviates the need for incisions and subperiosteal dissection in the growing skeleton of a child. When the patient is in the deciduous or early mixed dentition, adequate stability of arch bars using only circumdental ligatures may be difficult. Often arch bars and skeletal segments may be better stabilized using adjunctive maneuvers such as circummandibular, circumzygomatic and/or piriform aperture wires. Pediatric fractures

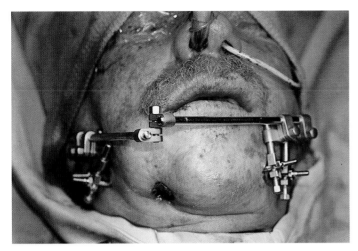

(a)

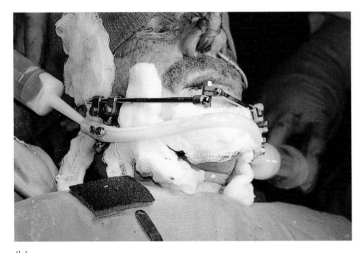

(b)

Fig. 15.6: **(a)** External fixator reduction apparatus prior to acrylic bar fabrication. **(b)** fabrication of acrylic bar with endotracheal tube and moist gauze to avoid thermal injury.

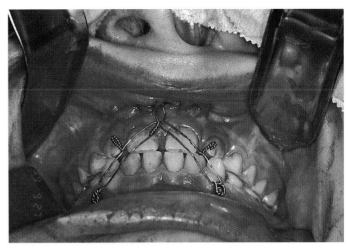

Fig. 15.7: Skeletal fixation in a pediatric patient in the mixed dentition with mandibular fractures. Piriform rim wires, circummandibular wires and slave maxillomandibular fixation wires are shown.

involving the mandibular arch form may be effectively managed utilizing a lingual splint and circummandibular wires (Fig. 15.7).

Open reduction

With the advent of miniplates and monocortical screws, it has become widely accepted that most fractures involving the craniomaxillofacial skeleton are best treated via open reduction, normally using the intraoral route, and internal fixation techniques. An open approach gives the surgeon the best visualization of the fracture ends and therefore allows for the best possible anatomic reduction. Fractures involving the mandibular symphysis, parasymphysis, body and angle regions may be successfully approached through a transoral incision and dissection. The rich blood supply of the maxillofacial skeleton allows for wide subperiosteal dissection and exposure of the mandible without compromising the vascularity and subsequent healing of the skeletal segments.

Transoral approaches begin with a vestibular incision where care is taken to preserve at least 5–7 mm of tissue from the mucogingival junction to avoid damage to the attached periodontal tissues and subsequent dehiscence. In the anterior mandible, the mentalis muscles are initially divided during the dissection towards the mandible. During closure, these paired muscles must be reapproximated using interrupted sutures as a separate layer. This avoids the 'witch's chin' deformity and covers the injured area with robust tissue for healing. Care should be taken to avoid the mental nerves as they exit the mental foramen near the bicuspid root tip region. Full exposure of the buccal surface of the inferior border is required to place adequate fixation.

The ramus, angle and body of the mandible are easily approached through a posterior vestibular incision. This incision starts along the inferior third of the external oblique ridge and courses approximately 5–7 mm below and parallel to the mucogingival junction. Full-thickness mucoperiosteal flaps are elevated to easily visualize these areas. Some medial ramus dissection and stripping of the temporalis tendon is sometimes helpful to fully expose the region and visualize the extent of the fracture morphology, but care must be taken to avoid the inferior alveolar neurovascular bundle as it enters the mandible on the medial surface. The transoral approach normally allows direct placement of hardware across most mandibular fracture sites; the combination of a transoral dissection with a percutaneous trocar usually allows treatment of the few other fractures, like condylar neck fractures, where the transoral routine alone is not possible. When used carefully, the trocar will often allow for placement of bone plates along the inferior border of the mandible, which of course is only exceptionally needed in rare grossly comminuted fractures.

There are also a number of techniques for approaching the mandible using cutaneous or extraoral incisions. While it is possible to approach the entire mandible from an external approach, approaches that require skin incisions are usually reserved for fractures involving the condylar neck, grossly comminuted fractures and a few severely atrophic fractures (<10 mm of mandibular height). Fractures in the anterior region can be approached through a submental incision but most are dealt with more effectively through an intraoral approach without the need for external scarring (Fig. 15.8a).

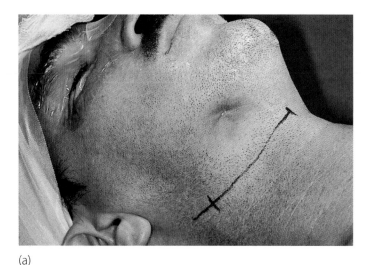
(a)

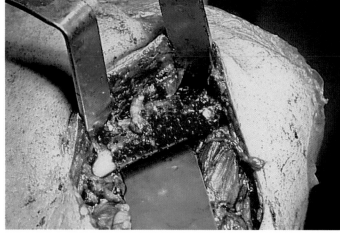
(b)

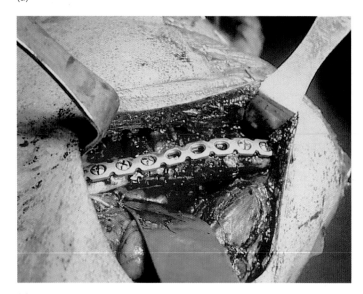
(c)

Fig. 15.8: (a) Patient with a non-union of the left mandibular body approached via a submandibular cervical incision.
(b) Exposure of the non-union site with placement of resorbable mesh for retention of a cortico-cancellous iliac crest bone graft.
(c) Placement of a reconstruction plate and iliac crest bone graft for treatment of a mandibular non-union site.

When the submandibular (Risdon) approach is utilized to place, for example, a lag screw for a condylar neck fracture, the incision is placed in the submandibular region approximately 1.5–2 cm below the inferior border of the mandible. This requires care to avoid the branches of the facial nerve that one may encounter during dissection. It is sometimes helpful to use a nerve stimulator to localize larger branches of the marginal mandibular or cervical branches of the facial nerve. The nerve is located along the undersurface of the superficial layer of the deep cervical fascia. Dissection is carried to the periosteum of the inferior surface of the mandible and an incision through periosteum exposes the fracture. Elevation of the periosteum will allow for the placement of rigid fixation plates (Fig. 15.8b,c).

A similar dissection can be performed in the retromandibular region to access ramus fractures or subcondylar fractures (Fig. 15.9). Again, care is taken not to injure the facial nerve branches. Pre-auricular or endaural incisions are utilized occasionally to expose high condylar neck fractures for rigid fixation or to remove foreign bodies from the joint space. This approach is not ideal as injury to one of the branches of the facial nerve is more common, and most subcondylar fractures are better accessed through retromandibular approaches without involving the joint space in the dissection.

Basic principles of mandible fracture repair using internal fixation

The basic components of mandibular fracture treatment can be summarized as reduction, stabilization and fixation. Open reduction and application of rigid internal fixation is carried out under general anesthesia and ideally a contoured nasal endotracheal (RAE) tube is utilized. The standard protocol for the use of miniplates is to have an assistant to stabilize the fragments and thus avoid even temporary mandibular maxillary wire fixation. In some complex cases, however, it may be helpful. Again, it is not necessary in well-reduced and stabilized mandibular fractures treated with miniplate fixation to use mandibular maxillary fixation postoperatively.

The authors' preferred approach, however, is to begin with the application of arch bars to the maxillary and mandibular arches using 25 G stainless steel circumdental ligature wires. Next, the transoral incision is marked and the soft tissues are injected with a local anesthetic solution containing vasocon-

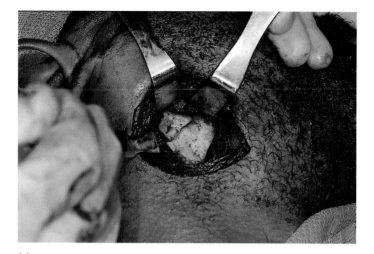

(a)

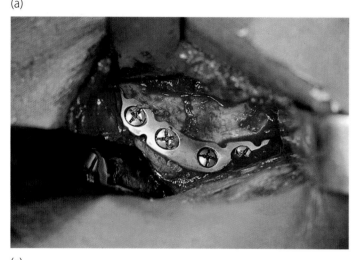

(c)

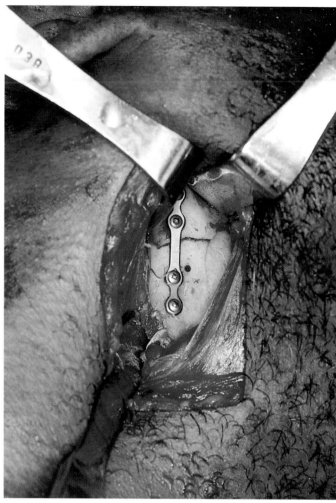

(b)

Fig. 15.9: **(a)** Retromandibular approach to the right mandibular subcondylar region. **(b)** Placement of a small rigid fixation plate with anatomic reduction of the subcondylar fracture. **(c)** Intraoperative view of right mandibular angle fracture exposed through a submandibular approach. The fracture was reduced and internal fixation was achieved using a 2.4 mm dynamic compression plate.

strictor. Exposure of the fracture is completed using transoral incisions and broad periosteal stripping to allow direct visualization of the fracture margins. The fracture is reduced and the mandible is placed into occlusion using the opposing maxillary arch form as a template for the fractured mandibular arch. Wire maxillomandibular fixation is applied to stabilize the mandible and is maintained during the placement of bone plates to fixate the fracture. In a situation where there is more than one fracture (e.g. body and ramus), it is appropriate to re-establish the mandibular arch form first and then apply the internal fixation to the fracture within the posterior mandible.

Once the bone plate and screws have been placed, the wound is packed and the wire maxillomandibular fixation is removed. This allows for examination of the occlusion and confirmation that the preinjury occlusal relationship and mandibular arch form have been restored. Releasing the maxillomandibular fixation also facilitates closure of the surgical wounds. We prefer to use heavy training elastics placed on the arch bars. The use of elastics limits the degree of mandibular movement but allows for better oral intake and hygiene and is

better tolerated by patients. Typically, the elastic use is continued for neuromuscular training only as long as is necessary to return patients to their normal range of motion and the arch bars are removed between 5 and 7 weeks postoperatively. In Europe, however, the use of even temporary mandibular maxillary fixation is not generally undertaken.

The primary advantage of rigid internal fixation is that it usually obviates the need for maxillomandibular fixation and allows for a faster return to function by the patient. Other advantages include better anatomic reduction, greater stability across the fractured segments, decreased mobility which reduces the incidence of infection and improved healing. The application of low-profile titanium-alloy plates with self-tapping screws requires less soft tissue stripping than was required in procedures for open reduction with the direct application of transosseous wires.

The introduction of fixation miniplates and monocortical screws described by Champy has revolutionized the treatment of mandible fractures. Systems used for rigid internal fixation of mandibular fractures now include plates and screws of a variety of sizes and configurations. The use of

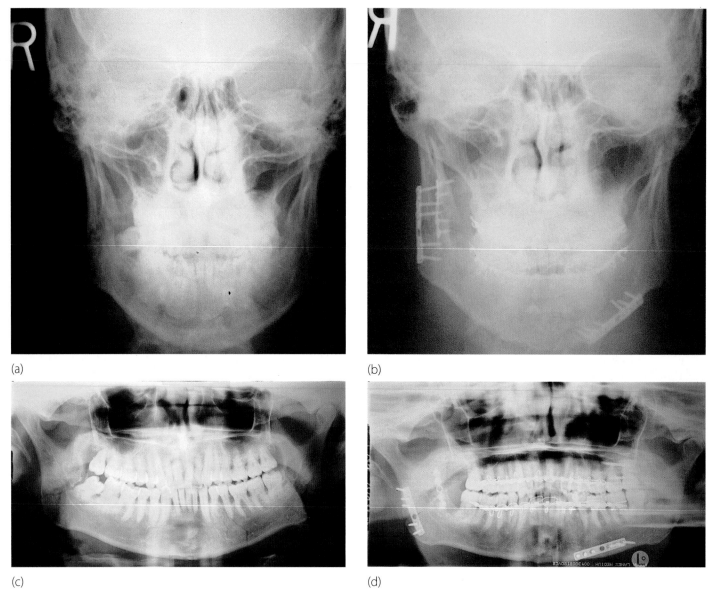

Fig. 15.10: Radiographic series of a patient with fractures involving the right mandibular ramus/angle and left mandibular body. **(a)** preoperative panoramic radiograph. **(b)** Postoperative panoramic radiograph. A trocar was utilized for placement of the internal fixation on the right side. Both fractures were repaired using transoral approaches. The right mandibular third molar was removed at the time of surgery. **(c)** Preoperative PA mandibular radiograph. **(d)** Postoperative PA mandibular radiograph.

heavy compression plates placed at the lower border using bicortical screws seems to have little to offer over miniplate fixation and a higher complication rate (Fig. 15.10).

The use of locking reconstruction plates has also been advocated in the repair of mandibular fractures. The concept of locking reconstruction plates is that the screw itself has a threaded head, which engages the hole within the plate. One technical advantage of this design is that, because the screw heads tighten down into the screw holes, the plate does not have to be ideally adapted against the bone. Other theoretical advantages of this system include the heavier, stronger design and the elimination of bone resorption, which may result from compression of the plate against the bony cortex. The application of these plates does rely on proper technique and proper anatomic positioning. There is at present scant evi-

dence that this more complex and expensive technique offers any advantage for the vast majority of patients. It may have a role in rare cases of gross comminution or continuity loss prior to formal reconstruction.

Recent investigations have examined whether larger sized plates or dynamic compression plates are superior to smaller miniplates used in fracture repair. Specifically, the question is, 'How much fixation is enough?'. Surgeons who advocate the use of two plates across the fracture and the use of larger (2.3 and 2.7 mm) bone plates feel that this is necessary to adequately stabilize the fractured segments and neutralize all forces that may occur during function.[31] In 1999, Potter & Ellis examined 46 patients with 51 fractures involving the mandibular angle who were treated using a malleable non-compression plate placed at the superior border of the

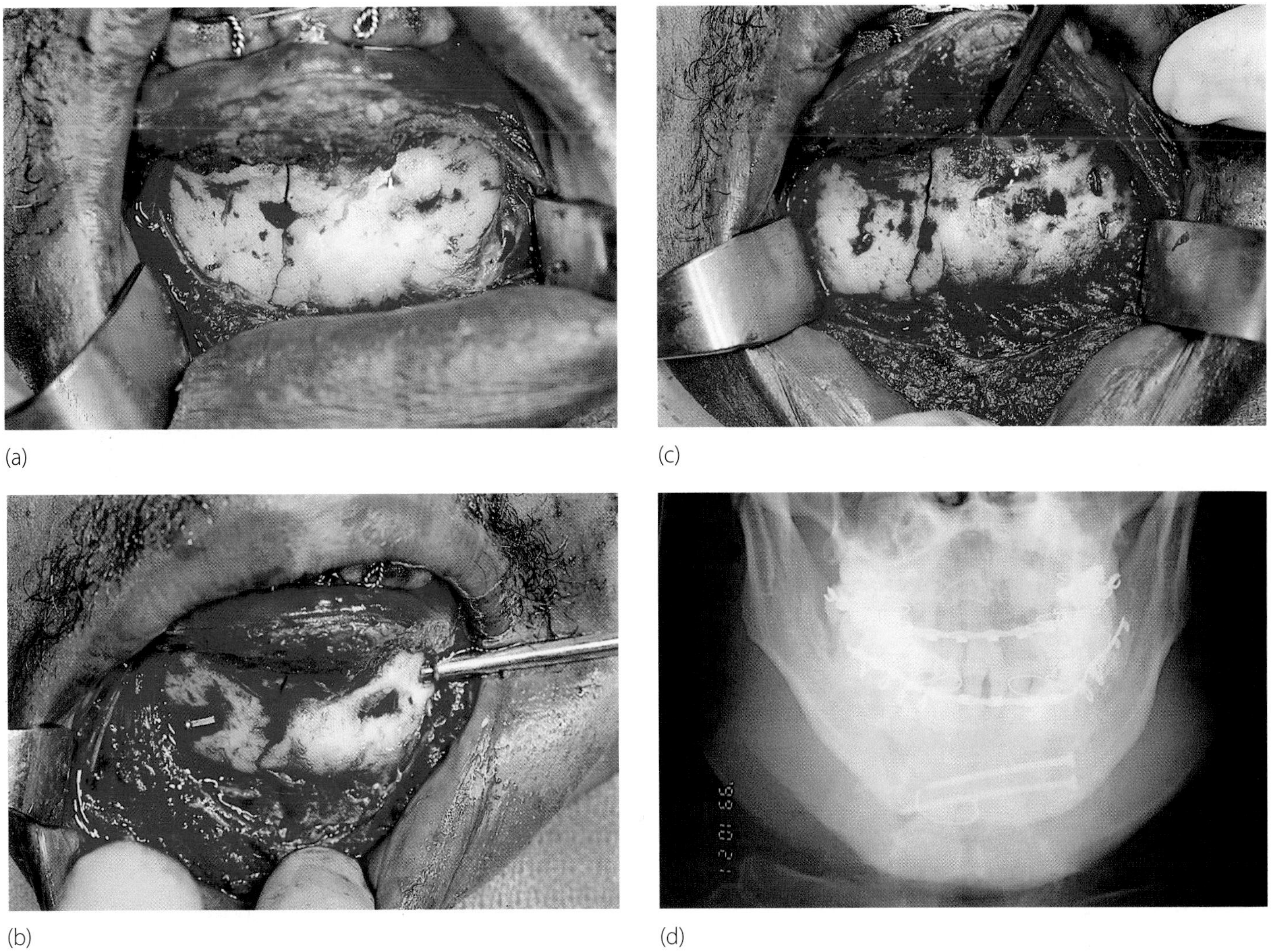

Fig. 15.11: **(a)** Intraoral approach to the right mandibular parasymphysis for placement of lag screw fixation. **(b)** The first screw hole is drilled and measured. **(c)** Both screws are placed at slightly different angulations to ensure optimal stability. **(d)** PA plain radiograph showing the reduction and fixation of the right mandibular parasymphysis fracture with two lag screws.

mandible. All the patients studied had uncomplicated healing of the fractures, suggesting that the level of fixation required for this type of injury is less than previously thought. The investigators also reported minor complications in seven cases and an unacceptably high (two patients) rate of fracture of the bone plate prior to fracture healing. The advantages of treating fractures with smaller bone plates include less dissection and morbidity. Some of these data show a decreased incidence of infection in patients who have undergone limited dissection and had a less rigid plate placed.[32] An inadequate amount of prospective data exists at this time to comment on which technique is best suited for each area of the mandible.

The use of lag screw techniques for fixation of mandibular fractures may be an excellent treatment alternative, especially in the anterior mandible. The first screw is placed furthest from the fracture segment to establish good stability. At least one additional screw in a different plane of space is required to resist rotational forces around the long axis of the

first screw. When used effectively, lag screws offer superb reduction and fixation. Lag screw fixation of fractures involving the posterior mandible and ramus regions is more technically demanding. Often, a trocar may be necessary to place the lag screw without damaging the inferior alveolar nerve or dental structures in the region. To place a lag screw effectively, the outer cortex is drilled slightly larger than the screw to be placed in the inner cortex. A countersink is utilized to allow flush adaptation of the screw head to the bony cortex. The screw head then reduces the inner and outer cortices together, offering a quick and very precise reduction (Figs 15.11, 15.12).

Outcomes

Complications of mandibular fractures

Complications following mandible fracture repair may be the result of the severity of the original injury, the surgical

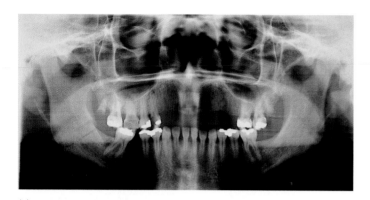

(a)

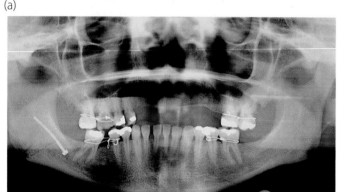

(b)

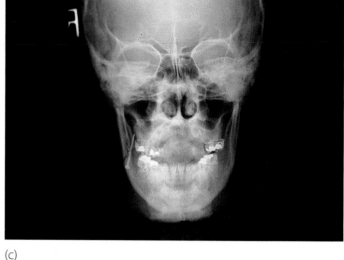

(c)

Fig. 15.12: (a) Preoperative panoramic radiograph of right mandibular angle fracture. **(b)** Postoperative panoramic radiograph after placement of a lag screw for fixation of the fracture. The placement of lag screw fixation in the mandibular body and ramus often requires the use of a percutaneous trocar. **(c)** Postoperative PA cephalometric radiograph of the same patient.

treatment or patient non-compliance with the postoperative regimen. Problems related to mandibular fractures present unique challenges to even the most experienced surgeon. The consequences of complications may include problems in anatomic form (cosmetic deformity) or residual functional disturbances. Complication rates have improved since the early days of wire fixation, but even the most sound fixation techniques can yield undesirable results (Fig. 15.13). Probably no other specific area of oral and maxillofacial surgery has been studied in more detail than the mandible fracture. Despite this fact, little prospective evidence is available regarding the outcomes of the various treatment modalities. Retrospective studies offer some evidence that certain techniques have independently done better than others, but better prospective studies are needed to further evaluate and compare these techniques.

Malunion non-union

The mandible is a site associated with a relatively high incidence of altered fracture healing (malunion, non-union). Mathog reported an incidence of 2.4% in his study of 577 patients.[33] There are a number of specific risk factors associated with mandibular fractures and their potential for non-union or malunion. Infection is the major contributing risk factor to unfavorable healing and mobility. Other risks include poor apposition of fracture segments, poor immobilization of segments, presence of foreign bodies, unfavorable muscle pull on the fracture segments, displacement of

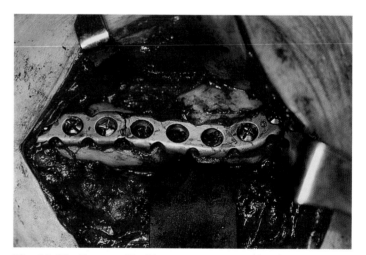

Fig. 15.13: Fractured locking reconstruction plate being removed after only 3 months of use due to spouse assault (courtesy of Dr David Stanton DMD, MD).

comminuted fracture segments (and the difficulty associated with adequately reducing them), aseptic necrosis of bony fragments, soft tissue interposition, malnutrition and debilitation (Fig. 15.14).

Residual arch form deformity following the surgical repair of a mandibular fracture is often the result of inadequate reduction. Failure to re-establish the anatomic configuration of the arch form result in occlusal prematurities and misalign-

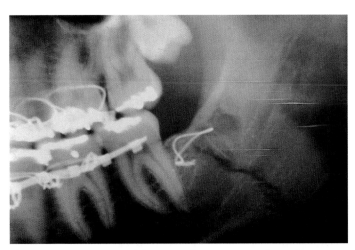

Fig. 15.14: Poor immobilization of segments with inadequate fixation of a superior border wire placed through an intraoral incision. This precipitated non-union healing in this patient.

ment which will compromise masticatory function. Clinicians treating mandibular fractures need to be familiar with dental anatomy and occlusion in order to balance the functional forces appropriately. Preoperative study models (with or without model surgery) and splint fabrication may aid in fracture reduction in some cases. Poor apposition of fracture segments may results from a delay in or an absence of treatment, inadequate treatment, inability to align segments secondary to the presence of a foreign body or loss of bony landmarks. Malaligned fracture segments noted early in the postoperative course may be corrected by returning to the operating room for removal of the hardware and repeat reduction with internal fixation. When the discrepancies are not caught early, the fracture segments will go on to heal in the improper anatomic position (malunion). Significant malunions of the mandible will produce asymmetry, facial convexity and/or functional disturbances and can only be resolved through carefully planned osteotomies for reconstruction of the mandibular arch form.

When a fracture occurs, the initial phase of healing is characterized by an inflammatory response and the formation of a hematoma between the bone fragments. Later, there is deposition of collagen fibers within the fracture site and the ingrowth of vascular elements. The resulting soft callus thus contains the elements of bone formation within the fracture gap and fracture healing. For these mechanisms to occur successfully, the fracture must be stabilized appropriately.

The most common cause of failure of fracture healing (non-union) is residual mobility across the fracture site. Movement of the bone ends will disrupt the fibrovascular structures, decrease the recruitment of osteoprogenitor cells and allow for fibrous tissue ingrowth instead of bony healing. Other contributors to fracture non-union include impaired healing capacity secondary to illness, tobacco use and infection. Non-union of mandibular fractures requires reoperation to excise any fibrous tissue within the fracture gap in combination with application of bone fixation. In some instances,

there may be loss of bone, producing a continuity defect which will require bone graft reconstruction. Treatment strategies vary from patient to patient and with each surgeon's experience in using different techniques. Potential reconstruction options for non-unions of the mandible are listed in Box 15.3.

Infection

Infection is the most common complication of surgical intervention. In the patient who undergoes repair of a mandible fracture, postoperative infection rates vary from less than 1% to 32%.[34-38] The potential for infection is always a consideration when treating fractures of the mandible, especially when there is communication with the oral cavity (e.g. compound fracture). Other risk indicators for increased chance of infection include active substance abuse and non-compliance with postoperative regimens.[39] A significant delay in treatment has also been associated with an increase in infection rates.[40] Other factors include gross contamination of the site, poor host healing potential, pre-existing dentoalveolar disease, teeth present in the line of fracture and atrophic architecture present in edentulous mandibles. Of the facial bones, the mandible is the most frequently infected region following surgical intervention for traumatic injury. This is likely due to instability of the segments from muscular actions on the proximal and distal segments and the density of the bone.

Manifestations of infection include cellulitis, abscess formation, fistula, osteomyelitis and rarely necrotizing fasciitis (Fig. 15.15). Management begins with clinical examination and plain radiographic studies to assess the status of the fractured segments and the hardware. Appropriate laboratory studies, including a complete blood count, should be obtained and provide useful information when systemic signs are present. The use of CT and MRI is appropriate when there is concern that the infection involves the surrounding soft tissues of the neck. Specimens for bacterial culture and sensitivity studies should be sent as early as possible in the patient's clinical course.

Most infections of the oral cavity and surrounding craniomaxillofacial region are polymicrobial. Early in the course of the infection, the bacterial population is largely aerobic and Gram positive. When an infection is more than a few days old or chronic, the composition of the organisms involved changes so that anaerobic, Gram-negative organisms predominate. Penicillin G, with its excellent Gram-positive coverage, is a good choice for treatment of early infections, while clindamycin, with broader Gram-negative coverage, is often the antibiotic of choice for chronic infections. It is important to note, however, that the antibiotic utilized does not need to cover all the organisms present within the infected site. It is well documented that the elimination of some of the causative organisms will successfully change the complex microenvironment enough to resolve infections in and around the oral cavity.[41] The use of broad-spectrum antibiotics in the initial management of infected fractures is usually reserved for severe infections or when the individual's host responses are compromised. When initial empiric antibiotic treatment fails

Box 15.3 Treatment options for reconstructing non-union fracture healing

- Maxillomandibular fixation
- Rigid internal fixation with a reconstruction plate
- External fixation
- Particulate bone grafting or cortical bone grafting to the defect
- Polyglycolic or polylactate mesh as a carrier for cancellous bone graft
- Nerve grafting
- Composite free flap reconstruction

If the infection is the result of a necrotic bony segment or non-restorable tooth, removal of the etiologic agent is required. When fluctuance is present, incision and drainage are necessary to establish prompt resolution. Often this is combined with pulsatile irrigation as an effective method of decreasing bacterial concentration within the wound. Patients with infected non-unions of the mandible require debridement and definitive stabilization using one of several methods available (maxillomandibular fixation, ORIF, external fixation, etc.).

The type of immobilization has been shown to be a factor in the incidence of complications associated with mandibular fractures. Passeri and colleagues found the incidence of infection in mandible fractures treated using closed reduction was about 14%.[39] Many infections treated with closed reduction are associated with teeth within the line of fracture and those compromised with caries and/or periodontal disease. Luhr examined mandible fractures treated with closed reduction, dynamic compression plating and wire fixation. He found a similar incidence of infection associated with closed reduction and open reduction with dynamic compression plating, but an increased incidence of infection when wire fixation was utilized.[42] This was hypothesized to be due to the mobility of the segments associated with wire fixation (Fig. 15.16). Ellis and his collaborators have examined multiple types of fixation methods utilized to treat mandible fractures. Ellis observed the highest rates of infection in patients who received two dynamic compression plates.[37] Wire fixation was associated with an infection rate approaching 25%.[40] Champy originally reported an incidence of only 3.8% associated with his technique of using a 2.0 mm tension band plate, placed with an intraoral approach.[15] Based upon these data, the old dictums that suggest the use of large plates with maximum rigidity and stability may not necessarily be the best treatment for all fracture scenarios. Unfortunately, each clinical setting and protocol differs significantly enough to

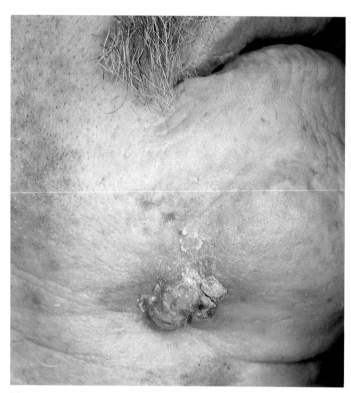

Fig. 15.15: Patient with a chronic draining fistula from a long-standing non-union of the right body of the mandible.

to resolve the infection, bacterial culture and identification studies help to redirect the surgeon's selection of antibiotics.

Perhaps the most common misconception in the management of infections is that they are treated with antibiotic coverage alone. In fact, successful resolution of most surgical infections requires three steps:

1. the development of adequate drainage
2. removal of the source
3. appropriate antibiotic coverage.

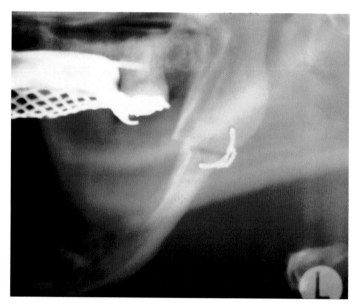

Fig. 15.16: Poor choice of fixation for an edentulous mandible fracture in a patient with severe atrophy.

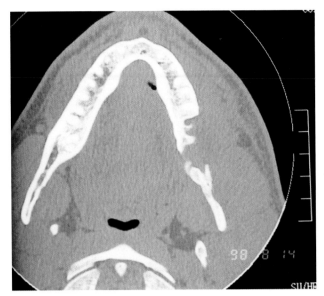

Fig. 15.17: Axial CT scan of the mandible with osteomyelitis from a long-standing unrepaired mandibular fracture.

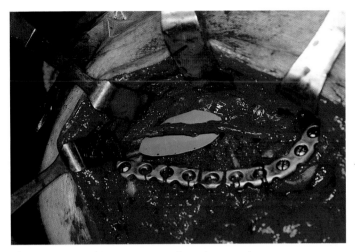

Fig. 15.18: Locking reconstruction plate used to reconstruct a large non-union site with iliac crest bone graft and a great auricular nerve graft.

make meaningful comparisons difficult. Prospective outcome trials comparing multiple modalities in similar settings are needed to properly evaluate these techniques.

Osteomyelitis warrants special attention. Osteomyelitis is an inflammatory reaction in bone with evidence of sclerosis, altered blood supply and dense scarring ultimately inhibiting the local tissues from mounting an adequate healing response. Clinically, it may be difficult to differentiate between osteomyelitis and simple non-union healing. Laboratory values such as a complete blood count, erythrocyte sedimentation rate and/or C-reactive protein levels may be helpful in both differentiating true osteomyelitis from simple infection and in following the effectiveness of therapy. Plain radiographs, CT and MRI have been used to visualize the site of infection and delineate the region of the mandible affected (Fig. 15.17). Radionucleotide scans have been helpful, but lack specificity.

The treatment of osteomyelitis includes obtaining cultures, surgical debridement, pulsatile irrigation of the site and long-term, directed antibiotic therapy. After adequate debridement and sequestrectomy the area should be immobilized and allowed to heal for several weeks prior to definitive attempts at reconstruction with bone grafts or other methods.

Nerve injury

Fractures that involve the mandibular body or angle will frequently result in injury to the inferior alveolar nerve. The degree of neurosensory disturbance depends on the degree of mandibular fracture displacement and the type of nerve injury that results. Patients with a paresthesia following a mandibular fracture should be observed during the postoperative period and the level of neurosensory return (subjective) is documented. In cases where patients report no improvement in their level of sensation after 6–8 weeks, the clinician may consider obtaining baseline nerve function data using objective testing. Objective neurosensory testing before

6 weeks may be of limited value because it is difficult to discern a Sunderland Class I injury (excellent prognosis without surgery) from a Sunderland Class V injury (poor prognosis without surgery) that early in the postoperative course. In the case of Sunderland Class IV and V injuries (equivalent to axonotmesis and neurotmesis) surgical repair is considered between 3 and 6 months.[43]

Immediate management of inferior alveolar nerve injury at the time of mandibular fracture repair has been advocated in situations where there is displacement at the fracture site and anesthesia.[44] Although a more aggressive approach may have merit, it would be limited to situations where there is an observed transection of the nerve. Immediate decompression and exploration are not necessary in less severe nerve injuries (Sunderland Class I, II, III) and surgical maneuvers used to expose the nerve trunk (decortication) may compromise subsequent fracture healing (Fig. 15.18).

Special considerations

Comminuted fractures

Comminuted fractures and their repair merit special consideration by the surgeon because they are technically difficult to repair and associated complications are more frequent. Reasons for this include:

- the increased force necessary to create this type of injury carries with it a higher degree of surrounding tissue injury
- there is increased difficulty with reduction and stabilization of multiple fragments
- comminution also places the patient at higher risk for ischemic compromise and avascular necrosis of fragments. Despite the rich vascular supply of the maxillofacial skeleton, small bony fragments seen in areas of comminution may be stripped of their blood supply and become non-viable. The result is fragment necrosis and sequestration, which may lead to non-union, infection and in some cases continuity defect.

Open treatment of severely comminuted fractures requires enough soft tissue dissection for adequate visualization while preserving as much periosteal and muscular attachment, and thus blood supply to the skeletal segments, as possible. In some situations, small bone fragments may be replaced as free bone grafts with the application of internal fixation. The authors' preference is to utilize a locking reconstruction plate in the repair of large comminuted fractures of the mandible. This type of fixation allows the surgeon to bridge the area of comminution and fix the plate to the proximal and distal intact bone segments. The comminuted fragments can then be reduced and stabilized using position screws.

Edentulous mandible fractures

Fractures of the severely atrophic edentulous mandible have always presented a difficult challenge. Mandibular atrophy is both a factor in the etiology of the fracture itself and a problematic consideration for the surgeon charged with repair of the injury. Previous methods of treatment have included the use of existing dentures with skeletal wiring, external fixators, internal wires, small plates and screws (both sub- and supraperiosteal), reconstruction plates and screws and lag screws. As our understanding of fixation methods improves and new techniques and materials surface, the ability to manage these difficult problems has become more predictable. These fractures warrant special attention and their management is controversial.

It is important to define more carefully 'edentulous' mandibles, since the literature shows that only those severely atrophic mandibles with a bone height less than 10 mm stand out as a 'difficult' or special problem. Above these heights, normal miniplate fixation may be effective.

Patients with severely atrophic edentulous mandible fractures may experience poor results for many reasons. As shown by Bradley, elderly patients have decreased vascularity to the mandible secondary to the decrease in flow from the inferior alveolar artery.[45] This study was based on patients having angiography for other reasons and could not be described as a 'normal' patient group. Unlike younger individuals, the blood supply to the edentulous mandible is primarily from the periosteal envelope. Elderly patients also have dense, sclerotic bone and decreased osteoblastic activity at an area with less bony contact than is present in the dentate mandible. Patients in this age group may have osteoporosis, vascular disease, renal insufficiency or failure, diabetes, malnutrition and calcium wasting disorders. All these factors contribute to poor healing potential at the fracture site and the increased rate of non-union, malunion and infection.[46,47]

Most edentulous mandible fractures occur at the body and condyle rather than the angle or parasymphysis regions (Fig. 15.19). The body of the mandible is generally weakest at the mid-body or saddle, as this is the most significant site of resorption. Without a dentition to stabilize the segments, the majority of edentulous segments will be significantly displaced as a result of the muscular pull on smaller and weaker bones.[46,47]

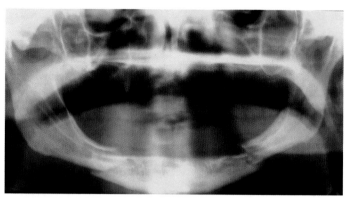

Fig. 15.19: Patient with bilateral edentulous mandible fractures in the typical 'saddle' region of greatest atrophy.

Box 15.4 Treatment methods for edentulous mandible fractures

- Closed reduction with the use of prosthetics (existing dentures or Gunning splints)
- External fixation
- Wire fixation
- Open reduction with internal fixation:
  1. reconstruction plates (2.3–2.7 mm diameter screws)
  2. mandible fixation plates (2.0–2.4 mm diameter screws):
     — dynamic compression plates
     — plates at both inferior and superior borders of the fracture
  3. bone grafting and miniplate fixation

Many treatment modalities have been used to treat severely atrophic edentulous mandible fractures (Box 15.4). This illustrates the difficulty in obtaining predictable results with any one method. The degree of atrophy in the mandible can be a factor when deciding which method is best for a given situation.

Closed reduction of edentulous mandible fractures has certainly been effective in some patients, but the best of conditions must be present (Fig. 15.20).[48] Patients should exhibit adequate bone quantity and quality, minimal swelling, good ridge form, adequate vestibular depth, favorable fracture angulations and good host healing potential and be compliant. Immobilizing the segments is difficult even if the prosthesis fits extremely well. This can be an option in the patient who is either unwilling or unable to undergo a surgical procedure. Longer periods of maxillomandibular fixation are recommended in the elderly patient to ensure adequate healing. Contraindications to maxillomandibular fixation include seizure disorders, psychiatric issues, significantly altered neurologic states and significantly compromised pulmonary or nutritional states.

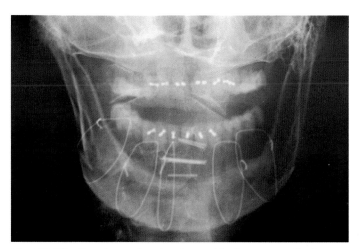

Fig. 15.20: Gunning splints in place with circummandibular wire utilizing the patient's own dentures.

An external fixation device can be used in patients who have grossly infected and/or massively comminuted mandible fractures. It is also useful in those patients with pathologic fractures due to osteoradionecrosis (ORN) or other bony lesions. In ORN patients this is useful stabilization while they receive hyperbaric oxygen therapy prior to surgical intervention that would require periosteal stripping and further devi-

talization of bone. External fixation is a very effective therapy despite its limited indications. However, if there is another option, patients will frequently not readily accept an external device due to its unsightliness. The external fixation device is often supported by an acrylic bar, which can be fashioned with the aid of an endotracheal tube. Great care must be taken when fabricating the bar due to the exothermic reaction associated with the acrylic resin. Diligent care of the transcutaneous pin sites is important to prevent infection and patients must be followed up regularly to assess the need for debridement and evaluate healing.

Open reduction of an edentulous mandible fracture is a viable treatment option in most cases, but the approach must be tailored to the individual patient, bony morphology of the mandible and type of fracture. Fixation of edentulous mandibular fractures using direct transosseous wiring is fraught with complications because of the degree of soft tissue stripping required and the lack of rigidity of such a technique. The use of arch bars and elastic traction to reduce functional forces on the mandible is not possible in these patients and so the wired segments must withstand displacement. Depending on the bone quality present and the degree of bone-to-bone contact at the fracture site, the same problem may result when very small bone plates are used to bridge an edentulous fracture (Fig. 15.21). Open reduction

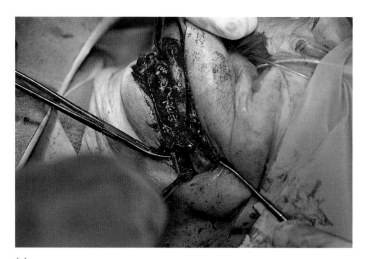

(a)

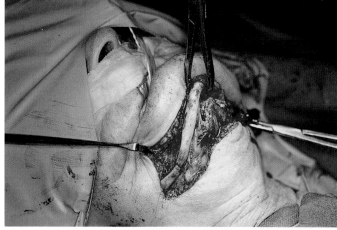

(b)

Fig. 15.21: (a) Intraoperative view of an edentulous patient with bilateral mandibular body fractures. The extreme atrophy resulted in pathologic fractures. The initial management (by another surgeon) consisted of open reduction and internal fixation using four-hole miniplates done through transoral approaches. The patient returned with mobility at the fracture sites and non-union resulting from failure of the hardware. **(b)** Intraoperative view of fracture site with previously placed miniplate. **(c)** Fixation of reduced fracture using a long span 2.0 mm universal fracture plate. Bone graft reconstruction of the severely atrophic mandible was carried out using autogenous bone graft obtained from the ilium.

(c)

with application of adequate-sized rigid internal fixation provides for stable repair and the most predictable healing of edentulous fractures.[49,50] Typically, this requires the use of at least 2.0 mm bone screws and plates with at least three screws on each side of the fracture. Larger reconstruction plates (2.7 mm diameter screws) have been used over large areas of the edentulous mandible to ensure rigid fixation of each segment. The disadvantages of this technique include a higher chance of nerve impingement, the need for excessive amounts of periosteal stripping (compromising the blood supply) and the use of large screws, which can fracture the severely atrophic mandible during placement. Smaller plates and screws (2.3 or 2.4 mm) can be used with less periosteal stripping and more precise screw placement.

In addition to adequate reduction and stabilization of the fractured segments, the successful management of fractures involving the edentulous mandible requires that consideration be given to the amount of bone present. When the mandible is severely atrophic, it is possible that healing will not occur even if open reduction and internal fixation principles are properly applied. In some circumstances, treatment consists of simultaneous bone graft reconstruction at the time of fracture repair. This is also appropriate treatment for patients presenting with non-union of an edentulous fracture. In most cases plans for definitive prosthetic reconstruction are delayed until full healing of the bony site has occurred. Some authors, however, do advocate early reconstruction with bone grafting and osseo-integrated implants.[51]

Key points

- Appropriate diagnosis
- Anatomic reduction
- Stabilization of the fractured segments using occlusion as a guide
- Stable internal fixation

Conclusion

The successful management of fractures of the mandible requires a firm cognitive understanding of its complex anatomy, developmental course, articulations, dental occlusion and related functional biomechanical forces. Modern state-of-the-art mandibular fracture repair is based on meticulous diagnosis, anatomic reduction, stabilization with a respect for pre-existing occlusal relationships and rigid internal fixation techniques. Continued research in diagnosis, materials and outcomes will further refine the treatment of mandible fractures and improve the quality of life for these patients.

References

1 Ellis E 1997 Advances in maxillofacial trauma surgery. In: Fonseca RJ, Walker RV, Betts NJ, Barber D (eds) Oral and maxillofacial trauma. WB Saunders, Philadelphia, pp 308–363

2 The Edwin Smith Surgical Papyrus 1930 (trans. Breasted JH). University of Chicago Press, Chicago

3 Lipton JS 1982 Oral surgery in ancient Egypt as reflected in the Edwin Smith Papyrus. Bulletin of the History of Dentistry 30: 108

4 Hippocrates 1928 Oeuvres completes (English trans. Withington ET). Cambridge, MA

5 Salicetti G 1275 Cyrurgia.

6 Prevost N 1492 Translation of Salicetti's Cyrurgia. Lyons, France

7 Gilmer TL 1887 A case of fracture of the lower jaw with remarks on the treatment. Archives of Dentistry 4: 388

8 Dorrance GM, Bransfield JW 1941 The history of treatment of fractured jaws. Army Medical Museum: Washington DC

9 Ivy RH 1915 Fracture of condyloid process of the mandible. Annals of Surgery 61: 502

10 Cole PP 1917 Dental surgery and injuries of the jaw. British Journal of Dental Science 60: 77

11 Heslop IH, Clarke PB, Becker R et al 1985 Mandibular fractures: treatment by open reduction and direct skeletal fixation. In: Rowe NL, Willams JL (eds) Maxillofacial injuries. Churchill Livingstone, Edinburgh, pp 293–336

12 Luhr HG 1968 Stable osteosynthesis in fractures of the lower jaw. Deutsche Zahnaertzliche 23: 754

13 Spiessl B 1976 New concepts in maxillofacial bone surgery. Springer-Verlag, Berlin

14 Michelet FX, Deymes J, Dessus B 1973 Osteosynthesis with miniaturized screwed plates in maxillofacial surgery. Journal of Maxillofacial Surgery 1: 79

15 Champy M, Lodde JP, Schmitt R et al 1978 Mandibular osteosynthesis by miniature screwed plates via a buccal approach. Journal of Maxillofacial Surgery 6; 14

16 Turvey TA, Bell RB, Tejera TJ, Proffit WB 2001 The use of self-reinforced biodegradable bone plates and screws in orthognathic surgery. Journal of Oral and Maxillofacial Surgery 60(1): 59–65

17 Suuronen R 1993 Biodegradable fracture fixation devices in maxillofacial surgery. International Journal of Oral and Maxillofacial Surgery 22: 50

18 Eppley BL, Prevel CD, Sarver D 1996 Resorbable bone fixation: its potential role in craniomaxillofacial trauma. Journal of Craniomaxillofacial Trauma 2: 56

19 Haug RH, Prather J, Indresano AT 1990 An epidemiologic survey of facial fractures and concomitant injuries. Journal of Oral and Maxillofacial Surgery 48: 926

20 Ellis E, Moos KF, El-Attar A 1985 Ten years of mandibular fractures: an analysis of 2137. Oral Surgery, Oral Medicine, Oral Pathology 59: 120

21 Olson RA, Fonseca RJ, Zeitler DR et al 1982 Fractures of the mandible: a review of 580 cases. Journal of Oral and Maxillofacial Surgery 40: 23

22 Adekey EO 1980 The pattern of fractures of the facial skeleton in Kaduna, Nigeria: a survey of 1447 cases. Oral Surgery, Oral Medicine, Oral Pathology 149: 491

23 Chayra GA, Meador LR, Laskin DM 1985 Comparison of panoramic and standard radiographs for the diagnosis of mandibular fractures. Journal of Oral and Maxillofacial Surgery 44; 677

24 Mokoena T, Abdool-Carrim AT 1991 Haemostasis by angiographic embolization in exsanguinating haemorrhage from facial arteries: a report of two cases. South African Medical Journal 80(11–12): 595–597

25 Sakamoto T, Yagi K, Hiraide A et al 1988 Transcatheter embolization in the treatment of massive bleeding due to maxillofacial injury. Journal of Trauma 28: 840–843

26 Cannell H, Silvester PC, O'Regan MB 1993 Early management of multiply injured patients with maxillofacial injuries transported to hospital by helicopter. British Journal of Oral and Maxillofacial Surgery 31: 207–212

27 Murakami WT, Davidson TM, Marshall LF 1983 Fatal epistaxis in craniofacial trauma. Journal of Trauma 23(1): 57–61

28 Komiyama M, Nishikawa M, Kan M et al 1998 Endovascular treatment of intractable oronasal bleeding associated with severe craniofacial injury. Journal of Trauma 44(2): 330–334

29 Chang CJ, Chen YR, Noordhoff MS et al 1990 Facial bone fracture associated with carotid-cavernous sinus fistula. Journal of Trauma 30: 1335

30 Blakey GB, Ruiz RL, Turvey TA 1997 Management of facial fractures in the growing patient. In: Fonseca RJ, Walker RV, Betts NJ, Barber D (eds) Oral and Maxillofacial trauma. WB Saunders, Philadelphia, pp 1003–1043

31 Shilli W, Stoll P, Bahr W et al 1998 Mandibular fractures. In: Prein J (ed) Manual of internal fixation in the craniofacial skeleton. Springer, New York, pp 57–93

32 Ellis E, Walker WR 1996 Treatment of mandibular angle fractures using one noncompression miniplate. Journal of Oral and Maxillofacial Surgery 54: 864–871

33 Mathog RH, Boies LR 1976 Nonunion of the mandible. Laryngoscope 86(7): 908–920

34 Bochlogyros PN 1985 A retrospective study of 1521 mandibular fractures. Journal of Oral and Maxillofacial Surgery 43: 597

35 Busuito MJ, Smith DJ, Robson MC 1986 Mandibular fractures in an urban trauma center. Journal of Trauma 26: 826

36 James RB, Kent JN 1981 Prospective study of mandibular fractures. Journal of Oral Surgery 39: 275

37 Ellis E, Sinn DP 1993 Treatment of mandibular angle fractures using two 2.4 mm dynamic compression plates. Journal of Oral and Maxillofacial Surgery 1989 51: 969

38 Theriot BA, Van Sickels JE, Triplett RG, Nishioka GJ 1989 Intraosseous wire fixation versus rigid osseous fixation of mandibular fractures: a preliminary report. Journal of Oral and Maxillofacial Surgery 47: 856

39 Passeri LA, Ellis E, Sinn DP 1993 Relationship of substance abuse to complications with mandibular fractures. Journal of Oral and Maxillofacial Surgery 51: 22–25

40 Moulton-Barrett R, Rubinstein AJ, Salzhauer MA et al 1998 Complications of mandibular fractures. Annals of Plastic Surgery 41: 258–263

41 Moenning JE, Nelson CL, Kohler RB 1989 The microbiology and chemotherapy of odontogenic infections. Journal of Oral and Maxillofacial Surgery 47(9): 976–985

42 Luhr HG 1982 Compression plate osteosynthesis through the Luhr system. In: Kruger E, Schilli W (eds) Oral and maxillofacial traumatology. Quintessence Chicago, p 319

43 Zuniga JR 1993 Advances in microsurgical nerve repair. Journal of Oral and Maxillofacial Surgery. 51 (suppl 1): 62–68

44 Thurmuller P, Dodson TB, Kaban LB 2001 Nerve injuries associated with facial trauma: natural history, management, and outcomes of repair. Oral and Maxillofacial Surgery Clinics of North America 13(2): 283–293

45 Bradley JC 1972 Age changes in the vascular supply of the mandible. British Dental Journal 132: 142–144

46 Bruce RA, Strachan DS 1976 Fractures of the edentulous mandible: the Chalmers J Lyons Academy study. Journal of Oral Surgery 34: 973–979

47 Bruce RA, Ellis E 1993 The second Chalmers J. Lyons Academy study of fractures of the edentulous mandible. Journal of Oral and Maxillofacial Surgery 51: 904–911

48 Gunning TB 1866 Treatment of fractures of the lower jaw by interdental splints. British Journal of Dental Science 9: 481

49 Krebs FJ 1988 Dynamic compression plating in treatment of the fractured edentulous mandible. Laryngoscope 98: 198–201

50 Luhr HG, Reidick T, Merten HA 1996 Results of treatment of fractures of the atrophic edentulous mandible by compression plating: a retrospective evaluation of 84 consecutive cases. Journal of Oral and Maxillofacial Surgery 54: 250–254

51 Eyrich GK, Gratz KW, Sailer HF 1997 Surgical treatment of the edentulous mandible. Journal of Oral and Maxillofacial Surgery 55: 1081–1087

16 Condylar Neck Fractures

Richard A Loukota, Patrick J McCann

Introduction

According to most large series reported in the literature, fractures of the mandibular condyle account for 26–57% of all mandibular fractures. The sex ratio (male:female) ranges from 3:1 to 2:1 depending on which population is studied. Between 48% and 66% of patients with condylar fractures will also have a body or angle fracture.

Approximately 84% are unilateral and etiology most commonly involves interpersonal violence, sport injury, falls and road traffic accidents. According to Silvennoinen,[1] approximately 14% are intracapsular, 24% condylar neck, 62% subcondylar and 16% associated with severe displacement. The highest incidence of fractures is seen in patients between 20 and 39 years of age.

Fractures may be classified according to their location, i.e. intracapsular, condylar neck and subcondylar. Further subdivision may be made according to deviation, displacement and dislocation of fragments in relation to the glenoid fossa. Classifications include those of Spiessel & Schroll:[2]

1. condylar neck fracture without serious dislocation
2. deep-seated condylar neck fracture with dislocation
3. high condylar neck fracture with dislocation
4. deep-seated condylar neck fracture with luxation
5. high condylar neck fracture with luxation
6. head or intracapsular fracture (dicapitular fracture)

and MacLennan[3] and Lindahl.[4]

Almost any direction of fracture propagation is possible and in general, the greater the displacement of fragments, the less favorable is the outcome. It should be noted that occasionally the reader may be confused when reading literature from continental Europe where 'displacement' (UK/USA) may be indicated by 'dislocation'. 'Dislocation' (UK/USA) may be indicated by 'luxation'. We shall use the UK/USA nomenclature.

Condylar fractures are complicated by their intimate relationship with the temporomandibular joint (TMJ). Direct fracture involvement of the joint or prolonged immobilization during treatment can lead to problems with deranged occlusion, internal derangement of the joint, ankylosis and reduced mandibular growth. Symptomatically these manifest as long-term pain, limitation of jaw movement and function, asymmetrical growth and malocclusion. TMJ ankylosis due to trauma is thought to account for only 0.4% of ankylosis cases.

Unlike mandibular body fractures, which are now almost universally treated with osteosynthesis plates, there exists considerable variation in the management of condylar fractures in patients over the age of 12 years. Protagonists of conservative (closed) treatment methods cite evidence in the literature of satisfactory outcome by closed fracture management. They believe that the risks of scar formation, seventh nerve injury and vascular compromise to the condylar head are not justified in the majority of simple condyle fractures.

With the lack of properly constructed high-powered prospective randomized trials, most of the literature on this topic is of a retrospective nature with agreed inevitable limitations. In an attempt to clarify everyday surgical practice, consensus studies and condyle management conferences, notably Budapest 1995 and Gronigen 1997, have been employed. These efforts are admirable but can only give an idea of current surgical practice based on personal experience and non-randomized, often retrospective studies. What is lacking is true evidence-based practice in the management of this complicated fracture type.

In this chapter we will attempt to draw on the published literature, consensus practice and our own unit policy to guide the reader in practical decision making when managing these patients.

Clinical Findings and Investigations

The majority of condylar fractures arise from blunt trauma to the anterior mandible. Forces are transmitted to the condylar region where posterior movement of the mandible is limited by the glenoid fossa, TMJ capsule and insertion of the lateral pterygoid muscles. When the force is sufficient to overcome the strength of the condylar region, fracture follows. Trauma involving the open mouth leads to flexion fractures of the condyle. Symmetrical impact is said to cause bilateral fractures. Unilateral impact causes contralateral condylar fractures and shearing forces are thought to produce intracapsular fractures. Closed mouth fractures tend to distribute some of the energy to the occlusal surface of the teeth and cuspal fractures are common.

Under the influence of the masticatory muscles the mandibular ramus may shorten vertically and produce premature occlusal contacts distally (Fig. 16.1). The condylar fragment can dislocate out of the fossa, usually in an anterior direction; however, it may displace laterally, medially or centrally into the middle cranial fossa. It should be appreciated that any combination of fractures is possible and that joint maceration poses considerable surgical and healing difficulties.

Direct trauma to the TMJ area is unusual but may be associated with fractures of the zygomatic complex.

The derangement of the occlusion may give an indication of the fracture pattern. A unilateral fracture with sufficient

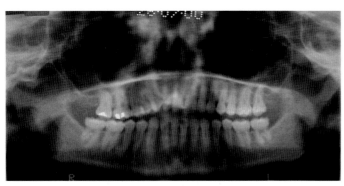

Fig. 16.1: Orthopantomogram demonstrating right condylar fracture with anterior and left-sided open bites.

fragment overlap/dislocation will result in premature posterior contact on the affected side and midline deviation to the affected side. Bilateral condylar fractures with overlap/dislocation will produce bilateral posterior premature contact, anterior open bite with little or no chin deviation.

Comminuted mandibular fractures with bilateral condyle fractures produce crossbites and tend to increase the interangular distance, making accurate reduction challenging. Failure to recognize and correct this increased interangular distance will lead to fixation of the body with a malocclusion (Fig. 16.2). Accurate reduction with the use of temporary IMF will insure this does not happen and is worth the time and effort prior to fixation of the body with miniplates.

Investigations

Radiological imaging in two planes is required. An orthopantomogram and a posteroanterior mandible are commonly used. Other views include reverse Towne's, lateral oblique and basic tomography.

If surgery is being considered computed tomography (CT) is recommended and may identify previously undiagnosed sagittal/dicapitular or comminuted fractures. If meniscus and capsular disruption are suspected, magnetic resonance imaging (MRI) is also advisable.

Management Strategies

The aims of condyle fracture treatment are to achieve:

1. pain-free mouth opening with interincisal distance greater than 40 mm
2. good movement of the jaw in all excursions
3. restoration of the preinjury occlusion
4. stable temporomandibular joints
5. good facial and jaw symmetry.

Indications for open reduction internal fixation (ORIF) in adult patients

Absolute

- Displacement into the middle cranial fossa or external auditory meatus.
- Inability to obtain adequate occlusion by non-surgical treatment.

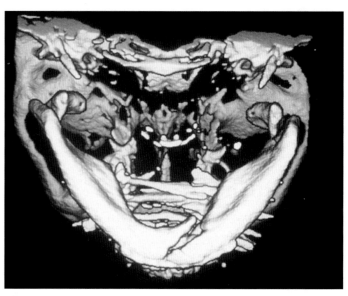

Fig. 16.2: Three-dimensional CT demonstrating symphyseal and bilateral condylar (Guardsman's) fractures in which the fixation of the symphyseal fracture has been inadequate with splaying of the lingual cortex and increase in the interangular distance.

- Invasion by foreign body or gross contamination.
- Lateral extracapsular displacement.

Relative

- Bilateral fractures in edentulous jaws.
- Intermaxillary fixation (IMF) contraindicated for medical reasons.
- Bilateral condyle fractures associated with comminuted midface fractures.

Other indications include those of Joos & Kleinheinz[5]:

- fracture types II and IV with an angle between fragments of >37°
- fracture types II and IV with longitudinal displacement of 4 mm.

The proposed Strasbourg Osteosynthesis Research Group (SORG) prospective randomized trial of ORIF versus conservative (10–45°) treatment has an angulation of >45° as an exclusion for randomization, as these fractures are thought to warrant internal fixation.

Indications for non-surgical treatment may include:

- condylar neck fractures in children <12 years
- high condylar neck fractures without dislocation
- intracapsular/dicapitular condylar fractures
- poor anesthetic risk.

Conservative closed functional treatment

Closed treatment definition

The treatment of condylar fractures by means other than surgical exploration, reduction and fixation of the fracture line, i.e. not involving an open surgical exposure of the fracture. Traditionally this has been achieved by arch bars, splints fitted over the remaining dentition, IMF screws or bonded brackets. Once reduction of the occlusion has been achieved, a period of immobilization may be required to encourage bony healing. Early mobilization is advised in order to minimize the risk of fibrous and bony TMJ ankylosis. This method of treatment is based on the principle that condylar non-union is unlikely despite mobilization.

Closed functional treatment definition

This involves the principles of closed treatment as above but followed by at least 3 months rehabilitation to include guiding elastics and mobilization regimes. It was found that when a full range of jaw movement was attained, normal jaw growth was not hindered. Adult muscles are more powerful than children's and commonly cause jaw shift, leading to malocclusion. The application of elastics to guide the occlusion will allow some degree of remodeling and articulation in its new position. Early mobilization will reduce the development of soft tissue scarring and promote increased mobility. Employing intermittent maxillomandibular elastic traction each night, followed by release in the morning for full daytime use, results in daily stretching of the soft tissues. The motion allows the linear and circumarticular healing of these tissues to be sufficient to allow a full range of joint and jaw movement. Scarring and tethering is inevitable but in this way it may be wide enough to allow full jaw mobility. Repeated holding of the jaw in occlusion at night results in a balance between remodeling of the condylar fracture and firm extension of the soft tissue healing. These are the principles of closed functional treatment.

In order to encourage mobilization, mechanical devices have been developed to provide continuous passive motion (CPM). However, they are cumbersome and expensive. An alternative is the use of wooden spatulas to achieve 40 mm of interincisal opening. The number of spatulas placed between the upper and lower molar and premolar teeth is gradually increased until the desired opening is achieved. They are then taped together to allow use 4–5 times per day during the 3 months of rehabilitation. Protrusive and excursive movements are equally important during this period.

The literature is inconclusive regarding the success of conservative treatment as series are often contradictory. Original work carried out by the Chalmers J Lyon Club[6] provides the basis for the conservative approach, citing good results in 120 cases treated conservatively. MacLennan[3] and Blevins & Gores[7] also published results supporting conservative treatment.

Based on research showing that bony union occurs in condylar fractures, whether intermaxillary fixation is applied or not, the restoration of occlusion in a unilateral or bilateral condylar fracture, by employing IMF and non-rigid immobilization for 7–10 days and 3–4 weeks respectively, provides a satisfactory functional outcome in many reported series.

In situations where there is gross displacement of the condylar fragment, IMF can achieve function by bony union of the fracture ends followed by pseudoarthrosis and re-education of the TMJ system over a 2–6 month period.

These early studies have been criticized heavily. In the case of the Chalmers J Lyon Club only 60 of the 120 patients were examined; the remainder were surveyed by post. In MacLennan's paper only 67 of the 120 patients were examined and Blevins & Gore used a postal questionnaire. Furthermore, there was no stratification of severity of injury and the caseloads spanned all ages. Subsequently it was found that bony remodeling and restoration of function varied with age, raising questions on the interpretation of these series.

Recent evidence supporting closed treatment of unilateral condylar fractures in adult patients

Over a 12-year period Marker[8] reviewed 348 patients who had closed treatment of mandibular condyle fractures. IMF was applied for 4 weeks in condylar fractures alone and for 6 weeks in combined body fractures. Patients were assessed for complaints, mouth opening, malocclusion and deviation after treatment and again after 1 year. In this series 72% of patients had unilateral fractures and 28% had bilateral condylar fractures. After 1 year 13% of patients stated that they had physical complaints, comprising one or a combination of symptoms which included: reduction in mouth opening, deviation on opening, malocclusion, clicking and limited chewing ability. In these 13%, there was no difference between the severity or frequency of symptoms according to whether a unilateral or bilateral fracture pattern was present. However, there was an association between cause of fracture and complaint. The unilateral fracture caused by sporting accidents and bilateral condylar fracture caused by road traffic accidents caused the most subjective complaints. This difference, however, was not statistically significant. Only 3% of the 348 complained of pain in the TMJ or muscles.

Mouth opening was recorded as abnormal immediately post treatment in 55% of cases whilst after 1 year this had fallen to only 10%. In these patients there was an almost equal distribution between unilateral and bilateral fracture pattern.

In cases with persistent limitation of movement at 1 year, 69% of patients were treated by IMF while the remainder had soft diet alone. Malocclusion was detected in only 2% of the 348 patients assessed. On review of the degree of dislocation and malocclusion it was found that 31% of patients with bilateral dislocations but only 5% of unilateral dislocations developed malocclusion. Of the overall 2% with malocclusion, most could be treated with simple occlusal grinding; the remainder of patients were not concerned and did not wish further treatment. Only one case required a sagittal split osteotomy to correct the malocclusion. Deviation on opening was recorded in 10% of cases and was more frequently associated with high forces of impact. The results were amalgamated to conclude that there were more complaints in the bilateral fracture group compared to the unilateral fracture group when measured objectively.

There was no record of the degree of angulation or overlap at presentation but Silvennoinen et al[1] estimate that 50% of condylar fractures would fall into the operative category, which when applied to this study should produce more dissatisfied patients. However, complaints were few. Marker et al therefore conclude that these 'rules' are by no means a definite criterion for surgery. They advocate closed treatment but are cautious in applying this treatment method to dislocation of the condylar head and bilateral fractures.

Joos & Kleinheinz[5] published a prospective study of 122 adult patients with 138 condylar fractures. Fracture types included were limited to type II and type IV low condylar neck fractures. The patients were allowed to choose between closed and open treatment. Assessment included clinical examination, three-dimensional axiography, radiographic assessment and ultrasound/TMJ evaluation. The results showed no significant differences in outcome.

In this paper the authors also try to predict mathematically the potential for vertical repair and angulation repair in the non-operated condyle. They conclude that 6° of angulation can resolve and 4 mm of height can be regained. However, angles greater than 37° can remodel little and give problems clinically.

Hidding et al[9] retrospectively analyzed 34 patients with unilateral dislocated fractures of the condylar neck; 20 were treated surgically by ORIF and 14 by closed treatment.

They assessed outcome subjectively and analytically by axiography, radiography and clinical and functional examination. They found some significant differences in measurement parameters but from the patients' own mastication ability they could not say one group recovered better than the other. One possible limitation to this paper is that it only looked at results 5 years from treatment and possible long-term sequelae are not predictable. However, Dahlstrom et al[10] suggested little long-term change in their series. The authors conclude that ORIF of the displaced condylar fracture should be undertaken on the grounds of better measurement criteria rather than subjective outcome.

Konstantinovic & Dimitrijevic[11] compared surgical versus non-surgical treatment of unilateral condylar process fractures. By computer-simulated graphic presentations of posteroanterior (PA) radiographs of the mandible, actual post-treatment condylar reduction was compared with ideal reduction as determined by the computer. Using standardized clinical evaluation to assess the two groups (maximal mouth opening, deviation and protrusion), no statistical difference was found between the open or closed group. However, the radiographic examination showed a statistically better position of the surgically reduced condyle process fracture. This study would seem to discourage open surgery on the grounds of overtreatment. However, the patient sample (26 open vs 54 closed) reveals that they did not randomize the patients' treatment and there was a much greater number of patients with severe condylar displacement in the surgical group, as stated in the article. If one assumes that the likelihood of post-trauma problems becomes greater as the degree of condylar displacement increases, then this study also tends to support open treatment because both groups had similar treatment results.

Dahlstrom et al[10] reported on a 15-year follow-up of conservatively treated condylar fractures in 36 patients. This series provides the best data available on the long-term outlook of closed treatment. In this study the patients who had sustained their injury in childhood had excellent results, with no growth restriction. Adults had some degree of restriction, as did the teenage group (12–19 years). Twice as many patients in the older group experienced symptoms of dysfunction compared to the younger group. Radiologically the younger group showed better ability to restore condylar morphology. Interestingly, in this study the symptoms and signs at 6 months were similar to those at 15-year follow-up, suggesting that long-term gradual improvement cannot necessarily be expected. Also from this we may conclude that future study design may not need to be protracted.

In order to guide the surgeon in the application of closed or open treatment, a number of measurable criteria have been advocated, including angulation of condyle by >37° and fragment overlap >5 mm. A recent study by Ellis et al[12] looked at the position of the condylar fragment when closed treatment was deemed appropriate only to find that the post-IMF condylar position was different to that at the outset of treatment. If the condyle position now falls into the operative criteria then should conservative treatment be abandoned for ORIF in the individual patient? In this study 65 patients were treated by closed treatment. Coronal and sagittal displacement was assessed pre IMF, immediately post IMF and at 6 weeks and a statistically significant difference (mean −5.5°) in the coronal position of the condylar process pre and post arch bars was found. The change in a sagittal plane was not statistically significant. Other planes of movement were noticed but did not reach significance. Further changes were noted at 6 weeks follow-up. The authors conclude that care must be taken in basing treatment decisions on the degree of displacement or dislocation of the condylar process in presurgical radiographs.

Studies supporting open treatment of unilateral fractures in adult patients

Palmieri et al[13] studied 136 patients with fractures of the condylar process; 74 were treated by closed methods and 62 by open methods. They were assessed for mandibular and condylar mobility at 6 weeks, 6 months and 1, 2 and 3 years post surgery. A jaw-tracking device was employed to assess mandibular motion. Radiographs were traced and digitized to assess condylar displacement and condylar mobility. It was accepted that patients treated by open reduction had significantly greater initial displacement of their condylar fractures compared to the closed group. As one would expect, condylar malposition persisted in the closed group compared with the open group. At 6 weeks, those patients treated by the closed method had some measures of mobility that were significantly greater than those in patients treated by open reduction and fixation. However, after that time there were minimal differences between the two groups and subsequently there was significant improvement in mobility in the open reduction group. No measure of presurgical displacement correlated with mobility measures in patients treated by open reduction. However, several measures of condylar displacement correlated with measures of mobility in patients treated by the closed method, indicating that the more displaced the condylar process, the more limited the mobility. The authors conclude that patients treated for fractures by open reduction had somewhat greater condylar mobility than patients treated by the closed method, even though the ORIF group had more severely displaced fractures before surgery. They believe ORIF can produce functional benefits in patients with severely displaced condylar process fractures.

Worsaae & Thorn[14] published a series in which they evaluated 52 patients (24 with dislocated fractures) who were randomized to ORIF (24 patients) or closed treatment (28 patients). All fractures were unilateral, the condyles were displaced from the fossa and/or overlapped at the fracture site and the patients were all 18 years or older and dentate. High condylar neck fractures were excluded from the study. The open treatment consisted of a submandibular incision and wire osteosynthesis followed by 6 weeks of IMF. The non-surgical (closed) treatment consisted of an average of 30 days IMF, with a range of 0–47 days. Both treatment groups had a median of 7 days of interarch training elastics following release of IMF. The mean follow-up period was 21 months for the ORIF group and 30 months for the closed (non-surgical) group, with each group having the same range of 6–64 months. The complication rate was 39% (11 of 28) in the non-surgical group and only 4% (one of 24) in the surgical group. The one patient with a problem in the surgical group had a collapse of the repositioned condyle and developed a malocclusion and muscle pain. In the non-surgical group, there were three patients with mandibular asymmetry, eight with malocclusions, three with reduced mouth opening (<35 mm), two with persistent headaches and six with muscle pain and impaired masticatory function. The median mouth opening for both groups was 45 mm, despite the relatively long periods in IMF. Thus, comparing mouth opening alone did not separate the two groups. This study could have produced better results if more rigid fixation had been used instead of wire osteosynthesis.

Eckelt[15] published a series of 103 patients treated by ORIF with 26 of these having bilateral fractures. The results were excellent compared with closed treatment. He reports normal anatomical alignment in 84% and limitation of protrusion in only 6% of cases.

Hidding et al[9] investigated 34 patients with dislocated fractures of the condylar neck of which 20 had been treated by open reduction and 14 by closed functional treatment. Assessment was by clinical, radiographic and axiographic means. The clinical results were nearly equal in both groups but instrumental registration and X-ray findings showed considerable deviation in the joint physiology in the closed group. Nineteen of 20 patients operated on showed near-anatomical reconstruction with good functional results. It may be reasonable to propose that these patients would do better in the long term.

Takenoshita et al[16] reported a comparison of open and closed reduction in 36 cases of condylar fracture with a 2-year follow-up. Sixteen of the cases were treated by open reduction and internal fixation via pre-auricular and short Risdon incision, followed by 3 weeks of IMF. The other 20 cases were treated by only 3 weeks of IMF. The two groups were not randomly selected. The open reduction group was selected for surgery because they had dislocated or severely displaced condylar processes. The authors' comparison showed that both groups had a similar result. If one assumes that severe condylar displacement is more likely to result in compromised jaw function, for which there is some evidence, then open reduction was beneficial for this surgical group.

Bilateral condylar fractures in adults

In the consensus study by Baker et al[17] bilateral undisplaced fractures of the condyle were generally managed similarly by surgeons throughout the world. The introduction of condylar displacement, dislocation and intracapsular fracture patterns showed great variation in treatment preference when dealing with bilateral condylar fractures.

The Gronigen Consensus Group[18] concluded that there was good evidence that displaced bilateral condylar fractures would benefit from *at least* one side being treated by open reduction and internal fixation. It was accepted that this may cause an increased risk of even further displacement of the other side. It was noted that some displaced bilateral fractures can be treated successfully by the closed method but predicting a favorable outcome is difficult.

Newman[19] published a series of 61 patients with bilateral condylar fractures; 51% of patients had bilateral condylar fractures alone, the remainder also had other fractures, mainly parasymphyseal. Nearly half the condylar fractures (46%) were undisplaced. Thirty nine patients (21%) were managed by the closed method with wire rigid IMF for a mean of 37 days, 13 were managed conservatively and nine (15%) with 10 fractured condyles were managed by open reduction and internal fixation. The most common complaint after treatment was persistent limitation in mouth opening, which was significantly less in the ORIF group (mean (SD) 44 mm (2 mm)) than in the IMF group (28 mm (2 mm), p<0.01).

More importantly, 10% of the patients treated by closed IMF required orthognathic surgery to correct a persistent anterior open bite, despite the long periods in rigid IMF. The authors also commented that most of this group requiring orthognathic surgery had minimal angulation at presentation. They concluded that the risk of complications from ORIF were minimal and that in the case of bilateral condylar fractures, ORIF should be undertaken at least on one side if displacement or angulation is present.

Our unit policy involves treating the patient with interarch elastic traction for a period of 1 week followed by further assessment. If the occlusion is found to be satisfactory and the condylar fragments are undisplaced on OPT and PA views, we treat the fracture by the closed method. If the fragments are seen on one side to be overlapped by >5 mm or angulation is >37° then we would select treatment by ORIF of the displaced fracture. If both sides show significant displacement and measurement of angulation and overlap are

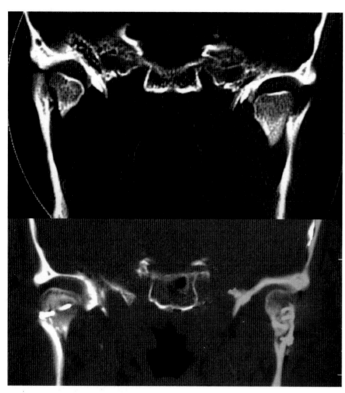

Fig. 16.3: Composite CT scan showing pre- and postoperative position following bilateral condylar fractures.

greater than the above values then we advise ORIF of both sides (Fig. 16.3), i.e. each side being assessed on its own merits.

Particular care is needed to achieve very accurate reduction of the fragments prior to fixation. This is necessary as it may not be possible to hold the teeth in occlusion during the procedure, as a downward distraction of the angle may be the only way to retrieve and reduce the condylar fragment. Once satisfactory fixation is achieved the patient can mobilize immediately postoperatively. To date we have not experienced any seventh nerve injury that would change this policy.

The benefits of ORIF are:

1. direct visualization of the fragments for accurate reduction and fixation
2. early mobilization of the mandible
3. early restoration of normal mouth and jaw activity.

Reported complications of open treatment include:

1. poor esthetic result following the skin incision. This is particularly relevant if keloid scarring is likely
2. neural damage, particularly the facial nerve
3. peroperative bleeding from the maxillary artery
4. loss of blood supply to the condylar head, leading to avascular necrosis.

Management of condylar fractures in panfacial injury

Panfacial injuries pose considerable challenges to the maxillofacial surgeon. The reduction and fixation of the facial

skeleton must be restored in the correct anteroposterior (AP), lateral (width) and vertical dimensions. In the case of severe comminution of the midface and mandible, the only point of reference from which to start reconstruction is the stable posterior area (temporal bone and proximal zygomatic arch), working sequentially to restore AP projection followed by reduction in width and restoration of the nasoethmoidal and orbital complex. Attention is then applied to accurate restoration of posterior vertical height by repositioning and fixation of the condylar ramus fracture. Access to the condylar fragment can be gained by extending the coronal incision used to access the zygomatic arch. Once posterior vertical height is restored then the anterior mandible can be fixed with accurate reduction in intercondylar width. Finally occlusion is attended to with fixation being applied lastly at the Le Fort I level, although some surgeons prefer to fix the occlusion at an earlier stage.

Surgical Approaches

Submandibular approach (Risdon approach) (Fig. 16.4)

This approach is best suited to low fractures of the condylar neck and ramus.

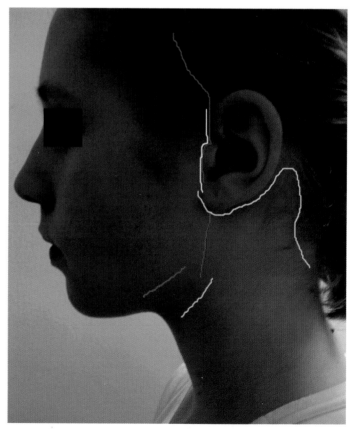

Fig. 16.4: Position of the various incisions. Blue = Bramley–Al Quayat; yellow = pre-auricular; turquoise = rhytidectomy; red = retromandibular; green = submandibular; purple = submandibular (continental).

Anatomical points of importance

The marginal mandibular branch of the facial nerve runs on the deep surface of the platysma and is most likely to be no lower than 1.5 cm below the lower border of the mandible. The facial artery runs vertically at the anterior border of the masseter muscle. The facial vein runs with the facial artery but posterior to it.

Preparation and draping

Conventional draping to allow exposure of the surgical field with the ear visible posteriorly and the corner of the mouth and lower lip anteriorly.

Incision marking and vasoconstriction

The proposed skin incision is marked before infiltration with vasoconstrictor (normal saline with 1:200 000 adrenaline). The incision should be 1.5–2 cm below the lower border of the mandible (if possible), employing the natural skin creases. These do not parallel the lower border but do provide ease of extension if required, with good cosmesis.

If there is shortening of the posterior mandibular height by telescoping of fragments, this should be taken into account when planning the site of the incision.

Dissection

The skin and platysma are incised, exposing the superficial layer of deep cervical fascia. Care must be taken to avoid cutting the facial artery and vein. If they limit access they can be tied and ligated or retracted. The marginal mandibular branch of the facial nerve lies superiorly and should be retracted gently with Langenback retractors. The dissection continues to the pterygomasseteric sling which is incised with a scalpel along the inferior border, its most avascular area. With the aid of a periosteal stripper the masseter is lifted off the lateral ramus. Dissecting superiorly, the entire lateral surface of the ascending ramus of the mandible can be exposed to the TMJ and the coronoid process. The fractured end of the proximal fragment is frequently embedded in the masseter and will need to be dissected free. Care must be taken not to shred the muscle or perforate the oral mucosa anteriorly.

Closure

It is possible to repair the pterygomasseteric sling with resorbable sutures. The insertion of a vacuum drain helps to reduce hematoma formation. Platysma can be closed by a running resorbable suture followed by interrupted subcuticular stitches. Finally the skin is closed with nylon.

Submandibular approach – continental

This incision is at the level of the lower mandibular border. Dissection is carried out above the masseter, identifying the seventh nerve branches. Medial dissection, splitting the masseter muscle to the ascending ramus, gives good exposure.

Retromandibular approach

This approach is more suitable for low condylar fractures (Fig. 16.5). There are a number of approaches which

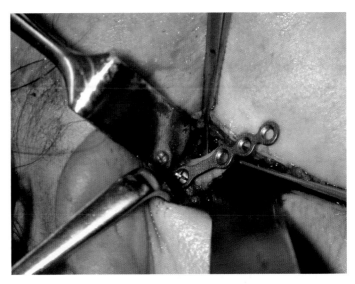

(a)

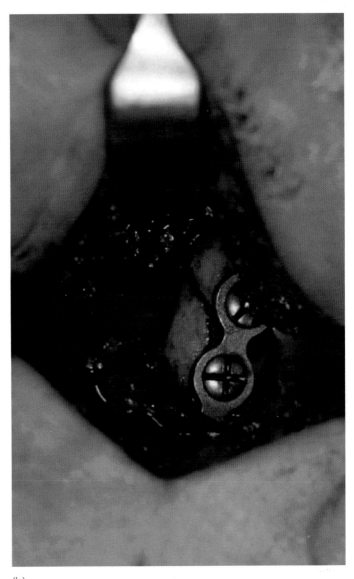

(b)

Fig. 16.5: Retromandibular approach demonstrating placement of fixation plate prior to **(a)** and after **(b)** reduction of the proximal fragment.

surgeons call 'retromandibular'. We shall initially deal with the most common.

Anatomical points of importance

The main trunk of the facial nerve divides into the temporofacial and cervicofacial divisions. The marginal mandibular branch courses obliquely inferiorly and anteriorly. It often arises from the main trunk behind the posterior border of the mandible, crossing the ramus at its lower border. This allows good access with relative safety between the buccal branch and the marginal mandibular nerve. The retromandibular vein courses through the parotid gland superficial to the external carotid artery.

Preparation and draping

Draping should expose the entire earlobe and the angle of the mandible. The mouth should also be visualized.

Incision marking and vasoconstriction

The incision line begins 0.5 cm below the earlobe and continues inferiorly for 3–3.5 cm. It is located behind the ascending ramus of the mandible and may be extended inferiorly. Normal saline with 1:200 000 adrenaline is injected into the operative field.

Dissection

Incise through skin and subcutaneous tissue. The parotid capsule is now seen. Before incising the capsule, undermine the skin to allow retraction. The superficial musculo-aponeurotic system (SMAS) and parotid capsule are now incised and blunt dissection directly onto the posterior edge of the mandible undertaken with a hemostat. The hemostat should be opened parallel to the anticipated direction of the nerve. The marginal mandibular branch may be directly encountered or can be sought with the aid of an electric nerve stimulator. Once the nerve is identified retraction can be performed in a superior or inferior direction. Placing a flat instrument behind the ascending ramus will hold the mandible steady to allow sharp dissection with a blade through the pterygomasseteric sling, subperiosteally. Blunt dissection superiorly, stripping periosteum, will expose the fracture ends. Care must be taken when disimpacting the condylar fragment from the masseter muscle.

Closure

It is possible to repair the pterygomasseteric sling with resorbable sutures. The insertion of a vacuum drain helps reduce hematoma formation. Closure of the parotid capsule and SMAS layer must be meticulous to reduce the chance of the formation of a salivary fistula. Platysma, once defined, can be closed by a running resorbable suture followed by interrupted subcuticular stitches. Finally the skin is closed with nylon.

Retromandibular approach – deep

Some surgeons dissect down to the sternocleidomastoid muscle then deep to the superficial lobe of the parotid gland and approach the posterior ramus from a deep angle, with the branches of the seventh nerve superficial to the dissection.

Retromandibular approach – horizontal through parotid

Some surgeons have advocated dissection above the parotid gland and incision horizontally through the parotid gland and masseter muscle, between the buccal and marginal mandibular branches of the seventh nerve, to gain access to the ascending ramus.

Modified Blair incision approach

This approach is suitable for both low and high condylar fractures. It combines the pre-auricular and the retromandibular approach and offers increased exposure. It is particularly good for demonstrating the upper TMJ as well as the meniscus. It is used for repositioning and fixing intracapsular and very high TMJ fractures.

Pre-auricular and auricular approach

This approach gives good access to the TMJ, allowing repair of capsular disruption, and is suitable for high condylar fractures. The facial nerve is preserved by using the Al Quayat and Bramley modification (Fig. 16.6). The incision is started superiorly through the scalp and the temporalis fascia is

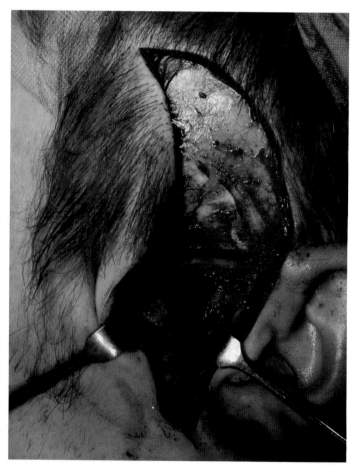

Fig. 16.6: Bramley–Al Quayat approach.

identified. Development of the flap in this plane is carried out anteroinferiorly to a point where the fat is visible through the superficial layer of temporalis fascia. This appears at about 2 cm above the zygomatic arch. The skin is dissected off the tragus and the cartilaginous external acoustic meatus. This plane is avascular and dissection ends with exposure of the postglenoid tubercle. The superficial layer of the temporalis fascia is incised at 45° anterosuperiorly to avoid the facial nerve. The periosteum of the arch is incised and raised as one flap with the outer layer of the temporalis fascia. Periosteum may be incised as far forward as is necessary to gain good exposure to the TMJ capsule. Ligation of the superficial temporal vessels is often required during this approach. The sharp condylar neck fragment often tears laterally through the capsule as it telescopes superiorly. Dissection of the condylar neck is performed by lateral capsular incision and periosteal stripping down the condylar neck to expose sufficient fixation surface.

The condylar head is usually deep and anteriorly sited and requires mobilization to deliver it laterally and upwards into accurate reduction. Kocher's bone-holding forceps or artery clips can grasp the condylar head fragment while the neck and ramus are pulled inferiorly by the assistant's fingers pushing intraorally on the molar region. A bone hook can help in moving the condylar neck but may risk splitting it if pulled too forcefully; we prefer the intraoral pressure method. Closure in layers is required to restore anatomy and a small vacuum drain prevents hematoma formation.

Rhytidectomy approach

Anatomical points of importance
In addition to the other structures mentioned above, the great auricular nerve courses at 45° to the sternocleidomastoid, anterosuperiorly just deep to the SMAS.

Preparation and draping
This should allow direct visualization of the corner of the eye and the mouth. The ear should be fully exposed along with the descending hair line and 2–3 cm of hair behind the ear.

Skin marking and vasoconstriction
The incision begins 1.5–2 cm superior to the zygomatic arch just behind the hair line and in front of the ear. The incision then curves inferiorly under the earlobe and about 3 mm onto the posterior surface of the auricle, which allows scarring to be less noticeable.

Incision and dissection
The incision is through the skin and subcutaneous tissue only, followed by wide blunt dissection deep to the subcutaneous tissue and the anterior surface is undermined widely. Once the lateral surface is exposed dissection continues as a standard retromandibular approach.

Closure
It is possible to repair the masseter and medial pterygoids with resorbable sutures. Closure of the parotid capsule and

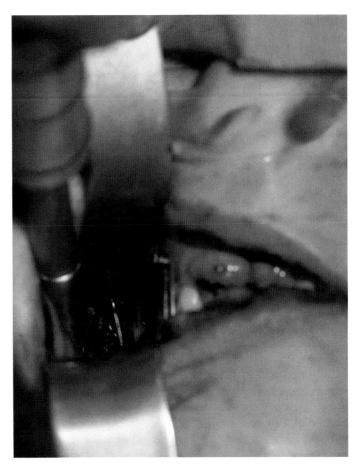

Fig. 16.7: Intraoral approach demonstrating use of right-angled drill.

SMAS layer must be meticulous to reduce the chance of a salivary fistula forming. Platysma can be closed by a running resorbable suture followed by interrupted subcuticular stitches. The insertion of a vacuum drain helps reduce hematoma formation. Finally the skin is closed with nylon.

Transoral approach

This technique has the advantage of avoiding facial scarring and risk of injury to the facial nerve. Facial nerve injury has, however, been reported during this approach and warnings should be included when obtaining patient consent.

The major disadvantage is limited access, making fragment control difficult and the procedure surgically more challenging. The introduction of right-angled instruments with illumination has promoted the use of this approach (Fig. 16.7). It should be reserved for fractures that involve the low condylar region. It may not be possible to align the posterior border perfectly and slight errors of reduction are therefore inevitable.

Technique
An incision is made over the anterior border of the vertical ramus, extending into the lower buccal sulcus. The temporalis muscle is stripped from the anterior ascending ramus and masseter is stripped by subperiosteal dissection. It is important to do this extensively as it allows easier retraction

and visibility. A Bauer retractor placed in the sigmoid notch can sometimes aid reduction. A LeVasseur Merrill fiberoptic retractor can be used to aid reduction while applying fixation.

A transbuccal trocar is introduced and drilling occurs transbuccally and the plate is introduced transorally. It may be difficult to maintain fixation in the posterior thick cortical bone and the drill may enter the fracture line or the weaker subsigmoid area.

Mokros[20] reported a series of 34 patients with low subcondylar fractures approached transorally. They employed a 90° drill and screw driver, special reduction hook and retractors.

Undt's[21] retrospective review of 55 patients who had 57 condylar neck fractures treated with transoral miniplate osteosynthesis concluded that satisfactory reduction and fixation can be achieved with avoidance of facial scarring.

Endoscopic approach

Endoscopically assisted reduction and fixation of fractures of the condyle have been described in the literature but are not widely employed in practice. Endoscopic approaches have been used for fixation of fractures of the wrist and tibial plateau regions and also in comminuted malar fractures. The advantages are reduced tissue trauma and reduced risk of facial nerve injury.

Lauer & Schmelzeisen[22] described an endoscopic approach in seven patients. In four cases standard endoscopic equipment was used via a pre-auricular/submandibular approach in conjunction with a transbuccal trocar through which the plates were introduced and fixed. They applied a new design of instrument in three cases, which allowed subperiosteal dissection as well as delivering the plate to the fracture site. However, one of the three cases required removal of the plate and screws due to loosening. They reported an operating time of 3.5 hours compared with 2–2.5 hours for their traditional open approach. No occurrence of facial nerve injury was noted.

The authors admit there are limitations to this technique: only straight plates can be placed, the overall view is restricted, there may be difficulties in the reduction of the condylar fragment and only experienced surgeons should try to use it. They also comment that it should not be applied to gross dislocations (displacement in UK/USA) or comminuted fractures.

Schmelzeisen & Wichmann[23] have also reported early work in endoscopic fixation of the condylar fracture (see Chapter 31).

Techniques of reduction

Reduction of the fractured condyle can be very difficult, especially when the condylar head is medially dislocated. In these cases surgical instruments must be employed to try to reposition the condyle (Fig. 16.8). The use of the curved elevator, Howarth's elevator and tracheostomy hook have all been advocated. Some surgeons have also drilled rigid fixation wires into the fragment to gain control. Kocher's boneholding forceps can be used to grasp and reduce fragments

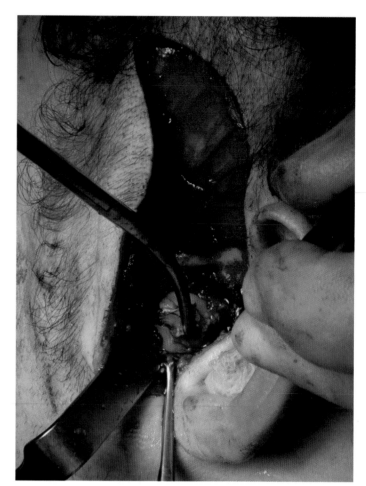

Fig. 16.8: Kocher's forceps being used to reduce the proximal fragment.

but can crush and split the condylar head so must be used with caution. In cases of severe and difficult reduction the lateral pterygoid insertion can be cut to give greater mobility and reducibility but preservation of the periosteal attachment to the condylar head is mandatory to preserve a blood supply to the proximal fragment. We do not agree with temporarily removing the condyle and replacing it as a free graft because the risk of avascular necrosis is high. Gross comminution in the non-compound/contaminated fracture of the condylar head should not be excised as this will result in loss of vertical height. We believe that leaving this in situ offers the potential to repair with non-rigid IMF. As in all fracture management, accurate reduction is mandatory and care must be taken in orientating the condyle, as this is not always obvious from the fracture ends.

Downward traction on the mandible can be achieved by double-gloved intraoral pressure in the molar region, temporary wiring or screw and wire traction on the lower border if surgical exposure allows. There is no substitute for practice to gain competence at reduction and surgeons will adopt instrumentation according to their own preference. We prefer the presence of two assistants during condylar surgery to ensure optimal exposure and reduction.

In cases of condylar fracture requiring ORIF with simultaneous fixation of body or symphyseal/parasymphyseal fracture, we fix the condyle first, thus giving greater mobility and easier reduction of the condyle. As mentioned earlier, bilateral fractures with body or sym/parasymphyseal fracture require particular attention to intercondylar distance when plating the non-condylar area. The tendency to open posteriorly can result in crossbite and malocclusion and external palm pressure applied simultaneously at the angles of the mandible will reduce this splaying, prior to the plating, and correct the crossbite.

Fixation

Historical methods of fixation include transosseous wire fixation, external fixation and Kirschner wire fixation. Current methods are discussed below.

Miniplate osteosynthesis

Condylar plate and screw systems are designed to withstand and overcome any biomechanical deforming forces that may arise, thereby minimizing micromotion of the bone ends. Under conditions of stability and perfect fracture reduction, the condition of primary bone healing will occur. In this situation new bone will form along the surface of the fracture without fibrous tissue intervening. High condylar fractures due to bony limitations may only accommodate one plate (Fig. 16.9). A 2 mm plate with two screws above and below the fracture parallel to the posterior border provides, in our opinion, adequate stability in most cases.

Hammer et al[24] reported inadequate stability leading to plate failure or screw loosening in more than one-third (35%) of cases treated with single adaptational plating. They questioned whether a period of maxillomandibular fixation was needed in combination with plating. Other authors have also reported fractures of plates used in condylar neck fractures and suggested that condylar plates should be stronger and thicker than the thinner adaptational plates.

Byung-Ho et al[25] studied the strengths of condylar plates in cadaver mandibles. They loaded the condyle to reproduce functional loading and fixation included miniplate (four screws), mini DCP (four screws), 2.4 mm plate (four screws) and double miniplate. They found that the only system able to withstand normal forces of loading was the double mini-

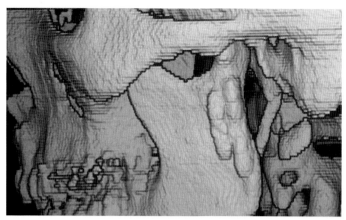

Fig. 16.10: Postoperative three-dimensional CT showing left condylar fracture following ORIF using two osteosynthesis plates.

plate method. This mechanical advantage stems from the neutralizing effect of the plates on the functional stresses in the condylar neck. In vitro strain measurements of the condylar process showed that the highest level of tensile strain occurred on the anterior and lateral surfaces and the highest compressive strain on the posterior surface. The two miniplates applied at the posterior and anterior border of the condylar neck seem to have the advantage of restoring the tension and compression trajectories.

In the case of low condylar fracture two plates may be required to achieve stability (Fig. 16.10). At least two screws should be placed in the condylar fragment and at least two in the main mandibular segment. The posterior plate should parallel the posterior ascending ramus and the anterior plate can be angulated across the fracture line.

Eckelt[27] has commented that a disadvantage of miniplating is the occasional need to remove these plates. This necessitates re-exploring the wound which involves a much greater risk of injury to the facial nerve due to its tethering and anatomical distortion. This has led to alternative minimal access techniques being developed, which we will discuss below.

Meyer (PhD thesis, University of Strasbourg) showed that in a comparative study of three methods of fixation of simulated condylar neck fractures using a mandibular model, 3D miniplates gave the most stable fixation. An Eckelt screw was next most stable and standard miniplates were the least stable of the three methods.

Dynamic compression plating

As the fractures are generally oblique any compression effect during plating could lead to overlap of the fragment ends and loss of ramus height. A review of current practice would indicate that dynamic compression plating has little place in condylar fractures, treatment is adequate with miniplates placed in the neutral mode.

Lag screw osteosynthesis

A true lag screw only has threads on the distal end, so that when these threads engage the far cortex, the screw head seats against the near cortex and on tightening, provides

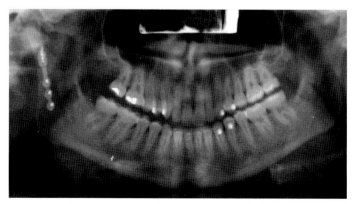

Fig. 16.9: Postoperative orthopantomogram following ORIF of right condylar fracture using a single osteosynthesis plate.

compression. This method is biomechanically advantageous because of the central location of the lag screw. The screw is placed in the interior of the condyle and there is therefore no need to open the joint capsule to place the fixation device. This permits a less traumatic operation than with miniplates, which may require the joint to be opened if the proximal fragment is short.

Lag screw osteosynthesis was first described in condylar fractures by Wackerbauer in 1962. Advantages of lag screws include rapid application of rigid fixation and close approximation of the fractured parts because of the large amount of compression generated. Contraindications to lag screw use are loss of bone in the fracture gap or comminution that would cause displacement and overriding of segments when compression is applied.

Many designs of lag screw are available but more simple designs rely on the spherical head of the screw acting as a wedge. Combining the screw with a washer or angled plate (e.g. Wurzburg lag screw plate) eliminates localized high stresses and transforms them into pressure which is better tolerated than crushing forces under the screw head. This prevents the screw head from penetrating the cortical bone. Lag screws with washers can be turned twice as tightly as those without washers before the surface bone begins to crack.[26] Authors have reported problems with lag screw systems, commenting that there is a tendency toward lateralization and rotation of the condylar head if the screw is not placed centrally. There is also a steep learning curve to this technique.

The Eckelt screw is one of the most popular lag screws in use today (Fig. 16.11). This technique involves an open approach with the preparation of a gliding canal between the buccal and lingual cortex of the larger fragment. This has a butt area at the lower border of the mandible that retains the device during tightening. The condylar head is reduced in one of three ways. First, by means of a thin elevator placed medially to the posterior border of the mandible and moved cranially, it is possible to push the fragment laterally and reduce it. Second, the reduction can be achieved by the use of specifically designed forceps to hold the condylar head on

its dorsal aspect. Third, the use of a reduction pin that is screwed into the condylar fragment and is manipulated to achieve reduction.

A gliding channel is drilled in the ramus of the mandible, parallel to the posterior border between the inner and outer cortices. The condylar fragment is then drilled with a narrow drill and a measuring gauge allows the correct screw length to be chosen. The lag screw is then inserted through the gliding channel into the condylar head and tightened with a nut. This provides good apposition of fragments and allows early mobilization. The screw can be removed under local anesthetic with a simple stab incision.

Eckelt[27] published a series of 230 patients who had undergone lag screw fixation over a 16-year period, showing an overall success rate of 90%. Fragment reduction and healing was present in 93.4% of cases. In 6.6% of cases healing occurred in a displaced position and incomplete reduction occurred in 3.5% of cases. Screw fracture or twisting after return to function occurred in 4.2% of cases. Stability of fixation allowing early mobilization was present in 91.1% of patients. In 5.8% there was instability attributed to extreme anatomical features and complicated fracture patterns. In these cases it was recognized peroperatively and additional methods of fixation were employed in conjunction with the lag screw. Surgical errors were reported: the screw too short to engage the condylar fragment in 3.1%; the screw being too long in 1.5% and anterior/medial malplacement of the screw in 4.2%. Once these errors were discovered postoperatively IMF was used for 2–3 weeks and the lag screw removed prematurely. Only three cases of screw fracture were encountered at the proximal end of the thread and screw bending occurred in only two cases. Screw migration may be caused by insufficient cooling of the drill, remodeling processes in the fracture gap or disturbed blood supply to the condylar fragment. Twenty-one percent of patients reported transient facial nerve weakness limited to the marginal mandibular branch and only one patient reported long-term problems with this nerve. The authors advocated supraplatysmal dissection to improve nerve protection. Krenkel[26] described a lag screw placed halfway up the ascending ramus. Welk et al[28] reported a contraindication rate to lag screws of 3.5% due to an extremely narrow or distorted ascending ramus and thin condylar neck. In another 9.3% they observed reduced loading capacity in the case of lateral bending forces due to considerable perforations of the lateral cortex after difficult screw placement. Teranobu[29] reported that certain racial differences of mandibular form may preclude lag screw use. Because of these potential problems, Hibi[30] has recommended a modified osteosynthesis method that combines miniplate and lag screw in atrophic mandibles. Kitayama[31] described the lag screw insertion via an intraoral approach but positioning in the condylar fragment can be eccentric, leading to displacement on tightening.

Pin fixation

Pin fixation uses 1.3 mm Kirschner wires placed into the condyle under direct vision. This technique requires an open

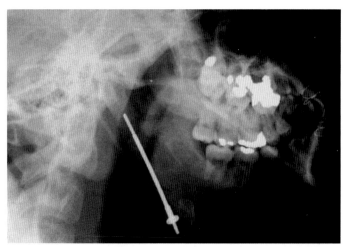

Fig. 16.11: Postoperative lateral oblique X-ray following ORIF of condylar fracture using Eckelt screw.

approach to the condylar head and traction applied to the lower border of the mandible. It is beneficial if the dorsal surface of the head can be seen, to enable reduction of the fracture to be assessed prior to fixation. Not all K-wires need to be passed through the surgical access site; a transbuccal approach can be used but this must be protected by a trephine. The direction of wire placement varies depending on the fracture configuration. Usually a minimum of three convergent K-wires is needed to ensure stability.

Resorbable plates and pins

The use of resorbable fixation devices is now well established in orthognathic and craniofacial practice. Authors cite good healing results with financial and psychological benefits. In particular, the use of resorbable materials during fixation of infected fractures is encouraging, as no foreign body persists to prolong the infection. However, resorption of the plate may take more than 2 years. Materials used include self-reinforced poly-L-lactide screws (SR-PLLA), polyglycolide pins and absorbable α-hydroxy polyesters. Report of their use in mandibular fractures is, however, limited to a few papers. Rass[32,33] described the replacement of the wires with resorbable polydioxanone pins giving good stability and avoiding the need for a second-stage removal procedure. Nehse & Maerker[34] also recommended polydioxanone, polylactide or autologous bone pins as temporary stabilization of subcondylar fractures but admitted that shortened IMF and functional therapy was mandatory with these fixation methods. They concluded that to date resorbable materials could not replace miniplate or traction screws, but enhanced the armamentarium available to the surgeon in the management of subcondylar fractures. Eppley et al[35] reported their experience of using polylactic-polyglycolic co-polymer plates in maxillofacial trauma and the results are encouraging, but to date no large series has been reported with regard to the mandibular condyle fracture.

Condylar Fractures in Children

Fractures of the facial skeleton in children account for only 5% of all facial fractures in a given population and are seen most commonly between the ages of 6 and 12 years. In most pediatric cohorts the most common maxillofacial fracture sites are the nose and dentoalveolar complex, followed by the mandible, orbit and midface. The male-to-female ratio is 2.4–2.9:1.0. Of the mandibular fractures, involvement of the condyle occurs in 43.3–72%.

In a retrospective analysis of 101 children under 16 years of age with condylar fractures, Thoren et al[36] found that 22% were intracapsular and 78% extracapsular. There was only a preponderance of intracapsular fractures (58%) amongst patients less than 6 years of age. In the older patients 78% of fractures were confined to the condylar neck. Subcondylar fractures accounted for only 4% of cases. They found displacement to be present in only 6% of cases but commented that dislocation of the condyle from the glenoid fossa was common in all ages. Sex of patient or etiology had no bearing on the fracture site.

Thoren[37] also published a series of 220 mandibular fractures in children in 1992 and found that condylar fractures were prevalent in those below 10 years of age. However, those children older than 10 years showed fracture patterns similar to the adult population, with body and angle fractures being more common.

As it is with adult patients, the management of childhood condylar fractures is controversial but consensus is now emerging that conservative treatment is the preferred method, especially in the younger patient. In the older age group and with severely displaced fractures, the debate continues. It is now accepted that the condylar cartilage and its 'condylar growth center', that traditionally was thought to provide the dominant growth impetus, is not as important as previously claimed. The mandible was likened to a long bone with the cartilage acting as an epiphyseal growth plate. Along with this growth center, appositional bone formation occurred at the sites of insertion of masseter at the angle of the mandible and temporalis at the coronoid. These sites lead to the development of the mandible in combination with alveolar margin stimulation.

Moss[38,39] proposed the functional matrix theory that the mandible develops in conjunction with the morphogenetic demands of the enveloping soft tissues, particularly muscle and ligaments, acting through their periosteal attachments. The theory states that the mandibular condyle is not the site of primary growth but has a secondary adaptive response, allowing the condylar head to stay in the fossa as the mandible develops. The predominant growth is downward and forward in response to the demand of the functional matrix. However, the condyle does have an important role in growth as condylectomy leads to reduced anteroposterior growth and trauma to the condylar region can result in unilateral or bilateral underdevelopment of the mandible.

If the condyle has lost its lead role in mandibular growth, how then are these findings explained? It is postulated that the matrix has been damaged in some way, possibly secondary to soft tissue trauma. The presence of ankylosis may also be significant in that it limits movement. Patients with juvenile arthritis (Still's disease) have been shown to have impaired anterior movement of the mandible by fibrous ankylosis. In these patients the condyle has lost its potential to remodel into the glenoid fossa.

As a result of this theoretical model it was commonly believed that the following patients/conditions would develop ankylosis and maldevelopment:

- children under 10 years of age
- fracture dislocations and intracapsular fractures of the condylar head
- compound fractures with comminution of the condylar head.

The treatment of condylar fractures in children is complicated by poor patient compliance, difficulty in applying IMF and crowded mandible and maxillae with developing teeth.

The methods employed to provide temporary immobilization include arch bars, acrylic splints, IMF screws and bonded brackets with heavy elastics. Fortunately the period of immobilization need only be for 1–2 weeks to allow early bone healing, followed by aggressive active mobilization of the mandible to prevent ankylosis. In addition, the use of guided elastics for up to 6–8 weeks will normally restore occlusion.

The 1999 Gronigen Consensus and a consensus study by Baker et al[17] confirm the practice of most units that ORIF has little or no role in the treatment of childhood condylar fractures. Numerous studies looking at the outcome of conservative fracture management in children confirm that closed functional treatment gives excellent results based on the growing patient's potential to remodel the condylar head and restore function.

Hovinga et al[40] studied 25 patients with childhood condylar fractures treated by the closed method over a 15-year period. They treated only five patients with IMF, the remainder being treated by early mobilization. The results were excellent with regard to masticatory function and patient satisfaction. High condylar fractures showed better regenerative tendency compared to intracapsular and low condylar fractures. Asymmetry was observed in only four patients by the trained observer and was not noticed by the patients. All deviations were distributed over all fracture types. The measurement of ascending ramus height did show some variation in 63.6% of cases but was usually not clinically significant. Only one case of intracapsular fracture had exhibited considerable growth disturbance and only one patient with persistent malocclusion required corrective osteotomy and in that case, the fracture was of a low condylar type. The findings of this series are in keeping with others who have assessed conservative closed functional treatment in children.

Other authors have assessed condylar repair by different methods: electronic computer-assisted recording of condylar movement, spiral computed tomography, nuclear magnetic resonance, plain radiographic assessment and orthopantomogram. Subtle findings including bony spurs, neo-arthrosis, bifid condyle, altered condylar angle, asymmetry and shorter condylar height are seen but these findings appear not to translate to functional problems and support the adaptive remodeling theory (see Fig. 16.10). This further confirms the role of conservative treatment in children.

Specific treatment strategies

Young patient <12 years with maximum remodeling potential

In this age group the adaptive mechanisms should restore function without a period of immobilization. We therefore advocate analgesia and early mobilization in all planes of mandibular movement.

Two patient groups need particular caution.

Where there is major disruption of occlusion
Significant occlusal disharmony consisting of open bite and possible retropositioning of the mandible may be seen after bilateral fracture dislocation. In these cases the potential for spontaneous correction by overeruption of teeth is limited.

Treatment in these instances should be by a conservative immobilization regime as in the case of an adult. In the case of a unilateral condyle fracture with major occlusal disruption, a period of immobilization for 10–14 days should be undertaken. Bilateral fracture may require immobilization for 3 weeks.

Young patients at risk of ankylosis and/or defective development

- Close proximity of the fractured condylar neck to the glenoid fossa, i.e. intracapsular fractures and fracture dislocation with telescoping
- Compound fractures with associated coronoid and zygomatic fractures

In these cases it must be assumed that there is damage to the meniscus and capsule. A conservative non-immobilization regime can be used if the patient has minimal symptoms. However, in the presence of severe pain a period of IMF, for no longer than 14 days, is recommended followed by active mobilization.

Adolescents 12–17 years of age

Similar principles apply to this age group as to the younger group, with slight modification. If a malocclusion is present, the capacity for spontaneous correction is less than in the younger age group. A malocclusion is therefore an indication for intermaxillary fixation for 2–3 weeks. The dentition at this stage tolerates simple islet wires or arch bars. The failure of conservative treatment would force the clinician to apply adult principles of treatment to the older members of this group.

Indications for open reduction and internal fixation

These are fortunately rare in the child patient and would include:

- failed conservative functional treatment
- where the fractured condyle directly interferes with jaw opening or movement
- where the fracture causes severe loss of ramus height with severe anterior open bite
- where the condylar fragment is dislocated into the middle cranial fossa.

It is important to appreciate that the best chance for full and functional recovery is obtained by causing as little trauma as possible to the surrounding tissues during the surgery. The authors would advise only experienced surgeons to undertake this procedure in the young patient.

Compound Fractures

Early operation with copious irrigation is indicated in both child and adult patients. In severe compound cases with gross comminution, removal of non-viable bone fragments is indicated at the time of exploration and closure. A swab for culture and sensitivity should be taken and followed by at least 5 days of broad-spectrum antibiotic. Early mobilization should be encouraged.

In the young patient cephalometric assessment should be performed postoperatively and repeated at follow-up to ensure adequate mandibular growth.

Complications

Malocclusion

Fractures close to the TMJ have a surprisingly favorable outcome. The bilateral condylar fracture causes the most malocclusions. Ellis[41] comments that despite accurate occlusion in these cases with rigid IMF and elastics, some patients will drift into anterior open bite after elastics have been removed for 12–24 hours. This is not a uniform finding. He postulates that the more displaced the condyles, the more adaptation is needed to maintain the normal occlusal relationship.

Most investigators conclude that the mandible functions as a class 3 lever system during biting. This means that the mean force vector of the elevator muscles is located between the fulcrum (TMJ) and the load (bite point). The loss of the fulcrum or displacement would significantly alter this relationship. In such cases the normal function of the elevators tends to raise the gonial angle further than normal, resulting in premature contact of the posterior dentition.

In Ellis' experience some patients can achieve normal occlusion despite displacement. He postulates that somehow the elevator muscles stay minimally active and do not contribute to the foreshortening. If they selectively activate the posterior temporalis muscle, the coronoid process is pulled posteriorly, allowing rotational closure of the mandible into occlusion with the maxilla. This results in inefficiency of the biting force but allows for the establishment of a new temporomandibular articulation by skeletal and dentoalveolar adaptations. Most patients cannot achieve this on their own and need IMF elastic traction to guide them. After non-surgical treatment a new temporomandibular articulation is established, resulting in restoration of the class 3 lever. As the mandibular plane becomes steeper the condylar stump approaches the skull base and once the remodeling is complete, the posterior vertical dimension stabilizes. Re-establishment is age related and younger patients may show normal TMJ morphology. Older patients show altered morphology with the new articulation being more inferior at the base of the articular eminence. The extrusion of anterior teeth and intrusion of posterior teeth restores the occlusion.

Persistent malocclusion can only be corrected by orthognathic surgery once the new articulation is stable. An asymmetrical anterior open bite can be corrected by a Le Fort I osteotomy. An asymmetric open bite or deviation of the mandible can be corrected by ascending ramus surgery.

Mandibular hypomobility

This is regarded as an interincisal opening of less than 40 mm. It is accepted that trauma is a cause of ankylosis. It is, however, rare after condylar fractures and has been estimated to occur in only 0.2–0.4%. Hypomobility has been reported to persist in between 8% and 10% of condylar fractures. Some patients function well at this reduced level of opening and some authors have found that masticatory dysfunction is higher in those patients who never regained a normal range of motion. Ellis recommends physiotherapy during recovery in the acute phase. Reducing the period of IMF can also help reduce hypomobility.

Asymmetry

Ellis comments that asymmetry in function is very common. Deviation towards the side of fracture has been reported in 50% of patients studied. It is presumed to be due to reduced lateral pterygoid function and/or pseudoarthrosis on the side of the fracture. The greater the condylar displacement, the greater the deviation. Asymmetry in mandibular growth has been shown to occur in approximately 25% of patients with fractures during the growing years. It is not always undergrowth – overgrowth has been reported to occur. From studies on patients with ankylosis we know that encouraging mobility leads to less growth disturbance. This principle should be applied to condylar fracture management.

Dysfunction/degeneration

Dysfunction and condylar degeneration have been shown to occur not only on the fractured side but also on the contralateral side. It is believed that fracture dislocation is most likely to give late problems. Ellis admits that it is difficult to determine the level of dysfunction but a literature review by him estimates it to occur in between 9% and 85%. Dysfunction has also been linked to long periods of fixation and increasing age. Condylar degeneration is not only limited to closed treatment but occurs in open cases too. Ellis estimates that 65% of patients are completely symptom free but the clinician may detect subtle symptoms and signs of dysfunction: deviation on opening, a long centric slide, TMJ clicking, popping and locking. The difficulty is that these are prevalent in the population and may have existed pre injury.

Iatrogenic injury

This includes:

- deterioration in oral hygiene secondary to IMF/elastics which may lead to decay of dentition
- injury to dentition by fixation methods
- malnutrition and weight loss due to IMF/elastics
- airway risk from fixation methods
- scars
- seventh nerve injury (reported incidence permanent 1%, transient 10–15%)
- salivary fistulae
- Frey's syndrome
- altered sensation of the ear/temple.

Esthetic Aspects

Mandibular asymmetry following trauma can be corrected by ramus osteotomy. Fortunately this is not frequently a major complaint of the patient. Minor subtle deviations may go unnoticed and can be treated expectantly.

The Future: Research Trends and Prospective Trials

In view of the literature accumulated over the last 50 years and the clear benefits of ORIF, a scientifically justified fully randomized comparative clinical trial between closed and open treatment at this stage would appear to be unethical. The only option would therefore seem to be a large prospective multicenter condylar fracture study with exclusion criteria. The Strasbourg Osteosynthesis Research Group has made plans to initiate this study but at this time progress has been slow, reflecting the scale of the organization required to coordinate this.

Conclusion

There now seems to be a sufficient body of evidence and consensus that bilateral condylar fracture with displacement is the fracture type that gives most long-term functional problems. The risks of surgical approaches are less than initially thought and should not preclude ORIF. Restoration of condylar height with adequate stabilization and restoration of the occlusion, followed by early mobilization, are the goals.

Adult unilateral fractured condyles should be opened and fixed if fragment displacement is >5 mm and/or angulation >37°. Displacement less than this should be given a trial of non-rigid IMF and radiological reassessment after 1 week, with surgery still being an option.

Bilateral condylar fractures should have at least one or both condyles opened and fixed at the time of presentation. Aggressive mobilization should help to restore jaw mobility. Children less than 12 years rarely if ever need ORIF and the surgeon must have clear justification to undertake it in this group.

References

1   Silvennoinen U, Lizyka T, Lindqvist C, Oikarinen K 1992 Different patterns of condyle fractures: an analysis of 382 patients in a 3-year period. Journal of Oral and Maxillofacial Surgery 50: 1032–1037

2   Spiessel B, Schroll K 1972 Gelenkfortsatzund gelenkkopfchenfrakturen. In: Higst H (ed) Spezielle frakturen-and luxationslehre BD.I/I. Thieme, Stuttgart

3   MacLennan DW 1952 Consideration of 180 cases of typical fractures of the mandibular condylar process. British Journal of Plastic Surgery 5: 122

4   Lindahl L, Hollender L 1977 Condylar fractures of the mandible. A radiographic study of remodelling processes in the temporomandibular joint. International Journal of Oral Surgery 6: 153–165

5   Joos U, Kleinheinz J 1998 Therapy of condylar neck fractures. International Journal of Oral and Maxillofacial Surgery 27: 247–259

6   Members of the Chalmers J Lyon Club 1947 Fractures of the mandibular condyle: a post-treatment survey of 120 cases. Journal of Oral Surgery 5: 45–73

7   Blevins C, Gores RJ 1961 Fractures of the mandibular condyloid process: results of conservative treatment in 140 patients. Journal of Oral Surgery 19: 392–406

8   Marker P, Nielson A, Lehmann Bastian H 2000 Fractures of the mandibular condyle. Part 2: results of treatment of 348 patients. British Journal of Oral and Maxillofacial Surgery 38, 422–426

9   Hidding J, Wolf R, Pingle D 1992 Surgical versus non surgical treatment of fractures of the articular process of the mandible. Journal of Craniomaxillofacial Surgery 20; 345–347

10 Dahlstrom L, Kalmberg KE, Lindhall L 1989 15 years follow-up of condylar fractures. International Journal of Oral and Maxillofacial Surgery 18: 18–23

11 Konstantinovic V, Dimitrijevic B 1992 Surgical versus conservative treatment of unilateral condylar process fractures: clinical and radiographic evaluation of patients. Journal of Oral and Maxillofacial Surgery 50: 349–352

12 Ellis E, Palmieri C, Throckmorton G 1999 Further displacement of condylar process fractures after closed treatment. Journal of Oral and Maxillofacial Surgery 57: 1307–1316

13 Palmieri C, Ellis E, Throckmorton G 1999 Mandibular motion after closed and open treatment of unilateral mandibular condylar process fractures. Journal of Oral and Maxillofacial Surgery 57: 764–775

14 Worsaae N, Thorn J 1994 Surgical versus non surgical treatment of unilateral dislocated low subcondylar fractures: a clinical study of 52 cases. Journal of Oral and Maxillofacial Surgery 52: 353–360

15 Eckelt U 1991 Zugschraubenosteosynthesebei unterkiefergelenkfortsatzfrakturen. Deutsche Zeitschrift fur Mund, Kiefer und Gesichts-chirurgie 15: 51–57

16 Takenoshita Y, Ishibashi H, Oka M 1990 Comparison of functional recovery after nonsurgical and surgical treatment of condylar fractures. Journal of Oral and Maxillofacial Surgery 48: 1191–1195

17 Baker AW, McMahon J, Moos KF 1998 Current consensus on the management of fracture of the mandibular condyle. A method by questionnaire. International Journal of Oral and Maxillofacial Surgery 27: 258–266

18 Bos R, Ward Booth P, de Bont L 1999 Mandibular condyle fractures: a consensus. Editorial British Journal of Oral and Maxillofacial Surgery 37: 87–89

19 Newmann L 1998 A clinical evaluation of the long-term outcome of patients treated for bilateral fractures of the mandibular condyles. British Journal of Oral and Maxillofacial Surgery 36: 176–179

20 Mokros S, Erle A 1996 Transoral miniplate osteosynthesis of mandibular condyle fractures-optimising the surgical method. Fortschrift fur Kiefer und Gesichtschirurgie 41: 136–138

21 Undt G, Kermer C, Rasse M, Sinko K, Ewers R 1999 Transoral miniplate osteosynthesis of condylar neck fractures. Oral Surgery, Oral Medicine, Oral Pathology, Oral Radiology and Endodontics 88(5): 534–543

22 Lauer G, Schmelzeisen R 1999 Endoscopic-assisted fixation of mandibular condyle process fractures. Journal of Oral and Maxillofacial Surgery 57: 36–39

23 Schmelzeisen R, Wichmann U 1997 Endoscopic fixation of condylar fractures. International Journal of Oral and Maxillofacial Surgery 26 (suppl): 65

24 Hammer B, Schier P, Prein J 1997 Osteosynthesis of condylar neck fractures: a review of 30 patients. British Journal of Oral and Maxillofacial Surgery 35: 288–291

25 Byung-Ho C, Kyung-nam K, Moon-Key K 1999 Evaluation of condylar neck fracture plating techniques. Journal of Craniomaxillofacial Surgery 27: 109–112

26 Krenkel C 1992 Axial anchor screw (lag screw with biconcave washer) or slanted screw plate for osteosynthesis of fractures of the mandibular condylar process. Journal of Craniomaxillofacial Surgery 20: 348–353

27 Eckelt U, Hlawitschka M 1999 Clinical and radiological evaluation following surgical treatment of condylar neck fractures with lag screws. Journal of Craniomaxillofacial Surgery 27: 235–242

28 Welk A 1997 Morphologische untersuchungen zur indikation der zugschraubenosteosynthese nach eckelt bei kiefergelenkfortsatzfrakturen. Med Diss, Geifswald

29 Teranobu O, Yamada K, Eide K 1997 Evaluation of lag screw osteosynthesis for condylar process fractures of the mandible. International Journal of Oral and Maxillofacial Surgery 26 (suppl): 239

30 Hibi H, Sawaki Y, Uede M 1997 Modified osteosynthesis for condylar neck fractures in atrophic mandibles. International Journal of Oral and Maxillofacial Surgery 26: 348

31 Kitayama S 1989 A new method of intra-oral open reduction using a screw applied through the mandibular crest of condylar fractures. Journal of Maxillofacial Surgery 17: 16–21

32 Rasse M 1993 Diakapituläre Frakturen der Mandibula. Die operative versorgung: tierexperiment und klinik. Habilitationsschrift Med Fakultat Universitat Wien, Vienna

33 Rasse M 1993 Diakapituläre Frakturen der Mandibula. Eine neue Operationsmethode und erste Ergebnisse. Zeitschrift fur Stomatologie 90: 413–428

34 Nehse G, Maerker R 1996 Indications for various reconstruction and osteosynthesis methods in surgical management of subcondylar fractures of the mandible. Fortschrift fur Kiefer und Gesichtschirurgie 41: 120–123

35 Eppley BL 2000 A resorbable and rapid method for maxillomandibular fixation in pediatric mandible fractures. Journal of Craniofacial Surgery 11(3): 236–238

36 Thoren H, Ilzuka T, Hallikainen D, Nurminen M, Lindqvist C 1997 An epidemiological study of patterns of condylar fractures in children. British Journal of Oral and Maxillofacial Surgery 35: 306–311

37 Thoren H, Ilzuka T, Hallikainen D, Lindqvist C 1992 different patterns of mandibular fractures in children. An analysis of 220 fractures in 157 patients. Journal of Craniomaxillofacial Surgery 20(7): 292–296

38 Moss M 1968 The primacy of functional matrices in orofacial growth. Dental Practitioner 19:65

39 Moss M, Saleentijn L 1969 The capsular matrix. American Journal of Orthodontics 56: 474

40 Hovinga J, Boering G, Stegenga B 1999 Long-term results of nonsurgical management of condylar fractures in children. International Journal of Oral and Maxillofacial Surgery 28(6): 429–440

41 Ellis E 1998 Complications of mandibular condyle fractures. International Journal of Oral and Maxillofacial Surgery 27: 255–257

17 Dentoalveolar Injuries

Richard R Welbury

Introduction

Dental trauma in childhood and adolescence is common. At 5 years of age 31–40% of boys and 16–30% of girls and at 12 years of age 12–33% of boys and 4–19% of girls will have suffered some dental trauma. Boys are affected almost twice as often as girls in both the primary and permanent dentitions.

The majority of dental injuries in the primary and permanent dentitions involve the anterior teeth, especially the maxillary central incisors. The mandibular central incisors and maxillary lateral incisors are less frequently involved. Concussion, subluxation and luxation are the commonest injuries in the primary dentition, while uncomplicated crown fractures are the commonest injuries in the permanent teeth.

The most accident-prone times are between 2 and 4 years for the primary dentition and 7 and 10 years for the permanent dentition. In the primary dentition, co-ordination and judgment are incompletely developed and the majority of injuries are due to falls in and around the home as the child becomes more adventurous and explores its surroundings. In the permanent dentition most injuries are caused by falls and collisions while playing and running, although bicycles are a common accessory. The place of injury varies in different countries according to local customs but accidents in the schoolyard remain common. Sports injuries usually occur in teenage years and are commonly associated with contact sports such as soccer, rugby, ice-hockey and basketball.

Injuries due to road traffic accidents and assaults are most commonly associated with the late teenage years and adulthood and are often closely related to alcohol abuse.

One form of injury in childhood that must never be forgotten is child physical abuse or non-accidental injury (NAI). More than 50% of these children will have orofacial injuries.

The exact mechanisms of dental injuries are largely unknown and without experimental evidence, but injuries can be the result of either direct or indirect trauma. Direct trauma occurs when the tooth itself is struck. Indirect trauma is seen when the lower dental arch is forcefully closed against the upper, e.g. blow to chin. Direct trauma implies injuries to the anterior region while indirect trauma favors crown or crown-root fractures in the premolar and molar regions as well as the possibility of jaw fractures in the condylar regions and symphysis. The factors which influence the outcome or type of injury are a combination of energy impact, resilience of impacting object, shape of impacting object and angle of direction of the impacting force.

Increased overjet with protrusion of upper incisors and insufficient lip closure are significant predisposing factors to traumatic dental injuries. Injuries are almost twice as frequent among children with protruding incisors and the number of teeth affected in a particular incident for an individual patient also increases.

The second major group of children with predisposition to traumatic injuries are the accident prone. They sustain repeated trauma to their teeth and frequencies have been reported to range from 4% to 30%.

Classification of Dentoalveolar Injuries

Correct and appropriate treatment demands accurate diagnosis. Box 17.1 summarizes the classification of dentoalveolar injuries based on the World Health Organization (WHO) system.

History and Examination

History specific to dentoalveolar injuries

- The exact nature of the accident gives information on the type and severity of dentoalveolar injury expected. In a minor a discrepancy between the history and the clinical findings should raise the clinician's suspicion of child physical abuse or non-accidental injury.
- Lost teeth or fragments should be accounted for. If there is a history of loss of consciousness and teeth/fragments cannot be found then a chest radiograph is essential. Similarly if there is a soft tissue laceration of either upper or lower lip then anteroposterior and lateral soft tissue views of the lips should be taken.
- The time interval between injury and treatment significantly affects both pulpal and periodontal ligament prognosis.
- A history of previous dentoalveolar trauma can affect pulpal sensibility tests and the recuperative capacity of the pulp and periodontum.
- In a minor a history of previous dentoalveolar trauma could raise one's suspicions about the possibility of child physical abuse or whether the minor is just accident prone.

Box 17.1   Classification of the nature of dentoalveolar injuries

Injuries to the hard dental tissues and the pulp

Enamel infraction:	Incomplete (crack) of enamel without loss of tooth substance
Enamel fracture:	Loss of tooth substance confined to enamel
Enamel-dentine fracture:	Loss of tooth surface confined to enamel and dentine not involving the pulp
Complicated crown fracture:	Fracture of enamel and dentine exposing the pulp
Uncomplicated crown-root fracture:	Fracture of enamel, dentine and cementum but not involving the pulp
Complicated crown-root fracture:	Fracture of enamel, dentine and cementum and exposing the pulp
Root fracture:	Fracture involving dentine, cementum and pulp. Can be subclassified into apical, middle and coronal third

Injuries to the periodontal tissues

Concussion:	No abnormal loosening or displacement but marked reaction to percussion
Subluxation (loosening):	Abnormal loosening but no displacement
Extrusive luxation (partial avulsion):	Partial displacement of tooth from socket
Lateral luxation:	Displacement other than axially with comminution or fracture of alveolar socket
Intrusive luxation:	Displacement into alveolar bone with comminution or fracture of alveolar socket
Avulsion:	Complete displacement of tooth from socket

Injuries to supporting bone

Comminution of mandibular or maxillary alveolar socket wall:	Crushing and compression of alveolar socket. Found in intrusive and lateral luxation injuries.
Fracture of mandibular or maxillary alveolar socket wall:	Fracture confined to facial or lingual/palatal socket wall
Fracture of mandibular or maxillary alveolar process:	Fracture of the alveolar process which may or may not involve the tooth sockets
Fracture of the mandible or maxilla:	May or may not involve the alveolar socket

Injuries to gingiva or oral mucosa

Laceration of gingiva or oral mucosa:	Wound in the mucosa resulting from a tear
Contusion of gingiva or oral mucosa:	Bruise not accompanied by a break in the mucosa, usually causing submucosal hemorrhage
Abrasion of gingiva or oral mucosa:	Superficial wound produced by rubbing or scraping the mucosal surface

---

Medical history specific to dentoalveolar injuries

- *Bleeding disorders*: close liaison with hematology physicians is crucial if soft tissues are lacerated or teeth are to be removed.
- *Allergies*: alternative antibiotics need to be prescribed.
- *Congenital heart disease or rheumatic fever*: these are not necessarily contraindications to reimplantation of teeth; however, the advice of the physician should be sought. If endodontic treatment is likely to be difficult or may involve a persistent necrotic focus then the risk of bacterial endocarditis will be significant and reimplantation may be contraindicated after a risk versus benefit analysis.
- *Severe immunosuppression*: this is a contraindication to any procedure that is likely to require prolonged endodontic treatment with a persistent necrotic focus.
- *Tetanus prophylaxis*: this should be checked with the physician. Generally if there is soil contamination of a wound then a tetanus toxoid booster will be required if one has not been given in the previous 5–10 years.

Extraoral examination

Severe facial swelling and bruising may indicate underlying bony injury. Lacerations will require careful debridement to remove all foreign material prior to suturing (Fig. 17.1). Antibiotics and/or tetanus toxoid may be required if wounds are contaminated. Limitation of mandibular movement or

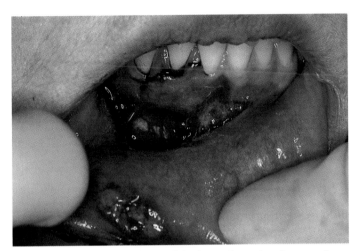

Fig. 17.1: Soft tissue injuries of the lip and gingiva that require thorough debridement.

mandibular deviation on opening or closing the mouth may indicate either a jaw fracture or dislocation.

Intraoral examination

This must be systematic and include the recording of:

1. laceration, hemorrhage and swelling of the oral mucosa and gingiva. All lacerations should be cleaned to remove any foreign bodies (Fig. 17.1). Any lacerations of lips or tongue require suturing but those of the oral mucosa heal very quickly and may not need suturing. Orofacial signs of child physical abuse may be present and will be discussed later
2. abnormalities of occlusion, tooth displacement, fractured crowns or cracks in the enamel.

The following signs and reactions to tests are particularly helpful.

- *Mobility*: degree of mobility is estimated in a horizontal and a vertical direction. When several teeth move together en bloc, a fracture of the alveolar process should be suspected. Excessive mobility may also suggest root fracture or tooth displacement.
- *Reaction to percussion*: in a horizontal and vertical direction and compared against a contralateral uninjured tooth. A duller note may indicate root fracture.
- *Color of tooth*: early color change is visible on the palatal surface of the gingival third of the crown.
- *Reaction to sensibility tests*: thermal tests with warm gutta percha or ethyl chloride are widely used. However, an electric pulp tester (EPT) in the hands of an experienced operator is more reliable. Nevertheless, vitality testing, especially in children, is notoriously unreliable and should never be assessed in isolation from the other clinical and radiographic information. Neither negative nor positive responses should be trusted immediately after trauma. A positive response does not rule out later pulpal necrosis and a negative response, while indicating pulpal damage, does not necessarily indicate a necrotic pulp. The negative reaction is often due to a 'shockwave' effect damaging

apical nerve supply. The pulp in such cases may have a normal blood supply. In all vitality testing always include and document the reaction of uninjured contralateral teeth for comparison. In addition, all teeth adjacent to the obviously injured teeth should be regularly assessed as they have probably suffered concussion injuries. In the future, advances in Doppler technology will allow the clinician to measure whether the vascular supply to individual teeth is intact. Doppler probes are currently too expensive for the general dental practitioner but research has shown them to be a reliable tool.

Radiographic examination

Three types of radiograph will allow the clinician to accurately diagnose and treat all dentoalveolar injuries.

- *Periapical*: reproducible 'long cone technique' periapicals are the best for accurate diagnosis and clinical audit. Two radiographs at different angles may be essential to detect a root fracture. However, if access and co-operation are difficult then one anterior occlusal radiograph rarely misses a root fracture. A small periapical film placed inside the upper or lower lip will detect tooth fragments or foreign bodies in the vertical plane.
- *Occlusal*: can detect root fractures and displacements when the mouth cannot open enough to accommodate a periapical film. An occlusal film held by the patient/helper at the side of the mouth can be used to detect tooth fragments or foreign bodies in the lateral plane (Fig. 17.2).
- *Dental panoramic tomograph*: this is essential in all dentoalveolar trauma cases and may detect an unsuspected underlying bony injury.

Photographic examination

Good clinical photographs are useful to assess treatment outcomes and for medicolegal purposes.

State-of-the-Art Management of Injuries to the Primary Dentition

During its early development the permanent incisor is located palatally to and in close proximity with the apex of the primary incisor. With any injury to a primary tooth there is a risk of damage to the underlying permanent successor (Fig. 17.3).

Parents should be advised that in all cases of trauma involving the primary dentition there is a 50% chance of developmental disturbances to the permanent successor teeth.

The most accident-prone time in the primary dentition is between 2 and 4 years of age. Realistically, this means that few restorative procedures will be possible and in the majority of cases the decision is between extraction or maintenance without performing extensive treatment. A primary incisor should always be removed if its maintenance will jeopardize the developing tooth bud.

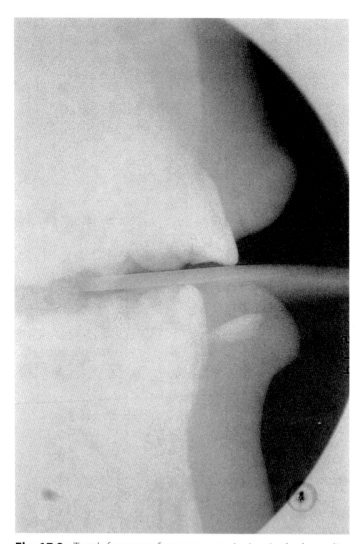

Fig. 17.2: Tooth fragment from an upper incisor in the lower lip.

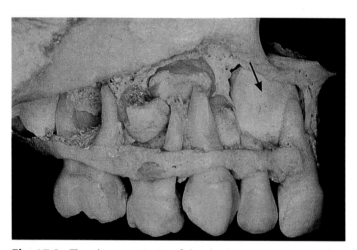

Fig. 17.3: The close proximity of developing permanent tooth germs to the roots of the primary dentition (arrow = permanent central incisor germ).

A traumatized primary tooth that is retained should be assessed regularly for clinical and radiographic signs of pulpal or periodontal complications. Radiographs may even detect damage to the permanent successor. Soft tissue injuries in children should be assessed weekly until healed. Tooth injuries should be reviewed every 3–4 months for the first year and then annually until the primary tooth exfoliates and the permanent successor is in place.

Uncomplicated crown fracture

The sharp edges should be smoothed or the crown morphology restored with a bonded restoration if co-operation allows.

Complicated crown fracture

Pulp extirpation, root canal obturation with resorbable zinc oxide cement and a bonded restoration to restore crown morphology can be achieved with reasonable co-operation. However, in many cases extraction of the tooth is the only realistic option.

Crown-root fracture

The pulp is invariably exposed and the fracture line extends well below the gingival margin. Restorative treatment would be extremely difficult to achieve and the tooth is best extracted.

Root fracture

Without displacement and with only a small amount of mobility the tooth should be kept under observation. If the coronal fragment becomes non-vital and symptomatic then it should be removed. The apical portion usually remains vital and undergoes resorption. Similarly with marked displacement and mobility only the coronal portion should be removed. Unnecessary searching for small apical root fragments runs the risk of iatrogenic damage to the permanent successor tooth.

Concussion, subluxation and luxation injuries

Associated soft tissue damage should be cleaned by the parent twice daily with 0.2% chlorhexidine solution using cotton buds or gauze swabs until healing occurs.

- *Concussion*: these require periodic review, observing closely for signs of non-vitality.
- *Subluxation*: if there is slight mobility then parents should be advised to keep the traumatized area as clean as possible and give the child a soft diet for 1–2 weeks.
- *Extrusive luxation*: these teeth are usually very mobile and require extraction.
- *Lateral luxation*: if the crown is displaced palatally the apex moves buccally and hence away from the permanent teeth germ. If the occlusion is not gagged then conservative treatment to await some spontaneous realignment is possible. If the crown is displaced buccally then the apex will be displaced towards the permanent tooth bud and extraction is indicated in order to minimize further damage to the permanent successor.

- *Intrusive luxation*: this is a common injury. The aim of investigation is to establish the direction of displacement by thorough radiographical examination. If the root is displaced palatally towards the permanent successor then the primary tooth should be extracted to minimize the possible damage to the developing permanent successor. If the root is displaced buccally then periodic review to monitor spontaneous re-eruption should be undertaken. Review should be weekly for a month then monthly for a maximum of 6 months. Most re-eruption occurs between 1 and 6 months. If re-eruption does not occur then ankylosis is likely and extraction is necessary to prevent ectopic eruption of the permanent successor.
- *Exarticulation (avulsion)*: replantation of avulsed primary incisors is not recommended due to the risk of damage to the permanent tooth germs. Space maintenance is not necessary following the loss of a primary incisor as only minor drifting of adjacent teeth occurs. The eruption of the permanent successor may be delayed for about 1 year as a result of abnormal thickening of connective tissue overlying the tooth germ.

Injuries to supporting bone

Most fractures of the alveolar socket in primary dentition do not require splinting due to rapid bony healing in small children. Jaw fractures are treated in the conventional manner, although stabilization after reduction may be difficult due to lack of sufficient teeth.

State-of-the-Art Management of Sequelae of Injuries to the Primary Dentition

Pulpal necrosis

Necrosis is the commonest complication of primary trauma. Evaluation is based upon color and radiography. Vitality testing is unreliable and of no clinical benefit in primary teeth. Teeth of a normal color rarely develop periapical inflammation but conversely, mildly discolored teeth may be vital. A mild gray color occurring soon after trauma may represent intrapulpal bleeding with a pulp that is still vital. This color may recede but if it persists then necrosis should be suspected. Radiographic examination should be 3 monthly to check for periapical inflammation. Failure of the pulp cavity to reduce in size is an indicator of pulp death. Teeth should be extracted whenever there is evidence of periapical inflammation, to prevent possible damage to the permanent successor.

Pulpal obliteration

Obliteration of the pulp chamber and canal is a common reaction to trauma. Clinically the tooth becomes yellow or opaque. Normal exfoliation is usual but occasionally periapical inflammation may develop and extraction is required. Annual periapical radiography is advisable to detect infection

and to check physiological root resorption. If resorption does not occur then the permanent successor will erupt in an ectopic position.

Root resorption

Internal resorption may be seen with concussion, subluxation and luxation injuries and external inflammatory resorption with intrusive injuries. Extraction is usually the preferred treatment for these types of root resorption.

Injuries to developing permanent teeth

Injuries to the permanent successor tooth can be expected in between 12% and 69% of cases of primary tooth trauma and 19–68% of jaw fractures. Intrusive luxation causes most disturbances. Avulsion of a primary incisor will also cause damage if the apex moved towards the permanent tooth bud before the avulsion. Most damage to the permanent tooth bud occurs under 3 years of age during its developmental stage. However, the type and severity of disturbance are closely related to the age at the time of injury. Changes in the morphology and mineralization of the crown of the permanent incisor are most common but later injuries can cause radicular anomalies. Injuries to developing teeth can be classified as follows.

- White or yellow-brown discoloration of enamel – injury at 2–7 years of age.
- White or yellow-brown discoloration of enamel with circular enamel hypoplasia – injury at 2–7 years of age.
- Crown dilacerations (Fig. 17.4) – injury at about 2 years of age.
- Odontoma-like malformation – injury at less than 1–3 years of age.
- Root duplication – injury at 2–5 years of age.
- Vestibular or lateral root angulation and dilaceration – injury at 2–5 years of age.
- Partial or complete arrest of root formation – injury at 5–7 years of age.
- Sequestration of permanent tooth germs.
- Disturbance in eruption.

The term 'dilaceration' describes an abrupt deviation of the long axis of the crown or root portion of the tooth. This deviation results from a traumatic non-axial displacement of already formed hard tissue in relation to developing soft tissue.

The term 'angulation' describes a curvature of the root resulting from a gradual change in the direction of root development, without evidence of abrupt displacement of the tooth germ during odontogenesis. This may be vestibular, i.e. labiopalatal, or lateral, i.e. mesiodistal. Evaluation of the full extent of complications following injuries must await complete eruption of all permanent teeth involved. However, most serious sequelae (disturbances in tooth morphology) can usually be diagnosed radiographically within the first year post trauma.

Injuries to the infant alveolus, even before the eruption of primary teeth, may cause disturbances in tooth morphology

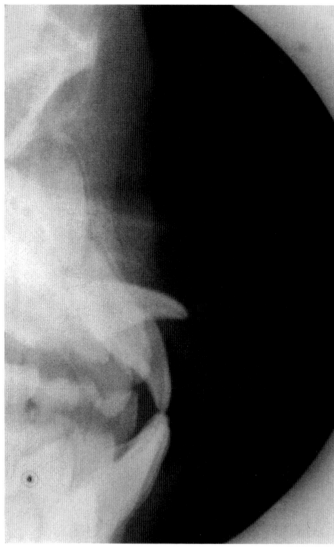

Fig. 17.4: Dilaceration of an upper permanent central incisor as a result of an intrusion injury to the primary incisor at the age of 2 years.

both to the primary teeth and more rarely to very early developing permanent teeth.[1]

Eruption disturbances of the permanent teeth may involve:

- delayed eruption due to connective tissue thickening over a permanent tooth germ as a result of early primary predecessor loss
- ectopic eruption due to lack of eruptive guidance due to either premature loss of the primary predecessor or failure of physiological resorption of the primary predecessor
- impaction and failure of eruption in teeth with malformations of crown or root.

Treatment of injuries to the permanent dentition

Yellow-brown discoloration of enamel with or without hypoplasia:

- acid-pumice microabrasion
- composite resin restoration: localized, veneer or crown
- porcelain restoration: veneer or crown (anterior): fused to metal crown (posterior).

Crown dilaceration:

- surgical exposure with or without orthodontic alignment
- temporary crown until root formation complete
- removal of dilacerated part of crown with or without one-stage root canal obturation
- coronal restoration.

Vestibular root angulation:

- combined surgical and orthodontic realignment.

Other malformations:

- extraction is usually the treatment of choice.

Disturbance in eruption:

- surgical exposure with or without orthodontic realignment.

State-of-the-Art Management of Injuries to the Permanent Dentition

Most traumatized permanent teeth can be treated successfully. Prompt and appropriate treatment instituted after correct diagnosis will improve prognosis.

The aims and principles of treatment can be broadly categorized into three parts.

1. Emergency:

   - retain vitality of fractured or displaced teeth
   - cover exposed dentine with a bonded restoration
   - treat exposed pulp tissue
   - reduction and immobilization of displaced teeth
   - antibacterial mouthwash, antibiotics and tetanus prophylaxis.

2. Intermediate:

   - may require pulp treatment
   - minimally invasive coronal restoration.

3. Permanent:

   - stimulated root end closure
   - root filling with or without root extrusion
   - may require gingival and alveolar collar modification
   - semi or permanent coronal restoration.

Trauma cases require painstaking follow-up to disclose any complications and institute the correct treatment. The intervals between examinations depend on the severity of trauma but the following schedule is a guide: 1 week, 3 weeks, 6 weeks, 3, 6 and 12 months and then annually for 4–5 years. At these times color, mobility, percussion and sensibility are routinely noted while radiographs are examined for periradicular conditions and changes within the pulp cavity.

Injuries to the hard dental tissues and the pulp

Enamel infraction

These incomplete fractures without loss of tooth substance and without proper illumination are easily overlooked. Periodic recalls are necessary as the energy of the blow may have been transmitted to the periodontal tissues or the pulp.

Enamel fracture

No restoration is needed and treatment is limited to smoothing of any rough edges and splinting if there is associated mobility. Periodic review as above.

Enamel-dentine fracture

Immediate treatment is necessary due to the involvement of dentine. The pulp requires protection against thermal irritation and from bacteria via the dentinal tubules. Restoration of crown morphology also stabilizes the position of the tooth in the arch.

Emergency protection of the exposed dentine can be achieved by:

1. a bonded composite resin or compomer bandage. Conventional glass ionomer cement alone will not be retained due to its poorer physical properties and bond strength
2. glass ionomer cement supported within either an orthodontic band or the incisal end of a celluloid crown former or stainless steel crown. These will serve as temporary retainers until further eruption occurs.

Intermediate restoration of most enamel-dentine fractures can be achieved by:

1. acid-etched composite either applied freehand or utilizing a celluloid crown former. With recent improvements in composite technology the majority of these restorations can be regarded as semi-permanent/permanent. Larger fractures should utilize more available enamel surface area for bonding by employing a complete celluloid crown former to construct a 'direct' composite crown. At a later age this could be reduced to form the core of a porcelain jacket crown preparation.
2. reattachment of crown fragment (Figs 17.5, 17.6). This method of restoration has become feasible since the development of dentine bonding agents. However, few long-term studies have been reported and therefore the longevity of this type of restoration is largely unknown.[2] In addition, there is a tendency for the distal fragment to become opaque or require further restorative intervention in the form of a veneer or jacket crown.

If the fracture line through dentine is not very close to the pulp then the fragment may be reattached immediately. If, however, it runs close to the pulp, then it is advisable to place

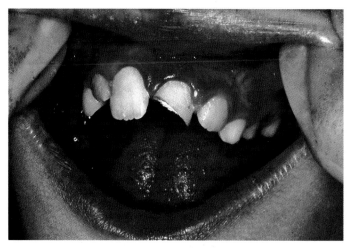

Fig. 17.5: An enamel dentine fracture of the upper left central incisor.

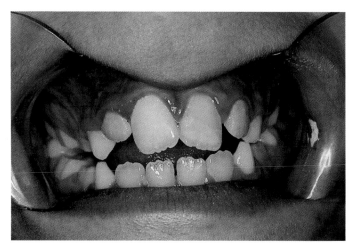

Fig. 17.6: After reattachment of the coronal fragment in Fig. 17.5.

a suitably protected calcium hydroxide dressing over the exposed dentine for at least 1 month while storing the fragment in saline, which should be renewed weekly.

- Check the fit of the fragment and the vitality of the tooth.
- Clean fragment and tooth with pumice-water slurry.
- Isolate the tooth with rubber dam.
- Attach the fragment to a piece of gutta percha to facilitate handling.
- Etch enamel for 30 s on both fracture surfaces and extend for 2 mm from fracture line on tooth and fragment. Wash for 15 s and dry for 15 s.
- Apply dentine primer to both surfaces and then dry for 15–30 s.
- Apply enamel-dentine bonding agent to both surfaces then lightly blow away any excess. Light cure for 10 s.
- Place appropriate shade of composite resin over both surfaces and position fragment. Remove gross excess and cure 60 s labially and palatally.
- Remove any excess composite resin with sandpaper discs.
- Remove a 1 mm gutter of enamel on each side of the fracture line both labially and palatally to a depth of

0.5 mm using a small round or pear-shaped burr. The finishing line should be irregular in outline.

■ Etch the newly prepared enamel, wash, dry, apply composite, cure and finish.

Enamel-dentine pulp fracture (complicated crown fracture)

In a tooth with an immature apex, the major concern is the preservation of pulp vitality in order to allow continued root growth. The injured pulp must be sealed from bacteria so that it is not infected during the period of repair. Partial pulpotomy or pulpotomy is the treatment of choice to try and retain vital radicular pulp. However, to have the best chance of success, treatment should be initiated within 24 hours of the injury. If radicular pulp vitality is not maintained or the pulpal exposure is wide, then total pulp extirpation (pulpectomy) is the only treatment choice. Non-setting calcium hydroxide is spun into the root canal and changed every 3 months in order to stimulate root end closure so a permanent root canal filling can be obturated against a closed apex. The average time for stimulated root end closure to occur with non-setting calcium hydroxide is between 9 and 12 months.[3,4]

In a tooth with a mature apex and a complicated crown fracture the treatment of choice is generally extirpation and obturation. However, if the exposure is very small then direct pulp cap can be attempted.

Uncomplicated crown-root fracture

After removal of the fractured piece of tooth, these vertical fractures are commonly a few millimeters incisal to the gingival margin on the labial surface but down to the cemento-enamel junction palatally. Prior to placement of a restoration, the fracture margin has to be brought supragingival either by gingivoplasty or extrusion (orthodontically or surgically) of the root portion.

Complicated crown-root fracture

As above, with the addition of endodontic requirements. If extrusion is planned then the final root length must be no shorter than the final crown length otherwise the result will be unstable. Root extrusion can be successful in a motivated patient and leads to a stable periodontal condition.

Root fracture

Root fractures occur most frequently in the middle or apical third of the root. The coronal fragment may be extruded or luxated. Luxation is usually in a lingual or palatal direction.

If displacement has occurred, the coronal fragment should be repositioned as soon as possible by gentle digital manipulation and the position checked radiographically. Mobile root fractures need to be functionally splinted to encourage repair of the fracture. Apical third fractures, in the absence of concomitant periodontal ligament (PDL) injury, are often firm and do not require splinting but need to be regularly reviewed to check pulpal status and treated endodontically if necessary.

Middle third and coronal third fractures must be splinted functionally[8]. A functional splint is one that includes one abutment tooth on either side of the fractured tooth and should remain in place for 2–3 weeks. The splint should allow color observations and sensitivity testing and access to the root canal if endodontic treatment is required. The splint design and placement techniques are discussed in the next section on splinting.

In about 80% of all root fractured teeth, the pulp remains viable and repair occurs in the fracture area. Three main categories of repair are recognized:

1. *repair with calcified tissue*: invisible or hardly discernible fracture line
2. *repair with connective tissue*: narrow radiolucent fracture line with peripheral rounding of the fracture edges
3. *repair with bone and connective tissue*: a bony bridge separates the two fragments.

In addition to these changes in the fracture area, pulp canal obliteration is commonly seen. Fractures in the cervical third of the root will repair as well as those in the middle or apical thirds as long as no communication exists between the fracture line and the gingival crevice. If such a communication exists then splinting is not recommended and a decision must be made to extract the coronal fragment and retain the remaining root, extract the two fragments or internally splint the root fracture. The latter option is unlikely to achieve long-term success.

If the coronal fragment is extracted and the root is retained then the remaining radicular pulp should be removed and the canal temporarily dressed prior to obturating with gutta percha. Three options are now available for the root treated radicular portion.

1. Post, core and crown restoration if access is adequate.
2. Extrusion of root either surgically or orthodontically if the fracture extends too subgingivally for adequate access. Rapid orthodontic extrusion over 4–6 weeks aiming to move the root a maximum of 4 mm is the best option. This is achieved by cementing a 'J' hook made from 0.7 mm stainless steel wire into the canal and using elastic traction applied over an arch wire cemented between one abutment tooth on either side of the injured tooth. Retention for 1 month at the end of movement is advised to prevent relapse.

   If esthetics are a particular concern then an orthodontic bracket can be bonded to a temporary crown made over the 'J' hook. The temporary crown length will need to be reduced as extrusion occurs.
3. Cover the root with a mucoperiosteal flap. This will maintain the height and width of the arch and will facilitate later placement of a single tooth implant.

Pulpal necrosis occurs in about 20% of root fractures and is the main obstacle to adequate repair. The amount of displacement of the coronal portion is significant in pulpal prognosis and presence of hard tissue union.

Table 17.1 Five-year pulpal survival data for injuries involving the periodontal ligament

Type of injury	Open apex (%)	Closed apex (%)
Concussion	100	96
Subluxation	100	85
Extrusive luxation	95	45
Lateral luxation	95	25
Intrusive luxation	40	0
Replantation	30	0

Table 17.2 Prevalence of resorption after periodontal ligament injury

Type of injury	Open apex (%)	Closed apex (%)
Concussion	1	3
Subluxation	1	3
Extrusive luxation	5	7
Lateral luxation	3	38
Intrusive luxation	67	100
Replantation	Frequent	Frequent

Most cases of necrosis are diagnosed within 3 months of a root fracture. A persistent negative response to electric stimulation is usually confirmed on radiography by radiolucencies adjacent to the fracture line.

The apical fragment almost always contains viable pulp tissue. In apical and middle third fractures any endodontic treatment is usually confined to the coronal fragment. After completion of endodontic treatment, repair and union between the two fragments with connective tissue is a consistent finding. In coronal third fractures that develop necrosis, either the radicular portion can be retained (see above), both portions extracted or the fracture internally splinted (see above).

Injuries to the periodontal tissues

As the severity of periodontal injury increases, there is a decrease in pulpal prognosis for the teeth involved (Table 17.1) and an increase in the amount of expected root resorption (Table 17.2). Table 17.1 demonstrates clearly that pulpal prognosis is superior for all the categories of injury in teeth with 'open' or immature apices. In these immature teeth the neurovascular bundle can survive some edema and movement around the 'open' apices, whereas in the mature tooth any mobility and edema within the narrow confines of the small apical foramen often lead to pulpal necrosis. Correct diagnosis and treatment of all periodontal tissue injuries aims to improve pulpal prognosis and decrease future resorption sequelae.[5]

Concussion

The impact force causes edema and hemorrhage in the PL fibers and the tooth is firm in the socket.

Subluxation

In addition to the above there is rupture of some PL fibers and the tooth is mobile in the socket, although not displaced. The treatment for both these injuries is:

- occlusal relief
- soft diet for 7 days
- immobilization with a splint if TTP is significant or the apex is closed
- chlorhexidine 0.2% mouthwash, twice daily.

In subluxation injuries, the immature apex tooth may not require splinting. However, the mature apex tooth should always be splinted to rest the periodontal tissues and protect the neurovascular bundle as it enters the small apical foramen.

Extrusive luxation

There is rupture of PL and pulp.

Lateral luxation

There is rupture of PL and pulp and damage to the alveolar plate(s) (Figs 17.7, 17.8). Treatment for both of these injuries is:

- atraumatic repositioning with gentle but firm digital pressure
- local anesthetic if there is an alveolar plate injury
- non-rigid functional splint for 2–3 weeks
- antibiotics, e.g. amoxicillin 250 mg three times daily (<6 years old 125 mg three times daily) for 5 days
- chlorhexidine 0.2% mouthwash twice daily while splint is in position
- soft diet 2–3 weeks.

Antibiotics may have a beneficial effect in promoting repair of the PL. They do not appear to affect pulpal prognosis.

After 2–3 weeks the teeth are radiographed. If there is no evidence of marginal breakdown, the splint can be removed.

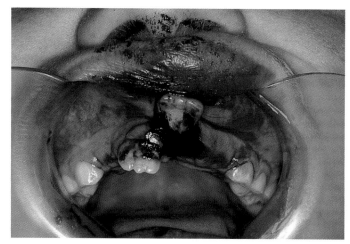

Fig. 17.7: Labial lateral luxation of upper left central incisor at age 8 years.

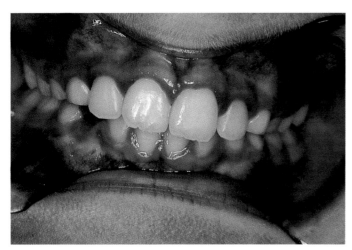

Fig. 17.8: The tooth in Fig. 17.7 at age 18 years after correct treatment.

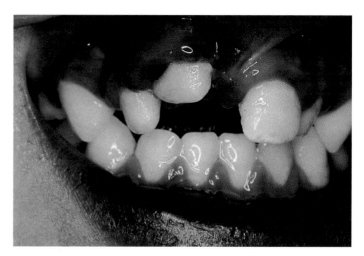

Fig. 17.9: Intrusive injury to the upper right permanent central incisor.

If marginal breakdown is present, then it should be retained for a further 2–3 weeks.

For extrusion and lateral luxation injuries the decision whether to progress to endodontic treatment depends on the combination of clinical and radiographic signs (see later). Five-year pulpal survival figures (Table 17.1) show that prognosis is significantly better for open apex teeth but nevertheless a proportion of mature teeth involved in luxation injuries will exhibit on radiographs a natural healing phenomenon known as 'transient apical breakdown' (TAB), which can mimic apical infection. Ambivalent clinical and radiographic signs should be given the 'benefit of the doubt' until the next review.

With more significant damage to the PL in both extrusive and lateral luxation injuries there is an increased risk of root resorption (Table 17.2). Thirty-five per cent of mature teeth that have undergone lateral luxation show subsequent evidence of surface resorption. This is because the PL has been irreversibly damaged by 'crushing' against the alveolar plates compared to 'tearing' in the extrusive luxation injury.

In cases of lateral luxation which present late, more than 2 days after the injury, the displacement cannot be reduced with gentle finger pressure. It is not advisable to use more force as this can further damage the PL. Orthodontic appliances, either a removable or a sectional fixed appliance, can be used to reduce the displacement over a period of a few weeks.

Intrusive luxation

These injuries are the result of an axial, apical impact and there is extensive damage to PL, pulp and alveolar plate(s) (Fig. 17.9).

Two distinct treatment categories exist: the open and closed apex.[6,7]

Open apex
Either:

- disimpact (with forceps if necessary) and allow to erupt spontaneously for 2–4 months. If there is no spontaneous movement start orthodontic extrusion

or

- disimpact and surgically reposition; functional splint for 7–10 days
- monitor pulpal status clinically and radiographically at 1, 3 and 6 months and start endodontics if necessary
- non-setting calcium hydroxide in root canal does not preclude orthodontic movement. Once apexification has occurred and orthodontic movement has ceased, obturate the canal with gutta percha.

Closed apex

- Elective orthodontic/surgical extrusion immediately
- Functional splint for 7–10 days after surgical extrusion
- Elective pulp extirpation at 7–10 days
- Maintain non-setting calcium hydroxide in root canal during orthodontic movement before obturation with gutta percha

If endodontic treatment is commenced within 2 weeks after an injury to the PL then some authors suggest that the initial intracanal dressing should be a polyantibiotic or antibiotic/steroid paste. This is because if non-setting calcium hydroxide is inadvertently spun through the apex before the PL fibers have healed then it can cause replacement resorption. Sixty per cent of PL fibers are healed 2 weeks after an injury.

At the outset, all intrusive luxation injuries should receive antibiotics, chlorhexidine mouthwash and a soft diet.

The risk of pulpal necrosis in these injuries is high, especially in the closed apex (Table 17.1). The incidence of resorption and ankylosis sequelae is also high (Table 17.2).

Avulsion and replantation

Replantation should always be attempted even though it may offer only a temporary solution due to the frequent occurrence of external inflammatory resorption (EIR).[9–13] Even when resorption occurs, the tooth may be retained for years, acting as a natural space maintainer and preserving the height and width of the alveolus to facilitate later implant placement.

Successful healing after replantation can only occur if there is minimal damage to the pulp and the PL. The type of extra-alveolar storage medium and the extra-alveolar time (EAT), i.e. the time the tooth has been out of the mouth, are critical factors. The suggested protocol for replantation can be divided into advice on phone, immediate treatment in surgery and review.

Advice on phone

- Do not touch root – hold by crown.
- Wash gently under cold tap water.
- Replace into socket or transport in a suitable medium to the surgery.
- If replaced then bite gently on a handkerchief to retain tooth and come to the surgery.

The best transport medium is the tooth's own socket. Understandably, non-dentists may be unhappy to replant the tooth and milk is an effective iso-osmolar medium. Saliva, the patient's buccal sulcus or normal saline are alternatives. The availability of normal saline has increased with increased use of contact lenses.

Immediate surgery treatment

- Do not handle root. If replanted, remove tooth from socket.
- Rinse tooth with normal saline. Note state of root development. Store in saline.
- Local analgesia.
- Irrigate socket with saline and remove clot and any foreign material.
- Push tooth gently but firmly into socket.
- Non-rigid functional splint for 7–10 days.
- Check occlusion.
- Baseline radiographs: periapical or anterior occlusal. Any other teeth injured?
- Antibiotics, chlorhexidine mouthwash, soft diet as previously.
- Check tetanus immunization status.

Review

- Radiograph – prior to splint removal at 7–10 days.
- Remove splint 7–10 days.
- Endodontics – commence prior to splint removal for categories (b) and (c).

  (a) Open apex EAT <45 min. Observe.
  (b) Open apex EAT >45 min. Endodontics.

   (i) Initial intracanal dressing – polyantibiotic or antibiotic/steroid paste.
   (ii) Subsequent intracanal dressings – non-setting calcium hydroxide.
   (iii) Replace calcium hydroxide 3 monthly until apical barrier (up to maximum 2–3 years).
   (iv) Obturate canal with gutta percha.

  (c) Closed apex. Endodontics.

   (i) Initial intracanal dressing – polyantibiotic or antibiotic/steroid paste.
   (ii) Subsequent intracanal dressing – non-setting calcium hydroxide.
   (iii) Obturate with gutta percha at 6–12 months as long as no progressive resorption.

- Radiographic review: 1, 3 and 6 monthly for 2 years then annually.
- If resorption is progressing unhalted keep non-setting calcium hydroxide in the tooth until exfoliation, changing it 6 monthly.

The immature tooth with an EAT of less than 45 min may undergo pulp revascularization (Table 17.1). However, these teeth require regular clinical and radiographic review because once EIR occurs it progresses rapidly.

Replantation of teeth with a dry storage time of greater than 1 hour

Mature teeth with a dry storage time of greater than 1 hour will have a non-vital PL. The PL and the pulp should be removed at chairside and the tooth placed in 2.4% sodium fluoride solution acidulated to pH 5.5 for 20 min. The root canal is then obturated with gutta percha and the tooth replanted and splinted rigidly for 6 weeks. The aim of this treatment is to produce ankylosis, allowing the tooth to be maintained as a natural space maintainer, perhaps for a limited period only. The sodium fluoride is believed to slow down the resorptive process.

Pulpal and periodontal status

Pulpal necrosis is the most common complication and is related to the severity of the periodontal injury (Table 17.1). Immature teeth have a better prognosis than mature teeth due to the wide apical opening where slight movements can occur without disruption of the apical neurovascular bundle.

Necrosis can be diagnosed in most cases within 3 months of injury but in some cases may not be evident for at least 2 years. A combination of clinical and radiological signs are often required to diagnose necrosis.

Sensitivity testing

The majority of injured teeth test negatively to electric pulp tester immediately following trauma. Most pulps that recover test positively within months but responses have been reported as late as 2 years after injury. A negative test alone therefore should not be regarded as proof of necrosis. Postpone endodontics until at least one other clinical and/or radiographic sign is present.

Tooth discoloration

Initial pinkish discoloration may be due to subtotal severance of apical vessels leading to penetration of hemoglobin from such ruptures into the dentine tubules. If the vascular system repairs then most of this discoloration will disappear. If the tooth becomes progressively gray then necrosis should be suspected. A gray color that appears for the first time several weeks or months after trauma signifies decomposition of necrotic pulp tissue and is a decisive sign of necrosis. Color changes are usually most apparent on the palatal surface of the injured teeth.

Tenderness to percussion

This may be the most reliable isolated indicator of pulpal necrosis.

Periapical inflammation

Radiological periapical involvement secondary to necrosis can be seen as early as 3 weeks after trauma. In mature teeth TAB may be mistaken for periapical inflammation.

Arrest of root development

If necrosis involves the epithelial root sheath before root development is complete, then no further root growth will occur. In an injured pulp, necrosis may progress from the coronal to the apical portion and hence residual apical vitality may result in formation of a calcific barrier across a wide apical foramen. Failure of the pulp chamber and root canal to mature and reduce in size on successive radiographs compared with contralateral uninjured teeth is also a reliable indicator of necrosis.

Inflammatory root resorption (external)

This is a pathognomic sign of necrosis and requires immediate endodontic treatment. Resorptive areas are usually evident within 3 weeks to 4 months after injury. External inflammatory resorption is most frequently associated with intrusive luxation and replantation. It is initiated by PL damage resulting in resorption cavities in cementum but is propagated and potentiated by infected necrotic pulpal products, stimulating an increase in inflammatory response in the PL via the dentinal tubules. 'Punched-out' areas of resorption on the external root surface are associated with adjacent bony radiolucencies. If EIR is not present within 1 year of injury it is unlikely to occur. If untreated, it will destroy the tooth completely within months and treatment consisting of extirpation, debridement and non-setting calcium hydroxide is necessary. The majority of cases will arrest and cemental repair occurs.

Inflammatory root resorption (internal)

This is an infrequent complication caused by chronic pulpal inflammation. It is often without clinical symptoms and is seen radiographically as a ballooning of the near parallel walls of the root canal. It progresses rapidly and perforation of the root surface will occur. Early endodontic treatment with extirpation, mechanical and chemical debridement and non-setting calcium hydroxide has a good chance of success.

Pulpal canal obliteration (PCO)

In up to 35% of injured teeth there can be progressive hard tissue formation within the pulpal cavity leading to a gradual narrowing of the pulp chamber and root canal and partial or total obliteration. There is a reduced response to vitality testing and the crown appears slightly yellow/opaque. The exact initiating factor which produces this response from the odontoblasts is unknown. It is more common in immature teeth and in luxation injuries than in concussion and subluxation injuries. Although radiographs may suggest complete calcification there is usually a minute strand of pulpal tissue remaining. Less than thirteen per cent of these teeth can give rise to periapical inflammation as long as 5–15 years after the initial injury. Instrumentation of these canals can be difficult and prolonged and may result in perforation. Current clinical opinion would support allowing PCO to occur rather than initiating prophylactic endodontic treatment.

Replacement resorption (ankylosis)

This is the most severe type of external root resorption and is significantly related to replantation of avulsed incisors with an extended extra-alveolar dry period. It is caused by extensive damage to the PL and the cementum resulting in bony union (ankylosis) being established between the alveolar socket and the root surface. The tooth then becomes essentially part of the bone and as such is constantly remodeled, resulting in continuous resorption of cementum and dentine. Radiographically, the periodontal space disappears and tooth substance is gradually replaced by bone. Most resorption is evident within 2 months to 1 year of injury and can be detected clinically by a high, metallic percussion note.

There is no effective treatment for ankylosis but as the rate of progression is relatively slow the tooth can be maintained for up to 10 years. However, such teeth can be a problem in the growing child as they may cease to 'move' or 'grow' with the rest of the jaws and cannot be moved orthodontically. Non-setting calcium hydroxide can increase replacement resorption if it is extruded through the apex of an injured tooth before PL healing has occurred. For this reason the initial intracanal dressing should be polyantibiotic or antibiotic/steroid for the first 2 weeks after injury to the PL.

Conclusion

The initial treatment of periodontal ligament injuries is often the easiest part of the management. All injuries should be seen by a specialist in pediatric dentistry or restorative dentistry within days of the initial injury so that appropriate endodontic and periodontal management is undertaken. Why go to the trouble of replanting a tooth in the middle of the night only to lose it 6 months later through external inflammatory resorption as a result of inadequate endodontic management?

Injuries to the supporting bone

The extent of the alveolar fracture should be verified clinically and radiographically (Figs 17.10, 17.11). If there is dis-

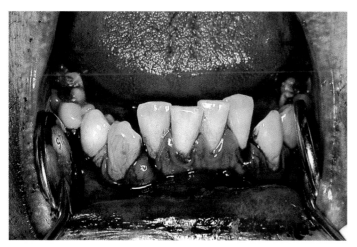

Fig. 17.10: Dentoalveolar fracture 'carrying' all lower incisors.

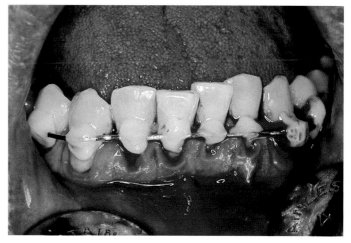

Fig. 17.12: Dentoalveolar fracture in Figs 17.10 and 17.11 after reduction showing rigid composite-wire splint.

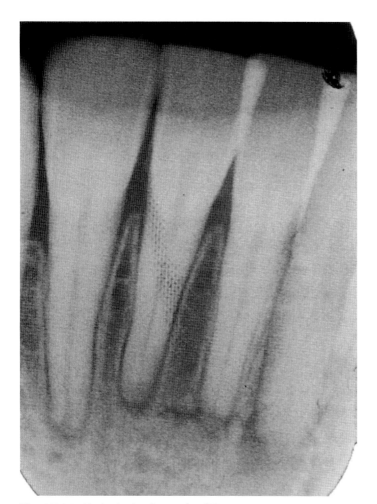

Fig. 17.11: Periapical radiograph of Fig. 17.10.

placement of the teeth to the extent that their apices have risen up and are now positioned over the labial or lingual/palatal alveolar plates ('apical lock') then they will require extruding first to free the apices prior to repositioning.

The segment of alveolus with teeth requires only 3–4 weeks of rigid splintage (composite-wire type) with two abutment teeth either side of the fracture (Fig. 17.12),

together with antibiotics, chlorhexidine, soft diet and tetanus prophylaxis check.

Pulpal survival is more likely if repositioning occurs within 1 hour of the injury. Root resorption is rare.

Splinting

Trauma may loosen a tooth either by damaging the PL or by fracturing the root. Splinting immobilizes the tooth in the correct anatomical position so that further trauma is prevented and healing can occur. Different injuries require different splinting regimes. A functional splint involves one and a rigid splint two abutment teeth either side of an injured tooth.

Splinting regimes

Periodontal ligament injuries

Sixty per cent of PDL healing has occurred after 10 days and it is complete within a month. The splinting period should be as short as possible and the splint should allow some functional movement to prevent replacement root resorption (ankylosis). As a general rule exarticulation (avulsion) injuries require 7–10 days and luxation (lateral luxation and extrusive luxation) injuries 2–3 weeks of functional splinting.

Root fractures

Recent research has shown that these injuries only require 2–3 weeks of functional splinting to encourage a repair with either calcified tissue or connective tissue. With a lot of mobility the fracture site becomes filled with granulation tissue and the tooth remains mobile.

Dentoalveolar fractures

These require 3–4 weeks of rigid splinting.

Types and methods of constructing splints

Acrylic resin

This method uses a thin 'sausage' of temporary crown material which is applied to the incisal half of the labial surfaces of the crowns after acid etching. It is the ideal 'single-handed opera-tor' splint for out-of-hours accident and emergency work.

Composite resin/acrylic resin and wire splint

This method uses either a composite resin or an acrylic resin temporary crown material. The composite resin is easier to place but the acrylic resin is easier to remove.

Technique for a functional resin-wire splint

- Bend a flexible orthodontic wire to fit the middle third of the labial surface of the injured tooth and one abutment tooth either side.
- Stabilize the injured tooth in the correct position with soft red wax palatally.
- Clean the labial surfaces. Isolate, dry and etch middle crown of teeth with 37% phosphoric acid for 30 s; wash, dry.
- Apply 3 mm diameter circle of unfilled then filled composite resin or of acrylic resin, to the center of the crowns.
- Position the wire into the filling material then apply more composite or acrylic resin.
- Use a brush lubricated with unfilled composite resin to mold and smooth the composite. Acrylic resin is more difficult to handle and smoothing and excess removal can be done with a flat plastic instrument.
- Cure the composite for 60 s. Wait for the acrylic resin to cure.
- Smooth any sharp edges with sandpaper discs.

For a rigid splint, use the same technique but incorporate two abutment teeth on either side of the injured tooth. These splints should not impinge on the gingiva and should allow assessment of color change and sensitivity testing.

Orthodontic brackets and wire

For displacement injuries and exarticulations these splints have the advantage of allowing a more accurate reduction of the injury by gentle forces.

Interdental wiring

Interdental 'figure of eight' wiring on an arch wire ligated to the teeth with ligature wire should not be used except as a temporary measure, as it compromises gingival health.

Foil/cement splint

A temporary splint made of soft metal (cooking foil or milk bottle top) and cemented with quick-setting zinc oxide-eugenol cement is an effective temporary measure, either as a single-handed operator or while awaiting construction of a laboratory-made splint.

Technique

- Cut foil to size, long enough to extend over two or three teeth on each side of the injured tooth and wide enough to extend over the incisal edges and 3–4 mm over the labial and palatal gingiva.
- Place foil over teeth and mold it over labial and palatal surfaces. Remove any excess.

- Cement the foil to the teeth with quick-drying zinc oxide-eugenol cement.

Laboratory splints

Thermoplastic and acrylic splints are used where it is impossible to make a satisfactory splint by the direct method, e.g. a 7-year-old with traumatized maxillary incisors, unerupted lateral incisors and either carious or absent primary canines. Both methods require alginate impressions and very loose teeth may need to be supported by wax, metal foil or wire ligature so they are not removed with the impression.

- *Acrylic*: there is full palatal coverage and the acrylic is extended over the incisal edges for 2–3 mm of the labial surfaces of the anterior teeth. The occlusal surfaces of the posterior teeth should be covered to prevent any occlusal contact in the anterior region. This also aids retention and Adams cribs may not be required. The splint should be removed for cleaning after meals and at bedtime.
- *Thermoplastic*: the splint is constructed from polyvinylacetate-polyethylene (PVAC-PE) co-polymer in the same way as a mouthguard with extension onto the mucosa. It should be removed like the acrylic splint after meals and at bedtime. However, with more severely loosened teeth it could be retained at night.

Both forms of laboratory splint allow functional movement and therefore promote normal periodontal healing. However, they may compromise general gingival health if oral hygiene is not maintained.

Child Physical Abuse (Non-Accidental Injury)

A child is considered to be abused if he or she is treated in a way that is unacceptable in a given culture at a given time. Non-accidental injury (NAI) is now recognized as an international issue and has been reported in many countries.[14-17] Each week at least four children in Britain and 80 children in the United States will die as a result of abuse or neglect. At least one child per thousand in Britain suffers severe physical abuse, for example fractures, brain hemorrhage, severe internal injuries or mutilation, and in the United States more than 95% of serious intracranial injuries during the first year of life are the result of abuse. Although some reports will prove to be unfounded, the common experience is that proven cases of child abuse are 4–5 times as common as they were two decades ago. In the United States a national emergency was declared in 1990 by the US Advisory Board in Child Abuse and Neglect because in 1989 there were 2.4 million cases of child maltreatment.

The significant scientific paper in this area was in 1962 when Henry Kempe, a pediatrician, and his co-workers published 'the battered child syndrome'. In this paper they concluded that previously unexplained fractures and head injuries must have been caused non-accidentally. The paper was a watershed and subsequently many health workers

Table 17.3 The incidence of orofacial injuries in child physical abuse

Type of injury		Incidence (%)
Extraoral	Contusions and ecchymoses	66
	Abrasions and lacerations	28
	Burns and bites	4
	Fractures	2
Intraoral	Contusions and ecchymoses	43
	Abrasions and lacerations (including frenal tears)	29
	Dental trauma	29

realized that children under their care had similar non-accidental injuries.

In the United Kingdom, the Children Act of 1989 defined four categories of abuse that could result in a child being placed on an 'at-risk' register[15]: physical abuse; sexual abuse; emotional abuse; neglect. Currently there are approximately 33 000 children on 'at-risk' registers in England and Wales. However, each category of abuse is not a diagnosis on its own, but merely a symptom of disordered parenting. The aim of intervention and placing a child on an at-risk register is to diagnose and cure the disordered parenting. Less than 4% of children who come to the attention of the Child Welfare Services are actually removed from the family environment because of significant risk. The greater majority of families receive help and guidance so that they function better. There is evidence that children do significantly better with their own parents rather than parental substitutes. Of those children who are severely abused, it has been estimated in the United States that 35–50% will receive serious re-injury and 50% could die if returned to their home environment without intervention.

At least 50% of cases diagnosed as child physical abuse have signs on the head, neck, face and mouth that are visible to the dental practitioner.[18–20] Indeed, the dental practitioner may be the first professional to see or suspect the abuse. Injuries may take the form of contusions and ecchymoses, abrasions and lacerations, burns, bites, dental trauma and fractures. The incidences of common orofacial injuries seen in child physical abuse are shown in Table 17.3. However, orofacial injuries are not limited to physical abuse alone. Up to 16% of sexual abuse and up to 33% of neglect cases may have signs on the head, neck, face and mouth.[16] Therefore a dental practitioner's awareness of the possibility of physical abuse may provide an opportunity for intervention. If this opportunity is missed, there may not be a further opportunity for many years.

The following 11 points should be considered whenever doubts or suspicions are raised.[17]

- Could the injury have been caused accidentally and if so, how?
- Does the explanation for the injury fit the age and the clinical findings?

- If the explanation of cause is consistent with the injury, is this itself within normally acceptable limits of behavior?
- If there has been any delay seeking advice, are there good reasons for this?
- Does the story of the accident vary?
- The nature of the relationship between parent and child.
- The child's reaction to other people.
- The child's reaction to any medical/dental examinations.
- The general demeanor of the child.
- Any comments made by the child and/or parent that give concern about the child's upbringing or lifestyle.
- History of previous injury.

Dental practitioners should be aware of any established system in their locality which is designed to cope with these cases. In the United Kingdom, each Local Authority Social Services Department is required to set up an 'Area Child Protection Committee'. Dental practitioners are advised how to refer and to whom, if they are concerned.[17]

Dental practitioners' awareness of child protection issues varies.[21–24] This is directly related to current undergraduate and postgraduate training programs with younger practitioners tending to have greater knowledge. In addition, specialist

Key points

- Boys experience dental trauma almost twice as often as girls.
- Maxillary central incisors are the most commonly involved teeth.
- Regular clinical and radiographic review is necessary to limit unwanted sequelae, institute appropriate treatment and improve prognosis.
- Injuries to the developing permanent dentition occur in half of all trauma to the primary dentition.
- Splinting for avulsion, luxation and root fractures should be functional to allow physiological movement and promote healing of the PDL and should not exceed 2–3 weeks.
- Splinting for dentoalveolar fractures should be rigid for 3–4 weeks.
- Endodontic management of some PDL injuries must start within 7–10 days of the injury. Referral to the pedodontic and restorative specialists is mandatory.
- In all luxation injuries the prognosis for pulpal healing is better with an immature apex.
- Root resorption increases with severity of damage to the PL.
- The prognosis for replantation of avulsed teeth is best if it is undertaken within 1 hour of injury, with a hydrated PL.
- Orofacial injuries are found in at least 50% of cases of child physical abuse.

training programs in pediatric dentistry now include child protection issues and in board exams in the United States, knowledge is essential for certification and recertification.

Since 1989, it has been mandatory for dental practitioners in the United States to report cases of child abuse. In addition, there is immunity from prosecution in all states as long as referrals are made in good faith. Despite these legislations, there is underreporting of suspected cases by dental practitioners and there is also evidence that similar underreporting may occur in the United Kingdom. The problem of underreporting would appear to be related both to the dental practitioner's knowledge of the physical signs of orofacial injury but probably more significantly to their lack of knowledge of how the Welfare Services work and what happens to a child and family after a referral is made. This defect in knowledge can only be addressed by the dental practitioner taking part in interagency training with all professionals involved in child protection.

In the United States, most states have a category of concern called 'Dental Neglect'. This is defined as: failure by a parent or guardian to seek treatment for visually untreated caries, orofacial infections and pain; or failure to follow through with treatment once informed that the above condition(s) exist, to ensure a level of oral health essential for adequate function and freedom from pain and care. However, to police this definition adequately would be very difficult as there are significant barriers to care including poverty, ignorance and lack of access to adequate care.

References

1 Cole BOI, Welbury RR 1999 Malformation in the primary and permanent dentitions following trauma prior to tooth eruption. Endodontics and Dental Traumatology 15: 294–296

2 Andreasen FM, Noren JG, Andreasen JO, Engelhardsten S, Lindh-Stromberg U 1995 Long-term survival of fragment bonding in the treatment of fractured crowns: a multicenter clinical study. Quintessence International 26: 669–681

3 Mackie IC, Bentley EM, Worthington HV 1988 The closure of open apices in non-vital immature incisor teeth. British Dental Journal 165: 169–173

4 Kinirons MJ, Srinivasan V, Welbury RR, Finucane D 2001 A study in two centres of variations in the time of apical barrier detection and barrier position in nonvital immature permanent incisors. International Journal of Paediatric Dentistry 11(6): 447–451

5 Andreasen JO, Andreasen FM 1994 Textbook and colour atlas of traumatic injuries to the teeth, 3rd edn. Munksgaard, Copenhagen

6 Kinirons MJ, Sutcliffe J 1991 Traumatically intruded permanent incisors: 'a study of treatment and outcome'. British Dental Journal 170: 144–146

7 Al-Badri S, Kinirons MJ, Cole BOI, Welbury RR 2002 Factors affecting resorption in traumatically intruded permanent incisors in children. Dental Traumatology 18: 73–76

8 Welbury RR, Kinirons MJ, Day P, Humphreys K, Gregg TA 2002 Outcomes for root-fractured permanent incisors: a retrospective study. Paediatric Dentistry 24: 98–102

9 Mackie IC, Worthington HV 1992 An investigation of replantation of traumatically avulsed permanent incisor teeth. British Dental Journal 172: 17–20

10 Andreasen JO, Borum MK, Jacobsen HL, Andreasen FM 1995 Replantation of 400 avulsed permanent incisors. Papers 1, 2, 3, 4. Endodontics and Dental Traumatology 11: 51–89

11 Barrett EJ, Kenny DJ 1997 Survival of avulsed permanent maxillary incisors in children following delayed replantation. Endodontics and Dental Traumatology 13: 269–275

12 Gregg TA, Boyd DH 1998 Treatment of avulsed permanent incisor teeth in children. International Journal of Paediatric Dentistry 8: 75–82

13 Kinirons MJ, Gregg TA, Welbury RR, Cole BOI 2000 Variations in the presenting and treatment features in reimplanted permanent incisors in children and their effect on the prevalence of root resorption. British Dental Journal 189: 263–266

14 Welbury RR 1994 Child physical abuse (non accidental injury). In: Andreasen JO, Andreasen FM (eds) Textbook and colour atlas of traumatic injuries to the teeth, 3rd edn. Munksgaard, Copenhagen

15 Murphy JM, Welbury RR 1998 The dental practitioner's role in protecting children from abuse: 1. The Child Protection System past and present. British Dental Journal 184: 7–10

16 Welbury RR, Murphy JM 1998 The dental practitioner's role in protecting children from abuse: 2. The orofacial signs of physical abuse. British Dental Journal 184: 61–65

17 Murphy JM, Welbury RR 1998 The dental practitioner's role in protecting children from abuse: 3. Reporting and subsequent management of child abuse by the Child Protection Service. British Dental Journal 184: 115–119

18 Becker DB, Needleman HL, Kotelchuck M 1978 Child abuse and dentistry: orofacial trauma and its recognition by dentists. Journal of the American Dental Association 97: 24–28

19 La Fonseca MA, Feigal RJ, Ten Bensel RW 1992 Dental aspects of 1248 cases of child maltreatment on file at a major county hospital. Paediatric Dentistry 14: 152–157

20 Jessee SA 1995 Physical manifestations of child abuse to the head, face and mouth: a hospital survey. Journal of Dentistry for Children 62: 245–249

21 Needleman HL, MacGregor SS, Lynch LM 1995 Effectiveness of a statewide child abuse and neglect educational program for dental professionals. Paediatric Dentistry 17: 41–45

22 Adair SM, Wray IA, Hanes CM, Sams DR, Yasrebi S, Russell CM 1997 Perceptions associated with dentists' decisions to report hypothetical cases of child maltreatment. Paediatric Dentistry 19: 461–465

23 Adair SM, Wray IA, Hanes CM, Sams DR, Yasrebi S, Russell CM 1997 Demographic, educational, and experimental factors associated with dentists' decisions to report hypothetical cases of child maltreatment. Paediatric Dentistry 19: 466–470

24 Welbury RR, Crawford MA, Macaskill SJ, Murphy JM, Evans D 2000 General dental practitioners perception of their role within child protection – a qualitative study. European Journal of Paediatric Dentistry 3: 114

18 Eyelid and Lacrimal Injuries

Anthony G Tyers

Introduction

The eyelids protect the eyes. Spontaneous blinking sweeps away microscopic debris and moistens the eyes with tears. A dust fragment or bright light stimulates reflex blinking and during sleep the eyes are protected by continuous eyelid closure. Without adequate eyelids the combined effect of desiccation and repeated minor trauma would soon lead to painful blindness. Neglected eyelid trauma can have the same disastrous result. The distress that inevitably accompanies facial trauma can be reduced considerably by a cosmetic and functional outcome that restores normality as far as possible, especially to the midface. This is achieved by careful assessment in the hours after trauma and appropriate early management with later adjustment if necessary. A multidisciplinary approach is appropriate for all but the most superficial injuries. Photographs add to the written record and aid in planning any late adjustments as well as providing an accurate graphical record for medicolegal purposes.

Anatomy

A sound knowledge of the anatomy of the periorbital region is essential for an accurate assessment and repair of eyelid and canthal trauma.

Surface anatomy (Fig. 18.1)

The upper and lower lids enclose the palpebral aperture and they join at the medial and lateral canthi. The average size of the palpebral aperture in an adult is 30 mm horizontally and 10 mm vertically between the centers of the lids. In the upper lid the delicate preseptal skin (inferior to the brow) and the pretarsal skin (superior to the lashes) meet at the upper lid skin crease, 6–10 mm from the lash line in an adult, lower in a child. The skin crease in the upper lid is formed by the insertion of the levator aponeurosis into the orbicularis muscle at this level. There is often redundant skin superior to the skin crease in the upper lid so that a skinfold is created which covers the skin crease when the eye is open. Superior to the skin crease, the 'fullness' in the upper lid is due to orbital fat. A less obvious skin crease may be visible in the lower lid, 4–5 mm from the lash line. Fullness in the lower lid is also due to orbital fat. The lateral canthus lies at a slightly higher position than the medial canthus and it rises further in upgaze.

Eyelid structure (Figs 18.2, 18.3)

An eyelid is conveniently divided into two anatomical lamellae. The anterior lamella includes the skin and the orbicularis muscle. The posterior lamella is formed by the tarsal plate and the conjunctiva. Any reconstruction of the eyelid must result in the restoration of an anterior covering lamella (skin) and the posterior lining lamella (mucosa) for the lid to function normally.

The skin of the eyelids is the thinnest in the body. It is attached loosely to the orbicularis muscle and more firmly in the region of the canthal tendons.

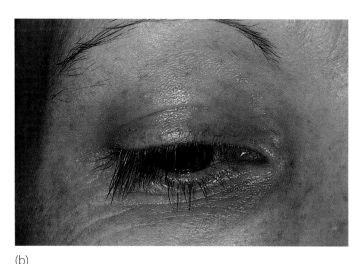

(a) (b)

Fig. 18.1: Surface anatomy of the eyelids in (a) the primary position and (b) downgaze.

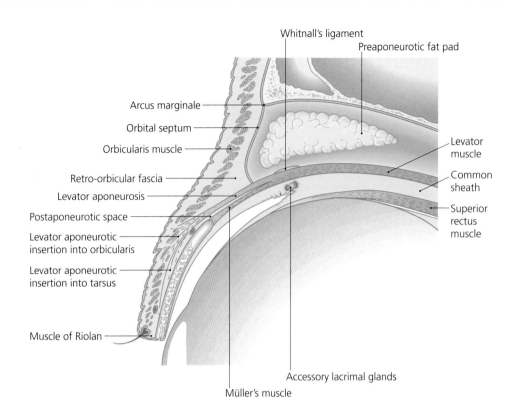

Fig. 18.2: Section through the upper eyelid.

Whitnall's ligament

Preaponeurotic fat pad

Arcus marginale

Orbital septum

Orbicularis muscle

Retro-orbicular fascia

Levator aponeurosis

Postaponeurotic space

Levator aponeurotic insertion into orbicularis

Levator aponeurotic insertion into tarsus

Muscle of Riolan

Levator muscle

Common sheath

Superior rectus muscle

Accessory lacrimal glands

Müller's muscle

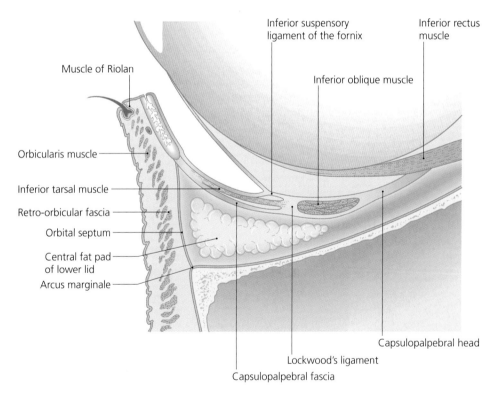

Fig. 18.3: Section through the lower eyelid.

Inferior suspensory ligament of the fornix

Inferior rectus muscle

Muscle of Riolan

Inferior oblique muscle

Orbicularis muscle

Inferior tarsal muscle

Retro-orbicular fascia

Orbital septum

Central fat pad of lower lid

Arcus marginale

Capsulopalpebral head

Lockwood's ligament

Capsulopalpebral fascia

The orbicularis oculi muscle is the main protractor of the eyelids (Fig. 18.4). It is a flat sheet of concentric fibers encircling the palpebral aperture and spreading out beyond the orbital rims. It is divided into concentric zones – palpebral and orbital. The palpebral part overlies the eyelids. It is subdivided into a pretarsal part overlying the tarsal plates and a preseptal part anterior to the orbital septum in the upper and lower lids. The orbital part of the orbicularis muscle lies peripheral to the palpebral part. Since the orbicularis muscle is supplied by the facial nerve, lacerations that damage the facial nerve may compromise eyelid closure.

The anatomy of the lymphatic drainage of the lids is important in facial trauma. Lacerations or surgical incisions that cut the lymphatic drainage may result in prolonged edema of the eyelid tissues. The lateral two-thirds of the upper lid and the lateral third of the lower lid drain to the

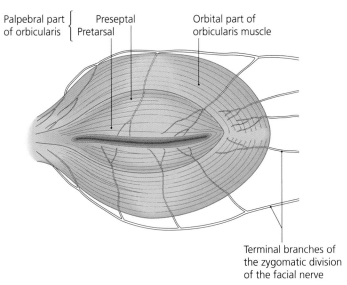

Palpebral part of orbicularis ∫ Preseptal ∫ Pretarsal

Orbital part of orbicularis muscle

Terminal branches of the zygomatic division of the facial nerve

Fig. 18.4: Orbicularis oculi muscle and terminal branches of the facial nerve.

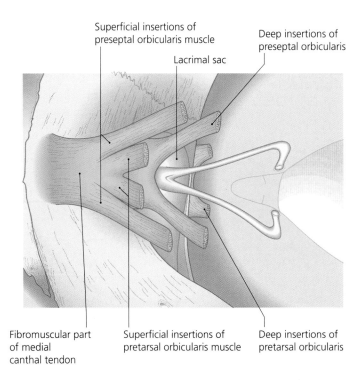

Superficial insertions of preseptal orbicularis muscle

Lacrimal sac

Deep insertions of preseptal orbicularis

Fibromuscular part of medial canthal tendon

Superficial insertions of pretarsal orbicularis muscle

Deep insertions of pretarsal orbicularis

Fig. 18.5: The medial canthus.

pre-auricular and parotid lymph nodes. The medial third of the upper lid and the medial two-thirds of the lower lid drain to the submandibular nodes.

Lateral canthal tendon

The pretarsal muscles join laterally and insert by a common tendon into Whitnall's tubercle, a bony prominence in the lateral orbital wall 5 mm posterior to the lateral orbital rim. The preseptal muscles join laterally to form a lateral raphé which is connected to the underlying tendon. Deep to the muscle insertions a Y-shaped fibrous thickening in the orbital septum joins the lateral ends of the tarsal plates to Whitnall's tubercle. These structures together form the lateral canthal tendon.

Medial canthal tendon (Fig. 18.5)

The medial canthal tendon is complex anatomically and some controversy still surrounds the detail of the anatomy. It has a fibrous and a muscular component – the muscular component being the insertions of the preseptal and pretarsal muscles. The fibrous component is attached laterally to the medial ends of the tarsal plates as two limbs of a Y. The stem of the Y inserts medially and it has an anterior and posterior component. The anterior component inserts on the frontal process of the maxilla just anterior to the anterior lacrimal crest level with the upper part of the lacrimal sac. The posterior part leaves the deep surface of the anterior part just lateral to the anterior lacrimal crest. It passes medially and posteriorly, lateral to the lacrimal sac, and inserts on the posterior lacrimal crest. The muscle insertions are divided into superficial and deep heads which also insert into the anterior and posterior lacrimal crests. Contraction of the preseptal orbicularis muscle during blinking activates the 'lacrimal pump' mechanism which facilitates the passage of tears from the palpebral aperture through the canaliculi into the lacrimal sac. In prac-

tice, the detailed anatomy of the medial canthal tendon is not evident at surgery. The fibrous part is clearly visible, especially the anterior component. The posterior components of the medial canthal tendon are the main anchor for the medial ends of the lids. It is important to reconstruct the posterior component, by reattaching the canthal tissues to the posterior lacrimal crest, if it has been divided by medial canthal trauma.

The upper and lower lid retractors
(see Fig. 18.2)

The levator palpebrae and Müller's muscles working together maintain the normal position of the upper lid when the eye is open.

The levator muscle arises from the roof of the orbit immediately anterior to the optic foramen. It passes forwards above the superior rectus muscle to end just posterior to the orbital septum as an aponeurosis. The aponeurosis passes forward into the lid and is inserted into the orbicularis muscle at the level of the upper lid skin crease and also into the lower third of the anterior surface of the tarsal plate. The orbital septum inserts into the anterior surface of the aponeurosis soon after its origin from the levator muscle. The aponeurosis expands medially and laterally to insert also into the region of the medial and lateral canthal tendons as the medial and lateral 'horns' of the aponeurosis (Fig. 18.6).

Müller's muscle lies deep to the levator aponeurosis between it and the conjunctiva. It arises from the deep surface of the levator muscle at the point of origin of the levator aponeurosis. It descends to insert into the superior border of the tarsal plate. Posterior to the septum and superior to the levator muscle lies the preaponeurotic fat pad. It is

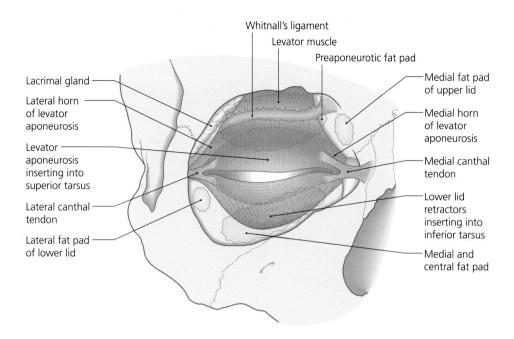

Lacrimal gland

Lateral horn of levator aponeurosis

Levator aponeurosis inserting into superior tarsus

Lateral canthal tendon

Lateral fat pad of lower lid

Whitnall's ligament

Levator muscle

Preaponeurotic fat pad

Medial fat pad of upper lid

Medial horn of levator aponeurosis

Medial canthal tendon

Lower lid retractors inserting into inferior tarsus

Medial and central fat pad

Fig. 18.6: The extraconal fat pads and insertions of the upper and lower lid retractors.

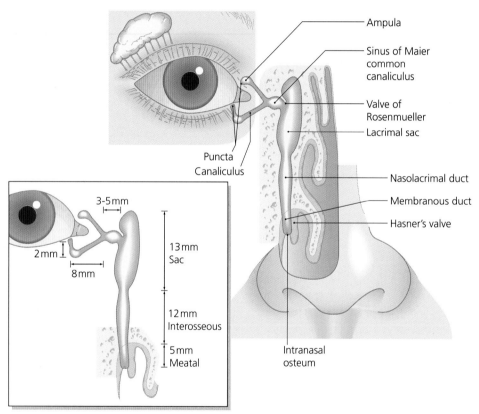

Ampula

Sinus of Maier common canaliculus

Valve of Rosenmueller

Lacrimal sac

Puncta

Canaliculus

Nasolacrimal duct

Membranous duct

Hasner's valve

3-5mm

2mm

8mm

13mm Sac

12mm Interosseous

5mm Meatal

Intranasal osteum

Fig. 18.7: The lacrimal drainage system.

this fat which gives the upper lid its 'fullness' and it is also an important surgical landmark.

The structure of the lower lid is similar. The lower lid retractors are vestigial but important in maintaining lower lid position. The central fat pad in the lower lid is similar anatomically to the preaponeurotic fat in the upper lid.

The lacrimal system (Fig. 18.7)

Tears are produced by the lacrimal gland which lies between the globe and the superior temporal quadrant of the anterior orbit, just within the orbital rim. The lateral edge of the levator aponeurosis, as it becomes the lateral horn, creates a deep cleft in the lacrimal gland, dividing it into two lobes – a larger orbital lobe above the lateral horn and a smaller palpebral lobe below the lateral horn. The palpebral lobe is just visible in the lateral end of the superior conjunctival fornix if the lateral end of the upper lid is lifted. Fine secretory ductules pass from the palpebral lobe to penetrate the conjunctiva of the superior fornix laterally.

Blinking spreads tears across the cornea and they move generally in a medial direction towards the lacrimal puncta situated in the upper and lower lids approximately 6 mm from the medial canthus. The puncta normally lie within the tear film and eversion of the puncta hinders the collection of tears. Canaliculi pass from the puncta medially to the lacrimal sac. The initial 2 mm of each canaliculus passes vertically into the lid before turning medially. At the medial canthal angle the canaliculi pass posterior to the anterior limb of the medial canthal tendon and usually join to form a common canaliculus 3–5 mm lateral to the lacrimal sac. The common canaliculus opens into the sac 2–3 mm behind the anterior limb of the medial canthal tendon. The lacrimal sac is situated within the fossa bounded by the anterior and posterior lacrimal crests. The sac empties inferiorly into the nasolacrimal duct that passes down through the bony naso-lacrimal canal, about 12 mm long, to open into the lateral wall of the nose under the inferior turbinate, approximately 15 mm from its tip, 30–35 mm from the external nares.

Assessment

History

An accurate account of the cause of the trauma allows a preliminary estimate of the depth and extent of the injury. Blunt trauma frequently leads to diffuse contusion with irregular wound edges while sharp objects cause wounds with smoother edges which are often deeper.

Examination

Tissue swelling or reduced conscious level may prevent a full assessment. A step-wise approach to the examination of the periocular soft tissues is helpful.

Obvious pathology

Note edema, ecchymosis, crepitus and the presence of hematoma. It is important to distinguish an orbital hematoma from preseptal hemorrhage. An orbital hematoma has a sharply limited edge (Fig. 18.8). The globe may be proptosed and eye movements reduced. In contrast, preseptal hemorrhage (Fig. 18.9) may be extensive, causing considerable local

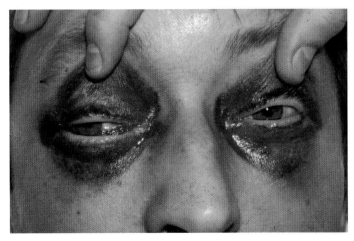

Fig. 18.8: Bilateral orbital hematomas.

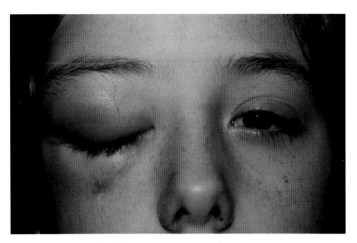

Fig. 18.9: Periorbital hematoma.

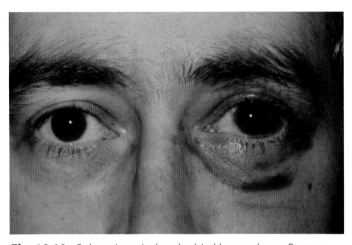

Fig. 18.10: Subconjunctival and orbital hemorrhage. Fracture of the zygoma.

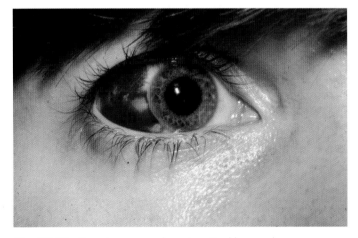

Fig. 18.11: Spontaneous subconjunctival hemorrhage.

swelling but without proptosis of the globe or limitation of eye movements. A subconjunctival hemorrhage arising from an orbital hemorrhage (Fig. 18.10) will have no posterior edge but disappears posteriorly around the equator of the globe. Subconjunctival hemorrhages due to direct trauma (Fig. 18.11) may be localized and with the whole edge visible

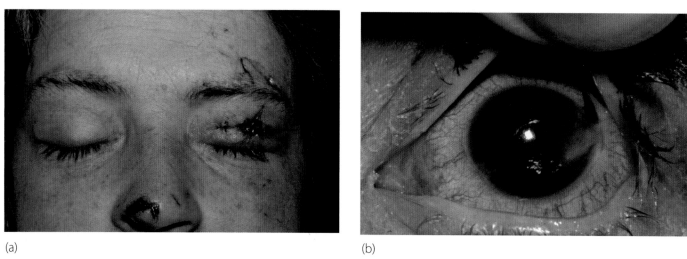

(a)   (b)

Fig. 18.12: **(a)** Upper lid laceration with **(b)** underlying penetrating eye injury.

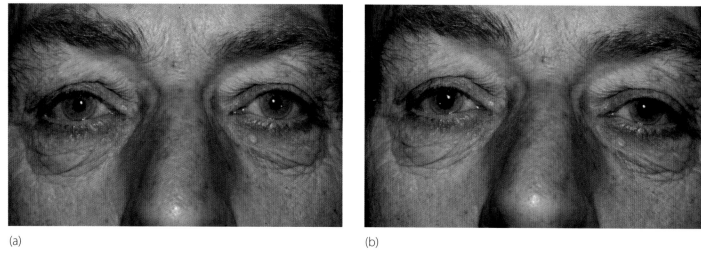

(a)   (b)

Fig. 18.13: Right relative afferent pupil defect (RAPD). **(a)** Light in front of normal left eye – both pupils constrict. **(b)** Light in front of abnormal right eye – both pupils dilate.

although the posterior edge is often well posterior and may not be visible.

Record entry wounds and estimate the depth of wounds. Note any possible loss of tissue.

Record whether the lid margins are involved in any laceration. Take particular note of lacerations involving the medial canthus and the presence of telecanthus. Note also lacerations in the upper lid that may have damaged the levator muscle or aponeurosis.

Exclude blunt or penetrating trauma to the eye. In particular, exclude penetrating injury of the globes if there is a laceration in the eyelids (Fig. 18.12). Check the visual acuity. Examine the pupils for their size at rest and also their reaction to light. The 'swinging flashlight' test (Fig. 18.13) is very valuable for identifying optic nerve trauma. To perform this test, dim the lights in the examination room and, if the patient is able to co-operate, indicate a distant target to look at. With a bright light, illuminate first one eye for 2 seconds then the other for 2 seconds. Swing the light backwards and

forwards in this fashion and observe the pupil reactions. In the absence of optic nerve trauma (or disease) or widespread retinal trauma, the pupils remain small in both eyes, apart from momentary dilatation during the transit of the light from one eye to the other. In the presence of unilateral trauma to the optic nerve or with widespread retinal trauma, the pupil on that side dilates, instead of remaining constricted, as the light is moved from the normal eye to illuminate that eye.

If the patient is mobile a slit-lamp examination with measurement of the intraocular pressures is important at this stage.

Eyelid position

Note the vertical position of the eyelids and the shape and position of the canthi. Although the vertical distance between the center of the upper and lower lids. The palpebral aperture (PA) is commonly used as a measure of the position of the lids,

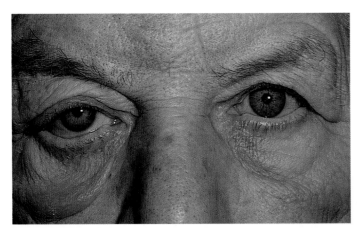

Fig. 18.14: The value of margin reflex distance (MRD). The asymmetrical lower lids provide poor reference points for measuring the relative positions of the upper lids.

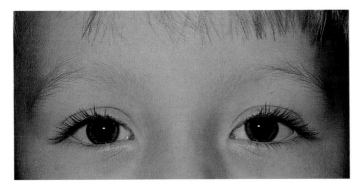

Fig. 18.15: Corneal light reflexes as reference points for measuring the position of the lids.

it has the disadvantage that the lower lid is used as the reference point for the position of the upper lid. In trauma and often in lid disease the lower lids themselves are not level (Fig. 18.14) so that a false impression of the lid positions is given. A better measure is the margin reflex distance (MRD). The patient is asked to look at a torch (Fig. 18.15). The dis-

tance from the corneal light reflex to each upper lid and each lower lid is recorded. This gives an accurate record of the position of all four lids. It remains reasonably accurate even if one eye is displaced by hemorrhage, swelling or an underlying squint.

The MRD is recorded as:

$$
\begin{array}{cc}
3 & 1 \\
\text{MRD} & \\
5 & 5
\end{array}
$$

In this case the right upper lid is 3 mm and the left upper lid is 1 mm above the corneal light reflexes. Both lower lids measure 5 mm from the light reflexes.

The distance between the medial canthi should be approximately half the distance between the centers of the pupils with the eyes in the primary position. Note any telecanthus. Note also any displacement of the lateral canthi. Disruption of the canthal tendons frequently leads to rounding of the angle of the canthi.

Eyelid movement

Estimate the function in the levator muscle of each upper lid. To do this, stabilize the brow with a thumb and hold a rule directly in front of the eyelids. Ask the patient to look up and down and measure the excursion of the upper lid in millimeters (Fig. 18.16). If there is no measurable levator function because of swelling or hemorrhage, look for any evidence of muscle action. The levator may cause only the slightest movement of the lid or dimpling of the upper lid skin. Bruising alone without transection of the levator can lead to a marked decrease in levator function (Fig. 18.17). Surgical emphysema causes a mechanical ptosis that resolves over several days as the emphysema disappears (Fig. 18.18).

Eye position

Measure the position of each globe in all three planes. A simple ruler is used to measure the vertical and horizontal position of the globes (Fig. 18.19). The center of the pupil

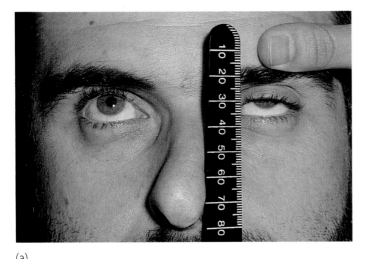

(a)

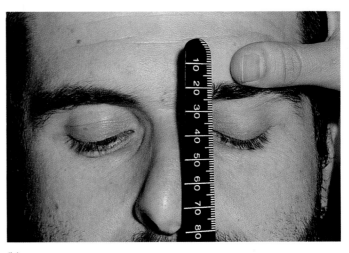

(b)

Fig. 18.16: With the brow fixed, measure the upper lid excursion in **(a)** upgaze and **(b)** downgaze.

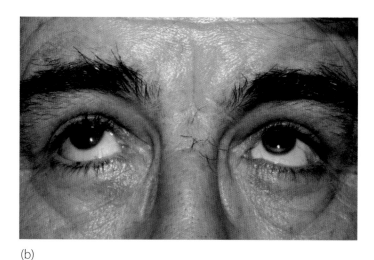

(a)

(b)

Fig. 18.17: **(a)** Orbital and periorbital hematoma with bruising of the levator muscle. **(b)** Full recovery after 2 months.

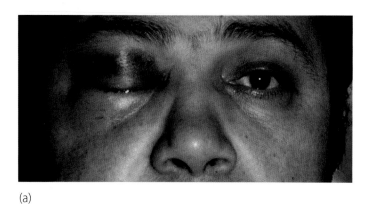

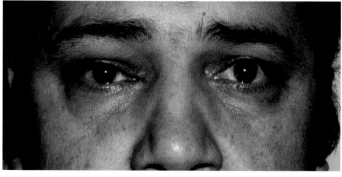

(a)

(b)

Fig. 18.18: **(a)** Extensive surgical emphysema. **(b)** Full recovery after 1 week.

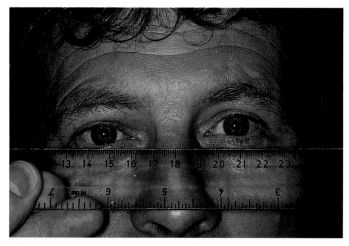

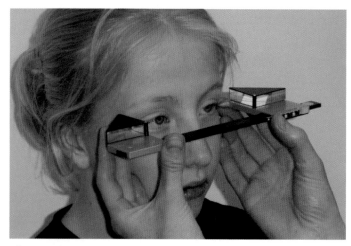

Fig. 18.19: Measuring vertical and horizontal displacement of the eye.

Fig. 18.20: Measuring proptosis with a Hertel exophthalmometer.

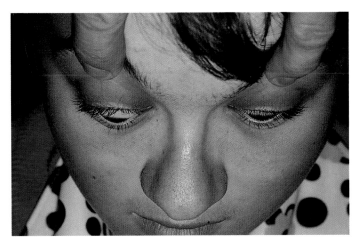

Fig. 18.21: Estimating proptosis by viewing from above.

and the medial limbus are useful reference points. A Hertel exophthalmometer is used to measure anteroposterior position (Fig. 18.20). The Hertel rests on the lateral orbital rims so in the presence of displacement of the zygoma, it is not accurate. A rough estimate of anteroposterior displacement can be made by looking over the patient's forehead from behind (Fig. 18.21). The relative positions of the eyes can be assessed quite easily.

Eye movement

Check that the eyes move together in horizontal and vertical directions. Record the presence of any diplopia and the direction of gaze in which the images are most widely separated.

Lacrimal system

Inspect the medial canthal areas and the nose. A fine probe (size OO) may be passed into the lacrimal puncta and along the canaliculi to assess continuity. Alternatively saline stained with fluorescein may be gently syringed through the canaliculi (Fig. 18.22). Note that as a result of naso-ethmoidal fractures that have damaged the walls of the nasolacrimal duct or sac the fluid may leak through a defect into the tissues and give the false impression of a patent

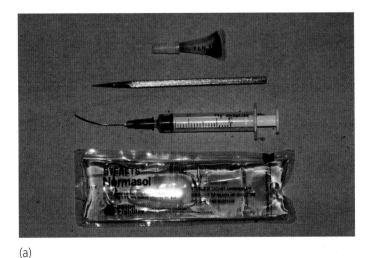

(a)

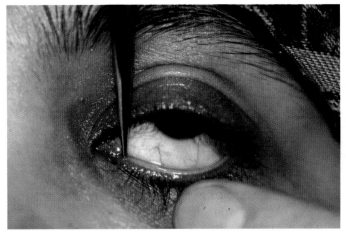

(b)

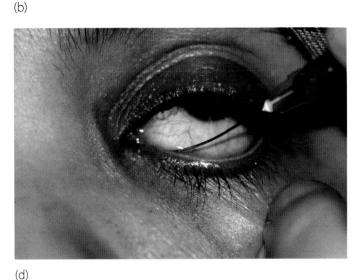

(c)

(d)

Fig. 18.22: **(a)** Equipment for syringing the lacrimal system. **(b)** After local anesthetic drops have been inserted, gently dilate the punctum, first vertically, then **(c)** horizontally a short distance along the canaliculus. **(d)** Pull the lid laterally to straighten the canaliculus and pass the lacrimal cannula along the canaliculus until the medial wall of the lacrimal sac can be felt as a 'hard stop'. Inject saline gently. In a patent system the patient feels the fluid in the throat.

nasolacrimal system. Patency of the lacrimal system is confirmed if fluid can be seen beneath the inferior turbinate. Fluid stained with fluorescein fluoresces green with a cobalt blue light.

Special investigations

It is important to exclude retained foreign bodies within the periocular tissues or globes. These are normally easily visible on a plain X-ray or CT scan.

Photography

A photographic record of the extent of the injuries at presentation is useful for medicolegal purposes but also for planning future treatment. The photographic department may not be available and it is helpful to have access to an alternative camera in the department. The most useful magnifications will be one eye (1:1), both eyes (1:3, 1:4) and full face (1:10). A suitable standard film (non-digital) camera would have a macro lens of approximately 100 mm focal length, a suitable flash and 100 ISO film speed. A digital camera should be capable of the same range of magnifications and a resolving power in excess of three megapixels.

Management Priorities

Complex periorbital trauma should be approached systematically. A suggested order of priority in addressing injuries in the emergency examination room and the operating theatre is as follows.

- Life threatening
- Decision on timing of any fracture stabilization
- Sight threatening (including corneal exposure)
- Lacrimal drainage system
- Medial canthal tendon
- Lid margins
- Lateral canthal tendon
- Levator muscle and aponeurosis
- Penetrating trauma of eyelids and periocular region

Anesthesia

General anesthesia is appropriate for children and most adults. However, local anesthesia may be particularly helpful in repairing the levator muscle or aponeurosis. In an adult patient with limited local swelling in whom general anesthesia is not required for other reasons, local anesthesia allows the levator to be identified more easily by asking the patient to look up and down during surgery. The lid level is also set more accurately if the patient is awake. 2% lignocaine (lidocaine) with 1:100 000 adrenaline (epinephrine) provides a good level of anesthesia as well as hemostasis. If local anesthesia is indicated because the patient is unfit for general anesthesia but local infiltration is difficult because of wide local contusion, a regional block such as a frontal block, infratrochlear block or infraorbital block avoids the injection of large volumes of local anesthetic.

Acute Management of Eyelid and Lacrimal Trauma

Sight-threatening trauma

The management of fractures affecting the optic canal and of penetrating ocular injury is considered elsewhere. Exposure of the cornea due to inability to close the lids requires immediate treatment. If the lids are intact chloramphenicol ointment should be put into the eye and the lids taped closed. If there is loss of lid tissue the cornea should be protected by creating a 'moist chamber'; eye pads are best avoided but a plastic 'Cartella' shield can be placed over the eye and the gaps sealed with tape. Alternatively, a fine plastic sheet such as 'Clingfilm' can be placed directly over the eye and lids and taped around the edges to the forehead and cheek to create a sealed moist space. If there is enough lid tissue to close the lids a temporary tarsorrhaphy suture of 4/0 Prolene placed over bolsters is an effective way of providing temporary protection of the cornea. If the loss of tissue does not allow a suture to be used then early reconstruction of the defect is required (see Reconstruction of full-thickness eyelid defects, p. 337).

Lacrimal drainage system

Lacerations of the inner canthus commonly damage the canaliculi. The lacrimal sac is less commonly damaged but nasoethmoidal fractures can cause complex medial canthal disruption. Bony nasolacrimal canal fractures can obstruct the nasolacrimal duct. The management of trauma to the lacrimal drainage system depends on the site of the trauma.

Canaliculus – laceration within 8 mm from the punctum

There is controversy about the need to repair a single divided canaliculus, especially the upper canaliculus. A single intact canaliculus is probably adequate in most patients to avoid watering and the risk of iatrogenic injury to the normal canaliculus, especially with a pigtail probe, is significant. However, most lacrimal surgeons now advise careful repair of any lacerated canaliculus whenever possible. The surgery is best undertaken within 24 hours of the injury – late repairs are less successful. A microscope is necessary for accurate repair.

The cut canaliculus can normally be identified easily, situated posteriorly within the lid close to the lid margin. If one canaliculus is damaged, a monocanalicular stent, e.g. Mini-Monaka stent (FCI; Novamed Ltd, Dundee, UK), is easy to place and it has the advantage over the Veirs rod that it is not easily dislodged during the healing period. If both canaliculi are damaged a single canalicular stent can be used in each canaliculus but a better alternative is bicanalicular silicone tubes, e.g. Ritleng tubes (FCI; Novamed Ltd, Dundee, UK). These are convenient and can be left in situ for 6 months or more. However, they can be difficult to insert. Most patterns of silicone lacrimal intubation tubes have probes attached to

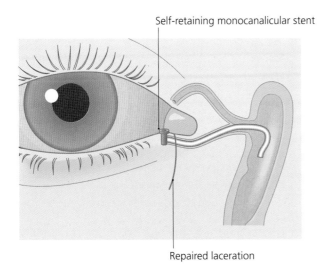

Self-retaining monocanalicular stent

Repaired laceration

Fig. 18.23: Position of the monocanalicular stent in lower canaliculus repair.

the tubes which are passed through the canaliculus in each lid and down the nasolacrimal duct to emerge below the inferior turbinate. Retrieving the probes can be difficult. The Ritleng tubes have a different system of intubation that is easier to insert.

Whatever system is used, once the tubes are in place the lower ends within the nose are knotted together or joined with a suture or Watzke sleeve and may be sutured within the ala of the nose with a 6/0 monofilament suture. However, the suture collects mucus and may gradually detach from the tissues. Silicone tubes can 'cheese-wire' through the puncta and canaliculi if they are too tight or alternatively abrade the cornea if they are too loose.

Insertion of monocanalicular stent
Technique

The Mini-Monaka stent is a silicone tube which is self-retaining within the canaliculus (Fig. 18.23). Its shape does not allow it to migrate down the canaliculus into the lacrimal sac. To insert it, pass the tube through the canaliculus and across the laceration into the distal canaliculus and lacrimal sac (Fig. 18.24). Locate the angle of the stent within the proximal canaliculus where it will be retained for 3 months or more without attention.

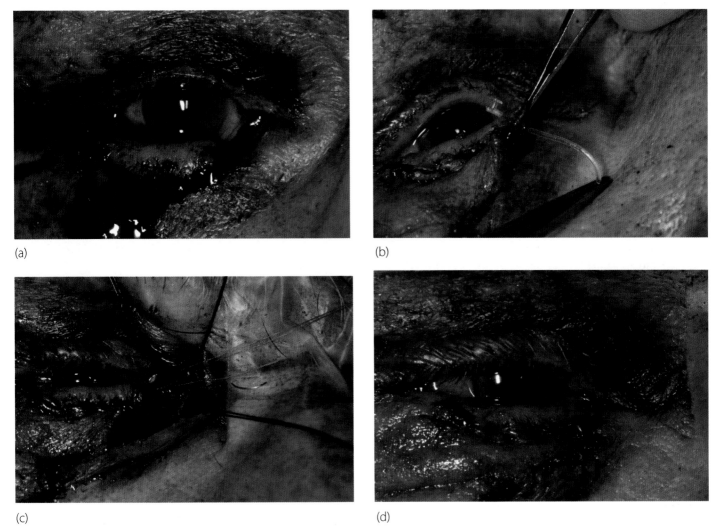

(a)

(b)

(c)

(d)

Fig. 18.24: (a–d) Insertion of a Mini-Monaka tube through the punctum, across the laceration and into the medial cut end of the canaliculus before the lacerations in the canaliculus and the lid are sutured.

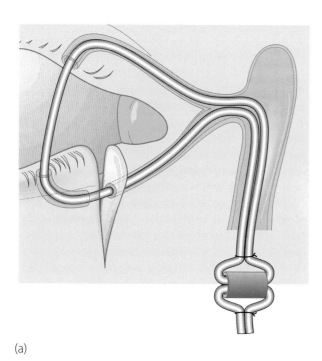

(a)

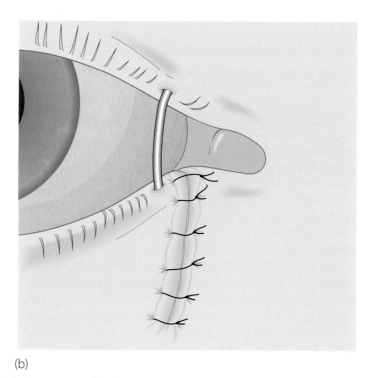

(b)

Fig. 18.25: **(a)** Bicanalicular intubation for single or double canalicular lacerations. **(b)** The wound is sutured in layers.

An alternative material is fine silicone tubing but it must be passed through both canaliculi because it does not have the angled self-retaining end for single canaliculus intubation.

Complications

The stent may fall out and can usually be replaced under local anesthetic. After removal of the stent it is common for the canaliculus to narrow or stenose and become non-functional. Little can be done to overcome this but a watering eye is not inevitable if the other canaliculus is patent.

Insertion of bicanalicular tubes
Technique

There are several systems for bicanalicular intubation. The commonly used Crawford tubes are more difficult to insert than the Ritleng system. The principle is the same: fine silicone tubing is passed through the upper and lower canaliculi, the ends are passed down the nasolacrimal duct and retrieved from the exit of the duct beneath the inferior turbinate (Fig. 18.25).

Complications

The loop of tubing may ride up within the nose and appear as a large loop within the palpebral aperture, abrading the cornea. It can be pulled down within the nose with the aid of a nasal endoscope and fine forceps. Alternatively, if it is too tight, the loop in the inner canthus may cheese-wire through the canaliculi. It should be loosened within the nose if this occurs.

Repair of canaliculus
Technique

Pass a silicone stent through the lacrimal punctum and across the laceration in the canaliculus. Place two or three fine sutures, e.g. 8/0–10/0 Vicryl or nylon, in the submucosal tissue surrounding the canalicular lumen to approximate the edges. Repair the lid tissues in layers (Fig. 18.26).

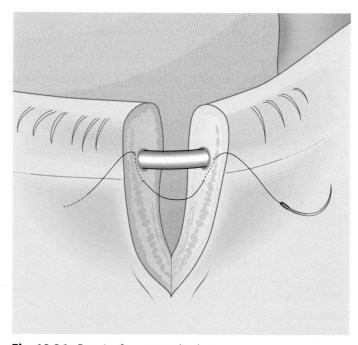

Fig. 18.26: Repair of a cut canaliculus.

Complications

Stenosis of the repair is common despite adequate stenting. Providing the other canaliculus is patent, watering of the eye is not inevitable.

The traditional alternative of a pigtail probe passed between the canaliculi via the common canaliculus is generally considered unsuitable because of the risk of iatrogenic damage and it is best avoided.

Canaliculus – laceration more than 8 mm from the punctum or in the common canaliculus

It is usually not possible to repair the distal canaliculus or common canaliculus directly. If the cut end of the canaliculus is visible the options are either to marsupialize the canaliculus into the conjunctival sac or to place a silicone stent. Lacerations more medially, through the common canaliculus, cannot be repaired and a Lester Jones tube (see below) may be required if watering is significant.

Marsupialization of the canaliculus
Technique

1. Identify the lower canaliculus in the medial cut edge (Fig. 18.27).
2. Cut the canaliculus longitudinally for about 5 mm (Fig. 18.28).
3. Separate the cut edges of the opened canaliculus (Fig. 18.29) and place two 7/0 absorbable sutures between the corners of the cut canaliculus and the adjacent conjunctiva. This will help to hold the canaliculus open (see Fig. 18.40).

Complications

The marsupialized canaliculus may not drain tears.

Silicone tubes introduced through the canaliculi and down the nasolacrimal duct as described above give the best chance of restoring patency. The medial canthal tendon is often damaged at the same time. If the posterior part of the tendon has been disrupted it must be repaired (see below).

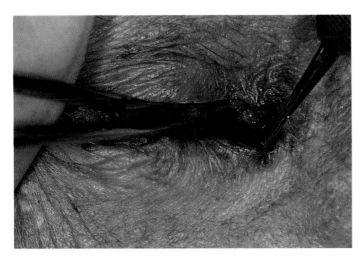

Fig. 18.27: Canaliculus identified medially.

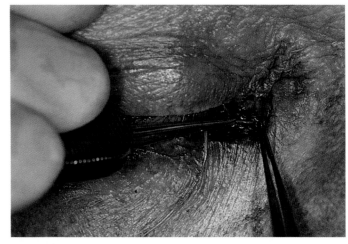

Fig. 18.29: The corners of the marsupialized canaliculus can be secured open with fine absorbable sutures.

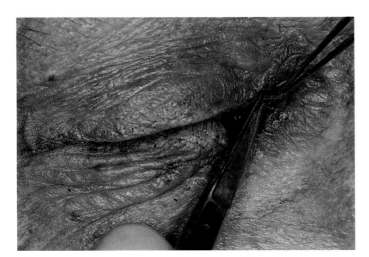

Fig. 18.28: Cut along the posterior wall to lay the canaliculus open for 5 mm.

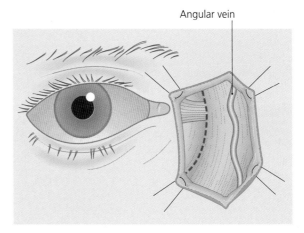

Fig. 18.30: Position of the incision into the periosteum of the anterior lacrimal crest. Medial canthal tendon laterally, angular vein medially.

Lacrimal sac

If the lacrimal sac has been damaged but the canaliculi and common canaliculus are intact a dacryocystorhinostomy with the insertion of silicone tubes is usually required. It may be appropriate to undertake this surgery at the time of the primary repair. However, in the presence of complex disruption in the region of the medial canthus it is preferable to defer definitive lacrimal surgery for several months until the tissues have healed. If the canaliculi and sac are both severely damaged it is unlikely that a patent lacrimal system can be achieved with any surgery. The tissues should be allowed to heal and a Lester Jones bypass tube should be inserted at a later date if watering is a problem.

Dacryocystorhinostomy
Technique
The principle of dacryocystorhinostomy (DCR) is that the bone between the lacrimal sac fossa and the middle meatus of the nose (cross-hatched shading in Fig. 18.31) is removed. The mucosa of the lacrimal sac and the mucosa of the nose are incised and anterior and posterior flaps respectively are anastomosed to create a direct connection between the lacrimal sac and the middle meatus.

1. Pack the nose and especially the region of the middle meatus with a nasal decongestant, e.g. 4% cocaine.
2. Make a straight incision about 15 mm in length and 8 mm medial to the inner canthus. One-third should be superior to the medial canthal tendon and two-thirds inferior. Deepen it through the orbicularis muscle to identify the anterior limb of the medial canthal tendon as it inserts into the anterior lacrimal crest.
3. Using a periosteal elevator, e.g. Rollet's rougine, cut through or disinsert the medial canthal tendon and the adjacent periosteum along the anterior lacrimal crest. Reflect it laterally to expose the lacrimal sac fossa as far as the posterior lacrimal crest. The angular vein may be encountered during this dissection (Fig. 18.30).
4. Using a small right-angled elevator, create a gap in the suture between the lacrimal bone and the frontal process of the maxilla in the floor of the lacrimal sac fossa. Fracture out a small piece of bone then reintroduce the right-angled elevator to push the underlying nasal mucosa away from the deep surface of the bone.
5. Using bone nibblers, enlarge the hole in the lacrimal sac fossa until the floor of the fossa has been removed. After the removal of each small piece of bone, reintroduce the right-angled elevator to separate the nasal mucosa from the leading edge of the enlarging rhinostomy. Extend the anterior edge of the osteum onto the anterior lacrimal crest. The final defect in the bone should be at least 15 mm in diameter (Fig. 18.31).
6. Pass a lacrimal probe through the lower canaliculus into the lacrimal sac to tent up its medial wall (Fig. 18.32). Make a vertical incision in the medial wall of the lacrimal sac to expose the tip of the lacrimal probe. Enlarge this vertically to the fundus of the sac superiorly and the nasolacrimal duct inferiorly.
7. Make a vertical cut in the nasal mucosa about one-third of the distance from the posterior edge of the bony defect. From the ends of this incision make transverse incisions to improve the mobility of the flaps (Fig. 18.33).

Fig. 18.31: Area of bone removal.

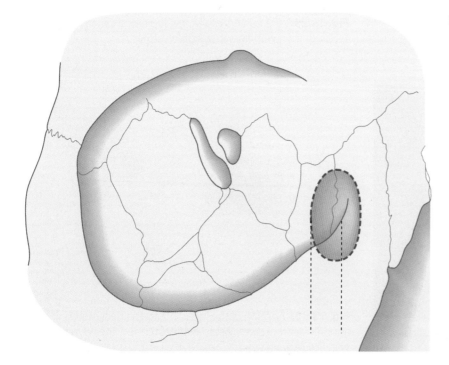

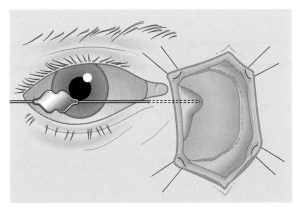

Fig. 18.32: Probe tenting the medial sac wall before opening it.

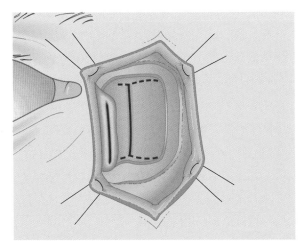

Fig. 18.33: Vertical cut into the lacrimal sac laterally and H-shaped cut into the nasal mucosa medially.

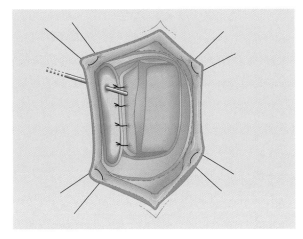

Fig. 18.34: Posterior flaps of the lacrimal sac and nose sutured.

8. Suture the posterior flap of the lacrimal sac to the posterior flap of nasal mucosa with three or four interrupted 6/0 absorbable sutures (Fig. 18.34). Introduce tubes at this point if necessary. To do this pass the metal introducers along the superior and inferior canaliculi into the lacrimal sac. Cut off the metal introducers. Tie a knot

5–10 mm from the point where the tubes enter the lacrimal sac or pass the tubes through a fine sleeve (e.g. watzke sleeve) located at the same point. Pass fine curved artery forceps up the nose into the DCR site and draw the ends of the tubes down the nose. A further knot or sleeve can be used to secure the lower ends of the tubes. Cut the tubes to leave their ends just within the nose.

9. Close the anterior flaps with three or four 6/0 absorbable sutures. Close the muscle and skin in two layers.
10. If tubes have been used they should be removed at 3 months.

Complications
DCR is successful in about 85% of patients although more than this achieve patency of the lacrimal drainage system but with residual watering of the eye. Repeat surgery can be difficult and the results are often disappointing.

Insertion of Lester Jones bypass tube
Technique
The principle of this technique is that a tube is passed from the medial canthus behind the medial end of the lower lid through the soft tissues and the bony rhinostomy of a DCR into the middle meatus of the nose.

1. Follow steps 1–8 as for a standard DCR.
2. Pass a fine pointed guidewire from the junction between the caruncle and the medial end of the lower lid in a downwards and posterior direction to pass through the lateral wall of the lacrimal sac and through the bony osteum into the middle meatus of the nose (Fig. 18.35).
3. Pass a 2 mm trephine over the guidewire to create a narrow channel. Remove the trephine and estimate the length of Lester Jones tube required to reach from the inner canthus to the middle meatus. Pass a Lester Jones tube of the correct length along the guidewire (Fig. 18.36). Check its position: the medial end should be 2–3 mm from the nasal septum (Fig. 18.37) and the lateral end should lie close to the lower fornix behind

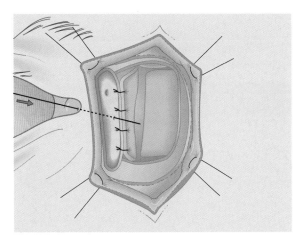

Fig. 18.35: Guidewire from the inner canthus to the osteum.

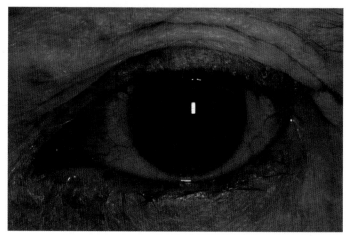

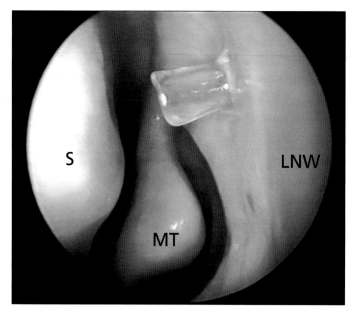

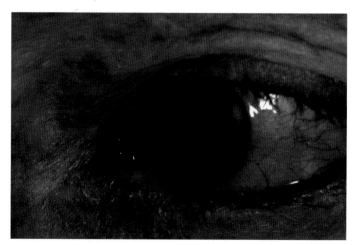

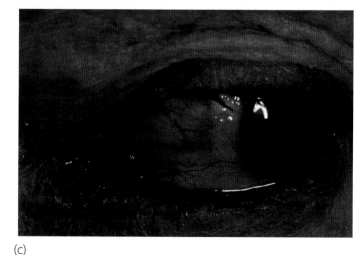

Fig. 18.36: Lester Jones tube over a guidewire at the inner canthus.

(a)

Fig. 18.37: Good tube position. S = septum, MT = middle turbinate, LNW = lateral nasal wall.

(b)

(c)

the medial end of the lower lid (Fig. 18.38; see also Fig. 18.41) so that tears can enter it easily. A 6/0 Prolene suture may be wound around the neck of the tube and through the adjacent lid to anchor it for the first week.

4. Close the lacrimal sac and the wound as for a DCR.
5. The tube should be irrigated twice daily by sucking saline drops through it.

Fig. 18.38: (a) Proximal end of the tube. **(b)** No tube–eye touch or **(c)** displacement with eye movement.

Complications

The tubes may become blocked or fall out. Regular cleaning by inhaling saline drops through the tube maintains patency in most patients. If the tube becomes blocked and cannot be cleared with syringing, or if it falls out, it must be replaced, usually under general anesthesia.

Nasolacrimal duct

If the nasolacrimal duct has been damaged by a fracture through the nasolacrimal canal but the lacrimal sac and canaliculi are intact a dacryocystorhinostomy is appropriate. This is usually deferred until the tissues have healed.

Extensive trauma with no reconstruction possible

Extensive damage to the lacrimal drainage system cannot be repaired with any significant chance of patency. The tissues are allowed to heal and if watering is a late problem, a Lester Jones bypass tube is inserted at a later date.

Medial canthal tendon

Disinsertion or disruption of the medial canthal tendon (MCT) may occur with nasoethmoidal and Le Fort II fractures or with local penetrating injuries. The anterior limb of the MCT can be ignored. The posterior limb, however, should be identified and reattached to the posterior lacrimal crest. The periosteum over the posterior lacrimal crest is slightly thickened and offers a good anchor point for a double-armed 5/0 non-absorbable suture which then passes forward to the severed tissues at the medial canthal angle. This repair is performed after any canalicular repair and care must be taken to avoid further damage or distortion of the canaliculi.

If it is not possible to achieve adequate fixation to the posterior lacrimal crest, alternative anchorage in the region of the posterior crest must be provided. This is achieved with either local wiring or a transnasal wire anchored to the MCT of the opposite side. A miniplate or microplate attached to the anterior lacrimal crest and angled back towards the posterior lacrimal crest can provide adequate posterior fixation. If there have been fractures in the region of the lacrimal fossa with loss of fixation points a transnasal wire may be preferred to attempted direct refixation of the MCT to the periosteum. A transnasal wire is also required for bilateral MCT disruption, especially if there is disruption of the normal bone anchor points. The wire must be passed through the floor of the lacrimal sac fossa as far posteriorly as possible. Care must be taken preoperatively to establish the position of the cribriform plate to avoid injury at surgery.

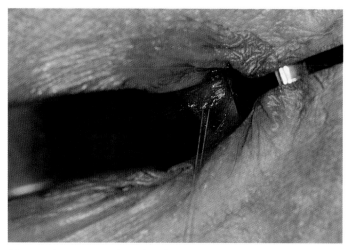

Fig. 18.39: Suture placed in the periosteum of the posterior lacrimal crest, right inner canthus.

Suture reattachment of the MCT to the posterior lacrimal crest
Technique

1. Using blunt dissection with scissors directed posteriorly and medially, lateral to the lacrimal sac, expose the posterior lacrimal crest at or just above the level of the medial canthus.
2. Place a malleable retractor gently against the globe to improve the exposure and insert both needles of a double-armed 5/0 non-absorbable suture, directed posteriorly through the periosteum of the posterior lacrimal crest (Fig. 18.39).
3. Pass one needle of the 5/0 suture through the edge of the tarsal plate in the lateral wound edge close to the lid margin, adjusting its position as necessary so that when the suture is tightened the lid is drawn medially and posteriorly to lie against the eye. Pass the second needle through the tarsal plate 2–3 mm inferior to the first (Fig. 18.40). Tie the 5/0 suture with a single throw to draw the lateral wound edge medially.

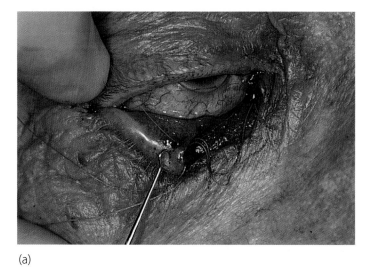

(a)

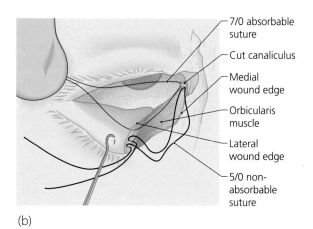

7/0 absorbable suture

Cut canaliculus

Medial wound edge

Orbicularis muscle

Lateral wound edge

5/0 non-absorbable suture

(b)

Fig. 18.40: (a,b) Posterior lacrimal crest suture passed through the cut medial edge of the tarsal plate. Note also the 7/0 absorbable suture anchoring the marsupialized canaliculus.

4. Close the conjunctiva to ensure that the 5/0 fixation suture is well covered. Tighten the 5/0 fixation suture further and tie it. Close the skin with 6/0 sutures.

Complications
The suture holding the medial canthus attached to the posterior lacrimal crest may become detached, resulting in migration of the canthus. It will need to be replaced.

Transnasal wire to fix the canthi
Technique (Fig. 18.41 and see p. 225)

Lid margins

Lid margin lacerations are common. Accurate repair, avoiding distortion or a notch, ensures comfort and corneal protection as well as good function with regard to the spread of tears. If the lid margin wound cannot be approximated because of limited local loss of tissue involving the lid margin, it may be necessary to release tissue in the region of the lateral canthus to allow direct closure. If tissue loss is more extensive, larger flaps and reconstruction of both eyelid lamellae may be required (see Reconstruction of full-thickness eyelid defects, p. 337).

Direct closure
Technique
The technique is identical for upper and lower lids (Fig. 18.42).

1. Place a 6/0 or 7/0 absorbable suture through the cut edges of the tarsal plate close to the lid margin but avoid including the conjunctiva (Fig. 18.43). Tie the knot on the anterior surface of the tarsal plate.
2. Place two more absorbable sutures through the edges of the tarsal plate in the same way to close the posterior lamella of the lid. Place a 6/0 suture through the gray line at the lid margin. Pass it across the wound and out through the gray line on the opposite side (Fig. 18.44). Tie the suture to support closure of the margin. Leave the suture ends long.

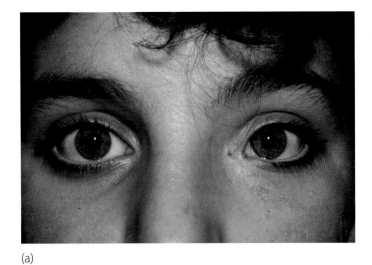

(a)

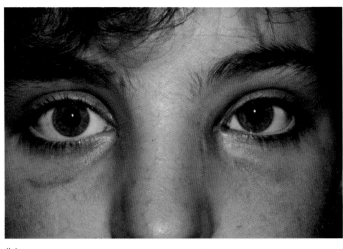

(b)

Fig. 18.41: (a,b) Traumatic telecanthus treated with a transnasal wire. A Lester Jones tube has been inserted at the same time.

(a)

(b)

(c)

(d)

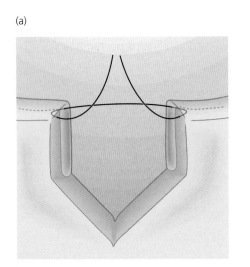
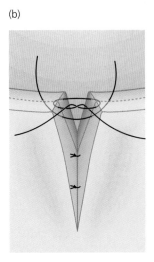
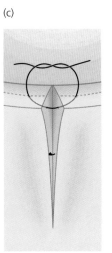
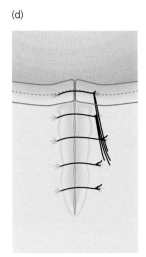

Fig. 18.42: (a–d) The principles of direct lid margin closure.

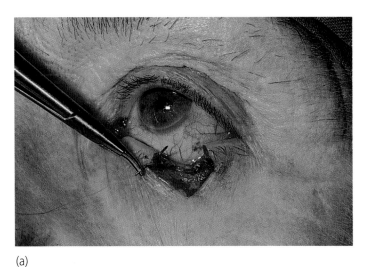

(a)

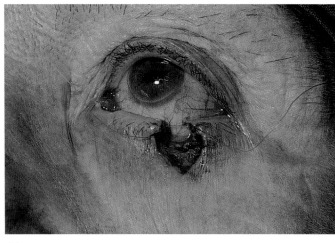

(b)

Fig. 18.43: (a,b) First suture placed through the tarsal plate at the posterior lid margin either side of the wound.

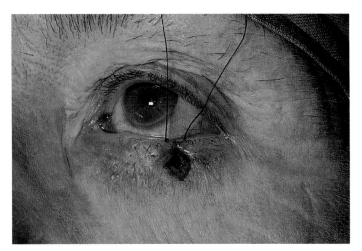

Fig. 18.44: Tarsal plate closed. Lid margin suture in situ through the gray line.

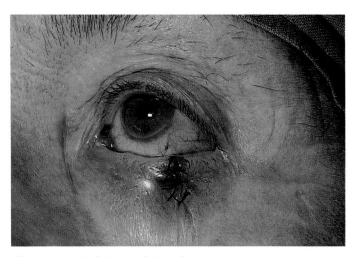

Fig. 18.45: Eyelid wound closed.

3. Close the orbicularis muscle within the wound with two or three 6/0 or 7/0 absorbable sutures. Close the skin with 6/0 or 7/0 sutures. Pass the long end of the lid margin suture beneath the skin closure sutures to prevent it damaging the cornea (Fig. 18.45). The lid margin and skin sutures can be removed at 1 week (Fig. 18.46).

Complications

A small notch may appear at the lid margin despite every effort to prevent it. It is best left alone. If an obvious notch or distortion of the lid margin is present (Fig. 18.47), allow the lid to heal for several months, excise the notch and resuture the lid. Occasionally the lid repair breaks down. Remove the sutures and allow the lid to heal without further attempt to suture it. The result is usually surprisingly good but if there is local distortion this area of the lid margin should be excised and the lid resutured.

Lateral canthal tendon

Disruption of the lateral canthal tendon leads to a rounded lateral canthal angle and displacement of the canthus medially and forward. The lateral canthal tendon should be reattached to Whitnall's tubercle. This is sometimes possible with a simple suture through the periosteum overlying Whitnall's tubercle. If this is not possible, a periosteal flap fashioned from the periosteum overlying the lateral orbital rim and based medially within the orbit provides adequate anchorage. Alternatively a wire passed through the lateral canthal tissues and through holes drilled in the lateral orbital rim provides secure fixation.

Periosteal flap
Technique (Fig. 18.48)
This technique is used to support the upper or lower lid, or both, laterally when the lateral canthal tendon is inadequate.

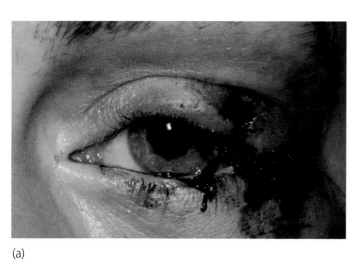

(a)

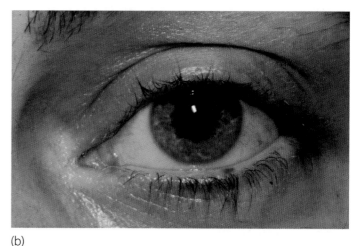

(b)

Fig. 18.46: **(a)** Upper lid lacerations with potential tattooing. **(b)** Repair following careful removal of debris from the skin and wounds.

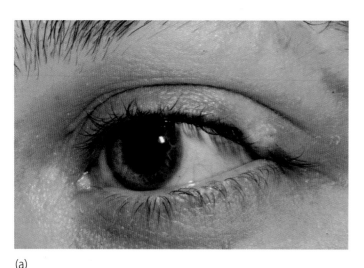

(a)

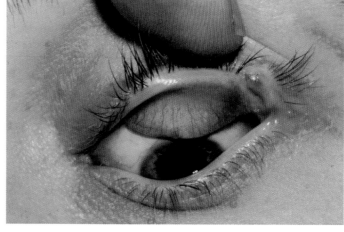

(b)

Fig. 18.47: **(a,b)** Upper lid margin distortion and tattooing due to inaccurate closure and incomplete removal of debris at the original operation.

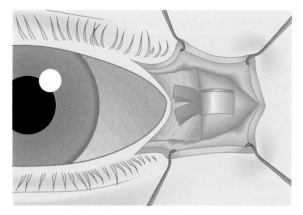

Fig. 18.48: Principle of a periosteal flap.

It is useful in lid reconstruction when lateral fixation of the posterior lamella is required or in any situation where the tendon is lax or absent and the lateral canthus has moved medially.

1. Make a horizontal incision from the lateral canthus to expose the lateral orbital rim. At the level of the proposed new lateral canthal tendon mark two horizontal lines on the periosteum, 8–10 mm apart, extending from the medial border of the lateral orbital rim to the temporalis fascia laterally. If support for both lids is required cut a broader strip of periosteum to allow it to be split later. Mark the lateral extent of the flap with a vertical line (Fig. 18.49).

2. Incise the edges of the flap, leaving the periosteum intact medially, and lift the flap of periosteum with a periosteal elevator. Leave the base of the flap attached to the periosteum within the lateral rim of the orbit (Fig. 18.50).

To attach the canthal tissues or the reconstructed posterior lamella to the periosteal flap, pass one or two double-armed 5/0 non-absorbable sutures through the lid tissues then pass both needles through the periosteal flap.

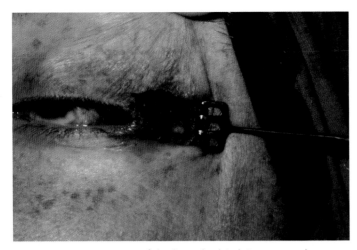

Fig. 18.49: Periosteum of the lateral orbital rim exposed.

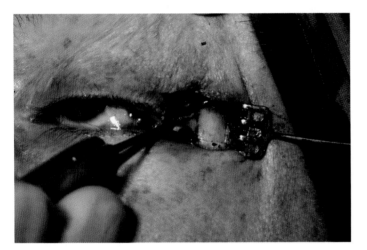

Fig. 18.50: Periosteal flap cut.

Tie the sutures to support the lid tissues. There should be minimal horizontal lid laxity. If a broader strip of periosteum has been cut for the support of both lids split it into an upper and a lower limb and attach them to the posterior lamellae of the upper and lower lids in the same way.

3. Close the incision in two layers (Fig. 18.51).

Complications
The canthus can drift medially again over several months. Resuture to the periosteal flap usually corrects this. Granuloma may form within the wound. Excise it and resuture the wound, taking care to cover the periosteal flap and sutures with orbicularis muscle during closure.

Levator muscle and aponeurosis

Laceration of the levator apparatus presents with ptosis. However, severe bruising and local swelling or surgical emphysema may also present with poor levator function and ptosis (see Figs 18.17, 18.18). Wounds in the upper lid must be explored to their depths and any damage to the levator identified. Fat visible within the wound in the upper lid is usually preaponeurotic fat and indicates that the septum has been cut. Brow fat that extends down from the brow on the anterior surface of the septum may also be visible. Preaponeurotic fat is lighter and more mobile than brow fat.

If a tear in the levator aponeurosis or muscle is found it should be repaired with 6/0 absorbable sutures. The septum should not be repaired. The levator can be repaired through the main wound in the upper lid if it is large. If it is not or if there is doubt about the adequacy of exposure, it is preferable to close the primary wound and make a second, formal incision within the upper lid skin crease to expose the levator and aponeurosis and repair it formally (Fig. 18.52).

If no damage to the levator is identified, the cause of the ptosis may be local bruising. The levator function and ptosis will then improve as the bruising subsides.

Penetrating eyelid and periocular trauma without tissue loss

Early repair of skin and orbicularis wounds within the first 8 hours is preferable. The repair may be delayed for 24–48 hours if circumstances demand although it becomes progressively more difficult due to edema. It may also be

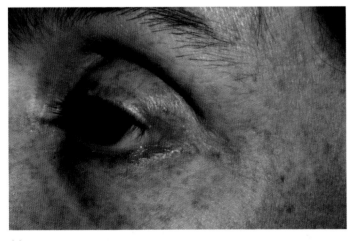

(a)

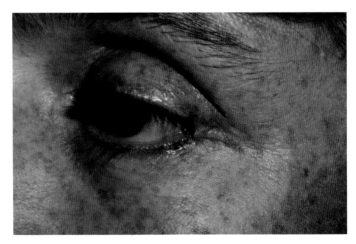

(b)

Fig. 18.51: (a) Rounded canthus due to detachment of the lateral canthal tendon. **(b)** Repaired with a periosteal flap.

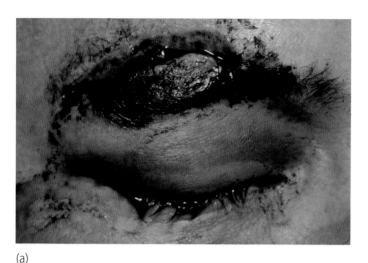

(a)

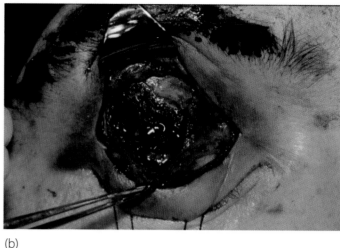

(b)

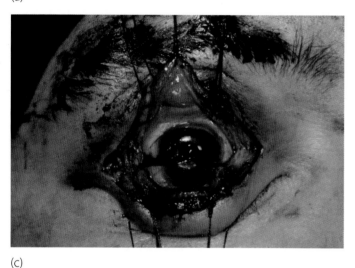

(c)

Fig. 18.52: (a–c) Oblique laceration above the brow, transecting the levator aponeurosis (exposed through a second incision at the upper lid skin crease) and penetrating the cornea.

more difficult to decontaminate the wounds adequately. The wound must be cleaned and irrigated and all visible foreign bodies removed. The skin must be cleaned meticulously of all embedded foreign material, with firm scrubbing with a brush if necessary to avoid tattooing (Figs 18.53, 18.54). Obviously dead tissue is excised but removal of tissue should be kept to a minimum.

The wounds should be explored carefully to determine the depth and nature of any damage. As mentioned above, fat visible within a wound may indicate laceration of the septum. This does not present a problem. The fat should be simply pushed back into position and the septum left open.

Close the wounds with absorbable sutures to the orbicularis muscle and 6/0 monofilament sutures to the skin. Closure of lid margin lacerations is described above.

Penetrating eyelid and periocular trauma with tissue loss

Check whether tissue loss has occurred. Distortion of the tissues due to edema or hemorrhage may give the impression of actual loss of tissue. This, however, is often not confirmed (Fig. 18.55).

The principles of reconstruction of defects in the lids and periocular tissues are the same as for reconstruction after tumor removal. A reconstructed eyelid must have an anterior covering layer (skin) and a posterior lining layer (mucosa). One of these layers must have a blood supply. There must also be adequate support for the lids medially and laterally. In planning the method of reconstruction, avoid excess tension or distortion. Try to match a skin graft color accurately with careful choice of donor site. A definitive repair in the hours following an injury should be considered only if adequate cleansing of the wounds has been possible and the viability of the tissues is certain.

Reconstruction of partial-thickness eyelid and periocular defects

Partial-thickness defects of the lids or periocular region may be closed directly or require reconstruction of the anterior covering layer with a skin graft or a skin flap.

Direct closure of wounds must be performed in a direction that does not cause distortion of the lid margin, e.g. ectropion or local retraction. In the lower lid this usually means a closure wound placed at right angles to the lid margin (Fig. 18.56).

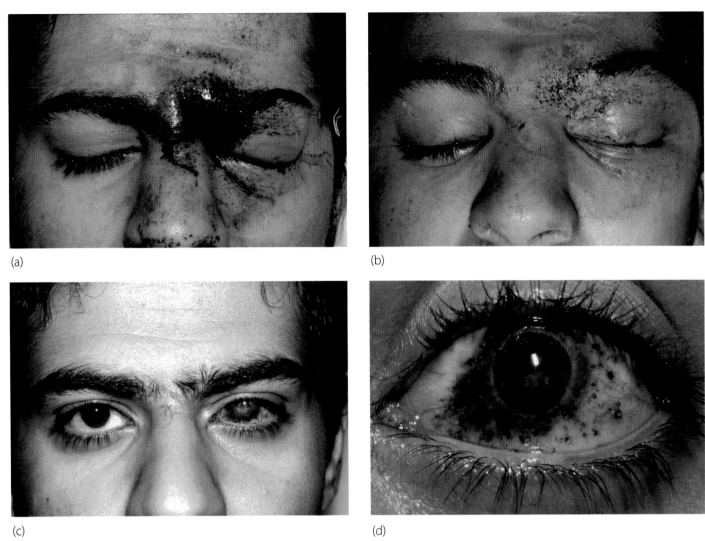

(a)

(b)

(c)

(d)

Fig. 18.53: **(a)** Embedded debris following a close-range shot with a blank. **(b)** Careful scrubbing removed as much foreign material as possible. **(c)** The appearance 1 year later. Tattooing of the cornea and conjunctiva cannot be avoided. **(d)** Note the corneal graft to restore clarity to the central cornea.

Closure with a skin flap or graft is indicated if the defect is too large for direct closure. Many different configurations of skin flap may be used in the periocular region. Local sliding or transposed flaps are common (Fig. 18.57).

Skin grafts may be partial or full thickness. Partial (split)-thickness grafts are usually reserved for large defects or those in the upper lid above the skin crease when skin from the opposite upper lid is not available. Full-thickness grafts are best taken from the upper eyelid – these give an excellent color match and good mobility. The graft is taken from the skin superior to the skin crease (Fig. 18.58). Alternative donor sites include the postauricular region and the supra-clavicular fossa.

Reconstruction of full-thickness eyelid defects

Full-thickness defects of up to a quarter of the lid length may be closed directly as described above. Defects up to about one-third of the lid require release of the upper or lower limb of the lateral canthal tendon – a lateral cantholysis – before they can be closed directly.

Full-thickness eyelid defects larger than about a third of the lid length (or up to a half in the elderly) require the reconstruction of the posterior lining layer as well as the anterior covering layer. When both of these layers have to be reconstructed at least one of them must have a blood supply. This means combining an anterior (skin) flap with a posterior graft or an anterior (skin) graft with a posterior flap. Alternatively, both may be flaps.

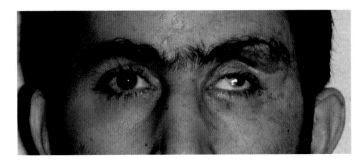

Fig. 18.54: Marked tattooing due to failure to remove debris at the original operation.

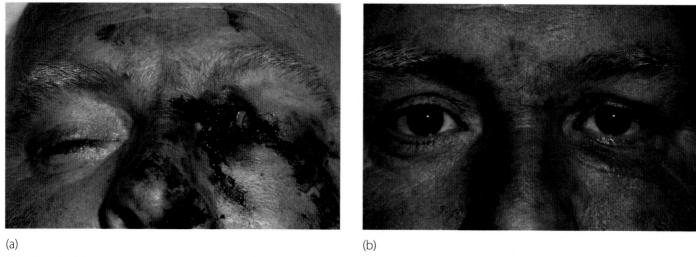

(a)   (b)

Fig. 18.55: (a) Apparent loss of tissue, not confirmed at operation. **(b)** The final result following a simple repair with careful attention to the restoration of anatomy.

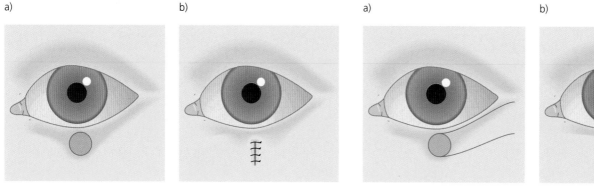

a)   b)   a)   b)

Fig. 18.56: (a,b) Direction of closure of small lower lid wounds to avoid vertical traction.

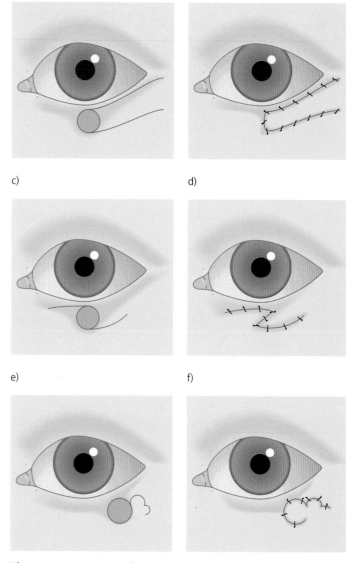

c)   d)

e)   f)

Fig. 18.57: Principle of **(a,b)** sliding, **(c,d)** O-Z and **(e,f)** bilobed flaps for reconstruction of lower lid defects.

Lateral cantholysis

This technique is used almost exclusively in the lower lid. In the upper lid, great care is needed when releasing the septum to avoid damage to the lacrimal gland. Up to one-third of the lid length can be reconstructed with the extra tissue made available by a cantholysis.

Technique (Fig. 18.59)

1. Make a horizontal cut from the lateral canthus to the orbital rim. Take care not to cut obliquely downwards or upwards through either limb of the lateral canthal tendon (Fig. 18.60).
2. Pull the lid medially to put the lateral canthal tendon on stretch. It can now be felt as a tight band just posterior to the orbicularis muscle, between the muscle and the conjunctiva. Expose this limb of the tendon by spreading scissors either side of it (Fig. 18.61).
3. Cut this limb of the tendon laterally (Fig. 18.62).
4. Close the lid defect in the usual way. Close the lateral wound in layers with 6/0 sutures (Fig. 18.63).

If the defect cannot be closed without undue tension, the orbital septum between the lateral tarsal fragment and the inferior orbital rim must be cut to allow the lateral tissues to

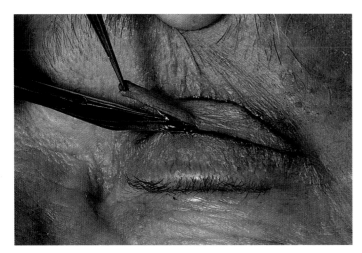

Fig. 18.58: Taking a full-thickness skin graft from the upper lid.

a)   b)

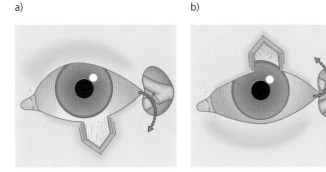

Fig. 18.59: **(a,b)** Principle of lateral cantholysis.

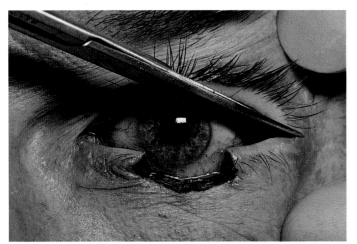

Fig. 18.60: Horizontal cut at the lateral canthus.

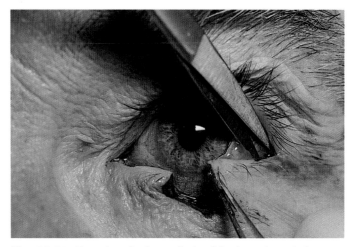

Fig. 18.61: Exposing the lower limb of the lateral canthal tendon. Note the traction on the lid to put the tendon on stretch.

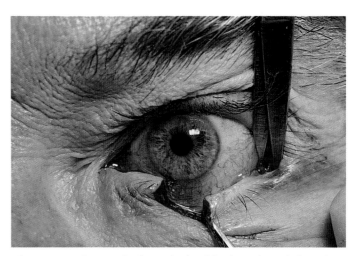

Fig. 18.62: Cutting the lower limb of the lateral canthal tendon.

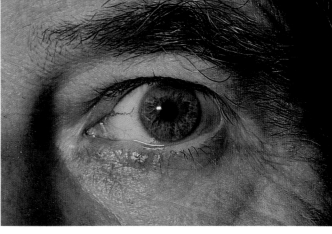

Fig. 18.63: The result 2 months after routine closure of the central defect with a cantholysis.

move further medially. To do this, grasp the medial cut end of the tendon and pull it laterally and slightly upwards to put the septum on stretch. Gently introduce scissors between the orbicularis muscle and the conjunctiva along the superior or inferior orbital rim and cut the septum as far medially as necessary to allow closure of the lid. With each cut into the septum, the lid will be felt to 'give' and become more mobile.

Complications
Slight notching of the lid margin at the outer canthus may occur if there has been excessive dissection to expose the

lateral canthal tendon. It is best left alone but, if marked, local resuturing will improve the profile of the lid margin.

Posterior graft + anterior flap

If the posterior layer is reconstructed with a graft the anterior layer must be reconstructed with a skin flap.

Grafts for the posterior (lining) layer include oral mucosa, tarsal plate or hard palate. Tarsal plate grafts are usually taken from the upper lid. Other grafts, e.g. donor sclera or ear cartilage, are less satisfactory because they do not have a mucosal lining so their use is generally restricted to the lower lid.

Taking tarsal plate grafts – technique

Full-thickness tarsal plate from the upper lid is an excellent posterior lamellar graft with a mucosal lining, when only a small area is required. It may be taken from the ipsilateral or the contralateral side.

1. Evert the upper lid over a Desmarres retractor and insert a stay suture close to the lid margin. Measure on the tarsal plate 4 mm from the lid margin at several points and mark off along this line the length of graft required (Fig. 18.64).
2. Incise the full thickness of the tarsal plate along the mark. Make vertical cuts from each end of the first incision to the superior border of the tarsal plate and extend them superiorly for 2 mm into the conjunctiva. Undermine and excise the graft with about 2 mm of conjunctiva attached (Fig. 18.65). Leave the donor site to granulate.

Complications

If the incision in the tarsal plate was made less than 4 mm from the lid margin, buckling of the lid may occur during healing. Once healed, the distorted area should be excised and resutured. Occasionally, lid retraction occurs with healing. Release of the upper lid retractors is necessary to correct this.

Many different flaps are used for the anterior (covering) layer. The small Tenzel flap and the larger McGregor flap are useful for defects up to about half the lid. A nasojugal flap medially or a transposed cheek flap laterally are commonly used for larger defects. These flaps are best for defects that

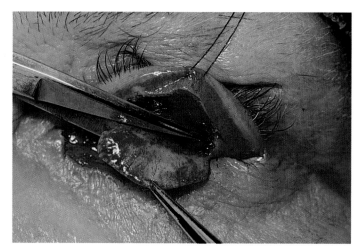

Fig. 18.65: Tarsal plate graft excised with 2 mm of conjunctiva superiorly.

do not extend far inferiorly into the cheek. Larger defects involving cheek skin often require a larger flap such as the Mustarde cheek rotation flap.

Tenzel flap – technique (Fig. 18.66)

This technique allows direct closure of upper or lower lid defects up to about one-half of the lid length.

1. Mark the semicircular flap approximately 22 mm in the vertical and 18 mm in the horizontal direction. Begin the mark as a lateral continuation of the line of the lid to be reconstructed. Continue more steeply upwards (for reconstruction of the lower lid) or downwards (for reconstruction of the upper lid), curving the line to achieve the correct dimensions. Finish level with the canthus and no further lateral than the end of the eyebrow (Fig. 18.67).

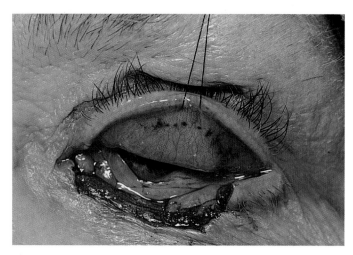

Fig. 18.64: Incision in tarsal plate marked 4 mm from the lid margin.

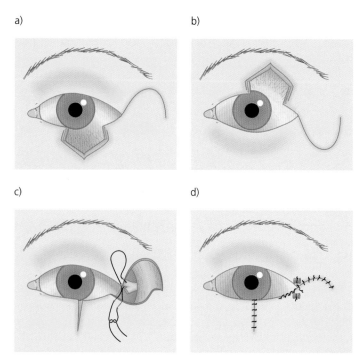

Fig. 18.66: (a–d) Principle of Tenzel semicircular flap.

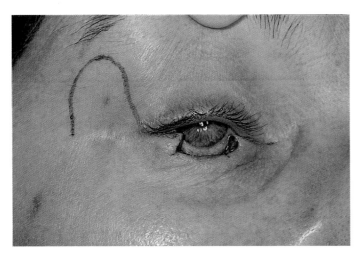

Fig. 18.67: Incision for Tenzel flap marked.

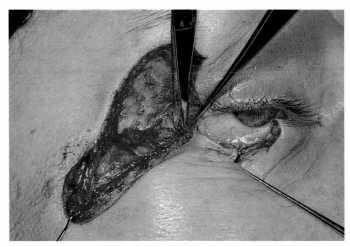

Fig. 18.68: Flap reflected; lower limb of the lateral canthal tendon being cut.

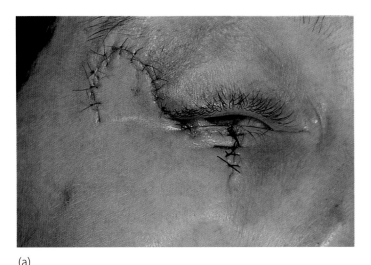

(a)

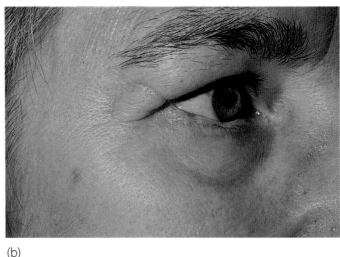

(b)

Fig. 18.69: (a) End of the operation and **(b)** 6 months later.

2. Make an incision along the mark and undermine the flap in the plane just deep to orbicularis muscle. Reflect the flap to expose the lateral canthus. Cut the appropriate limb of the lateral canthal tendon (Fig. 18.68).
3. For closure of a lower lid defect, free the septum. Close the eyelid defect in the usual way. Pull the lid gently laterally to remove any horizontal lid laxity. Support the flap with a 4/0 non-absorbable suture to the deep tissues. Where the flap edge crosses the lateral canthus, fix it to the opposite limb of the lateral canthal tendon with a 4/0 long-acting absorbable suture to create a new canthus.
4. Close the edge of the flap in two layers with 6/0 catgut and a 6/0 non-absorbable suture to the skin. Remove the surface sutures at 5 days (Fig. 18.69).

Complications
Shallow notching of the lid margin at the outer canthus may occur. If marked, resuture the affected lid to correct the notch.

McGregor flap – technique
This flap utilizes a Z-plasty which helps to avoid a dog-ear in the superior edge of the wound and partly hides the scar by breaking the line.

1. Mark an incision from the lateral canthus towards the ear with a gentle curve convex upward (for the lower lid) or downward (for the upper lid). Mark a Z with the stem along the main incision, placing the more lateral limb of the Z on the same side of the main incision as the lid to be reconstructed (Fig. 18.70).
2. Reflect the flaps, keeping deep to the orbicularis muscle while medial to the orbital rim but superficial to orbicularis, within the subcutaneous fat, lateral to the orbital rim. Undermine beyond the flaps. Cut the appropriate limb of the lateral canthal tendon and mobilize the lateral part of the lid.
3. Close the defect in the lid. Transpose the flaps in the usual way and close the skin (Figs 18.71, 18.72).

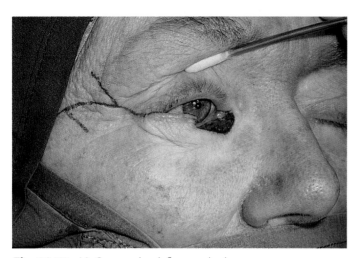

Fig. 18.70: McGregor cheek flap marked.

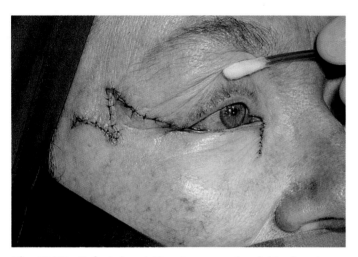

Fig. 18.71: Defect closed. Flaps transposed and skin closed.

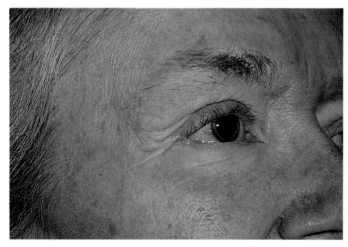

Fig. 18.72: Four months after McGregor cheek flap.

Complications

Shallow notching of the lid margin at the outer canthus may occur. If marked, resuture the affected lid to correct the notch.

Nasojugal flap – technique (Fig. 18.73)

This flap is used for medial lower lid defects.

1. Reconstruct the posterior lamella with a suitable graft. The flap should be almost vertical in the nasojugal area with its base just inferior to the medial canthus. Care is needed in the design of the flap to ensure that it is long enough to fill the defect (Fig. 18.74).
2. Raise the flap, staying superficial to the facial muscles, within the fat layer.
3. Close the cheek wound first. Transpose the flap into the defect and trim it to fit. Close the skin with interrupted 6/0 sutures (Fig. 18.75).
4. Close the lid margin with a continuous 6/0 suture which unites the skin and the mucosa of the posterior lamellar reconstruction.

Complications

Nasojugal skin is thicker than eyelid skin and the reconstruction may be rather bulky. Later debulking is possible if nec-

a)

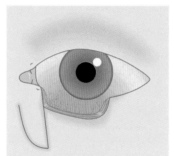

b)

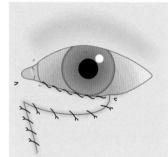

Fig. 18.73: **(a,b)** Principle of nasojugal flap.

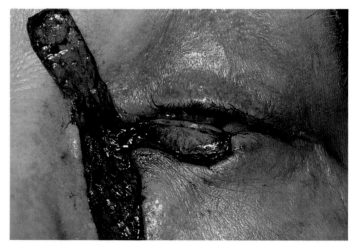

Fig. 18.74: Nasojugal flap. Posterior lamella reconstructed with a tarsal plate graft.

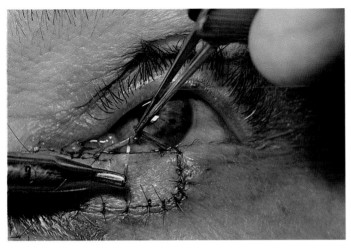

Fig. 18.75: Nasojugal flap – end of operation.

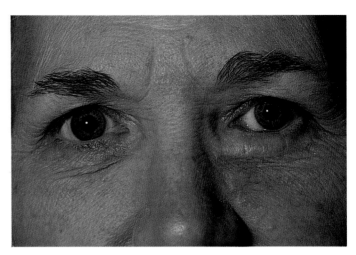

Fig. 18.76: Nasojugal flap after 6 months.

a)

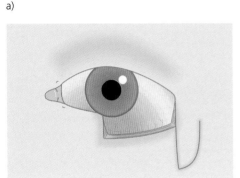

b)

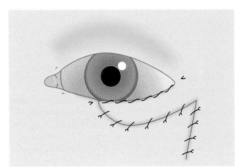

Fig. 18.77: (a,b) Principle of transposed cheek flap.

a)

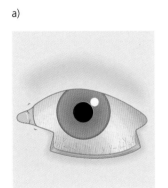

b)

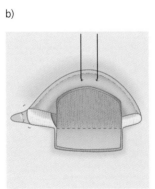

c)

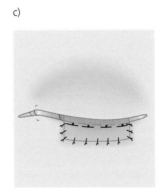

Fig. 18.78: (a) Principle of Hughes reconstruction of central lower lid defect. **(b)** Posterior lamella reconstructed with a flap of tarso-conjunctiva from the upper lid. **(c)** Anterior lamella reconstructed with a full-thickness skin graft.

essary (Fig. 18.76). Necrosis of the tip of the flap is unusual. If it occurs, wait to see how much of the flap survives then reconstruct the defect that remains if necessary.

Transposed cheek flap – technique (Fig. 18.77)
Large lower lid defects which extend to the lateral canthus can be reconstructed with a transposed flap based near the outer canthus, extending down into the cheek. Take care to design the flap with sufficient length and width to fill the defect. It must be lined, usually with oral mucosa. To close the secondary defect, undermine the edges of the wound.

Complications
Cheek skin is thicker than eyelid skin and the reconstruction may be rather bulky. Later debulking is possible if necessary. Necrosis of the tip of the flap is unusual. If it occurs, wait to see how much of the flap survives then reconstruct the defect that remains if necessary.

Posterior flap + anterior graft
If the posterior layer is reconstructed with a flap of tarsus and conjunctiva with its blood supply intact (Hughes procedure), a skin graft is usually used to fill the anterior defect although a flap may be used.

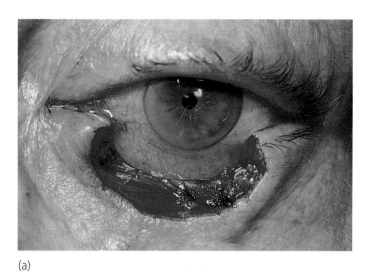

(a)

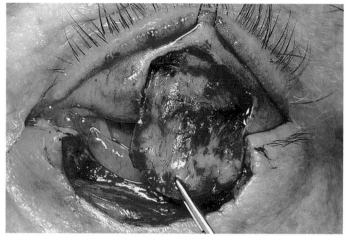

(b)

Fig. 18.79: (a) Large lower lid defect. **(b)** Tarso-conjunctival flap cut for reconstruction of the posterior lamella.

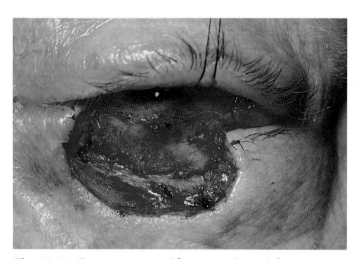

Fig. 18.80: Tarso-conjunctival flap sutured into defect.

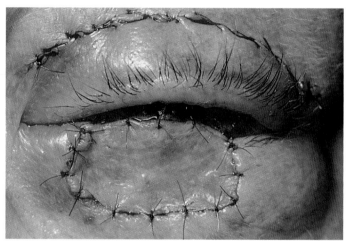

Fig. 18.81: Skin graft from upper lid.

Hughes procedure – technique (Fig. 18.78)
This is a two-stage technique to reconstruct full-thickness defects in the lower eyelid. A broad strip of upper tarsal plate on a pedicle of conjunctiva is used to reconstruct the posterior lamella of the lid. It may be covered with a skin graft or flap. The pedicle is divided after a few weeks. The use of the Hughes flap is restricted to relatively shallow lower lid defects which do not extend much beyond the inferior border of the tarsal plate.

1. Insert a stay suture of 4/0 silk through the tarsal plate close to the lid margin and evert the lid over a Desmarres retractor. Mark a line 4 mm from and parallel to the lid margin. Mark on this line the horizontal length of tarsal plate required. From these marks draw vertical lines to the superior tarsal border to delineate the flap. Incise the tarsal plate through its full thickness along the marks. Raise the flap of tarsus by dissection in the pretarsal space as far as the superior border of the tarsal plate (Fig. 18.79).

2. Suture the flap into the defect with 6/0 catgut sutures. Begin by suturing the ends of the superior border of the upper tarsal plate to the lower lid margins at the edges of the defect. Suture the remaining edges of the tarsus to the conjunctiva (Fig. 18.80).

3. Reconstruct the anterior lamella with a full-thickness skin graft or a local flap of skin and muscle (Fig. 18.81).

4. After about 3 weeks divide the pedicle 2–3 mm superior to the tarsal plate and the skin graft (Fig. 18.82). Suture the free edge of the conjunctiva to the skin with a continuous 6/0 monofilament suture. Remove this suture at 5 days. The upper lid retractors will have been advanced by the procedure and must be recessed to prevent upper lid retraction. To do this, dissect between the conjunctiva and the retractors until the lid is at a satisfactory level. Allow the proximal conjunctiva to retract. A downward traction suture on the upper lid for 24 hours may be needed.

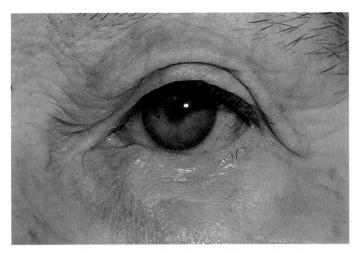

Fig. 18.82: Three months after division of the bridge of conjunctiva.

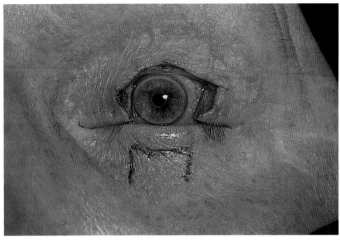

Fig. 18.84: Defect in the upper lid. Cutler–Beard bridge flap marked.

Complications

Retraction of the upper lid may follow the second stage if the upper lid tissues have not been freed sufficiently. Dissect further between the conjunctiva and the upper lid retractors until the lid is at the correct level.

Closure with flaps for both lamellae

Both anterior and posterior lamellae may be reconstructed with flaps, i.e. a tarso-conjunctival flap posteriorly and a local skin flap anteriorly.

Composite flaps (e.g. Cutler–Beard bridge flap), which include all layers of the lower lid inferior to the tarsal plate, are useful for larger central upper lid defects.

Cutler–Beard bridge flap – technique (Fig. 18.83)
This is a two-stage technique for reconstruction of large full-thickness defects in the upper lid.

1. Draw a horizontal line 5 mm inferior and parallel to the lash line of the lower lid. On this line mark the width of flap required to fill the defect in the upper lid and draw two vertical lines as far as the inferior orbital rim (Fig. 18.84).
2. Incise along the lines. Perforate the full thickness of the lid at the corners of the flap and with a pair of scissors inserted between the stab incisions, complete the horizontal full-thickness incision. Extend this inferiorly along

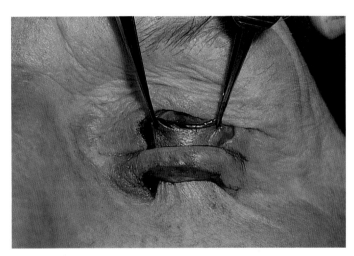

Fig. 18.85: Flap cut and placed into the defect.

the vertical lines to the inferior conjunctival fornix to create an inverted U-shaped flap. Pull the flap up posterior to the lower lid margin (Fig. 18.85).

3. Suture it into the upper lid defect in three layers: conjunctiva to conjunctiva, and orbicularis muscle of the lower lid to the levator aponeurosis and orbicularis muscle of the upper lid, with interrupted 6/0 absorbable sutures. Finally, skin to skin with 6/0 interrupted

a)

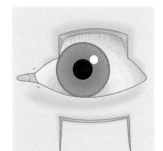

b)

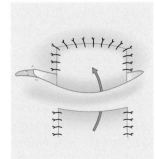

c)

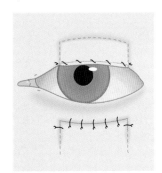

Fig. 18.83: (a) Principle of Cutler–Beard reconstruction of an upper lid defect. **(b)** A full-thickness flap from the lower lid is sutured into the defect and **(c)** the bridge is divided after 6 weeks.

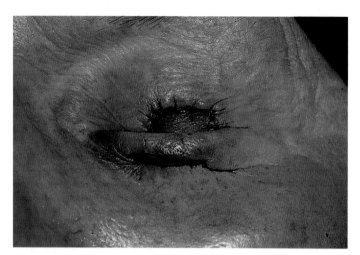

Fig. 18.86: Flap sutured into the defect in layers.

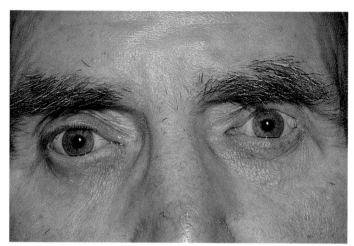

Fig. 18.88: Six months after left upper lid reconstruction with a Cutler–Beard flap.

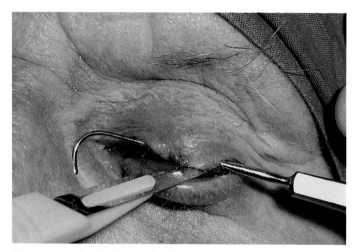

Fig. 18.87: Bridge being divided at 6 weeks.

non-absorbable sutures. Remove the sutures at 5 days (Fig. 18.86).

4. After 6 weeks estimate whether the flap has stretched enough to reduce the tension. If it is still tight leave it another 3 weeks. If it has stretched and feels less tight divide the bridge to restore the upper lid margin. To do this pass a squint hook posterior to the flap and carefully incise the layers of the flap, making the initial incision convex downwards to allow for retraction. Leave an excess of conjunctiva (Fig. 18.87).

5. Suture the conjunctiva to skin, over the new lid margin, with a 6/0 continuous monofilament suture. Remove this at 5 days. Replace the pedicle of the bridge into the lower lid defect and repair it in layers to avoid a fistula through the lid (Fig. 18.88).

Complications

The reconstructed upper lid margin is relatively unstable and may develop entropion. If this occurs a graft of donor sclera or ear cartilage may need to be inserted between the lamellae of the reconstructed lid. The margin may be irregular at the edges of the bridge flap. Allow the lid to heal and excise

the notches if necessary. Skin hairs may cause irritation and they can be treated with cryotherapy.

Reconstruction of full-thickness periocular defects

Small defects can be closed directly or with small local skin flaps. It is important to avoid vertical tension in the upper or lower lids. It is better to allow a scar to cross the relaxed skin tension lines rather than close with vertical tension. Larger defects require a local flap or skin graft.

Medial canthus

A medial canthal defect that cannot easily be closed directly is usually reconstructed with a skin flap, e.g. a glabellar flap, if it is mainly above the medial canthal tendon, especially if it is relatively deep, or a skin graft below the medial canthal tendon. A deep defect below the canthal tendon may also be closed with a local flap. Vertical tension spanning the tissues above and below the canthus and within 8 mm medial to the canthus will have a tendency to form a web. It is preferable to use a small skin graft.

In reconstruction of the medial canthus it is important to perform any lacrimal drainage system repair first, then reconstruct the medial canthal tendon and finally the overlying soft tissue defect.

Glabellar flap – technique (Fig. 18.89)

A full-thickness skin graft may be used for superficial defects at the inner canthus. If the defect is deep, a glabellar flap is preferred. It does not require a posterior lamellar reconstruction. An inverted V is created in the glabellar region and converted to a Y to allow the flap to be transferred to the inner canthus. If the defect is small the flap is used as a sliding flap, the excess being trimmed off. If the defect is large the flap may be used as a transposed flap with little trimming necessary. If the defect extends into the upper or lower eyelid supplementary procedures may be needed to reconstruct the residual lid defect.

a)

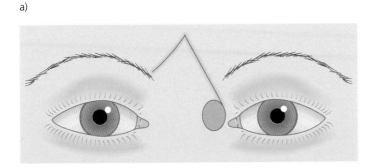

b)

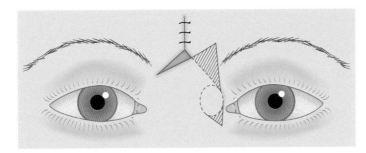

c)

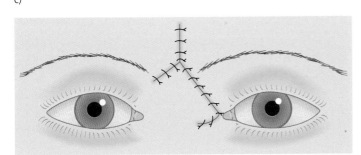

Fig. 18.89: (a–c) Principle of glabellar flap. A V-shaped flap in the glabella is converted to a Y to allow the flap to slide into a medial canthal defect.

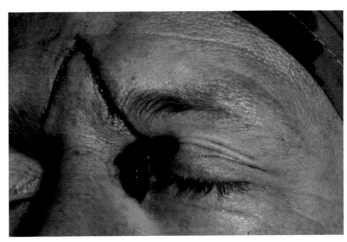

Fig. 18.90: Glabellar flap marked.

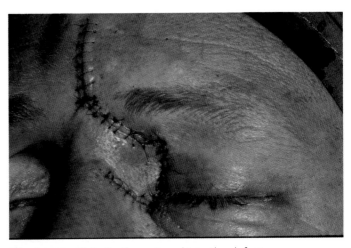

Fig. 18.91: Glabellar flap sutured into the defect.

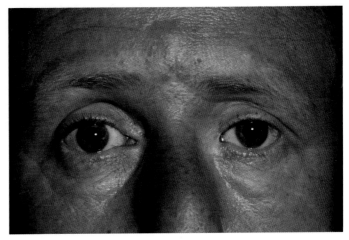

Fig. 18.92: One year after repair of a large medial canthal defect with a glabellar flap.

1. Mark an inverted V, centered in the midline of the forehead. One limb of the V is drawn to the lateral border of the canthal defect, the other is drawn to the medial end of the opposite brow (Fig. 18.90). Undermine the flap, dissecting in the layer of subcutaneous fat. Extend the dissection beyond the boundaries of the flap to allow it to be placed without tension into the canthal defect.
2. Once the position is satisfactory insert one or two 4/0 non-absorbable sutures between the deep surface of the flap and the tissues of the canthus to anchor the flap. Undermine either side of the forehead defect to allow closure with minimal tension. Close the forehead in two layers to just above the brows.
3. Trim the excess tissue from the glabellar flap. Suture the flap into the canthal defect with 6/0 absorbable sutures to the subcutaneous tissues and 6/0 non-absorbable sutures to the skin. Complete the closure of the forehead (Fig. 18.91). Remove all skin sutures at 1 week (Fig. 18.92).

Complications
A fold or dog-ear commonly occurs on the bridge of the nose, especially if the defect is large. Leave it for 6 weeks then trim it if necessary. Poor application of the flap to the hollow

at the inner canthus, and the appearance of telecanthus, can be avoided by careful placement and suturing of the flap at operation.

Larger upper or lower lid defects extending into the medial canthus

Occasionally, an upper or lower lid defect extends into the inner canthal area and a more complex combination of reconstructive techniques is needed. In the canthus a glabellar flap is usually a good choice for deeper defects that are mainly superior to the medial canthal tendon; other local flaps are used for deep defects below the medial canthal tendon. Skin grafts are appropriate for shallow defects. The residual defect in the lid is closed with one of the techniques described above in Reconstruction of full-thickness defects of the eyelids (Figs 18.93, 18.94).

Medial and lateral support

A reconstructed lid must have adequate medial and lateral support to prevent the lid drooping. This is especially important in the lower lid. A defect that includes the medial or lateral canthal tendon must be reconstructed in such a way that the support is restored. Medially the tissues of the reconstructed lid should be attached to the posterior lacrimal crest; this will ensure that the lid is pulled posteriorly as well as medially and is well applied to the globe.

Laterally there should be an attachment in the region of Whitnall's tubercle, either directly to the periosteum or with a periosteal flap or with a wire. If the lid droops despite all attempts to support it, a sling of autogenous fascia lata may be needed. This is attached to the medial canthal tendon and, having traversed the lid close to the lid margin, it is passed through holes in the lateral orbital rim (Fig. 18.95).

Lateral canthus

Having corrected any disruption of the lateral canthal tendon, defects at the lateral canthus are closed either directly, if small, or with a local flap.

Cheek or temple

Assess facial nerve function. Close small defects directly, avoiding vertical tension, especially in the lower lid. Local flaps are used to close larger defects. The O-Z plasty is particularly useful in these areas. Alternatively a full-thickness skin graft may be needed.

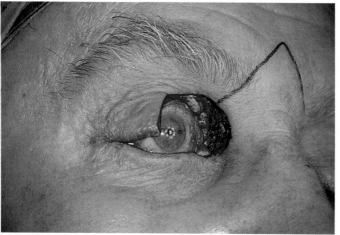

(a)

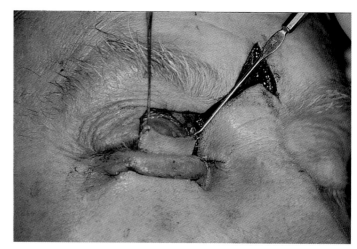

(b)

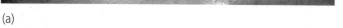

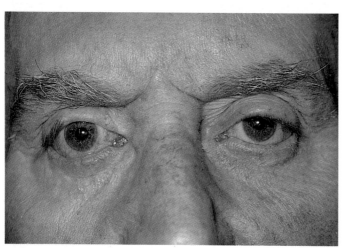

(c)

Fig. 18.93: (a) Large upper lid and medial canthal defect reconstructed with **(b)** a combined glabellar flap and Cutler–Beard flap. **(c)** One year postoperative.

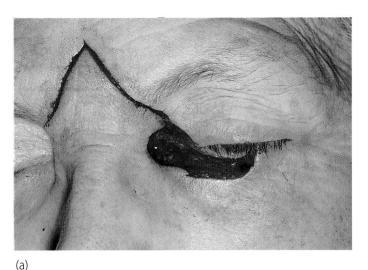

(a)

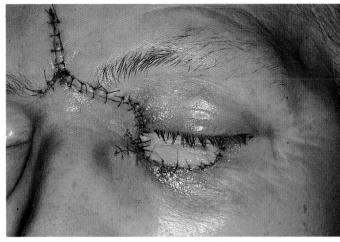

(b)

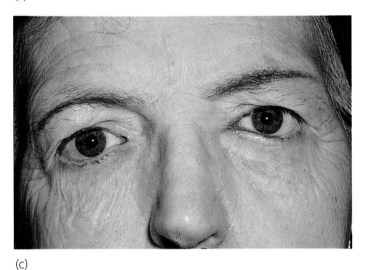

(c)

Fig. 18.94: **(a)** Large lower lid and medial canthal defect reconstructed with **(b)** a glabellar flap and a Hughes flap. **(c)** Three months postoperative.

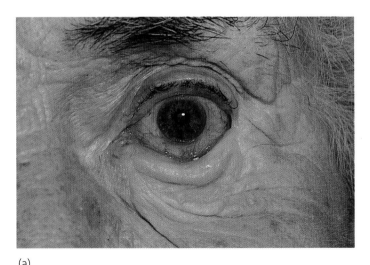

(a)

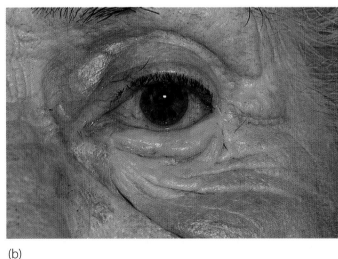

(b)

Fig. 18.95: **(a)** A lax lower lid after multiple reconstructions. **(b)** Supported with a sling of autogenous fascia lata.

Late Repair of Eyelid and Lacrimal Trauma

If the initial repair of an eyelid injury is unsatisfactory but the eye is adequately protected, revision can be deferred for 6 months to allow the scars to mature. In planning any revision ophthalmic plastic surgeons would normally collaborate with maxillofacial colleagues in case any revision of the fractures is required at the same time. It is easier to make appropriate adjustments if the initial repair is anatomically correct. If it is not, the tissues should be dissected to reconstruct the injury and display the anatomy. The lid is then reconstructed and the appropriate adjustment made.

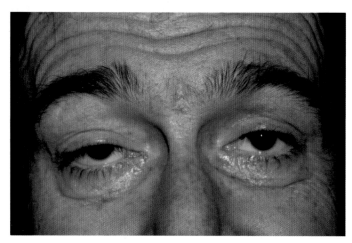

Fig. 18.96: Bilateral ptosis with poor levator function after severe head injury.

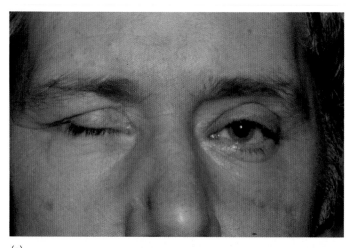

(a)

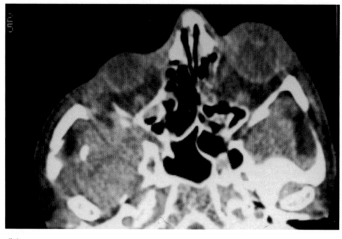

(b)

Fig. 18.97: (a,b) Severe injury to the right orbit with complex ptosis.

Lids

Common late deformities of the lids include cicatricial ectropion or entropion, lid retraction, distortion or notching of the lid margins and ptosis.

Cicatricial ectropion is due to a shortage of skin in the lower lid. If this is caused by a contracted linear scar, it is corrected with a Z-plasty. If there is a more diffuse shortage of scarred skin, a full-thickness skin graft is used.

Cicatricial entropion is due to shortening of the posterior lining lamella of the lid. Choice of the appropriate operation for the degree of scarring is important and the surgery can be difficult. In the lower lid it is corrected either by fracturing the tarsal plate and inserting everting sutures or by inserting a graft of oral mucosa to release the contraction. In the upper lid several different operations are used depending on the degree of scarring and amount of associated upper lid retraction. The principle is that the anterior lamella of the lid is moved up in relation to the posterior lamella, everting the lid margin. In more severe scarring it may be necessary to divide the tarsal plate to evert the scarred lid margin.

Retraction of the upper or lower lid is usually due to shortening of the upper or lower lid retractors, possibly combined with scarring in the anterior or posterior lamellae. The retracted lid is explored and the retractors released. The surgery can be difficult. If it is necessary to release the anterior or posterior lamella at the same time in order to achieve a satisfactory lid position the defect is reconstructed as outlined above for cicatricial ectropion and entropion.

Notching and distortion of the lid margin are usually due to inaccurate initial closure (see Fig. 18.47). It is usually easiest to excise the initial repair scar and close the lid margin accurately.

Ptosis may be due to trauma to the levator apparatus or adhesion within the lid between the upper lid retractors and adjacent structures, e.g. the orbital rim periosteum. Brain injury can result in bilateral ptosis with reduced levator function (Fig. 18.96). Ptosis is assessed as described above by measuring the degree of ptosis (margin reflex distance), the function in the levator muscle and the adequacy of the eye movements.

The surgery can be complex and the anatomy difficult in severe lid injuries (Fig. 18.97) The upper lid is explored through a skin crease incision and the anatomy displayed. Adhesions are divided. The preaponeurotic fat can conveniently be used to provide a barrier to prevent readhesion of the tissues. If the levator function is good the levator aponeurosis is shortened and advanced to the tarsal plate to correct the ptosis (Fig. 18.98). If the levator function is poor, despite the division of any adhesions, it may be necessary to consider a brow suspension procedure. Particular care is needed to avoid corneal exposure postoperatively.

Medial canthus

Persistent telecanthus requires reattachment of the medial canthal tendon to the posterior lacrimal crest or adjustment to a unilateral or transnasal wire if it was inserted at the original surgery. Any webbing of the skin at the medial canthus should be corrected with a Z-plasty or possibly a skin graft

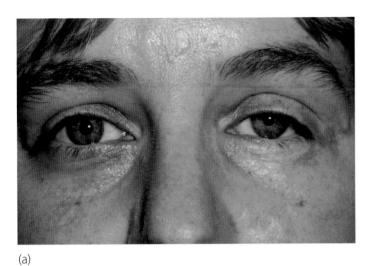

(a)

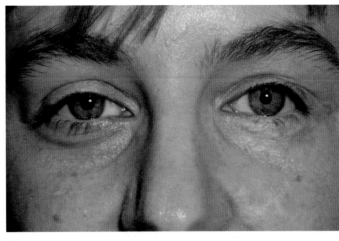

(b)

Fig. 18.98: **(a)** 'Simple' traumatic ptosis with moderate levator function **(b)** corrected with a skin approach levator resection.

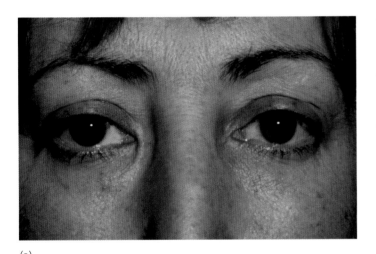

(a)

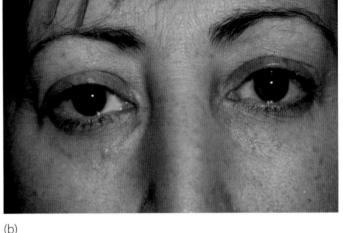

(b)

Fig. 18.99: **(a,b)** Web at inner canthus corrected with a Z-plasty.

(Fig. 18.99). If the canthus has been displaced vertically a Z-plasty may be required to correct the position (Fig. 18.100). Care should be taken to preserve the lacrimal drainage apparatus if it is patent and functioning. It is better to leave the medial canthus with slight distortion rather than risk damage to the lacrimal apparatus.

Lateral canthus

Displacement with rounding of the canthus requires re-establishment of the attachment to the region of Whitnall's tubercle with a periosteal flap or a wire. Displacement of the canthus in a vertical direction may require a Z-plasty to correct the position.

Lacrimal drainage system

Narrowing of the punctum can be improved with a 'one-snip' procedure that opens the vertical 2 mm of proximal canaliculus. Eversion of the punctum can be corrected with retropunctal cautery if slight or with the excision of a diamond of tarsoconjunctiva inferior to the punctum and closure with 7/0 absorbable sutures. More severe degrees of eversion may be associated with shortage of skin, with an ectropion, and will require a full-thickness skin graft.

Blockage in the canaliculi is difficult to treat. If a block is found in both canaliculi within 8 mm of the puncta it is not possible to reconstruct the connection with the lacrimal sac. A Lester Jones bypass tube is indicated if watering is significant.

Distal block in both canaliculi more than 8 mm from the puncta can be reconstructed by excision of the scarred canaliculi and anastomosis of the patent proximal canaliculi directly to the lacrimal sac. A DCR is normally also performed. This 'canaliculodacryocystorhinostomy' is not always functional even if the system is patent on syringing.

Scarring at the distal end of the common canaliculus at its entry into the lacrimal sac can be excised. A DCR is performed and silicone tubes are inserted for 3 months. If the lacrimal sac and adjacent tissues are disrupted it may not be possible to re-establish patent drainage. A Lester Jones bypass tube will then be required.

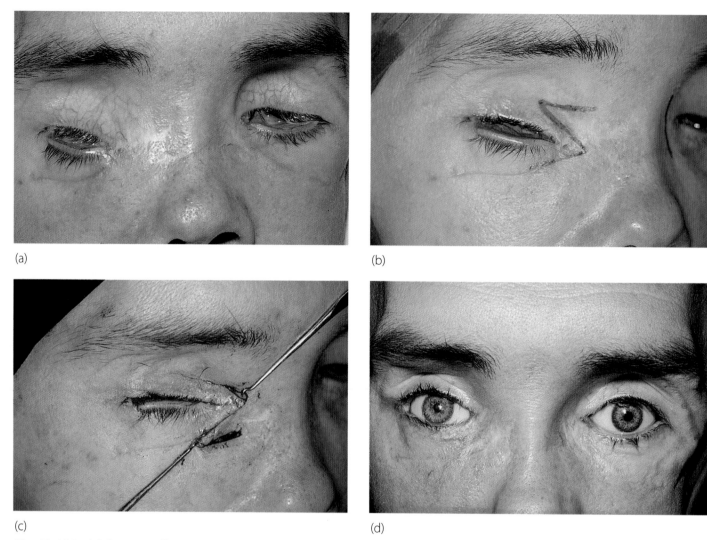

(a)

(b)

(c)

(d)

Fig. 18.100: (a) Severe midface trauma with loss of both eyes. **(b)** Z-plasty and **(c)** transnasal wire to correct the position of the medial canthi. **(d)** Result, with artificial eyes.

Further Reading

Bartley GB. Acquired lacrimal drainage obstruction: an etiologic classification system, case reports and review of the literature. Ophthalmic Plastic and Reconstructive Surgery 1992;8:237, and 1993;9:11

Beyer RW, Levine M. A method for repositioning or extraction of lacrimal system tubes. Ophthalmic Surgery 1986;17:496

Borges AF. Relaxed skin tension lines (RSTL) versus other skin lines. Plastic and Reconstructive 1984;73:144

Bosniak S. Principles and practice of ophthalmic plastic and reconstructive surgery (2 vols). Philadelphia; WB Saunders, 1996

Collin JRO. Immediate management of lid lacerations. Trans Ophthalmology Society of UK 1982;102:214

Collin JRO (ed). A manual of systematic eyelid surgery, 2nd edn. Edinburgh: Churchill Livingstone, 1989

Crawford JS. Intubation of obstruction in the lacrimal system. Canadian Journal of Ophthalmology 1977;12:289

Cutler NL, Beard C. A method for partial and total upper lid reconstruction. American Journal of Ophthalmology 1955;39:1

Guzek JP, Ching AS, Hoang TA, et al. Clinical and radiologic lacrimal testing in patients with epiphora. Ophthalmology 1997;104:1875

Harrington JN. Reconstruction of the medial canthus by spontaneous granulation (laissez faire): a review. Annals of Ophthalmology 1982;14:956

Harvey JT, Anderson RL. Transcanalicular removal of prolapsed Silastic tubing after nasolacrimal intubation. Journal of Ocular Therapy and Surgery 1982;2:294

Hawes MJ, Segrest DR. Effectiveness of bicanalicular silicone intubation in the repair of canalicular lacerations. Ophthalmic Plastic and Reconstructive Surgery 1985;1:185

Jones LT. An anatomical approach to problems of the eyelids and lacrimal apparatus. Archives of Ophthalmology 1961;66:111

Jones LT. The cure of epiphora due to canalicular disorders, trauma and surgical failures on the lacrimal passages. Trans American Academy of Ophthalmology and Otolaryngology 1962;66:506

Levine MR. Manual of oculoplastic surgery. Boston: Butterworth Heinemann, 1996

Linberg JV. Contemporary issues in ophthalmology, vol.5: lacrimal surgery. Edinburgh: Churchill Livingstone, 1988

Maurice DM. The dynamic drainage of tears. International Ophthalmology Clinics 1973;13:103

McGregor IA. Fundamental techniques of plastic surgery, 8th edn. Edinburgh: Churchill Livingstone, 1989

McNab AA. Manual of orbital and lacrimal surgery. Edinburgh: Churchill Livingstone, 1994

Moss ALH. Medial canthal tendon reconstruction. Journal of Maxillofacial Surgery 1984;12:131

Mustarde JC. Repair and reconstruction in the orbital region, 3rd edn. Edinburgh: Churchill Livingstone, 1991

Olver J. Colour atlas of lacrimal surgery. Oxford: Butterworth Heinemann, 2002

Patrinely JR, Anderson RL. A review of lacrimal drainage surgery. Ophthalmic Plastic and Reconstructive Surgery 1986;2:97

Rodriguez RL, Zide BM. Reconstruction of the medial canthus. Clinical Plastic Surgery 1988;15:255

Salasche SJ, Grabski WJ. Flaps for the central face. Edinburgh: Churchill Livingstone, 1990

Shore JW, Rubin PAD, Bilyk J. Repair of telecanthus by anterior fixation of cantilevered miniplates. Ophthalmology 1992;99:1133

Smit TJ, Mourits M. Monocanalicular lesions: to reconstruct or not. Ophthalmology 1999;106:1310

Spoor TC, Nesi FA. Management of ocular, orbital and adnexal trauma. New York: Raven Press, 1988

Stranc MF. The pattern of lacrimal injuries in nasoethmoid fractures. British Journal of Plastic Surgery 1970;23:339

Tenzel RR. Reconstruction of the central one half of an eyelid. Archives of Ophthalmology 1975;93:125

Tyers AG, Collin JRO. Colour atlas of ophthalmic plastic surgery; 2nd edn. Oxford: Butterworth Heinemann, 2001

Veirs ER. Malleable rods for the immediate repair of traumatically severed canaliculus. Trans American Academy of Ophthalmology and Otolaryngology 1962;66:262

Welham RAN. Immediate management of injuries of the lacrimal drainage apparatus. Trans Ophthalmology Society of UK 1982;102:216

Welham RAN, Henderson PH. Results of dacryocystorhinostomy: analysis of the causes of failure. Trans Ophthalmology Society of UK 1973;93:601

19 Primary Repair of Facial Soft Tissue Injuries

Barry L Eppley

Introduction

The complex and specialized anatomical regions of the face have significant influence on facial appearance and merit unique consideration. The requirement for many secondary soft tissue procedures, which can prove considerably more difficult, can be obviated by good primary surgery.[1] Special considerations are given to injuries of the scalp, forehead and brow, eyelid, nose, lips and ear as well as the important deeper structures of the facial nerve, lacrimal gland and the parotid duct.

It is important that the initial care is undertaken as has been mentioned in Chapter 6:

- primary ATLS care and evaluation of injuries
- control of hemorrhage
- early intervention for soft tissue injuries
- careful evaluation of damage to nerves, ducts and blood vessels
- careful evaluation of any ocular injuries
- identification of foreign bodies
- clinical and radiological examinations to exclude bone fractures.

The following text assumes that these principles have been adhered to.

Scalp and Forehead

The scalp, with its well-defined five layers, represents a single anatomical unit which, including the forehead, extends from the supraorbital margins anteriorly to the superior nuchal line posteriorly. The musculoaponeurotic galea not only provides a source of vascular perforators to the skin but its fibrous composition makes it a good anchor for deep sutures. The galea is readily mobilized, facilitating wound closure and the development of local flaps. The subgaleal fascia is the plane in which scalp avulsions almost exclusively occur (Fig. 19.1).

Scalp injuries, particularly avulsions, often bleed profusely and patients presenting in hemorrhagic shock require aggressive fluid resuscitation and blood replacement. Blood loss can be minimized with the application of pressure dressings and/or ligation of the galeal vessels and temporary suturing or stapling of the wounds. The vigorous blood supply of the scalp enhances the viability of tissue fragments that would not survive elsewhere. Near-complete avulsions of scalp segments may survive on small bridges of tissue or even as isolated islands. Only debridement of obvious devitalized tissue should be performed. Scalp tissue that appears to have only a very tenuous blood supply should be given the benefit of the doubt and retained, as the hair that it contains is a valuable resource. Subsequently any non-viable tissue can be readily removed and is not normally a source of infection. The robust blood supply serves as an adjunct in the

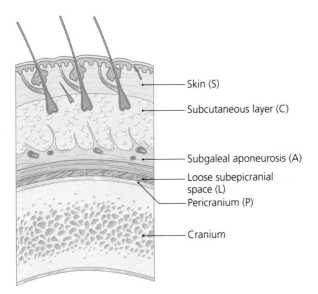

(a)

Skin (S)

Subcutaneous layer (C)

Subgaleal aponeurosis (A)

Loose subepicranial space (L)

Pericranium (P)

Cranium

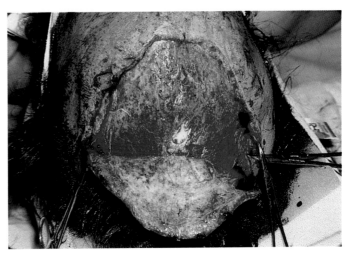

(b)

Fig. 19.1: (a) The five layers of the scalp include the skin (S), subcutaneous tissue (C), subgaleal aponeurosis (A), loose subepicranial space (L) and pericranium (P). **(b)** Scalp avulsions commonly occur in the subgaleal plane.

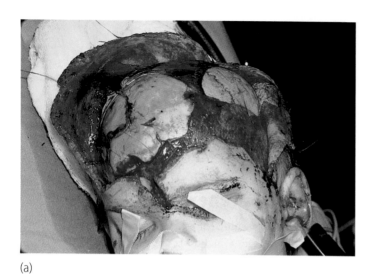
(a)

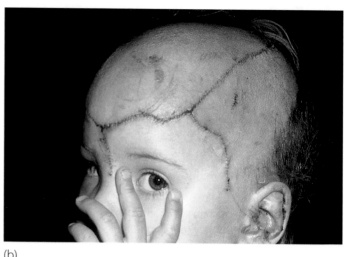
(b)

Fig. 19.2: Extensive scalp lacerations with degloving in a 4-year-old involved in a motor vehicle accident (unrestrained passenger). **(a)** Intraoperative view. **(b)** Seven days postoperative view.

prevention of infection. Scalp infections are uncommon even in contaminated wounds and such resistance to infection makes it unnecessary to clip or shave hair from the wound edges, unless doing so aids the alignment of the tissues.

Primary closure is the method of choice where there is no significant tissue loss (less than 3 cm). The wound edges tend to contract and what initially may appear to be a large defect may be relatively easily closed with subgaleal undermining (Fig. 19.2). Wounds on the vertex of the scalp are usually more difficult to close because of the decreased tissue mobility in this region. Scoring of the galea on its deep surface is a well-described procedure to facilitate closure and consists of transverse incisions made perpendicular to the axis of advancement. Care should be taken not to damage the more superficial subcutaneous vessels.

A layered primary closure is carried out if the galea has been lacerated. The galea is tightly adherent to the overlying skin and its approximation facilitates skin closure. Failure to repair this layer may result in cosmetic deformity, ranging from a depressed scar to asymmetric brow contraction. Closure of the galea also prevents the spread of wound contaminants to the intracranial cavity via the emissary veins, which connect the skin to the venous sinuses. A satisfactory galeal closure prevents the development of most potential problems, from osteomyelitis to meningitis. The galea is approximated with interrupted 2–0 or 3–0 slowly resorbable sutures.

As a noticeable scalp scar is determined primarily by the presence of alopecia, maximal care should be paid to follicular viability. Dermal sutures are used sparingly, if at all, to reduce the possibility of hair follicular damage. Restoring the continuity of the galea obviates the need in most cases for dermal sutures, relieving tension on the skin sutures so they may be removed early. Closure of the skin is carried out using non-interlocking continuous sutures of 3–0 nylon or Prolene in adults and 4–0 in children (Fig. 19.3). Metallic staples may also be used.

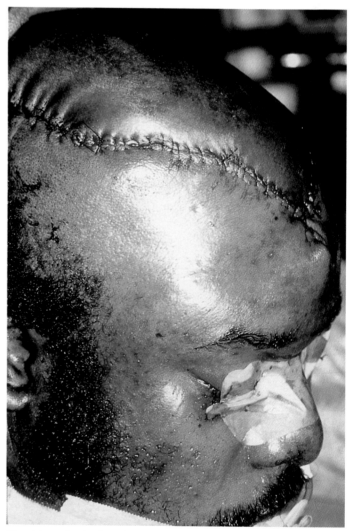

Fig. 19.3: Scalp skin closure can be done expeditiously with a running suture or staples.

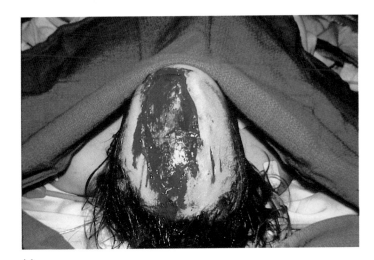

(a)

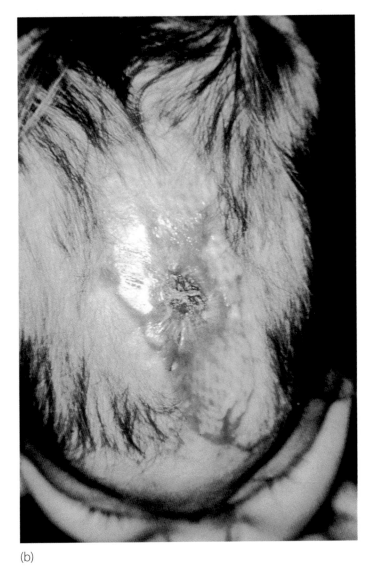

(b)

Fig. 19.4: Split-thickness skin grafting on the scalp. **(a)** Partial scalp avulsion in a 3-year-old male due to a dogbite, with underlying pericranium intact. **(b)** Ten days after split-thickness skin grafting with approximate 90% take. Small central eschar represents only area of non-take which will heal secondarily.

Split skin grafting

Placement of a split-thickness skin graft is the treatment of choice for the majority of larger scalp defects not amenable to primary closure. The pericranium must be intact, as grafts will not 'take' on denuded bone. Split-thickness skin grafts provide a rapid and very reliable method for wound coverage in the acute setting (Fig. 19.4). They are harvested at 0.14 inch to 0.20 inch thickness with a dermatome, usually from the lateral thigh, and can be placed either as sheet grafts, if encroaching on the forehead, or more usually meshed in a 1.5:1 ratio and placed with minimal expansion. The purpose of meshing the graft is twofold: first, they take better without bolstering by allowing fluid egress and second, result in greater wound contracture, which is subsequently beneficial. As scalp skin grafts are ultimately esthetically undesirable due to contour depression and alopecia, they are usually serially excised about 6 months after placement. Because split-thickness skin grafts contract by between 20% and 40%, the reduction in size of the defect aids secondary excision and closure. In grossly contaminated wounds or those where the viability of the pericranium is questionable, a homograft (cadaveric) or xenograft (porcine) may be used as a temporary biological dressing until the placement of an autograft is considered appropriate.

As previously noted, the lack of a pericranium obviates the successful take of a skin graft. In the absence of a pericranium, it is traditionally recommended to remove the outer table of the cranium, exposing the well-vascularized diploe, which is an excellent bed for grafting. This can be done by either burring away the outer table or drilling multiple holes through the outer table; either method allows granulation tissue to cover the exposed bone. After about 3 weeks there should be a satisfactory covering of healthy granulation tissue on to which the graft can be placed. Whilst an effective method to achieve epithelial coverage, it does require a considerable delay between the bone removal and the placement of the graft and is likely to leave a poorly contoured defect.

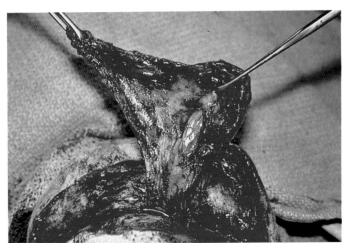

Fig. 19.5: Pericranial flaps usually must have a defined vessel to ensure viability. A frontal pericranial flap based on the supraorbital/supratrochlear vessels is one option.

Flaps

Unless there are contraindications, a flap procedure would provide a more expedient solution. Either a locally based pericranial flap, if the defect is small, or a free tissue transfer, when larger defects are present, could be used. Pericranial flaps allow for the transfer of a thin vascularized cover onto which a skin graft can be placed. Although originally thought to be random in nature, these flaps derive much of their blood supply from the overlying subgaleal fascia, which is usually elevated with the flap. To be effective and reliable, the pericranial flap should be centered over a major vascular territory with minimal dissection close to the pedicle (Fig. 19.5). The blood supply is extremely sensitive and postoperative graft dressings should be very lightly applied.

Use of local flaps

Flaps using local scalp tissue are appropriate for relatively small partial or full-thickness defects (3–5 cm wide). Local flaps are advantageous in that they permit closure of the defect with hair-bearing skin of similar thickness. Their use is appropriate for the cover of clean, sharp lacerations when surrounding tissue viability is not compromised. Many traumatic scalp wounds are the result of either crush or avulsion injuries where adjacent tissue damage is inevitable and as flap elevation may further compromise an already tenuous blood supply, the raising and rotation of local flaps have only limited use in such circumstances (Fig. 19.6).

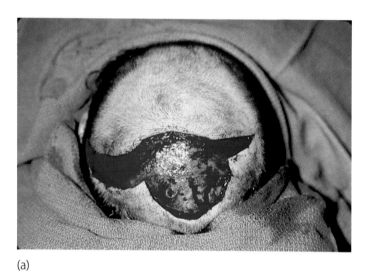

(a)

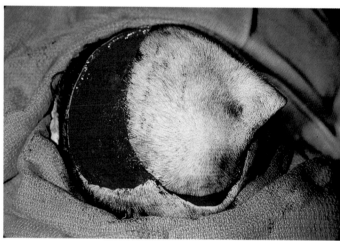

(b)

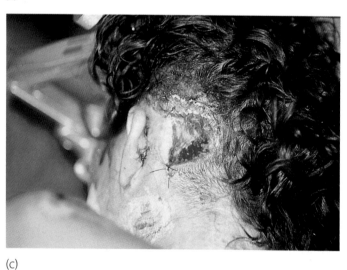

(c)

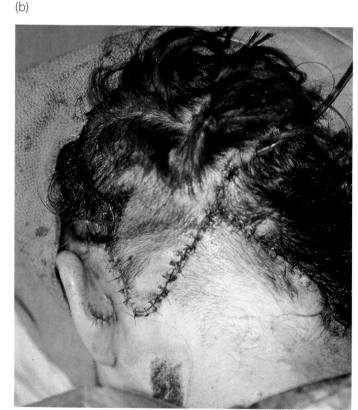

(d)

Fig. 19.6: Coverage of avulsed scalp defects with rotational flaps. **(a)** Debrided scalp avulsion defect from dogbite in 4-year-old male child. **(b)** Rotational flap coverage with the wake of the flap to be covered with a skin graft. The flap was needed due to the exposed bone underneath the avulsion. **(c)** Small occipital scalp defect seen 8 days after avulsive injury from a roll-over motor vehicle accident in 21-year-old female. **(d)** Coverage of exposed bone with a scalp transpositional flap.

Use of free tissue transfer

Embarking on free vascularized flaps is a long and potentially demanding procedure and timing of this must be considered with care. It is not a procedure to start late at night with tired or inexperienced surgeons and anesthetists; it should be a planned, semielective procedure. Wet-dry dressings can be applied to large denuded defects until free vascularized tissue transfer can be arranged. Flaps should generally be muscular for bulk and maximal vascularity and the flap of choice is almost always the latissimus dorsi due to its large surface area, relatively long pedicle and ease of harvest (Fig. 19.7). Other options include the rectus abdominis muscle, scapular or parascapular flaps and the omental fat flap.[2] Almost all of these options require a simultaneously placed split-thickness skin graft for outer coverage of the flap.

Replantation

Microsurgical scalp replantation is the treatment of choice for total or near-total scalp avulsion. These are fortunately very uncommon injuries but classic in their presentation and are usually caused by the entanglement of long hair in rotating machinery. The separation occurs in the subgaleal, loose areolar plane at the peripheral margins of the scalp where the galea is less resistant to applied force. Partial avulsion injuries are rare and the scalp and forehead are generally removed as a single anatomic unit (Fig. 19.8). The upper eyelids and portions of the ears may also be included in the avulsed segment because of the intimate relationship between the muscular segments of the galea and these structures.[3]

Microsurgical replantation, if successful, is esthetically and functionally superior to any other method of wound closure or coverage. It restores normal hair growth in unscarred areas and a large amount of the avulsed segment, such as eyelids and ears, can be expected to survive (Fig. 19.8c). Provided that the avulsed segment is not severely crushed and mutilated and the warm ischemia time is not greater than 12 hours, every effort should be made for replantation.[4]

Successful replantation is largely dependent on emergency access to the operating theater finding suitable recipient vessels in the surrounding temporal scalp or neck (which is always possible) and finding suitable vessels in the avulsed segment (which may not always be possible). Vein grafts may be needed to move the microvascular repair out of the zone of injury and reduce tension along the vessels and across the anastomoses. Although the scalp can survive with only one arterial anastomosis, it is preferable to identify at least two vessels suitable for repair. If possible (although rare), bilateral superficial temporal and occipital arteries should be identified and repaired. As venous congestion is the predominant cause of most postoperative flap failure, it is extremely important to ensure adequate venous outflow. If no suitable veins are available, venous outflow can be achieved by anastomosing a scalp artery directly to a recipient vein. The use of medicinal leeches is an option but a large scalp replant would require multiple (4–6) leeches concurrently and the patient would need extensive transfusions until venous outflow was re-established. Once

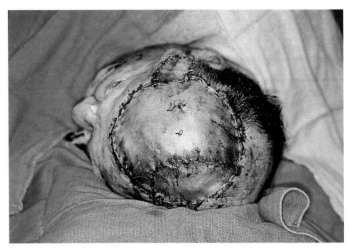

(a)

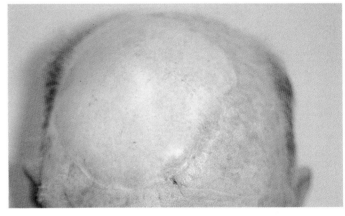

(b)

Fig. 19.7: Coverage of a large scalp wound with a free latissimus muscle flap covered with a skin graft. **(a)** Intraoperative view with the free muscular flap sewn into the defect. The microvascular anastomoses are in the right neck and the muscle is covered with unmeshed split-thickness skin grafts. **(b)** Six months postoperative view with healed flap and no contour deformity.

established, most scalp replants will require secondary revision of the scars, eyelids, ears and any large remaining areas of alopecia.[5]

If it is not possible to replant the scalp then coverage may be obtained using one of the methods previously described (Fig. 19.9).

When avulsion occurs in the forehead region primary closure can be a problem because of the difficulty in recruiting local tissue to cover the defect. Extensive mobilization and release of the galea can help but only to close defects of several centimeters. Reduction of the width of the forehead causes problems with medial or superior eyebrow transposition and frontal hairline disturbances, neither of which is easy to restore secondarily without recreating the original defect. Initial repair is usually best managed by coverage with a split or full-thickness skin graft. If the avulsion is only partial thickness, with preservation of some or all of the frontalis muscle, a full-thickness graft or unmeshed thick split-

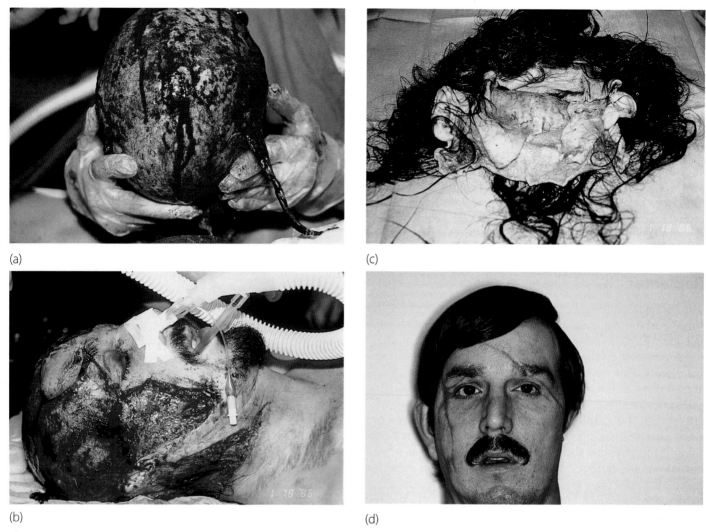

(a)

(b)

(c)

(d)

Fig. 19.8: Microsurgical scalp replantation. **(a)** 33-year-old male who sustained a complete scalp avulsion due to hair becoming entangled in machinery. **(b, c)** Total scalp avulsion including ears and eyebrows. **(d)** Successful scalp replantation with survival of the eyebrows and most of both ears (courtesy of A Michael Sadove MD, Indianapolis, Indiana).

thickness graft may produce a reasonable result without significant contour deformity (Fig. 19.10a,b). Where only pericranium is left, a split-thickness skin graft produces a healed but depressed wound that will then require secondary reconstruction through tissue expansion and or local flaps (Fig. 19.10c,d).

The eyebrow is the most valuable esthetic structure of the forehead. Preservation of hair-bearing skin and accurate realignment of the eyebrow unit is essential (Fig. 19.11). It is important never to shave the eyebrow hairs because firstly, they may not fully regrow and secondly, it increases the likelihood of secondary eyebrow deformities should they in fact regrow. Once a portion of the eyebrow is lost, the remaining portion of the eyebrow should be put back together along its preinjury arc even if this creates a larger forehead defect. Closing the wound with the eyebrow canted up or down can make secondary reconstruction more difficult, although a Z-plasty will often provide a simple solution. Significant eyebrow loss will ultimately require free scalp grafts or micrograft hair transplants for reconstruction (Figs 19.10**d**, 19.11**d**).

Eyelids

Of primary consideration in the management of injury to the eyelids is the exclusion of associated trauma to the underlying globe. If the cornea has been exposed care should be taken that the cornea remains moist by regular saline irrigation or placement of a saline-soaked dressing. At the time of repair it is good practice to protect the cornea with a soft lens/shield. If injury is not seen or suspected an ophthalmology opinion is not immediately necessary and visual acuity can be assessed by simple tests. If an injury is suspected then an expert evaluation is mandatory. A common error is to miss a foreign body. Lifting the lids away and carefully inspecting the depths of the fornices is a simple but important procedure. Corneal abrasions are common in facial trauma; pain and irritation of the injured eye are typical findings. Definitive diagnosis requires ophthalmology assessment with fluorescein dye and slit-lamp examination and with appropriate treatment, healing is usually rapid and uncomplicated. In rare cases, devastating infection with pseudomonas can occur which warrants immediate ophthalmology intervention.

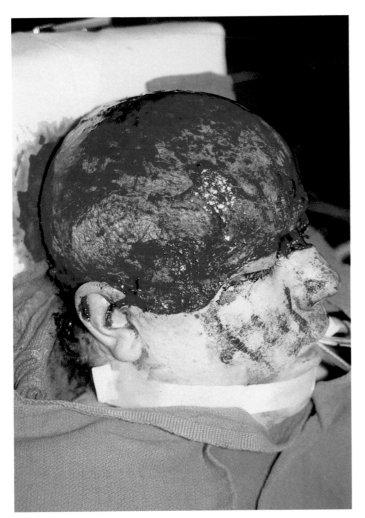

(a)

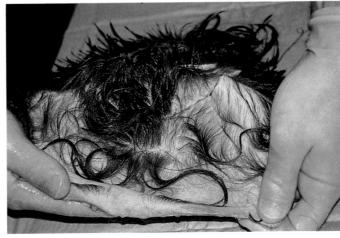

(b)

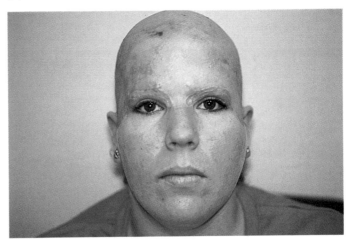

(d)

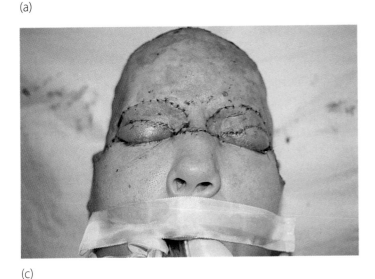

(c)

Fig. 19.9: Total scalp avulsion covered with skin grafts.
(a) 28-year-old female with complete scalp avulsion after hair became entangled in machinery. **(b)** Avulsed scalp segment. **(c)** As the scalp was not replantable due to poor vessel quality, immediate coverage was done with meshed and unmeshed (forehead and upper eyelid) split-thickness skin grafts. **(d)** Near 100% graft take seen 3 weeks after initial surgery.

For practical purposes the eyelid has two layers: an inner layer comprising the tarsal plate and conjunctiva and an outer layer of skin and orbicularis muscle (Fig. 19.12a). Apposition of skin, muscle and tarsal plate is important, as conjunctival lacerations frequently heal adequately on their own. Lacerations in the upper eyelid may disrupt the levator aponeurosis and result, if not properly repaired, in postoperative downward positioning of the upper eyelid (ptosis). Downward positioning of the lower eyelid (ectropion) is usually the result of lacerations that run perpendicular to the lid margin and is caused by poor anatomical realignment, tissue loss or canthal disruption.

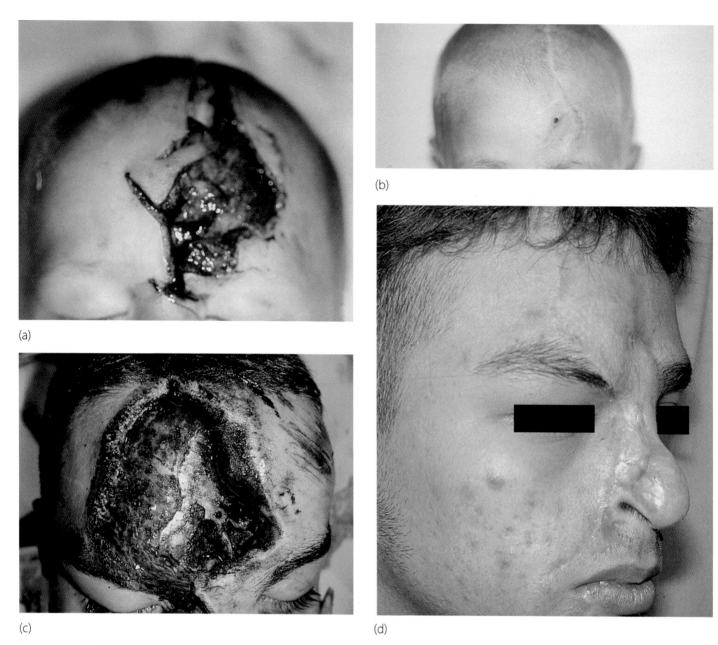

Fig. 19.10: Forehead avulsion with skin graft coverage. **(a)** Four-year-old male with dogbite avulsion of the central forehead, leaving pericranium and galea intact. **(b)** Three-month postoperative result with an unmeshed split-thickness skin graft coverage with minimal contour deformity. **(c)** Large forehead and eyebrow (partial) avulsion in a 24-year-old male secondary to motorcycle accident with only pericranium intact. **(d)** Postoperative result at 1 year. Multiple revisions of the forehead, eyebrow and nose will be needed.

Full-thickness eyelid lacerations should have the lid margin approximated first by lining up the gray line (squamous–mucosal junction) or the meibomian gland orifices with a 7–0 Vicryl with the tail of the suture left long so it may be sewn down by the adjacent sutures. The remainder of the laceration is repaired in layers with 6–0 Vicryl for the tarsus and muscle, 6–0 plain or chromic gut, with the knots inverted to prevent corneal irritation, for the conjunctiva and 6–0 or 7–0 nylon or Prolene for the skin (Fig. 19.12b,c). Approximating the tarsus and the ciliary margin are the crucial steps provided there is no significant tissue loss.[5] With partial-thickness injuries with skin loss, full-thickness skin grafts from the avulsed segment (if available) or the opposite upper eyelid or postauricular area can be used. In small full-thickness defects involving less than one-third of the lid, primary closure can be carried out. Defects up to one-half of the lid may be able to be primarily closed with the release of the lateral canthus (Fig. 19.13). Defects any larger than one-half will require the use of either a cheek advancement (Mustarde) or an upper lid switch procedure. Use of these more extensive flap procedures, which are often only one-time use techniques, is not advised in the acute trauma setting. In some cases with more superficial loss, a full-thickness graft from the other upper eyelid is desirable.

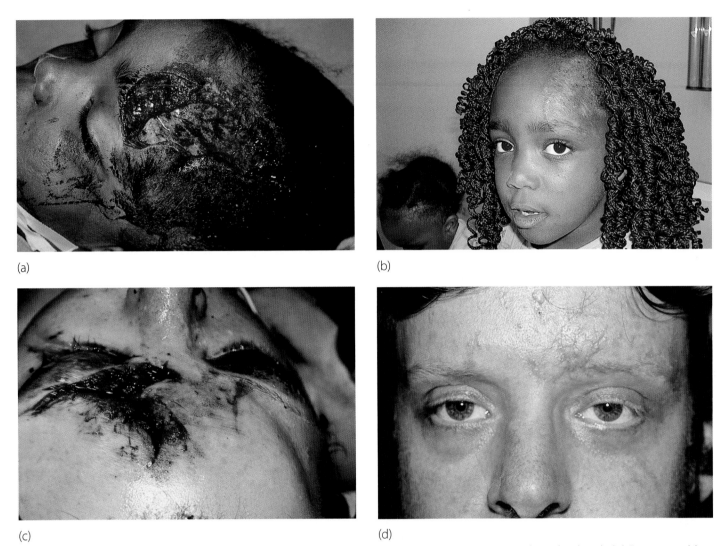

Fig. 19.11: Realignment of the eyebrow in forehead lacerations re-establishes a very important esthetic landmark. **(a)** Four-year-old female with an extended scalp-to-eyelid laceration due to a motor vehicle accident. **(b)** Six-week postoperative result. Despite healing scars, the alignment of the eyebrow produces a good early result. **(c)** Deep forehead lacerations with partial eyebrow loss in 31-year-old male from motor vehicle accident. **(d)** Proper alignment of the eyebrow, even if deficient, has been satisfactorily done. This can now be secondarily grafted without the need for further skin surgery.

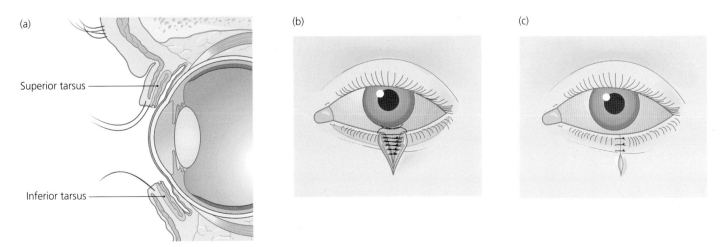

Fig. 19.12: **(a)** The eyelid consists essentially of two layers: an inner lamella of conjunctiva and tarsus and an outer lamella of skin and orbicularis muscle. **(b)** Closure of the inner lamella. **(c)** Closure of the outer lamella.

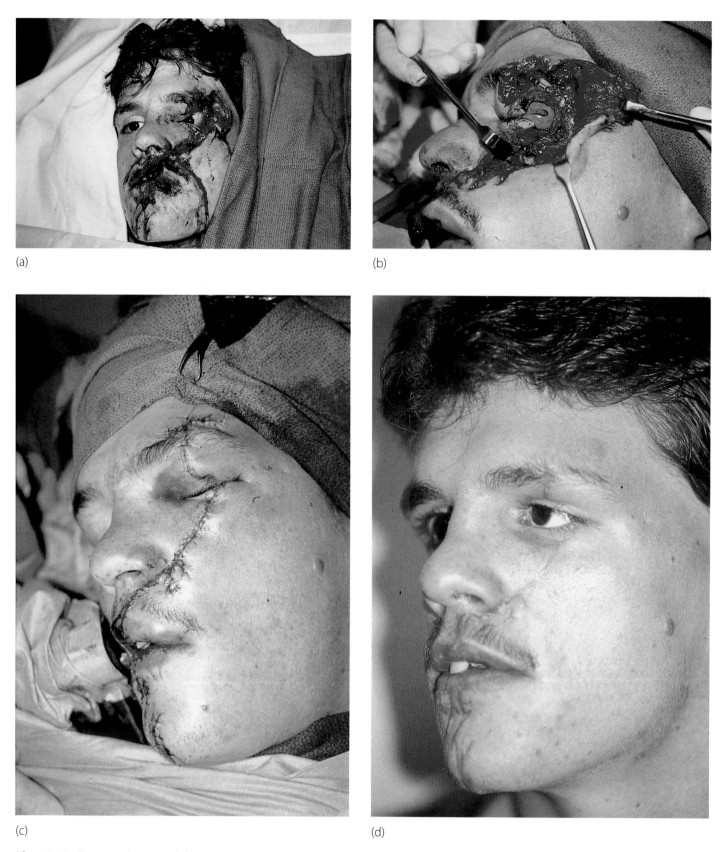

(a)

(b)

(c)

(d)

Fig. 19.13: Extensive lower eyelid laceration repair. **(a)** 26-year-old male with a severe laceration secondary to a chainsaw belt injury with loss of about one-fifth of the lower eyelid. **(b)** Bony repair of the periorbital skeleton prior to eyelid reconstruction. **(c)** Immediate postoperative result requiring lateral canthotomy for lower eyelid closure. **(d)** Three-month postoperative result without lower eyelid notching.

Lacrimal apparatus

Any injury to the medial aspect of the eyelids, particularly the lower, may involve the lacrimal system (Fig. 19.14). Inspection and cannulation of the punctum with probes will confirm the injury (Fig. 19.14a–c). Repair is usually carried out by loop intubation with the punctae being initially cannulated with silastic stents that pass into and through the lacrimal duct into the nose, where they are tied[6] (Fig. 19.14d,e). Repair of the canaliculae, sac or duct can then be done with 9–0 nylon but this is often more theoretical than practical. A combination of the remainder of the lid repair and keeping the stents in place for at least 3 months will often result in adequate tear drainage. Injury to the upper canaliculus alone rarely causes a tearing problem. Retrograde probing is an alternative to loop intubation. The specialized probes are passed through the uninjured punctum

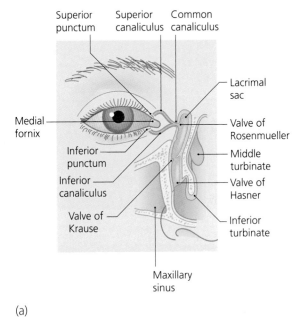

(a)

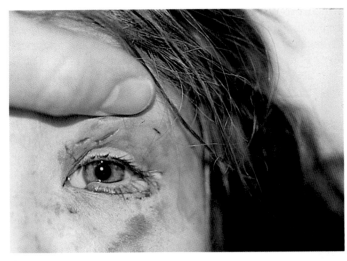

(b)

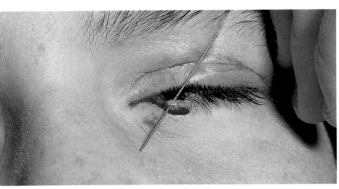

(c)

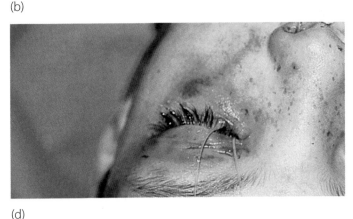

(d)

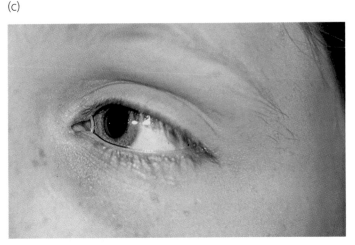

(e)

Fig. 19.14: Repair of lacrimal duct injuries. **(a)** Anatomy of the nasolacrimal system. **(b)** Medial laceration of lower eyelid in a 9-year-old female due to a dogbite. **(c)** Cannulation with probe confirms the lacrimal transection (not the same patient). **(d)** Anterograde cannulation of nasolacrimal system through upper and lower eyelid punctum with Crawford tubes. **(e)** The tubes are kept in place for 3 months after laceration repair. The silastic loop can be seen in the medial aspect of the eye between the puncta.

into the common canaliculus and then into the proximal end of the cut canaliculus. This can be of use when the punctum proximal to the laceration cannot be entered.

Canthal ligaments

Disruption of the canthal ligaments is not common but when present, an attempt should be made to reattach them to the orbital walls. Untreated, this produces a very ugly deformity. So long as a small fragment of bone remains attached to the ligament the result is reasonably predictable. Small microplates can be used to hold the bone fragment and canthus in the correct position. If the canthus is completely free it is difficult to restore its position. Wires passed through these small canthal stumps look fine in diagrams, but frequently cut through the fine tissues, especially if treated late and more force is needed. A useful way to prevent this is to place a clear acrylic (so any skin necrosis can be detected) button over the canthal skin and run the wire through the button as well as the ligament. This way the acanthus is 'pulled' and 'pushed' into position. The wire canthopexy has to be fixed to an artificial anchorage which, in the medial canthal area, can be provided by placement of a small miniplate (Fig. 19.15). In the lateral canthal area, a small hole placed through the lateral orbital wall works well. Where the soft tissue injury is associated with underlying skeletal injury it is common to find comminution of the bone and transnasal fixation may be required.

Nose

Lacerations to the nose are usually uncomplicated but may involve the underlying cartilaginous or bony structures which if not suspected may be overlooked (Fig. 19.16). The rich vascular supply of the nose through the septum and enveloping skin makes it difficult for any portion of the nose not to survive providing some pedicle remains. Full-thickness lacerations should be closed in three layers: the mucous membrane

(4–0 chromic); torn cartilages (5–0 or 6–0 PDS, clear nylon); the overlying skin (6–0 nylon). Once the cartilaginous and bony framework is anatomically aligned, the nasal skin usually approximates provided there is no significant loss. Dermal sutures are often not necessary which is fortuitous as the thick sebaceous skin with its high bacterial content is prone to suture abscesses. When there has been cartilaginous loss consideration should be given to the placement of a primary cartilage graft to resist postoperative contracture and depression of the scar although the need for this technique is not that frequent.

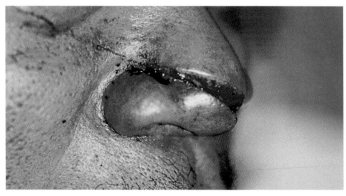

(a)

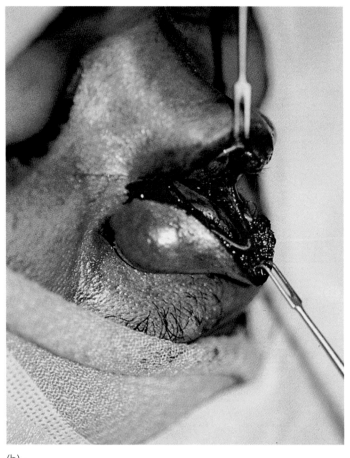

(b)

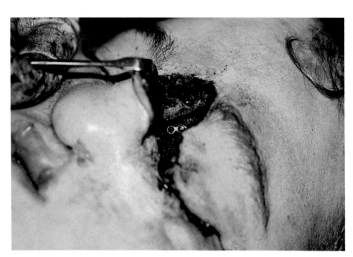

Fig. 19.15: The placement of a metallic plate on the inner orbital wall for medial canthal reattachment during orbital repair from injuries sustained from a motor vehicle accident in a 15-year-old female.

Fig. 19.16: Nasal laceration secondary to knife wound. **(a)** Apparent superficial laceration across the distal nose in 47-year-old male. **(b)** Intraoperative evaluation of the laceration shows its complete transection through the alar cartilages and septum.

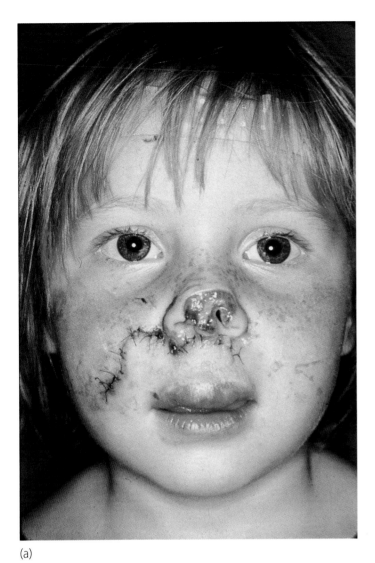

(a)

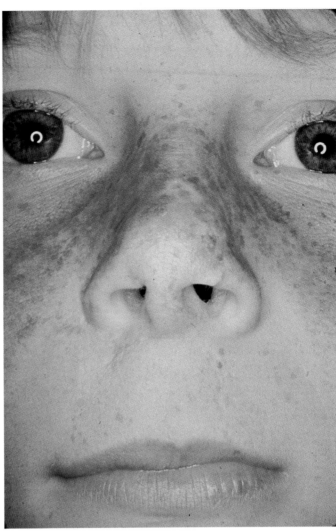

(b)

Fig. 19.17: Reconstruction of the nasal tip with a full-thickness skin graft. **(a)** One week after nasal tip avulsion in a 4-year-old male due to a dogbite. **(b)** One year after secondary reconstruction with a full-thickness skin graft and secondary cartilage grafting.

Abrasion/avulsion injury

Abrasion/avulsion injuries are common and this prominent facial structure is frequently exposed to abrasive tangential forces. Partial-thickness avulsions are best left alone and treated topically as they have a remarkable ability to heal. With deeper lesions that penetrate the dermis, full-thickness skin grafts from either the pre- or postauricular areas provide the best color match and prevent significant depression of the healed wound. Split-thickness grafts produce a translucent contracted appearance and should only be considered in partial-thickness avulsions where some dermis remains. Full-thickness grafts should be secured with a tie-over dressing for at least 5–7 days, as the revascularization may not be complete for at least 1 week after placement. The timing of the graft placement may be delayed from the acute setting to allow for an improved recipient bed if the risk of contamination is high or there is exposed underlying cartilage (Fig. 19.17). The survival of the nasal skin can be remarkable even with very large avulsive injuries attached by a narrow

pedicle. As long as there is bleeding from the dermal edges of the cut tissue, the nasal flap should be replaced and can be expected to survive (Fig. 19.18).

Amputation injury

Amputation injuries are dramatic and management is dependent upon the size of the separated part. With nasal segments 2.5 cm or less, replacement as a composite graft may be successful (Fig. 19.19). Complete revascularization through existing vascular channels may occur and though it may initially appear that the segment is non-viable, it may 'pink up' 10–14 days later. Patience and patient reassurance are necessary before deciding that it has not survived. Systemic anticoagulants do not improve the success of the composite replacement although topical vasodilators (e.g. nitroglycerin paste) have been reported to be helpful. If the amputated part is not available consideration should be given, especially for small clean defects of the nostril margin, to composite grafting, the ear being a suitable donor site. Success is variable but may

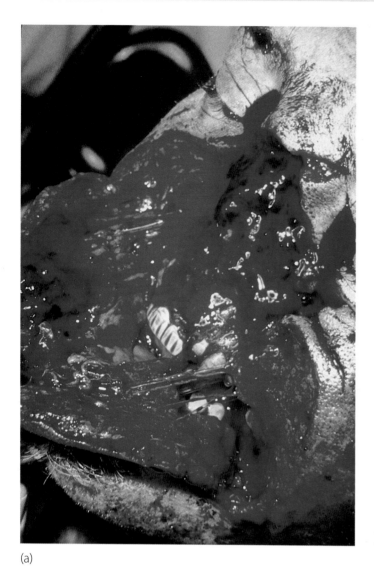

(a)

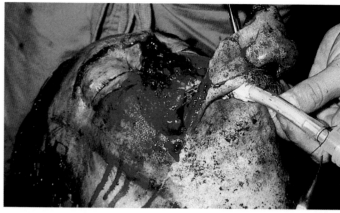

(b)

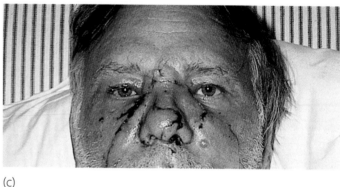

(c)

Fig. 19.18: Large nasal avulsion in 53-year-old male secondary to motor vehicle accident. **(a, b)** Entire nose and midfacial tissue avulsed, being attached by the upper lip only. **(c)** Reattachment of the pedicled nasal flap with complete survival 1 week after the injury.

avoid a prominent disfigurement. In larger nasal amputations, non-vascularized replantation will not succeed and the segment will need to be discarded. In children, the size limitation of the replanted nasal segment may be increased as composite grafts are more forgiving and the difficulty in reconstructing a growing nose justifies the risk. In a few instances, the amputated nose has been successfully replanted using microvascular techniques but this requires a very clean amputation of the part and a short warm ischemia time.[7]

Septal hematomas/hemorrhage

The nose also presents two relatively unique problems: septal hematomas and bleeding. Septal hematomas usually present as an anterior nasal swelling that is both obstructive and tender. Drainage should be performed without delay to prevent both abscess formation and avascular necrosis of the septal cartilage. Treatment is best carried out using a

hemitransfixion incision and mucosal approximation with 4–0 plain gut transseptal sutures. Plastic septal stents can also be used and secured with large transseptal Prolene sutures.

Most nasal bleeding stops spontaneously but on occasion, it persists and requires active management. Although not invariably, underlying skeletal injury may be the cause and should be suspected in such instances. If the bleeding is arising from the anterior aspect simple packing may suffice. If the bleeding is arising from the posterior aspect postnasal as well as anterior packing may be required. A number of adjuncts, including balloon catheters, are commercially available (Fig. 19.20). Very occasionally operative intervention is required to establish the source of bleeding and tie off the regional vessels. It should be remembered that the blood supply to the nasal cavity below the middle turbinate arises from the external and that above from the internal carotid systems. Exploration of the medial orbital wall to identify the anterior and posterior ethmoidal arteries may occasionally be necessary.

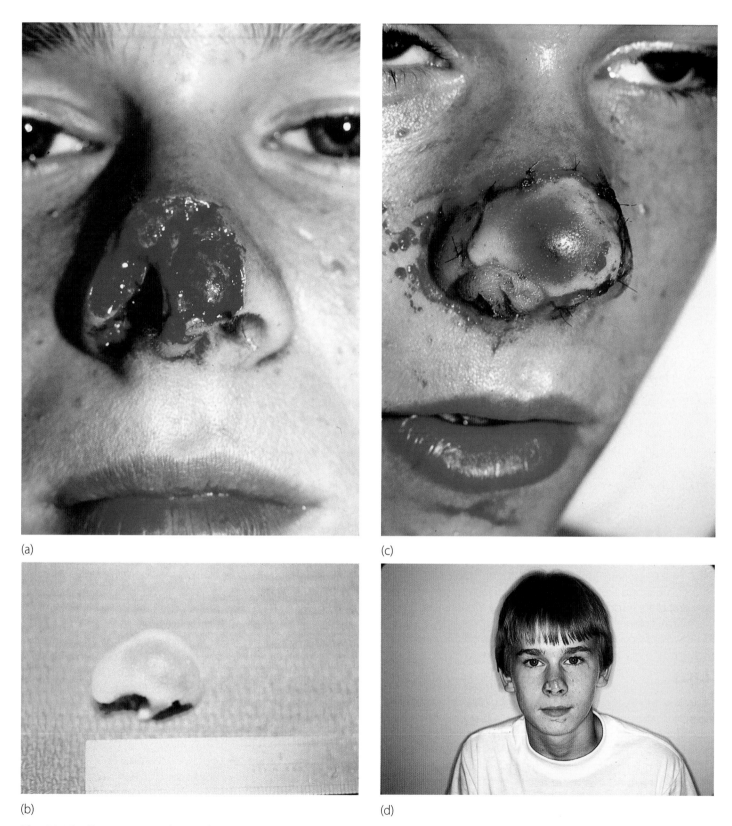

(a)

(b)

(c)

(d)

Fig. 19.19: Composite nasal tip replantation. **(a)** 12-year-old male with nasal tip avulsion secondary to a dogbite. **(b)** Avulsed nasal tip segment. **(c)** Replantation of composite piece. **(d)** One year postoperative result with survival of much of the replanted skin (courtesy of A Michael Sadove MD, Indianapolis, Indiana).

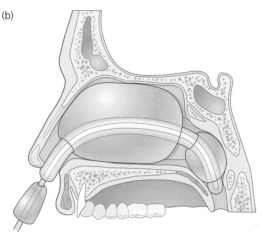

Fig. 19.20: Treatment of nasal epistaxis by silicone catheters. **(a)** A Foley catheter is a simple and very effective device in the management of posterior epistaxis. While inflated posteriorly, Vaseline gauze is then packed anteriorly. **(b)** More sophisticated double-balloon designs obviate the need for anterior gauze packing.

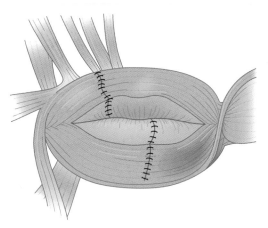

Fig. 19.21: Layered lip anatomy and closure. The circumoral musculature puts a near circumferential pull on lip wounds. The key points are muscle reapproximation and alignment of the vermilion–cutaneous junction.

Lips

The key to successful repair of the lips is ensuring correct approximation and alignment of the orbicularis oris muscle and the vermilion border. The orbicularis muscle should be repaired with 4–0 or 5–0 Vicryl or Dexon and enough sutures should be placed to prevent dehiscence of the muscle. If not properly repaired, loss of lip height, notching and an incompetent sphincter may result. It is helpful at this stage to accurately align the vermilion border, using 5–0 nylon or Prolene, before proceeding to closure of either the mucosal or skin surfaces (Fig. 19.21). The intraoral mucous membrane is then closed with either 4–0 chromic or plain gut. Finally, the skin is closed using 5–0 chromic for the dermis and 6–0 nylon or Prolene for the skin. Ideally, the laceration should cross the vermilion border at 90° to facilitate correct alignment but most lacerations do not and removing tissue to make this conversion is of uncertain merit in the acute setting.[8]

Avulsion injuries are managed depending upon the size of the defect. In rare cases of very small vermilion loss, the recovered piece may be successfully replaced as a free composite graft (Fig. 19.22). Usually, however, it is best to complete a wedge excision as this can be performed, with up to one quarter of the lip lost or removed, without any real functional or esthetic defect other than the scar (Fig. 19.23). In larger defects, where the loss extends to 50% of the lip, primary closure can still be carried out but some degree of microstomia will result. Postoperative lip-stretching exercises will help but the total circumoral surface area will be decreased. With defects greater than 50% primary closure is not possible. In such circumstances a skin-to-mucosal closure will be the treatment of choice, with secondary surgery to recreate the oral aperture. Some form of rotational flap will be required. In rare cases, an amputated lip segment may be capable of being replanted, as the labial vessels in both the remaining and avulsed lip are fairly easy to locate due to their predictable position.[9] The avulsed nature of most lip amputations, however, usually makes it very difficult to re-establish flow in stretched vessels with significant intimal damage (Fig. 19.24).

Intraoral Wounds

Mucosal lacerations of the cheek, vestibules, floor of mouth, tongue and palate commonly occur. They most often result from compression or shearing of the mucosa against the dentition (natural or otherwise) or underlying bone but can occur as a result of penetrating injury or in association with mandibular/maxillary fractures.

Palate

Injuries to the palatal mucosa most commonly occur either, in children, as a result of a fall whilst sucking a foreign body (toothbrush, pencil, etc.), in which case the injury tends to

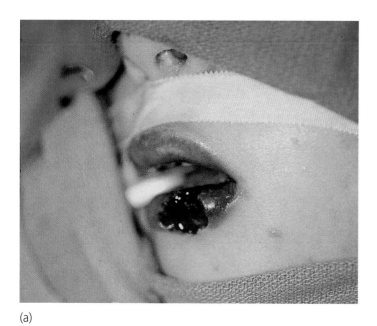
(a)

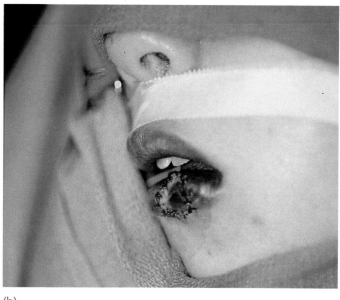
(b)

Fig. 19.22: Vermilion avulsion of lower lip. **(a)** Four-year-old female with small vermilion avulsion due to a dogbite. Primary closure would require extending a wedge excision into the skin. **(b)** Preservation and replant of avulsed vermilion segment with ultimate complete take.

be towards the posterior aspect, crescentic with the convexity anterior and likely to involve the soft palate, or in association with maxillary fracture and most likely to be associated with a split palate and lying in the sagittal plane. In the former scenario care should be taken to ensure that no foreign bodies are retained and, dependent upon the extent of the laceration, the wound may be 'tacked' closed or not. Occasionally a 'through-and-through' wound results along the posterior edge of the maxilla, separating the soft palate from its anterior attachment. In such an instance both the nasopharyngeal and oral surfaces should, if practicable, be repaired. In the presence of underlying maxillary fracture the initial requirement is to stabilize and fix the fracture and repair the soft tissues of the nasal floor (if required) and palate in order to avoid the possibility of an oronasal fistula developing.

Cheeks and lips

Lacerations to the cheek or mucosa along the inner lip surface should be closed with either 4–0 chromic or plain sutures with, depending upon the depth of injury, dermal sutures as required. Care should be taken in the cheek to ensure that the parotid papilla/duct is not compromised.

Floor of mouth

In the majority of instances lacerations in the floor of mouth can remain unsutured. Inexperienced suturing in this area may result in damage to either the submandibular/sublingual salivary ducts or the lingual nerve. 'Through-and-through' wounds require exploration and suturing in layers to avoid fistula formation.

Tongue

Significant tongue lacerations should be closed in layers, to prevent notching and marginal deformities, with loosely tied 3–0 chromic or Vicryl sutures in anticipation of muscular edema. Although rare, profuse bleeding can obstruct the airway and early intubation is recommended in these cases.

Degloving injury

Degloving injuries in the anterior mandibular region occur when significant compression and downward shearing forces are applied to the lower lip and chin. Often the mental nerves and vessels remain intact and a variable amount of the alveolar mucosa is stripped from the anterior mandible, commonly exposing the outer table from the alveolus to the chin point as far back as the mental foramina. The wound is often contaminated with particulate debris (the injury is commonly caused by patients hitting their chin and lower lip against the ground, having fallen off a bicycle/skateboard, etc.) and requires thorough cleaning before 'tacking' the mucosa back to its original position. Commonly it is not possible to approximate the tissues back to their original position and exposed areas subsequently heal by secondary intention. External strapping/bandaging is recommended for the first 48 hours after repair.

Finally mucosal injury may be the first indication of child abuse, which should be considered if the explanation appears incompatible with the injury.

Ear

The ear is similar to the nose in that there is a potential for disruption of a complex cartilaginous framework. Only the lobule,

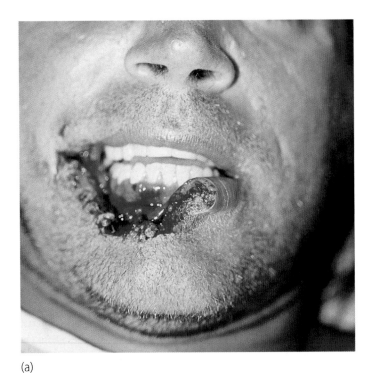

(a)

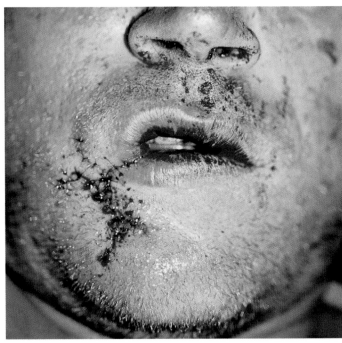

(b)

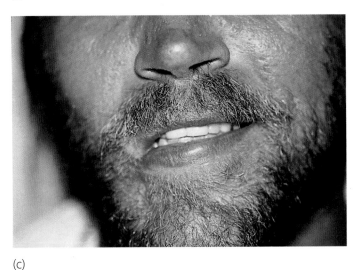

(c)

Fig. 19.23: Loss of one-half of lower lip due to a dogbite. **(a)** Extent of lip loss in a 34-year-old male. **(b)** Primary closure after unsuccessful microvascular replant attempt. **(c)** Six-month postoperative result with some degree of microstomia.

made up of skin and adipose tissue, is devoid of cartilage. The large area of perichondrium and cartilage predisposes to hematoma formation after blunt injury. An enlargement of the ear with loss of definition is usually an indication of hematoma and warrants immediate incision and drainage to prevent subsequent cartilaginous and fibrous disfigurement – a cauliflower ear. Following incision and drainage, bolsters should be placed and tied through and through onto both the anterior and posterior surfaces of the ear to prevent reaccumulation of the hematoma, a more reliable and comfortable method than circumferential tight pressure dressings (Fig. 19.25).

The unique structures of the ear warrant conservative debridement as their replacement can be difficult. The blood supply is extensive and many large ear segments can survive on narrow skin flaps. The cartilage must be approximated before closing the overlying skin. The elastic cartilage of the ear does not heal by cartilaginous ingrowth but by the

development of a fibrous scar between the cut edges and should be sutured with an undyed, slowly resorbing or clear permanent suture for a more secure closure.[10] As the shape and position of the ear are determined primarily by the support provided by the outline of the helical rim and antihelix, the repair of the cartilaginous components is critical. Repair of the cartilage within the concave hollows of the ear, such as the concha and triangular fossa, is less critical as unsupported soft tissue healing alone will maintain the concavity. Notching of the helical rim is common after transection and repair and is particularly noticeable to the eye. Particular attention should be paid to cartilage realignment and skin closure in this area with the use of vertical mattress sutures to evert the skin if necessary. Suturing of the dermis is rarely necessary as the cartilaginous repair generally relieves any likely tension across the skin closure and the dermis is usually quite thin anyway (Fig. 19.26).

Avulsion injuries vary greatly but the majority involve some degree of tearing and crushing. Replacement of small avulsions as composite grafts may be considered and there is usually little risk other than that of secondary removal and reductive closure with delayed reconstruction. Only the smallest segments (less than 1.0–1.5 cm) are likely to survive and, dependent upon the components involved, it may be more expedient, and with little detriment, to complete a wedge excision and close primarily. For injury involving segmental avulsions of the upper two-thirds of the helix, the retained cartilage may be denuded of skin and buried in the postauricular area with the torn/cut skin edges of the ear sutured into the same area, facilitating the subsequent use of a postauricular flap for secondary reconstruction and saving both an operative stage and a donor site.

Most large incomplete avulsions, even if attached by a very narrow pedicle, will survive with simple reattachment. However, whilst the skin pedicle will usually offer adequate vascular inflow, the venous outflow may not be sufficient. This will be made evident, in the immediate postoperative period, by bluish discoloration and sluggish to non-existent capillary refill, classic signs of venous congestion. Leeches used for several days will often salvage the situation. One or two leeches, changed twice daily, combined with the typical ooze after removal will allow the venous system rapidly to re-establish itself. There can be surprisingly significant blood loss using this technique and daily monitoring of the hematocrit is a requirement. A broad-spectrum antibiotic active against aeromonas, a common gut bacterium of the leech, should be prescribed. Despite the nursing care needed and its unappealing nature, the salvage of tissue from venous congestion with leech therapy can be remarkable. (Fig. 19.27).

When the ear avulsion is complete, a microvascular repair provides the best hope for successful replantation (Fig. 19.28). The success is low due to the very small size of the vessels (0.5 mm or less), difficulty in finding recipient vessels in the remaining wound bed and donor vessels in the amputated segment and the intimal damage to the vessels that occurs with the more common avulsive injury. However, the arterial inflow from a single arterial anastomosis combined with post-operative leech therapy for venous outflow makes success possible, particularly in children.[11] Every large avulsed ear segment with a limited amount of warm ischemia time should have a microvascular replant attempt. When micro-vascular replantation is not possible, placing the cartilage in a postauricular subcutaneous pocket (pocket principle) should be considered.[12] It is uncovered weeks later and used as part of the secondary reconstruction.

Facial Nerve

Because lacerations of the lateral face, involving an area from the temporal region to the neck, may involve branches of the facial nerve, facial nerve function must be assessed as part of the examination. Injuries to the nerve anterior to a vertical line from the lateral canthus or the midpupillary line do not require repair and do not result in permanent loss of muscle

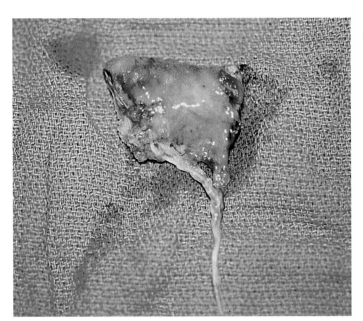

Fig. 19.24: Avulsed lower lip segment from patient in Fig. 19.23. Such avulsions severely injure the labial vessels, making re-establishing vascular flow very difficult. The strand of tissue coming from the lip segment is a branch of the mental nerve.

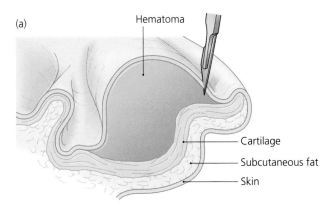

(a)

Hematoma

Cartilage

Subcutaneous fat

Skin

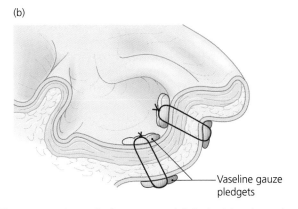

(b)

Vaseline gauze pledgets

Fig. 19.25: Auricular hematoma. **(a)** An incision is made over the hematoma and the clot is evacuated. **(b)** After evaluation, pressure is applied by through-and-through chromic sutures tied over a bolster placed on the side of the hematoma to prevent reaccumulation.

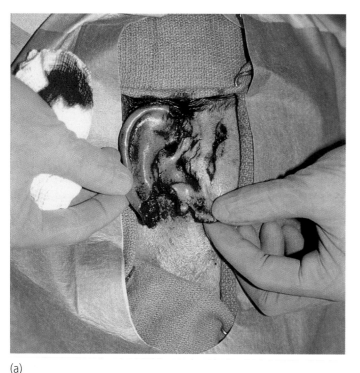

(a)

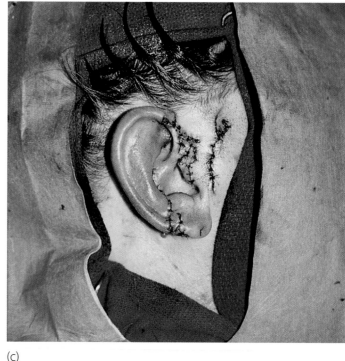

(c)

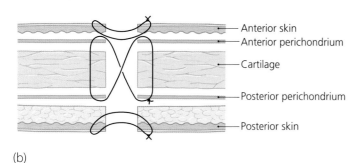

— Anterior skin
— Anterior perichondrium

— Cartilage

— Posterior perichondrium

— Posterior skin

(b)

Fig. 19.26: Closure of ear lacerations requires careful attention to cartilage repair. **(a)** Partial ear transection. **(b)** Figure-of-eight sutures through the cartilage prevents the edges from overriding each other. The skin is closed with either simple sutures or everting mattress sutures. **(c)** Partial ear transection closure.

function because the superficial facial muscles are innervated via their posterior aspects (Fig. 19.29). Posterior to these vertical lines, severed branches of the facial nerve should, if possible, be repaired under microscopic guidance within the first 24 hours of injury. In this early period, the distal nerve ends remain capable of being stimulated and identified.[13,14]

Whether carrying out an epineural or a fascicular repair, surgery should always be done using appropriate magnification, either loupes or the operating microscope. Where large branches are involved an epineural repair may be adequate if a reasonable alignment and orientation of the fascicles within the sheath can be achieved. After cleaning and trimming of the nerve ends simple interrupted sutures are placed using 10–0 nylon or Prolene on a 75–100 micron needle. Only 3–5 sutures are usually needed (Fig. 19.30). In the smaller more distal branches, the fascicles may be directly repaired with 11–0 suture material. There is some dispute as to which method of repair, epineural alone or fascicular, produces the better functional outcome.[15] This argument often becomes moot as the size of the nerve and its number of fascicles usually dictate the repair technique used.

When there has been loss of nerve tissue and continuity cannot be restored without unacceptable tension across the anastomosis, a primary nerve graft using the sural nerve should be considered (Fig. 19.31). The nerve graft is quick to harvest and is associated with minimal morbidity (lateral plantar anesthesia) at the donor site.

Severe functional deficits arise from transections of the peripheral single nerve branches, the frontal and marginal mandibular nerves. They have no cross-innervation with other branches and motor function will therefore never recover without their anastomosis. Unfortunately, they tend to be the hardest to find and the least forgiving of a poor repair (Fig. 19.32).

Transection of the main nerve trunk as it exits from the stylomastoid foramen poses a difficult problem. Whilst the nerve trunk at this level is large, a sufficient proximal segment may not always be available to facilitate a repair. Mastoid bone can be removed and this may expose enough of the proximal segment to complete the repair. In rare circumstances, a proximal segment may not be available and consideration should be given to a primary crossfacial nerve graft.

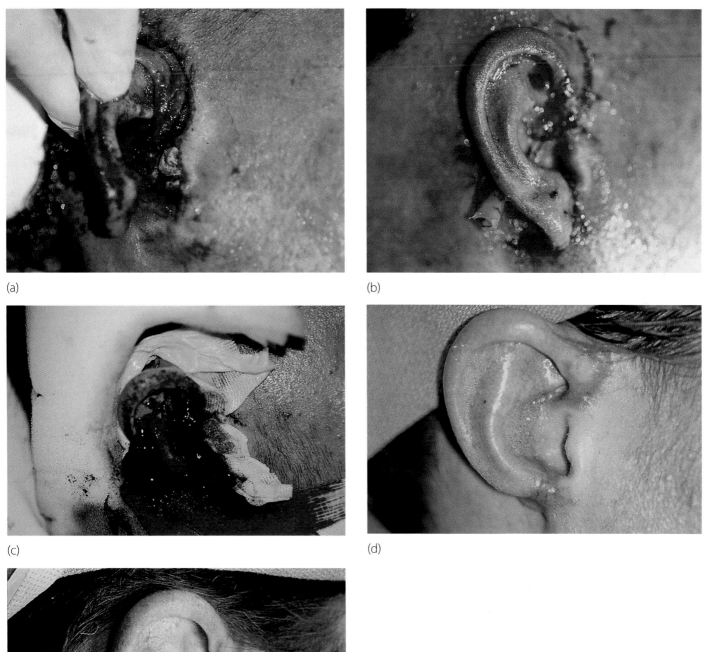

(a)

(b)

(c)

(d)

(e)

Fig. 19.27: Partial ear avulsion. **(a)** Near complete ear avulsion in 27-year-old male due to a roll-over motor vehicle accident. Only a small skin bridge remains at the superior helix. **(b)** Primary reattachment without microvascular anastomoses. **(c)** Use of postoperative leeches for 5 days was necessary for venous outflow. **(d)** All of the ear survived with the exception of the lobule. **(e)** Secondary reconstruction was then done with a cartilage graft and release.

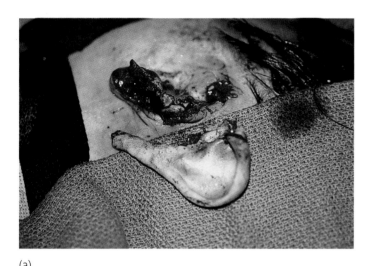

(a)

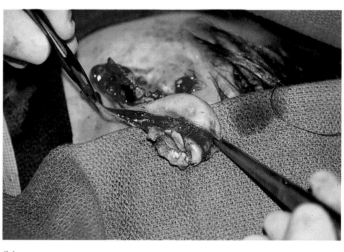

(b)

Fig. 19.28: Total ear amputation from roll-over motor vehicle accident (unrestrained passenger) in an 18-year-old female. **(a)** Complete transection through the concha. **(b)** The severe crush mechanism of the avulsion made the small (0.25 mm) vessels found for a microvascular replant attempt unusable.

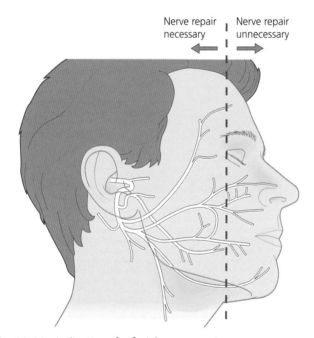

Nerve repair necessary

Nerve repair unnecessary

Fig. 19.29: Indications for facial nerve repair.

The sural nerve graft, usually about 16–20 cm in length, is anastomosed to the distal branches of the normal nerve on the opposite side of the face and then tunneled across the upper lip to the site of injury (Fig. 19.33). There is no advantage in delaying the repair under these circumstances unless the wounds are severely contaminated. Primary crossfacial nerve grafting offers the best hope for return of spontaneous and symmetrical facial expression. Should the graft not restore function to the remaining distal nerve branches, it can be used for a gracilis muscle transfer for smile reanimation.

Parotid Duct

Because the parotid duct runs parallel to the buccal branch of the facial nerve, traversing the middle third of a line drawn from the tragus to the midpoint of a line drawn between the alar of the nose and the vermilion border of the upper lip, lacerations in this area may potentially sever both it and the nerve branch. Saliva is rarely present in the wound after transection; a high index of suspicion must exist for it not to be missed (Fig. 19.34**a**). Retrograde cannulation of Stenson's will either confirm or refute transection of the duct (Fig. 19.34**b**). The duct is large, usually 4–5 mm in diameter, which makes finding the proximal portion a simple procedure under loupe magnification. The injection of colored dyes from the distal end is often recommended but this seems unnecessary and only serves to color and obscure the operative field. The proximal portion can be found by expressing saliva from the parotid gland. The repair is carried out with either 6–0 or 7–0 nylon or Prolene over a plastic stent; the silastic tubing from an angiocatheter of a similar size to the duct will suffice. The stent is allowed to extend from the papilla for about 1 cm and is sutured to the mucosa with a 4–0 chromic suture. The stent is retained for about 2 weeks and then removed if it has not already become dislodged.[16]

If a section of the duct is missing and there is not enough residual duct to satisfactorily reconstitute the lumen, there are three practical options. First, to reconstruct the duct with

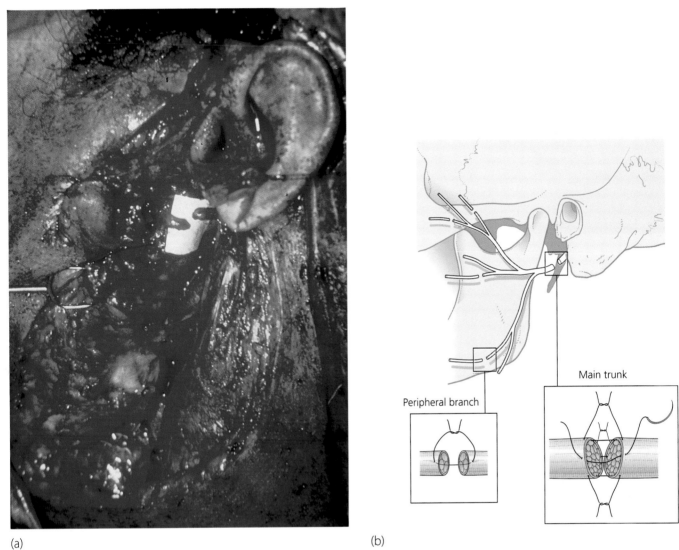

(a)

(b)

Fig. 19.30: Primary repair of facial nerve transection. **(a)** Typical location of nerve branch transections at the lateral face. **(b)** Suture technique of epineural repair of facial nerve transections.

a vein graft, second, to create a new oral opening by diverting the proximal stump through the oropharyngeal wall and third, to ligate the duct and hope for eventual atrophy without creating a source of chronic infection.

Lacerations to the parotid gland itself should be repaired in layers (capsule, subcutaneous tissue, dermis and skin) to avoid fistula formation. Generally lacerations involving the substance of the gland do not pose a problem unless there is obstruction to the adequate drainage of saliva. If saliva collects within the wound and persists after multiple aspirations the wound needs to be further explored to ensure that neither a transection has been missed nor a repair failed. Persistent collection of saliva in the presence of a restored duct may benefit from a more recent technique using botulinum toxin to block the parasympathetic innervation.[17]

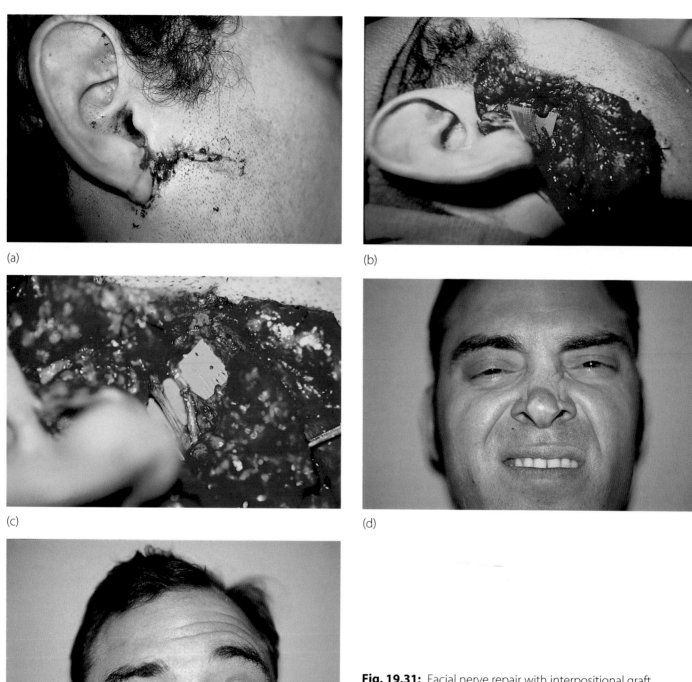

(a)

(b)

(c)

(d)

(e)

Fig. 19.31: Facial nerve repair with interpositional graft. **(a)** Laceration sustained from a hook (artificial arm) in a 34-year-old male with near complete facial paralysis, sparing only the marginal mandibular branch. **(b)** Intraoperative view of main branch transections with a gap. **(c)** Interpositional sural nerve grafts. **(d)** One year postoperative result with complete return of buccal innervation. **(e)** One year postoperative result with lack of frontal innervation.

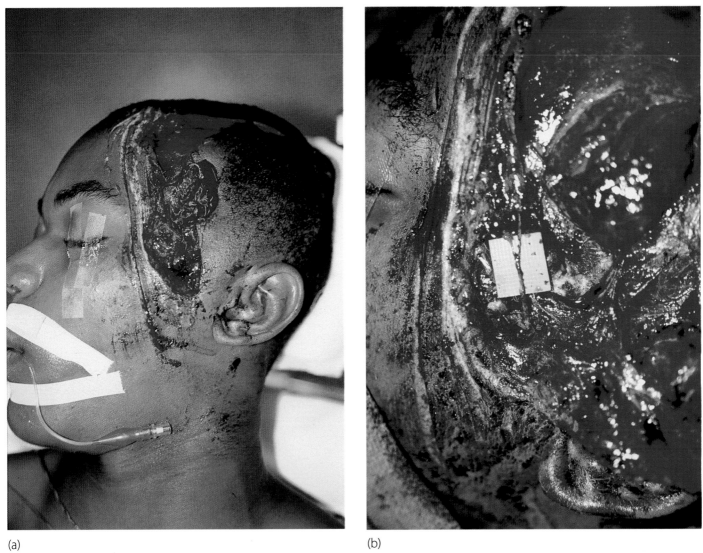

(a)(b)

Fig. 19.32: Transection of terminal frontal branch of the facial nerve. **(a)** Severe left temporal lacerations from motorcycle accident in a 16-year-old male. **(b)** Identification and repair of the frontal nerve branch transection. These facial nerve branches are usually only one or two fascicles in size.

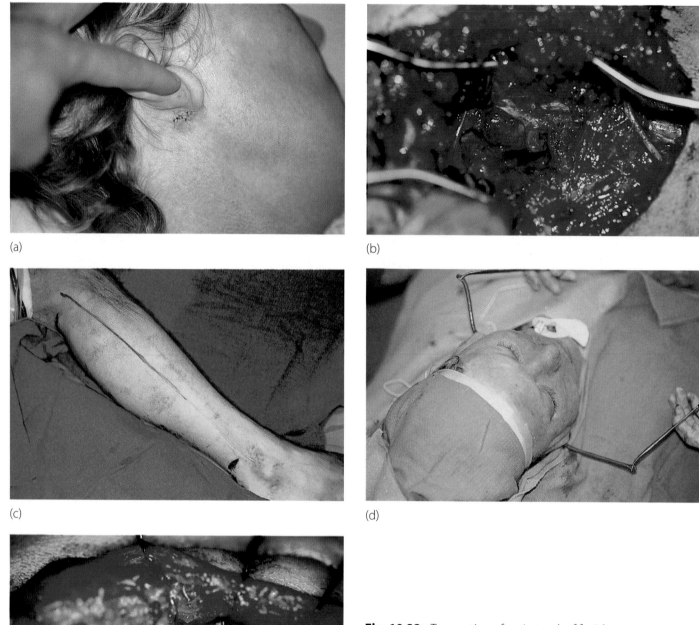

Fig. 19.33: Transection of main trunk of facial nerve.
(a) Entrance site of small glass shard from a fall (push) through a glass door with immediate and complete facial paralysis.
(b) Transection of main trunk of facial nerve at the level of its exit from the bone. Distal end of trunk is seen. Primary repair to proximal end was not possible. **(c)** Sural nerve graft harvest done with an endoscope. **(d)** Nerve graft tunneled from the uninjured side, where it was anastomosed to the buccal branches, to the injured side through a catheter. **(e)** Number of fascicles available for anastomoses to distal end of the facial nerve trunk from the nerve graft.

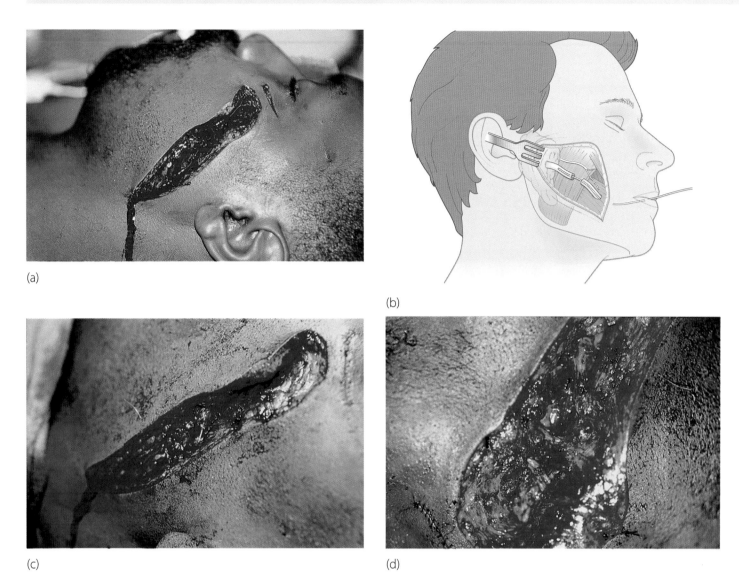

(a)

(b)

(c)

(d)

Fig. 19.34: Parotid duct repair. **(a)** Transfacial laceration due to knife wound in a 27-year-old male with a high suspicion of parotid duct laceration. **(b)** Diagram of probing of the parotid duct laceration. **(c)** Intraoperative probing of parotid duct laceration. No facial nerve branches were injured. **(d)** Repair of parotid duct laceration over stent.

References

1   Holt GR 1990 Concepts of soft tissue trauma repair. Otolaryngology Clinics of North America 23: 1019–1030

2   Sadove AM, Eppley BL 1990 Major craniomaxillofacial reconstruction aided by microsurgical transfer. Journal of Craniofacial Surgery 1: 77–87

3   Sadove AM, Moore TS, Eppley BL 1990 Total scalp, ear, and eyebrow avulsion: aesthetic adjustment of the replanted tissue. Journal of Reconstructive Microsurgery 6: 323–328

4   Thomas A 1998 Total face and scalp replantation. Plastic and Reconstructive Surgery 102: 2085–2087

5   Schultz RC 1991 Treatment of soft tissue injuries to the face. In: Smith JW, Aston SJ (eds) Plastic Surgery. Little, Brown, Boston, pp 325–345

6   Osguthorpe JD, Hoang G 1991 Nasolacrimal injuries: evaluation and management. Otolaryngology Clinics of North America 24: 59–73

7   Hammond DC, Bouwese CL, Hankins T, Maxwell-Davis CS, Furdyna J, Capraro PA 2000 Microsurgical replantation of the amputated nose. Plastic and Reconstructive Surgery 105: 2133–2136

8   Zide BM 1990 Deformities of the lips and cheeks. In: McCarthy JG (ed) Plastic Surgery, vol 3, part 2. WB Saunders, Philadelphia, p 2014

9   Wong SS 1999 Successful replantation of a bitten-off lower lip: case report. Journal of Trauma 47: 602–604

10   Templer J, Renner GT 1990 Injuries of the external ear. Otolaryngology Clinics of North America 23: 1003–1018

11   Concannon MJ, Puckett CL 1999 Microsurgical replantation of an ear in a child without venous repair. Plastic and Reconstructive Surgery 102: 2088–2093

12   Pribaz JJ, Crespo CD, Orgill DP, Pousti T, Bartlett RA 1997 Ear replantation without microsurgery. Plastic and Reconstructive Surgery 99: 1868–1872

13   Zuker RM, Eppley BL 2000 Facial reanimation. In: Coleman III JJ (ed) Plastic surgery: indications, operations, and outcomes, vol III. Mosby, St Louis, pp 1611–1623

14   Kelly KJ 1998 Soft-tissue injury to the face. Operative Techniques in Plastic and Reconstructive Surgery 5: 246–256

15   Baker DC 1990 Facial paralysis. In: McCarthy JG (ed) Plastic surgery, vol 3, part 2. WB Saunders, Philadelphia, p 2258

16   Dumpis J, Feldmane L 2001 Experimental microsurgery of salivary ducts in dogs. Journal of Craniomaxillofacial Surgery 29: 56–62

17   Marchese RR 1999 Management of parotid sialocele with botulinum toxin. Laryngoscope 109: 344–346

20 Reconstruction of Large Hard and Soft Tissue Loss of the Face

Barry L Eppley, John J Coleman

Introduction

The distinctive features of the human face and its obvious visibility to other people pose major challenges in facial reconstruction. When large or massive defects of the face are present, these challenges become truly great. Fortunately, situations that induce extensive injury with such large losses of facial tissue are infrequent. The most common cause, outside wartime, are gunshot wounds of either accidental, self-inflicted or criminal origin. This mechanism of traumatic injury often produces unpredictable patterns of facial injury which result in large composite defects that may severely compromise multiple orofacial functions including breathing, eating, speaking and seeing. Rarely, a severe motor vehicle, industrial or home accident may cause extensive damage but this is usually of a more blunt nature with the crushing and comminution of facial structures rather than large tissue loss. Glass or metal may produce long and deep lacerations with underlying bone fractures but this is usually a less complicated problem than the tissue loss that occurs with high-energy penetrating missiles and the blast effect from discharge close to the face.

When first presented with a patient that has sustained severe injury or loss of facial tissues, it can be bewildering to know where to begin after the initial resuscitation, control of the bleeding and systemic stabilization. The successful reconstruction of these facial defects involves replacement of much of the missing tissue before significant scarring and contracture have occurred. Such an approach demands early surgical intervention and the knowledge and application of every known, and often creatively designed, reconstructive procedure.

Gunshot pathophysiology

While large composite facial defects can occur from numerous etiologies, they are most consistently produced by firearms. This problem is most significant in the United States. Currently, the continued upward trend in firearm injuries will soon eclipse motor vehicles as the leading cause of traumatic death in the United States.[1] As such, the morbidity and mortality from firearms are likely to worsen in the near future, particularly as the availability and sophistication of these dangerous weapons increase. As more of these facial insults occur, their management would benefit from a basic understanding of ballistics and their mechanisms of tissue injury.

The study of the interaction of penetrating projectiles into body tissues has a significant history of scientific investigation

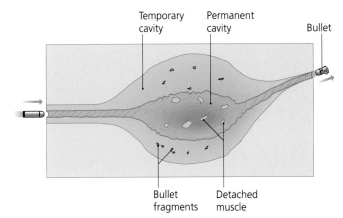

Fig. 20.1: Characteristic wound profile of a bullet traveling through tissue. Note the large amount of tissue destruction (detached muscle) and the size of the temporary cavity compared to the permanent cavity. The false belief that a bullet damages tissue in direct proportion to its velocity is widespread. Tissue destruction is as much based on bullet shape and construction as on its velocity.

but is often misunderstood in the medical literature. While a large number of gun and bullet types exist, the mechanisms by which the projectile disrupts tissue are quite basic and are purely mechanical in nature. Initially, the bullet crushes sufficient tissue to make a hole (entrance) through which it penetrates the underlying tissue (permanent cavity). Depending upon the speed at which it is traveling and the bullet caliber, the walls of the permanent cavity radiate outward to form a temporary cavity (Fig. 20.1). The permanent cavity has obvious tissue destruction but the damaging effect of the temporary cavity is variable. A third mechanism, powder gases that follow the bullet out of the barrel being forced into the tissues, occurs only in wounds in which the gun is in close contact with the skin at the time of firing.[2]

The tissue damage produced by a projectile depends on numerous factors including its shape, construction and mass and not just its velocity alone. This is best illustrated by comparing three well-known bullets which all travel at about the same projectile velocity. From a distance of 15 feet, the tissue damage caused by a 22 caliber bullet is less significant than that caused by a 44 Magnum hollow-point bullet. The increased size and deformation of the 44 Magnum bullet on impact account for the greater tissue damage. Both pale, however, compared to the tissue disruption caused by a load of 00 buckshot from a 12 gauge shotgun. The pellets from a shotgun hit so close together that they shred tissue for a

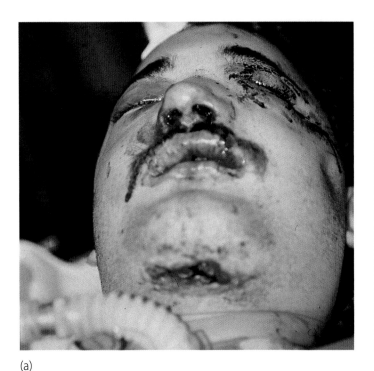

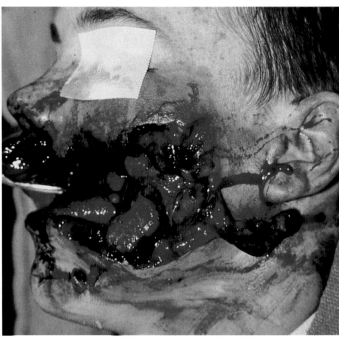

(a)   (b)

Fig. 20.2: Differences in facial damage caused by two different bullet types that travel at roughly the same velocity at roughly the same distance from the face at firing. **(a)** .38 caliber handgun. **(b)** 20 gauge shotgun.

diameter of up to 10 cm, causing the greatest harm of any small arm[2] (Fig. 20.2).

What makes the face unique in most gunshot injuries is that an unimpeded through-and-through bullet wound occurs only in the minority of cases. The facial bones make up much of the volume of the face and bone is almost always struck within 1–2 cm of entering any facial area. This anatomic difference from the trunk and extremities accounts for two distinct considerations in evaluating and treating gun wounds to the face. As the resultant damage caused by projectiles is a function of tissue density (decreased elasticity), facial bones when hit suffer significant damage as they have the second highest specific gravity of any body tissue (exceeded only by the enamel of teeth). Second, when bullets entering the face hit bone, they deform or yaw. Yaw causes them to change direction, altering their original straight path. Yawing deformed bullets are unpredictable in their path but nonetheless produce a large temporary cavity and damage more tissue. (Fig. 20.3). Such behavior demands that a thorough search for potential injury be made of all craniofacial areas, not just the structures between the entrance wound and the exit site, if an exit site exists at all (Fig. 20.4).

Wound Classification

Certain patterns of facial injury due to penetrating missiles have been reported in the literature over the past decade. These are based on either the path of the missile (entrance and exit wound) or the pattern of tissue injury/loss that occurs. The four general patterns of involvement for gunshot wounds have been described as the frontal cranium, the orbit, the lower midface and the mandible (Fig. 20.5). The location of the exit wound provides a rough guide to the pattern,

which is most accurately predicted by the location of the entrance and exit wounds. In general, skin and bone complications are less severe in the upper face and cranial area. In the lower face, greater comminution of fractures and damage to intraoral lining is present.[3]

More clinically useful is an appreciation of the zones of facial tissue injury and tissue loss based on the patterns of gunshot wounds. These include the central face, the lateral mandible, the lateral midface and orbit, and the lateral cranium and orbit (Fig. 20.6). In each case, a wide zone of hard and soft tissue injury surrounds a smaller zone of actual

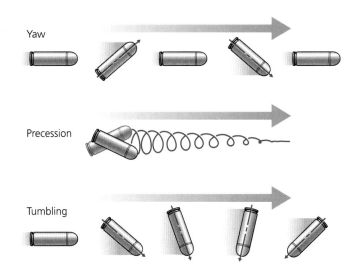

Yaw

Precession

Tumbling

Fig. 20.3: Different variations in the motion of bullets which lead to greater tissue damage. These are usually caused by striking facial bones after entering the skin and can radically change their straight-line course through the face.

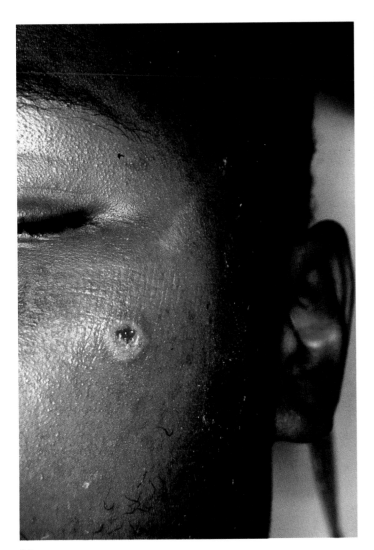

(a)

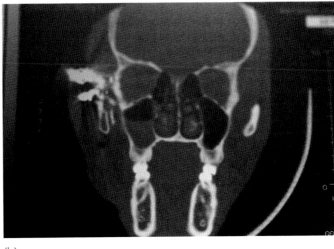

(b)

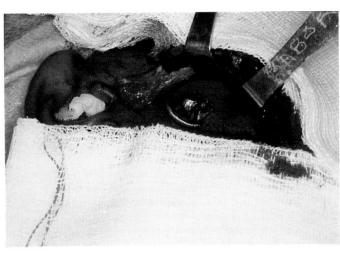

(c)

Fig. 20.4: Dramatic change of bullet path by striking facial bone. Patient was shot on one side of the face (malar area) and the bullet ended up on same side of the face (temporal area). **(a)** Left malar entrance site. **(b)** Axial CT image of left temporal location of bullet. **(c)** Location of bullet in left temporal area which was removed due to masticatory pain.

hard and soft tissue loss. The important point is to appreciate that the zone of injury is more expansive than that of tissue loss and must be factored into the reconstructive plan.

State-of-the-Art Management

Principles

The historic approach to the early management of ballistic injuries to the face included multiple debridements, daily dressing changes and delayed reconstruction. This was fostered and appeared rational based on the rate of complications which developed when early reconstruction was undertaken which included infection, wound breakdown with necrosis and ultimate collapse of the reconstructed facial segments. The application of craniofacial surgical and diagnostic techniques has revolutionized the management of blunt facial injuries but will still frequently fail in the gunshot facial wound if the fundamental differences between these two types of facial injuries are not appreciated. Recognition

of the absence of tissue and the devascularized, compromised quality of some of the remaining hard and soft facial tissues is paramount in choosing the appropriate reconstructive techniques as well as the timing of their application.

The facial gunshot wound, first and foremost, must be controlled by debridement of necrotic non-viable tissue, elimination and/or evacuation of hematoma or infection, obliteration of dead space with vascularized tissue and the recreation of adequate skin and mucosal lining.[1] In addition to understanding this most important conceptual approach, the initial management of facial gunshot wounds should take into account several basic principles based on the combination of the unique anatomy of the face and the behavior of penetrating missiles.

Treat the wound, not the weapon

The exact gun type and circumstances that caused the facial wound, while of interest, do not guide or alter one's subsequent surgical management. Victims as well as ob-

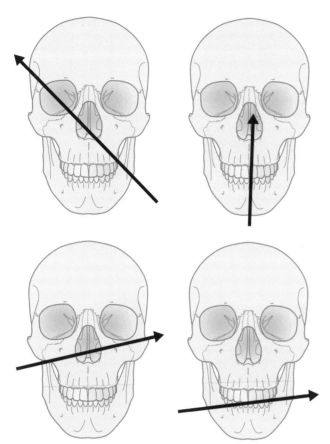

Fig. 20.5: General patterns of facial gunshot wounds. These include the frontal cranium, the orbit, the midface and the mandible. The locations of the entrance and exit wounds are a rough guide as to the type of pattern (adapted from Clark N, Birely B, Robertson B et al 1996 Plast Reconstr Surg 98:583–601).

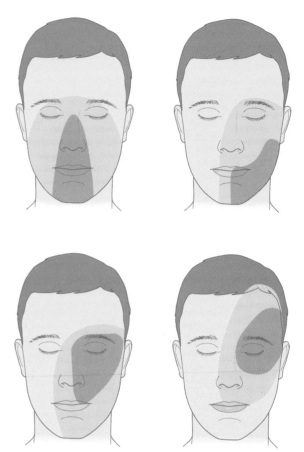

Fig. 20.6: Zones of facial involvement based on the pattern of the facial gunshot wound. These include the central face (upper left), the lateral face and mandible (upper right), the midface and orbit (lower right) and the orbit and skull (lower right). Zones of tissue loss (entrance/exit wounds) are blacked out and surrounding zone of tissue injury has diagonal lines (adapted from Clark N, Birely B, Robertson B et al 1996 Plast Reconstr Surg 98:583–601).

servers of gunshot wounds are unreliable and frequently misrepresent many of the events of the shooting, particularly the type of weapon and distance of fire. Focus on the facial damage present and do not concern yourself with the details of the gun. The only gun specific that really matters is whether it was a single bullet or multiple pellet firearm. The facial wound itself, however, usually makes this obvious. Much is made of whether the penetrating missile is high or low velocity but this does not usually change the required treatment.

The primary care of facial gunshot wounds follows basic trauma resuscitation

In significant injuries where facial tissue damage is severe, management of the airway is of supreme importance. Intubation, or preferably tracheostomy, should be liberally done. In addition to solving issues of early airway patency and obstructive bleeding, the need for numerous subsequent reconstructive procedures is facilitated. Oral and nasal intubation often hinders proper access for the reconstruction, even when done many months later. Keeping a tracheostomy or feeding tube in place for up to 1 year after the injury in severe facial tissue loss is not uncommon. Patients tolerate airway and feeding tubes well and they do not preclude breathing around the tracheostomy tube or orally feeding between reconstructive surgeries.

Provide adequate antibiotic coverage in the immediate injury state

A bullet is not sterilized by being fired. Penetrating projectiles carry bacteria into the wound. When combined with the presence of devitalized tissues and open wounds, a near ideal bacterial culture medium may exist that can overcome even the superior blood supply of the face. Group A β-hemolytic streptococcus and clostridia have been historically reported from battlefield gunshot wounds but have been nearly eliminated since the development of antibiotics since World War II. A broad-spectrum cephalosporin or penicillinase-resistant antibiotic should be given. Subsequent surgeries are obviously covered as one would for any other facial reconstructive procedure.

A high level of suspicion for vascular injury should exist

By definition, most facial gunshot wounds are classified as being in either zone II (between the cricoid cartilage and mandibular angle) or zone III (between the mandibular angle and the skull base). Vascular injury in this zone may be obscure and not easily diagnosed by clinical examination. CT evaluation is especially helpful for assessment of major vessels as well as the cranial and orbital contents. When in doubt, consider carotid angiography.

Initial surgical treatment should be in the operating room with minimal debridement and as much primary closure as possible

After patient stabilization, the patient should be taken to the operating room as soon as possible. This permits a thorough wound exploration and determines what type of reconstruction will be subsequently needed. At this time, the following can be accomplished:

- removal of loose teeth and bone
- removal of obvious bullet fragments but do not dissect and retrieve fragments that lie deep
- debride only obviously non-viable tissue
- irrigate copiously with saline
- close as much soft tissue as possible, going from the inside out
- stabilize facial bones by either direct plate and screw fixation and maxillomandibular fixation if enough teeth and jaw structures are present or use an external mandibular or cranial halo (midface) fixator if large bone segments lack continuity and are flail segments.

Plan for early reconstruction, when possible, and think tissue replacement

This is the cornerstone of contemporary reconstruction of large facial defects. Early replacement of missing hard and soft tissue deficits provides the best long-term results. Until recently, treatment consisted of initial wound debridement, packing of extensive defects and serial dressing changes followed by subsequent surgical debridement procedures until soft tissue closure could be achieved. Concerns about contamination and lack of reliability of local tissues were overriding themes. It is now clear that there is no facial advantage to allowing the wound to heal by secondary intention or skin grafting open wounds prior to initiating reconstruction. The historic approach allows a tremendous amount of scar formation and contracture to occur, making the formal reconstruction attempts much more difficult and often ending up in partial or patchwork results. Facial tissue should be replaced as soon as the patient is stable and the margins of wound viability are clear.[5] Neurologic and ophthalmologic injuries may frequently cause the initial reconstruction to be delayed but often it can still be performed within the first weeks after the injury. A pre-reconstructive CT scan, preferably 3D, can be very informative as to the extent of missing bone.[6]

This contemporary approach employs the liberal use of microvascular tissue transfers to replace missing bone, oral lining and cutaneous cover, often in a single operation. While a single free flap alone cannot provide the complete facial reconstruction, it does introduce healthy, unscarred tissue which can be manipulated in subsequent procedures.

Reconstructive Flap Options

The concept of early tissue replacement in extensive traumatic facial wounds is very similar to the reconstruction of facial defects from oncologic resection. The knowledge of a variety of tissue flaps, some of which must be transferred as free tissue and others as pedicled in design, provides very powerful reconstructive options that permit early facial intervention. These include flaps composed of free bone with or without a skin paddle, free fasciocutaneous, free muscular and pedicled fasciocutaneous options. Several superb texts are available on this topic that provide detailed descriptions of the entire scope of tissue flap anatomy and the reader is referred to these for descriptive detail and operative guidance.[20] The following flap options are not meant to be all-inclusive but describe those flaps that are commonly used for the majority of facial gunshot wounds.

Free fibular flap

The fibula is the longest bone which can be transferred by microsurgical techniques. It is often described as an ideal mandibular replacement in terms of bony stock but this is not entirely accurate. It has very similar cross-sectional thickness but lacks adequate vertical height, usually less than half of a normal dentate mandible. Its available length, up to 24 cm, does allow it to be used for long bone defects. The pedicle is large and very reliable and septocutaneous branches make a significant skin paddle possible. It is a truly expendable long bone with little donor morbidity other than an external scar if properly harvested.

Fibular transfer depends upon the endosteal and periosteal blood supplies from the peroneal artery. The endosteal circulation is supplied through a nutrient artery which typically enters the middle third of the fibula. The pedicle of the peroneal artery is actually fairly short, usually about 6–8 cm at best. A single central artery with a diameter of 2–3 mm is surrounded by two venae comitantes. In addition to the nutrient and periosteal vessels to the fibula, the peroneal artery gives off multiple branches to all of the surrounding muscles of the leg and to the lateral leg skin. There are 2–6 cutaneous perforating branches of the peroneal artery which travel along the posterior crural septum and through the soleus and flexor hallucis longus muscles. They supply a longitudinally oriented area of skin which can be raised as a septofasciocutaneous flap with the central axis along the posterior crural septum (Fig. 20.7**a**).

The fibular free flap is most commonly used for mandibular reconstruction, particularly of the symphysis and angle where osteotomies may be required to provide a three-dimensional reconstruction. When used with a skin paddle, it offers replacement of the external skin, lip or lining of the buccal mucosa or floor of the mouth[7,8] (Fig. 20.7b,c). When only a small amount of bone is needed, such as in reconstruction of the anterior maxilla, a long vascular pedicle can be created by using the more distal end of the bone.

Free scapular flap

The scapular flap has gained utility over the past decade as it provides good bone stock with a large pedicle that is long and relatively easy to find. The circumflex scapular pedicle is a branch of the subscapular system with a pedicle length of 5–6 cm and vessel diameters up to 2.5 mm. There is direct vascular connection between the circumflex scapular artery and the periosteum of the scapula, which makes osseous transfer possible. The lateral border of the scapula provides a 10–14 cm segment of straight bone located between the glenoid fossa and the tip of the scapula.[9] The lateral inferior axillary border of the scapula also receives a periosteal pedicle (angular) from a branch of the thoracodorsal artery and associated venae comitantes. If the thoracodorsal branch is included with the circumflex scapular pedicle, a second vascularized bone segment may be designed with the scapular flap.[10] The overlying soft tissue can be harvested with the bone transfer either with or without the overlying skin. The skin is thick, hairless and with only a thin layer of subcutaneous fat, which is usually advantageous in the face. The donor site can be closed primarily, even when a skin paddle is used, and the back scar is often wide but acceptable. One of its most significant advantages is in the wide arc of movement between the skin paddle and the osseous portion of the flap which is due to the differing transverse (skin paddle) and descending branches (bone) of the circumflex scapular pedicle (Fig. 20.8).

The scapular region also provides an excellent source of vascularized fasciocutaneous tissue which was used long before its potential for bone transfer was recognized. The soft tissue is based on the horizontal or descending branch of the circumflex scapular artery either in a horizontal (scapular) or vertically oriented (parascapular) design. This provides thin pliable tissue, up to 10 cm in width with skin attached, or larger when only the fascial component is required.

The one disadvantage to the scapular flap is the necessity to have significant arm rotation to properly visualize and dissect the pedicle through the triangular space. This precludes a two-team approach with simultaneous flap elevation and facial recipient site preparation.

The scapular free flap has been described for both mandibular and maxillary bone reconstruction. It is a good choice when a straight piece of bone is required. The use of a skin paddle with bone makes it useful for a variety of composite defects about the orofacial and orbitomaxillary regions. The use of its fascial or fasciocutaneous component alone provides an excellent source of vascularized soft tissue fill.

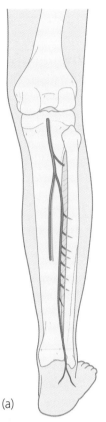

(a)

Fig. 20.7: Fibular free flap. **(a)** Peroneal blood supply. **(b)** Large segments of mandible can be replaced which requires multiple osteotomies and shaping of the fibula. **(c)** The need for shorter bone lengths creates a longer vascular pedicle by using the distal end.

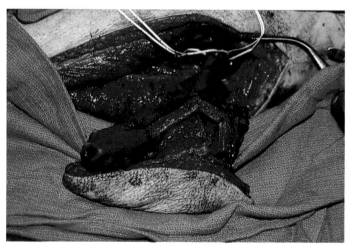

(b)

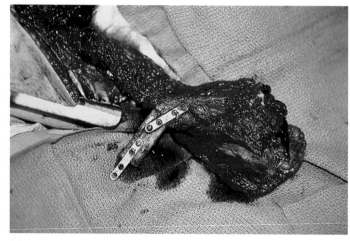

(c)

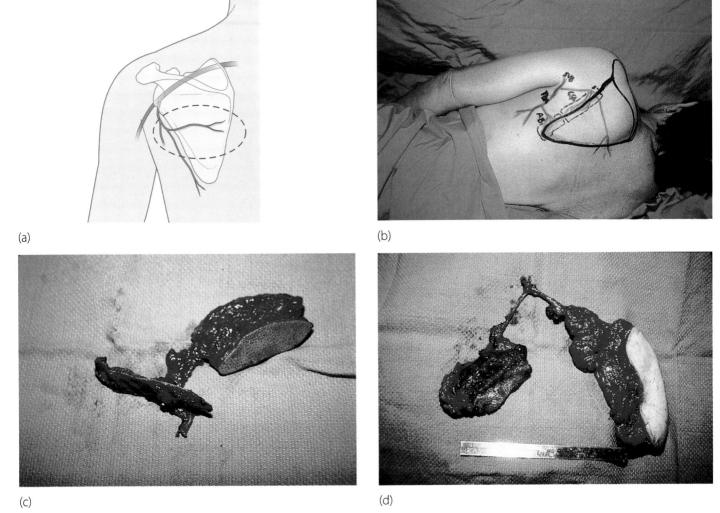

(a)

(b)

(c)

(d)

Fig. 20.8: Scapular free flap. **(a,b)** Subscapular blood supply with two distinct branches to the lateral border of the scapula. **(c)** Lateral scapular bone graft with skin island (common scapular artery). **(d)** Bipedicled design with the inferior edge of the scapula based on the ascending branch.

Free radial flap

The radial forearm provides a potentially large, thin fasciocutaneous free flap on the ventral surface of the forearm. While historically described as a useful osteocutaneous flap, the radius is a poor source of good bone stock and places the donor bone at a significant risk of postoperative fracture. If bone is needed, other free flap options such as the fibula or scapula are usually better. Therefore, the forearm should be restricted to a source of thin soft tissue only.

Almost all or any part of the skin and fascia extending from the antecubital fossa to the wrist may be elevated based on the radial artery and its septocutaneous branches. The more distal the skin flap is designed, the longer the pedicle will be. The radial artery is of good size (2.5 mm), has a very consistent anatomy and courses between the bellies of the brachioradialis and pronator teres in the upper forearm and between the tendons of the brachioradialis and flexor carpi radialis in the lower forearm. Most of the septocutaneous-fasciocutaneous branches are in the distal half of the radial artery and are easily identified emerging from the intermuscular septum, which must be preserved during harvest, at the radial border of the flexor carpi radialis muscle[11] (Fig. 20.9).

The radial forearm flap has numerous advantages as a soft tissue source including a large amount of thin tissue, a long and large pedicle and ease of harvest. These qualities make it particularly well suited for lining of intraoral defects or external skin cover.[12] However, the harvest of a flap from an extremity requires several precautions to avoid significant donor site complications. It is absolutely essential that the inflow to the hand be preoperatively evaluated with an Allen's test to confirm that circulation through the ulnar artery is sufficent for survival of the hand. This should also be reconfirmed during the flap dissection by placing a microvascular clamp distally and releasing the tourniquet prior to division of the radial artery. The peritenon covering the tendons of the flexor carpi radialis, brachioradialis and finger flexors must be preserved to avoid skin graft failure and possible loss of the tendons postoperatively.

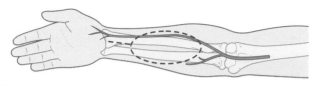

(a)

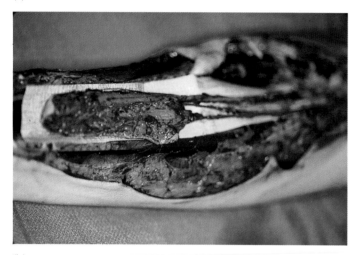

(b)

Fig. 20.9: Radial forearm flap. **(a)** Radial blood supply. **(b)** Thin fasciocutaneous components of the flap (turned over).

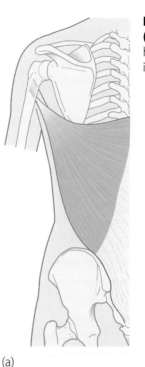

Fig. 20.10: Latissimus dorsi flap. **(a)** Muscle location. **(b)** Size of muscle harvested through a lateral thoracic incision.

(a)

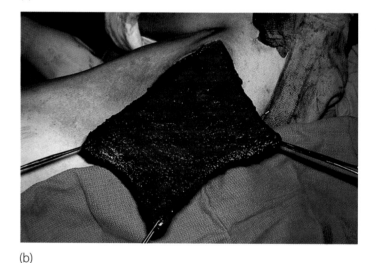

(b)

Free latissimus flap

The latissimus dorsi is a large, flat, triangular muscle that offers the largest source of well-vascularized soft tissue in the body, measuring up to 25 × 35 cm in size. Its tendon attaches to the humerus proximally with broad attachments to the lower thoracic and sacral vertebrae, posterior iliac crest and the external abdominal muscles. While it is responsible for adduction, extension and rotation of the humerus, it is a completely expendable muscle in most patients as long as they have intact synergistic shoulder girdle musculature. Its dominant pedicle is the thoracodorsal artery and venae comitantes which is a major branch off the subscapular. The thoracodorsal pedicle (2.5 mm in vessel size) offers reasonable length, around 8 cm, but this can be significantly extended if the distal portion of the muscle is the only tissue required. A reliable, large skin paddle can also be obtained as there are extensive vascular communications to the overlying back skin.[13] When a skin paddle is taken, the donor site can almost always be primarily closed. While rotation of the muscle into the head and neck area can be done around the axilla and tunneling on top of the pectoralis muscle, it will only extend to the lower face and may suffer potential compromise by compression of the overlying tissues. It is of far greater utility when transferred as a free microvascular flap (Fig. 20.10).

The latissimus dorsi free flap has numerous applications in reconstruction of the face. It has been equally applied to the midface as well as the mandible over the past 20 years with great reliability.[14] Its wide muscular expanse makes it uniquely suited for extensive scalp replacement and calvarial coverage when combined with skin grafting. The reliability of its skin paddle can provide for reconstruction of large defects of external skin cover, particularly those of the lateral face. The patient position necessary for harvest does make it difficult for a simultaneous two-team approach but the speed at which the flap can be raised makes this of little significance.

Free rectus flap

The paired, vertically oriented rectus muscles of the abdomen provide another reliable donor source for vascularized tissue. This long flat muscle, measuring about 6 cm in width and 25 cm in length, is easy to harvest due to its constant anatomy and can be done simultaneously with facial work as a two-team approach. It lies within an anterior and posterior fascial sheath and its dissection is only complicated by the release of the tenacious attachments of three sets of horizontal inscriptions. While having dual dominant pedicles, the inferior

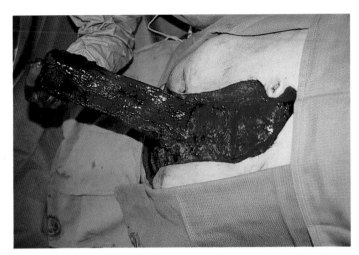

Fig. 20.11: Rectus muscle flap. This is the muscle raised on the superior pedicle which is not used for for free tissue transfer (inferior pedicle). The length and width of the muscle can be appreciated, however.

epigastric is always used due to its larger size, longer length and easier dissection. Entering at the underside of the lateral surface of the muscle, the inferior epigastric is about 2.5 mm in diameter with a fairly short pedicle length of around 4–5 cm.[15] The length of the muscle usually makes the usable pedicle length 'longer' than that of the actual vessels. A vertical or horizontally oriented skin paddle can be taken but this is rarely used in facial reconstruction. The donor site, even if a skin paddle is taken, can always be primarily closed. Previous abdominal surgery with any horizontal scar across the rectus territory will preclude its use.

The musculocutaneous territories supplied by the inferior epigastric have their greatest use in breast reconstruction, but also have significant value in a variety of head and neck sites.

When combined with a skin graft, it can be used for outer cover of scalp and skull defects[16] as well as vascularized fill for a wide variety of lower facial wounds. The long length of the muscle rarely makes its short pedicle length a problem (Fig. 20.11). However, extending the pedicle into the neck for anastomosis requires a very wide subcutaneous tunnel to avoid postoperative venous congestion of the flap.

Free serratus flap

The free serratus flap provides a very long pedicled musculofascial flap that has excellent utility for facial applications.[17] Its long pedicle (15–20 cm) combined with the length of muscle and fascia can easily reach the midface when anastomosed into the neck. It can be raised with both skin and muscle but the amount of rib obtained is usually not sufficient for most facial reconstructive needs. The serratus is a thin broad muscle that originates from the outer surface of ribs 8 and 9 and inserts on the ventral surface of the scapula. It has a dual blood supply from both the lateral thoracic artery and branches of the thoracodorsal artery. Most commonly, it is based on the thoracodorsal branch as it emanates from the undersurface of the latissimus dorsi as it is easier to elevate. It has very predictable anatomy and is easy to identify and dissect out between the lateral borders of the latissimus and pectoralis muscles, tracing the pedicle up into the axilla (Fig. 20.12).

Pedicled forehead flap

The median forehead flap is primarily used for nasal coverage and reconstruction. The forehead is the single best source of external nasal skin replacement with similar color and thickness as those of the nose. The supratrochlear vessels are the dominant pedicle and supply the entire central forehead skin, including the frontalis, corrugator and procerus. These vessels are a terminal branch of the ophthalmic artery, are 1 mm in size and have a short 1–2 cm pedicle length. Since this a rotational flap, these vessel dimensions are of no significance

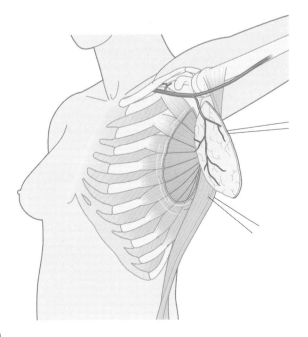

(a)

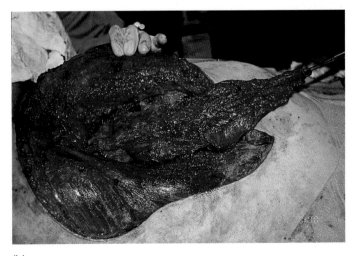

(b)

Fig. 20.12: Serratus muscle flap. **(a)** Thoracodorsal blood supply of the serratus muscle. **(b)** The muscle can be long and narrow with a very long vascular pedicle.

other than to appreciate that it emerges over the supraorbital rim deep to the frontalis and may easily be injured during dissection of the flap. The supraorbital vessels are a minor pedicle but should be preserved if possible. The base of the flap can be fairly narrow compared to the distal end and may be skeletonized down to the vessels to aid the 180° of flap rotation that is usually required. The flap length is determined by the height of the frontal hair line and at least 7–8 cm is usually necessary to cover the most distal nasal defects. With low hair lines, an oblique flap orientation will improve flap length.

In extensive defects involving the nasal tip, columella and upper lip, a 'gull-wing' design at the distal end of the flap design is often used.[18] In large nasal defects, tissue expansion of the flap itself should be avoided due to unfavorable postoperative contraction. Preoperative tissue expansion lateral to the flap, however, can aid greatly in donor site closure[19] (Fig. 20.13).

Regional Considerations

Central face

Lower face and mandible

The lower face and mandible is the most frequently affected area in severe gunshot wounds, usually due to their self-inflicted nature. This typical injury is produced when the patient fires under the chin with the neck hyperextended (Fig. 20.14). In this manner, only the anterior lower and midface is blown off, ending commonly in a non-lethal injury. Usually the lateral mandible with the attached masseter and temporalis muscles are sufficiently posterior and internal that they will be spared and continue to provide excursion to the lower jaw. The loss of the anterior mandible and lip and their

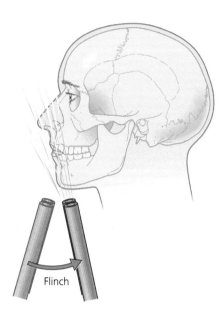

Fig. 20.14: Classic angle of gunshot impact from a self-inflicted injury. The flinch makes it a non-lethal wound but often eliminates much of the anterior facial structures.

Flinch

importance in breathing, speech and mastication make destruction of this orofacial region a serious functional handicap. The functional abnormalities may be further aggravated if significant damage has occurred to the tongue and surrounding muscles that are attached to the anterior mandible. Bony reconstruction of the anterior mandible helps provide a stable suspension of the hyocervical musculature while soft tissue reconstruction of the lip and chin allows oral continence to be restored. If significant tongue muscle is lost or severe scarring has occurred on the floor of the mouth, the dynamic nature of this soft tissue complex will sorely be missed and can only poorly, if at all, be replaced or reconstructed. At best, we can only currently replace the lining defect and possibly provide a mechanical dam that can aid in speech and deglutition in these circumstances.

The reconstruction of this submental injury includes restoring the continuity of the three major components which are usually lost, namely the lining, bony structures and external cover. During the first procedure after the initial injury, obvious devitalized soft tissue should be debrided and bony stabilization of the flailed lateral mandibular segments carried out. This can be done with a reconstruction plate (preferably) or an external fixator. It is perfectly acceptable to have the reconstruction plate exposed in the immediate postoperative period as the chin tissues may be missing. This poses no significant increase in the risk of infection and its exposure will shortly be remedied by a free flap reconstruction. We prefer this to an external fixator as this creates additional scarring in the uninjured lateral facial skin and is usually in the way for the placement of the free flap and neck microvascular anastomoses.

Almost always, the use of free vascularized bone for anterior mandibular reconstruction is desired as the second stage of reconstruction. This may follow the initial debridement and stabilization as soon as the patient is able. Often this can be within the first 10–14 days of hospital admission. Even in small segmental bone loss (less than 6 cm), vascularized bone offers numerous advantages over any other method. It can be performed immediately and regardless of the amount of soft

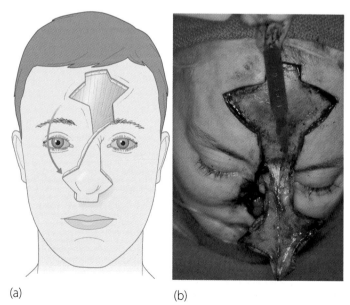

(a)   (b)

Fig. 20.13: Median forehead flap. **(a)** Maximal flap design of forehead flap. **(b)** Raising of the flap design based on the supratrochlear vessels (red arrow).

tissue present, it does not rely on surrounding tissue vascularity for survival, it does not disturb other local anatomy and can offer a single-stage solution to the tissue loss problem. Bone donor options are essentially three: radius, scapula and fibula. The fibula is preferred as it has ample bone, a long pedicle of good vessel caliber (particularly if only the distal portion is used), can be shaped to some degree by selective osteotomies and is fairly easy to harvest as its anatomy is consistent with no significant postoperative morbidity. The radius has much thinner bone in more limited quality

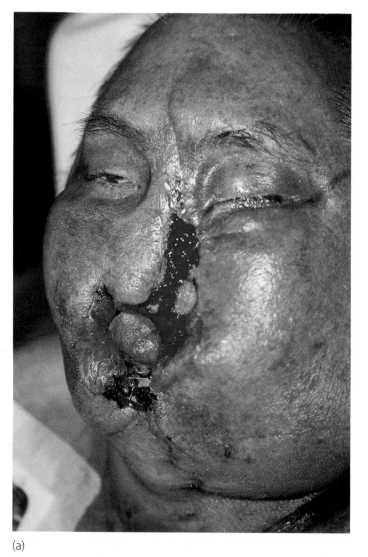

(a)

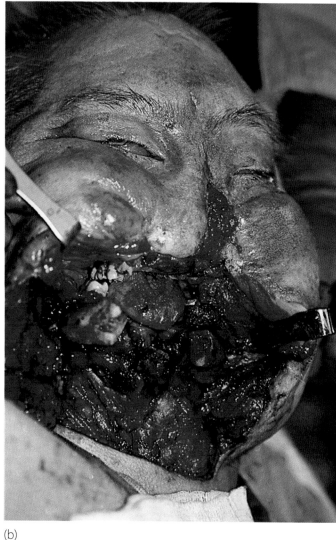

(b)

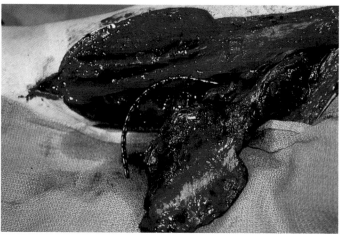

(c)

Fig. 20.15: Free fibular flap reconstruction of composite lower facial defect secondary to self-inflicted gunshot wound.
(a) Patient transferred in with loss of mid- and lower facial structures; the mandibular defects had a spanning reconstruction plate in place. **(b)** Lower facial defect exposed and 'old' reconstruction plate removed. **(c)** Fibular donor site with composite flap with bone osteotomized and shaped according to a template from a new reconstruction plate.

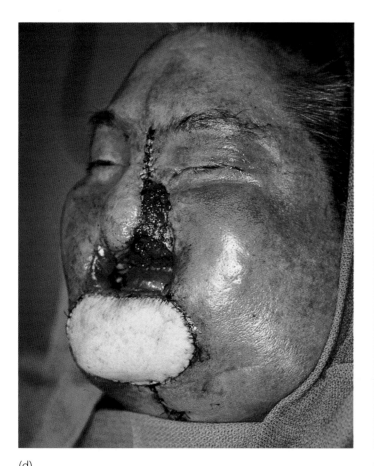

(d)

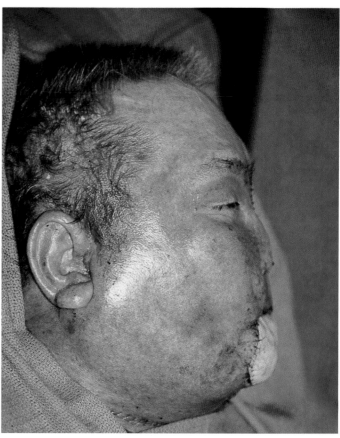

(e)

Fig. 20.15: (d) Frontal view of free fibular flap in position with leg skin used for chin/submental skin replacement. The skin color and texture never match and this has to be accepted. **(e)** Lateral view of reconstruction.

and creates a very noticeable donor site. The scapula is also an excellent source of vascularized bone but can be more difficult to harvest and precludes simultaneous work on the face and back due to positioning needs (Fig. 20.15).

Repairing the lining deficit is often ignored or not considered important but is a frequent cause of late functional disturbances. The loss of lining between the lip and anterior mandible is usually the greatest and poses great problems in the long-term stability of any reconstructed vertical lip height as well as a pliable separation from the alveolus where dental restoration must be done and hygienically maintained. In theory, elevation and rotation of surrounding oral and buccal mucosa can provide some coverage. In reality, these flaps look good in drawings but cannot reach the midline and often do not survive after transfer. The use of tongue flaps is appealing as they can easily be drawn up over a reconstruction plate or anterior bony reconstruction but should be avoided as they lead to speech and deglutition problems and induce the potential for future restriction in tongue mobility. For these reasons, the skin paddle of a vascularized bone transfer offers a versatile and robust fascial and skin composite reconstruction. All of the commonly used free bone flaps previously described can be composite flaps with fascia and skin if desired.

Midface

The midface is often impacted obliquely from an inferior etiology due to a submentally directed gunshot injury. It is rare that a direct midface impact is seen as this is often a lethal injury (Fig. 20.16). Thus, these wounds are frequently

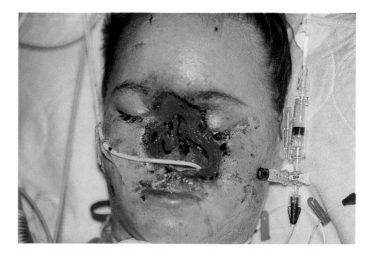

Fig. 20.16: Midfacial avulsion secondary to being struck by a flying tire cleat from a racecar which struck the wall. Such a non-lethal but composite midfacial avulsion injury is very rare.

part of a concomitant pattern of tissue loss which includes the anterior mandible, lip and chin as well as the upper lip, anterior maxilla and nose.

Such injuries to the midface are the most difficult of all facial injuries to reconstruct because of the shape and contour of the component parts. Many small and delicate bone and soft tissue elements are present, as are a labyrinth of air spaces, cavities and canals. Lining of these delicate structures can, at times, be an impossible task. While the lining of the upper aerodigestive tract can fill in rather quickly with granulation tissue from neighboring areas, this leads to collapse of the overlying soft tissue and complete obliteration of nasal breathing and sinus drainage. The presence of these air-filled cavities throughout the midface also imposes an increased risk of postoperative infection and makes it very difficult to build anatomical structures on top of such cavities. These reconstructive efforts are finally complicated by the prominent position of the midface with the protruding and individualized nose which is such an important element in the recognition of one's face.

The typical gunshot wound creates a cone of injury which, after cautious debridement, leaves a large central facial defect without support. In smaller defects where the soft tissue loss is limited, immediate reconstruction with free bone grafts and local coverage can be done. However, this is usually the exceptional case. Most of these defects have significant tissue loss that makes this approach impractical. Even those midfacial defects that appear small will almost always be missing important lining of either the mouth or nose which is certain to ultimately compromise any 'limited' approach. The absence of lining and the presence of the sinuses and open communication with the mouth and nose make it mandatory to both control the wound and replace lining and bone. This is best done simultaneously, or through various stages, with vascularized tissue.

In smaller facial gunshot wounds, the entrance wound is usually more diminutive than the amount of internal hard and soft tissue loss. In these cases, the nose is often mercifully spared and the defect is primarily intraoral. The thin bone of the maxilla and the tight tissue of the alveolus and vestibule make transfer of any local tissue difficult. The use of vascularized fibula works well for the replacement of missing maxilla (Fig. 20.17). It offers a long pedicle which is ideal to reach the neck vessels by tunneling subcutaneously from the facial wound into the neck. A skin paddle is usually not necessary as the muscle cuff on the fibular bone will rapidly become covered with mucosa (Fig. 20.17**d**). When more lining is needed, a skin paddle of more than adequate dimensions can be carried with the bone although this is often quite bulky in the limited confines of the midface and mouth. This bone also provides excellent bone stock into which endosseous implants can be eventually placed (Fig. 20.17**f**).

In moderate tissue loss from midfacial gunshot wounds, some portion of the upper or lower lips are usually involved or missing. This would be far more common than a midfacial injury without lip involvement. This now creates a composite midfacial wound in which the reconstruction must provide not only bone and lip replacement but also a vestibule as well. Hopefully, one lip is left relatively unaffected and ideally it would be the lower lip. This then would provide for an eventual cross-lip transfer which would be the best solution to any upper lip and vestibular problem. Reconstruction of these composite midfacial tissue losses essentially takes place in two major stages: an initial microvascular bone flap for replacement of the missing maxilla followed by a regional cross-lip transfer (Fig. 20.18). When the amount of missing upper lip is significant (>50%) or the lower lip is concomitantly damaged, lip reconstruction may have to be done by incorporating the lip replacement from the skin paddle from the microvascular transfer.

In larger midfacial defects, particularly when portions or all of the nose are missing, the provision of lining may present a tremendous challenge in reconstruction of this area. Failure to provide adequate lining may leave areas of bone exposed, increasing the chance of infection and loss of tissue; it can increase the scarring and resorption of normal cavities and overlying tissue; and it can produce unwanted retraction and contraction of the midface, which may later prove difficult to resolve. Local flaps and skin grafts may be effective in some more limited cases but the amount of lining required usually makes these a poor option.

In these cases of severe midfacial tissue loss, one should think about either vascularized obliteration of the base of the midfacial defect or extensive vascularized replacement of missing bone and soft tissue. In vascularized obliteration, the sinuses and nasal airway are replaced with vascularized muscle or fat to initially control the wound and allow it to heal (Fig. 20.19). The previous placement of a tracheostomy tube obviates any need for a patent nasal airway, in the short term anyway. This also allows bones to heal whether it be the fixation of fractures or the placement of bone grafts across the maxilla, zygoma or orbital floors or rim.

The latissimus dorsi or rectus muscles provide excellent fill of the midface but the sheer bulk of muscle mass requires that the facial skin be split for passage of the muscle and its pedicle into the neck (Fig. 20.19**c,d**). The length of pedicle needed to traverse the midface to the neck limits the number of free flap tissue options. The omentum is also an excellent choice for fill and its very pliable amorphous form allows it to fill all midfacial cavities. Its slender pedicle permits a subcutaneous tunnel to be created into the neck without a facial split. With these flaps, the risks of infection are dramatically reduced, if not nearly eliminated, and a vascularized base is established onto which the anterior maxilla, upper lip or nasal reconstruction can be based. This does not mean that a future free or pedicled flap reconstruction will still not be needed. It simply provides early control of the open facial wound until secondary facial reconstruction can be carried out (Fig. 20.20). This is particularly useful in very large facial wounds and in those patients whose mental status is not yet clear. Attempts to re-establish a nasal airway can eventually be done secondarily as the very last midfacial reconstructive procedure through the use of a nasal stent or trumpet around which a skin graft is wrapped and passed through the vascularized muscle or fat to the posterior choana.

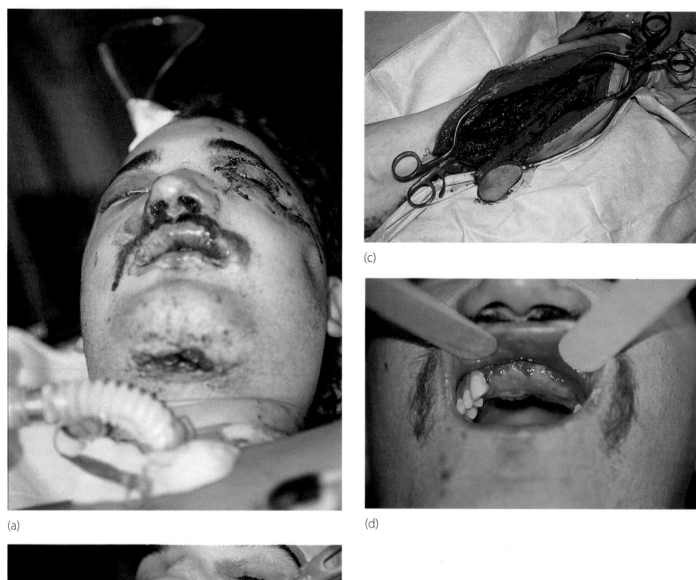

(a)

(b)

(c)

(d)

Fig. 20.17: Loss of anterior maxilla with large oronasal communication from a submentally directed handgun (.38 caliber) injury. An anterior mandibular fracture resulted but without any significant bone loss. The bullet lodged in the frontal sinus without intracranial injury. **(a)** Entrance site of bullet wound on day of injury. **(b)** Missing anterior maxilla and oronasal communication 10 days after debridement of lost bone and teeth. **(c)** Free fibular bone transfer using the very distal end of the bone and discarding the skin paddle, thus creating a very long vascular pedicle. **(d)** Three months after reconstruction with the muscle over the bone completely covered with mucosa.

In other patients, a more anatomically based free flap reconstruction of the midface can be done early. This is best done in midfacial defects that are not massive, in which the facial wounds are quite clean, the viability of adjacent tissue margins is quite clear and the mental status of the patient is more defined. Free flap reconstruction of midfacial defects often involves very clever flap designs and thought-out patterns for tissue replacement[21–23] (Fig. 20.21). Much of this has been learned from oncologic resection of the midface where one flap does not fit all defects. The composite creation of palatal/maxillary/orbital bone and soft tissue fill and/or lining requires preoperative design of the flap compo-

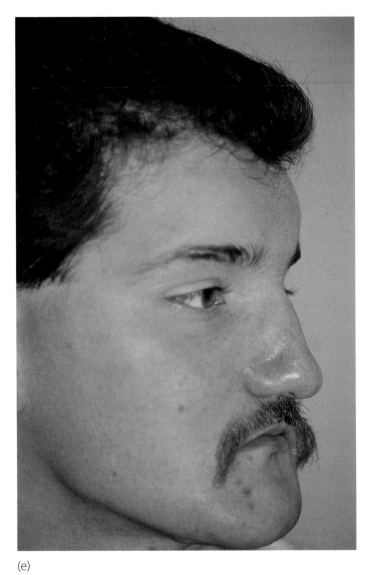

(e)

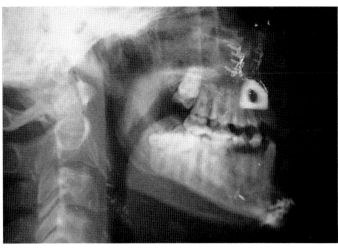

(f)

Fig. 20.17: (e) Three month postoperative lateral facial view with reasonable horizontal projection. **(f)** Two-year postoperative X-ray showing cross-section of fibular bone in the anterior maxilla.

nents which must then be properly traced out for the flap harvest. This design must be done with the location and orientation of the vascular pedicle in mind to avoid a major surprise when the tissue is transferred to the face. While no one flap can be universally applied, either scapular or fibular osteocutaneous composite flaps are most commonly used.[21] They offer adequate bone and attached soft tissue which can have a different arc of rotation from that of the bone. This is a particular asset in the scapular flap where a bipedicled flap design can be created.

The re-establishment of a nose depends on recreating a support framework of cartilage and/or bone and an external skin cover. With the severe loss of lining, the placement of these structures is highly dependent upon having a vascularized base onto which they can be placed. The rebuilding of the nasal framework is fairly straightforward and either bone or cartilage can be used to make an L-strut with lateral support (Fig. 20.22). Lateral alar support is important to prevent the eventual method of skin coverage from contracting completely around the tip of the framework. Due to decreased resorption potential, we prefer cartilage rather than bone for the majority of the framework when possible. This requires rib harvests from the free floating ninth and eighth ribs which are easy to harvest. It is important to recruit or wrap any surrounding vascularized tissue around the framework to eliminate any non-vascularized 'dead space' underneath the graft reconstruction.

The more difficult challenge is in the reconstruction of the nasal skin cover, which frequently includes portions or all of the upper lip also. In smaller defects of nasal cover, the pedicled forehead flap remains the most ideal option. It has the best color match, is fairly similar in skin texture and thickness (albeit slightly thicker in most patients) and is easy to harvest, with a very predictable survival. It frequently involves a three-stage procedure: a first-stage transfer, a second-stage separation of the pedicle weeks later and an eventual revision of the transferred tissue and/or donor site (Fig. 20.23). It is almost always available in facial gunshot wounds as the forehead is usually spared from the blast. The donor site certainly leaves a vertical scar which initially seems undesirable given that it may be one of the few esthetic facial units that has not been violated by the initial injury.

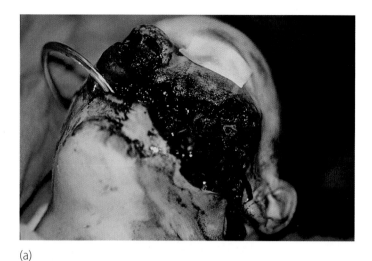

(a)

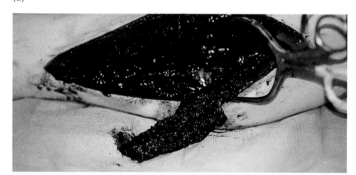

(c)

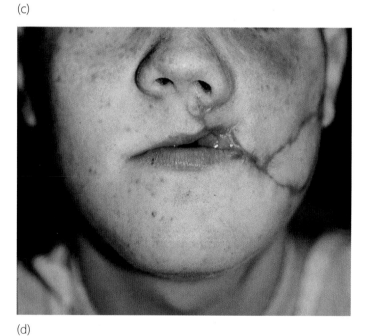

(d)

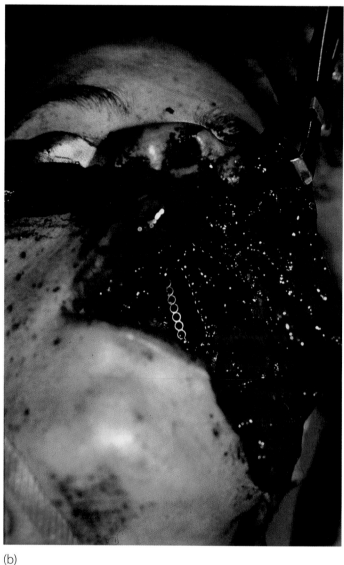

(b)

Fig. 20.18: Loss of left hard and soft tissue midfacial tissue from an accidental gunshot wound from a tangential direction. Reconstruction was done in three stages consisting of an initial debridement and bone stabilization, a second-stage microvascular bone flap and a third-stage cross-lip transfer. **(a)** Facial injury in emergency room. **(b)** First-stage debridement and stabilization of remaining maxillary segments. **(c)** Second-stage (7 days later) free fibular bone flap using only the distal end with no skin paddle. **(d)** Six months postop frontal facial view.

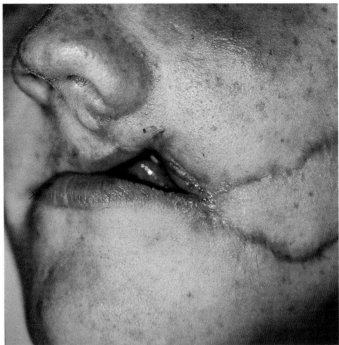

(e)

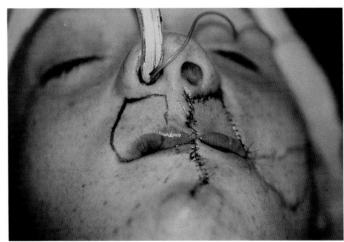

(f)

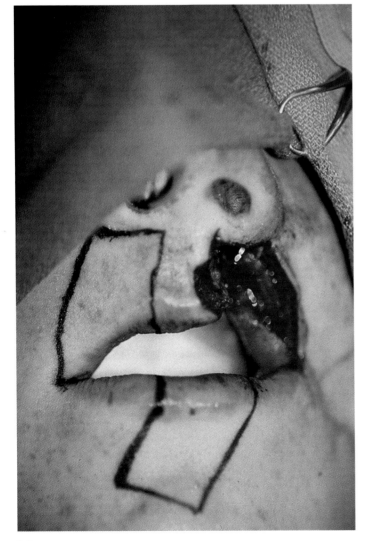

(g)

(h)

Fig. 20.18: (e) Adequate reconstruction of maxilla and coverage with mucosa. **(f)** Residual missing upper lip. **(g)** The missing upper lip segment is excised as an esthetic unit. **(h)** Intraoperative flap placement with separation of the pedicle 2 weeks later.

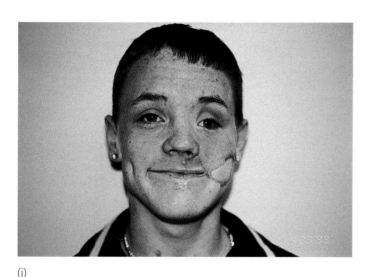
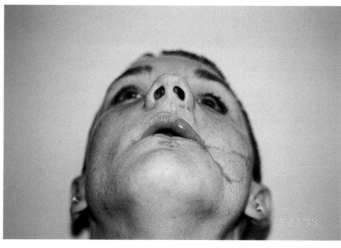

(i)   (j)

Fig. 20.18: (i) One year after injury, facial view. **(j)** Submental view 1 year after reconstruction demonstrating midfacial projection and restoration of lip contours. Further orbital and scar revision work is planned.

However, the eventual fading and blending of the scar usually looks surprisingly good, even if the forehead donor wound cannot be completely closed after harvest.

One helpful manuever is the use of tissue expansion prior to forehead flap transfer. However, this is not to create more tissue for transfer but rather to help close the midline forehead defect. Pre-expanding the forehead flap itself intuitively seems helpful but will only result in a nasal skin reconstruction that will ultimately undergo significant contraction. Tissue expanders should be placed outside the outline of the flap to expand the residual forehead tissue. This will allow a very large flap to be taken and still permit primary closure of the forehead. This is particularly useful in total nasal reconstruction. It is very important also not to forget the importance of nasal lining and coverage of the framework from an intranasal standpoint. Failure to do so will result in eventual extrusion, infection and loss of the framework.

When the need for total nasal reconstruction exists, particularly when portions of the upper lip are also missing, the amount of tissue from the forehead can be inadequate. In these circumstances, coverage of a nasal framework with a free tissue transfer is often the only option. Donor requirements are a thin fasciocutaneous or muscle flap (which will require a skin graft) and a long vascular pedicle which must reach into the neck. Minimum pedicle lengths of 12–15 cm are needed. The radial forearm fasciocutaneous free flap is probably the first choice as it best fulfills these requirements. Despite the color match and texture differences, it produces good coverage of nasal frameworks (Fig. 20.24). Multiple revisions will ultimately be necessary for shaping, contouring and the placement of nostrils if desired. Other available free flap options exist, such as serratus muscle and scapular fascial flaps, but these will require skin grafts as their cutaneous components are too large and bulky to be useful for nasal cover.

With orbital involvement, the reconstructive problems are typically either the recreation of orbital lining after enucleation due to a penetrating injury to the globe or the

secondary correction of vertical dystopia due to loss of bony support from missing floor or walls. With loss of the globe in most gunshot wounds, the eyelids are still frequently present and the issue is to provide some vascularized fill of the intraorbital space which will eventually accommodate a prosthesis. If the intraorbital defect is fairly isolated, options include either a pedicled temporalis musculofascial flap (Fig. 20.25) or a small free tissue transfer such as the radial forearm flap (see Fig. 20.24). The temporalis flap is appealing due to its proximity and ease of harvest but it only provides a limited amount of tissue fill as the very distal end of the flap is only fascia, usually only sufficient for creating lateral orbital lining. This may be enough in many cases, however, to line the orbital floor, cover bone grafts and allow a skin or mucosal graft to be placed and may provide enough vascularized lining to allow an orbital prosthesis to be made. The donor site morbidity is minimal other than the temporal scar from the coronal incision and the potential for temporal hollowing if a large amount of muscle is taken with the fascia. In larger defects or when the ipsilateral temporal region is also damaged, free vascularized tissue will be needed. The radial forearm flap can provide more than adequate soft tissue and skin for the orbit and is the preferred choice in many of these more complex orbital cases (Fig. 20.26).

In vertical dystopia, repositioning and/or reconstruction of the bony box is the main method of correction. This is usually accomplished by completely rebuilding the orbital floor and rim, best done with autologous cranial bone or alloplastic materials. Proponents exist for each method but the patient's anatomy and problem must be carefully considered. If there is good vascularized tissue around the orbit and the sinus is obliterated, any autologous or alloplastic method will likely work and will have a low infection risk. The use of titanium mesh is common as it is easily adapted and can be secured to the surrounding bone. Autologous cranial bone may or may not be combined with it although the need for bone grafting with a rigid titanium mesh that re-establishes and secures the intraorbital volume is not completely obvious.

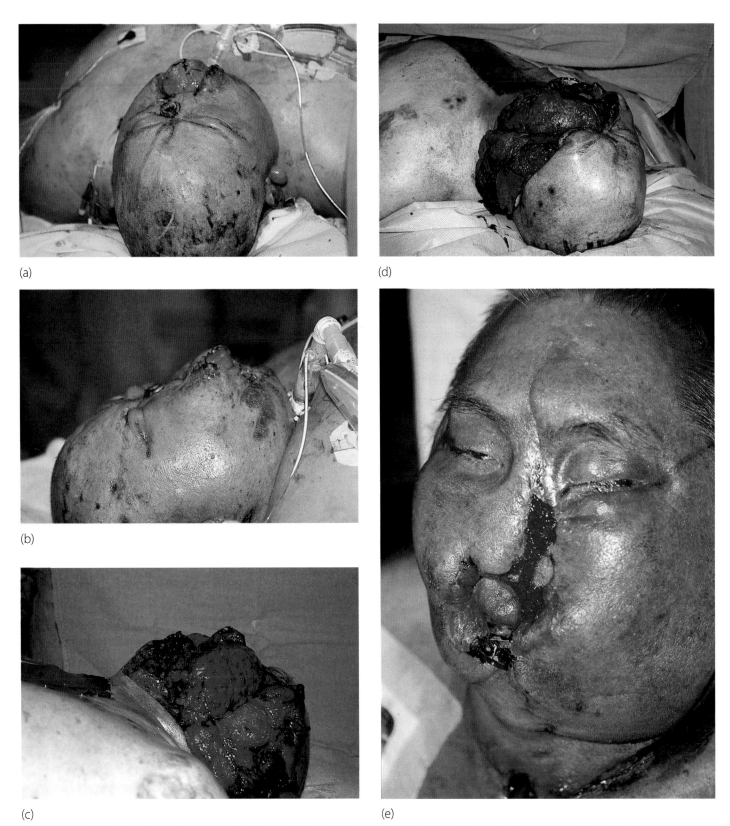

Fig. 20.19: Self-inflicted gunshot wound to face with loss of all central midfacial and lower facial structures. The patient was transferred in with a nasal trumpet in place and the skin closed around it. First-stage reconstruction was done with a vascularized muscle fill of the entire midface. **(a)** Preoperative frontal facial view. **(b)** Preoperative lateral facial view. **(c)** Facial split with latissimus muscle flap in place with vascular anastomoses in the neck. **(d)** Superior view of vascularized muscle fill of midface. **(e)** Healed midfacial wound now ready for more definitive reconstruction of the mid- and lower face.

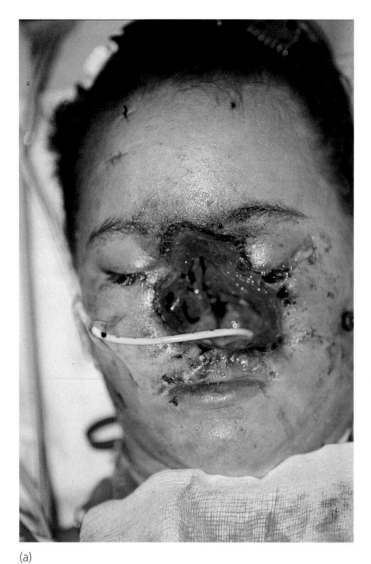

(a)

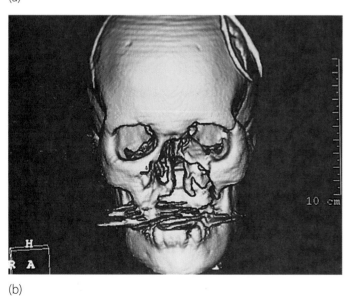

(b)

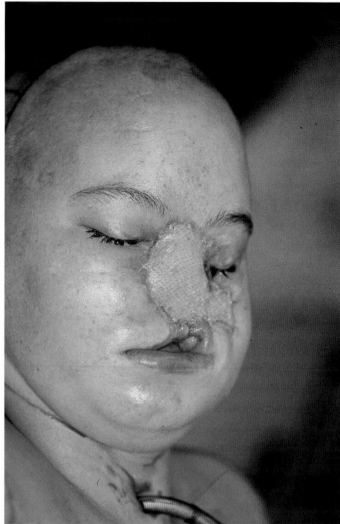

(c)

Fig. 20.20: Vascularized obliteration of midfacial avulsive defect. **(a)** Preoperative frontal facial view, Fig. 16 also. **(b)** 3D CT scan demonstrating extent of midfacial bone loss. **(c)** One month postoperative facial view with well-healed skin graft overlying the muscle flap.

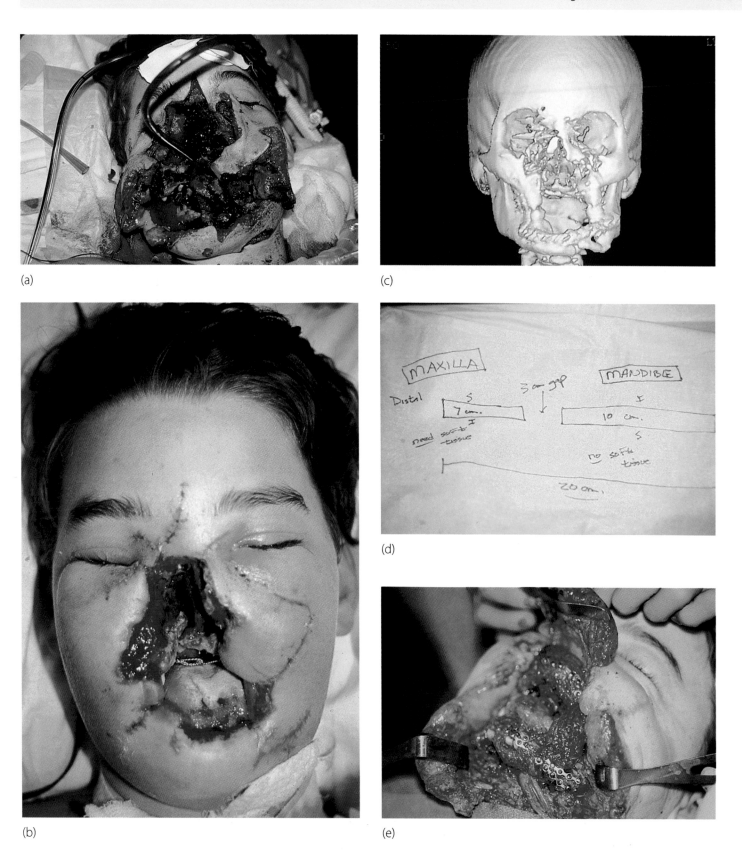

(a)

(c)

(b)

(d)

(e)

Fig. 20.21: Accidental shotgun wound to central face in a teenager initially reconstructed with a composite free flap for concomitant maxillary and mandibular reconstruction. **(a)** Appearance in emergency room. **(b)** After initial debridement and bone stabilization. **(c)** 3D CT scan demonstrating extent of midfacial bone loss. **(d)** Design of first-stage free flap reconstruction using a long fibular flap creating a bone gap in the middle so it can be turned to fill both the maxillary and mandibular defects with the skin paddle covering the external nasal skin defect. **(e)** Intraoperative flap positioning with vessels anastomosed into the neck.

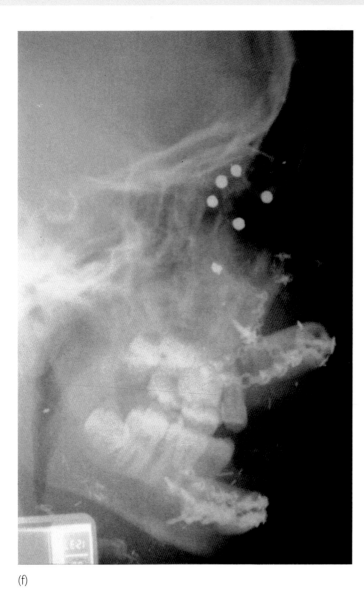

(f)

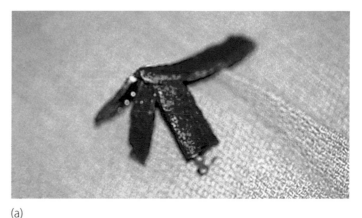

(a)

(b)

Fig. 20.22: Nasal framework reconstruction using either cranial bone **(a)** or rib cartilage **(b)**.

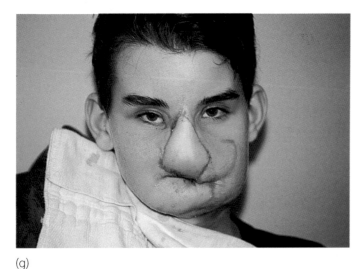

(g)

Fig. 20.21: (f) One month postoperative X-ray appearance of bone placement. **(g)** Three month postoperative facial view. The patient will still require nasal framework placement, skin shaping, and upper and lower lip reconstruction.

Bone grafting is another viable method but the amount of graft needed can often be deceiving and some form of graft fixation is still required. In orbital defects of poor tissue quality with an underlying open sinus exposure, titanium mesh is probably best as it is very well tolerated even when exposed and it will predictably maintain elevation of the globe. In certain cases where the gunshot has passed through the maxilla and obliterated the pillars, the entire orbital box may have shifted down as a result of orbitomalar displacement. In these patients, an osteotomy and repositioning, with or without bone grafting, may be done (Fig. 20.27). This would be superior to globe elevation only by floor reconstruction as it more effectively addresses the lack of malar projection and lower eyelid support.

One specific issue with orbital reconstruction in facial gunshot wounds is the frequent need for eyelid repositioning and reconstruction. As the globe elevates, the eyelid will often not follow due to scar contracture or actual loss of lid tissue. The liberal use of canthal reconstructions and release and full-thickness skin grafting to the lower lid is often needed. One should resist the temptation to simply pull up the lower eyelid through the medial or lateral canthus only, particularly if the amount of movement is significant. This will only result in postoperative ectropion. Most significant movements will require more lower eyelid tissue through the use of full-thickness skin grafting or the interposition of more tissue through a temporalis fascial flap.

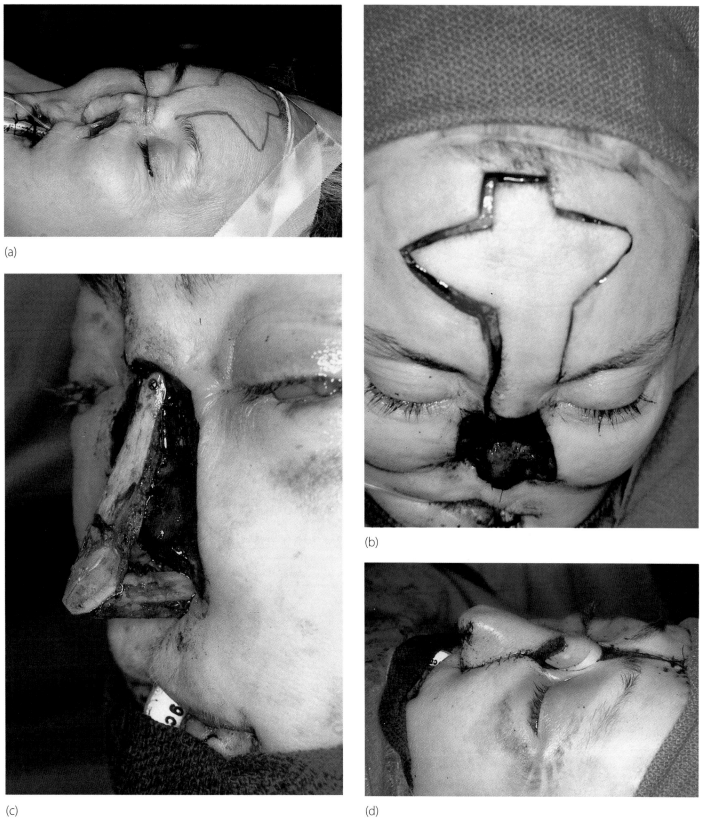

(a)

(b)

(c)

(d)

Fig. 20.23: Total nasal reconstruction with a forehead flap from loss due to a self-inflicted gunshot wound. **(a)** Preoperative appearance 6 months after the initial injury. **(b)** Forehead flap design. **(c)** Rib graft nasal framework reconstruction. **(d)** Flap coverage of the nasal framework with turning the pedicle 180°.

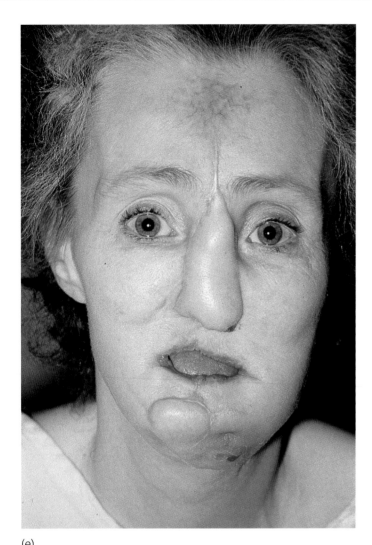

(e)

Fig. 20.23: **(e)** Three month postoperative result with secondary healing of the central forehead defect and the need for further revisions.

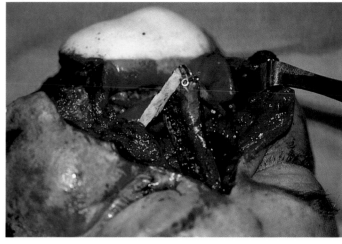

(a)

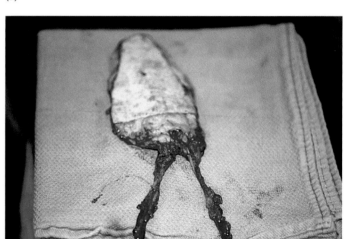

(b)

Fig. 20.24: Total nasal reconstruction using vascularized fasciocutaneous cover. **(a)** Nasal framework fabricated from rib cartilage. **(b)** Radial fasciocutaneous free flap harvested with vascular pedicle located at the inferior end.

Lateral face

The side of the face provides a less complicated array of anatomical structures and contours and the resultant tissue loss is somewhat simpler to reconstruct. Many single bullet gunshot wounds to the face do not result in large hard or soft tissue loss. Shortly after skin entrance the bullet strikes bone, causing a comminuted fracture and changing the path of the bullet. Reconstruction in these cases focuses on bony reduction and stabilization as the entrance and exit sites are small (Fig. 20.28). Small amounts of tissue loss, either intra-oral lining or external skin cover, can be tolerated as local tissue rearrangement can be done which may permit the placement of free bone grafts (Fig. 20.29). Loss of intraoral lining, however, is less well tolerated than external skin cover. Oral lining loss results in scar contracture, decreased oral opening and difficulty with subsequent dental rehabilitation. External skin loss results in undesirable visible scarring but does not usually result in serious functional handicaps.

The mass of bone to soft tissue is greater on the side of the face and for this reason bullets do not often traverse the entire width of the face, particularly the lower third due to the presence of the mandible. Shotgun wounds, however, spare little in their path. As almost all of these occur at close range, the amount of composite destruction is significant. Even when large soft tissue loss has not occurred, the blast effect from the bullet will frequently damage surrounding bones as well, including the maxilla and zygomatico-orbital complex (Fig. 20.29a, 20.31b).

Many lateral facial defects involve through-and-through wounds with moderate to large mandibular bone defects. The loss of inner and outer lining obviates any successful efforts at free bone grafting. The use of free fibular or scapular flaps with a skin paddle oriented to the side with the greatest lining loss is the most common method of immediate reconstruction in these cases. While the skin paddle does not produce a good color match with the surrounding facial skin, it provides ample coverage for most defects (Fig. 20.30).

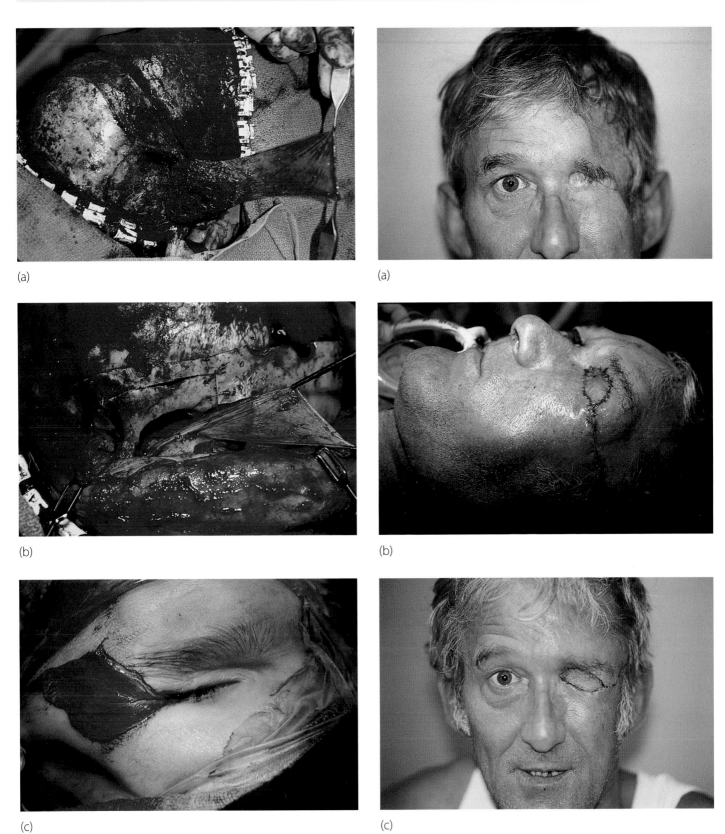

(a)

(b)

(c)

Fig. 20.25: Pedicled temporalis fascial flap for orbital lining. **(a)** Harvest of the temporalis fascial flap. **(b)** Extent of fascial reach through the orbit. **(c)** Amount of thin fascial tissue that can be gained for intraorbital lining.

(a)

(b)

(c)

Fig. 20.26: Orbital reconstruction with vascularized skin. **(a)** Preoperative appearance of healed temporo-orbital gunshot wound with significant hard and soft tissue loss. **(b)** Intraoperative placement of small radial fasciocutaneous flap into orbit after fronto-temporal cranioplasty. **(c)** Three-month postoperative result.

The relatively flat contour of the lateral face makes shaping and positioning the flap almost two-dimensional, rather than a three-dimensional effort. In very large composite defects, the amount of internal and external lining needed may make even these free flaps inadequate (Fig. 20.31). In these cases, a large soft tissue flap can be initially placed to establish external coverage which usually has the greatest amount of surface area loss. Once the wound is controlled, a second free flap can be placed to reconstruct the lost bone and internal lining.

Many lateral facial wounds result in direct injury to facial nerve branches. This typically involves the buccal and marginal mandibular branches, sparing innervation to the frontal and orbital areas. Primary nerve repair is usually impossible due to the blast injury and early nerve grafting is difficult without adequate soft tissue coverage and an ability to find the distal ends of the nerve. Secondary nerve or muscular reconstruction is rarely done as restoration of facial movement in the injured area is prohibited by the transplantation of reconstructed tissue and the resultant surrounding scar.

Prosthetic Reconstruction

The severity of tissue loss and the complexity of facial structures, particularly in the midfacial area, make reconstruction of extensive defects an almost overwhelming challenge. The practicalities of access to experienced and expert surgical care, the economics and physical stamina required to undergo a large number of surgical procedures, and age and medical/mental status of the patient raise certain philosophical questions. Most pertinently, how far should one go in providing autogenous reconstruction? Unfortunately, autogenous tissue has limitations in the formation and detail that can be obtained in certain facial features. Prostheses, when fabricated by skilled anaplastologists, provide an unparalleled artistic replication of the patient's lost facial features. The development and refinement of osseo-integrated implant techniques have enabled prosthetic replacement to be a viable alternative or, more commonly, an adjunct to the reconstruction of complex facial loss. Osseo-integrated prosthetic reconstruction has certain advantages, such as a more limited surgical burden on the patient, but is not without its own level of demand for a good outcome. Most importantly, there must be an adequate amount of bone volume and density at key locations to allow implants of proper length and orientation to be placed so the prosthesis is stable and does not produce any significant amount of rocking or torque on the bone fixtures. There is also the need for adequately thin attached tissue around the abutments as well as adequate access for maintenance.

It is important to point out that prosthetic reconstruction of severe facial defects is, in most cases, not a simple choice between reconstruction with autogenous tissue or a prosthesis supported by osseo-integrated implants. While each has its own obvious advantages and disadvantages, the combination of both is frequently needed and combined in stages. The defect is usually initially reconstructed with a vascularized osseous or osseocutaneous flap followed secondarily by implant placement.[25,26]

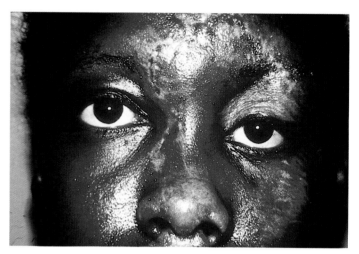

(a)

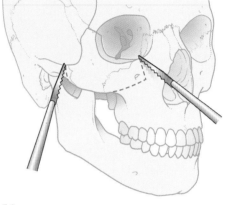

(b)

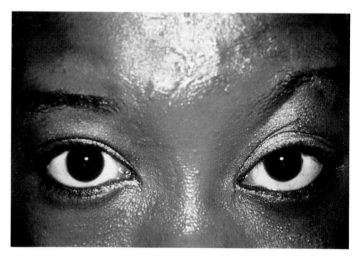

(c)

Fig. 20.27: Repositioning of the orbital box through osteotomies. **(a)** Preoperative facial view of severe orbital dystopia due to loss of left maxillary support from gunshot wound. **(b)** Osteotomy design, cranial bone grafting, and plate and screw fixation. **(c)** Six month postoperative result.

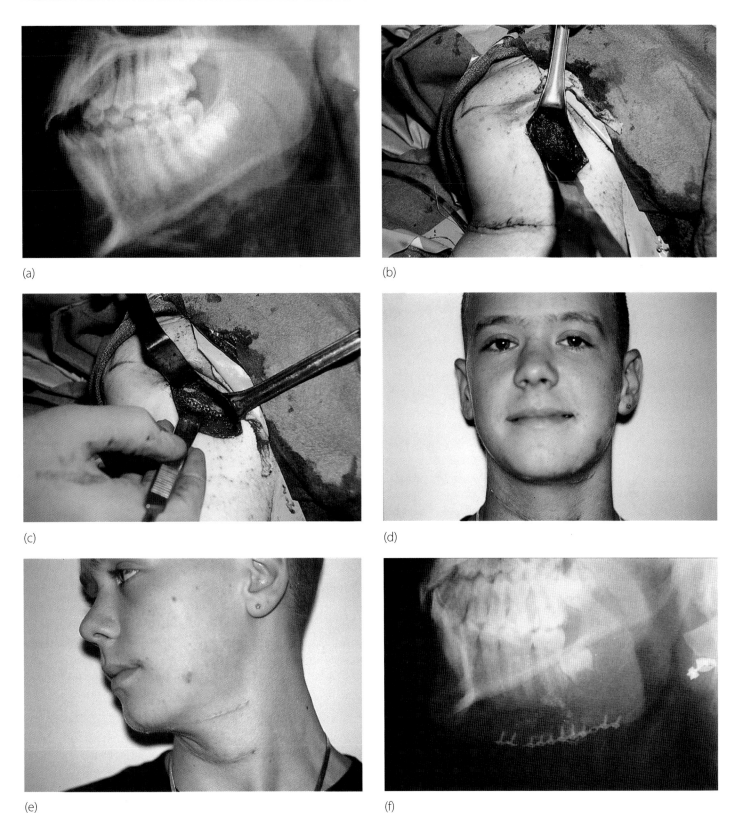

(a)

(b)

(c)

(d)

(e)

(f)

Fig. 20.28: Gunshot wound to the lateral face striking the mandible with no soft tissue deficit. **(a)** Preoperative lateral facial film. **(b)** Comminution and loss of inferior bone of mandibular body. **(c)** Due to good soft tissue cover, immediate reconstruction with bone fragments and iliac marrow. **(d)** Three month postoperative frontal facial view. **(e)** Three month postoperative lateral facial view. **(f)** Three month postoperative X-ray appearance.

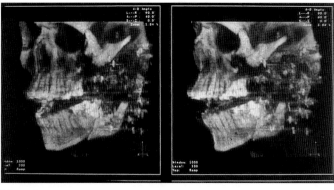

(a)

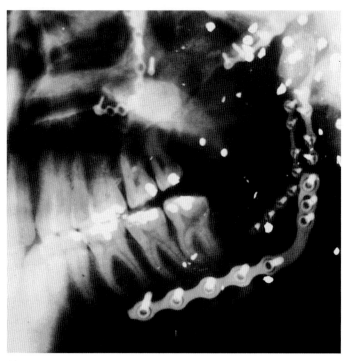

(c)

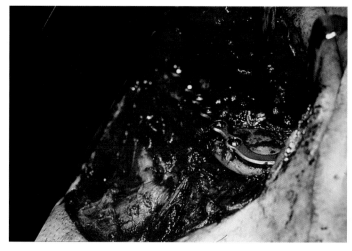

(b)

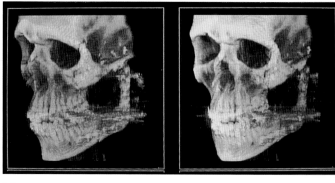

(d)

Fig. 20.29: Gunshot wound to lateral face with minimal loss of overlying soft tissue. **(a)** 3D CT scan with obliteration of left ramus of mandible. **(b)** Reconstruction with plate and iliac marrow. **(c)** Postoperative panorex. **(d)** Postoperative 3D CT scan with good alignment of the condyle and ramus (courtesy of Dr Anders Westermark, Stockholm, Sweden).

Controversies

The concept of reconstruction of severe facial wounds that have large tissue loss with vascularized tissue is well accepted and commonly used today due to the absence of any other satisfactory method of reconstruction in these cases. Some controversy exists, however, in the timing of this reconstructive procedure. Should the procedure be done early, such as within the first few days to weeks, or delayed for several weeks to months? Given the risk of a large operation with the limited use of available flap options in the body, the argument can be made for delaying vascularized reconstruction until a more 'ideal' time. What this timing is, however, is not often defined. Given that the majority of these facial injuries generally occur on healthy patients with non-compromised necks (lack of previous surgery and no irradiation), the initial vascularized reconstructive procedure should probably be done when the patient is stable, the viability of the tissue margins fairly obvious and the status of vital functions within the field (brain function and vision) fairly well defined. In

some cases, these issues will be known within the first few days after the injury.

In large composite tissue loss in the face, little controversy exists as to the use of microsurgical techniques given the lack of other viable treatment options. In smaller defects, particularly those that involve small mandibular segments, the issue of non-vascularized versus vascularized reconstructive techniques is often encountered. As most large traumatic facial wounds have non-compromised tissues (i.e. non-irradiated) prior to their injury, the use of bone grafts should have the potential for near normal healing. The type of bone graft required, however, is usually determined by the amount of soft tissue loss. Without an adequate soft tissue cover, free bone grafts will frequently become exposed and partial or complete graft loss will occur. The soft tissue issue is principally to do with intraoral lining. In small losses of mucosal lining, it may be possible to recruit enough local tissue to obtain reconstructive cover. Even if this results in loss of vestibular depth, secondary correction through release and skin grafting can be done when the free graft has revascular-

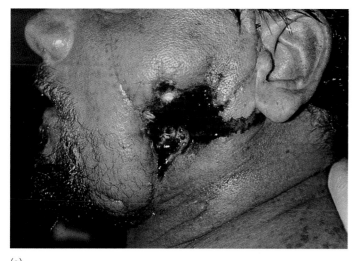

(a)

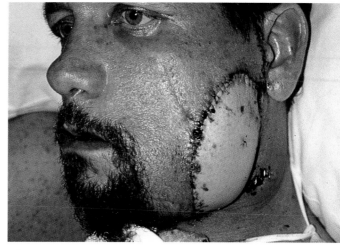

(c)

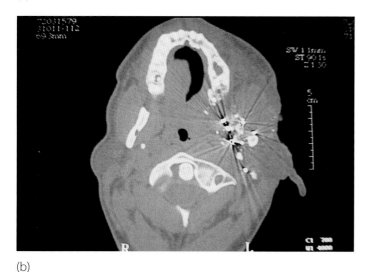

(b)

Fig. 20.30: Gunshot wound to the lateral face with loss of posterior body and ramus of the mandible with external skin loss. **(a)** Preoperative appearance 2 weeks after injury. **(b)** Preoperative CT appearance. **(c)** Reconstruction with free fibular osteocutaneous flap. (Courtesy of Jeffrey Wagner M.D., Indianapolis.)

ized and undergone osseous healing. This approach becomes increasingly inadequate as the amount of missing lining increases.

The concept of prefabrication of flap transfer is based on the use of delay procedures and interposition of specialized vascularized tissue to certain areas of the body from which a frame or pattern can be made that will simulate the complete tissue needed in another region of the body. This is best illustrated for nasal replacement in which the nose complete with lining, bone and skin can be initially constructed on the forehead, forearm, back or abdomen. After maturity the nose is harvested on a vascularized pedicle that has been relocated into the area and is then transplanted to the face by microvascular surgery. This concept has obvious appeal as the complex anatomy of the nose can be put together in pieces at a distant site first before being transferred to the face where such manipulations can be more difficult. This concept has also been clinically done for other complex facial areas such as in extensive midfacial defects.[24] Despite its theoretical advantages and reported successes in select clinical cases, the actual use of this concept is more difficult and often less satisfactory than one would envision. It is a concept which clearly has merit but is not yet ready for universal application. Many composite tissue free flaps, if properly designed, can achieve the desired reconstructive goals in one operation versus two. Furthermore, the reverse of prefabrication can be done very successfully; that is, the placement of vascularized soft tissue first followed by free bone grafting secondarily.

Lastly, the role of prosthetic (alloplastic) reconstruction as opposed to autogenous reconstruction must be considered, in both primary as well as secondary efforts. The tremendous surgical effort and expertise, patient endurance and tolerance of numerous operations over a prolonged period, the economic and resource cost, and the esthetic quality of the final facial result make a prosthetic replacement a viable option in select patients. The use of endosseous implants for attaching oral and facial prostheses overcomes the traditional problems associated with glues and dental anchorage methods. Which patients should receive this therapy in large facial defects is open to debate and numerous factors must be considered in addition to the defect size and location.

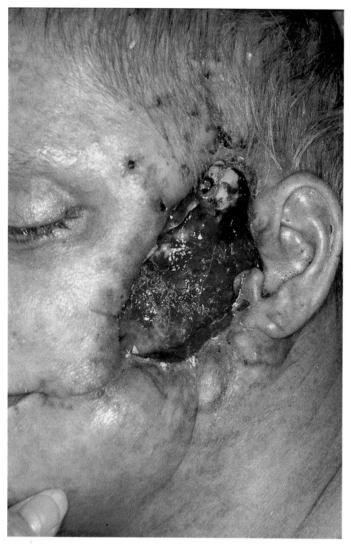

(a)

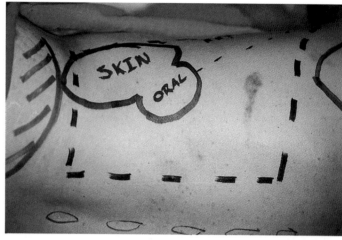

(c)

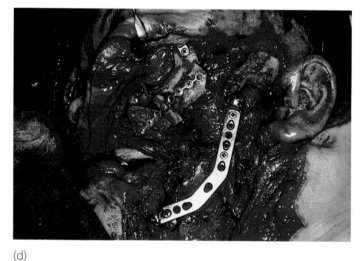

(d)

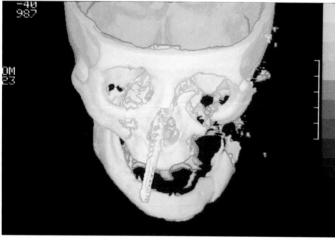

(b)

Fig. 20.31: Gunshot wound to the left face with the entrance site intraoral. **(a)** Preoperative appearance 2 weeks after injury at time of transfer. **(b)** 3D CT showing loss of entire ramus of mandible and disruption of the zygomatic complex. **(c)** First-stage reconstruction with free latissimus musculocutaneous flap (design on back). **(d)** Plate fixation of fractures and temporary alloplastic (metal) reconstruction of mandibular segment prior to flap inset.

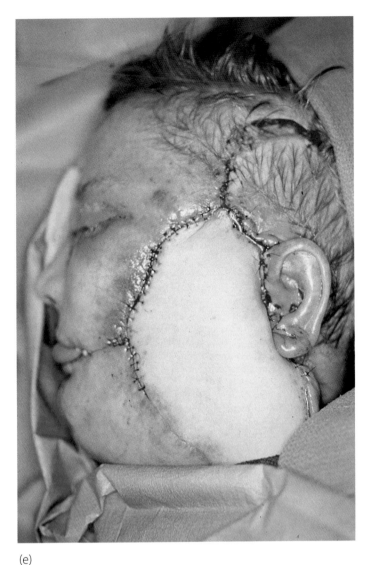

(e)

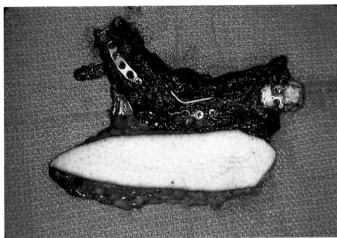

(g)

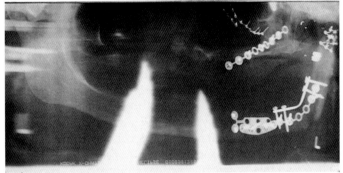

(h)

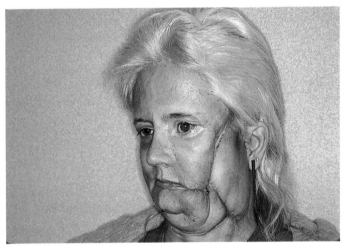

(i)

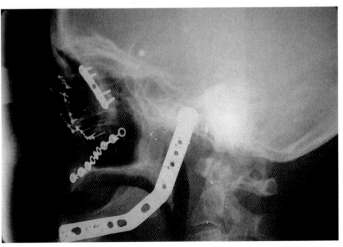

(f)

Fig. 20.31: (e) Latissimus flap inset over bony reconstruction. **(f)** Immediate postoperative X-ray appearance. **(g)** Second-stage mandibular reconstruction 6 months later with free fibular osteocutaneous flap (skin is used for inraoral lining. **(h)** Postoperative panorex. **(i)** Nine months after second free flap reconstruction, scar revisions and skin flap adjustments are needed but good well-vascularized tissue is present.

Conclusion

Large defects of the midface and lower face result in loss of many specialized tissues. As initially described in 1965, 'massive compound facial injuries create a sense of dismay, which may lead to therapeutic inertia'.[27] To overcome this potential treatment stagnation, successful reconstruction of these defects entails early action which involves replacement of the tissues before significant scarring and contracture have occurred. There are no specific algorithms of reconstruction that will apply to all patients as each facial gunshot wound creates a unique set of tissue requirements. Thorough evaluation of the facial wound, including radiographic assessment, preferably with three-dimensional CT scans, will delineate the extent of the missing tissue. Lining, bony structures and soft tissue cover are the three basic elements that need to be replaced in almost all of these injuries. Immediate or early repair, usually with the aid of microsurgical tissue transfer, will not only provide for a facial wound that heals more quickly but will maintain the relationship of the remaining key landmarks that serve as the scaffold for future facial revision and reconstruction. In large defects, more than one free tissue transfer may be necessary to provide enough tissue to restore some semblance of facial form. Realistic counseling with the patient who has sustained a large facial tissue loss and their family is paramount. This is not only to bring in psychological evaluation and support but also to help them to understand that a large number of reconstructive procedures will be necessary, up to 10–15 not being uncommon, over an extended period of time (1–2 years) for the maximal benefit of reconstructive facial surgery to be obtained. Complete preinjury restoration of facial form and function is almost never achieved in large composite facial defects but reasonable function and facial proportions can be obtained. In select patients, oral and facial prostheses in conjunction with osseointegrated implants for anchorage provide an alloplastic alternative and/or adjunct to autogenous reconstructions.

References

1 Centers for Disease Control and Prevention 1994 Deaths resulting from firearm and motor vehicle-related injuries – United States, 1986–1991. Journal of the American Medical Association 271: 495

2 Fackler ML 1998 Civilian gunshot wounds and ballistics: dispelling the myths. Emergency Medicine Clinics of North America 16: 17–28

3 Robertson B, Manson PN 1998 The importance of serial debridement and 'second-look' procedures in high-energy ballistic and avulsive facial injuries. Operative Techniques in Plastic and Reconstructive Surgery XX: 236–245

4 Clark N, Birely B, Manson PN et al 1996 High-energy ballistic and avulsive facial injuries: classification, patterns, and an algorithm for primary reconstruction. Plastic and Reconstructive Surgery 98: 583–601

5 Vasconez HC 1991 Management of massive bone and soft tissue defects of the midface and lower face. Problems in Plastic and Reconstructive Surgery 1: 466–481

6 Manson PN 1991 Dimensional analysis of the facial skeleton. Avoiding complications in the management of facial fractures by improved organization of treatment based on CT scans. Problems in Plastic and Reconstructive Surgery 1: 213–237

7 Hidalgo DA 1991 Aesthetic improvement in free flap mandible reconstruction. Plastic and Reconstructive Surgery 88: 574–589

8 Schusterman MA, Rees GP, Miller MJ, Harris S 1992 The osteocutaneous free fibula flap: is the skin paddle reliable? Plastic and Reconstructive Surgery 90: 787–798

9 Swartz WM, Banis JC, Newton ED, Ramasastry SS, Jones NF, Acland R 1986 The osteocutaneous scapula flap for mandibular and maxillary reconstruction. Plastic and Reconstructive Surgery 77: 530–538

10 Coleman III JJ, Sultan MR 1989 The bipedicled osteocutaneous scapula flap: a new subscapular system free flap. Plastic and Reconstructive Surgery 84: 71–79

11 Timmons MJ 1986 The vascular basis of the radial forearm flap. Plastic and Reconstructive Surgery 77: 80–87

12 Soutar DS, McGregor IA 1986 The radial forearm flap in intraoral reconstruction: the experience of 60 consecutive cases. Plastic and Reconstructive Surgery 78: 1–10

13 Bartlett SP, May JW Jr, Yaremchuk MJ 1981 The latissimus dorsi muscle: a fresh cadaver study of the primary neurovascular pedicle. Plastic and Reconstructive Surgery 67: 631–639

14 Yamamoto K, Takagi N, Miyashita Y, Hirabayashi M, Gota A 1987 Facial reconstruction with latissimus dorsi myocutaneous island flap following total maxillectomy. Journal of Craniomaxillofacial Surgery 15: 288–295

15 Taylor GI, Corlett RJ, Boyd JB 1984 The versatile deep inferior epigastric (inferior rectus abdominis) flap. British Journal of Plastic Surgery 37: 330–338

16 Miyamoto Y, Harada K, Kodama Y, Takahashi H, Okano S 1986 Cranial coverage involving scalp, bone and dura using free inferior epigastric flap. British Journal of Plastic Surgery 39: 483–489

17 Inoue T, Ueda K, Hatoko M, Harashina T 1991 The pedicled serratus anterior myocutaneous flap for head and neck reconstruction. British Journal of Plastic Surgery 44: 259–267

18 McCarthy JG, Lorenc ZP, Cutting C, Rachesky M 1985 Median forehead flap revisited: the blood supply. Plastic and Reconstructive Surgery 76: 866–893

19 Burget GC, Menick FJ 1986 Nasal reconstruction: seeking a fourth dimension. Plastic and Reconstructive Surgery 77: 824–833

20 Mathes SJ, Nahai F (eds) 1997 Reconstructive surgery: principles, anatomy and techniques. Churchill Livingstone, New York

21 Foster RD, Anthony JP, Singer MI, Kaplan MJ, Pogrel MA, Mathes SJ 1997 Reconstruction of complex midfacial defects. Plastic and Reconstructive Surgery 99: 1555–1565

22 Holle J, Vinzenz K, Wuringer E, Kulenkampff K-J 1996 The prefabricated combined scapula flap bony and soft-tissue reconstruction in maxillofacial defects – a new method. Plastic and Reconstructive Surgery 98: 542–552

23 Thomas WO, Harris CN 1997 Subtotal midfacial/total nasal reconstruction following shotgun blast to the face employing composite microvascular serratus, anterior rib, muscle, and scapula tip. Annals of Plastic Surgery 38: 291–295

24 Keller K, Vasconez HC 1998 Customized composite reconstruction of extensive midfacial defects. Annals of Plastic Surgery 40: 291–296

25 Stevens MR, Heit JM, Kline SN, Marx RE, Garg AK 1998 The use of osseointegrated implants in craniofacial trauma. Journal of Craniomaxillofacial Trauma 4: 27–34

26 Harris L, Wilkes GH, Wolfaardt JF 1996 Autogenous soft-tissue procedures and osseointegrated alloplastic reconstruction: their role in the treatment of complex craniofacial defects. Plastic and Reconstructive Surgery 98: 387–392

27 Moore AM, Winslow P 1965 Initial care of shotgun wounds of the face. Report of 2 cases. American Surgeon 31: 321–328

21 Facial Nerve Injuries

Henning Schliephake, Jarg-Erich Hausamen

Introduction

Traumatic injuries of the facial nerve are uncommon compared to other causes of facial nerve dysfunction such as tumors, cerebral ischemia or idiopathic nerve palsy. When the facial nerve is damaged in head and neck trauma, it is often associated with a potentially life-threatening pattern of injuries. Thus the focus of therapy is towards life-saving measures and stabilization of the patient's general condition. Although a traumatic lesion of the facial nerve may therefore not appear to be of primary importance in the emergency room, permanent facial paralysis subsequent to traumatic injury nevertheless severely affects the patient's life thereafter. Not only is the loss of facial movement and insufficient eye closure a considerable burden to the patient with respect to function, but in addition, the social consequences of disfigurement and loss of facial expression are particularly distressing. Both sequelae are likely to impair the patient's personal relationships and social life in a profound manner.

Adequate management of the traumatic injuries of the facial nerve requires not only thorough knowledge of the complex anatomy of the course of the nerve but also sophisticated diagnostic means and, even more, surgical skills in microsurgical nerve repair. It is up to the surgeons who are performing primary surgical care to provide the conditions for successful recovery or repair of a traumatic nerve damage. The basis of diagnostic and therapeutic strategies covering features at initial presentation, diagnostic measures, timing and techniques of nerve repair will be highlighted in this chapter.

Epidemiology

Traumatic damage to the facial nerve can be indirect or direct. **Indirect** damage may be encountered after intracerebral bleeding. As intracerebral lesions of the facial nerve nucleus or its fascicles are unlikely to be subject to direct surgical repair, they are omitted from this chapter. **Direct** trauma to the nerve can occur on its intratemporal and extratemporal routes.

The most common site of direct traumatic lesions is the **intratemporal** route, caused by temporal bone fractures (86%).[1] However, as only 7% of all temporal fractures account for facial nerve damage,[2] this indicates that direct facial nerve injuries in head and neck trauma are relatively rare. The second most frequent cause for traumatic damage to the facial nerve is gunshot wounds to the temporal bone,[3] although only 8% of all gunshot wounds in the head and neck

were found to be associated with facial nerve injury.[4] Damage to the nerve on the **extratemporal** route is even less frequent. Blunt injuries, stab wounds, severely dislocated mandibular fractures, gunshot wounds and birth trauma are reported to account for facial paralysis. In gunshot wounds, traumatic damage may occur through blast injury even though the trunk or the large branches have not been directly severed.[5] Obstetric reasons for a facial nerve lesion are rare (approximately 0.07% of all deliveries), but facial nerve damage is nevertheless the second or third most frequent injury due to obstetric trauma.[6,7]

All in all, 6.3% of all facial nerve disorders result from direct traumatic injuries.[1] Occasionally, late damage to the facial nerve may occur in association with posttraumatic vascular malformations.[8,9]

State-of-the-Art Management

Diagnosis of facial nerve damage in acute trauma is commonly impaired by anesthesia required to manage the patient in the emergency room. Facial nerve damage has therefore often to be 'assumed' from the location and extent of soft tissue wounds. However, even if direct damage to parts of the facial nerve appears to be very likely from clinical inspection, not every traumatic lesion of the facial nerve is inevitably followed by complete paralysis of the facial muscles. Even in extensive lacerations of facial soft tissues, nerve function may not be damaged or, after initial weakness, recovers to adequate function (Fig. 21.1). There are several reasons for these observations.

First, the nerve is completely embedded in soft tissue and has considerable longitudinal elasticity, which accounts for its amazing resistance against mechanical damage even during direct impact. Second, there is an extensive system of anastomotic parallel nerve supplies to every region of the facial muscles (with the exception of the mandibular branch). Such multiple nerve supplies, with mutual exchange between fibers of different branches, almost always exist between the zygomatic and buccal branches. Therefore, isolated damage to one of these branches commonly does not result in a paresis of the corresponding facial muscles. Ironically, on the other hand, clinical evidence of nerve dysfunction from weakness of the facial muscles is not necessarily associated with severing and irreversible damage to corresponding nerve fibers.

The severity of nerve damage in general has been classified into three categories: neurapraxia, axonotmesis and neurotmesis. Although these categories refer to structural alterations

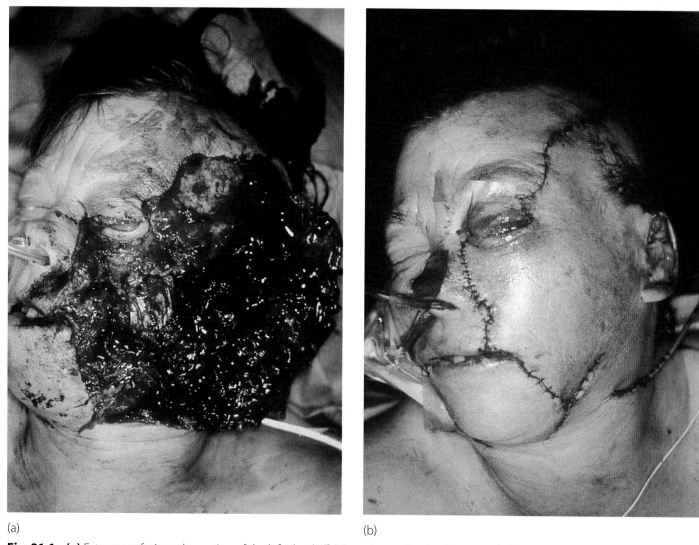

(a)   (b)

Fig. 21.1: (a) Extreme soft tissue laceration of the left cheek. **(b)** State immediately after wound closure.

of the nerve at a microscopic level, they have a direct relationship with the prognosis and the clinical outcome for the patient.

Neurapraxia is the simplest type of injury to the nerve and its clinical manifestation is only temporary. The axons of the nerve remain undamaged, but injury has occurred to the myelin sheath, for instance due to compression or hyperextension of the nerve. The resulting edema of the myelin sheath causes temporary dysfunction from which the nerve recovers within days to weeks.

In **axonotmesis**, continuity of the nerve is still preserved. However, damage has been more severe due to prolonged compression or a localized ischemic lesion of the nerve. It therefore affects both the myelin sheath and the axons. Both components degenerate but regeneration of axons is guided by the fibrous structures of the nerve which are still intact. In electromyographic recordings, axonotmesis is characterized by degenerative reactions, retardation of muscle twitching and complete interruption of nerve conduction. However, because the continuity of the fibrous framework of the nerve has been maintained along the entire length of the whole nerve, regeneration can proceed to the distal end of the

nerve. First, the axons and the myelin sheath undergo Wallerian degeneration after which their debris is digested by Schwann cells and invading macrophages. Concurrently, Schwann cells proliferate within the basal membrane and arrange themselves into chains known as Hanken–Büngner bands. Regeneration of axons then commences proximal to the site of damage and follows the Hanken–Büngner bands to the periphery. Thus regeneration of the normal nerve fiber pattern is possible resulting in more or less complete functional restoration.

In **neurotmesis**, continuity of the nerve is completely severed and its ends are separated by retraction due to the longitudinal elasticity of the nerve. Clinically and electromyographically, axonotmesis and neurotmesis are identical. The morphological alterations during degeneration of axons and myelin sheath are likewise the same in axonotmesis and neurotmesis. However, in the latter case, spontaneous regeneration in the peripheral nerve segment is impossible as it depends on bridging of the gap between the two retracted nerve ends. This requires surgical intervention to establish continuity of the nerve by direct suturing or grafting.

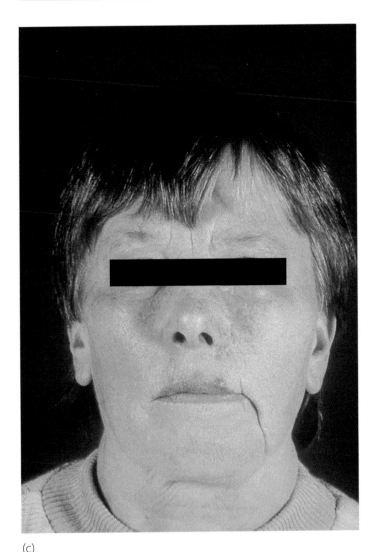

(c)

Fig. 21.1: (c) Facial appearance approximately 6 months later.

Diagnosis and Timing of Treatment

In conscious and co-operative patients, function of the facial muscles is easily tested by asking the patient to sequentially activate his frontal, periorbital, buccal and perioral muscles.

In injuries with suspected intratemporal damage to the nerve, diagnostic imaging is required. In temporal bone fractures, CT scans are preferable to plain films as only 20–30% of temporal fractures can be visualized by the latter technique.[10] MRI scans provide additional information of facial nerve damage by showing abnormal nerve enhancement, particularly in distal intrameatal nerve segments.[11] Enhancement of MRI scans by gadolinium-diethyl-triamine-pentaacetic acid (Gd-DTPA) produces even more informative MRI studies for the evaluation of facial nerve pathology and thus can help to define lesions to the nerve more accurately.[12–14]

Electrodiagnostic tests such as evoked electromyography or electroneuronography play an important role in the objective assessment of facial nerve damage and provide indications for decision making with respect to surgical intervention.[15–17] However, most electrodiagnostic tests are focused on exam-

ination of the nerve distal to the stylomastoid foramen and cannot evaluate the nerve across the injury site in intratemporal lesions.[17,18] Pathologic findings in the results of electrodiagnostic nerve testing can only be seen if Wallerian degeneration of the axons distal to the damaged site has occurred in the meantime. Therefore, these diagnostic tools are only useful for late assessment of posttraumatic facial nerve damage.

In order to provide earlier information about the severity of facial nerve lesions, transcranial magnetic stimulation of the facial nerve after non-traumatic damage has been studied in Bell's palsy patients.[19,20] This technique has also been applied successfully in immediate examination of traumatic facial nerve lesion in an experimental setting.[17] However, contradictory results in clinical and experimental studies preclude recommendation of its use in clinical routine at the current time.

If deep lacerations of facial soft tissues in the buccal or pre-auricular area indicate damage on the extratemporal route of the nerve and if there is clinical evidence of paresis, meticulous inspection and identification of severed nerve ends is often the only way to positively identify nerve damage. Because the definite functional sequelae of evident damage to individual nerve branches is difficult to predict due to the above-mentioned reasons, primary nerve reconstruction after identification of nerve ends is not always indicated. From the experience with cross-face nerve grafts for facial reanimation, it is known that 50% of facial nerve fibers are sufficient to provide both satisfactory muscle tonus at rest and symmetric movement under voluntary function. Therefore, primary repair is recommended only if there is morphological proof that the trunk of the facial nerve itself has been severed. Only in this case should further dissection of the nerve segments be performed. However, if it is not possible to do a primary repair, because of soft tissue swelling, bleeding, lack of operation time or in a seriously injured patient, repair can be delayed. Reconstruction after 3–4 weeks may be preferable in many cases when the patient's condition has become stable and soft tissue swelling has gone down. In order to identify the severed nerve ends in the secondary approach, they have to be marked during primary care, using non-resorbable atraumatic marker sutures, which are fixed to the skin.

If an extratemporal traumatic facial nerve lesion is present and the surgeon is uncertain whether the injury is only of minor severity (i.e. neurapraxia) or whether the nerve has been completely severed, no more than 3 months should elapse. In this time the nerve function has to be monitored electromyographically and the decision has to be made whether or not to perform a reconstruction. If no signs of regeneration are seen during this time, revision and reconstruction should no longer be delayed. Physical therapy such as electrostimulation of the facial muscles and massaging should be administered in the meantime.

The interval for secondary nerve repair is limited by the progressive atrophy of the facial muscles on the paretic side of the face. If reconstruction of the nerve is considered, it has to be performed at least within the first year postoperatively, as after this period muscle function, even with reinnervated facial nerve fibers, will be insufficient to accomplish satisfactory movement of the face on the paretic side. Beyond this interval reanimation of the paralysed face has to be performed by revascularized transfer of neuromuscular segments. In these procedures, a vascularized segment from the gracilis muscle or the latissimus dorsi muscle with a branch of the supplying nerve is transferred to the face to augment the atrophic facial muscles and allow for innervated function of the transferred muscle.[21–26]

Surgical Repair

Surgical intervention for repair of traumatic damage to the facial nerve differs according to the location of the nerve injury. In intratemporal lesions, decompression surgery of the nerve in the osseous canal through the temporal bone has to be considered. In extratemporal lesions, the decision for microsurgical repair of the nerve has to be made. While the former procedure is more a domain of otolaryngology or neurosurgery, the maxillofacial surgeon will be involved in the latter.

Microsurgical repair of the extratemporal portion of the facial nerve requires a high standard in both technical equipment and surgical training. A surgical microscope with continuously adjustable magnification between 2 and 40 and foot control should be available. Suture material of 25 µm diameter (10-0) is recommended and forceps with smooth non-serrated ends are preferable to avoid trauma to the delicate perineural tissue.

Nerve suturing

Basic surgical techniques for repair of the extratemporal part of the facial nerve have been contributed by Conley[27] and Miehlke.[28] Before the use of the microscope for surgical nerve repair, nerve suturing was commonly performed by suturing the epineurium. This was often unsuccessful, mainly due to inadequate preparation of the cross-sectional surface of the nerve ends and insufficient adaptation of the individual fascicles. This has dramatically improved since the introduction of the microscope which allowed for atraumatic handling and precise adaptation of the nerve ends and individual fascicles.[29,30] The poor results obtained with epineural suturing in the premicroscopic era were initially attributed to the epineural location of the suture as such and new concepts of perineural suturing with adaptation of individual fascicles were developed. Today, numerous studies have shown that both techniques can achieve similar results as long as they are performed with the same accuracy and atraumatic handling of the nerve ends and fascicles.

The differential indication for epineural versus perineural suturing is dependent on the fascicular structure of the nerve. The pattern of fascicles has been categorized into three different types:[31] monofascicular, oligofascicular (<5 fascicles) and polyfascicular structure (Fig. 21.2). While epineural suturing is considered to be appropriate in mono- and oligofascicular nerve ends, perineural sutures are required only in

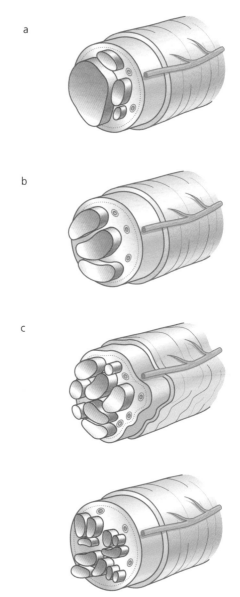

Fig. 21.2: (a) Cross-section of a monofascicular nerve. **(b)** Cross-section of an oligofascicular nerve. **(c)** Cross-section of a polyfascicular nerve.

polyfascicular nerves. Because the facial nerve has a mono- or oligofascicular structure at the nerve trunk and its first divisions into peripheral branches, epineural suturing is supposed to be adequate for suturing in most areas of the nerve.

The aim and strategy of microsurgical intervention are defined by the timing of the surgery and the degree of damage to the nerve. In **primary repair** and any other microsurgical repair procedure, the nerve ends are dissected free of epineural connective tissue (Fig. 21.3a), because the greatest hazard for axon proliferation from the central nerve end into the peripheral segment is the proliferation of connective tissue at the site of suturing. Intervening connective tissue can prevent axons from further elongation into the distal segment or can even turn down already regenerated axons. Possible factors that account for this fibrosis are traumatic dissection of the nerve during preparation for suturing or suturing of the nerve ends whilst under longitudinal tension.

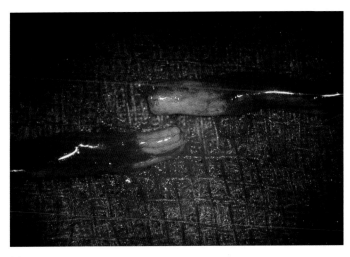

(a)

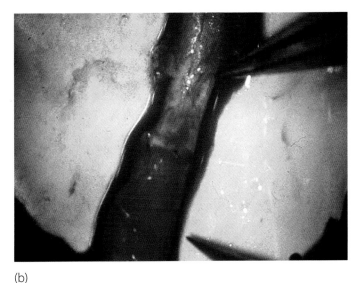

(b)

Fig. 21.3: (a) Removal of epineural tissue. **(b)** Fascicles protruding from the perineural tissue.

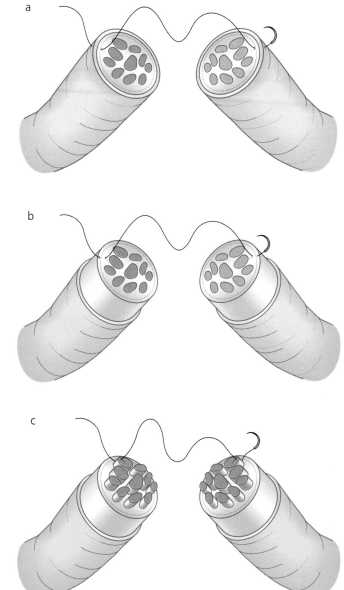

Fig. 21.4: (a) Microsurgical suturing of the epineurium. **(b)** Microsurgical suturing of the perineurium. **(c)** Interfascicular microsurgical suturing.

Tension-free suturing of the nerve ends and atraumatic dissection therefore are mandatory.

Because the epineural fibroblasts proliferate more rapidly than the fibroblasts and Schwann cells of the endoneural space, the epineural tissue should be removed from the nerve ends both to reduce the proportion of connective tissue in nerve cross-section and to allow for more precise adaptation of the fascicles (Fig. 21.3b). However, removal of the epineurium in facial nerve repair is only feasible at the trunk, as it becomes very thin on the more peripheral branches and is hardly discernible from their remaining parts.

Before suturing the nerve ends in primary repair after trauma, they are dissected free of their surrounding tissue and trimmed with serrated scissors until the cut ends look completely undamaged. Subsequently, the epineurium is opened and removed on both ends for a length of 5–10 mm with the scissors at 10-fold microscope magnification. This reveals the location and structure of fascicles at the cross-section of the nerve. After trimming, axons tend to prolapse due to the endoneural pressure and the longitudinal retrac-

tion of the perineural tissue. These protruding axons should be removed to gain a smooth cross-sectional area which facilitates adaptation and suturing of the nerve ends. Protruding axons are grasped with the forceps, pulled forward and cut with serrated scissors at the level of the epi- or perineural annulus. Suturing can be performed by epineural, perineural or interfascicular suturing (Fig. 21.4).

The choice between the three techniques is not as important as the precise adaptation of the nerve ends and their fascicles. In order to ensure mechanically stable and reliable adaptation, three to four sutures are recommended around the complete circumference of the nerve. When microsurgical repair is performed at the nerve trunk, correct reorientation of the fascicles in distal nerve ends corresponding to the proximal end is of importance to ensure restoration of the functional organization of the nerve plexus.

In late **secondary repair** of lacerated nerves, the nerve ends commonly have to be identified in the scar tissue of the former injury. In many cases the scar tissue may serve as a landmark of dissection and orientation to identify the nerve ends. When the nerve ends have been marked with sutures during primary care, it is often useful to excise the scar completely and to locate the nerve ends distally and proximally of this area along the suture marks. If no marking has been performed, dissection and identification of the severed nerve ends are a lot more difficult using the scar tissue as a starting point. In this case it is often preferable to start with the exposure of the nerve trunk at the stylomastoid foramen and to proceed along its main branches until the scar area is reached. In the same way, the peripheral branches are identified distal to the scar area and followed proximally (Fig. 21.5a,f).

If the severity of injury to the nerve is unclear, microsurgical neurolysis should be considered first by isolating the nerve from scar tissue and removing the epineurium in order to examine the fascicles for intact or severed continuity under the microscope. For this purpose, the nerve is located outside the area of former injury and dissected free of scar tissue at magnifications of 10–25 X. Frequently, a neuroma is encountered, which may disguise interruption of nerve continuity, but occasionally only increased intraneural scar formation of the fibrous sheath may be found, with underlying individual fascicles exhibiting undisturbed continuity. In any case, the epineurium has to be removed to examine the intraneural situation. If an endoneural neuroma is found, it is removed and the nerve ends are treated as described above for primary nerve repair. If intraneural fibrosis is encountered, an interfascicular neurolysis is required with careful removal of the compromising scar tissue between the fascicles to free the intact nerve components.

Cable grafting

Direct end-to-end repair of traumatic facial nerve damage is possible in only a few selected cases. This is where the nerve has had a straight cut in the area of the trunk or larger peripheral branches without crushing or tearing trauma. Commonly, even in primary nerve repair, trauma to the nerve

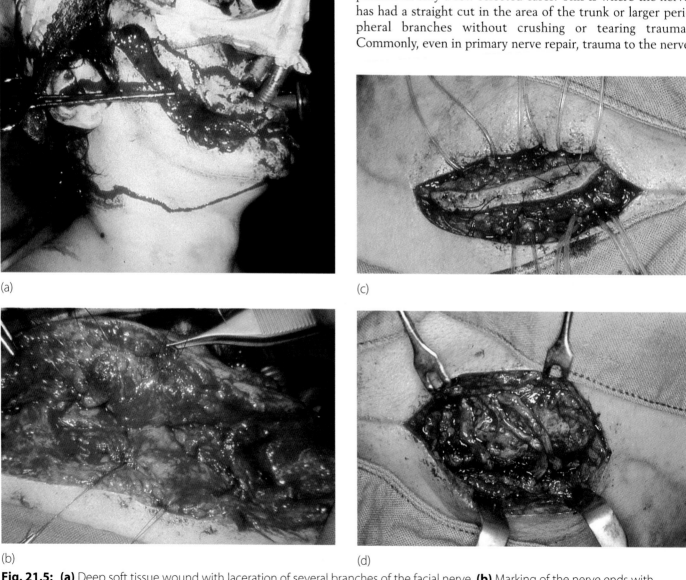

(a)

(b)

(c)

(d)

Fig. 21.5: **(a)** Deep soft tissue wound with laceration of several branches of the facial nerve. **(b)** Marking of the nerve ends with non-resorbable, atraumatic sutures. **(c)** Removal of scar tissue and identification of the individual branches (rubber bands). **(d)** Bridging of the defect by cable grafts.

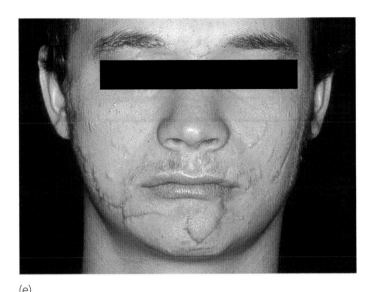

(e)

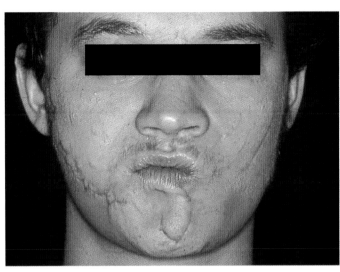

(f)

Fig. 21.5: (e,f) Postoperative function of the facial nerve.

requires removal of the damaged nerve tissue during trimming. This precludes tensionless suturing of the nerve ends during suturing. Therefore, both in primary repair of traumatic nerve damage and in secondary reconstructions, when scar formation has separated the nerve ends, use of a cable graft will be necessary to bridge the continuity defect of the nerve. In general, autogenous nerve grafts are the method of choice, although allogenic nerve grafts have proved to be functional as well. However, low-dose immunosuppression is necessary with the use of allogenic grafts and the hazard of transmitting infectious diseases is much more serious than the hazard of donor site morbidity from harvesting autogenous grafts. This has precluded allogenic grafts from clinical use so far.[32] The possibility of vascularized nerve transfer using the saphenous nerve or the sural nerve has also been subject to a number of clinical and experimental approaches. So far no clear advantage of the increased surgery of vascularized nerve transfer has been shown over non-vascularized nerve grafting with respect to axonal morphology or postoperative nerve function.

Suitable donor sites for non-vascularized nerve grafts include the branches of the cervical plexus in the neck and the sural nerve from the calf. The great auricular nerve from the cervical plexus has been employed for cable grafting because its anatomy provides a suitable number of branches that can be connected to the peripheral branches of the facial nerve plexus, while its thicker proximal end is sutured to the central stump of the facial nerve. The sural nerve also provides a similar morphology of branches.

The branches of the cervical plexus are easily identified on the outer surface of the sternocleidomastoid muscle vertically below the auricle. For exposure, an incision parallel to the course of the muscle or an extended submandibular incision is used. Both the great auricular nerve and the transverse cervical nerve appear at the lower border of the sternocleidomastoid muscle at the so-called punctum nervosum. The great auricular nerve courses upwards to the auricle while the transverse cervical nerve runs medially and branches off shortly after the punctum nervosum.

The sural nerve is often preferred, if longer or multiple grafts are required. This cutaneous nerve can been conveniently exposed through a horizontal incision behind the lateral malleolus (Fig. 21.6a). During dissection the lateral saphenous vein may be encountered, which overlies the sural nerve and is commonly preserved. After isolation of the nerve its proximal course can be identified by gently pulling the nerve and palpating approximately 6–8 cm upwards of the first incision. At this point a second horizontal incision is performed and the nerve exposed. The nerve runs from the ankle joint to the back of the calf so that the more proximal incisions should be placed further backwards. In this way the nerve can be followed up to the knee joint where it joins the lateral sural cutaneous nerve. From the knee to the ankle joint the sural nerve has a length of 30 cm. It is important for the reconstruction of the facial nerve that the sural nerve sends off branches in the distal part that allow for reconstruction of large parts of the facial plexus and are easily accessible (Fig. 21.6b). Preference is often given to the sural nerve over the cervical nerve branches because the former provides longer and stronger grafts.

If there is a discrepancy between the cross-sectional area of the facial nerve and the procured nerve graft, two or even more grafts can be connected to the thickest nerve ends (Fig. 21.6c). In the periphery of the plexus it is very often the reverse, with thin and tiny branches of the facial nerve for suturing with much thicker grafts.

The aims of suturing of nerve grafts to the facial nerve are exactly the same as those for primary repair. Suturing has to be absolutely tensionless and atraumatic preparation and handling of the nerve graft are mandatory. Therefore, the cable nerve grafts clearly have to be longer than the length of the nerve defect.

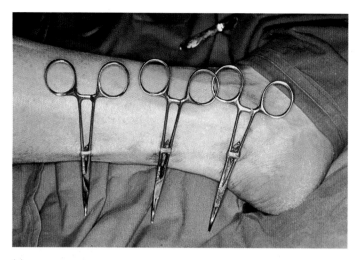

(a)

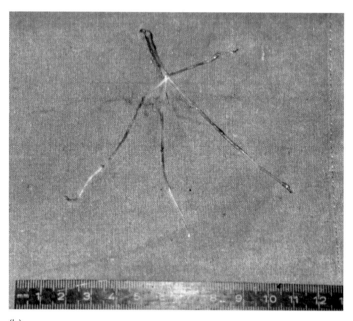

(b)

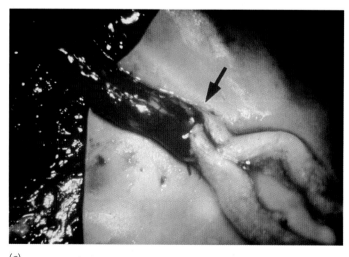

(c)

Fig. 21.6: (a) Identification of the sural nerve. **(b)** Sural nerve procured. **(c)** Suturing of two nerve ends from the sural nerve to fit a larger cross-section of the recipient nerve.

Nerve crossovers

Indications for crossover anastomoses in facial nerve repair have been considerably reduced due to the great advances in extracranial and intracranial treatment of these lesions. However, if the proximal part of the trunk of the facial nerve has been destroyed during trauma, direct suturing or cable grafting will be unsuccessful for nerve repair. Innervation of the facial muscles then has to be provided by connecting another cranial motor nerve, such as the hypoglossal, gloss-opharyngeal or accessory nerve, to the peripheral facial nerve supply or by providing nerve supply from the opposite uninjured side by a cross-face nerve graft.

Nerve crossovers using cranial motor nerves have been employed for many years.[33-37] In particular, the hypoglossal nerve and the accessory nerve have been used for this procedure. The nerves that 'lend' their supply to the facial nerve are exposed and cut at a convenient length to reach the facial nerve and anastomosed with the distal end of the facial nerve trunk. Axonal regeneration and neurotization of the previously denervated facial nerve then occurs quickly, originating from the hypoglosssal or accessory nerve. However, this method occasionally has resulted in unco-ordinated movements through the contralateral nerve and was always associated with functional loss of muscles of the donor nerve supply. Therefore, today hypoglossal–facial crossover is the only crossover anastomosis that is performed using other cranial motor nerves. The unilateral functional loss of tongue muscles is commonly more easily compensated for by the patient than the unilateral limitation of shoulder function in an accessory–facial nerve crossover procedure.

The hypoglossal–facial crossover is a relatively simple operation that can achieve restoration of very good function with regard to both muscular tone of the facial muscles and soft tissue symmetry at rest. It also improves lag-ophthalmos and permits voluntary movement of the facial muscles to a limited extent. Patients with hypoglossal–facial crossover, however, require a high degree of postoperative muscular training to learn to activate the facial muscles without concurrently activating the tongue muscles. Therefore, although voluntary contraction of facial muscles can be accomplished on command, symmetric affective or emotional expression of the face is not restored in full. Occasionally, moderate intraoral dysfunction, mass movement and hypertonia of the face can occur. However, these untoward effects are infrequent and generally well accepted by the patients.

If a hypoglossal–facial crossover is intended after the central part of the facial nerve was lost due to trauma, the distal part of the facial nerve trunk is located in a secondary procedure in the retromandibular fossa, as is done during removal of parotid tumors. From a pre-auricular incision the dissection proceeds medially and inferiorly along the outer surface of the cartilage of the external auditory canal. This cartilage forms a triangular prominence before it links up with the osseous part of the canal. Approximately 7–10 mm medially and inferiorly to this point, the nerve trunk can be located and exposed (Fig. 21.7a). Electrostimulators are indispensable during the final stage of dissection for identification of the nerve. The

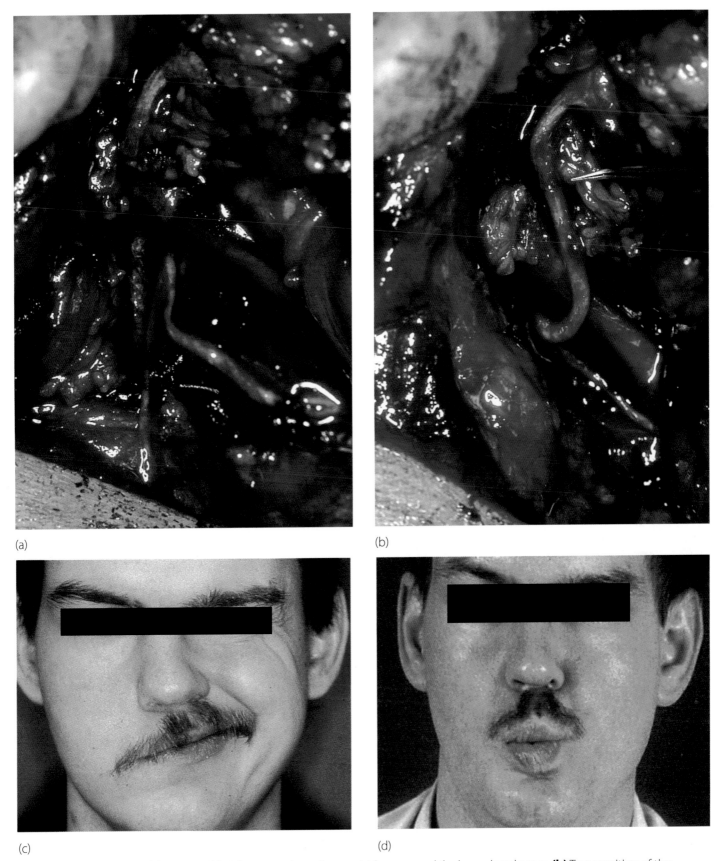

(a)

(b)

(c)

(d)

Fig. 21.7: **(a)** Exposure of the severed facial nerve at the stylomastoid foramen and the hypoglossal nerve. **(b)** Transposition of the hypoglossal nerve and crossover with the peripheral end of the facial nerve trunk. **(c)** Preoperative facial nerve function. **(d)** Postoperative facial nerve function.

pre-auricular approach is then extended into the submandibular region and the hypoglossal nerve is located beneath the intermediate tendon and the posterior belly of the digastric muscle. From this point, the hypoglossal nerve is followed proximally until it passes over the bifurcation of the carotid arteries. The nerve is then cut distal to the exit of the descending branch on the level of the digastric tendon and transposed cranially over the digastric muscle where suturing with the facial nerve is performed (Fig. 21.7**b–d**).

Another type of crossover anastomosis is the facio–facial crossover or cross-face anastomosis, which was already developed in 1971. The principle of this procedure is a theoretically ingenious concept, enabling specific facial nerve fibers to reanimate the paretic facial muscles without loss of function of one of the other cranial nerves, and provides symmetric facial movement also in emotional expression. The concept is based on the knowledge that approximately 50% of the facial nerve fibers are sufficient for undisturbed function of the facial muscles, so that almost 50% of the neural fibers can be used to reinnervate the paretic side. In order to connect the paretic side with the uninjured side, a nerve graft of 10–15 cm length is required, which is passed through a subcutaneous tunnel in the upper lip to reach the contralateral side (Fig. 21.8**a**). The zygomatic branch of the healthy side is commonly selected as the source for innervation of the contralateral side as it contains 40% of the total number of facial nerve fibers and has an intimate exchange of fibers with the buccal branch (Fig. 21.8**b**). Because of this extensive system of anastomoses, transection of the zygomatic branch on the uninjured side does not result in paralysis of the periorbital muscles on the healthy side. Stimulation of the contralateral side through the nerve graft to the paretic side then allows for satisfactory contraction of both the orbicularis oculi and the orbicularis oris muscles if it is connected to the zygomatic branch of the severed facial nerve.

The zygomatic branch of the facial nerve is exposed on both sides through a vertical pre-auricular incision that is located centrally over the parotid gland. For suturing of the zygomatic branch on the paretic side, the distal end of the nerve has to be reversed by 180° (Fig. 21.8**c–e**).

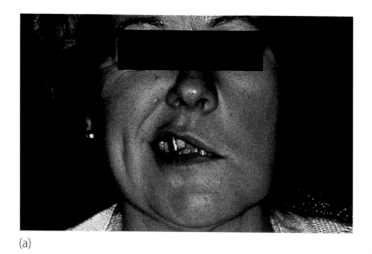

(a)

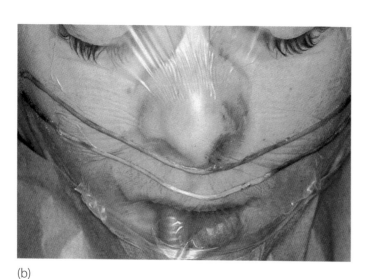

(b)

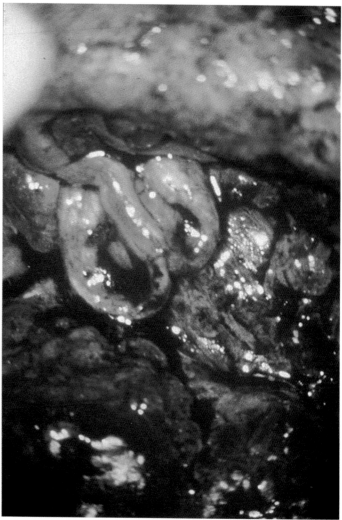

(c)

Fig. 21.8: (a) Preoperative facial nerve function. **(b)** Positioning of two sural nerve grafts on the upper lip on their cross-face route. **(c)** Suturing of the grafts to the zygomatic branch on the healthy side.

The time schedule for cross-face nerve grafting varies considerably according to the result required. If cross-face grafting is intended for repair of the contralateral facial nerve, it can be performed as a one-stage or two-stage procedure. In the latter case, the graft is connected to the zygomatic branch on the healthy side and led through the subcutaneous tunnel. Suturing with the zygomatic arch on the paretic side is, however, done only 3–4 months later after proliferation of axons from the non-paretic side into the grafted nerve has commenced. If the cross-facial nerve graft is employed to reinnervate a revascularized muscle segment for facial re-animation after long-standing facial paralysis, the second procedure is performed 10–12 months later at which time the regenerating axons should have reached the contralateral end of the nerve graft.

Nerve conduits

A new technique in nerve repair has evolved during recent years, which uses the regenerative capacity of the nerve and its inherent growth potential to restore its original morpho-logy. As in many other fields of reconstructive surgery, the use of tissue barriers has also been introduced into nerve reconstruction, employing tubes of synthetic, organic and biologic material that serve as conduits for regenerating axons across a gap of up to several centimeters. The aim of this concept is to avoid sacrifice of autogenous donor nerves in nerve reconstructions across a gap.

A large number of studies on this topic have been published using both clinical and experimental settings.[38-43] The range of results reported in these studies is as wide as the experimental approaches used so far. While some authors describe positive experience with the experimental use of collagen or fibronectin nerve guides,[44] others report no or hardly any advantage of using conduits.[45,46] Biologic conduits such as amnion tubes, veins or avascular muscle grafts showed regeneration in experimental settings across a gap of up to 10 mm that was comparable to that of autogenous nerve grafts.[41,42,47] However, clinical results with gaps of 40–58 mm in nerve reconstruction of the upper extremity were poor.[48]

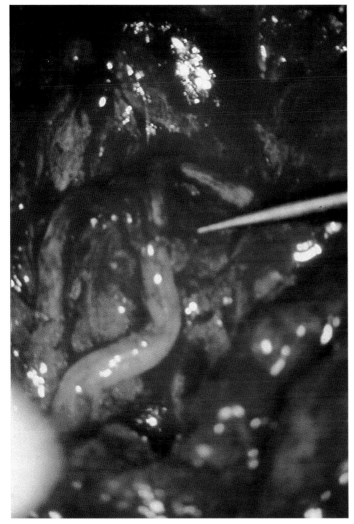

(d)

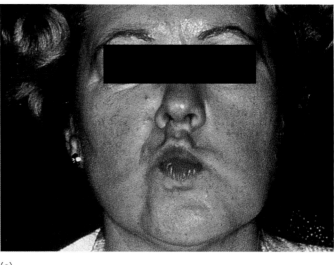

(e)

Fig. 21.8: (d) Suturing of the graft ends to the zygomatic branch on the paretic side. **(e)** Postoperative facial nerve function.

The application of synthetic conduits appears to be the most widely researched approach, with numerous types of resorbable and non-resorbable polymers in use.[49–51] However, polymeric conduits have not shown an advantage in nerve regeneration when compared to nerve grafts or epineural suturing of nerve ends.[52,53] Healing in nerve gaps of up to 10 mm was even worse or not present at all.[46,51,52] Experimental bridging of large gaps of 80 mm by polyglycolic acid tubes resulted in some degree of regeneration but obvious functional deficits.[40] The conduit material as such does not seem to have a profound effect on outcome,[43] but advances in biological approaches with the additional application of nerve growth factors or cultivated Schwann cells in these conduits may extend the gap that can be regenerated by the nerve on its own.[39,54,55] So far there are only very few studies that elucidate the complex effects of this topic in a randomized clinical setting. Weber et al[38] have shown that when a polyglycolic acid conduit is used for repair of nerve gaps of 4 mm or less, improved sensation resulted 1 year postoperatively compared with end-to-end repair of digital nerves. Repair of larger gaps also produced results superior to those obtained with nerve grafts in this area. The use of these conduits, therefore, may hold some promise in the repair of traumatic facial nerve damage.

Problems and Pitfalls

One so far unresolved problem in facial nerve reconstruction is the occurrence of uncontrolled or spontaneous (synkinetic) mass movement of the facial muscles. These disturbing effects are not only prevalent during nerve healing but can also affect the facial movements permanently thereafter. One of the most frequent synkinetic movements is the synchronous elevation of the oral commissure which is associated with considerable loss of emotional expression. Mass movements can result from poor regeneration of fascicles and from the difficulty to accurately readapt individual fascicles with high precision even under microscopic control. Several ways to solve this problem have been suggested.

Miehlke & Stennert[36] have divided the facial muscles into two functional units: the upper face and the lower face. They concluded that synkinetic movements of the upper and lower functional units could be eliminated by separate reinnervation. Therefore, they advocated two different sources of the reinnervation of the facial muscles. For the repair of the part of the facial nerve plexus that supplies the upper facial muscles, autogenous nerve grafts that connected the peripheral ends with the trunk of the facial nerve were used. The facial nerve supply to the lower face was accomplished through suturing the hypoglossal nerve to the peripheral nerve ends of this part of the plexus.

Another solution has been suggested by Millesi,[56] who used a sophisticated system of interfascicular anastomoses based on anatomic studies about the topographic orientation of certain sectors of the facial nerve cross-section to different groups of facial muscles. To avoid misinnervation in short defects of the trunk of the facial nerve, the use of three to four small nerve grafts is recommended, which connect corresponding groups of fascicles in the proximal and peripheral cross-section of the trunk. Bridging of defects between the trunk and peripheral nerve ends can be accomplished by eight nerve grafts that connect these groups of fascicles with the peripheral supply. However, misinnervations can also occur even with this technique due to variations in the course of the individual fascicles.

Postoperative Care

Postoperative treatment should commence as early as possible and be continued until normal facial motion is gained. In general, three treatment modes are available: 'neurotrophic' vitamins, physical therapy and electrotherapy.

Neurotrophic vitamins have frequently been recommended for enhancement of neural regeneration after nerve trauma. However, apart from severe general metabolic disorders due to alcohol abuse or malabsorption, so-called neurotrophic vitamins have no reliable or reproducible effect on nerve regeneration.

Physical therapy is administered to the paretic face in order to reduce the atrophy of the facial muscles. Massaging increases the local perfusion and percutaneously applied electrical current can enhance this effect. Electrotherapy cannot accelerate reinnervation and does not completely prevent muscular atrophy of the paretic muscle. It is useful in cases of complete paresis and should be continued after reconstruction until the first signs of reinnervation occur. The use of so-called exponential currents has proved to be effective, through which a distinct contraction of paretic muscles can be induced.

After onset of clearly visible voluntary contraction, active co-operation of the patient is of great importance. Electrotherapy is now replaced by active muscular exercises. The patient is instructed to voluntarily contract all facial muscles several times per day in front of the mirror. Massaging of the face should be continued at this stage.

Results

The results of facial nerve reconstruction are commonly assessed using a mixture of subjective patient criteria and observer-rated criteria.[21,61] While most observer-rated scales are semiquantitative or provide a summated score of subjective ratings,[24,57] electromyograms provide objective data on voluntary muscle contraction.

Isolated reports on the results of facial nerve reconstruction after trauma, however, are scarce. The prognosis of intratemporal lesions is strongly dependent on the severity and the delay of onset. While incomplete and delayed-onset palsies show good recovery, patients with immediate onset of complete paralysis have a poor prognosis.[2] Decompression surgery is considered to be beneficial only during the first 24 days in patients with 95% or more degeneration on electroneurograms. Blunt injuries to the extratemporal route have been reported to have a good prognosis without surgical intervention, in contrast to those to the intratemporal course.[58,59] Results of reconstruction of the facial nerve in the extratemporal part vary considerably on an individual basis according to both the techniques used and the time elapsed between trauma and repair. The most favorable results are obtained from direct nerve suturing as a primary procedure. However, this is not always possible and the second best results are achieved by using cable grafts which are interposed between the severed nerve ends.

The results of nerve crossover procedures are controversial. While some prefer cross-facial nerve grafts,[60] others advocate the hypoglossal–facial nerve crossover.[62] However, the results of nerve crossover procedures are clearly inferior to those of direct facial nerve reconstruction. In all cases an attempt should be made to perform suturing of severed nerve ends either directly or by using an interposed nerve graft.

The duration of the period of reinnervation is quite variable after complete severing of the nerve and subsequent reconstruction. Depending on the extent of the damage, return of function can be expected after 6–12 months. The function of the facial muscles continues to improve thereafter for another year. After this period the final result is commonly achieved. In long-standing facial palsy with atrophy of the muscles, neurovascular reanastomized muscle grafts (i.e. gracilis muscle) have to be considered (see Chapter 28).

References

1 May M 1986 The facial nerve. Thieme, New York, pp 181–216

2 Brodie HA, Thompson TC 1997 Management of complications from 820 temporal bone fractures. American Journal of Otology 18: 188–197

3 Qiu WW, Yin SS, Pate WE, Hardjasudarma M, Stucker FJ 1999 Neurotologic evaluation of facial nerve paralysis caused by gunshot wounds. Ear Nose and Throat Journal 78: 270–272

4 Stack BC, Farrior JB 1995 Missile injuries to the temporal bone. Southern Medical Journal 88: 72–78

5 Telischi FF, Patete ML 1994 Blast injuries to the facial nerve. Archives of Otolaryngology Head and Neck Surgery 111: 446–449

6 Bhat V, Ravikumara M, Oumachigui A 1995 Nerve injuries due to obstetric trauma. Indian Journal of Pediatrics 65: 207–212

7 Hughes CA, Harley EH, Milmoe G, Bala R, Martorella A 1999 Birth trauma in the head and neck. Archives of Otolaryngology Head and Neck Surgery 125: 193–199

8 Lalak NJ, Farmer E 1996 Traumatic pseudoaneurysm of the superficial temporal artery associated with facial nerve palsy. Journal of Cardiovascular Surgery 37: 119–123

9 Roland JT, Hammerschlag PE, Lewis WS, Choi I, Berenstein A 1994 Management of traumatic facial nerve paralysis with carotid artery cavernosus sinus fistula. European Archives of Otorhinolaryngology 251(1): 57–60

10 Turetschek K, Czerny C, Wunderbaldinger P, Steiner E 1997 Temporal bone trauma and imaging. Radiologe 37: 977–982

11 Sartoretti-Schefer S, Scherler M, Wichmann W, Valavanis A 1997 Contrast-enhanced MR of the facial nerve in patients with postraumatic peripheral facial nerve palsy. American Journal of Neuroradiology 18: 1115–1125

12 Koike Y, Tojima H, Maeyama H, Aoyagi M 1994 Contrast-enhanced MRI of the facial nerve in patients with Bell's palsy. European Archives of Otorhinolaryngology (suppl): S346–348

13 Orloff LA, Duckert LG 1995 Magnetic resonance imaging of intratemporal facial nerve lesions in the animal model. Laryngoscope 105: 465–471

14 Kumar A, Mafee MF, Mason T 2000 Value of imaging on disorders of the facial nerve. Topics in Magnetic Resonance Imaging 11: 38–51

15 Nosan DK, Benecke JE, Murr AH 1997 Current perspective on temporal bone trauma. Archives of Otolaryngology Head and Neck Surgery 117: 67–71

16 Chang CY, Cass SP 1999 Management of facial nerve injury due to temporal bone trauma. American Journal of Otology 20: 96–114

17 Har-El G, McPhee JR 2000 Transcranial magnetic stimulation in acute facial nerve injury. Laryngoscope 110: 1105–1111

18 Metson R, Rebeiz E, West C, Thornton A 1991 Magnetic stimulation of the facial nerve. Laryngoscope 101: 25–30

19 Schriefer TN, Mills KR, Murray NMF, Hess CW 1988 Evaluation of proximal facial nerve conduction by transcranial magnetic stimulation. Journal of Neurology Neurosurgery and Psychiatry 51: 60–66

20 Parisi L, Coiro P, Valente G et al 1994 Neurophysiological evaluation of Bell's palsy: electroneurography and transcranial magnetic stimulation. European Archives of Otorhinolaryngology (suppl): 253–257

21 Schliephake H, Schmelzeisen R 2000 Free revascularized muscle transfer for facial reanimation after long standing facial paralysis. International Journal of Oral and Maxillofacial Surgery 29: 243–249

22 Harii K, Ohmori K, Torii S 1976 Free gracilis muscle transplantation with microneurovascular anastomoses for the treatment of facial palsy: a preliminary report. Plastic and Reconstructive Surgery 57: 133–156

23 Kärcher H 1990 Die Reanimation der langbestehenden Facialisparese. Fortschritte der Kiefer und Gesichtschirurgie 35: 144–147

24 Harii K, Asato H, Yoshimura K, Sugawara Y, Nakatsuka T, Ueda K 1998 One-stage transfer of the latissimus dorsi muscle for reanimation of a paralyzed face: a new alternative. Plastic and Reconstructive Surgery 102: 941–951

25 Terzis JK, Noah ME 1997 Analysis of 100 cases of free muscle transplantation for facial paralysis. Plastic and Reconstructive Surgery 99: 1905–1921

26 Ueda K, Harii K, Yamada A 1994 Free neurovascular muscle transplantation for the treatment of facial paralysis using the hypoglossal nerve as a recipient motor source. Plastic and Reconstructive Surgery 94: 808–817

27 Conley J 1955 Surgical treatment of tumors of the parotid gland with emphasis on immediate nerve grafting. Western Journal of Surgery 63: 534

28 Miehlke A 1960 Die Chirurgie des Nervus facialis. Urban & Schwarzenberg, Munich

29 Millesi H 1972 Die operative Wiederherstellung verletzter Nerven. Langenbecks Archiv fur Chirurgie 332: 347–355

30 Samii M 1975 Modern aspects of peripheral and cranial nerve surgery. In: Krayenbühl H (ed) Advances and technical standards in neurosurgery, vol 2. Springer, Vienna

31 Millesi H 1980 Looking back on nerve surgery. International Journal of Microsurgery 2: 143–155

32 Lassner F, Becker MH, Fuhrer S, Walter GF, Berger A 1996 Time limited immunosuppression in allogenic nerve transplant in the rat. Handchirurgie, Mikrochirurgie, Plastische Chirurgie 28: 176–180

33 Stennert E 1979 Hypoglossal facial anastomosis: its significance for modern facial surgery. Clinics in Plastic Surgery 6: 471–482

34 Conley JJ, Baker DC 1979 Hypoglossal-facial nerve anastomosis for re-innervation of the paralyzed face. Plastic and Reconstructive Surgery 63: 63–72

35 Evans DM 1974 Hypoglossal-facial anastomosis in the treatment of facial palsy. British Journal of Plastic Surgery 27: 251–260

36 Miehlke A, Stennert E 1981 New techniques for optimum reconstruction of facial nerve in its extratemporal course. Acta Otolaryngologica 91: 497–505

37 Hausamen JE 1981 Principles and clinical application of micronerve surgery and nerve transplantation in the maxillofacial area. Annals of Plastic Surgery 7: 428–437

38 Weber RA, Breidenbach WC, Brown RE, Jabaley ME, Mass DP 2000 A randomized prospective study of polyglycolic acid conduits for digital nerve reconstruction in humans. Plastic and Reconstructive Surgery 106: 1036–1045

39 Hadlock T, Sundback C, Hunter D, Cheney M, Vacanti JP 2000 A polymer foam conduit seeded with Schwann cell promotes guided peripheral nerve regeneration. Tissue Engineering 6: 119–127

40 Matsumoto K, Ohnishi K, Sekine T et al 2000 Use of newly developed artificial nerve conduit to assist peripheral nerve regeneration across a long gap in dogs. ASAIO Journal 46: 415–420

41 Fansa H, Keilhoff G, Forster G, Seidel B, Wolf G, Schneider W 1999 Acellular muscle with Schwann-cell implantation: an alternative biologic nerve conduit. Journal of Reconstructive Microsurgery 15: 531–527

42 Mohammad J, Shenaq J, Rabinovsky E, Shenaq S 2000 Modulation of peripheral nerve regeneration: a tissue-engineering approach. Plastic and Reconstructive Surgery 105: 660–666

43 Strauch B 2000 Use of nerve conduits in peripheral nerve repair. Hand Clinics 16: 123–130

44 Kitahara AK, Nishimura Y, Shimizu Y, Endo K 2000 Facial nerve repair accomplished by the interposition of a collagen nerve guide. Journal of Neurosurgery 93: 113–120

45 Whitworth IH, Brown RA, Dore C, Green CJ, Terenghi G 1995 Orientated mats of fibronectin as a conduit material for use in peripheral nerve repair. Journal of Hand Surgery 20: 429–436

46 Vasconelos BC, Gay-Escoda C 2000 Facial nerve repair with expanded polytetrafluoroethylene and collagen conduits: an experimental study in the rabbit. Journal of Oral and Maxillofcial Surgery 58: 1257–1262

47 Di Benedetto G, Zura G, Mazzucchelli R, Santinelli A, Scarpelli M, Bertani A 1998 Nerve regeneration through a combined autologous conduit (vein plus acellular muscle). Biomaterials 19: 173–181

48 Tang JB, Shi D, Zhou H 1995 Vein conduits for repair of nerves with a prolonged gap or in unfavourable conditions: an analysis of three failed cases. Microsurgery 16: 133–137

49 Nicoli Aldini P, Perego G, Cella GD et al 1996 Effectiveness of a bioresorbable conduit in the repair of peripheral nerves. Biomaterials 17: 959–962

50 Giardino R, Nicoli Aldini P, Perego et al 1995 Biological and synthetic conduits in peripheral nerve repair: a comparative study. International Journal of Artificial Organs 18: 225–230

51 Evans GR, Brandt K, Widmer MS et al 1999 In vivo evaluation of poly(L-lactic acid) porous conduits for peripheral nerve repair. Biomaterials 20: 1109–1115

52 Francel PC, Francel TJ, Mackinnon SE, Hertl C 1997 Enhancing nerve regeneration across a silicone tube conduit by using interposed short-segment nerve grafts. Journal of Neurosurgery 87: 887–892

53 Ljungberg C, Johansson-Ruden G, Bostrom KJ, Novikov L, Widberg M 1999 Neuronal survival using resorbable synthetic conduit as an alternative to primary nerve repair. Microsurgery 19: 259–264

54 Whitworth IH, Terenghi G, Green CJ, Brown RA, Stevens E, Tomlinson DR 1995 Targeted delivery of nerve growth factor via fibronectin conduits assists nerve regeneration in control and diabetic rats. European Journal of Neuroscience 7: 2220–2225

55 Mohammad JA, Warnke PH, Pan YC, Shenaq S 2000 Increased axonal regeneration through a biodegradable amnionic tube nerve conduit: effect of local delivery and incorporation of nerve growth factor/hyaluronic acid media. Annals of Plastic Surgery 44: 59–64

56 Millesi H 1979 Nerve suture and grafting to restore the extratemporal facial nerve. Clinics in Plastic Surgery 6: 333–341

57 Fisch U, Rouleau M 1980 Facial nerve reconstruction. Journal of Otolaryngology 9: 487–492

58 Simo R, Jones NS 1996 Extratemporal facial nerve paralysis after blunt trauma. Journal of Trauma 40: 306–307

59 Guerrissi JO 1997 Facial nerve paralysis after intratemporal and extratemporal blunt trauma. Journal of Craniofacial Surgery 8: 431–437

60 Samii M 1981 Zur Indikation, Technik und zu den Ergebnissen der facio-facialen Anastomose. Neurochirurgie 24: 90–104

61 Hausamen JE, Schmelzeisen R 1996 Current principles in microsurgical nerve repair. British Journal of Oral and Maxillofacial Surgery 34: 143–157

62 Hausamen JE 1987 Microsurgery of the facial nerve trauma. In: Stark RB (ed) Plastic surgery of the head and neck. Churchill Livingstone, New York

22 Facial Burns

Barry L Eppley, Rajiv Sood

Introduction

Nearly half the patients who are admitted to a burn unit have some degree of facial burns. Fortunately, most facial burns are superficial injuries with typical etiologies of flash or splatter mechanisms. Extensive facial burns are more uncommon and are usually the result of engulfing flame injuries from large explosions or housefires or scald injuries in children. In either case, the treatment of facial burns has numerous considerations that are different from other systemic locations. Facial tissue that is burned affects esthetic appearance and has a potential negative influence on surrounding orifices such as the eyes, nose, mouth and ears. Skin grafts are often a poor substitute for native facial skin and such specialized structures as the eyelids or lips, for example, simply can never be completely restored to their native state. The primary management of facial burns has a major role to play in their outcome and is the subject of this chapter. Secondary burn reconstruction is a much larger topic that is not within the scope of this review.

Burn etiology and classification

The head, face and neck are the most frequent anatomical sites to sustain thermal injury. The most common cause of facial thermal injury is flash burns and the least common occurs with exposure to hot surfaces.[1] The severity of burns to the face depends on the duration of exposure to and the intensity of the burning agent. As time and temperature are the prime determinants of the severity of thermal injury, at temperatures between 44°C (110°F) and 51°C (124°F), the rate of cellular destruction doubles with each degree of increase in temperature. At temperatures above 51°C (124°F) less than 3 minutes is required for a full-thickness burn and above 70°C (158°F), less than 2 seconds is required for complete epidermal necrosis.[2]

The specific burning agent (heat source) also has an effect on the extent of the facial burn. Non-combustible hot liquids, such as water, are frequently encountered but are usually less than 70°C (158°F) and their duration of exposure is very short (less than 2 seconds) as they descend inferiorly over the body surface. Such scald burns therefore typically result in only partial-thickness facial burns. Combustible hot liquids, such as grease, are usually heated to much higher temperatures (greater than 100°C) and due to their viscous nature have a much longer duration of exposure. This often creates contact areas of full-thickness burns. Flash burns to the face cause only a brief exposure to the heat source, resulting in a superficial or partial-thickness burn. The singed eyebrow or nasal hairs from flash burns may make one suspicious of an inhalation injury but the absence of carbonaceous soot or difficulty in breathing as well as the location of the injury will make it unlikely that an inhalation injury has occurred. Bronchoscopy should be carried out in all these patients. Flame burns, particularly with ignition of clothing, have a longer exposure to intense heat and make a full-thickness injury more likely.[1]

Burns are traditionally classified into first-, second- and third-degree injuries depending upon the depth and completeness of dermal involvement. A better anatomic classification is that of superficial, partial-thickness (superficial and deep) and full-thickness burn injuries. All superficial and most partial-thickness burns maintain some dermal circulation and are usually capable of going on to heal without excision or grafting. This can be clinically confirmed by the appearance of blisters and pain and the presence of capillary refill. In the face, this is the most common type of burn as this area is often involved in external burn etiologies (e.g. flash, explosions) rather than direct flame contact (Fig. 22.1). Withdrawal or turning of the face is a natural protective reaction and frequently serves to spare the face from more severe thermal damage.

Full-thickness burns irreversibly damage the epidermis, papillary and reticular dermis and result in thrombosis of the subdermal plexus. Clinically, the skin appears pale with minimal to no refill. Removal of the hair shafts occurs easily. This degree of facial burn is commonly due to prolonged flame contact from bed or house fires where the victim is disabled by smoke, alcohol or drugs (Fig. 22.2). Extensive full-thickness burns, often called fourth-degree injuries, also exist in which tissues and structures beneath the skin are involved. The skin is usually charred and insensitive and etiologies include electricity greater than 1000 volts, molten metal or prolonged contact with hot metal or flames. This degree of burn injury is rare in the face.

While the four degrees of burn classification are embedded in the literature, it is better to describe burns as either partial or full thickness, particularly in the face. This provides a simpler classification which is more physiologically based and directly reflects what should be done from a subsequent management standpoint. While classifying the location and perceived depth of the burn is important, it is critical to also understand the evolving nature of thermal injuries after their occurrence. It may take several days before the full extent and depth of a burn is apparent. Therefore, any early thoughts about surgical excision should be delayed until the

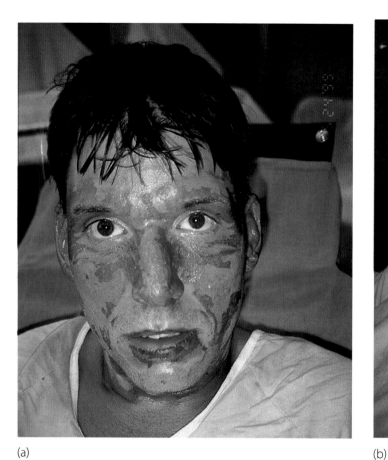

(a)

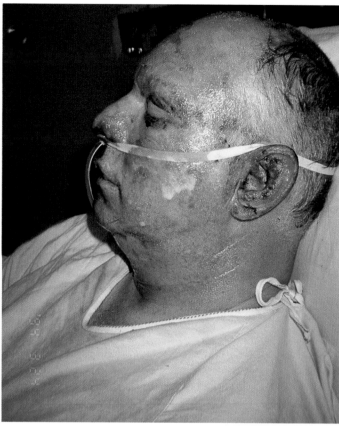

(b)

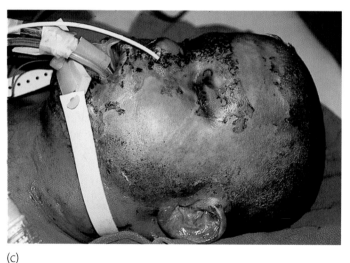

(c)

Fig. 22.1: Partial-thickness facial burns. **(a)** Flash burn from gas grill. **(b)** Flash burn from throwing gasoline on burning wood. **(c)** Deeper partial-thickness burn from flames from house fire.

burn depth and margins are clear. All interventions directed toward burn care, such as resuscitation, antibiotics, etc., help to prevent 'conversion' of the burn to deeper levels.

Role of topical antimicrobials

The necrotic non-viable tissue that covers the surface of a burn wound is a fertile medium for bacterial growth. While excision of the burned tissue is the ultimate treatment for this potential problem, this is not done until the demarcation of the burn is evident and the patient is adequately resuscitated and stabilized. In the interim, the use of topical anti-

microbials is the mainstay of the prevention of infection. Although numerous bacteria, fungi and viruses have been associated with primary infection of burn wounds, the most devastating are the Gram-negative bacteria, particularly pseudomonas. In the face of infection, burn wounds may easily progress in depth and extent. Intravenous systemic antibiotics are often of little value as they cannot reach the site of inoculation due to vascular thrombosis.

The most commonly used topical agents include bacitracin, 1% silver sulfadiazine, mafenide acetate (Sulfamylon) and collagenase (Santyl) (Fig. 22.3). For superficial burns to the face, bacitracin, regular or ophthalmic (E. Fougera, Melville,

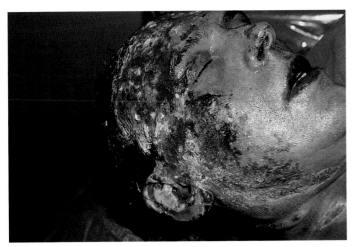

Fig. 22.2: Full-thickness facial burn from house fire involving the forehead, cheek and ear.

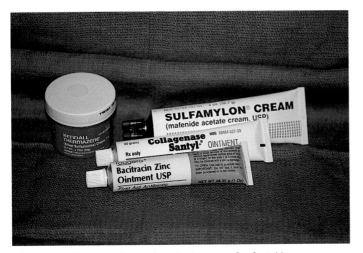

Fig. 22.3: Commonly used topical agents for facial burns (Bacitracin, Silvadene, Sulfamylon and collagenase).

NY), is the preferred mode of treatment. It contains 500 mg/g of active agent and is a well-tolerated topical antimicrobial agent that causes minimal tissue reactivity. It offers no penetration of burn eschar, however, which is why its use is limited to superficial burns. In deeper partial-thickness and full-thickness burns, 1% silver sulfadiazine (Silvadene or Thermazene, Kendall Company, Marsfield, MA) is commonly used as it has the advantages of good penetration of burn eschar and is painless on application. It combines the antimicrobial action of silver ions with sulfadiazine. The use of silvadene, however, tends to produce a 'pseudoeschar' if not used appropriately and this may confuse assessment of the depth of burn. Mafenide acetate (Sulfamylon 85 mg/g, Butek Pharmaceuticals, Morgantown, WV) is a potent antimicrobial, has the best eschar penetration but is associated with pain after application. Both Silvadene and Sulfamylon must be kept away from the periorbital region as corneal ulceration, conjunctival edema and chemosis and visual damage may result. In facial burns, all three antimicrobial agents are used but in selective applications. Around the periorbital area, bacitracin ophthalmic

ointment is preferred, regardless of the depth of the burn, as it poses no risk to the eye. In the remainder of the face and scalp, 1% silver sulfadiazine may be liberally applied. Due to the known risk of cartilage exposure and suppurative chondritis from burns, Sulfamylon is used almost exclusively on the ear.

Recently, we have started to use an enzymatic debriding agent, collagenase (Santyl Ointment, Knoll Pharmaceutical, Whippany, NJ), for superficial to deep partial-thickness burns. Santyl is a product of the bacterium *Clostridium histolyticum* which is able to digest native and denatured collagen in devitalized tissue. In prospective studies, it has been shown to improve healing and re-epithelization times in partial-thickness burns when compared to Silvadene.[3] Since the majority of the dry weight of necrotic and viable tissue consists of collagen, a debriding collagenolytic enzyme would seem to be an appropriate choice. It offers the ability of chemically discriminating between viable and non-viable tissue, thereby preserving more viable tissue. This is of particular value in the face where every square millimeter of tissue has esthetic value. Antibiotic powders may be mixed with the ointment to add an antibacterial benefit. Other newer debriding ointments are also available such as Accuzyme (Healthpoint Medical, San Antonio, TX), a papain-urea preparation (1 100 000 units of papain and 100 mg/g of urea). This debriding ointment is stronger than collagenase with some significant pain on application. For this reason, we do not use it on the face.

State-of-the-Art Management

In the acute phase of facial burn management, it is medically important to initially rule out the presence of heat injury to the upper aerodigestive passages and lungs. The location of the burn injury is the single greatest determinant of inhalational injuries. Burns that have occurred outdoors or in open environments are unlikely to cause internal heat injuries. In closed environments, particularly house fires, suspicion should be high (Fig. 22.4). Inhaled hot air can directly damage mucous membranes with resultant edema. Swelling occurs within the first 24–48 hours and, if severe, may lead to

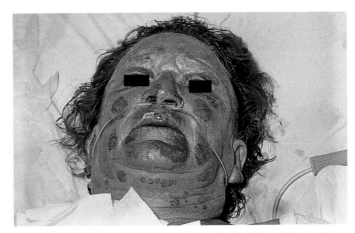

Fig. 22.4: Patient with high suspicion of inhalation injury with perinasal/perioral burns from a housefire. Bronchoscopy is mandatory.

airway obstruction and pulmonary insufficiency. In these cases, early endotracheal intubation should be performed. Nasotracheal intubation is preferred to the oral route as it can be easier to perform, is more comfortable when used for longer periods and can be firmly secured. Fixation of the nasal tube is best done by transseptal suturing (2-3 or 3-0 silk) which not only provides good security but also eliminates the need for tape on the face. When orally placed, the tube can be secured with interdental wires or sutures. If respiratory insufficiency is due to heat injury, it is usually possible to extubate the patient after several days.

On admission, facial burns are debrided of all loose blisters and eschar. While much debate occurs about whether to leave or open blisters, in general leaving fluid-filled blisters in the face may be an impediment to wound evaluation and healing. In very superficial burns, particularly involving the periorbital area, bacitracin ophthalmic ointment without dressings is used. Deeper burns may require more aggressive treatment which is influenced by the anatomic location of the facial burn.

Tetanus prophylaxis is given to all burn patients unless a booster has been received in the past 5 years. Since routine administration of antibiotics does not protect against burn wound cellulitis and burn wound sepsis, its use in the acutely burned patient is not recommended. Unless specifically indicated by obvious wound infection or positive cultures, the liberal use of antibiotics contributes to the development of resistant organisms, a not uncommon problem in hospital burn units.

Scalp

The scalp is protected from burn injury by a combination of a covering of hair, a thick dermis and a rich vascularity through an extensive network of subdermal vessels. Most scalp burns, therefore, can be treated conservatively. The dermal appendages of hair and sweat glands, from which much epithelial regeneration emanates, extend very deeply and allow most burns of the head to heal. They generally do so with minimal hypertrophic scarring as they are stretched out over a tight skull and maximal hair follicles can be preserved (Fig. 22.5). If you feel that the scalp burn will heal within 2 weeks, then conservative management is warranted. In deeper scalp burns, the easy removal of hair follicles is one indicator of a complete irreversible dermal injury. When early excision is needed, usually indicated by the unmistakable white leathery appearance, the underlying galea, pericranium or developing granulation tissue makes an excellent bed for skin graft acceptance (Fig. 22.6). Tangential excision in the scalp can result in rapid and significant blood loss even though its surface area is relatively small. It may be helpful to tumesce the scalp with a dilute epinephrine (1 : 1 000 000) solution prior to excision to control the blood loss and reduce the tendency for excessive electrocoagulation of bleeders, which adds another thermal insult.

The occipital scalp burn presents a difficult problem as the skin is both burned and is exposed to continuous pressure with the patient in the supine position on the bed. This

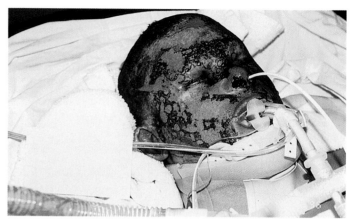

Fig. 22.5: Superficial scalp burn from house fire which will heal on its own.

combination increases the risk of full-thickness tissue necrosis down to the galea and bone. Soft head support and frequent changes in patient positioning are helpful in controlling progression of the burn injury in this area. Pressure relief mattresses and beds are often used in the more severely burned patients.

In very deep scalp burns, the calvarium can become exposed which is a difficult problem. Small areas will heal by the enveloping development of granulation tissue which may take several weeks. This may occasionally require mechanical burring of the outer table of the calvarium to induce the formation of granulation tissue. When larger areas of the calvarium are exposed, local or free vascularized flaps may be necessary for coverage (Fig. 22.7). However, this does not need to be done acutely as the exposed calvarium does not add any significant risk to the recovering burn patient and may be covered with moist dressings for some time until the patient is in an improved metabolic state for a more major surgical procedure.

Eyelids and eyebrows

Any patient with periorbital burns must be assumed to have corneal injury until proven otherwise. Corneal injury can be a direct result of the burn injury or from the presence of a foreign body. Patients with flame burns will usually not have a corneal injury but those exposed to explosion or chemical burns often will. Chemicals are particularly destructive to the cornea, particularly alkaline fluids such as sodium hydroxide. The alkali combines with protein and fat to form soluble soaps which penetrate and then irreversibly damage the epithelial and stromal cells of the cornea. Acid burns are better tolerated in the eye than alkali burns due to the natural acid-buffering capacity of living tissue. Initial emergency treatment is copious continuous irrigation with water or saline. Low pressure (<1 psi) with 0.9% saline with the lids retracted helps ensure complete flushing of the entire conjunctival sac.

It is important for an ophthalmologist to perform a fluorescein dye examination within the first hours after injury to detect the presence of a corneal injury. As the eyelids will

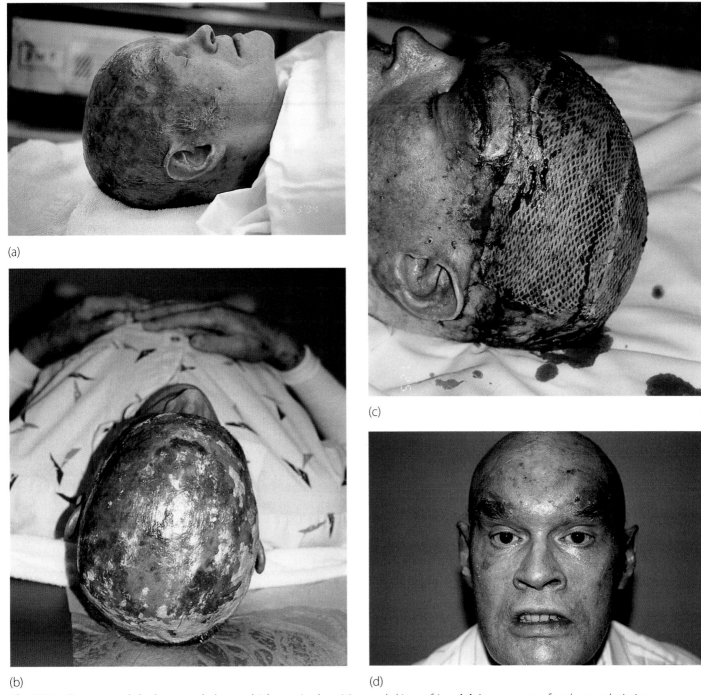

(a)

(b)

(c)

(d)

Fig. 22.6: Deep partial-thickness scalp burn which required excision and skin grafting. **(a)** Appearance of scalp on admission. **(b)** Non-healing scalp burn 10 days later with topical Silvadene treatment. **(c)** Tangential excision and meshed split-thickness skin grafting. **(d)** Healing result 10 days later.

swell very quickly, an examination may not be possible the next day. When present, many corneal injuries will heal by topical therapy which usually includes antibiotic ointments and 1% atropine drops to prevent ciliary and iris sphincter spasm.

When the cornea is exposed, it must be kept lubricated to prevent desiccation. If the surrounding tissue has only minor burns, ophthalmic lubricating ointment with an overlying occlusive film may be adequate. In more severe burns when this is not possible, a scleral lens can be placed. In clinical

practice, however, corneal coverage in the first few days or week after eyelid burns is not a problem due to the resultant edema, a natural patching mechanism for the next 48–72 hours. The issue of corneal protection becomes relevant as the edema subsides and the globe is again visible. Historically, the use of a tarsorrhaphy is often described as a temporary method of eyelid closure but contemporary burn care has moved away from its use as it is often ineffective at lid closure, is prone to separation and causes damage to the lid margin which may make future reconstruction difficult.

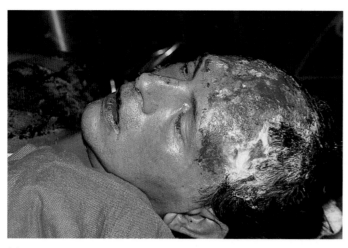

(a)

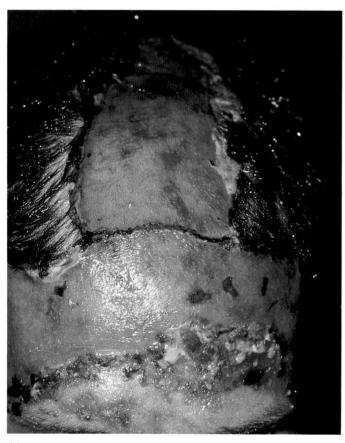

(b)

Fig. 22.7: Full-thickness anterior scalp and forehead burn. **(a)** Three days after admission. **(b)** Ten days after sheet split-thickness skin grafting.

Therefore, we do not currently advocate its use. If some lid apposition is desirable, it would be preferable to use a temporary suture of 4-0 or 5-0 nylon placed between the gray lines of the lid margin off the corneal axis. In more severe cases of exposure, a conjunctival flap (Gunderson procedure) can aid in preservation of the integrity of the globe (Fig. 22.8).[4]

Most burns of the eyelids are partial thickness and will heal spontaneously without significant scarring. In deep partial-thickness or full-thickness burns involving extensive skin loss

of the eyelids, skin grafting will be necessary as soon as the eschar separates and a healthy bed of granulation tissue develops. Unlike other facial areas, the concept of eyelid burn excision is more theroetical than practical. It is easy to remove the underlying orbicularis and levator muscles, rendering the eyelid immobile if not already so from the depth of the burn. Therefore, direct excision of the burn wound is rarely performed. If skin gafting is necessary, our preference is to use full-thickness facial or neck skin on a delayed basis for reconstruction. A full-thickness skin graft of upper eyelid skin is ideal but both eyelids are usually burned in most cases, eliminating this option. Following application of the autograft, maximal immobilization of the graft to the eyelids must be done. The grafts are best secured by tie-over bolster dressings which remain in place for 5–7 days.

Although postponement of eyelid grafting permits it to be done under more favorable wound-healing conditions, exposure of the cornea or significant lid deformity may develop in severely burned cases. In such cases, early skin grafting can be performed with the realization that subsequent contraction and the development of ectropion may require further graft reconstruction. Fortunately, complete loss of significant eyelid tissue (lid margins and large amounts of upper and lower eyelid tissues) is rare. In these cases, an early masquerade technique is needed in which the upper and lower eyelid conjunctiva is sewn together and overlaid with a skin graft.[4]

The development of burn ectropion of the eyelids, particularly the lower, is a common sequel of significant periorbital burns, whether they are primarily grafted or not. This occurs due to either an intrinsic mechanism from actual eyelid contracture, from an extrinsic mechanism due to surrounding periorbital tissue contracture, or both. In either case, secondary reconstruction with release and skin grafting are necessary and this potential need must be appreciated from the onset of the burn injury. The dynamic nature of the eyelids combined with their thin tissue quality makes their function very unforgiving of deep partial-thickness and full-thickness burns.

Eyebrows are frequently singed in flash and explosive type injuries. In these circumstances, regrowth almost always occurs. In severe burns of the eyelids, significant full-thickness injury to the eyebrows may occur as well. Although most follicles lie within the subdermal level, a full-thickness skin injury will usually irreversibly damage them. In these cases, even if a few follicles survive, they are of no value as the overlying skin must be completely debrided and grafted. Secondary eyebrow reconstruction is delayed until the patient is well recovered and is often one of the last reconstructive procedures performed.

Nose

Burns to the nose are frequent due to its prominent position on the face, occurring in a large majority of facial burns. The thick dermis of the nose, particularly in men, and its rich blood supply make for a high incidence of partial-thickness injuries (Fig. 22.9). Unlike the eyelid, burns of the nose usually do not impose the risk of significant functional

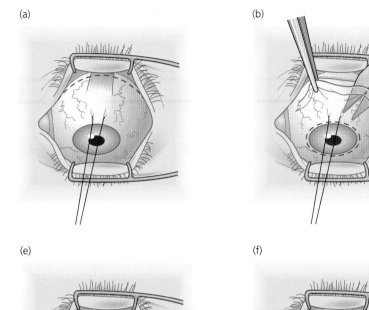

(a) (b) (e) (f)

Fig. 22.8: In severe full-thickness eyelid burns, the globe can be protected by the raising and closure of upper and lower conjunctival flaps which are then covered by a skin graft.
(a) Outline of conjunctival flaps, **(b)** sharp elevation of conjunctival flaps, **(c)** suturing together of upper and lower conjunctival flaps for corneal coverage, **(d)** vascularized conjunctival bed for skin graft placement.

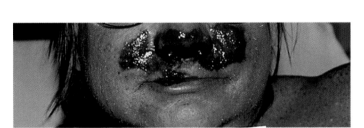

Fig. 22.9: Partial-thickness perinasal burn which will heal on its own with topical therapy.

deformity as the underlying structural framework of the cartilage, bone and mucosal lining is spared. However, the nose has a profound effect on the patient's self-image and a well-healed, non-deformed nose is desirable.

The main goal of primary nasal burn treatment is to conserve as much tissue as possible and prevent further injury by iatrogenic means. The initial treatment is to apply bacitracin ophthalmic ointment for more superficial burns and 1% Silvadene for deeper burns. Debridement should be minimal and excision of the burn can be delayed for 2–3 weeks to allow maximal time for demarcation and skin survival. In severe burns with more extensive systemic involvement where pulmonary management is necessary, endotracheal and nasogastric tubes must be secured so they do not cause further skin injury through pressure necrosis or adhesive tape.

This may be done through transseptal suturing of nasal tubes or the use of the oral route if tube placements are likely to be of short duration. If it appears that the patient is at risk for nostril stenosis due to significant alar involvement, splints can be fabricated and placed early.[5]

Ear

Like the nose, a large majority of facial burns will have involvement of the ear. Unlike the nose, however, the skin overlying the auricular cartilage is very thin and is quite susceptible to full-thickness thermal injuries. Even if not severely burned, a suppurative chondritis may develop weeks after the initial burn as a complicating factor. Furthermore, pressure from pillows and any circumferential dressings may further extend the damage to the ear.

With prevention in mind, the inital treatment of burned ears has changed significantly over the past 30 years. The original concepts employed early debridement and grafting. While this technique is effective, significant ear deformities were common. Given that 75% of burned ears heal without grafting, less radical excision of only obviously necrotic skin and exposed cartilage is now performed (Fig. 22.10).[5] A regimen of minimal debridement and twice-daily application of Sulfamylon, due to its better penetration of relatively avascular cartilage, is used in most centers. Sulfamylon is

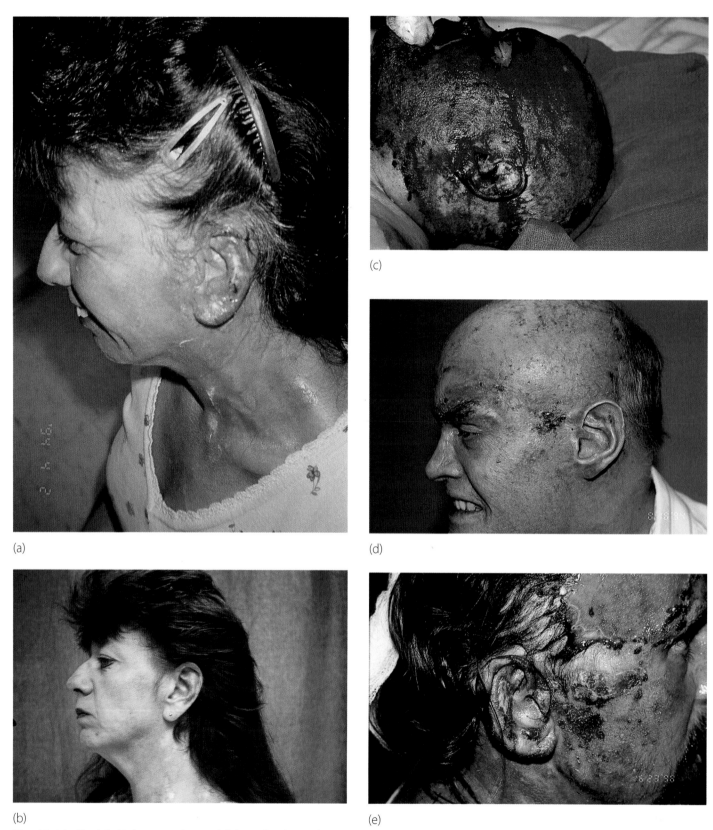

(a)

(b)

(c)

(d)

(e)

Fig. 22.10: Partial-thickness ear burns. **(a)** Superficial partial-thickness ear burn 3 days after injury. **(b)** Three months post injury with spontaneous healing. **(c)** Deeper part-thickness ear burn on admission. **(d)** Complete healing by one month after injury. **(e)** Combination partial and full-thickness ear burn 3 days after admission.

applied thickly and often enough to prevent desiccation of the ear. When the cartilage is exposed, allow time for granulation tissue to develop first from the normal skin edges, which may take weeks. This will allow a better bed for later skin grafting. If the cartilage remains exposed, skin grafting is ultimately performed over its cut edges after debridement back to bleeding tissue. In rare cases, the cartilage from an isolated severely burned ear can be covered by a temporal ascial flap based on the temporal vessels.

Some burn centers employ a topical treatment of antibiotic iontophoresis in place of or in addition to Sulfamylon topical cream in the burned ear. Iontophoresis involves applying gentamicin sulfate antibiotic (5–10 mg/ml) as either a cream or soaked on gauze to the ear with the subsequent application of a direct electrical current (positive electrode of 10–15 mA for gentamicin). A ground (negative pole) is placed somewhere else on the body. This technique has good experimental evidence for antibiotic penetration into cartilage and clinical reports support its effectiveness.[6,7] However, it is not clear that it prevents suppurative chondritis and is clearly more cumbersome than Sulfamylon cream alone. Its greatest benefit may be as an adjunctive treatment in established chondritis as it may minimize the need for significant amounts of cartilage resection.

Avoiding pressure on the ear is another important aspect of primary management. The patients should not be allowed to use pillows as this is an unappreciated source of potential pressure. If necessary, but rarely used, foam can be placed around the pinna to prevent further pressure. No external wound dressings are needed for ear coverage as antibiotic cream is sufficient.

All burned ears have the potential for suppurative chondritis which is often not seen until weeks after the initial injury. The symptoms of infectious chondritis are a red, hot, tender, swollen ear. Purulence is uniformly present, is often green in color and usually cultures out to be *Pseudomonas aeruginosa* (mostly) or *Staphylococcus aureus*. Interestingly, the burn to the ear may be healed at this time and cartilage exposure may never have been initially present. Prompt treatment is necessary to prevent loss of all ear cartilage. The abscess is opened through a limited bivalving incision and cartilage is debrided as necessary. Systemic antibiotics are given in conjunction with topical Sulfamylon. With the cartilage debridement and subsequent wound contracture, the esthetic outcome is usually poor and some patients may lose most of their ear. Therefore, prevention is paramount and aggressive early treatment, including antibiotic iontophoresis if available, is essential.[8,9]

Lips and mouth

The constant motion of the lips and exposure to contaminated salivary fluids make care of burn injuries in this area uniquely different from the rest of the face. As a result, this area commonly develops hypertrophic scarring and contracture after being burned. As the mouth provides access for eating, hygiene and intubation, early treatment is often directed to the prevention of microstomia. The risk of microstomia is

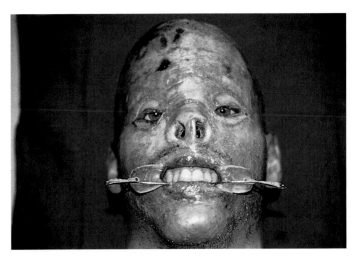

Fig. 22.11: Splinting of the oral commissure is an important treatment for perioral burn care. The splints are applied early after grafting when the wound is stable. They may be used for months to conteract sphincteric contractures. In this case, the splint is an extraorally based device with a circumferential strap.

usually either from severe burns about the perioral area, which cause subsequent narrowing of the mouth, or the oral commissure electrical burn. In either case, the use of splinting devices is the mainstay of primary treatment.

Oral splinting devices should be fabricated and inserted as soon after the burn as possible. Except for the most severe injuries, tangential excision or excision of the lip burns is rarely done or necessary. Lip burns are generally allowed to demarcate and heal on their own. Therefore, early and continual resistance of contracture for months is usually the best treatment approach as successful reconstruction of microstomia can be difficult.

Splints fundamentally are of three types based upon their point of anchorage: external such as head and neck straps, self-retaining lip splints and dental or orthodontic appliances (Fig. 22.11). When possible, a dental-based splint is preferred as it attaches to the maxillary teeth and palate intraorally and is less obtrusive than other devices. However, this requires adequate intraoral access for dental impressions which frequently may be difficult, even in the operating room. The other types of microstomia splints do not have to be 'custom made' and are easier to apply even if they are more visible.

The oral commissure burn deserves special mention as it is not uncommon and is easily treated. This injury typically occurs in toddlers under 5 years of age and involves the small child placing an electric cord in his mouth. Through chewing and violation of the cord's plastic cover, the saliva creates an electrical short and an arc is created. This arc produces high heat, up to 3000°C, and chars the portion of the mouth in contact with the arc.[10] This causes extensive local tissue destruction at the commissure with a zone of full-thickness burn (Fig. 22.12). There is no treatment that needs to be done immediately other than the application of bacitracin ointment and to warn the parents that bleeding from the labial artery may occur several weeks after the injury as the

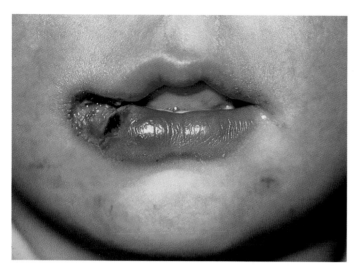

Fig. 22.12: Classic example of an electrical oral commissure burn which is a full-thickness injury with a well-demarcated eschar.

eschar separates. While initially frightening when seen, the bleeding is easily controlled by manual compression. Provided that the child can take fluids and nourishment, there is no need for acute hospitalization. After allowing several weeks for eschar separation and healing, a palatal splint is fabricated

and worn ideally for up to 6 months after the injury on a near continual basis. When compliance is good, subsequent surgical correction is usually not necessary (Fig. 22.13).[11]

Neck

The neck is frequently involved when the face is burned, although it is unusual to have extensive involvement if there are not significant upper trunk burns as well. The neck is often spared in flash burns due to clothing but, conversely, can be deeply burned in flame injuries when clothes are ignited. Significant deep neck burns signify greater systemic involvement and these patients often require fluid resuscitation and intubation as well. As the neck is the rotational mechanism for the head, deep burns can lead to contracture and a functional deformity of restriction of movement.

Superficial and partial-thickness burns of the neck are liberally covered with Silvadene until the demarcation of the wound is clear. Partial-thickness wounds, particularly in men due to the re-epithelialization capabilities of hair-bearing skin, are allowed to heal on their own. In patients with full-thickness neck burns, early excision of the wound is accompanied by either the application of homograft (if the wound bed is uncertain) or large sheets of relatively thick (0.018–0.020 inch) split-thickness skin grafts. Not meshing and expanding the skin graft helps to prevent postoperative

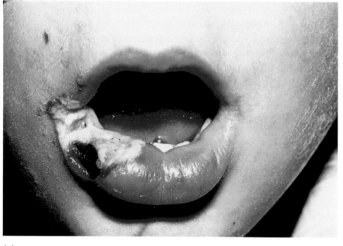

(a)

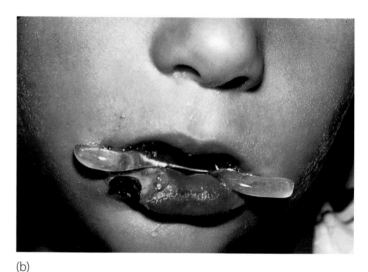

(b)

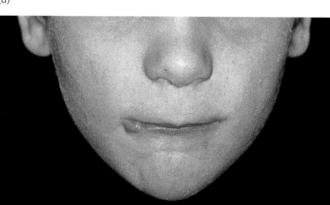

(c)

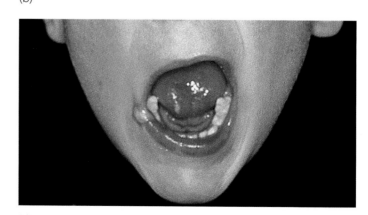

(d)

Fig. 22.13: Electrical oral commissure burn result without surgery. **(a)** Extent of injury. **(b)** Use of splint appliance for 3 months. **(c)** Healed result after one year. **(d)** Oral opening after one year.

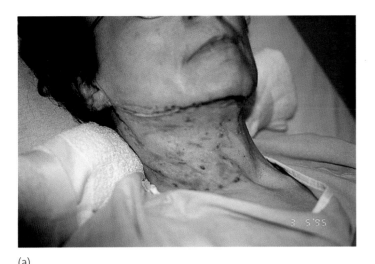
(a)

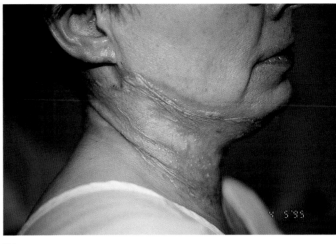
(b)

Fig. 22.14: Skin grafting to the neck is usually done as sheet (unmeshed split-thickness) grafts to both decrease the risk of contractures and improve the esthetic result. **(a)** One week after grafting. **(b)** One month after grafting.

contracture and gives a better esthetic result, but graft take is often poorer due to the inevitable postoperative movements of the neck that occur and the build-up of subgraft fluid. Therefore, a good compromise is to use meshed split-thickness skin but with no minimal expansion (Fig. 22.14). An overlying compression dressing or bolster is preferred but this is usually not practical in most burned patients with significant skin involvement.

Early excision and coverage of deep neck burns is particularly important in patients with inhalation injury requiring extended mechanical ventilatory support (more than 2–3 weeks). Once the neck is successfully grafted and healed, placement of a tracheostomy through healthy surrounding or intact skin graft can be done.

The rest of the face

Treatment of burns to areas other than the eyelids, ears, nose and lips differs somewhat from these previously discussed regions. These are areas of high esthetic significance but have a more favorable geometry, being more flat and covering greater surface areas. Furthermore, they do not impinge significantly on most of the important facial functions. Like all reconstructive facial surgery, the esthetic unit principle applies when managing burns to these areas (Fig. 22.15).

Facial burns in these areas are initially treated as previously described by debridement of loose blisters, daily cleaning and coverage with topical antibacterials. The critical management difference is that if the burns are not healed or expected to heal within 3 weeks of the injury on their own, primary excision and grafting is done. This more 'aggressive' approach to burns in these facial areas has been shown to yield a better appearance and function than that obtained by allowing spontaneous healing over more than 3 weeks or grafting on granulation tissue. In addition, the magnitude and number of subsequent reconstructions are decreased.[12] Those esthetic facial units judged to be incapable of healing within 3 weeks are excised; occasionally small unburned or healed areas must be included in the excision to preserve the esthetic unit (Fig. 22.16). Excised areas are initially covered with homo-

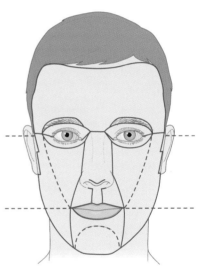

Fig. 22.15: Esthetic facial units.

graft for 48 hours until the egress of serum and blood decreases. Thereafter, thick split-thickness (0.018–0.025 inch) grafts are harvested and placed in an unmeshed fashion according to the esthetic unit outlines (Fig. 22.16).[13] In smaller surface area burns, a better color match is obtained from scalp, neck or inner upper arm skin. If the entire face is to be grafted, color match becomes an irrelevant issue. Some form of postoperative compression of the grafts is important (e.g. foam or compression garments) and the grafts must be carefully inspected postoperatively several times daily to check for subgraft fluid. Any hematomas or seromas are removed through small graft incisions placed in the relaxed skin tension lines. Once healed, pressure garments or masks must be worn to lessen the incidence of hypertrophic scarring.

Early excision and grafting of facial burns produces better results than delayed excision or spontaneous healing. Subsequent reconstruction is often limited to junctures, seams and smaller areas. However, most patients that require such therapy have either extensive or deep facial burns and will therefore rarely have a normal appearance to the burned areas (Fig. 22.16). As such, this approach should be reserved

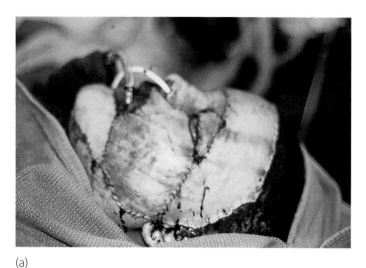

(a)

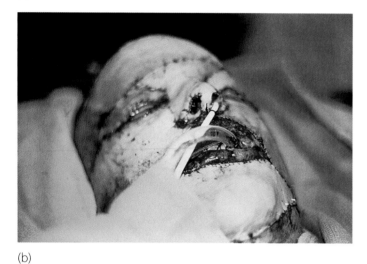

(b)

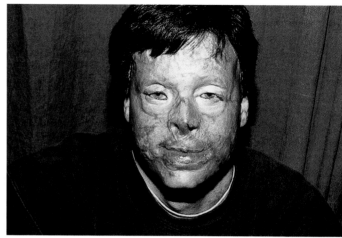

(c)

Fig. 22.16: Sheet grafting (unmeshed split thickness) to the face as done by esthetic units. **(a)** Lateral view. **(b)** Frontal view. **(c)** One year post grafting.

only for these more difficult facial burn problems. Again, if the facial burn will heal spontaneously within 3 weeks, it is better left alone.

Controversies

Many controversies still exist regarding facial burn management. These include the potential choice of topical agents, early versus late excision and closure of the wound, options for limited coverage of the face versus full facial coverage, and ultimately the timing of reconstruction.

For the choice of topical agents, most burn centers are evolving away from the routine use of Silvadene and being more aggressive with enzymatic debriding ointments. Our current approach is directed toward the prevention of pseudoeschar formation which is particularly critical in preventing a subeschar proliferation of bacteria, a known mechanism for converting burn wounds to a greater depth. Preventing eschar formation potentially improves the speed of healing, leading to earlier closure of the wound and decreased likelihood of hypertrophic scarring. Without eschar formation, one is also better able to assess whether the wound will be able to heal. For the face, this usually translates to a mid-to late execution of tangential excision. In our

burn center, we typically wait at least 5–7 days before carrying out tangential excision of the face. At this point the potential for the wound to heal on its own should be evident.

Controversy still exists regarding choice of options for more limited facial burns. In general, it is traditionally better to excise and cover esthetic facial units as a whole. However, this is often somewhat impractical, such as in a hemi-forehead burn. Does one really want to sacrifice this much normal tissue? In this circumstance, we prefer to think of how primary grafting can be improved by secondary reconstruction. Primary excision and grafting of a subesthetic unit may be eliminated or improved by secondary reconstruction through the use of tissue expansion or other local flap techniques. The esthetic unit concept is not completely valid in all cases. If only a small amount of normal skin exists as part of the esthetic unit, then it is probably better to remove these areas.

The best donor match for facial burns is from the neck but this is a limited source. Other options must be considered including upper arm or upper chest skin. In larger burns in which full facial coverage may be needed, a large thick (between 15 and 18 one-thousandths of an inch) sheet graft from the upper back is very useful. The color and texture may not be ideal but it will be homogenous throughout the grafted skin.

Lastly, the timing of contracture/hypertrophic scar releases is undergoing a conceptual change. Historically, contracture releases were not carried out until scar maturation had occurred which may take up to 18–24 months. In facial contractures, either of the eyelid or neck, this is not ideal due to the functional restrictions imposed. Most burn centers are now moving toward earlier releases and coverage to shorten the period of functional impairment. This is particularly useful for eyelid and oral burn scar restrictions.

References

1   Morgan RF, Nichter LS, Haines PC, Kenney JG, Friedman HI, Edlich RF 1985 Management of head and neck burns. Journal of Burn Care and Rehabilitation 6: 20

2   Moritz AR, Henriques FC Jr 1947 Studies of thermal injury II. The influence of time and surface temperature in the causation of cutaneous burns. American Journal of Pathology 23: 695

3   Hansbrough J 1995 Wound healing: special considerations in the burn patient. Wounds 7 (supplA): 78A

4   Achauer BM, Adair SR 2000 Acute and reconstructive management of the burned eyelid. Clinics in Plastic Surgery 27: 87

5   Bernard SL 2000 Reconstruction of the burned nose and ear. Clinics in Plastic Surgery 27: 97

6   Purdue GF, Hunt JL 1986 Chondritis of the burned ear: a preventable complication. American Journal of Surgery 152: 257

7   Kaweski S, Baldwin RC, Wong RK et al 1993 Diffusion versus iontophoresis in the transport of gentamicin in the burned rabbit ear model. Plastic and Reconstructive Surgery 92: 1342

8   Rigano W, Yanik M, Barone FA et al 1992 Antibiotic iontophoresis in the management of burned ears. Journal of Burn Care and Rehabilitation 13: 407

9   Mills DC, Roberts LW, Manson AD et al 1988 Suppurative chondritis: its incidence, prevention, and treatment in burned patients. Plastic and Reconstructive Surgery 82: 267

10 Luce EA 2000 Electrical burns. Clinics in Plastic Surgery 27: 133

11 Niazi ZBM, Salzberg CA 1999 Thermal, electrical, and chemical injury to the face and neck in children. Facial Plastic Surgery Clinics of North America 7: 185

12 Engrav LH, Heimbach DM, Walkinshaw MD, Marvin JA: 1986 Excision of burns of the face. Plastic and Reconstructive Surgery 77: 744

13 Warden GD, Saffle JR, Schnebly A, Kravitz M 1986 Excisional therapy of facial burns. Journal of Burn Care and Rehabilitation 7: 24

Section 3
Secondary Surgery

23 Facial Scar Management

Edward Wai Hei To, Man Kwon Tung, Chi Wang Peter Pang

Introduction

The face is essential for the expression of emotion and physical state. Scars on the face, in particular, are a stigma in human society and can isolate a person from social contacts.

Facial wounds are commonly the results of road traffic accidents, windscreen injuries, assaults, animal and human bites and occasionally war injuries.

Facial wounds should be aggressively treated to avoid the consequence of an unsightly scar. The presence of separate esthetic units and the combined injury of bone, skin and vital structures will require special attention in the assessment and treatment of facial wounds and subsequent scars.

Background

Although facial scar management is an elective procedure, the appropriate management of acute facial wounds will dramatically affect the quality and quantity of scar tissue formation, thus affecting the need for and results of secondary scar revision procedures. It is therefore essential to understand and make use of the principles of wound healing.

Principles of wound healing[1–3]

Acute inflammation

As soon as tissue is damaged, the wound is filled by a coagulum. Nerve impulses are generated at the injured site and the substances released by the damaged cells cause local hyperemia and increase permeability of the vessel wall. This acute inflammatory reaction is the initial step and cornerstone of the healing process. Platelet degranulation and activation of the complement and clotting cascade form a fibrin clot for hemostasis. Chemotactic agents including epidermal growth factor (ECF), insulin-like growth factor-1 (IGF-1), platelet-derived growth factor (PDGF) and transforming growth factor-β (TGF-β) are released during platelet degranulation. Recruitment of neutrophils, macrophages, epithelial cells, mast cells, endothelial cells and fibroblasts follows. Inflammatory cells proliferate and differentiate for phagocytosis with further release of cytokines and form granulating tissue.

The second phase, known as the proliferative phase, starts from the fifth day post injury to 2 weeks. Capillaries and fibroblasts invade the coagulum in the wound. This new tissue is known as granulation tissue. Blood supply to the area remains high but permeability of the vessel walls is restored to normal and edema resolves. However, prolonging the inflammatory process as a result of infection, the presence of foreign bodies and delay in treatment would increase the activity of fibrogenic cytokines such as TGF-β and ICF-1, thus increasing the chance of hypertrophic scar development.

During the maturation phase of the wound the collagen scaffold is being remodeled, resulting in increase of the tensile strength. This process continues for about 1 year under normal conditions.

Scar formation

In a scar the type I collagen is laid down by the fibroblasts. Its appearance ranges from an inconspicuous line to keloid which overgrows the original wound. This process begins on day 4 of wound healing when the fibroblasts start synthesizing extracellular collagen. The activity of the fibroblasts is increased by the fibroblast activation factor liberated by the macrophages. Capillaries develop from the vascular endothelium and form a dense vascular network within the newly formed connective tissue. Myofibroblasts differentiate into fibroblasts and produce type I collagen, giving the scar stability. Capillaries are obliterated and the original multitude of cells is reduced to a few cell types. Various factors cause persisting stimulation of the wound, resulting in enhanced cicatrization. Therefore care is needed to remove all foreign bodies and prevent infection. Adequate debridement should remove all necrotic tissue and further trauma should be avoided by use of an atraumatic suturing technique.

Factors Affecting Wound Healing

General factors

The process of healing is generally more rapid in young patients. Patients with protein, vitamin or trace elements deficiency will heal more slowly. Chronic illness such as anemia, uremia, uncontrolled diabetes or immunosuppressive states will decrease wound-healing capacity. The long-term use of steroids or immunosuppressives for other medical illnesses could change the inflammatory phase of the wound and lead to delayed formation of new tissue.

Local factors

Blood supply

A healing wound needs energy and building materials such as oxygen, glucose, amino acids, vitamins and trace elements. The blood supply to the wound affects the oxygen availability to the tissue. Blood supply is decreased in the state of shock, arteriosclerosis and diabetes. Hematoma underneath the wound will raise the skin flap, resulting in an impaired blood supply to the tip of the flap via the reticular dermal plexus and causing necrosis of the wound edge and also secondary infection. Though the face is rich in blood supply, necrosis of wound edges will result in undesirable scars.

Necrotic tissue

The facial skin has a rich blood supply and debridement should be minimal because most of the tissue will survive and heal.

However, necrotic tissue at the wound edges, as a result of direct trauma to the skin, can harbor bacteria. It should be trimmed off before suturing, because devitalized tissue provides an anaerobic medium for the multiplication of anaerobic microbes as well as other micro-organisms.

Foreign bodies

Depending on the mechanism of injury, foreign bodies are common in certain trauma scenarios. Organic foreign bodies, such as wooden splinters and soil, and inorganic foreign bodies such as glass or metallic chips should be removed thoroughly during the acute treatment of wounds. These materials not only provide a nidus for bacteria, they also prolong the inflammatory response of the wound, causing scars, recurrent infection and traumatic tattooing.

Previous irradiation

The head and neck area may have been irradiated for the treatment of cancer or other clinical conditions. The radiation effect to the skin will be permanent if the radiation exceeds 15–20 Gy over a relatively short time. Radiation-induced atrophy is usually noted from weeks to months after the initial exposure, although further atrophic changes may evolve over 1 or 2 years. The skin is thinned, dry and hyperkeratotic. Telangiectasia, hyper- or hypopigmentation are usually prominent features. In the upper dermis, capillaries are reduced in number and the capillaries, venules and lymphatics are often widely dilated. Wound healing of the irradiated skin is usually slower than normal skin and complications such as infection and dehiscence are usually more common. Irradiated skin wounds are usually inelastic and the edges are difficult to approximate in the usual manner.

Infection

Infection of the wound causes an inflammatory reaction and edema. There is an increased number of inflammatory cells, fibrinolysis and breaking down of collagen and hence the the tensile strength of the wound is affected.

Common bacteria causing skin infection are commensals such as staphylococcus and streptococcus. Wounds communicating with the nasal or oral cavities may potentially be contaminated with anaerobes. Antibiotics are usually not necessary with adequate debridement and cleaning of the wound. Booster tetanus immunization is mandatory in appropriate cases.

Types of Wound

The nature of the wound is the most important determining factor for the final result of wound healing. The orientation of the wound in relation to the resting skin tension line (RSTL), its location, pattern, degree of tissue trauma, presence of foreign bodies, degree of contamination and individual tissue response will determine the final scar appearance.

Every wound that involves the dermal papilla will produce a scar. The most important prognostic factor for the final appearance of the scar is how the wound was inflicted rather than how it was sutured. Surgical technique is important in alleviating the damage caused by the injury but cannot totally reverse it.

Lacerated wound

Laceration causes the minimum tissue loss. Contamination is usually limited. However, the deep structures such as nerves and underlying organs should be examined for any injury.

Crush wound

Crush injury is caused by blunt trauma. The wound edges are often irregular and tissue is lost (Fig. 23.1). All obviously devitalized tissue should be debrided. Traumatized tissue may be left behind as the blood supply of the facial skin is rich and the chance of recovery is high. Unjustified debridement of facial skin would lead to disfigurement, deformity, loss of function and creation of a bigger scar.

Contaminated wound

Contaminated wounds must be cleansed thoroughly. Deep-seated debris will encourage inflammation, allergic reactions and infection whereas debris embedded within the superficial

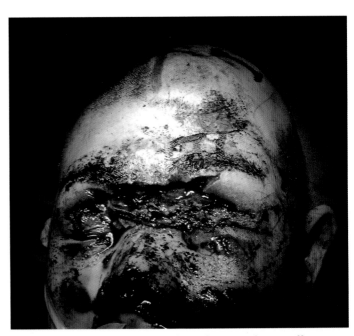

Fig. 23.1: Badly crushed open facial fracture after a traffic accident.

dermis will become an unsightly 'traumatic tattoo' if left unattended. Thorough scrubbing with a brush under general anesthesia is necessary in the acute stage of wound treatment. This can avoid further treatment after the wound has healed.

Potentially contaminated wound

Wounds that communicate with the nasal or oral mucosa are potentially contaminated by the presence of normal flora, secretions and anaerobes. They should be closed as soon as possible (i.e. within 6 hours) and patients should be prescribed antibiotics for Gram-positive cocci and anaerobic bacteria.

Penetrating wound

Care should be taken in treating penetrating wounds and deep lacerations as important structures can be damaged. A thorough examination should be carried out and a plan for wound exploration prepared if necessary.

Management of Acute Wounds

Timing

Treatment should be undertaken as early as possible and preferably under general anesthesia in order to reduce the patient's discomfort and speed up healing. Delay in wound closure increases the risk of infection. In wounds with a low risk of infection, the 'golden period' is within 12–24 hours after injury. In contaminated wounds or immunocompromised patients, primary closure should be achieved within 6 hours. In wounds that carry a high risk of infection, delayed primary closure should be used. However, poor cosmetic outcome, prolonged patient discomfort and inconvenience are negative factors of this treatment modality and should be thoroughly discussed with the patient.

Debridement with scrubbing

Particles of dark color such as dirt, sand or gunpowder will result in a traumatic tattoo if they remain in the wound. Such discoloration tends to be permanent. This can be easily dealt with by debridement or scrubbing in the acute stage and these preventive measures cannot be overemphasized (Figs 23.2, 23.3).

Thorough irrigation to remove foreign bodies

'The solution to pollution is dilution.' Normal saline irrigation remains the best, most economical and most readily available solution. Other antiseptics such as povidone-iodine or hydrogen peroxide are sometimes used; however, these agents can induce tissue reaction, inflammation and possibly toxicity and should be avoided.

Pressurized irrigation is used in contaminated wounds in order to remove soil or small foreign bodies. The optimum pressure for irrigation remains debatable as too high a pres-

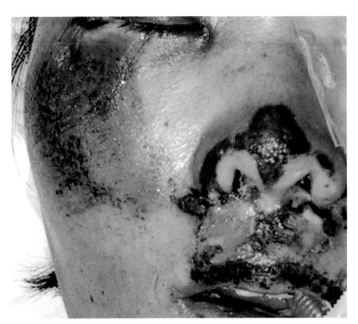

Fig. 23.2: Fine foreign bodies embedded in an abraded wound.

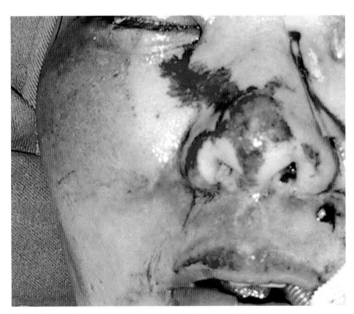

Fig. 23.3: Clean abraded wound after scrubbing.

sure will increase tissue trauma. The recommended pressure of 5–8 lb per square inch can be achieved by using a 16 or 19 gauge needle.

Trimming of necrotic tissue

The potential for skin recovery in blunt facial trauma is great as the blood supply of the face is abundant. Trimming should therefore be limited to obviously dead tissue. The trimming of other tissue such as muscle and nerve should be minimal as this would lead to depressed scars and loss of function.

Functional and anatomical repair in layers

Facial appearance and expression depend on the integrity and function of the underlying musculature. Failure of functional and anatomical repair would lead to depressed scars, tethering of the overlying skin or facial asymmetry.

Damage to facial structures[12]

Deep laceration is liable to damage underlying or adjacent organs or structures. Early identification and surgical repair is necessary to avoid unnecessary complications.

The facial nerve emerges from the skull base via the stylomastoid foramen. It emerges into the parotid gland from the posteromedial surface and divides into two main trunks, the temporozygomatic and cervicofacial branches. They are further divided into five branches: temporal, zygomatic, buccal, marginal mandibular and cervical. They remain under the superficial musculo-aponeurotic system (SMAS) until the line shown in Figure 23.4. The function of the facial nerve should be tested if the clinical situation allows. Wounds superficial to the SMAS behind the line are unlikely to have injured the facial nerve and need not be explored.

Parotid duct injury should be suspected if the wound is situated at the anterior border of the parotid gland or if there is salivary leak. The duct should be repaired with absorbable sutures. Untreated parotid injury would lead to fistula formation.

The nasolacrimal duct connects the lacrimal sac at the medial canthus, slopes downwards and laterally and drains to an opening in the inferior meatus. Its injury should be suspected if there is a wound or previous suturing at or below the medial canthus. Cannulation of the duct with a fine probe is necessary before exploring or suturing the wound at that area.

Appropriate use of antibiotics and suturing materials[10]

Routine systemic antibiotics are not necessary. The use of antibiotics should be tailored on the basis of host defense status, degree of contamination, the mechanism of injury and the likelihood of wound infection. Debridement is the most important step in 'cleaning up' the wound and antibiotics should not be a substitute.

Prophylactic antibiotics are necessary when the wound is expected to be contaminated, such as animal bites or wounds that communicate with the oral cavity. In medical conditions such as rheumatic heart disease or when host resistance is compromised, as in patients with uncontrolled diabetes, taking steroids or immunosuppressive agents, antibiotics should also be commenced systemically and early. Commonly encountered organisms are streptococcus, staphylococcus and Gram-positive bacteria. Penicillin and cloxacillin are the drugs of choice. Patients who are sensitive to the penicillin group should be given erythromycin.

Topical antibiotics, e.g. chloramphenicol ointment, are definitely beneficial. (It should be noted that very rarely, significant side effects of chloramphenicol haved been reported, even when used topically. In some hospitals, its use is prohibited.) Elimination of local infection can reduce the chance of keloid and hypertrophic scar formation.

It is best not to leave any foreign bodies, even stitches, in the wound. If stitches are required at the subcuticular level, the first choice was plain catgut. Synthetic absorbable sutures such as vircyls are now commonly used to avoid the potential problem of Cruetzfeldt–Jakob Disease. Stitches that are dissolved by hydrolysis rather than by inflammation have a lower chance of causing keloid and hypertrophic scars. The best result comes from using non-absorbable monofilament stitches that are removed on day 3–7.

Tetanus passive immunization should be given if necessary. A booster dose should be given if previous immunization was more than 10 years ago. Active immunization should be given in heavily contaminated wounds.

Assessment of Existing Scar

Types of scar

Good scar

A desirable scar should be inconspicuous with the face at rest as well as in the dynamic situation. It should be flat, the same color as the surrounding skin, soft, narrow and orientated in the same direction as the RSTL.

Bad scar

A bad scar causes disfigurement and catches the observer's eye. It is usually raised or depressed, hyper- or hypopigmented, wide and crossing the RSTL. However, the disfigurement may also be exaggerated by the mind of the patient. This largely depends on the patient's gender, cultural background, profession and attitudes. Therefore, before deciding upon the best method of revision of the scar deformity, it is important to communicate clearly with the patient and forestall any disappointment. It should be emphasized to the patient that a scar can only be improved or reduced and not completely erased.

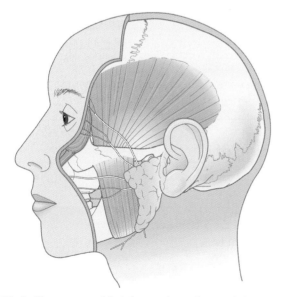

Fig. 23.4: The course of facial nerve branches and the maximal extent of dissection deep to the SMAS.

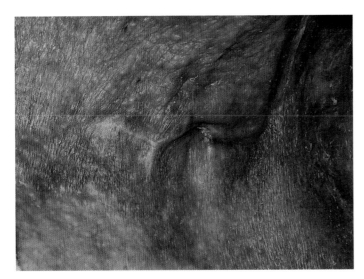

Fig. 23.5: Depressed scar after previous tracheostomy.

Depressed scar

A depressed scar commonly occurs running perpendicular to the RTSL as a result of wound closure under tension (Fig. 23.5). Hematoma formation, wound infection and inverted wound closure are the common causes of a depressed scar. It may also result from initially deep injury with loss of subcutaneous tissue and contracted fibrous tissue adhering to underlying fascia and muscle. Meticulous layered closure of the wound is important in preventing depressed scars. Tissue augmentation or dermabrasion or laser resurfacing can achieve recontouring of smaller depressed scars. Z-plasty or W-plasty is used to correct the underlying tension problem, excise and elevate the scar in the same operation. Depression due to adherence of scar tissue to underlying structures requires excision of the scar, undermining the subcutaneous tissue and closure in layers in order to avoid recurrence.

Curved scar

Healing of a curved scar will produce contraction along the scar, causing a purse-string effect (Fig. 23.6). This produces a 'trapdoor' appearance of the scar. Small trapdoor scars can be excised and primarily closed but larger trapdoor scars are best revised with Z-plasty or multiple W-plasty in order to realign the scar to the RSTL. Wider undermining peripheral to the trapdoor flap may also help to oppose the trapdoor deformity.

The possible mechanism of this is the outward pulling force acting on the scar after the revision.

Pigmented scar

Hyperpigmentation is not a common problem in Caucasians but occurs more frequently in Asians and dark-skinned people. During the scar maturation process, exposure to sunshine and smoking are the risk factors identified with causing the pigmentation. Topical tretinoin is useful in the treatment of hyperpigmentation but avoidance of sunshine till the scar matures is the best way to combat this condition. Laser has been used to treat hyperpigmentation with limited success.

Stitch marks

Tensionless suturing is the best way to avoid stitch marks. In order to minimize stitch marks, the use of skin hooks other than forceps and a subcuticular method of suturing are desirable. If a simple interrupted suturing technique is adopted, fine sutures (i.e. 7/0) should be used and early removal (i.e. 3 days) is preferred.

Step-off deformities

Step-off deformities are the result of inaccurate epidermal closure. Dermal abrasion and resurfacing with laser are commonly used techniques for this kind of scar. Generally, excision and resuturing is necessary if the step is more than 1 mm (Fig. 23.7).

Painful scar

Entrapment of a nerve ending in a healing wound results in a painful or tender scar. If conservative treatment with oral analgesic is not effective, the wound should be re-explored. The nerve should be clean cut and allowed to retract away from the wound and into muscle, if possible.

Patient's tissue response

The patient should be examined to detect the presence of other scars in order to determine whether they have a tendency to form keloid or hypertrophic scars. However, the presence of a well-healed scar may be misleading as the formation of hypertrophic or keloidal scars depends heavily on

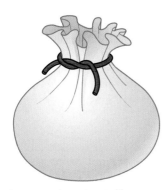

Fig. 23.6: A circular wound contracts like a purse string.

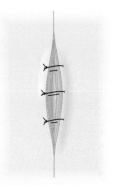

Fig. 23.7: Improper alignment of wound edges resulting in step deformity.

other factors including the degree of tissue crushing during trauma, orientation of the wound and site of the scar.

The mechanism of initial injury is the single most important factor in determining the formation of a scar. Those with blunt trauma and crushed wound edges do badly when compared with those with cleancut wounds. The presence of foreign bodies would prolong the inflammatory reaction and increases the likelihood of bad scar formation. Tissue loss and healing by secondary intention will lead to an unsightly scar.

Hypertrophic scar or keloid

A simple hypertrophic scar is limited to the tissue that constitutes the wound, whereas a keloid overgrows the wound and invades into the surrounding tissue. Keloid grows slowly and may relapse for years before it becomes static. Hypertrophic scars will become softer and paler as time passes. Histologically, both types of scar have the same appearance and it is a problem distinguishing the two in the initial year after wound healing.

Esthetic units

The face is divided into six esthetic units (Fig. 23.8), namely forehead, eye, nose, cheeks, mouth and ears. Each can be further subdivided into small units.

Forehead

Scars in this region can usually be improved with simple procedures. Forehead skin has a very rich blood supply and so suction apparatus should be ready when operating in this area. When revising forehead scars, special attention should be paid to anatomical reconstitution of different layers such as frontalis muscle and skin. Preoperative documentation of the sensation status of the supratrochlear and supraorbital nerves should be made.

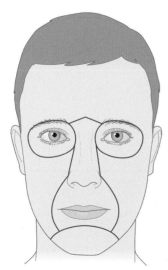

Fig. 23.8: Cosmetic units consist of forehead, nose, periorbital area, perioral area and chin.

Eye

Eyebrows

It is important to recognize the fact that injury to hair follicles will result in bald patches. Therefore dissection in this area should be carried out with extreme caution with the incision parallel to the direction of hair follicles so as to avoid damage. Small segments of alopecia should be removed if feasible and larger areas may require hair-bearing skin graft. The direction of the skin incision should be oblique to avoid transection injury to the hair follicles. Perfect alignment of the eyebrow is critical, as step-off deformity is very obvious.

Eyelids

Scar contracture over the eyelids can cause ectropion or entropion and it should not be tackled as a linear scar contracture. Adding of new tissue, either by free skin grafting or local flaps, is necessary in order to achieve good results. Damage to the tarsal plate would result in notching. The upper and lower eyelids consist of the thinnest skin of the body and should be grafted with paper-thin (less than 0.5 mm) skin for good results. The crows feet at the lateral canthus provide a good area for disguise in scar revision. Multiple W-plasty to realign the scars along the crows feet results in an inconspicuous scar. The degenerative laxity of the lower eyelid requires special attention, as this would precipitate ectropion if the procedure creates downward tension.

Nose

The skin of the nose is strongly adherent to the underlying muscle and cartilage. Because of the underlying naris muscle pull, the skin has limited directions of movement. Excision of scars and closure of defects should always be undertaken with great care and may be helped by borrowing nearby tissue such as a bilobed flap.

Cheeks

The cheek is a flap with minimal wrinkles except in the older patient. Scars crossing this area are extremely difficult to hide. Laser resurfacing has a particularly important role in the treatment of scars over this area.

Mouth

The mucocutaneous vermilion border of the lip should be perfectly restored in the revision of scars crossing the lip. Other anatomical borders such as the red line and white line should be accurately restored. A three-layer closure of mucosa, muscle and skin must be performed.

Ears

The ears themselves are not prone to any special scarring except keloid formation at the earlobe after earring puncture. The pinna provides an invaluable composite skin-cartilage-

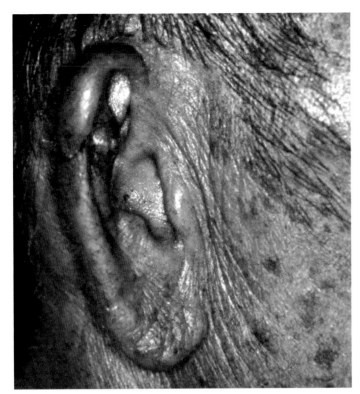

Fig. 23.9: Composite graft harvested from the pinna consisting of skin and cartilage.

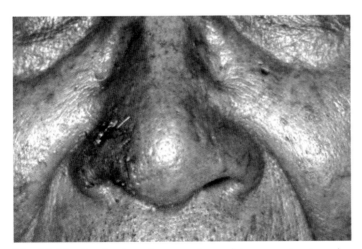

Fig. 23.10: Application of composite graft to reconstruct an alar defect.

skin graft for reconstruction of alar tissue loss (Figs 23.9, 23.10).

Factors affecting scar quality

Age

The older the patient, the better the scar and the results of revision. Younger people have a greater overall skin tension, which causes the scar to spread and become hypertrophic. Skin tension is one of the most important factors for the esthetic outcome of scar surgery.

Relaxed skin tension lines (RSTL)

The skin is draped over the body in a fashion that permits mobility, retraction, extension, expansion and flexion to occur. Areas allowing greater movement, such as the perioral area, will stretch and create excess skin to accommodate the movement of muscles. Over time, the excess skin, in conjunction with the loss of elastic tissue, creates wrinkles and age lines. These wrinkles often coincide with relaxed skin tension lines (Fig. 23.11).

Practical Management of Facial Scars

Early scar management

History of the injury

The patient's history should be recorded clearly on how, when and where the injury occurred and the chance of foreign bodies being present in the wound. This may indicate the possibility of other vital organ injury and degree of tissue damage.

Psychological support for the patient

Every injury results in a more or less obvious scar. A scar may stigmatize a person and possibly affect social contact so psychological counseling should be started as soon as possible.

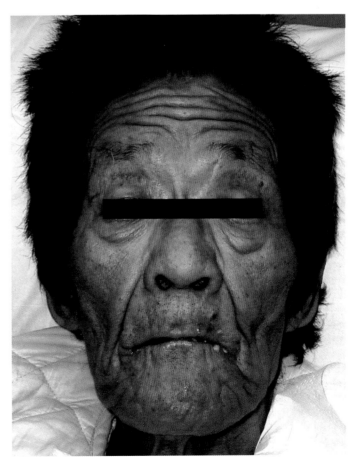

Fig. 23.11: Wrinkles on the elderly face.

Anticipation is the key to success in minimizing long-lasting emotional injury and 'scars' in the mind.

Communication

Good rapport with the patient and adequate explanation are necessary for the patient to understand the unavoidable scar formation. Reassurance should be given concerning the expected progress of the scar, the time sequence of the treatment and possible future revision measures.

Documentation

Documentation is the surgeon's second-best defense against legal claims. The first defense is, of course, good patient communication and surgery. It is important to document the essence of all communications with the patient. Particular attention should be paid to the factors affecting wound healing. Host factors include ethnic group, extremes of age, diabetes mellitus, chronic renal failure, obesity, malnutrition and the use of immunosuppressive therapy. The tendency of the patient to form keloid should be assessed, as this may predict the formation of a poor scar.

The site and degree of contamination and tissue trauma should be clearly documented. The size, depth of wound and the injury of deep structures such as tendons, nerves and vessels should be accurately recorded for possible future legal purposes.

A history of drug allergy, especially to local anesthetic agents and antibiotics, should be determined as these are the agents likely to be administered in the acute stage of the injury.

Photographic record

A photographic record for pre- and postoperative comparison and legal aspects is necessary. Recording the initial wound and subsequent wound progress is mandatory for legal purposes. Though digital cameras are widely used nowadays, images are only accepted as a method of documentation for legal purposes if produced as hard copies.

Thorough discussion with the patient about the possible outcome

The patient's contribution plays an important part in producing a good scar. A motivated patient is necessary for good compliance in scar management in the first 6–9 months post injury. This starts in the immediate postoperative period. Keeping the head above the heart level to reduce wound edema is necessary for the initial 24 hours. The wound should be observed for any signs of infection such as erythema, warmth, swelling and discharge. The patient should be advised to seek prompt medical attention if infection sets in or doubt arises.

After the wound is healed, the patient needs to accept responsibility for sun avoidance and protection from UV light. Sunlight exposure increases the risk of scar hyperpig-mentation. High sun-protective factor sunscreens must be used appropriately. Possible alterations in the patient's outdoor occupational and recreational activity may be necessary.

Surgical options

The simplest method of primary wound closure should be used, unless there is substantial tissue loss that renders primary wound closure impossible. A local flap is the best choice in cases of significant tissue loss. Adjacent skin usually provides the best replacement in terms of color and texture. Full-thickness skin grafting should be the last option and a graft harvested from the postauricular and supraclavicular areas provides the best color match to the facial skin.

Silicone sheet[6,8]

A silicone gel sheet can be used as a conservative treatment for hypertrophic scar or keloid (Fig. 23.12). The sheet should be worn for as long as 24 hours per day. The mechanism is largely unknown but a possible effect exerted by the silicone gel is that it increases the local temperature of the scar and therefore enhances the collagenase activity. Another postulated mechanism is its pressure effect, causing a lowering of oxygen tension and occlusion of the scar. A direct chemical effect of silicone on the scar is unlikely, as there is no evidence of silicone entering the scar tissue.

There are drawbacks. The sheet cannot be worn for long periods in hot and humid conditions. Sweat can cause skin excoriation and eczema and the scratching in response to the itchiness causes further damage. As a result, the keloid or hypertrophic scar can become more severe. The application of silicone gel on the face is much less acceptable cosmetically than on other parts of the body.

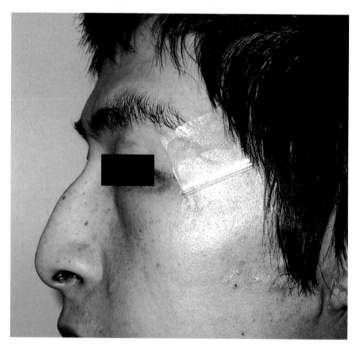

Fig. 23.12: Application of silicone gel sheet on facial hypertrophic scar.

Corticosteroid intralesional injection

Intralesional injection of triamcinolone in combination with local anesthesia and other therapies has been used to control scars. It was reported to have a 50% response rate in keloid treatment over 5 years in terms of flattening and decrease in discomfort. Various regimens with different concentrations (10, 20, 30, 40 mg/ml) at an interval of 4 weeks were used. The improvement of scars is brought about by the inhibition of transcription of matrix protein genes ($\alpha 1(I)$ and $\alpha 1(III)$ procollagen, fibronectin, TGF-β and other cytokines) and the collagenase activity by $\alpha 2$-macroglobulin synthesis.

Pain is substantial in intralesional steroid injection so local anesthesia should be infiltrated around the scar before treatment. Telangiectasia, infection and necrosis of the skin are the possible complications of steroid injection. Incorrect injection of the steroid into the subcutaneous tissue would lead to subcutaneous fat atrophy and formation of a depressed scar.

The systemic effects of steroids can be avoided by spacing the interval of injection. Female patients should be asked about pregnancy as this treatment should not be given. It is also important to mention possible irregularity of periods and the increased amount of flow after steroid injection. Other relative contraindications to the use of steroid include a previous history of breast or endometrial cancer.

Intralesional injection of calcium channel blocker[5] (verapamil hydrochloride) is an effective alternative in treating hypertrophic scarring. It possibly behaves like trifluoperazine, a calmodin inhibitor that causes cells to round up through an unknown intracellular, calcium-independent process involving the alternation or rearrangement of the actin cytoskeleton. Surgical excision and intraoperative perilesional injection of verapamil is effective to prevent keloid recurrence.

Pressure dressings[9]

Constant compression (Fig. 23.13) of a hypertrophic scar has proven to be beneficial in preventing excessive growth of scar tissue. To be effective, a constant pressure of 15–40 mmHg for at least 18 hours per day for 4–6 months is necessary. This can be used in conjunction with silicone gel. It should be tailor made to fit the involved parts of the body such as elasticized cervical collars, elastic ski masks or spring-pressure earring devices for post earlobe keloidectomy. This treatment modality should be explained carefully to the patient beforehand. Pressure sensors should be used to monitor the efficacy of the pressure garment at follow-up consultations.

Delayed scar revision

Timing of scar revision[11]

Complete scar maturation takes about 2–3 years. There is a common consensus that scar revision should be delayed until the scar has reached full maturation. However, during the scar maturation process, its appearance is worst during the 2 weeks to 4 months post injury. If the orientation of the scar crosses the RSTL, it will never heal in an optimal manner.

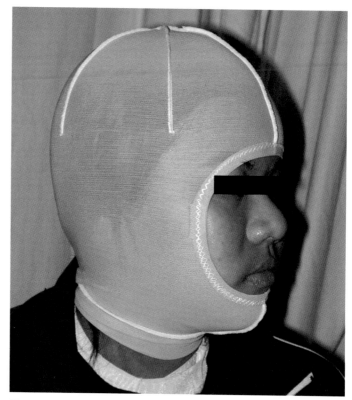

Fig. 23.13: Tailor-made pressure garment for facial scar.

Borges therefore advocated that an interim scar revision and reorientation should be carried out at 2 months post injury so as to achieve the best result in the process of delayed scar revision. However, the average timing for scar revision ranges from 6 months to 1 year.

Technical aspects[13]

The main objective of scar revision is to make it less conspicuous. This can be achieved by excision of scar tissue and rearrangement to maximize the length and reorientate the scar along the RSTL. This enables the scar to heal with minimum tension and in the optimum direction.

Simple excision

The oldest and simplest technique in scar revision is fusiform scar revision (FSR). This is done by excision of the scar followed by direct closure of the wound. This is possible if orientation of the scar is approximately along the RSTL. This is very effective in treating a wide scar or a scar tethered to underlying structures. In FSR, it may not be necessary to excise the whole scar; partial treatment (Fig. 23.14) can still achieve marked improvement to the scar.

The drawback in this technique of FSR is the formation of a deep furrow caused by the vertical contraction of scar tissue. Excision of all the underlying scar tissue and closure in layers can reduce the chances of this result.

Serial excision

When the scar is too wide and a single FSR would result in undue tension for wound closure and unfavorable conditions

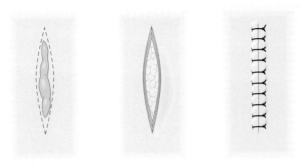

Fig. 23.14: A linear scar was excised in a fusiform manner and closed primarily.

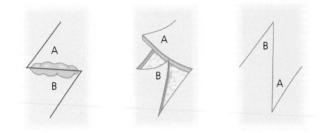

Fig. 23.15: Z-plasty.

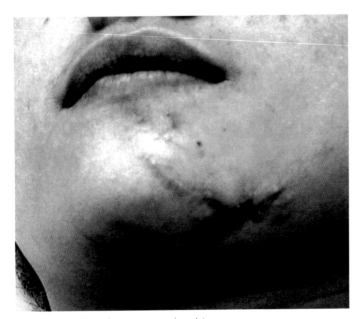

Fig. 23.16: Trapdoor scar on the chin.

by lengthening and, more importantly, by changing the direction of scar tissue in order to align it more closely to the RSTL. Z-plasty should be undertaken when the scar is slanted 60° or less from the RSTL (Fig. 23.15). In multiple Z-plasties with limbs following the RSTL, the direction of each postoperative oblique scar (diagonal) is the same as that of the original scar. The adjoining tissues must be elastic enough in order to make Z-plasty possible. Often following the release of the scar contracture and undermining the flaps of the Z-plasty, the flaps will automatically realign to the final configuration.

It is convenient to wait until the scar has matured before performing the Z-plasties in order to avoid unnecessary sacrifice of tissue. Early Z-plasty is indicated in selected cases where the wound can only be worsened as the scar contracts, e.g. circular-shaped wound and malalignment of the vermilion border. Trapdoor deformity (Fig. 23.16) is inevitable. So multiple Z-plasty should be undertaken as soon as the wound has healed.

W-plasty

W-plasty is used either in the initial incision in elective surgery to prevent later contracture or to convert a scar to a less apparent one. The latter is done by zigzag excision of scars, producing a shortened, acutely angulated incision that can be closed by advancement without rotation of tissue to produce a scar that aligns along the RSTL (Figs 23.17–19).

W-plasty is used to break up a long scar and realign it along the RSTL as far as possible. One can eliminate a depressed

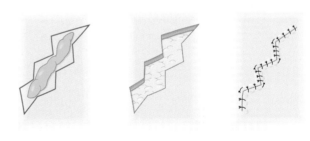

Fig. 23.17: Realignment of scar to relaxed skin tension lines with W-plasty.

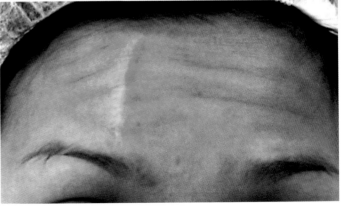

Fig. 23.18: Forehead scar oriented across the relaxed skin tension lines.

for subsequent wound healing, serial intralesional excision of the scar could be used in order to give time for the nearby skin and tissue to expand and allow a tensionless wound closure.

Z-plasty

The main function of Z-plasty is to prevent thickening and contraction and for reorientation of the scar. This is achieved

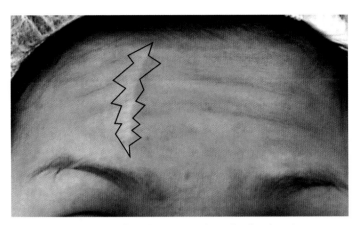

Fig. 23.19: Design of W-plasty to realign the forehead scar.

scar by advancing V-shaped arms of tissue across the field of the scar.

Dermabrasion[14]

This can be carried out with a high-speed dermabrator with a diamond fraise. Fraises are stainless steel wheels with industrial-grade diamonds bonded to them. The scar should be pretreated with 0.05% tretinoin cream to shorten the re-epithelialization time and reduce the incidence of postoperative milia formation and hyperpigmentation. The procedure can be carried out with local or regional block together with sedation.

Laser[15]

Laser is used in the treatment of scars as its precise cutting and welding properties cause less tissue damage than other methods. Its photochemical reaction may also provide a beneficial effect in altering metabolic function within the keloid. Superpulsed CO_2 laser causes a significant increase of keloid dermal fibroblast FGF-β secretion and inhibits the secretion of TGF–β. These stabilize the cellular phenotype and inhibit excess collagen secretion. It also causes thermal contraction of collagen, resulting in dermal tightening. Nd:YAG laser is noted to have a suppressive effect on collagen synthesis without changing DNA synthesis or causing loss of viability. Clinically it is useful in moderate reduction of keloid size and consistency. 585 nm flashlamp-pumped pulsed-dye laser is used for its specific hemoglobulin absorption characteristic.

Laser is used for its ablative nature and specific wave length for the vascular component of the hypertrophic scar.

Pulsed-dye laser (585 nm) has been shown to be effective in the treatment of microvascular lesions such as telangiectasia and port-wine stains. Studies have shown that it reduces the erythematous component and scar height and increases pliability. Posttreatment scar biopsy showed sclerotic collagen bundles and local mast cell proliferation is also noted.

The mechanism of laser action is selective photothermolysis. Selective absorption of light by hemoglobin leads to local heating of cutaneous blood vessels; the vessels are then thrombosed and vasculitis follows. There is gradual local

repair with neovascularization. Microvascular destruction leads to ischemia of the scar and affects collagen synthesis and the release of collagenase. The heat produced is conducted via the blood vessels to the surrounding dermis and alters the collagen composition of the scar.

Tissue expander

Nearby tissue offers the best esthetic outcome in terms of color match and texture for facial skin reconstruction, yet the supply is always limited. Tissue expansion is invaluable in the reconstruction of extensive scars with inadequate tissue nearby. Previously expanded skin flaps have an improved survival rate when compared with similar flaps developed in non-expanded skin.

Scar alopecia can be treated by expanding the remaining scalp. As much as half of a hair-bearing scalp defect can be reconstructed with tissue expansion (Fig. 23.20). Similarly, expansion of forehead skin for a forehead defect is feasible (Fig. 23.21). The innervation of the forehead frontalis muscle should be preserved to avoid later brow ptosis. The expansion of forehead skin can also provide extra good-quality thin skin for reconstruction of the nasal area.

To reconstruct the cheek area, the tissue expander is best placed in the pre-auricular area, superficial to the superficial aponeurosis muscle. Further dissection superficial to the platysma muscle at the neck is necessary for placing the tissue expander and expanding the neck skin. Extra skin can then be acquired by a rotational flap. Neck skin is expanded for the reconstruction of cheek and perioral scars and defects.

Skin grafting

Skin grafting usually cannot provide a satisfactory cosmetic result for facial scars and defects. However, it is invaluable in wound coverage in the acute stage so that later flap recon-

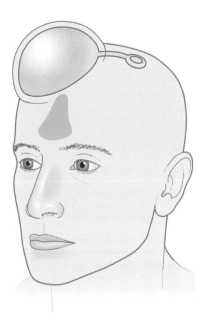

Fig. 23.20: Placement of the forehead tissue expander for reconstruction of a forehead scar.

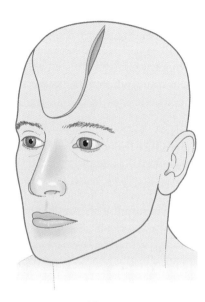

Fig. 23.21: Reconstruction of forehead with the expanded skin.

struction may be planned, such as tissue expansion. Split-thickness skin grafts can be harvested from the thigh or scalp. Full-thickness skin grafts can be harvested from the pre- and postauricular, neck, nasolabial and supraclavicular areas.

Soft tissue augmentation

The ideal material should be safe, easy to apply, permanent and non-allergenic.

Collagen injection[7]

Injectable bovine collagen has been used for depressed scars. This xenogenic substance has the problem of allergenicity, which needs to be evaluated before treatment with a small test dose. The FDA approved the Zyderm collagen implant for clinical use in 1981, which is marketed as Fibrel. It consists of three types of collagen depending to the composition: Zyderm I (35 mg/ml type I collagen), Zyderm II (65 mg/ml type I collagen) and Zyplast (glutaraldehyde cross-linked collagen). Each has different physical properties and different uses. Zyderm I is indicated for shallow scars or fine wrinkles, Zyderm II is for intermediate deep depressed scars and Zyplast is for deep scars and deep dermal defects. However, intermittent swelling, vascular and necrotic changes of the overlying skin are possible complications. This is caused by the heavy suspension of the Zyplast collagen which results in infarction of larger subdermal vessels and local tissue necrosis.

The injection should be carried out with a 30 G needle with a multiple puncture or fanning technique, at a 35° angle to the skin. Care must be taken to avoid both implant extrusion through pores or around the needle orifice or injection deep to the subcutaneous tissue. In dealing with fibrotic scars, one has to undermine the scar with a needle to create a pocket for the injected collagen. Local anesthesia by regional block is necessary for the possible pain caused by the undermining.

Injection treatment is contraindicated if there is history of keloid formation, sensitivity to gelatin, bleeding disorder, history of cardiac, renal or herpetic disease or autoimmune disease.

With skillful injection, the depressed scar can be leveled off (Figs 23.22, 23.23). However, the difference in surface texture of the scar and the surrounding skin cannot be altered with this treatment. The most important thing is to prevent a depressed scar in the first instance by layered closure of underlying muscle, preventing the separation of muscle and adherence of scar to the underlying structure.

Silicone injection

Silicone microdroplet technique is used for the injection to stimulate an encapsulating ring of collagen that elevates depressed scars. Silicone is a foreign, non-physiological material with serious concerns about its safety. Following the complications arising from the use of silicone breast implants, the FDA withheld approval for the use, distribution and promotion of silicone injection for skin augmentation.

Fat injection

Autologous adipose tissue acquired during liposuction is used to correct skin and soft tissue contour defects. It is a viable graft and should be harvested with care. A 14-gauge needle with limited negative pressure has been advocated for harvesting. The tissue is used in the replacement of subcutaneous tissue lost but not as a dermal filler or to rebuild dermal defects. The complications of lipoinjection are bruis-

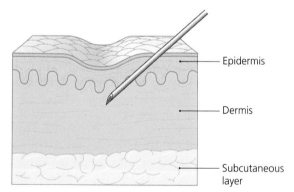

Fig. 23.22: Depressed scar as a result of deficient dermis.

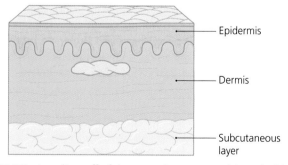

Fig. 23.23: Leveling off of depressed scar was achieved with the injection of augmentation material.

ing, prolonged inflammation, induration, local infection and hematoma formation. An unsolved problem with lipo-injection is gradual graft loss; it is estimated that only 30–40% of the graft remains after 1 year.

Tissue transfer (flaps)

Tissue transfer can be local random flaps, local pedicled flaps and distant free flaps. The choice of flap depends on the availability of local tissue, which is the best choice with best texture and color match; distant free flaps depend on available surgical expertise and resources.

Radiotherapy

Radiotherapy is an efficient and time-honored method of treating resistant keloid. The mechanism of radiotherapy involves fibroblast destruction without replacement. A common concern is the potential risk of radiation-induced malignancy and immunosuppression in various degrees.[4] Various types of radiotherapy have been used in treatment, including kilovoltage irradiation (including superficial X-ray), electron beam and interstitial radiotherapy. Sarcoma is the most likely radiation-induced tumor, usually developing 8–10 years post treatment.

Isotretinoin

Isotretinoin is used in the treatment of keloid. There is a raised T-lymphocyte count found in keloid tissue and it has been postulated that sebum that leaks from the pilosebaceous structure acts as an antigenic stimulus in triggering T-lympho-cyte migration, proliferation and activation, causing production of lymphokines which all influence fibroblasts to produce more collagen. Isotretinoin eliminates sebocytes and causes sebum suppression.

Wound care

Finally, although it is neither 'high tech' nor surgically exciting, the role of wound care is extremely important. Good appropriate dressings certainly help wound healing. A moist environment speeds cell migration while negative pressure dressings speed up healing, especially in the presence of infection, silicone dressings may reduce hypertrophic scar formation and adhesives may reduce tension across a wound. In a busy unit great benefits can be obtained from fully involving wound care specialists and the reader is directed to the appropriate literature.

Innovations

Skin closure material

Usage of subcutaneous absorbable sutures to relieve the tension of the overlying skin is a standard procedure to minimize scar formation. Fine non-absorbable monofilament sutures are often used to minimize stitch marks. Stitches are generally removed early, on postoperative day 3.

Cyanoacrylate adhesives have been used as an alternative for skin closure in Canada and Europe for over 20 years with no adverse effects reported. They are effective in closing superficial lacerations under low tension and can also be used in closing surgical wounds, e.g. parotidectomy, thyroidectomy. Various studies show that they give comparable results to using monofilament sutures. However, they are superior in their ease of application and cost-effectiveness and they have obvious advantages in children. Major limitations of butyl-cyanoacrylates include low early breaking strength and a brittle consistency when dry. Therefore their use should be avoided over skin creases. The proper usage (Figs 23.24, 23.25) is necessary to achieve optimal results.

Scarless healing[16–23]

Healing in the early gestation fetus is by regeneration, which is rather different from that in the adult which happens by fibrosis. This phenomenon will have a profound impact in clinical practice and is now being extensively investigated. The repairing process requires extracellular matrix turnover

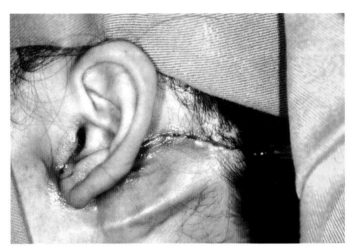

Fig. 23.24: Post parotidectomy with facelift incision closed with glue.

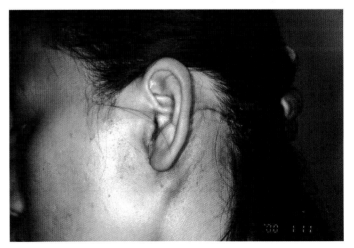

Fig. 23.25: Post-parotidectomy wound 2 weeks after the operation.

and fetal skin is found to have a higher matrix metallopro-teinase level when compared with that in the adult. These proteinases are responsible for matrix degradation and are released by various cell types as zymogens and activated by removal of N-terminal propeptides. TGF-β1 level is noted to be deficient in the fetus. Its function is to stimulate the deposition of collagen and other matrix components by fibroblasts, inhibit collagenase, block plasminogen inhibitor, enhance angiogenesis and have a chemotactic effect on fibroblasts, monocytes and macrophages. Addition of TGF-β1 to a fetus will make the fetal wound heal with scarring. The injection of TGF-β1 neutralizing antibodies into the wound may encounter antigenicity problems which limit the clinical potential. The application of sugar mannose-6-phos-phate blocks the insulin-like growth factor type II/ mannose-6-phosphate receptor which in turn decreases the activation of TGF-β1. The anti-TGF-β1 therapeutic strategies would be a way of reducing scarring during wound healing.

References

1 Bernstein EF, Mauviel A, Uitto J et al 1996 Wound healing. In: Lask GP, Moy RL (eds) Principles and techniques in cutaneous surgery. McGraw-Hill, New York

2 Muir IFK 1990 On the nature of keloids and hypertropic scars. British Journal of Plastic Surgery 43: 61–69

3 Niessen FB, Spauwen PH, Schalkijk J, Kon M 1999 On the nature of hypertropic scars and keloids: a review. Plastic and Reconstructive Surgery 104(5): 1435–1458

4 Darzi MA, Chowdri S, Kaul SK, Khan M 1992 Evaluation of various methods of treating keloids and hypertropic scars: a 10-year follow-up study. British Journal of Plastic Surgery 45: 375–379

5 Lee RC, Doong H, Aileen F 1994 The response of burn scars to intralesional verapamil. Archives of Surgery 129: 107–111

6 Fulton JE Jr 1995 Silicon gel sheeting for prevention and management of evolving hypertrophic and keloid scars. Dermatologic Surgery 21(11): 947–951

7 Coleman WP, Lawrence N, Sherman R et al 1993 Autologous collagen? Lipocytic dermal augmentation: a histologic study. Journal of Dermatology and Surgical Oncology 19: 1032–1040

8 Lindsey WH, Davis PT 1997 Facial keloids: a 15-year experience. Archives of Otolaryngology Head and Neck Surgery 123(4): 397–400

9 Carr-Collins JA 1992 Pressure techniques for the prevention of hypertropic scar. Clinics in Plastic Surgery 19(3): 733–743

10 Haas AF, Grekin RC 1995 Antibiotic prophylaxis in dermatologic surgery. Journal of the American Academy of Dermatology 32: 155–176

11 Borges AF 1990 Timing of scar revision techniques. Clinics in Plastic Surgery 17(1): 71–76

12 Seckel BR, Greene AB 1994 Facial danger zones: Avoiding nerve injury in facial plastic surgery. Quality Medical Publishing, St Louis.

13 Harahap M 2000 Surgical techniques for cutaneous scar revision. Marcel Dekker, New York.

14 Coleman WP 1991 Dermabrasion and hypertropic scars. International Journal of Dermatology 30: 629

15 Nowak KC, McCormack MB, Koch RJ 2000 The effect of superpulsed carbon dioxide laser energy on keloid and normal dermal fibroblast secretion of growth factors: a serum-free study. Plastic and Reconstructive Surgery 105(6): 2039–2048

16 Adzick NS, Longaker MT 1991 Scarless wound healing in the fetus: the role of the extracellular matrix. In: Barbuk A et al (eds) Clinical and experimental approaches to dermal and epidermal repair: normal and chronic wounds. Wiley-Liss, New York, pp 177–192

17 Bullard KM, Cass DL, Banda MJ, Adzick NS 1997 Transforming growth factor beta-1 decreases interstitial collagenase in healing human fetal skin. Journal of Pediatric Surgery 32(7): 1023–1027

18 Massague J 1990 The transforming growth factor-beta family. Annual Review of Cell Biology 6: 597–641

19 Wikner NE, Persichitte KA, Baskin JB et al 1988 Transforming growth factor β stimulates the expression of fibronectin by human keratinocytes. Journal of Investigative Dermatology 91: 207–212

20 Vassalli P 1992 The pathophysiology of tumour necrosis factors. Annual Review of Immunology 10: 411–452

21 Sullivan KM, Lorenz HP, Meuli M, Lin RY, Adzick S 1995 A model of scarless human fetal wound repair is deficient in transforming growth factor beta. Journal of Pediatric Surgery. 30(2): 198–203

22 Singer AJ, Clark RAF 1999 Mechanisms of disease: review article. New England Journal of Medicine 738–746

23 Singer AJ, Hollander JE, Quinn JV 1997 Current concepts: evalution and management of traumatic lacerations. New England Journal of Medicine 337(16): 1142–1148

24 Secondary Osteotomies and Bone Grafting

David Richardson, David Carl Jones

Introduction

Modern techniques of fracture management allow easy access to the whole craniofacial skeleton, accurate fracture reduction, internal fixation with mini and microplating systems and primary bone grafting where necessary to replace missing bone. The goal of primary treatment is to restore normal anatomy and therefore normal form and function of the craniofacial complex. However, patients may present with posttraumatic deformity for a variety of reasons. They may fail to present in the acute phase or injuries may go undiagnosed if specialist expertise is not available. Other serious injury or medical conditions may preclude or compromise immediate treatment of facial injuries and the results of primary treatment may be unsatisfactory if the extent of the injury is underestimated or in the more severe comminuted panfacial fractures (Fig. 24.1).[1]

Classification

There is no entirely satisfactory system for classification of posttraumatic facial deformity which incorporates the necessary mix of hard and soft tissue deficits or takes account of resultant esthetic or functional difficulties. Tessier[2] proposed a system based on the major esthetic aspects of the disfigurement and included an orbital syndrome with enophthalmos

(Fig. 24.1), a craniofacial syndrome including stigmata of residual frontal and nasoethmoidal fractures, a maxillary syndrome with occlusal abnormalities, and a nasal syndrome characterized by naso-orbital dislocation. Other workers such as Manson[3] and Gruss[4] have devised systems related to the previous location of bone fractures, comprising frontobasilar, Le Fort I, II and III fractures of the maxilla, naso-orbitoethmoid, zygomatic, nasal, mandibular, complex and panfacial deformities.

Principles of Management

The principles underlying management of secondary post-traumatic skeletal deformity include:

■ accurate assessment by history, clinical examination and special investigations
■ treatment planning
■ surgery, utilizing a variety of techniques for management of soft and hard tissue deficits or deformities, including osteotomies and bone grafting.

Assessment

Assessment of any deformity requires a detailed history, examination and special investigations.

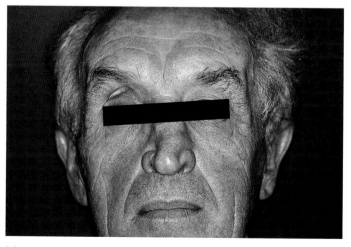

(a)

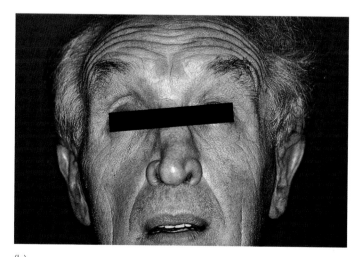

(b)

Fig. 24.1: Residual nasal and zygomatic deformity with enophthalmos and restricted ocular motility following untreated midfacial injury. **(a)** Facial appearance. **(b)** Restricted eye movement.

History

A full history is essential in diagnosis of secondary post-traumatic deformity. Of particular importance is documentation of the patient's complaints or concerns. A number of potentially correctable deformities may be present, but it is important to assess which of these require correction in order to address the concerns of the patient. A brief assessment of the psychosocial effect of the deformity may help to highlight important areas, since relatively minor physical abnormalities may give rise to significant psychological, social or occupational problems. The history of the original injury, whether any primary surgery was carried out and if so what this involved are important in order to plan secondary surgery and anticipate potential difficulties or complications (e.g. previous craniotomy with or without dural repair will make subsequent craniotomy more difficult due to dural adhesions, thus predisposing to increased risk of dural tear and subsequent CSF leak. Eye injury or visual loss will increase the significance of the risk to vision in operating on the contralateral orbit). Time elapsed between the original injury or its primary management and presentation of secondary deformity may be significant because timing of secondary surgery may be important. Some problems are better corrected early, whilst in others the timing may be less critical (e.g. correction of enophthalmos and orbital and nasal reconstruction).

Examination

A comprehensive clinical examination of the craniofacial complex is mandatory and should include assessment of both hard and soft tissues.

Soft tissues

Whilst not directly the subject of this chapter, mention must be made of the soft tissues. The presence of cutaneous scars, soft tissue deficiency and distortions or subcutaneous fat atrophy may limit the extent of bony movement and/or the degree of soft tissue response to the underlying bony movement and leave a persisting esthetic or functional deficit even

if a perfect underlying skeletal position can be achieved. This should be appreciated in the planning phase so that soft tissue adjustment can be carried out at the appropriate time, usually subsequent to the skeletal reconstruction.[1,4] In addition, what may seem to be a bony asymmetry may be solely due to soft tissue problems and surgical technique for correction is likely to be different from that chosen where the underlying problem is truly skeletal in nature. When considering complaints of orbitozygomatic deformity, soft tissues of the bony orbit are of paramount importance. Globe displacement in the vertical or anteroposterior plane needs to be accurately assessed and the presence of characteristic stigmata of enophthalmos, such as pseudoptosis, implies a degree of displacement of the orbital tissues (Fig. 24.1).

Examination of eye movement and forced duction test will allow assessment of tethering of the extraocular muscles (Fig. 24.2) and traction on the insertions of the medial and lateral recti (usually under general anesthetic prior to surgery) will give an indication of the potential for improvement in anteroposterior eye position following enophthalmos correction. On occasion, intraorbital fibrosis may preclude anterior eye repositioning despite good orbital volume correction. The position of the lateral and medial canthi should be assessed, intercanthal distances measured and note made of any abnormality of eyelid position such as retraction or ectropion.

Hard tissues

A thorough assessment of any bony distortion, deficiencies or asymmetry must be carried out by inspection and palpation. Techniques used for assessing the bony (and cartilaginous) craniofacial skeleton are well documented in the craniofacial, rhinoplasty and orthognathic literature. Assessment should be applied in a logical way and must include all areas of the craniofacial skeleton, including the calvarium and forehead, frontal sinus, orbits, zygomas, external and internal nose, temporomandibular joints, mandible, upper and lower dental arches and dental occlusion. Assessment should be made of displacements in each area examined in the three planes of

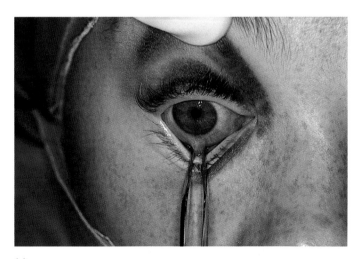
(a)

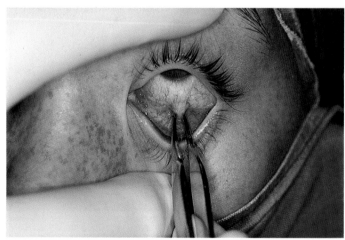
(b)

Fig. 24.2: Forced duction test. **(a)** Tethering of inferior rectus. **(b)** Normal contralateral eye.

space, anteroposterior, vertical and transverse, and should include assessment of asymmetries in each of these three planes.

Special investigations

These may include plain films, dental study models, photographs and CT or MR scanning, with three-dimensional stereolithographic modeling where appropriate.

Plain films

Plain films will demonstrate the site and extent of the original injuries, the presence of bone plates and grafts used in primary treatment. Detailed measurements to assess malposition and asymmetries, including AP and lateral cephalometry, may be useful both in delineating the underlying problem and in planning surgical correction. This particularly applies to fractures of the mandible where plain films will demonstrate a fibrous or non-union, the direction and extent of displacements and major occlusal abnormalities such as anterior open bite or mandibular asymmetry.

Dental study models

Dental study models are mandatory for assessment of posttraumatic deformity involving the tooth-bearing segments of the maxilla or the mandible. Where a posttraumatic malocclusion exists, an assessment can be made of the achievable occlusion and whether any secondary dentoalveolar compensatory changes have occurred, which may result in a need for orthodontic or restorative correction or segmental surgery. Face bow recording and anatomical articulation may be useful particularly in cases of bilateral condylar malunion, where vertical face height changes are planned and mandibular autorotation is anticipated.

CT scanning

CT scanning in the axial and coronal planes yields very useful information, particularly in complex midface and orbitozygomatic deformity and calvarial defects. Two-dimensional imaging is useful in delineating areas of deformity or deficiency and, as with plain films, accurate measurements taken from stable and unaffected portions of the craniofacial skeleton can give an assessment of degree of displacement or deformity. However, an additional benefit of CT scanning is its ability to generate three-dimensional images which allow the surgeon to visualize all aspects of the deformity at the same time and can sometimes reveal the underlying cause of a deformity or discrepancy, which is difficult to assess by two-dimensional scans (Fig. 24.3). In addition, the recent introduction of stereolithographic modeling allows direct visualization of the defect. Direct measurement of required bony movements or augmentation is possible and if necessary, surgical simulation may be carried out. It also facilitates prefabrication of alloplastic implants and production of templates as a guide for size and shape of bone grafts, as well as prebending of plates or mesh for graft fixation. Stereolithographic modeling has been a major advance in the management of patients with complex posttraumatic bony deformity.

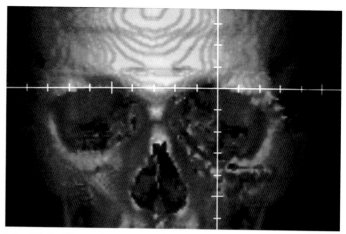

Fig. 24.3: Three-dimensional CT scan of malunited fracture of left zygoma with measurement of displacement.

Treatment planning

Having identified the concerns of the patient, established treatment goals and documented all areas of anatomical and functional abnormality, detailed operative planning is required. If a portion of a craniofacial skeleton is malpositioned or deficient and is giving rise to patient concerns or complaints, it should be restored to its normal anatomical position, shape or volume. However, in planning treatment, it must be borne in mind that correction of one deformity may result in accentuation of another, which may not have been previously noticed by the patient, e.g. malar osteotomy may make a previously mild enophthalmos more obvious or correction of mandibular asymmetry may exaggerate an ipsilateral mild nasal deviation. In this situation, the milder unnoticed defects may require simultaneous or subsequent correction even though they may not be of direct concern to the patient initially.

Detailed planning of surgical interventions and movements depends on the information gathered from the history and examination, but in particular the special investigations. When planning bony surgery, it is essential that an accurate plan of surgery and movements is established prior to operation. This entails a detailed assessment of the extent of movement required in the three planes of space, i.e. anteroposterior, vertical and transverse. If onlay grafts are to be used, the site and extent of augmentation should be similarly established preoperatively. Intraoperative judgment of the extent of necessary bone movement or augmentation to achieve symmetry is extremely difficult, due to distortion of overlying soft tissues as a result of the surgical access, edema, presence of an endotracheal tube and inaccessibility of normal reference points beneath sterile drapes. Where three-dimensional modeling is available, prebending of plates, preforming of implants or production of bone graft templates helps to facilitate accurate correction of the deformity and may reduce operating time.

It is important to ensure a co-ordinated approach to the correction of both bony and soft tissue abnormalities. This usually means correcting the bony abnormality first and then carrying out any necessary soft tissue revision subsequently.

It is essential to discuss with the patient the proposed correction and ensure a realistic expectation of outcome, including both the positive and negative effects of any proposed surgery.

Treatment Techniques

Surgical access

Surgical access to the entire craniofacial skeleton is afforded by bicoronal flap, lower eyelid or transconjunctival and intra-oral buccal sulcus incisions. In addition, a variety of intra- and extraoral incisions are available for access to the mandible, in particular the vertical ramus and condyle.

Coronal flap

A coronal flap gives excellent surgical exposure of the upper craniofacial skeleton. Pre-auricular extension of the incision and dissection in the temporal region immediately adjacent to the deep temporal fascia allow excellent exposure down to and including the zygomatic arches. If the dissection is kept on the surface of the deep temporal fascia, there is no need to pass deep to the superficial layer of the deep temporal fascia and the frontal branch of the facial nerve is elevated with the flap, resulting in little risk of nerve injury and easy dissection in a single surgical plane (subgaleal), leaving pericranium attached to the outer table of the skull. Once the flap is raised to within a centimeter of the supraorbital margins the pericranium can be incised along the temporal crest each side and across the vertex of the skull posteriorly. The pericranial flap pedicled anteriorly can be raised to expose the underlying skull and is available as vascularized tissue for dural repair if needed. Freeing the supraorbital nerves from their foramina can be carried out using small osteotomies medial and lateral to the nerves. The calvarium, forehead, supraorbital rim, orbital roof and lateral orbital rim are exposed and after mobilization and reflection of the temporalis muscle, access is gained to the lateral wall of the orbit and the temporal fossa.

At the end of the operation, the temporalis muscle must be anchored to the lateral orbital rim with sutures, if necessary following anterior mobilization of the muscle, to prevent postoperative retraction and temporal hollowing (Fig. 24.4). Access to the infraorbital margin and orbital floor is possible through a coronal flap but is limited and fixation of osteotomy cuts or grafts can be difficult from this approach without a lower eyelid incision. In addition, if at the start of the operation the medial canthal ligament is intact and attached to the anterior lacrimal crest, it should never be detached during elevation of the flap, since this requires the use of a transnasal canthopexy on closure, the results of which are often disappointing. The attachment of the medial canthal ligament can therefore limit access to the medial orbital wall. If full access to the medial orbital wall is necessary, a lower eyelid incision is required in addition to access gained via the orbital roof exposure of the bicoronal flap.

Lower eyelid incision

Transconjunctival, subciliary or midtarsal incisions, with retro-orbicular preseptal dissection, all give excellent access to the infraorbital rim, orbital floor, infraorbital foramen and anterior surface of the maxilla. We avoid the infraorbital incision for cosmetic reasons. Occasionally, postoperative lower eyelid retraction and increased scleral show may occur but this is unusual and amenable to correction if it fails to resolve spontaneously (Fig. 24.5).

Intraoral buccal sulcus incisions

A horseshoe incision in the upper buccal sulcus gives excellent access to the lower half of the maxilla and zygomatic buttress, and limited access to the infraorbital rim. It should be placed at the height of the sulcus, extending from first

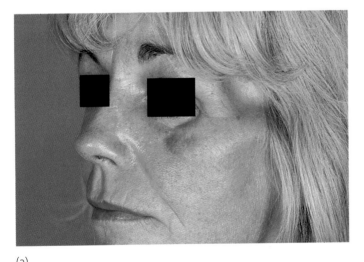

(a)

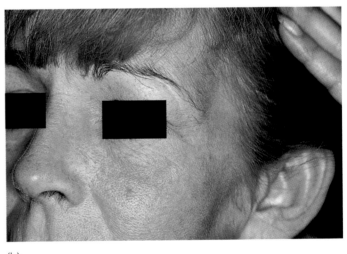

(b)

Fig. 24.4: Postoperative retraction of temporalis muscle. **(a)** Before treatment. **(b)** After treatment by onlay augmentation of temporal fossa and correction of lower eyelid tethering.

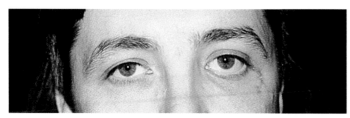

(a)

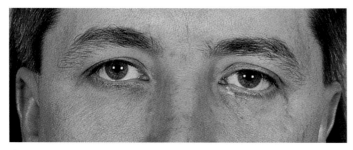

(b)

Fig. 24.5: Postoperative lid retraction. **(a)** Before treatment. **(b)** Following correction by placement of auricular cartilage graft.

molar to first molar, and be directed out into the cheek posteriorly to avoid tearing and ensure maintenance of a good vascular pedicle to the maxilla. Repair of the paranasal muscles at the end of the procedure may reduce the risk of alar flaring postoperatively.[5]

Extraoral approach to the mandible

While lower buccal sulcus incisions give good intraoral access to the horizontal ramus and angle of the mandible, on some rare occasions avoidance of the transoral route is necessary. In addition, intraoral access to the vertical ramus and mandibular condyle is poor and surgical procedures on these areas of the lower jaw often require an extraoral approach.

The submandibular approach gives good access to the horizontal ramus and angle and allows limited access to the vertical ramus of the mandible. The marginal mandibular branch of the facial nerve must be protected, either by dissection deeply on the cervical fascia or by dissection on the deep surface of platysma and formal identification of the nerve in the subplatysma fascial layer. Excessive traction may result in temporary paralysis of the lower lip due to stretching of the marginal mandibular branch of the facial nerve but permanent weakness should be uncommon through this approach. However, nerve injury is more likely if the submandibular approach has been used previously, with fibrosis, loss of surgical planes and distortion of the local anatomy.

Retromandibular incision with blunt dissection between the buccal and marginal mandibular branches of the facial nerve can give excellent access to the vertical ramus and condylar neck and a pre-auricular incision with temporal extension allows access to the condylar head and temporomandibular joint. As with the bicoronal flap, dissection on the surface of the temporalis fascia will avoid injury to the frontal branch of the facial nerve.

Other incisions

Other local incisions such as the upper eyelid blepharoplasty incision, lateral eyebrow incision or use of existing scars may be indicated in selected cases, where more extensive exposure is not necessary.

Correction of deformity

Correction of bony deformity may be carried out by using osteotomy, onlay grafting or a combination of both techniques. If an individual component of the facial skeleton is of normal morphology but in abnormal position (**displacement**), osteotomy is usually the technique of choice. If the bulk of the bone is in normal position but there is abnormal morphology, e.g. localized contour deficit (**deficiency**) then onlay grafting may be appropriate.[4] If both displacement and deficiency exist, then both techniques may be required. However, the choice of technique must take account of the concerns of the patient, as well as the nature and degree of deformity, the extent of surgery required, potential complications and a realistic assessment of the likely outcome. These considerations may necessitate a departure from or modification of the basic principles outlined above.

Osteotomy

A variety of osteotomies are available and are well documented.[1-4] These effectively recreate the original fracture pattern in the area of concern. Secondary osteotomies for trauma patients are usually carried out using conventional surgical techniques with use of interpositional bone grafting if required to fill gaps created by the bony movements, to ensure primary bone healing, stability of the bony movement and support for overlying soft tissues. Osteogenic distraction of the craniofacial skeleton is becoming more widespread and may offer another treatment option in selected cases.[6] However, its role in the correction of posttraumatic deformity has yet to be established.

Onlay grafting

Onlay grafting to correct bone deficiencies may be carried out using a number of materials. Autografts, homografts, heterografts and alloplastic materials have been described and each has its advantages and disadvantages. The 'ideal' characteristics of onlay grafts have been outlined by a number of authors but include the following: biocompatible, no risk of disease transmission, resistant to infection, dimensionally stable, easy to shape or mold, amenable to skeletal fixation, long shelf life, cheap.

Bone

Autogenous bone may be used as an interpositional graft or for onlay augmentation. It has several advantages over other materials, including its biocompatibility and lack of risk of disease transmission. Resistance to infection is good, particularly if the bone is vascularized.[7] Dimensional stability is variable and depends on the vascularity (vascularized being better than non-vascularized),[8,9] embryological origin (membranous bone being better than cartilaginous bone),[10] fixation (rigid fixation better than non-rigid fixation),[10] graft site (interpositional graft better than onlay) and functional loading (functional loading is better than no functional loading). A number of donor sites including tibia, iliac crest, mandible and calvarium are available. The author's preferred donor site is iliac crest for cancellous or corticocancellous bone grafting to mandibular non-union and calvarial bone grafting for almost all other situations where osteotomy gaps or bony deficiency exist, where masticatory loading is expected and where dimensional stability is important.

The use of non-vascularized grafts requires a healthy, well-vascularized graft bed. This is usually present in secondary posttraumatic deformity patients, but occasionally the graft bed may be of sufficiently poor quality to require vascularized bone grafts. Vascularized calvarial bone pedicled on temporalis muscle or the superficial temporal vessels and temporoparietal fascia provide an excellent source of vascularized bone for midface and mandibular reconstruction.[11] A disadvantage in mandibular reconstruction is the possibility of postoperative restriction in mouth opening. In cases where a large bulk of vascularized bone is required, microvascular free flap transfer is the treatment of choice, with a variety of potential donor sites, including iliac crest (deep circumflex iliac artery) and fibula. In selected cases, bone regeneration by distraction osteogenesis may be an option[6] but has currently not been widely applied to treatment of posttraumatic deformity.

The disadvantages of autogenous bone grafting include prolongation of operating time and the creation of a graft donor site, with its potential associated morbidity. Variability of calvarial thickness may result in inadvertently cutting into the intracranial space during graft harvesting,[12] but complications are rare.

Cartilage

Autogenous cartilage is an excellent material for reconstruction in some situations.[13] It is biocompatible, maintains its viability, is dimensionally stable and is easy to carve and shape. It can be fixed with wires or sutures. Although its resistance to infection is limited, it has been proved to be a reliable material when implanted into a vascular bed, especially when used in the orbit and nose. It is an excellent space filler but not rigid and therefore unsuitable for load bearing. Potential donor sites are auricular concha and nasal septum, which give a relatively thin sheet with limited area and volume, or costal cartilage, which has an abundant supply and can provide large volume. As with autogenous bone, prolongation of operating time and donor site morbidity, particularly if costal cartilage is used, are relative disadvantages.

Other materials

A variety of homografts, heterografts and alloplastic materials are available and the reader is referred to Chapters 8 and 31 for discussion of these. In principle, we prefer to use auto-

genous materials in most situations to minimize the risk of disease transmission, peri-implant infection or late extrusion. Exceptions to this are large calvarial defects, where sufficient autogenous bone may not be available, temporal or forehead contour defects, where bone graft substitutes (e.g. tricalcium phosphate) may be used, and minor malar deficiencies where alloplastic onlay grafts are an option.

Follow-up

Postoperative follow-up is essential, not only to monitor the results of treatment but to assess the need for further procedures. It is not uncommon for several reconstructive procedures to be necessary in order to achieve the best possible result. Cohen & Kawamoto[1] presented a series of complex posttraumatic deformity cases, with an average of 3–4 procedures per patient in order to obtain optimal correction and a range of 1–15. It is also important to appreciate the limitations of corrective surgery and to accept that some patients cannot be restored to complete normality. There is a danger that unrealistic expectations of outcome on the part of the patient or the surgeon may result in increasing numbers of surgical interventions yielding diminishing returns. If this point is reached, psychological counseling may be appropriate in order to help the patient accept and cope with any residual deformity.

The principles of secondary correction of posttraumatic deformity will be discussed in the following areas.

- Cranial vault deformity
- Orbitozygomatic injuries
- Nasoethmoidal injuries
- Posttraumatic malocclusion
- Complex cases involving bone deficiency

Defects and deformity of the skull

These will be discussed under the headings of calvarial defects, frontal sinus fractures and orbital roof fractures.

Full-thickness calvarial defects

Background

Full-thickness calvarial defects may be seen in a number of situations such as following gunshot wounds, after loss of osteoplastic craniotomy flaps or as a result of a growing skull fracture. Growing skull fracture is a specific and unusual variant on the full-thickness calvarial defect. These may be linear or non-linear skull fractures, which enlarge with time and are usually seen in children below the age of 3 (Fig. 24.6).[14] Ninety percent occur under the age of 3 years but the process may be observed in older children and adults.[15] The incidence of 'growth' as a delayed complication of skull fracture is rare and occurred in only 0.6% of the cases in one large series.[16] They present with soft swelling in the region of a previous skull fracture with clinical and radiographic evidence of increased width and length of a

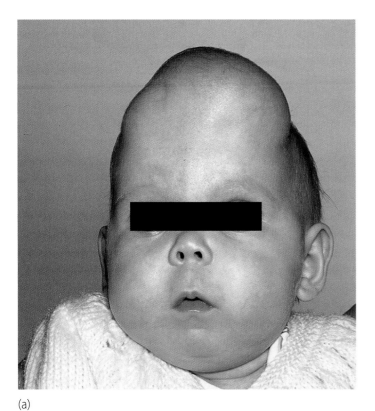

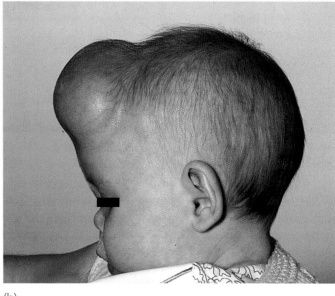

(a)   (b)

Fig. 24.6: Clinical presentation of growing skull fracture. **(a)** Frontal. **(b)** Lateral.

previous fracture. The predominant factor responsible for increase in the size of the fracture seems to be a dural defect[17] with abnormal growth of the underlying cerebral tissues,[18] usually in the form of a leptomeningeal cyst but also from herniated cerebrum or dilated underlying ventricle with porencephalic cyst.

Full-thickness calvarial defects may require treatment for a number of reasons. The patient may be at risk from further trauma, either from blunt injury or penetrating objects, and a significant cosmetic defect may be apparent (Fig. 24.6). In addition, infections of the scalp present a significant risk of intracranial spread due to loss of the natural barrier of the calvarial bone, with potentially serious consequences.[19]

Reconstruction using alloplastic prostheses has historically been the most commonly used method for correction of the larger full-thickness calvarial defect. In the early 20th century active interest developed in autogenous cranioplasty from various donor sites, such as tibia, ilium, ribs or skull. More recently, however, the trend has been to use split-thickness calvarial bone grafting. Calvarial bone grafts have become more popular because of their greater dimensional stability and lower donor site morbidity compared with other bone graft donor sites. However, harvesting of these grafts still involves small risks of dural tears, meningitis, brain abscess, encephalitis and sagittal sinus tears. These risks depend upon the size of the graft harvested and whether full-thickness or split-thickness grafts are used,[20] the location of the donor site and the skill and experience of the operator.

Assessment

A full history of the cranial defect should be established together with previous surgical details, including any prior attempts at reconstruction, in order to anticipate potential surgical complications such as dural tears or the need to remove plates or other implants placed previously. As always, a thorough clinical examination is required. Special attention should be given to the site and size of the skull defect. The position of previous surgical scars should be noted and the quality of the soft tissues overlying the bony defect assessed.

Plain X-rays show a characteristic irregular oval or elliptical skull defect which may be demonstrated on anteroposterior and lateral films. However, more detailed images are gained from CT scans, which in addition give useful information about the underlying brain. This is of special relevance where growing skull fractures are being managed and an MRI study is often used in addition because of its excellent soft tissue imaging characteristics. Reformatting of axial and coronal CT images can be performed to create three-dimensional images which give excellent visualization of the cranial defect. Modern software allows the milling of an exact model of the skull and defect. This is particularly useful for very large defects as it allows the fabrication of a custom-made alloplastic cranioplasty implant (Fig. 24.7).

Treatment planning

The decision to reconstruct a full-thickness calvarial defect depends on a number of factors including age, risk of injury, size of defect, any underlying pathology and the cosmetic consequences of the defect. The decision to operate is taken

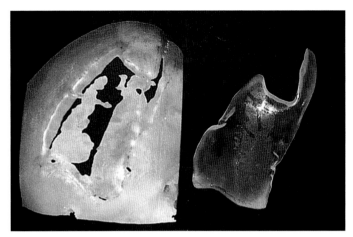

Fig. 24.7: Three-dimensional model of skull defect and prefabricated implant.

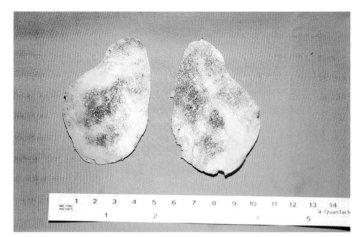

Fig. 24.8: Split calvarial bone graft showing outer and inner tables separated.

on the merits of each individual case. Whether calvarial bone graft or alloplastic implant is used depends largely on the size of the defect and the availability of sufficient calvarial bone to cover the defect, without leaving a deficiency in the donor area. Large full-thickness calvarial defects therefore are usually reconstructed using acrylic or titanium implants, whilst smaller defects are amenable to the use of split calvarial bone grafts.

Operative technique

Surgery is performed using a standard coronal flap approach. Great care is needed when elevating the flap in the region of the bony defect in order that a dural tear is not produced. The margins of the defect are carefully exposed by subpericranial and extradural dissection and any soft tissues within the fracture line or defect are excised or replaced. Excision of non-viable cerebral tissue and dural repair is carried out where necessary.

If calvarial bone graft is to be used, a template of the defect is cut out using sterile paper to aid in accurate harvesting of the graft. The exact form of the calvarial bone graft depends on the size of the defect being reconstructed. Shave

grafts consist of fine strips of bone harvested from the outer table with osteotomes. Their advantage is that multiple grafts can be harvested from a wide area without leaving a significant donor defect. However, their small size means that they cannot be rigidly fixed in their new position.

Sliding bone grafts are in many ways analogous to the advancement flaps used in skin surgery. An area of bone is exposed adjacent to the defect and a bone graft somewhat larger in size than the defect is marked out using saws or burrs. The outer table of the skull is then harvested through the diploic layer as a partial-thickness graft. The bone graft is then slid across the defect in such a manner that it still partially lies across the inner table of the donor site. Such overlap allows increased primary stability and may possibly lead to earlier bony union.

Transposition calvarial bone grafts are now the most widely accepted method of reconstructing sizeable full-thickness skull defects.[20] Following complete exposure of the edges of the bony defect, a temporary template is fashioned and a suitable area for the harvest of calvarial bone is identified. This is most usually in the parietal region on the contralateral side to the pre-existing defect. A full-

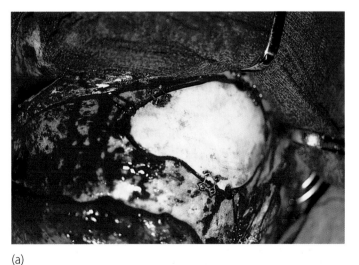

(a)

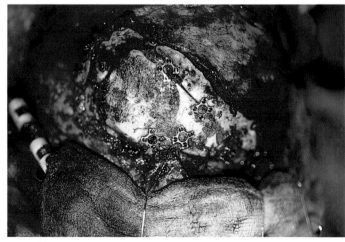

(b)

Fig. 24.9: Split calvarial bone graft. **(a)** Outer table replaced at donor site. **(b)** Inner table reconstructing defect.

thickness piece of calvarial bone slightly larger in dimensions than the template is removed, taking great care not to damage the underlying dura. Once this has been achieved the bone graft is split using fine osteotomes and saws along the diploic layer, thus producing two similarly sized pieces of bone consisting of the inner and outer table respectively (Fig. 24.8). Once this has been done, the outer table bone graft can be returned to the donor site, leaving the inner table graft which can then be adapted to reconstruct the bony defect.

Fixation is achieved for the bone at the donor and the grafted sites using micro or miniplates (Fig. 24.9). In growing skull fractures in pediatric patients, consideration should be given to use of resorbable plates to avoid drift of the plate from the outer to the inner aspect of the calvarium with continued skull growth. The donor site should be covered with a layer of Surgicel, the pericranial layer closed and the scalp repaired over a suction drain if necessary.

Outcome of calvarial defect reconstruction

The outcome of reconstruction of simple calvarial defects using split calvarial bone grafts is excellent. In a follow-up study of 27 patients, Posnik et al[21] found minimal complications with no infections, graft exposures or intracranial injuries. However, a growing skull fracture is a different clinical entity. In a study of 41 patients with growing skull fractures Gupta et al[16] reported a death rate of 7%, postoperative CSF leaks in 7% and local wound infection in 14%. In a review of 132 cases reported in the literature, Pezzota et al[22] found a high incidence of seizures and focal neurological deficit, with functional recovery being linked to the clinical presentation and early diagnosis. Reconstruction of simple calvarial defects is therefore associated with a better outcome than growing skull fractures, in which the postoperative morbidity is largely related to abnormalities of the underlying brain.

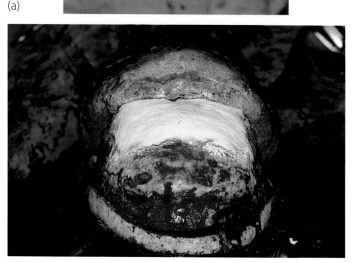

(a)

(c)

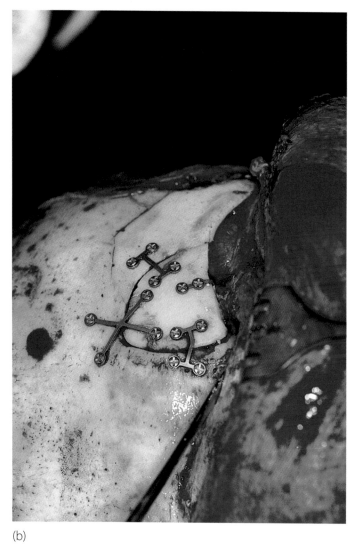

(b)

Fig. 24.10: Frontal sinus fracture. **(a)** Bicoronal flap. **(b)** Osteotomy and fixation of fragments. **(c)** Augmentation with tricalcium phosphate bone cement.

Frontal sinus fractures

Background
Frontal sinus fractures are most commonly managed in the acute setting where open reduction and internal fixation of the disrupted bone is performed together with any necessary maxillofacial or neurological surgery.[23] Where the posterior wall of the frontal sinus is fractured, cranialization of the sinus and stripping of the lining mucosa together with obliteration of the frontonasal duct with muscle, fat or cancellous bone chips are necessary to prevent late complications of CSF leakage, mucopyoceles, osteomyelitis and meningoencephaloceles.[24] A dural repair is generally required where the posterior wall is fractured. On occasion, however, patients may present for late correction of a depressed fracture of the frontal bone, usually for reasons of cosmesis.

Assessment
A thorough history of the injury and its subsequent management should be taken. If the posterior table was involved in the original fracture it is important to know if a cranialization procedure was performed as this will have important consequences for the reconstruction of the bony defect. In this situation, fibrosis and adhesions will increase risk of further dural tear and avoidance of extradural dissection is desirable. Onlay bone graft or use of an alloplastic filler material may be more appropriate than osteotomy in order to reduce risk of complications.

Examination of the frontal bone contour together with the condition of the overlying skin is performed. The sensation subserved by the supraorbital and supratrochlear nerves should be assessed prior to raising the coronal flap.

Plain films can give useful information especially with regard to the presence and location of metalwork from previous surgical procedures. CT scans are required to show greater detail of the anatomy of the anterior and posterior walls of the frontal sinus. The presence or otherwise of active frontal sinus disease can also be assessed and if present, should be treated prior to reconstruction.

Treatment planning
There are two principal methods of management, both usually through a coronal approach. First, the bone may be re-osteotomized along the previous fracture lines and the bone fragment(s) fixed in their original position with miniplates or microplates. If the posterior table has been involved this is likely to involve a formal craniotomy. Alternatively the defect can be masked with an onlay bone graft or, if the contour defect is minor, it may be corrected more simply using a calcium triphosphate bone replacement material keyed to the bone with microscrews or fine titanium mesh.

Operative technique
Figure 24.10 illustrates the operative technique.

Outcome
Outcome of secondary osteotomy or bone grafting for displaced anterior wall fractures is excellent. Most complications are associated with the original injury and are dependent on whether the posterior wall is involved with dural tear, CSF leaks, involvement of the nasofrontal duct and whether adequate treatment including, where necessary, dural repair, cranialization or obliteration of the sinus and nasofrontal duct were carried out. In a series of 33 patients with frontal sinus fracture,[25] long-term complications occurred in four patients, with only two being cosmetic. The requirement for secondary surgery is therefore small in well-managed frontal sinus fractures.

Orbital roof fractures

Background
Orbital roof fractures are a consequence of severe trauma and are associated with a considerable likelihood of neurological and ophthalmological injury. In general such injuries are managed in the acute phase but where they are not treated or where treatment is inadequate, the patient may present with a significant secondary deformity. Below the age of 3, the orbital roof may be the site of a growing skull fracture.[15]

Assessment
A full history of the original injury is taken together with a history of previous treatment. Original notes, X-rays and scans are of great help in shedding light on previous treatment and planning surgery.

A full assessment of the external bony contour should be made. Irregularity or asymmetry of the supraorbital rims should be noted. An assessment of enophthalmos or exophthalmos (including pulsating exophthalmos indicative of orbital roof defects) should be made. Sensory function of the supraorbital and supratrochlear nerves should be assessed. As with any orbital reconstruction, an ophthalmological opinion should be sought before any surgery is performed to document vision and ocular motility preoperatively to identify problems and to act as a baseline for postoperative follow-up. Where the orbital roof itself has been depressed, ocular dystopia with inferior displacement of the globe is a common finding (Fig. 24.11). Larger defects of the orbital roof put the patient at risk of dural herniation which may result in pulsating exophthalmos and disturbance of ocular function.

Special investigations
Fine cut axial and coronal CT scans should be obtained to give detailed images of the orbital roofs of both orbits (Fig. 24.12). This allows accurate surgical planning and measurements can be made of bony displacement, deficiency or asymmetry.

Operative technique
In the great majority of cases a coronal flap will be the most appropriate approach. Occasionally it may be possible to access the surgical area via an existing scar and for small defects confined to the supraorbital rim, this approach may be adequate. However, more major deformities and any significant displacement or deficiency of the orbital roof

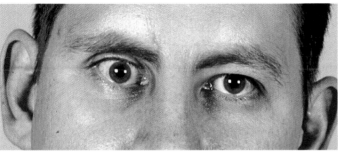

(a)

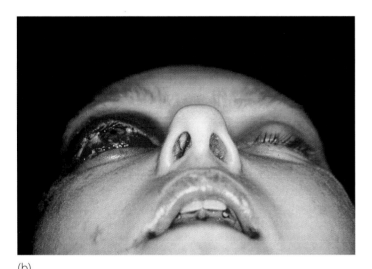

(b)

Fig. 24.11: Orbital roof fracture. **(a)** Inferior displacement of eye. **(b)** Proptosis.

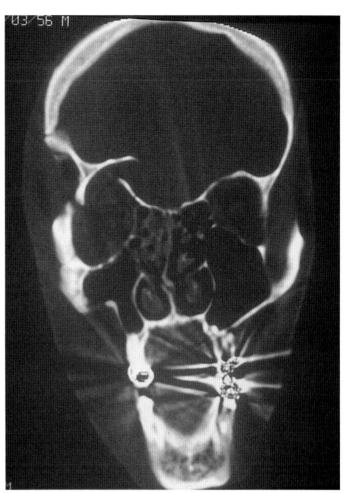

Fig. 24.12: CT scan of orbital roof fracture showing significant displacement of fracture segment.

will require a transcranial approach with unilateral frontal craniotomy, retraction of frontal lobe and on occasion may require removal of the supraorbital bar. This obviously requires joint neurosurgical/maxillofacial management.

Where small depressions or contour irregularities exist they may be masked by bony recontouring with burrs and by the application of small onlay bone grafts or alternatively one of the proprietary bone cements now available. Large displacements or defects in the orbital roof require accurate reduction or reconstruction with split-thickness calvarial bone graft, if necessary following dural repair. Where a frontal craniotomy has been performed, the graft can be harvested from the inner table of the frontal bone flap, thus avoiding any visible or palpable donor site defect.[26]

Outcome

There is very little in the literature regarding secondary correction of orbital roof fractures.[27] With accurate reconstitution of the anatomy, the outcome should be good in both pediatric and adult patients. However, some inaccuracy in vertical and AP globe partitioning may occur, as well as postoperative diplopia.

Deformity of the zygomaticoorbital region

Background

The treatment of fractures of the orbit and fractures of the zygoma will be dealt with together due to the great overlap of these topics. Injuries to this area can produce complex deformities and careful planning is required when secondary corrective surgery is contemplated. In general, deformity is due to inadequate primary surgery[28] and is related in part to the underlying bony skeletal abnormality and in part to the soft tissue component including scarring, thickening and incorrect draping of the soft tissue envelope on the facial bones. Deformities of upper and lower eyelids may be seen, often as a result of the initial trauma but also occasionally resulting from a previous surgical approach. Patient complaints may be related to the cosmetic or functional deficit that they are experiencing or both. It is important to establish from the outset the specific concerns of the patient and his expectation of the outcome of treatment. This will allow surgery to be tailored to the patient's concerns rather than the surgeon's view of the deformity and will give the opportunity to dispel any unrealistic expectations that the patient may have.

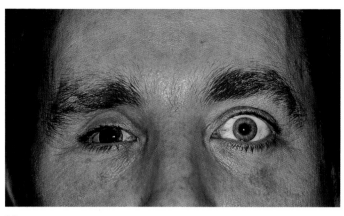

(a)

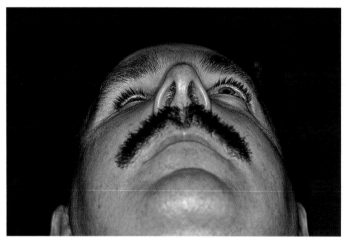

(b)

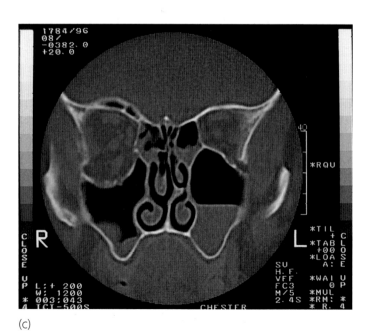

(c)

Fig. 24.13: Enophthalmos. **(a,b)** Clinical appearance. **(c)** CT scan showing large floor blow-out.

Assessment

A full history should be taken including the mechanism of the original injury, the treatment previously received and the current concerns of the patient. A number of factors contribute to unsatisfactory appearance following orbito-zygomatic injuries and give rise to cosmetic complaints.

Enophthalmos is common due to increased orbital volume or herniation of orbital contents through defects in the orbital walls, usually inferior or medial (Fig. 24.13). Ocular dystopia may occur with inferior displacement of the globe when Whitnall's tubercle is inferiorly displaced as a result of zygomatic malunion following an inferiorly displaced fracture. Loss of zygomatic prominence leading to cheekbone asymmetry is common and increased facial width due to bowing of the zygomatic arch may occur secondary to an inadequately reduced posteriorly displaced zygomatic fracture. Telecanthus may be present if the original fractures involved the portion of bone bearing the medial canthal ligament or if the ligament has been detached during surgical access for primary treatment.

Esthetic concerns with regard to the periorbital soft tissues are frequently related to the position of the eyelids and canthi. Lid retraction and/or true ectropion may be seen, usually as a result of previous treatment (see Fig. 24.5).

Functional deficits following orbital trauma frequently relate to injury to the globe itself and are thus within the preserve of the ophthalmological surgeon. Tethering and scarring of the periorbita and extraocular muscles may cause diplopia which, if severe, can be disabling (see Fig. 24.1). Epiphora is a frequent complaint and may be due to damage to the bony or soft tissue component of the lacrimal drainage apparatus, including abnormalities of lower lid and therefore lacrimal punctum position. Where epiphora persists, corrective surgery may be necessary.

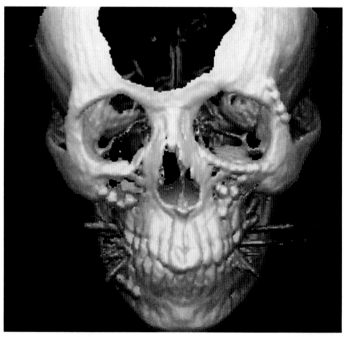

Fig. 24.14: Three-dimensional CT scan showing overreduction of the fracture of the left zygoma.

Clinical examination should include assessment of the degree of enophthalmos, which should be assessed subjectively by clinical examination and objectively by exophthalmometry. The classic signs of enophthalmos, including obvious ocular retrusion, hypoglobus, deep supratarsal fold, pseudoptosis and narrowing of the palpebral fissure, may be apparent (Fig. 24.13). Normal anterior projection of the globe relative to the lateral orbit rim is between 12 and 16 mm. Whilst formal exophthalmometry would seem likely to give a more objective assessment than clinical examination, it should be remembered that it is comparing the position of the globe with that of the lateral orbital wall and if this bony landmark has been altered by the original trauma, the subsequent reading may be unreliable.

Any asymmetry of the malar prominences should be noted. The malar eminence on the injured side may be displaced medially, posteriorly or inferiorly or combinations of these. Rarely, if previous surgery has overreduced the zygomatic complex, it may be lateral to its normal position and therefore overprominent (Fig. 24.14). Facial width should be assessed by comparing the relative prominence of the zygomatic arch on the injured and uninjured side. If the zygoma is displaced posteriorly, this results in a 'bowing out' of the zygomatic arch, thus increasing the facial width on the injured side.

An assessment of the overlying soft tissues should be made. The quality and thickness of the tissues should be noted.

Scarred, contracted tissues may require correction either at the time of osteotomy or subsequently. Loss of sensation in the distribution of the infraorbital nerve is common following orbital trauma, whilst loss of supraorbital and supratrochlear nerve sensation is less frequently seen. There is no evidence to suggest that secondary surgery will have a beneficial effect on compromised nerve function and indeed, the patient should be aware that surgery carries the risk of further nerve damage.

Special investigations

Plain X-rays have a limited role in surgical planning of midface deformity. They are useful in identifying the type and position of internal fixation used in previous operations, as this will almost certainly need to be removed if further surgery is performed. A submento-vertex radiograph will show the form of the zygomatic arches. Subtle variations in the shape of the zygomatic arches can have a profound effect on facial width and overall facial balance.

CT scans are invaluable in surgical planning. Images should be obtained in the coronal and axial planes and 3D images can be particularly useful in orbitozygomatic injuries. By taking measurements from unaffected fixed points such as the pterygoid plates or contralateral uninjured orbit, a quantitative measurement of the bony deformity can be established with respect to the contralateral uninjured side. These

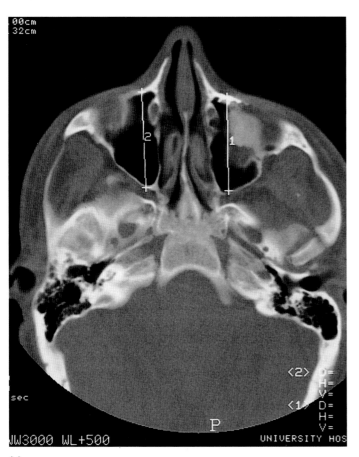

(a)

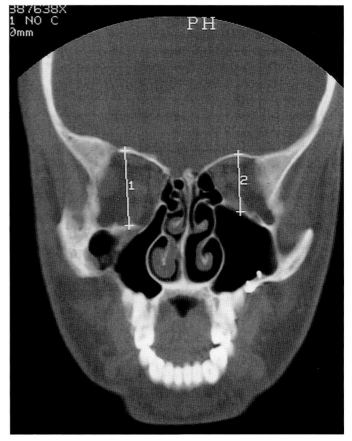

(b)

Fig. 24.15: Surgical planning on CT scans. **(a)** Anteroposterior measurement. **(b)** Vertical measurement.

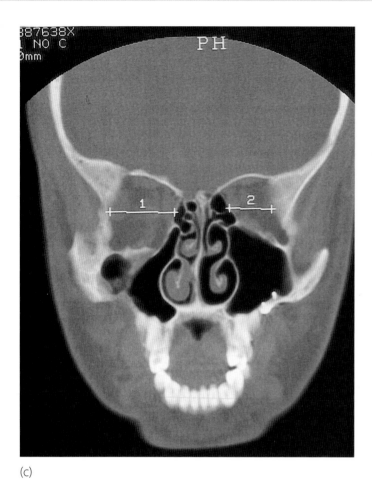

(c)

Fig. 24.15: (c) Transverse measurement.

measurements should be established in three planes so that the necessary movements or augmentations of the zygomatico-maxillary complex can be predicted in the vertical, mediolateral and posteroanterior planes. These movements should be accurately established before surgery is undertaken (Fig. 24.15).

MR scans are little used in the planning of facial bone osteotomies at the present time but they do have a role in assessing the nature and quality of the overlying soft tissues and may be a useful investigation in difficult cases. The degree of herniation of tissues through the medial, inferior and to a lesser extent the lateral orbital walls may be assessed with MRI scanning. It may also be possible to image trapping or tethering of extraocular muscles.

Dental study casts have little role to play in the management of zygomatico-orbital deformity unless there is going to be a simultaneous osteotomy of the maxilla or mandible to correct a malocclusion. The advent of computer-generated 3D models of the bony facial skeleton milled or cast using information derived from CT scans has been a major step forward in this regard. Exact measurements can be made on the models and the surgery accurately pre-planned. If alloplastic materials are to be used they can be custom made on the 3D models. Recent advances in computer software are likely to allow much more specific surgical planning in relation to the hard or soft tissue movements.

Sinus endoscopy is a relatively recent innovation and may be useful to assess the condition of the orbital floor. In the acute situation, some success with definitive fracture management has been achieved but whether endoscopically assisted surgery will have any role in the management of the secondary deformity is unclear. One case has been reported of correction of enophthalmos secondary to a medial wall defect using alloplastic material inserted via an endoscopic approach medial to the lacrimal caruncle.[29]

Where surgery is being considered a full ophthalmic and orthoptic assessment is required as a baseline. This is especially important in those cases where the patient is experiencing diplopia.

Surgical technique

For successful correction of the zygomatico-orbital deformity, complete regional exposure is required[28] although some authors advocate a more conservative approach.[30,31] This is performed through a bicoronal flap, combined with a lower eyelid incision, and an upper buccal sulcus incision. The bicoronal flap gives excellent access to the orbit and zygomatic arch and body and permits harvesting of calvarial bone graft. Stripping of the temporalis muscle facilitates exposure of the lateral orbital wall. Lower eyelid approach gives access to the infraorbital rim and orbital floor and allows visualization and protection of the infraorbital nerve. It may be through a skin incision (blepharoplasty, midtarsal or infraorbital) or via a transconjunctival incision. The transconjunctival incision, which is usually combined with a lateral canthotomy, is technically more difficult to perform but has the advantage of leaving less facial scarring compared with the cutaneous approaches and may be associated with a lower incidence of lid retraction. The combination of bicoronal flap and lower lid approach allows circumferential subperiosteal dissection within the orbit. The lateral canthal ligament should be tagged and reattached at the end of the procedure. Conversely, the medial canthal ligament, which is notoriously difficult to reattach, should have its origin carefully preserved.

The orbital floor must be dissected with great care as the infraorbital nerve is frequently embedded in dense scar tissue and may easily be damaged. A similar situation applies where gaps in the bony skeleton, for example in the lateral orbital wall, have led to fusion of the intra- and extraorbital soft tissues. The buccal sulcus incision gives access to the anterior surface of the maxilla, zygomatic buttress and, via the maxillary sinus, the inferior aspect of the orbital floor.

Correction of bony deformities in the zygomatico-orbital area is dependent upon the performance of several key maneuvers. Zygomatic osteotomy will reproduce the fracture lines of the original injury. Following exposure, bone cuts are made from the infraorbital rim just lateral to the nerve extending down the anterior maxillary wall, passing posteriorly, to the zygomatic buttress. The bone cut is continued around the lower extent of the buttress onto its posterior face. Within the orbit the cut passes from the infraorbital rim posteriorly to the anterior end of the inferior orbital fissure. The cuts are then continued superiorly through or just anterior to the greater wing of the sphenoid and continued to the zygomatico-frontal suture. Completion of the osteotomy at the posterior aspect of the buttress is best performed using a fine, curved osteotome, inserted via the coronal approach behind the lateral orbital rim within the temporal fossa, and extends from the anterior end of the inferior orbital fissure to join with the cut already made in the inferior part of the buttress. The root of the zygomatic arch is sectioned, resulting in complete freeing of the zygoma from its bony attachments. For the less experienced operator, appreciation of the exact three-dimensional anatomy is enhanced if a dry skull or a three-dimensional model is available in the operating theater.

Before the zygoma is mobilized, the bony movements should be marked at the infraorbital rim, the zygomatico-frontal suture and the zygomatic arch. The most common posttraumatic displacement of the zygoma involves impaction posteriorly, inferiorly and medially. Usually, bone removal is required at the zygomatico-frontal suture to permit superior repositioning of the zygoma, whereas advancement and lateral movement will create bony gaps. The zygoma is fixed into its new position with microplates. Repositioning of the body of the zygoma will often produce contour deformities and steps in the zygomatic arch and the arch itself may require local osteotomies to allow it to be recontoured.

Anterior, lateral and superior movement of the osteotomized zygoma will create bony gaps and step deformities at several sites and these require bone grafting in order to ensure bony union, stability and soft tissue support and to avoid palpable irregularities and edges beneath the thin periorbital skin. Gaps occur at the infraorbital margin, orbital floor, the frontozygomatic cut, lateral orbital wall, zygomatic arch and zygomatic buttress. In addition, the zygomatic repositioning may have created an orbit larger in volume than before and allow herniation of periorbital tissues through bony defects of the orbital walls. Considerable widening of the inferior orbital fissure may occur as a result of repositioning. This increased orbital volume predisposes towards the development of enophthalmos. The inferior orbital fissure should be exposed and the soft tissues divided (no significant structures pass through it) and it should be obliterated with a graft. Bone grafting is essential to treat pre-existing enophthalmos and to prevent its occurrence

following osteotomy. Contoured calvarial bone is used for this purpose. Calvarial bone graft exhibits considerably less tendency for resorption than the previously used rib or iliac crest grafts, particularly when rigid fixation techniques are utilized.[10] Calvarial bone should now be considered as the 'gold standard' for grafting in and around the orbit. The bone is readily available and does not require a separate incision for its harvest. Enough bone is available for the great majority of cases and the morbidity associated with its harvest has been shown to be very low.[32] The technique has been described elsewhere but the bone is usually obtained as thin rectangular strips, which are ideally suited for grafting orbital defects.

For the correction of enophthalmos it is important that the bone graft is largely situated behind the equator of the globe in order that the eye is displaced forwards. Hypoglobus may be corrected if the bone graft is placed in the orbital floor beneath the globe, but care must be taken in placing orbital bone grafts not to produce unwanted elevation in globe position. Bone grafts placed posteriorly within the orbit do not generally require fixation although a number of specifically designed plates are available for this purpose. Where grafts are more anteriorly placed, fixation is recommended to minimize the amount of resorption and prevent migration. Where possible, the metalwork should be placed within the orbital margin so that it is not subsequently palpable through the thin infraorbital skin. A forced duction test is performed immediately before and after placement of bone graft to ensure that ocular motility has not been jeopardized (see Fig. 24.2).

In cases where a bone graft is being placed to correct a pre-existing enophthalmos, overcorrection is advisable at the time of surgery in order to allow for swelling and a degree of bone graft resorption.[28] Bone graft is carefully placed until a degree of exophthalmos has been achieved. Some authors have recommended incisions within the scarred periorbital tissues in order to allow the globe to take up a more anterior position. It is likely, however, that the scarring will recur and this maneuver is not recommended. Advancement of the displaced zygoma and orbital rim is dependent on the ability to simultaneously correct the enophthalmos as otherwise the appearance of the enophthalmos itself may be worsened (Fig. 24.16).

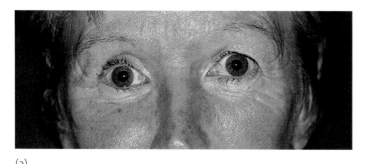
(a)

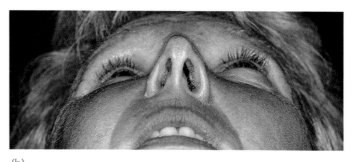
(b)

Fig. 24.16: Zygomatic osteotomy with calvarial bone graft to orbit. **(a,b)** Preoperative photographs showing enophthalmos, hypoglobus and loss of zygomatic prominence.

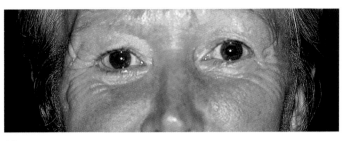

(c)

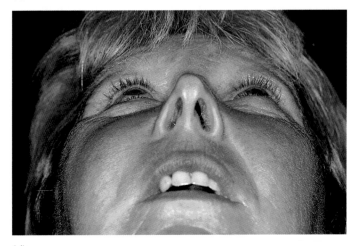

(d)

Fig. 24.16: (c,d) Following operative correction.

Onlay grafting

Onlay grafting may be used in mild cases of malar asymmetry and can usually be carried out easily through a lower eyelid incision. Calvarial bone, bone substitutes or alloplastic implants may be used (Fig. 24.17).

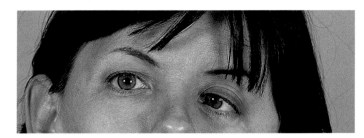

(a)

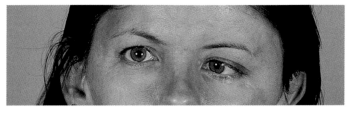

(b)

Fig. 24.17: Onlay augmentation of left zygoma utilizing vascularized calvarial bone pedicled on temporalis muscle. **(a)** Preoperative. **(b)** Post operative.

Nasoethmoid fractures

Detachment of the medial canthal ligaments together with their bony insertion is relatively common following orbital and nasoethmoidal fractures. Inadequate primary management leads to telecanthus and blunting of the medial canthal angle. Osteotomy and repositioning of the naso-ethmoidal segment may be required. Complete correction of the medial canthal position is notoriously difficult and overcorrection should be the aim. In those cases where the medial canthal ligament is not attached to an identifiable bone fragment, a transnasal canthopexy is required (Fig. 24.18). Where a nasoethmoidal fracture has been a

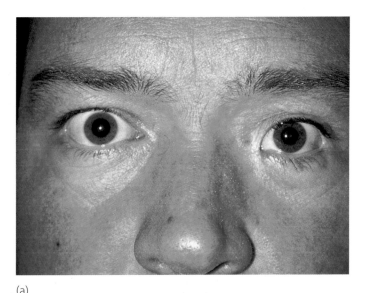

(a)

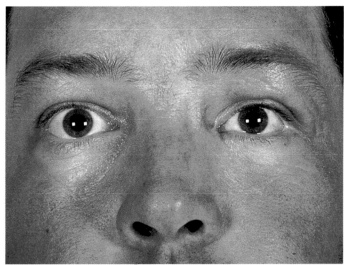

(b)

Fig. 24.18: Secondary deformity following nasoethmoidal injury. **(a)** Medial canthal detachment. **(b)** Appearance following transnasal canthopexy.

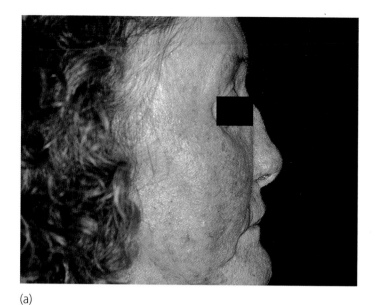

(a)

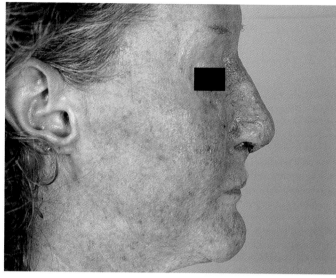

(c)

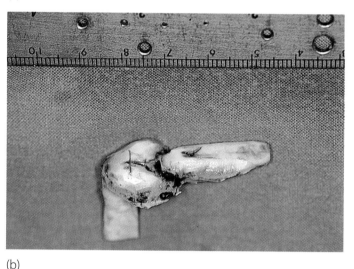

(b)

Fig. 24.19: Nasal reconstruction following comminuted midfacial trauma. **(a)** Preoperative lack of nasal projection. **(b)** Carved costal cartilage graft. **(c)** Postoperative improvement in nasal projection.

significant part of the orbital injury a graft will almost invariably be needed to the dorsum of the nose to recreate the degree of nasal projection present before the injury. Calvarial bone has been widely used in the past but although it gives a satisfactory appearance, its 'feel', especially towards the nasal tip, is too solid to be natural and a nasal dorsal graft of carved costal cartilage may be preferred (Fig. 24.19).

Outcome

Long-term outcome depends on the extent of the secondary deformity, on detailed planning, choice of technique and meticulous surgery. In a series published by Freihofer & Borstlap,[33] osteotomy was found to give superior results compared with onlay techniques. In 16 posttraumatic cases, 14 were assessed as good or satisfactory, with only two being rated as unsatisfactory, due to undercorrection, overcorrection or persistence of enophthalmos. They found no decrease in visual acuity and in five cases with associated posttraumatic enophthalmos, two were corrected fully whilst three were

only partially corrected. Infraorbital nerve sensory loss occurred in approximately half of the group. In a series of four cases, Perino et al[34] reported good results and low complication rate. However, both these had a significant requirement for further procedures to ensure optimum outcome and in Cohen & Kawamoto's series[1] including 14 cases of orbitozygomatic deformity, the average number of operations required was 3.76. Further procedures may be required to reduce overcorrected malar position, to correct medial and lateral canthal dystopias, recurrence of enophthalmos and abnormalities of eyelid position.

Hammer[28] reported good or satisfactory esthetic results following secondary zygomatico-orbital reconstruction in 20 out of 26 patients. Where diplopia was present prior to secondary correction, improvement occurred in just over half of the group. There was a complication rate of 15% including visual loss due to displacement of bone graft, endophthal-0mitis, orbital abscess and exposure of a nasal bone graft.

Freihofer[35] reported a series of patients who underwent secondary correction of fractured zygomas, with a good result obtained in 80%. Medial canthopexy was carried out in

19 patients. Three required further procedures but all 19 achieved satisfactory or good final outcome.

Posttraumatic malocclusion

Background

Posttraumatic malocclusion may present following malunion of any fracture that directly or indirectly involves the alveolar segments of the maxilla or mandible. These include isolated dentoalveolar fractures of maxilla or mandible, maxillary fractures including Le Fort I, II or III with or without palatal split, and mandibular fractures.

Before the introduction of miniplating, stabilization of the occlusion by intermaxillary fixation (IMF) was the primary aim of treatment of facial fractures. The introduction of internal fixation makes direct anatomical segment reduction the primary aim. If this is achieved, a normal occlusion should automatically follow. This is indeed the case in the majority of cases. However, in some comminuted maxillary or mandibular fractures, a perfect occlusion may be difficult to achieve and most fractures of the mandibular condyle tend to be managed by closed techniques, with the potential for displacement following removal of the intermaxillary fixation. In addition, large muscle forces in the mandible may cause movement of the fracture site, resulting in fibrous or non-union. Infection of mandibular fractures, particularly those involving the tooth-bearing segment of the mandible or angle, may result in non-union and segment displacement with malocclusion.

Diagnosis

In the presence of small displacements of segments, patients usually complain of functional difficulties in biting and chewing and the inability to find a positive, comfortable intercuspal position. In large displacements, an effect on facial appearance may be added, particularly increases in mandibular angle causing anterior open bite, and mandibular asymmetry, both usually due to mandibular condylar fracture malunion. Complaints related to temporomandibular joint dysfunction may follow malunion of condylar fractures and mechanical joint derangement may result in severe deviation or limitation of mouth opening.

Assessment of temporomandibular joint function is mandatory, since restriction of mouth opening or severe deviation may necessitate surgery to the temporomandibular joint in addition to osteotomies or bone grafting. It is important to check for mandibular displacement and ensure that when the malocclusion is assessed, the mandible is fully retruded. Occasionally, a patient will present with occlusal complaints but will apparently show a good occlusion. This may be due to a minor mandibular displacement, indicating a discrepancy between the retruded condylar position of the mandible and intercuspal position. In addition, fibrous union of a body fracture, allowing a very small degree of movement between segments, may allow good intercuspation but only at the expense of bone movement at the site of the fibrous union. It may be difficult to see obvious fracture mobility in this

situation by standard clinical examination but careful inspection of the fracture site whilst occluding and discluding the teeth may demonstrate movement. The use of articulating paper may help assessment in cases where the discrepancy is small.

Investigation usually includes study models and plain radiographs. CT scans may occasionally help, particularly in assessment of condylar injuries.

Dental study models are necessary to assess whether segmental surgery or whole-jaw surgery should be undertaken. If the pretraumatic occlusion is obtainable with the existing arch form, then one-piece jaw surgery is indicated. If an acceptable occlusion is not obtainable, it may be indicative of a malunited segmental fracture or a degree of dentoalveolar compensatory change secondary to the altered occlusion and jaw position. In this situation, one-piece jaw surgery alone will not establish the pretraumatic occlusion and adjunctive treatment is necessary. If the occlusal discrepancy is slight, selective occlusal grinding may allow a reasonable seating of the occlusion. If this is considered undesirable or will not achieve a satisfactory occlusion, then orthodontic treatment may be considered. However, a number of patients will be unsuitable for orthodontics due to lack of anchorage, poor oral hygiene or dental condition or lack of sufficient motivation. If orthodontics is precluded for any of these reasons, occlusal rehabilitation by restorative techniques may also be considered but may also be limited by existing dental condition, oral hygiene or patient motivation. In this situation segmental surgery may be the only viable option.

Face bow recording and anatomical articulation are useful in planning treatment for correction of anterior open bite. They allow accurate assessment of the degree of posterior maxillary impaction required and an approximate assessment of the degree of mandibular autorotation. This is helpful in planning the need for mandibular osteotomy to correct anteroposterior jaw relationships.

Plain X-rays, particularly OPG and lateral cephalogram, will demonstrate fibrous union, gross segment displacement, site of previously inserted metalwork and if orthognathic techniques are being used, provide a basis for orthognathic work-up.

Treatment planning

It is important to consider the need for multidisciplinary involvement before treatment is undertaken. This may involve an orthodontist and occasionally a restorative dental surgeon, since some occlusal discrepancies may be amenable to occlusal adjustment, restorative or orthodontic treatment. As discussed above, other patients may require a joint orthodontic and surgical approach using standard orthognathic techniques, particularly if a pre-existing malocclusion or dental crowding existed or if sufficient time has elapsed since the injury to allow some compensatory dentoalveolar changes to occur. On occasions, the amount of movement required at osteotomy is relatively small and this gives only a small acceptable margin of error in jaw and segment positioning at surgery. If positioning errors occur, then elastic traction may be adequate for correction in the early postoperative phase but should this prove inadequate, an assessment of the feasibility of orthodontic or restorative solutions is useful.

With regard to the detailed surgical movements, these are of course dictated by the establishment of an acceptable dental occlusion. Intraoperative occlusal wafers to assist accurate jaw and segment positioning are essential. Preformed arch bars facilitate intraoperative intermaxillary fixation and if significant edentulous areas exist, especially posteriorly, then acrylic saddles should be incorporated within the arch bars to facilitate jaw positioning and should be left in situ postoperatively to improve jaw stability and prevent loss of posterior ramus height in the early postoperative period.

Osteotomies

Maxilla

Indications
In order to correct occlusal abnormalities due to maxillary malunion, Le Fort I osteotomy is indicated. Osteotomy at Le Fort II or III level, or variations of these procedures tailored to the individual needs of the patient, may be required in some instances where simultaneous correction of midface deformity is necessary. However, primary treatment by open reduction with internal fixation and primary bone grafting have substantially reduced the need for more extensive maxillary osteotomies in the treatment of secondary posttraumatic deformity. Le Fort I osteotomy is therefore indicated for most cases of maxillary occlusal abnormality, when segmental or one-piece maxillary repositioning is necessary. In addition, maxillary osteotomy may be required in order to close an anterior open bite following bilateral condylar malunion.

Operative technique
Standard Le Fort I down fracture is carried out via a horseshoe-shaped buccal sulcus incision. Bone cuts of lateral maxillary wall, zygomatic buttress, lateral nasal walls, pterygomaxillary dysjunction and nasal septum are carried out in a similar way to standard orthognathic surgery. Following down fracture, the maxilla is mobilized and if indicated, segmentation of the maxilla can be carried out from the nasal aspect by making a horseshoe-shaped cut in the bony palate and extending this cut radially between the roots of the teeth either side of the site of the desired segmental cut. After segmentation, an acrylic palate retained with Adams cribs helps to control the segments and temporary intermaxillary fixation is applied using a prefabricated occlusal wafer to establish the desired position of the maxilla relative to the mandible. Any areas causing interference with establishment of the desired position of the maxilla are removed. This is particularly important in the nasal septum to avoid postoperative septal deviation and at the posterior maxilla in cases of maxillary impaction. The maxilla is then fixed with miniplates, at the piriform apertures and zygomatic buttresses.

Once the maxilla is fixed, the intermaxillary fixation is removed in order to check the newly established dental occlusion. This must be exactly as planned and must be achievable by gentle upward pressure on the chin point, ensuring that no distraction of the mandibular condyles out of the glenoid fossae has occurred. If this happens, an anterior open bite will be detectable following removal of intraoperative intermaxillary fixation. If undetected at this stage, it would certainly become apparent in the early postoperative period. If on careful checking of the occlusion, any discrepancy, in particular anterior open bite, is detected, then the occlusal wafer and intermaxillary fixation must be reapplied and the maxilla repositioned and replated, following the removal of any persistent bony interferences, especially in the region of the maxillary tuberosity and pterygoid plates.

Once the correct maxillary position is established, any significant bony gaps or deficiencies are bone grafted. This is particularly important at piriform and zygomatic buttresses and at the anterior maxillary wall. These ensure union, stability and support for the overlying soft tissues of the cheek. However, the use of bone grafts in Le Fort I osteotomies to correct posttraumatic occlusion is uncommon due to the relatively small movements involved.

If segmental surgery is necessary to reposition a dentoalveolar segment only, then this is best carried out via a full Le Fort I down fracture in the manner described above. This approach facilitates access for bone cuts, particularly in the palate, and removal of bony interferences between segments. Care must be taken to avoid injury to the dental roots adjacent to segmental bone cut, especially if preoperative orthodontic treatment has not been carried out. If palatal expansion is carried out then bone graft may be placed in the palatal osteotomy gaps to improve transverse stability.[1] Previously described local segmental maxillary osteotomies have largely been superseded by the Le Fort I down fracture technique.

Outcome
There is very little literature devoted to the outcome of maxillary osteotomies for the correction of posttraumatic deformity, either one-piece or segmental procedures. Stability following osteotomies for posttraumatic deformity will be dependent to an extent on the nature of the original injury, its treatment and subsequent secondary procedures and the presence of soft tissue scarring which, if present, is likely to increase relapsing forces, a phenomenon well known in cleft osteotomy. Cohen & Kawamoto[1] reported the results of 25 patients with severe posttraumatic facial deformities, including 10 Le Fort I osteotomies. Although they present no detailed analysis of long-term outcome, they take the view that malocclusion following secondary correction should be rare. However, any adult non-orthodontic, orthognathic surgery demands meticulous technique and accurate positioning of segments.

Mandible
Patients presenting with malocclusion following mandibular injuries may present with non-union, fibrous union or malunion.

Non-union/fibrous union

Non-union and fibrous union may occur following fracture of any part of the mandible but most commonly affect fractures of the mandibular angle.[36] In a study of 1432 mandibular fractures, Mathog et al[37] found an incidence of non-union of 2.8%. They reported increased incidence in men, in fractures affecting the body of the mandible and in patients with multiple fractures. Inadequate stabilization or reduction and osteomyelitis were found to be common. Other contributory factors included lack of prophylactic antibiotics, delay in treatment, presence of teeth in the line of the fracture, alcohol and drug abuse, an inexperienced surgeon and lack of patient compliance.[37] Moreno et al[38] found that the overall complication rate, postoperative infection and postoperative malocclusion were significantly correlated with the severity of the original fracture and similar risk factors were identified by Haug & Schwimmer.[39]

Treatment

Treatment requires debridement of the fracture site and eradication of infection, with accurate reduction and fixation. In the absence of significant bone deficit this treatment should result in successful union. Since infected non-unions present with a mandibular continuity gap, temporary fixation of fragments is desirable to allow resolution of infection prior to bone grafting. Where there is intact overlying mucoperiosteum, this may be achieved by rigid internal fixation. However, in long-standing severe cases, the quality and availability of mucosal cover for the fracture may be poor. If internal fixation is used in these cases, dehiscence of the intraoral wound may occur with resultant plate exposure. In this situation immobilization is best achieved by use of an external fixator (Fig. 24.20). Once infection is eradicated and mucosal healing has occurred, cancellous or corticocancellous bone graft and internal fixation in the form of mesh or plates is carried out usually via an extraoral approach to avoid contamination of the bone graft by intraoral bacteria.

Operative Technique

The fracture site is approached by a standard intraoral or extraoral incision. The fracture is mobilized, bone ends cut back to healthy bleeding bone and segments repositioned with the aid of temporary intraoperative intermaxillary fixation and use of an occlusal wafer for accurate location of the teeth. Where little or no bone gap is present, bone grafts may be unnecessary but in most cases cancellous or corticocancellous bone harvested from the iliac crest will restore mandibular continuity defects and ensure bony union.

Outcome

Outcome is usually good although sensory loss in the region of the inferior dental nerve is common due to inevitable scarring and damage as a result of the original injury, primary treatment and subsequent secondary bone grafting.

Malunion

Malunion may occur in the horizontal or vertical ramus of the mandible.

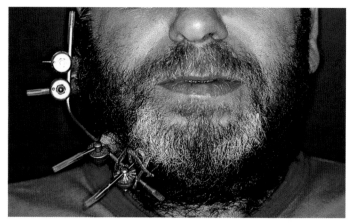

(a)

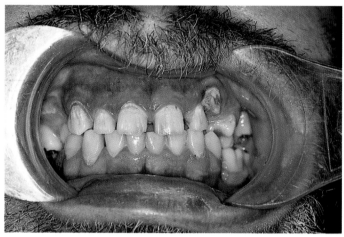

(b)

Fig. 24.20: Infected non-union of fractured mandible. **(a)** External fixator in place. **(b)** Maintenance of occlusion with fixator.

Horizontal ramus

Malunion of a fracture of the horizontal ramus usually requires direct osteotomy to recreate the fracture, mobilization and repositioning of the segments and placement of internal fixation, with the expectation of an excellent outcome.

Background

Angle, ramus and condylar fractures
Malunion of fractures behind the tooth-bearing segment of the mandible result in displacement of the whole dentoalveolar arch. Uncomplicated angle and ramus fractures rarely result in malunion because they are amenable to open reduction with internal fixation. However, mandibular condyle fractures are often treated non-surgically by closed methods of reduction, intermaxillary fixation and elastic traction. Displacement of the mandible and resulting malocclusion may occur for a variety of reasons. Severe condylar malposition with dislocation allows vertical shortening of the ascending ramus and this may be associated with restricted mouth opening or deviation on opening due to mechanical disruption of the temporomandibular joint. The functional status of the temporomandibular joint is an important factor in the choice of technique adopted for correction of the

occlusal deformity. If temporomandibular joint function is significantly compromised, reduction of the dislocation may be necessary, along with disc repositioning. If temporomandibular joint function is acceptable, ramus osteotomy is indicated in order to avoid joint surgery and the possibility of surgically induced limitation of mouth opening. Vertical ramus shortening may also occur following angular displacement of the condylar neck without dislocation if telescoping of the proximal and distal fragments occurs, particularly if the molar teeth are absent and there is lack of posterior occlusal support. It may also be seen following condylar resorption.[39]

In unilateral condylar fractures, malunion results in shortening of the ipsilateral ramus height, transverse cant of the lower occlusal plane, gagging of the occlusion on the ipsilateral posterior molars and contralateral open bite. In addition, there may be posterior displacement of the ipsilateral mandible resulting in obvious chinpoint asymmetry, as well as cross or scissors bite. If bilateral malunion occurs, then both ascending rami shorten, with an increase in mandibular and lower occlusal plane angle, bilateral occlusal gagging on the posterior molars, anterior open bite, with class II jaw relationship and, if severe, lip incompetence (Fig. 24.21).

Unilateral treatment
The aim of treatment in unilateral cases is to restore the pretraumatic ramus height and correct posterior mandibular displacement if present. This corrects the occlusal plane cant and restores a normal occlusion and can be achieved by either performing an osteotomy at the site of the original fracture, repositioning and if necessary interpositional bone grafting to maintain lengthening of the ramus, or by a ramus osteotomy distant from the fracture site, e.g. vertical subsigmoid, inverted L or sagittal split osteotomy. Direct fracture line osteotomy is appropriate where the fracture site involves the angle or ascending ramus. However, if the fracture involves the condylar neck, direct osteotomy and grafting can be difficult and carry significant risk of postoperative trismus or ankylosis. In this situation vertical subsigmoid osteotomy, inverted L or sagittal split osteotomy is indicated where temporomandibular joint function is adequate. Where temporomandibular joint function is compromised, reduction of the condylar fragment and disc repositioning may be necessary despite the surgical difficulty and risk of surgically induced restriction of mouth opening postoperatively.

Where temporomandibular joint surgery or condylar reduction is not necessary, the particular type of osteotomy chosen is governed by the direction and extent of displacement. Rubens et al[40] recommend that when horizontal movement is the primary goal, sagittal split osteotomy is appropriate. Where vertical correction is required, they recommend use of an intra- or extraoral ramus osteotomy. However, they also point out that other factors such as facial scarring, ease of condylar segment manipulation and available bone influence the approach selected.

Bilateral treatment
Bilateral condylar malunion usually results in anterior open bite and class II jaw relationship. This is best treated in the

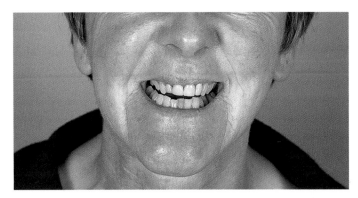

(a)

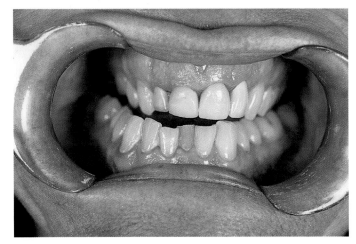

(b)

Fig. 24.21: Bilateral condylar malunion. **(a)** Obvious chinpoint asymmetry. **(b)** Occlusal derangement with open bite.

same way as a developmental high angle class II anterior open bite, utilizing standard orthognathic and if necessary orthodontic techniques. This approach effectively accepts the reduced ramus height and therefore a reduced posterior face height. The correction is achieved by adjusting the maxilla to accommodate this reduced posterior face height by carrying out a posterior maxillary impaction. This results in an increase of the occlusal plane angle, but this is of little significance and will result in a stable correction of the anterior open bite component of the deformity, as a consequence of mandibular autorotation. Mandibular autorotation will also result in a degree of anterior mandibular projection and this may be sufficient to correct the mild class II skeletal relationship. The degree of anterior projection as a result of autorotation may be assessed preoperatively by surgical simulation using an anatomical articulator. If autorotation is insufficient to correct anteroposterior discrepancy, then bilateral sagittal split mandibular advancement is indicated. As in orthognathic cases, in some patients addition of advancement genioplasty may enhance the esthetic result and improve lip competence where needed.

Unilateral operative technique
Access is gained via a posterior intraoral buccal sulcus incision or submandibular, retromandibular (see Fig. 24.22b) or pre-auricular extraoral incisions.

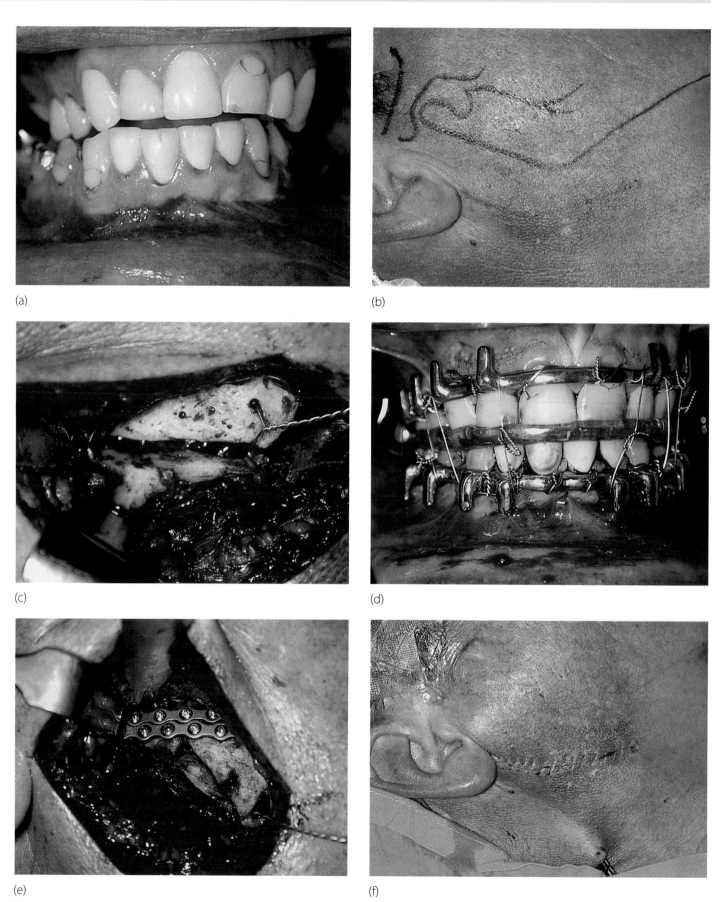

(a)

(b)

(c)

(d)

(e)

(f)

Fig. 24.22: Vertical ramus osteotomy to correct posttraumatic malocclusion. **(a)** Preoperative malocclusion. **(b)** Retromandibular incision marked. **(c)** Vertical ramus osteotomy performed. **(d)** Temporary intermaxillary fixation with occlusal wafer. **(e)** Fixation of osteotomy. **(f)** Wound closure.

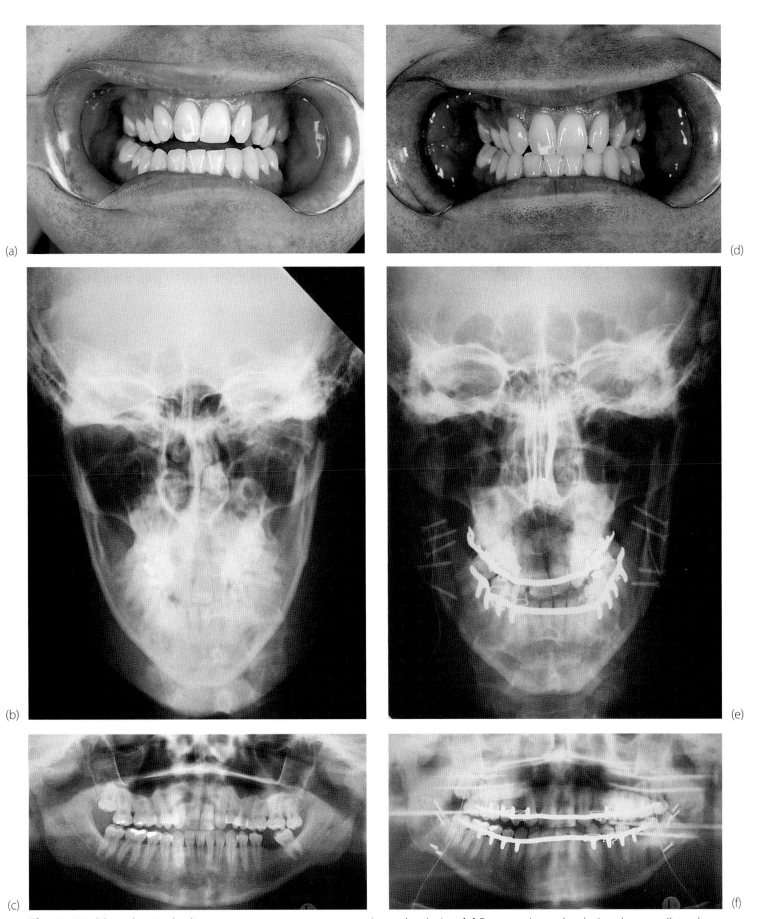

Fig. 24.23: Bilateral sagittal split osteotomy to correct postoperative malocclusion. **(a)** Preoperative malocclusion due to unilateral condylar fracture. **(b)** Preoperative cephalogram. **(c)** Preoperative OPG. **(d)** Postoperative occlusion following osteotomy. **(e)** Postoperative PA cephalogram. **(f)** Postoperative OPG.

Depending on the technique chosen, the old fracture line is osteotomized or a ramus osteotomy carried out distant from the fracture site (see Fig. 24.22c). Once this has been done, temporary, intraoperative intermaxillary fixation with an occlusal wafer is applied (see Fig. 24.22d). Following this, posterior and upward traction on the proximal fragment will keep the condyle in its retruded position. The condyle may be located outside the confines of the glenoid fossa if dislocated. In this situation, intraoperative judgment of the correct condylar position is a little more difficult but the surgeon should err on the side of overcorrection if doubt exists. This maneuver will reveal the extent of the ramus height deficit. If direct fracture osteotomy or inverted L osteotomy has been carried out, a suitably sized bone graft is inserted into the osteotomy gap and internal fixation applied. If vertical ramus osteotomy or sagittal split has been carried out, no bone graft is necessary and having repositioned the proximal segment, fixation is applied (see Fig. 24.22e). In some cases of unilateral injury, a contralateral sagittal split osteotomy may be required in order to achieve the preplanned occlusion. This can be assessed preoperatively using an anatomical articulator and intraoperatively, when the occlusion can be assessed following osteotomy on the injured side. If a satisfactory occlusion is achieved, contralateral osteotomy may be unnecessary. If satisfactory occlusion cannot be achieved contralateral osteotomy must be carried out (Fig. 24.23).

Bilateral operative technique

Posterior maxillary impaction, mandibular autorotation and advancement are well described in the orthognathic literature and the use of these techniques in a posttraumatic situation usually demands little or no modification (Figs 24.24).

Outcome

The techniques described are effective in correcting the esthetic and functional problems associated with posttraumatic malocclusion. In a study of 21 patients, Becking et al[41] reported stable dental and cephalometric results in 20 patients. Similarly, Spitzer et al[42] reported occlusal correction and normal mandibular movement in a group of 14 patients. Rubens et al[40] presented four cases with successful outcome, including correction of occlusion and resolution of temporomandibular joint and muscle pain.

Traumatic tissue loss

Severe posttraumatic tissue loss is uncommon in civilian practice. It may occasionally be encountered following gunshot wounds, high-speed road traffic accidents or industrial accidents. Often there is a combination of hard and soft tissue loss demanding a variety of primary and secondary reconstructive techniques with multiple operations in order to restore lost form and function. Initial management usually follows traditional principles of trauma management and subsequent correction may involve pedicle or free tissue transfer to replace hard and soft tissue. The recent development of osteogenic distraction in the craniofacial skeleton gives another option for replacement of bony deficits along with their closely associated soft tissues. Each case will be different and must be planned and treated on its own merits, but Figure 24.25 shows a case which illustrates many of the principles and problems involved in these patients.

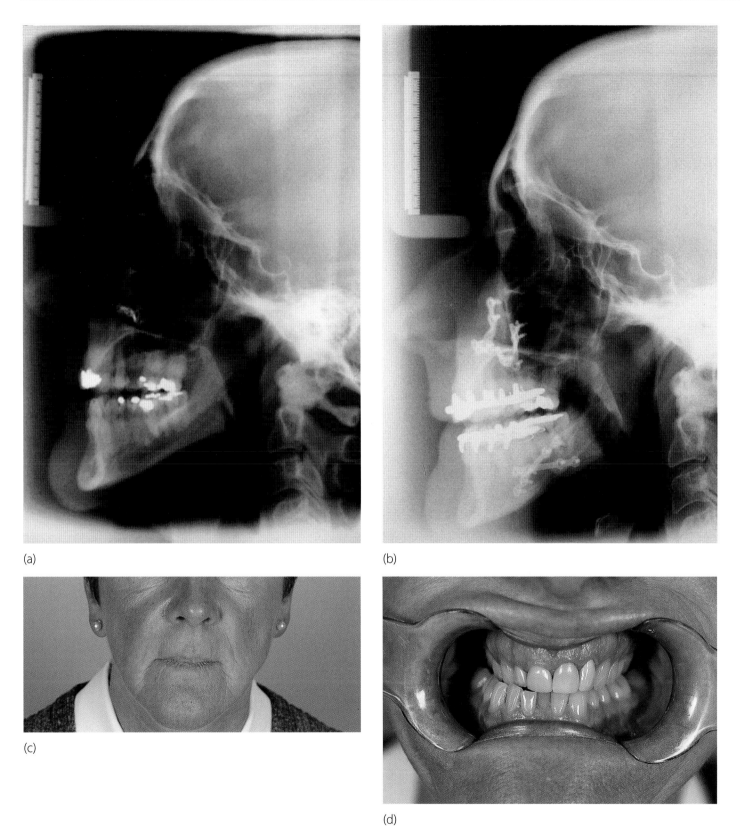

(a)

(b)

(c)

(d)

Fig. 24.24: Bimaxillary osteotomy to treat anterior open bite and mandibular asymmetry following bilateral condylar fracture. See Fig. 24.21 for preoperative clinical appearance. **(a,b)** Pre and postoperative lateral cephalograms. **(c,d)** Postoperative facial appearance and occlusion.

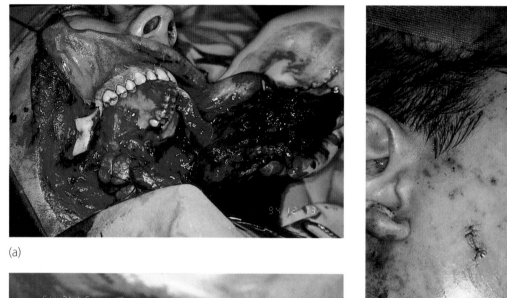

(a)

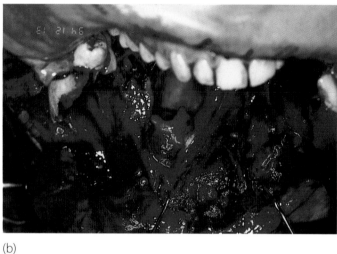

(b)

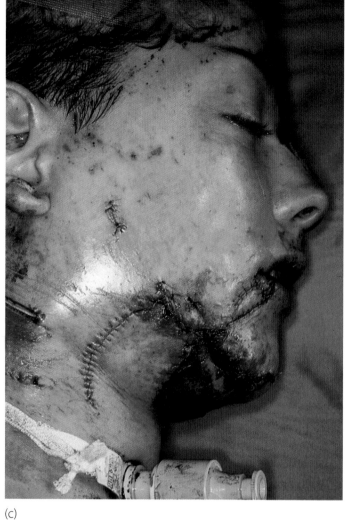

(c)

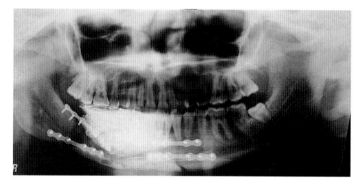

(d)

Fig. 24.25: Road traffic accident with severe lower third facial injury involving bilateral mandibular fracture, severe soft tissue disruption and complete traumatic glossectomy. **(a,b)** Appearance on presentation. **(c)** Tracheotomy, plating of fracture and soft tissue repair, defect in floor of mouth dressed with Whitehead varnish pack. **(d)** OPG showing mandibular fixation.

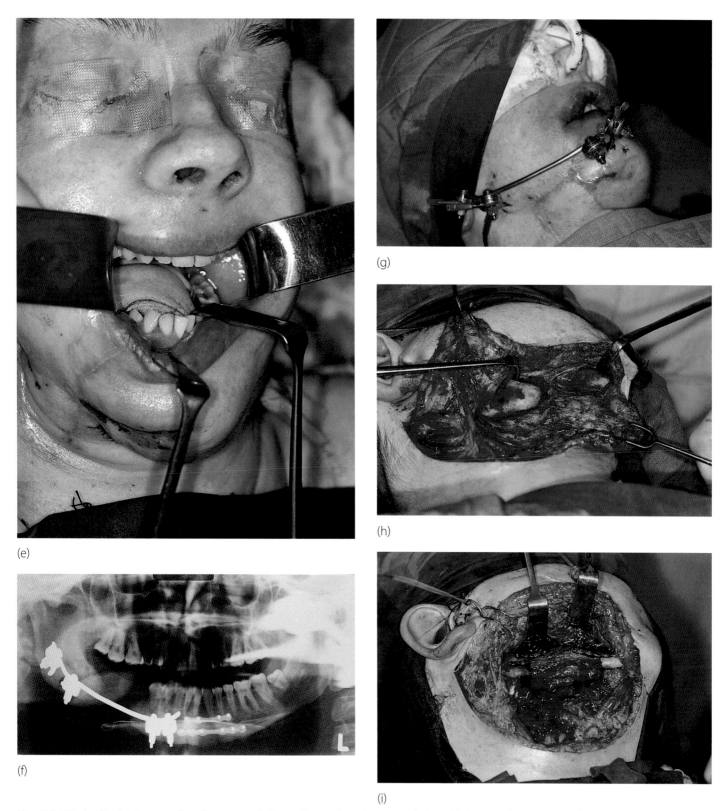

Fig. 24.25: **(e)** Radial forearm free flap to repair floor of mouth and tongue defect. **(f,g)** Avascular necrosis of right mandibular body treated by removal of fixation, debridement and application of external fixator. **(h)** Mandibular defect following non-union. **(i)** Reconstruction with DCIA free vascularized bone flap.

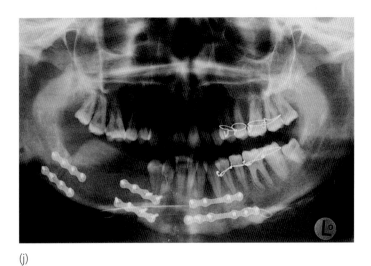

(j)

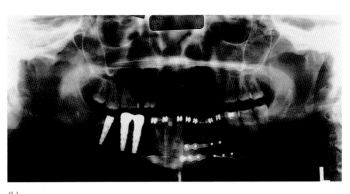

(k)

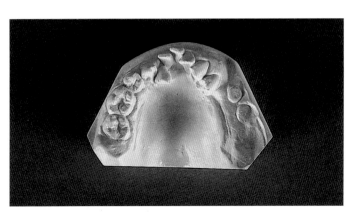

(l)

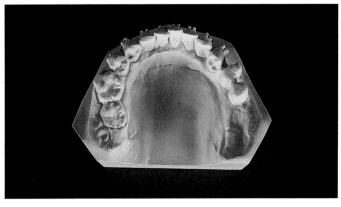

(m)

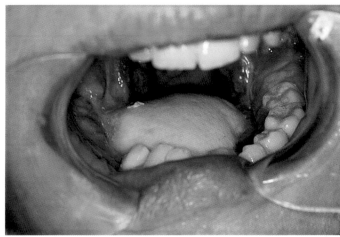

(n)

(o)

Fig. 24.25: (j) OPG showing mandibular reconstruction.
(k) Endosseous implants placed into DCIA bone graft (Courtesy Mr J I Cawood). **(l)** Lingual movement of lower incisors due to lip pressure following loss of tongue. **(m)** Appearance following orthodontic treatment using implants as anchorage (Courtesy of Mr S J Rudge and Mr S Chadwick). **(n)** Intraoral appearance of radial forearm flap. **(o)** Facial appearance at commencement of orthodontic treatment.

References

1 Cohen SR, Kawamoto HK 1992 Analysis and results of treatment of established post traumatic facial deformities. Plastic and Reconstructive Surgery 90(4): 574–584

2 Tessier P 1971 Total osteotomy of the middle third of the face for faciostenosis or for sequelae of Le Fort III fractures. Plastic and Reconstructive Surgery 48: 533

3 Manson PN 1990 Facial injuries. In: McCarthy JG (ed) Plastic surgery. WB Saunders, Philadelphia, pp 867–1141

4 Gruss JS 1982 Frontonaso-orbital trauma. Clinics in Plastic Surgery 9: 557

5 Schendel SA, Lewis W, Williamson DDS 1983 Muscle reorientation following superior repositioning of the maxilla. Journal of Oral and Maxillofacial Surgery 41: 235–240

6 Shvykov MB, Shamsudinov AK, Sunarckov DD, Shvyrkova II 1999 Non-free osteoplasty of the mandible in maxillofacial gunshot wounds; reconstruction by compression-osteodistraction. British Journal of Oral and Maxillofacial Surgery 37(4): 261–267

7 McCarthy J, Zide BM 1984 The spectrum of calvarial bone grafting: introduction of the vascularised calvarial bone flap. Plastic and Reconstructive Surgery 74: 10

8 Berggren A, Weiland AJ, Dorfman M 1982 Free vascularized bone grafts: factors affecting their survival and ability to lead recipient bone defects. Plastic and Reconstructive Surgery 69: 19

9 Paskest JP, Yaremchuk MJ, Randolph MA et al 1987 Prolonging survival in vascularised bone allograft transplantation: developing specific immune unresponsiveness. Journal of Reconstructive Microsurgery 3: 254

10 Zins JE, Whitaker LA 1983 Membranous versus endochondral bone autografts: implications for craniofacial reconstruction. Plastic and Reconstructive Surgery 72(6): 778–785

11 Yaremchuk MJ 1989 Vascularised bone grafts for maxillofacial reconstruction. Clinics in Plastic Surgery 16(1): 29–39

12 McCarthy JG, Cutting CC, Shaw WW 1987 Vascularised calvarial flap. Clinical Plastic Surgery 14(1): 37–47

13 Zalzal GH, Cotton RT, James McAdams AMD 1986 Cartilage grafts – present status. Head and Neck Surgery 8(5): 363–374

14 Yen CP, Cheung CM, Loh JK, Jong YJ, Howng SL 1999 Growing skull fracture. Kaohsiung Journal of Medical Sciences 15(3): 175–181

15 Colak A, Akbasak A, Biliciler B, Erten SF. Kocak A 1998 An unusual variant of a growing skull fracture in an adolescent. Paediatric Neurosurgery 29(1): 36–39

16 Gupta SK, Reddy NM, Khosla VK et al Growing skull fractures: a clinical study of 41 patients. Acta Neurochirurgica 139(10): 928–932

17 Sener RN 1995 Growing skull fracture in a patient with cerebral hemiatrophy. Paediatric Radiology 25(1): 64–65

18 Scarfo GB, Mariottini A, Tomaccini D, Palma L 1989 Growing skull fractures. Child's Nervous System 5(3): 163–167

19 Hunter PD, Pelofsky S 1995 Classification of autogenous skull grafts in cranial reconstruction. Journal of Craniomaxillofacial Trauma 1(14): 8–15

20 Hunter D, Baker S, Sobol SM 1990 Split calvarial grafts in maxillofacial reconstruction. Otolaryngology Head and Neck Surgery 102(4): 345–350

21 Posnick JC, Goldstein JA, Armstong D, Rutka JT 1993 Reconstruction of skull defects in children and adolescents by the use of fixed cranial bone grafts: long-term results. Neurosurgery 32(5): 785–791; discussion 791

22 Pezzota S, Silvani V, Gaetani P, Spanu G, Rondini G 1985 Growing skull fractures of childhood. Journal of Neurosurgical Sciences 29(2): 129–135

23 Ionnides Ch, Freihofer HP, Friens J 1993 Fractures of the frontal sinus: a rationale of treatment. British Journal of Plastic Surgery 46: 208–214

24 Luce EA 1987 Frontal sinus fractures: guidelines to management. Plastic and Reconstructive Surgery 80(4): 500–510

25 Gonty AA, Marciani RD, Adornato DC 1999 Management of frontal sinus fractures: a review of 33 cases. Journal of Oral Maxillofacial Surgery 57(4): 372–379; discussion 380–381

26 Penfold CN, Lang DD, Evans B 1992 The management of orbital roof fractures. British Journal of Oral Maxillofacial Surgery 30: 97–103

27 Horowitz JH, Persing JA, Winn HR, Edgerton MT 1984 The late treatment of vertical orbital dystopia resulting from an orbital roof fracture. Annals of Plastic Surgery 13(6): 519–524

28 Hammer B, Prein J 1995 Correction of post traumatic orbital deformities: operative techniques and review of 26 patients. Journal of Craniomaxillofacial Surgery 23: 81–90

29 Barone CM, Gigantelli JW 1998 Endoscopic repair of posttraumatic enophthalmos using medial transconjunctival approach: a case report. Journal of Craniomaxillofacial Trauma 4(1): 22–26

30 Watzinger F, Wanschitz F, Wagner A et al 1997 Computer-aided navigation in secondary reconstruction of post traumatic deformities of the zygoma. Journal of Craniomaxillofacial Surgery 25(4): 198–202

31 Jones RH, Ching M 1995 Intraoral zygomatic osteotomy for correction of malar deficiency. Journal of Oral Maxillofacial Surgery 53(4): 483–485

32 Frodel JL, Marentette LJ, Quatela VC et al 1993 Calvarial bone graft harvest – techniques, considerations and morbidity. Archives of Otolaryngology Head and Neck Surgery 119(1): 17–23

33 Freihofer PM, Borstlap WA 1989 Reconstruction of zygomatic area. A comparison between osteotomy and onlay techniques. Journal of Craniomaxillofacial Surgery 17 (6): 243–248

34 Perino KE, Zide MF, Kinnebrew MC 1984 Late treatment of malunited malar fractures. Journal of Oral and Maxillofacial Surgery 42(1): 20–34

35 Hans PM, Freihofer P 1995 Effectiveness of secondary post-traumatic periorbital reconstruction. Journal of Oral and Maxillofacial Surgery 23: 143–150

36 Ellis E 3rd 1999 Treatment methods for fractures of the mandibular angle. International Journal of Oral and Maxillofacial Surgery 28(4): 243–252

37 Mathog RH, Toma V, Clayman L, Wolf S 2000 Nonunion of the mandible: an analysis of contributing factors. Journal of Oral and Maxillofacial Surgery 58(7): 746–752; discussion 752–753

38 Moreno JC, Fernadez A, Ortiz JA, Montalvo JJ 2000 Complication rates associated with different treatment for mandibular fractures. Journal of Oral and Maxillofacial Surgery 58(3): 273–280; discussion 280–281

39 Haug RH, Schwimmer A 1994 Fibrous union of the mandible: a review of 27 patients. Journal of Oral and Maxillofacial Surgery 52(8): 832–839

40 Rubens BC, Stoelinga PJW, Weaver TJ, Biijdorp PA 1990 Management of malunited mandibular condylar fractures. International Journal of Oral and Maxillofacial Surgery 19: 22–25

41 Becking AG, Zijerveld SA, Tuinzing DB 1998 Management of post traumatic malocclusion caused by condylar process source. Journal of Oral and Maxillofacial Surgery 56(12): 1370–1374; discussion 1374–1375

42 Spitzer WJ, Vanderborght G, Dumbach J 1997 Surgical management of mandibular malposition after malunited condylar fractures in adults. Journal of Craniomaxillofacial Surgery 25(2): 91–96

25 Distraction Techniques

Alexander C Kübler, Joachim E Zöller

History of Distraction

The first clinical application of bone distraction was described in 1905 by Codivilla who performed a bone distraction of the lower leg.[1] This distractor was fixed via a plaster at the upper and lower leg, providing only minor stability, and severe soft tissue problems like necrosis occurred. Thereafter various experimental studies followed regarding the rate and distance of distraction as well as the effect of the periosteum and the soft tissue on the distraction process. In 1927 Rosenthal reported the first distraction of the mandible.[2] He treated a patient with a mandibular retrognathism by bone distraction and fixation of the distractor along the teeth. In 1952 Anderson et al described the first use of cortical bone pins for the fixation of the distractor.[3] This was a milestone in the technique of bone distraction as it enabled rigid fixation of the bone fragments.

The real 'father of bone distraction' was a Russian orthopedic surgeon named Ilizarov who popularized the technique more than 30 years before it became known in the West. In the late 1980s he published in America for the first time his research and clinical results on bone distraction, causing a wave of developments in bone distraction techniques worldwide.[4]

Principle of bone distraction

The aim of bone distraction is to obtain new bone tissue and gain bone length by slow distraction of the callus. Moreover, the basic principle of bone distraction is the process of bone fracture healing. There are two different methods of performing the osteotomy. In the original method, described by Ilizarov, a corticotomy is performed in which only the cortex of the bone is separated and the cancellous stays untouched. Another method, which is more often used in head and neck surgery, is to split both the cortex and the cancellous of the bone in order to facilitate the process of distraction. By using this technique, the forces needed to distract the bone are significantly lower, allowing use of smaller distractors which can be placed under the skin or the mucosa.

After the osteotomy and a latent period of about 5–7 days, the bones at both sides of the osteotomy line are slowly pulled apart in order to stretch the fracture cleft and the newly formed callus.[5,6] A latent period between the osteotomy and the start of the distraction process allows callus formation and soft tissue healing. Also a higher activity of the osteoblasts and blood vessel growth within the osteotomy line and the callus can be achieved.[7] Various

experimental and clinical studies have reported a latent period ranging from 0 to 14 days between the osteotomy and the start of the distraction, depending on the individual situation.[7] In the field of head and neck surgery an average waiting period of about 5–7 days seems to be advisable. However, patient age, bone size or soft tissue coverage may change the latent period.

The process of distraction has to take place slowly in order to achieve new bone formation within the callus. An average distraction rate of about 1–1.5 mm per day provides the best clinical results.[6] At a lower rate of 0.5 mm per day or less, an early ossification process will take place whereas at a higher rate of 2 mm per day or more, no bone formation will occur.[8] Another important fact is the frequency of distraction. The ideal situation is a continuous distraction of callus[6] but as this is rather difficult, repeated distraction once or twice a day seems to be useful, totalling 1–1.5 mm per day.

Numerous experimental and clinical studies have investigated the effect of bone distraction and the progress of bone formation during distraction. It has been shown that the gap between the distracted bone edges is first occupied by fibrous tissue.[9] As distraction proceeds, the fibrous tissue becomes longitudinally oriented in the direction of distraction. Early bone formation advances along the fibrous tissue, starting from the cut bone edges. Bone is formed predominantly by intermembranous ossification.[10,11] Histological observations showed a gradual change from an amorphous matrix to a fibrous matrix and, finally, an osseous like tissue.[10] Bone columns crystallize along longitudinally oriented collagen bundles, expanding circumferentially to surrounding bundles.[11] While the distraction gap increases, the bone columns increase in length and in diameter, while the fibrous interzone remains constant at a few millimeters.[6] Data from animal experiments as well as clinical data have shown that distraction osteogenesis provides unlimited new bone formation that remodels at a daily rate ranging from 200 to 400 microns.[8,11]

Most of these experimental data were obtained from orthopedic studies, therefore only limited detailed information for indications in maxillofacial surgery is available.

Various methods are described for fixation of the distractor.[12] The easiest way of fixation is to use bone pins which are placed in the bone near the osteotomy line and through the skin. The pins are fixed externally to the distractor which can be slowly expanded. These external distractors are easy to fix and very stable but most of them are rather bulky and the transcutaneous pins may cause scars.[11] These factors encouraged the development of smaller devices which can be placed intraorally. Today mini- or microdistractors are used which are small enough to be placed completely subcutaneously or under the mucosa. Only the screw for the activator of the distractor is visible.

Another distractor for the midface is the halo frame.[13] This frame is fixed at the skull by screws and attached to the midface.

A very important aspect of all distractors is their stability and stiffness. It has been shown in experimental studies that mobility during the process of distraction will cause micro-movements, resulting in impaired bone formation.[8] Therefore distractor size is limited by physical stability and rigidity.

After reaching the intended bone length, the distractor (or plate fixation) has to stay in place for many weeks until mineralization and ossification of the newly formed callus has been completed and a sufficient bone strength has been reached.[14] Again, the length of this period depends on various individual factors like the location of the osteotomy, the bone length gained and the age of the patient.[15,16] A retention period of 8–12 weeks seems to be sufficient for the facial skeleton. Some surgeons remove the distractor and use plates to provide stabilization for the consolidation period.

Timetable for bone distraction

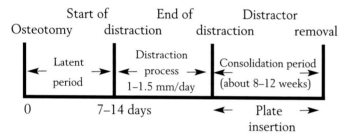

Indications and Techniques for Bone Distraction

At first congenital malformations of the mandible were the most frequent indications. McCarthy first described the use of a miniaturized distractor as an extraoral device to lengthen the malformed mandible.[17] Soon smaller distractors were developed which were placed completely intraorally in order to avoid scars and hide the distractors. Today the distraction of the mandible can be classified as distraction of the horizontal mandible ramus, the vertical mandible ramus, the mandible symphysis and the distraction of the alveolus.

Horizontal or vertical distraction of the ramus, or angle of the mandible

Malformations of growth of the ramus horizontally or vertically are the most frequent indications for distraction in head and neck surgery. In less severe orthognathic surgery cases, unilateral or bilateral sagittal split can be performed followed by bone distraction until the intended occlusion is reached.[18,19] By osteotomies of the cortex alone, the risk of nerve injury is less likely. It may also have a role after severe trauma.

Other special indications are young children with a congenital, traumatic or infection-induced hypoplasia of the mandible (Figs 25.1–25.3) which can impair airway. By distraction of the mandible, the space for soft tissues like the tongue and the floor of the mouth increases, improving air flow.[20] This indication can avoid a permanent tracheotomy and can be applied from the age of 6 months when ossification of the mandible allows fixation of the distractor.

Which part of the mandible has to be distracted depends on the location of bone growth deficit.[21] As some distractors have only one vector of distraction, the bone will be advanced in one direction, and the position of the distractor is critical for the final clinical result. The placement of the distractor parallel to the occlusal plane, will result in a horizontal mandibular advancement. If the distractor is placed at an angle to the occlusion plane, the result will be a mandibular advancement and a tendency for an open bite. Finally if the distractor is set vertically in relation to the occlusion plane, a mal-occlusion of the molars will result. Therefore the position and the angle between the distractor and the occlusal plane have to be determined carefully preoperatively by a cephalometric analysis and/or by model surgery. In some cases a bilateral osteotomy and distraction may be necessary.

The operation is usually performed under general anesthesia. After local disinfection and injection of a vasoconstrictor, the mucosa is opened and the mandible is exposed subpe-

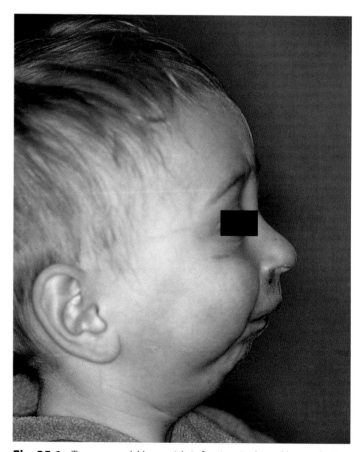

Fig. 25.1: Two-year-old boy with infection-induced hypoplasia (osteomyelitis) of the mandible with severe breathing problems prior to distraction of the mandible.

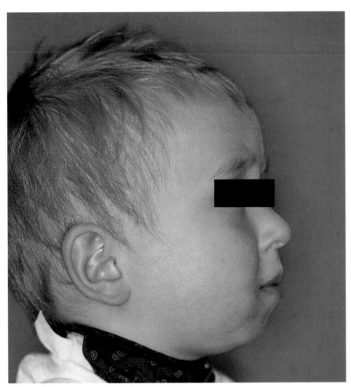

Fig. 25.2: Three months after distraction of the mandible on both sides near the mandibular angle for about 15 mm. Breathing problems disappeared completely.

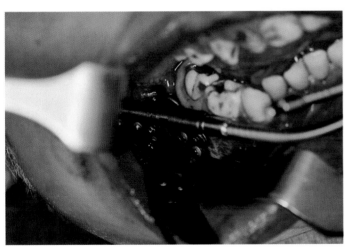

Fig. 25.3: Intraoperative view at the osteotomy line and the placement of the distractor near the mandibular angle on one side.

riosteally. Then the distractor is placed at the intended position and fixed temporarily with two monocortical screws. The osteotomy line is marked on the buccal side of the mandible using a drill. The distractor and the screws are removed and the osteotomy is performed. The lingual side of the osteotomy is achieved very carefully in order to prevent exposure of the lingual periosteum as this is important for the blood supply. The osteotomy is mobilized and the distractor is fixed using the holes drilled earlier and the remaining screws. Finally the soft tissue is closed so that the thread of

the distractor is visible and can easily be reached by the patient. After a waiting period of about 5–7 days, the distraction can be started at a rate of 0.5 mm twice per day until the intended mandible length is obtained. The retention period lasts about 12 weeks before the distractor can be removed under local or general anesthesia. Some surgeons replace the distractor with plates to complement the consolidation period.

Distraction of the mandible symphasis

In patients with a congenital or a trauma-induced narrow mandible (e.g. after mandible fracture), surgical widening might be necessary (Figs 25.4–25.6). Vertical osteotomy of the mandible between the incisors followed by horizontal distraction will result in a significant increase in width. Due to the principle of distraction, the condyles will be rotated but this causes no permanent problems.

Under general anesthesia the vestibular mucosa between the canines is opened and the mandible exposed. The distractor is temporarily placed using two monocortical screws. It is important that the upper arms of the distractor are placed anteriorly to the teeth. Therefore only the lower arms of the distractor are fixed at the bone using monocortical screws. Then the osteotomy line is marked using a drill and the distractor removed. Thereafter the mandible is separated between the two first incisors. The lingual periosteum is not exposed as the depth of the cut can be felt with the finger. After mobilization of the fragments the distractor is fixed using screws for the lower arms. The upper arms of the distractor are fixed at the teeth using wires or dental composite.

The dental anchorage of the upper arms of the distractor is important in order to avoid twisting of the segments; by fixing both arms of the distractor at the bone, an uncontrolled rotation of both sides of the mandible may occur. The mucosa is closed and the distraction can start at a rate of 0.5 mm twice per day after a waiting period of about 1 week. Again, a retention period of 12 weeks for mineralization and ossification of the newly formed callus has to be observed.

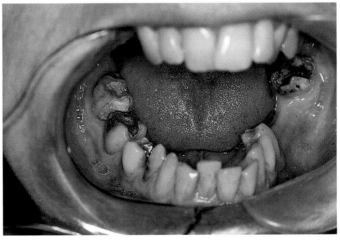

Fig. 25.4: Forty-year-old patient with a narrow mandible prior to distraction.

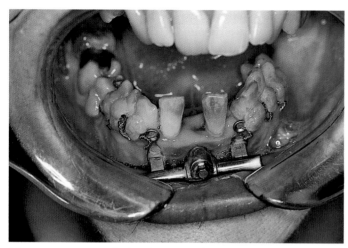

Fig. 25.5: One week after the start of the distraction process. Separation of the incisors becomes obvious.

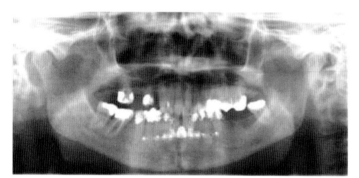

Fig. 25.6: X-ray during distraction.

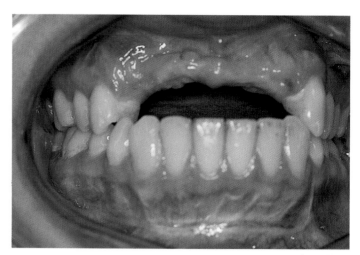

Fig. 25.7: Twenty five-year-old patient with traumatic loss of the upper incisors and a significant lack of vertical height of the alveolar ridge prior to therapy.

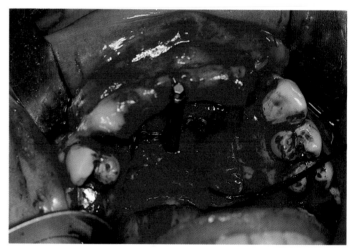

Fig. 25.8: Intraoperative view at the placement of the distractor for vertical distraction of the alveolar ridge.

Vertical distraction of the alveolar ridge

Since the development of mini- and microdistractors, vertical distraction of the alveolar ridge of the mandible and maxilla has become very popular[22] (Figs 25.7–25.16). There are a wide range of indications[23] for this technique which can be used in edentulous parts of the mandible after segmental resection in tumor surgery or following trauma, instead of bone transplantation. Also, patients who lose their teeth due to periodontal diseases or those with badly fitting dentures often suffer from reduced bone volume. In these cases vertical distraction of the alveolar ridge can improve the bone volume to enable the placement of dental implants or to provide a prosthesis. A residual mandible height of at least 7 mm is necessary in order to enable horizontal splitting and rigid fixation of the distractor.

The osteotomy and placement of the distractor can be carried out under general anesthesia and smaller segments under local anesthesia. The mucosa is opened on the buccal side and the alveolar ridge is exposed. First the distractor is placed and fixed temporarily using two monocortical screws. Then the osteotomy line is marked using a drill and the distractor is removed. The osteotomy is carried out using a drill or a small saw, ensuring the lingual mucosa and periosteum are not injured. After osteotomy the segmented cranial

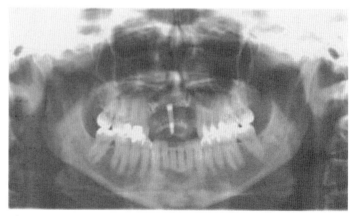

Fig. 25.9: X-ray during distraction.

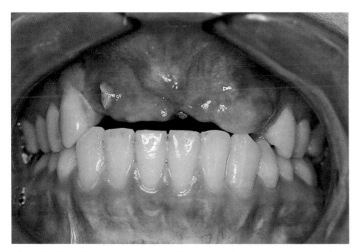

Fig. 25.10: Clinical situation with the newly gained height of the alveolar ridge following vertical distraction during the process of retention.

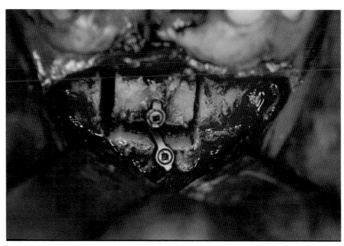

Fig. 25.13: Intraoperative view during placement of the distractor (implant distractor).

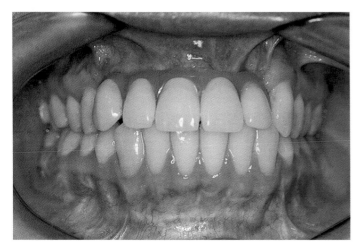

Fig. 25.11: Clinical situation after insertion of dental implants and prosthetic rehabilitation.

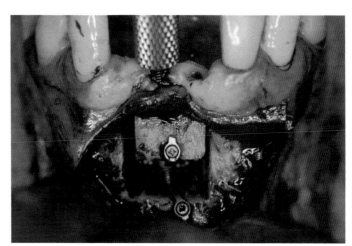

Fig. 25.14: Intraoperative view; the bone segment is temporarily distracted for testing.

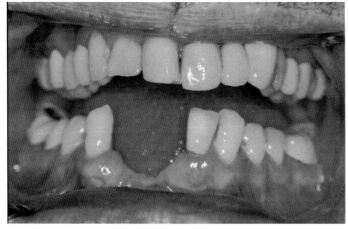

Fig. 25.12: Thirty two-year-old man with traumatic loss of the lower front teeth. (Courtesy of University Clinic, Freiburg).

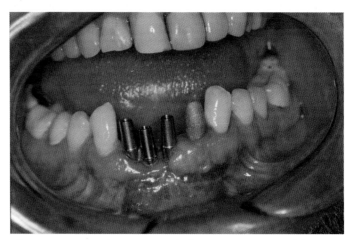

Fig. 25.15: After distraction and after the placement of three implants.

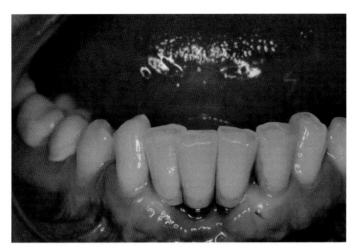

Fig. 25.16: Clinical situation after distraction and prosthetic rehabilitation with implant of single crowns.

part of the bone segment of the mandible is mobilized. The survival of this segment depends on the preservation of the lingual mucoperiosteal flap. The distractor can then be attached by screws and the bony segment is stabilized for 7 days. Again the distraction is performed at a rate 0.5 mm twice every day. Within 15 days a vertical increase of 15 mm can be obtained. After reaching the required bone height, the thread of the distractor can be removed for patient comfort using a drill. The distractor stays in place for another 10–12 weeks. Four weeks after the end of the distraction process, there is mineralization of the new bone and reunion of the transported bone in the alveolar ridge. Early mineralization studies suggest that insertion of dental implants is possible after 3 months at the time of removal of the distractor under local anesthesia.

In tooth-bearing areas of the mandible or maxilla, vertical distraction of the alveolar ridge to transport tooth-bearing segments is possible. This may be indicated in patients with an open bite, with vertical deficiencies of the alveolar ridge caused by ankylosed teeth or for orthopedic reasons. The principle of distraction is similar for edentelous regions of the alveolar ridge and can be performed under local or general anesthesia. Via a vestibular approach, the distractor is placed and the osteotomy lines are marked. After removal of the distractor the segment is osteotomized using a small saw or a Lindemann burr. Again the lingual mucoperiosteum ensures vitalization of the tooth-bearing segment and wound healing. The lingual cortex must be separated using a small chisel. After mobilization of the tooth-bearing segment, the distractor is fixed and the wounds are closed. The schedule for distraction is the same as for edentelous segments. If necessary, the distractor can be removed after 4 weeks. In order to prevent a relapse of the segment, a bracket stabilization of the distracted segment to the neighboring teeth with an orthopedic wire is advisable for another 4–8 weeks. During distraction, the vitality of the mobilized teeth remains intact and no damage to neighboring teeth appears. There are few limitations to the size of the distracted segment. If necessary, several teeth can be distracted simultaneously within one segment.

Bone transportation distraction technique of the mandible

This technique of bone distraction was first described by Ilizarov in 1988.[3] In patients with a traumatic or operative defect of the continuity of the mandible, this horizontal distraction technique can be used in order to regain bone contact. The principle of this technique is based on bone distraction but due to technical problems this is still rather experimental.[24,25]

Under general anesthesia both ends of the mandible near the continuity defect are exposed. A distractor is placed between the two ends and a 1.5–2 cm wide section of the mandible is split off near the defect using a saw. Subsequently this piece of bone is slowly moved from one end of the mandible defect to the other end until bone contact is obtained. Therefore both ends of the mandible as well as the separated piece of mandibular bone have to be fixed by a distractor which enables movement of this part. By moving this separated segment of bone according to the principles of bone distraction with regard to waiting periods and distraction speed, new mandible bone can be gained and the defect can be closed by obtaining a new mandibular continuity. This technique has also been successful after radiotherapy of the mandible. Importantly, it also 'transports' good quality attached mucosa.

Distraction of the maxilla arc

The principle of opening the palatal suture by surgery followed by orthopedic expansion of the maxilla was described in 1961 by Haas.[26] There are various surgical techniques described, focusing on the surgical weakening of the maxilla suture.[27]

The procedure should be performed under general anesthesia but local anesthesia is possible. The maxilla suture is exposed by an incision through the mucosa from the back of the hard palate up to the canalis incisivus (Fig. 25.17). The suture is separated by using a small drill from the back of the hard palate up to the incisive canal. Usually there is no need to open the suture anterior to the incisive canal. If the suture will not split a small vestibular incision above the incisors followed by separation of the suture with a small chisel is necessary. Weakening the zygomatic buttress by using a drill is advisable (Fig. 25.18). For expansion of the suture an orthopedic device is used, which is individually manufactured and anchored at the teeth (Figs 25.19, 25.20). The distraction rate is 0.5 mm twice every day. A retention of about 10 weeks has to be followed in order to prevent a relapse. Orthopedic treatment can be continued 4 weeks later.

Distraction of the midface

The main reasons for distraction of the midface are congenital growth disorders but also posttraumatic situations with insufficient primary osteosynthesis or wrong bone or midface placement. Midface distraction is undertaken for cosmetic motives as well as functional reasons like restricted air flow, malocclusion or visual problems.

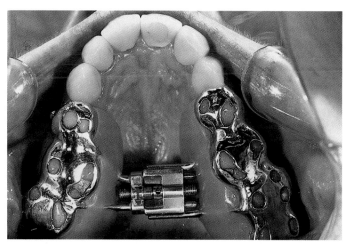

Fig. 25.17: Twenty two-year-old patient with a narrow maxillary arc. Intraoperative view to the maxilla. The maxilla suture is exposed and separated.

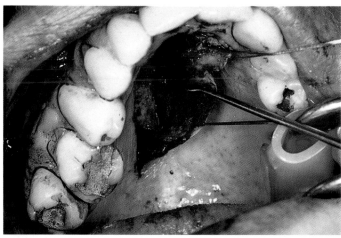

Fig. 25.18: Intraoperative view to the crista zygomaticus. The crista is exposed and separated for distraction of the maxilla arc.

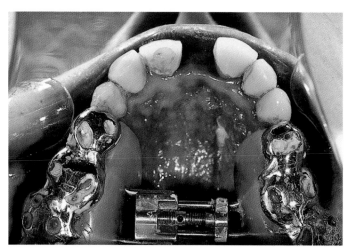

Fig. 25.19: Clinical situation after the separation of the suture with the distraction device in place, before the start of the distraction.

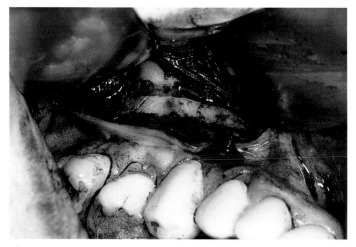

Fig. 25.20: Clinical situation after distraction of the maxilla arc. The incisors are separated.

Distraction of the midface can be classified by the lines of osteotomy and can be performed at the Le Fort I, II or III level depending on the indications. Also the zygoma can be distracted separately.

For distraction at the Le Fort I level, an external distraction device, the halo frame, is mainly used[28,29] (Fig. 25.21). A conventional Le Fort I osteotomy is performed first under general anesthesia using a vestibular approach. After osteotomy, the maxilla is distracted using a dental anchored device which is fixed to the skull via the halo frame. There are also intraoral distractors available but those are difficult to place and the determination of the distraction vector is rather difficult and cannot be altered after the operation. In comparison, using a halo frame, the direction and the vector of distraction can be altered during the process of distraction in order to obtain a perfect occlusion. An average distraction speed of about 1–2 mm per day is advisable.

After completing the distraction process a retention period of about 8 weeks has to be observed after which the halo frame can be removed under local anesthesia however in cleft patients, longer stabilization is needed. This has to be followed by treatment with an orthodontic device which maintains the occlusion for another 2 months.

For the Le Fort II and III levels, external distraction using the halo frame seems to be the most effective modality[28,29] (Figs 25.22, 25.23). Osteotomy of the midface is carried out under general anesthesia using a bicoronal approach and standardized operation techniques. After osteotomy and mobilization of the midface within the Le Fort II or III level, two wires are fixed at the inferior orbital rims. One of the wires has to be fixed at the center of the lower orbital brim and the other is fixed near the nose towards the center of the midface. The wires are pulled through a hole at the orbital rim, directed through the skin by a small incision and fixed to the halo frame which is located in front of the face.

After a waiting period of about 5 days, distraction starts by pulling the wires at a rate of 1–2 mm per day. During the process of distraction the direction of advancement and the distraction vector can be adjusted according to the intended position of the midface and the dental occlusion.

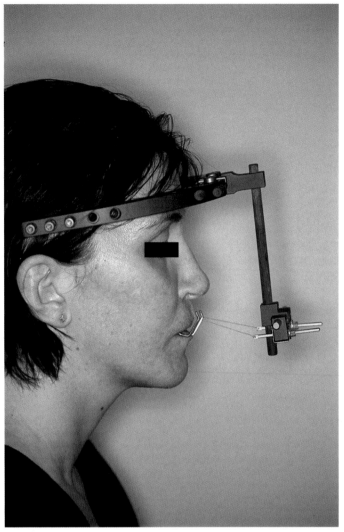

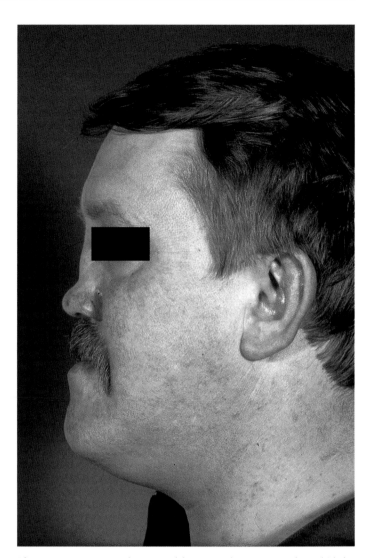

Fig. 25.21: Twenty eight-year-old patient with trauma-induced posterior position of the maxilla during the process of distraction on the Le Fort I level. The halo frame is fixed to the skull and the dental anchored device is attached to the maxillary teeth.

Fig. 25.22: Forty eight-year-old man with trauma-induced 'dish face'.

For distraction of the Le Fort III level subcutaneous distractors fixed at the zygoma do not offer the possibility to change the direction of advancement and the distraction vector[30,31] (Fig. 25.24). Furthermore, these distractors have to be removed under general anesthesia.

By following the rules of distraction a midface advancement of up to 3 cm can be obtained if necessary. After achieving the final position of the midface a retention period of 8 weeks has to be observed after which the halo frame can be removed under local anesthesia. This has to be followed by treatment with an orthopedic device which maintains the obtained occlusion for another 2–3 months.

Distraction of the skull sutures

There are also techniques described for distraction of the skull sutures[32,33] but these are mainly experimental and seldom used in clinical practice. Currently surgical widening is still the technique of choice.

Preoperative Planning

Each distraction treatment requires a careful preoperative planning. Besides clinical examination a two-dimensional X-ray is a basic requirement. If feasible, CT with three-dimensional reconstruction offers the best option for a successful planning and distraction treatment. Here the osteotomy lines as well as the placement of the distractor can be planned and simulated. There are also software programs available which enable the surgeon to plan and simulate the movement of the bone under the distraction procedure. The location of the osteotomy lines and the direction of distractor placement determine the direction of the distraction vector and bone movement. With the exception of the halo frame, the direction of distraction cannot be changed after placement of the distractor and the end of the operation. Care must be taken to avoid compound fractures, nerve damage, or ischemic necrosis. Furthermore vertical distraction of the mandible has to take into account the placement of implants into the new bone.

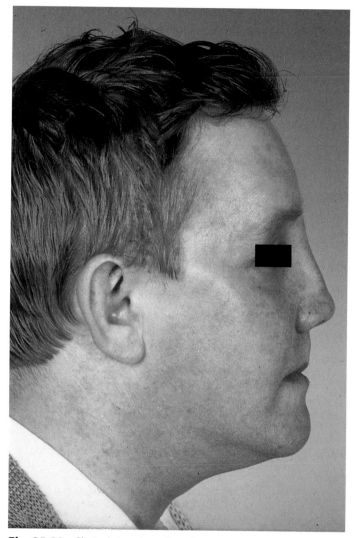

Fig. 25.23: Clinical situation after distraction of the midface on the Le Fort III level using a halo frame.

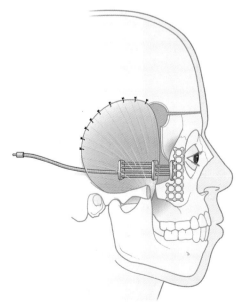

Fig. 25.24: Principle of distraction at the Le Fort III level by using subcutaneously implanted distractors on both sides.

In some cases, like the distraction of the hypoplastic mandible in younger children, the placement of the distractor can be difficult due to the small size and reduced space. Here it might be useful to manufacture a lithography model based on the CT data, followed by a simulated operation of the model and the experimental placement of the distractor. By this technique not only can the placement of the distractor be planned, but the procedure of distraction itself and the final clinical situation after the distraction can also be simulated.

Another important aspect of the planning procedure is the location of the distractor's thread. This has to be placed so that it does not harm the soft tissues but is easily reached for the patient who has to activate it once or twice every day.

Complications

One of the most frequent mistakes is the incorrect placement of the distractor and incorrect distraction vector. Only when using the halo frame can the distraction vector be altered during the process of distraction. If an error becomes obvious, the complication can be managed according to the principle of 'floating bone'. The distractor has to be removed as soon as the complete distance of distraction is reached. At this stage the callus is still soft and malleable as the process of mineralization and ossification is not complete. The direction of the newly formed bone can easily be corrected. For intra-oral devices special orthognathic devices such as plates or activators can be used. For extraoral devices, often the forces of the soft tissue might be responsible for a partial relapse or reshaping of the new bone.

Soft tissue problems with exposure of the new bone or the distractor may occur. In cases with intraorally placed distractors this is not a problem. Mostly the process of distraction can be continued and the soft tissue will heal.

Fractures of the distractor or the distractor thread seldom occur and are mainly a sign of an inadequate osteotomy, wrong selection of distractor or very strong soft tissue forces. In these cases only an exchange of distractor can help.

A lack of ossification can be seen if the distraction process is performed too fast. By exceeding a distraction speed of 1.5 mm per day, the gap between the bone ends will not be remodeled by newly formed bone but by fibrous tissue. Sometimes a callus compression can be tried but surgical removal of the soft tissue and a new, slower redistraction has to be performed.

A relapse of the newly formed bone to the preoperative position can be seen after midface distraction and too early removal of the distractor. Therefore frequent clinical examinations must be performed after removal of the midface distractor. At these examinations the clinical results must be checked carefully. Therapeutically either orthognathic devices like the Delaire mask have to be used, or the distractor must be replaced.

References

1 Codivilla A 1905 On the means of lengthening in the lower limbs, the muscles and tissues which are shortened through deformity. American Journal of Orthopedic Surgery 2: 353–369

2 Rosenthal W 1949 Kiefergelenksankylose und Mikrogenie. Deutsche Zahnarztliche Zeitschrift 4: 786–793

3 Coleman SS, Noonan TD 1967 Anderson's method of tibia lengthening by percutaneous osteotomy and gradual distraction. Journal of Bone and Joint Surgery 49: 263–279

4 Ilizarov GA 1988 The principle of the Ilizarov method. Bulletin of the Hospital for Joint Diseases 48: 1–11

5 Ilizarov GA 1989 The tension-stress on the genesis and growth of tissues: Part I. The influence of stability of fixation and soft-tissue preservation. Clinical Orthopaedics and Related Research 238: 249–281

6 Ilizarov GA 1989 The tension-stress on the genesis and growth of tissues: Part II. The influence of the rate and frequency of distraction. Clinical Orthopaedics and Related Research 239: 263–285

7 White SH, Kenwright J 1991 The importance of delay in distraction of osteotomies. Orthopedic Clinics of North America 22: 569–579

8 Aronson J 1994 Experimental and clinical experience with distraction osteogenesis. Cleft Palate Craniofacial Journal 31: 473–481

9 Karp NS, McCarthy JG, Schreiber JS, Sissons HA, Thorne CH 1992 Membraneous bone lengthening: a serial histological study. Annals of Plastic Surgery 29: 2–7

10 Califano L, Cortese A, Zupi A, Tajana G 1994 Mandibular lengthening by external distraction: an experimental study in the rabbit. Journal of Oral and Maxillofacial Surgery 52: 1179–1183

11 Aronson J, Good B, Stewart C, Harrison B, Harp J 1990 Preliminary studies of mineralization during distraction osteogenesis. Clinical Orthopedics 250: 43–49

12 Sproul JT, Price CT 1992 Recent advances in limb lengthening. Part I: Clinical advances. Orthopedics Review 21: 307–314

13 Polley JW, Figueroa AA 1997 Management of severe maxillary deficiency in childhood and adolescence through distraction osteogenesis with an external, adjustable, rigid distraction device. Journal of Craniofacial Surgery 8: 181–185

14 DeBastini G, Aldegheri R, Renzi-Brivio L, Trivella G 1987 Limb lengthening by callous distraction (callostasis). Journal of Pediatric Orthopedics 7: 129–134

15 Paley D 1990 Problems, obstacles and complications of limb lengthening by the Ilizarov technique. Clinical Orthopedics 250: 81–104

16 Fischgrund J, Paley D, Suter D 1994 Variables affecting time to bone healing during limb lengthening. Clinical Orthopaedics and Related Research 301: 31

17 McCarthy JG, Schreiber J, Karp N et al 1992 Lengthening the human mandible by gradual distraction. Plastic and Reconstructive Surgery 89: 1–8

18 Wangerin K, Gropp H 1997 Multidimensional intraoral distraction osteogenesis of the mandible – 4 years of clinical experience. International Journal of Oral and Maxillofacial Surgery 26 (suppl 1): 14

19 Gropp H, Wangerin K, Paello F et al 1998 Skeletal stability following distraction osteogenesis of the mandible with transorally applied devices. Journal of Craniomaxillofacial Surgery 26 (suppl 1): 64

20 Janette AJ, Vicari FA, Bauer BS et al 1995 Treatment of upper airway obstruction secondary to mandibular deficiency by distraction osteogenesis. Journal of Oral and Maxillofacial Surgery 53 (suppl 4): 96

21 Wangerin K, Gropp H 1999 Mandibular distraction osteogenesis using intraorally applied devices. In: Härle H, Champy M, Terry B (eds) Atlas of craniomaxillofacial osteosynthesis. Thieme Stuttgart, pp 148–152

22 Block MS, Chang A, Crawford D 1996 Mandibular alveolar ridge augmentation in the dog using distraction osteogenesis. Journal of Oral and Maxillofacial Surgery 54: 309–314

23 Hidding J, Zöller JE 1999 Alveolar bone distraction. In: Härle H, Champy M, Terry B (eds) Atlas of craniomaxillofacial osteosynthesis. Thieme, Stuttgart, pp 139–140

24 Costantino PD, Friedman CD, Shindo ML et al 1993 Experimental mandibular regrowth by distraction osteogenesis. Long term results. Archives of Otolaryngology Head and Neck Surgery 119: 511–516

25 Annino DJ, Goguen LA, Karmody CS 1994 Distraction osteogenesis for reconstruction of mandibular symphyseal defects. Archives of Otolaryngology Head and Neck Surgery 120: 911–916

26 Haas AJ 1961 Rapid palatal expansion of the maxillary dental arch and nasal cavity by opening the midpalatal suture. Angle Orthodontist 31: 73–76

27 Hidding J, Breier M 1997 Distraction-osteogenesis of the maxilla. International Journal of Oral and Maxillofacial Surgery 26 (suppl 1): 76

28 Molina F, Ortiz Monasterio F, Paz A et al 1998 Maxillary distraction: aesthetic and functional benefits in cleft lip-palate and prognathic patients during mixed dentition. Plastic and Reconstructive Surgery 101: 951–963

29 Polley JW, Figueroa AA 1998 Rigid external distraction: its application in cleft maxillary deformities. Plastic and Reconstructive Surgery 102: 1360–1372

30 Chin M, Toth BA 1997 Le Fort III advancement with gradual distraction using internal devices. Plastic and Reconstructive Surgery 100: 819–830

31 Cohen SR. Craniofacial distraction with a modular internal distraction system: evolution of design and surgical techniques. Plastic and Reconstructive Surgery 103: 1592–1607

32 Persing JA, Babler WJ, Nagorsky MJ et al 1986 Skull expansion in experimental craniosynostosis. Plastic and Reconstructive Surgery 78: 594–603

33 Tschakaloff A, Losken HW, Mooney MD et al 1994 Internal calvarial bone distraction in rabbits with experimental coronal suture immobilization. Journal of Craniofacial Surgery 5: 318–326

26 Secondary Rhinoplasty for Traumatic Nasal Deformities

Barry L Eppley, Mark M Hamilton

Introduction

The nose is the most frequently traumatized structure on the face due to its prominent central location and its elevation from the relatively flat frontal facial plane. The composite osteocartilaginous structure and its complex interconnections make the nose easily deformed when exposed to blunt trauma. Primary treatment of traumatic nasal deformities is presented in Chapter 13 but secondary treatment may be required due to the high incidence of persistent deformities following primary treatment. Some report a very high failure, up to 80%,[1] mainly due to failure to correct the septum, not just in the immediate postoperative period but over a longer time.

There are numerous reasons for the high incidence of secondary deformities of the nose after trauma. These include inadequate initial treatment due to a failure to appreciate the deranged anatomy, unstable bony and cartilaginous anatomy due to fracture lines and dislocations, insufficient postoperative stabilization, delayed presentation for treatment and recurrent trauma in the early postoperative period. Regardless of the reason, patients need to be informed of the potential need for secondary rhinoplastic surgery.[2]

Secondary nasal deformities are associated with a variety of cosmetic and functional issues. Typically the nose is either deviated or depressed, or both. Nasal breathing is often impaired, usually being unilateral on the side of the deviation. Surgical correction of such nasal deformities can present some of the most difficult challenges in rhinoplasty. This chapter will discuss the various deformities that may be found and some common techniques for their correction.

Anatomic Deformities and Evaluation

The effects of trauma to the nose and central face have been well described.[2,3] With initial low-velocity trauma, the nasal tip alone can become malpositioned. Typically, the lower portion of the fracture rotates inward and the upper portion is pushed upward and outward. This action causes a supratip depression with a small more cephalic hump (Fig. 26.1). With increasing force, the cartilaginous and bony dorsum becomes fractured. Often, however, there is an incomplete fracture, which leads to a late deviation. This is often confused with a dislocation of the septum from the groove in the palatal shelf.

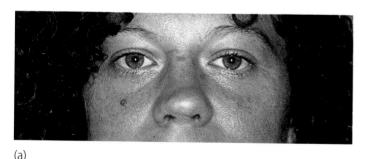

(a)

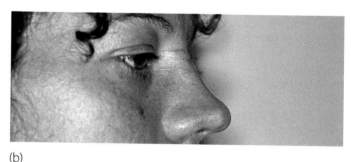

(b)

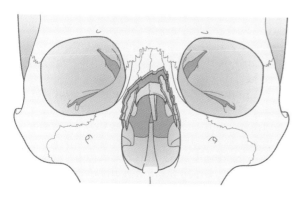

(c)

Fig. 26.1: Secondary nasal deformity from old fracture with depression of the end of the right nasal bone and middle vault displacement. **(a)** Frontal view. **(b)** Right lateral view. **(c)** Diagrammatic representation of fracture pattern.

Clinical Examination

With experience and careful examination it is possible to evaluate the external deformity and understand the underlying structural deformity. It is, however, important to have a logical approach to the clinical examination of the nose. The variables are:

- symmetry
- depression of nasal saddle
- nasal skin scars
- internal examination.

Symmetry

Asymmetry of the face is very common and examination of the nose for asymmetry must be undertaken in context with the whole face. Preinjury photographs are important to exclude long-standing asymmetry. Nasal symmetry is best assessed by looking from above the patient, with the head tilted back. This allows the nasal form to be examined 'afresh' with the eyebrows and chin point being the reference points. Once these key landmarks have been evaluated then by further tilting, the cupid's bow of the upper lip can be brought into the visual field to relate that to the nasal tip. In many cases the symmetry will vary as the eye 'runs' down the nose and the deviation should be noted along the length of the nose. Deviation of the upper third of the nose most likely reflects nasal bone deformation while the lower two thirds reflect the symmetry of the septum. This should give a clear understanding about the extent and position of any asymmetry. The columella should be examined from below, to confirm any tip deviation and symmetry of the nares and domes. Finally the nasal spine should be palpated. Traumatic displacement of this can make alignment of the nose impossible.

Depression of the nasal saddle

To appreciate the position of the nasal saddle, both lateral and anterior views must be evaluated. Laterally the nose should come off the nasion and frontal bone at an angle of about 135°. This line should continue until the slight rise at the nasal tip, to give the characteristic tip break. The columella should make an angle with the upper lip of 90–108°. From these normal values an appreciation of the defect should be possible and allow an appropriate plan to obtain, for example, the correct size of implant necessary.

In the anterior or full face examination any broadening of the nasal ridge and or alar base should be evaluated. The alar width should fall on a vertical line from the inner canthi. In trauma cases, however, it is important to be sure the injury did not extend into the nasoethmoid complex as this can produce a traumatic telecanthus. The normal width in a Caucasian adult is about 34 mm.

Any pseudo elevation of the tip, caused by a saddle deformity, should be distinguished from a true traumatic elevation caused by upward displacement of the nasal spine.

Nasal skin scars

Any lacerations or abrasions should be carefully noted, as they should not be confused with planned surgical incisions for, say, an open rhinoplasty. Of course, if any scars by chance are in the correct position they should be utilized. Any scarring may also be a potential weakness and can reopen at secondary surgery, especially early on after trauma. It may also be an opportunity to revise any scar.

Internal examination

This is probably the most important part of the examination. For this to be useful it needs a good head light speculum of appropriate length to examine the whole nose or a fiberoptic endoscope. The clinical examination should first test function, that is, the nasal airway, ideally obtaining and documenting flow studies. The effect of opening the internal nasal airway by pulling the soft tissue on the lateral nose laterally and the effect of vasoconstrictors, which reduce post-traumatic edema, may help to focus on the cause of any obstruction.

Observation of the internal nose will aim to identify:

- deviated septum
- resolving septal hematomas
- mucosal hyperemia and or edema
- conchal hyperplasia
- displacement of lateral nasal bones
- evidence of nasal valve trauma.

Radiologically they look similar as the fracture or incomplete fracture occurs low in the septum, as the nose is distorted on impact and the palatal shelf is a solid fixed point. In children, of course, a missed septal hematoma will also lead to a late delayed deviation, as the result of impairment of symmetrical growth as well as distortion caused by the organizing hematoma.

Accompanying this fracture pattern, septal fracture and dislocation may occur. Initially the dorsum may be merely deflected to one side but with increased force comes a more retro-displacement of both cartilage and bone (Fig. 26.2). The septum is central to correcting the symmetry and prominence of the nasal bridge. Guyuron has described six typical variations of septal positions in over 1000 revision procedures;[16] 40% had a simple tilt of the septum, which probably indicates no fracture. Other common presentations include a C-shaped deformity, either horizontally or vertically, and an S-shaped deformity, normally horizontally. These more extensive deformities reflect severe distortion with likely fracture or partial fracturing of the septum. It is of course the healing of these fractures which generates tensions leading to late deformation of the septum which is reflected in a distorted nose.

Initial fracture of the nasal bones may extend to involve the nasal process of the frontal bone, the nasal process of the maxilla, the lacrimal bone and the lamina papyryacea. In larger blunt forces which occur directly over the bridge of the nose or from an inferior direction, naso-orbitoethmoid

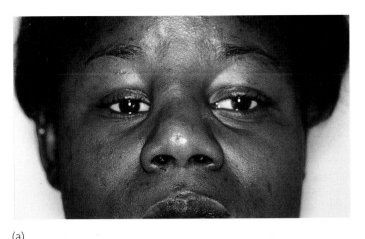

(a)

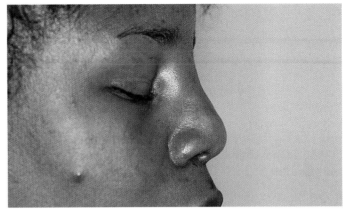

(b)

Fig. 26.2: Secondary nasal deformity with more significant impaction of nasal bones, shortening of septum and superior tip rotation. **(a)** Frontal view. **(b)** Lateral view.

(NOE) fractures occur with telecanthus. This results in a flat, wide nasal dorsum with decreased nasal length, decreased nasal projection and support and columellar retraction (Fig. 26.3). NOE fractures are frequently part of more extended midfacial type fractures. While an understanding of these common fracture patterns aids in the assessment of the secondarily deformed nose, the need for a thorough preoperative evaluation is not obviated.

Unlike primary esthetic rhinoplasty, the deformed traumatized nose is more often associated with some degree of nasal obstruction, reflecting the damage to the septum or, less commonly, damage to the intranasal valve. This is more commonly seen in cases with lacerations or penetrating injuries. Its correction requires identification of both fixed and dynamic components of the obstruction. This requires a thorough examination of the nasal passages before and after the topical application of a vasoconstrictive agent. The shrinkage of the mucosa aids in identifying surgically reversi-

ble causes of nasal obstruction. With a nasal speculum, the position of the septum, size of the turbinates and the internal and external valves should be assessed.[3] The septum when fractured is often found to be either displaced off the maxillary crest to one side or telescoped upon itself. Nasal valve obstruction is frequently found with either upper lateral cartilage displacement medially or collapse. This may be confirmed by performing the Cottle maneuver which should improve with lateral displacement of the cheek on the obstructed side. Enlarged turbinates, especially with lateral wall displacement medially, can also contribute to further nasal obstruction.

Esthetics

A trauma patient seeking revision is no different from a patient seeking a cosmetic rhinoplasty. Clearly some trauma patients fit into the 'warrior class' and have little regard for

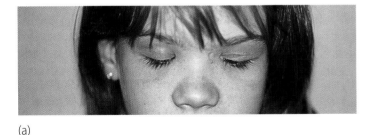

(a)

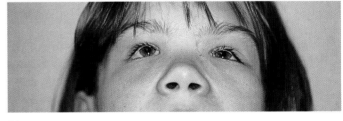

(b)

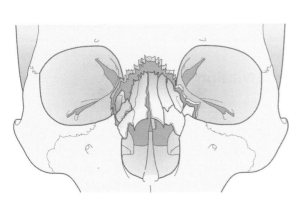

(c)

Fig. 26.3: Secondary deformity from naso-ethmoidal orbital fracture pattern with nasal impaction and telecanthus. **(a)** Frontal view. **(b)** Submental view. **(c)** Diagrammatic representation of fracture pattern.

appearance or social behavior, but they are unlikely to seek revision surgery. Some patients who have been injured in a domestic dispute may in fact be more demanding than a patient seeking a cosmetic rhinoplasty, as their deformity carries much more 'baggage', as a great deal of anger may be associated with the injury.

As with any cosmetic aspect, the patient's wishes not only guide the surgical process but can guide the surgeon about the patient's psychological make-up. This is discussed in Chapter 30 but trauma patients are just as likely to be dysmorphic as any other group. The two important 'warning signs' are:

- vague non-specific comments about appearance
- concerns about appearance which seem inappropriate to your clinical findings.

It is also important to determine just how the nose looked prior to injury and exactly how that compares to the fractured nose. Old pictures may be beneficial in determining which deformities have always been present and which are secondary to the nasal trauma.

Investigations

After a history and thorough examination, radiographic assessment is often helpful to:

- exclude other facial fractures
- better plan any bony surgery.

Plain X-rays are, however, even less useful than they are in primary nasal fracture repair (Fig. 26.4**a,b**). They simply do not provide an anatomic assessment of the internal nasal airway which is often the ambiguous issue. Computed tomographic (CT) scans are the most helpful in this regard and their axial and coronal slices provide the most complete view of the internal nasal airway (Fig. 26.4**c,d**). They are not particularly helpful for evaluation of external nasal morphology. Some controversy exists as it is often felt that a thorough intranasal examination makes them superfluous. In certain cases, this is probably true but the traumatized nose superimposes variable anatomic derangements on top of the patient's native nose, which may or may not have been normal before the injury. If the intranasal examination is not clear, a paranasal CT scan is warranted. In rare cases, usually those with untreated or undertreated NOE fracture patterns, a 3D CT reconstruction may be useful to assess surrounding facial skeletal morphology as well (Fig. 26.4**e**), although with the thin fine bones in this area, the computer reconstruction may create artefacts.

Summary of preoperative examination

- What are the patient's concerns?
- Careful external examination of the nose and face for symmetry and deformity, from lateral and full face. Examination of the whole face and nose from above is the most reliable method of determining symmetry of the face and nose.
- Careful internal examination with speculum and endoscope.
- Airway examination.
- Radiological examination in some cases.

Common Traumatic Nasal Deformities

While traumatic nasal rearrangement can produce a wide variation of deformities, a pattern of nasal dysmorphologies can be identified. These include the expected alterations which can occur with any projected tripod structure:

- loss of height
- deviation
- asymmetries.

Most traumatized noses have a component of all of them and the anatomic contribution to each component must be understood if an ideal correction is to be achieved.

Saddle nose

A saddle nose deformity leaves the patient with a lack of structure in the nasal dorsum, either of bone and/or cartilage.[1,2] This defect leads to a scooped-out appearance from the lateral view and an appearance of a flattened nasal bridge from the frontal view. An illusion of tip rotation accompanies the depression and in some cases in which significant middle vault collapse has occurred, this may be real as well. Also noted is an apparent widening of the nasal vault on frontal view without displacement of the nasal bones or cartilage. Loss of height and lack of a light reflex lead to this illusion.

Short nose

The short nose deformity is characterized by a decreased distance from the nasion to the tip defining point, a low ratio of tip projection to nasal length and a more obtuse than normal nasolabial angle.[1] Overall the nose appears overrotated and deprojected. This nasal deformity can be caused by multiple factors including weakening of the lower lateral cartilages, shortening of the septum or destabilization/detachment of the upper lateral cartilages from the nasal bones. This is of course the characteristic appearance of a depressed nasoethmoid fracture and this should be excluded. In well-pneumatized frontal sinuses, a minimal injury is needed to depress the whole complex.

Nasal deviation

Blunt trauma from a lateral direction may cause the nasal dorsum or tip to become deviated. This is seen as a portion or all of the nose being deviated off a straight line drawn from the glabella down through the central aspect of the cupid's bow. This is most often due to displacement of one or both nasal bones, but may extend down through the structures of the middle vault as well. Illusions of deviation of the nose

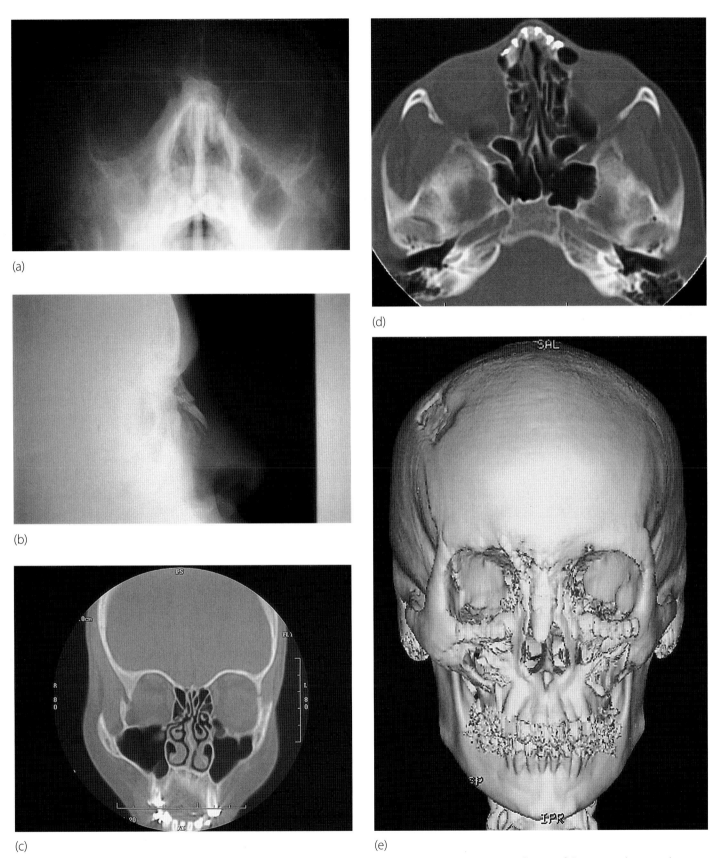

(a)

(b)

(c)

(d)

(e)

Fig. 26.4: Radiographic assessment of secondary nasal deformities. Plain X-ray assessment is even less useful in secondary nasal deformities than in primary nasal fractures. Plain films of an old nasal fracture in a patient who presents with a secondary depressed nasal deformity. **(a)** Submental view. **(b)** Lateral view. The bony pattern of an old nasal fracture can be appreciated in these plain X-rays but they do not add to what a good physical examination would show. CT scans are more useful, particularly axial and coronal paranasal views, and occasionally a 3D reconstruction as can be appreciated in this older teenager with severe nasal depression and airway obstruction after the primary treatment of an NOE injury. **(c)** Coronal view. **(d)** Axial view. **(e)** 3D reconstruction. The internal nasal derangement as well as the surrounding facial bone treatments can be visualized.

may also be seen with collapse of an ipsilateral upper lateral cartilage and bone, leading to shadowing along one side.

There is no doubt, however, that deviation and/or damage to the cartilaginous septum is extremely important as a cause of nasal deviation. Its importance is as much about the difficulty in correcting the damage as making the diagnosis.

In children it has been recognized for a long time that a resolving hematoma on the septum produces deviation which deteriorates as the nose grows. The resultant deviation and nasal obstruction are extremely significant. It is made all the worse since diagnosis of the hematoma and drainage largely prevents the problem.

In adults the problem is controversial not because of the well-recognized effects of a deviated septum but because of the etiology. At one time it was suggested that the deviation was entirely due to the septum being displaced from the palatal groove or from its position between the crura anteriorly. It has been shown experimentally and clinically that the deviation developed from small linear fractures of the cartilage just superior to the palatal groove. This healing fracture then produced the deviation. Localized submucous resections are advocated acutely to prevent long-term deviations.

Columellar retraction

The normal distance from the nasal ala to the base of the columella is 2 mm on lateral view. With nasal trauma, the amount of columellar show can change depending upon the direction of the displacing force and the nasal structures disrupted. It can be decreased or become non-existent due to retro-displacement of the caudal septum which pulls the columellar skin posteriorly. This usually occurs from a direct blow directed at the base of the nose. With upper and middle vault collapse, the tip may rotate superiorly which can result in increased columellar show.

State-of-the-Art Management

Timing

The timing of a secondary corrective rhinoplasty is not critical in most patients. The deformities encountered, while distressing to the patient and often restrictive of some nasal air flow, are not life threatening and good healing of the nasal structures should have occurred before manipulation is attempted. For some patients, timing is not an issue as their injury had occurred months to years previously and the present surgeon was not involved in the management of the original problem.

When the secondary deformity is an extension of the original treatment or it is a primary nasal injury that has presented late (months), the decision as to when to operate can be more difficult. Ideally, nasal mucosal swelling and inflammation should have resolved and the deformities of the osteo-cartilaginous structures completely apparent by resolution of cutaneous edema. The surgical axiom of 6–12 months after the injury is often quoted but operating earlier may be indicated based upon the patient's desires, a full appreciation of the aberrant anatomy and the type of surgical approach.

Approaches

Deciding whether to use the open or closed approach depends on both the surgeon and the defect. It is reasonable to use the open approach for all secondary rhinoplasties unless the surgeon has complete confidence in both his diagnosis of the nasal deformities and his ability to correct them through the more limited exposure of the closed approach. For many surgeons, the use of an endonasal approach in secondary surgery usually requires either a more limited nasal problem or an extensive experience in rhinoplastic surgery on the part of the surgeon. Many secondary nasal deformities, however, can be adequately treated through a closed approach involving the use of traditional marginal and intercartilaginous incisions as has been well described in the past (Fig. 26.5). In more extensive correction, which almost always involves the placement of cartilage grafts, the open approach provides superior visualization of the nasal structures and better facilitates graft placement onto the upper and middle vaults as well as the nasal tip. (Fig. 26.5).

Surgical techniques

Grafting of the nasal dorsum

Nasal dorsal grafting is a common technique used for repair of the saddle nose deformity. Which material is best for augmentation in this area has been a source of controversy over the years and could occupy the entire text of this chapter. The materials available for nasal augmentation are similar to those used elsewhere in the face and can be divided into autografts, homografts and alloplastic biomaterials.

Autograft materials and both bone and cartilage may be appropriate, offer the advantage of incorporation into the recipient site and a lack of any risk of rejection. They do have to be harvested which takes time and, in certain donor sites, has some limited morbidity. Bone or cartilage are the choices and many surgeons make that choice based on the amount of

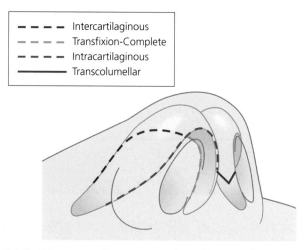

Fig. 26.5: Diagrammatic representation of incisional options in nasal approaches (1 = intercartilaginous, 2 = complete transfixion, 3 = infracartilaginous (marginal rim), 4 = transcolumellar).

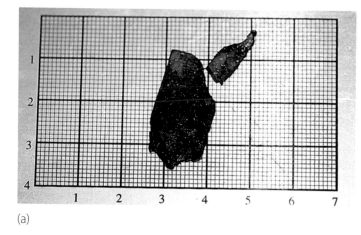

(a)

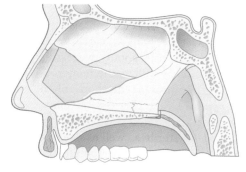

(b)

Fig. 26.6: Septal harvest, when it is relatively undamaged, can provide a large amount of graft tissue. **(a)** It is very important, however, to maintain enough dorsal and caudal septum to ensure external support of the dorsal line, tip and columella. **(b)** The lined area indicates the maximum amount of septum that should be harvested.

augmentation needed. In small to moderate-sized dorsal grafts, cartilage is usually chosen as it is fairly easy to harvest and shape. The most common donor sites are the underlying septum, ear and rib.

Septal cartilage has the advantage of being right in the operative field and can offer a large amount of graft material as only a centimeter of dorsal and caudal cartilage must be retained for adequate dorsal support in a traditional septal harvest (Fig. 26.6). With a previous nasal injury, however, this cartilage is usually less than optimal and straight pieces of sufficient length may not be harvestable due to previous fractures and potential shortening of vertical septal height. This cartilage, when relatively undamaged, is easy to sculpt, often matches the deficient structure and is usually the first choice of most surgeons.[4] With increasing graft thickness, septal cartilage must be stacked and sutured together which requires some skillful crafting. In the thin-skinned patient, this may result in some palpable edges.

Auricular cartilage is also in the same operative field and harvest of the concha through a postauricular incision is rapid and causes little morbidity. The curved shape of this cartilage may or may not be beneficial depending on the defect. For smaller dorsal defects where a long length is not required, conchal cartilage may be adequate (Fig. 26.7). For nasal tip work, its inherent curved shape is often useful. For long straight line grafts of the dorsum, however, it can be problematic in both shape and length.

Costal cartilage offers the advantage of a large amount of donor tissue but it has some inherent disadvantages that may be difficult to overcome. Of all the cartilage donor sites, rib is the most likely to warp or curl. This is because the eighth and ninth rib harvest sites are curved and cannot provide a long

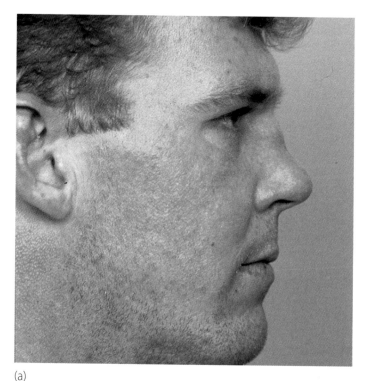

(a)

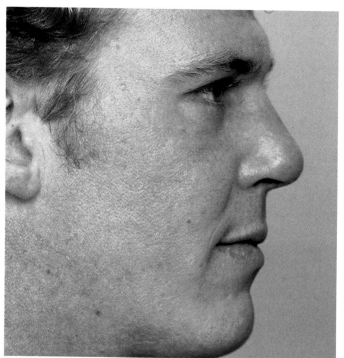

(b)

Fig. 26.7: Dorsal reconstruction with a combination of conchal cartilage and acellular human dermis (Alloderm) in a depression of the upper and middle vaults. **(a)** Preoperative. **(b)** Six months postoperative.

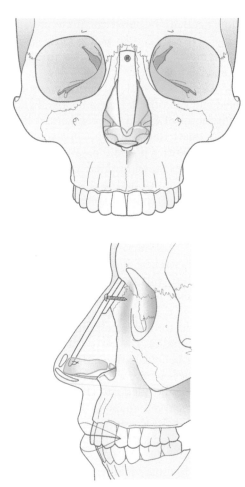

Fig. 26.8: Augmentation of the nasal dorsum with a cranial bone graft placed deep to the cartilage domes, lag screw fixation and cartilage grafts to the columella and tip.

straight graft. Bending the graft by scoring the perichondrium or removing it completely may make it straight intraoperatively but postoperative memory or recoil may often occur. Some surgeons have attempted to overcome this tendency by placing a K-wire through the center of the graft prior to dorsal placement and this appears to be effective. Besides warping, the other concern with all types of cartilage grafts is resorption. Most cartilage grafts do undergo some resorption with an unpredictable change in graft volume. Whether this is significant for the dorsal profile is dependent on graft size and source and the amount of augmentation needed.

Autogenous bone grafts offer the advantage of greater support and augmentation that may be required in larger defects. The most common donor sites are rib, iliac crest and calvarium. Calvarial bone offers the advantages of being close to the operative field and of greater maintenance of volume over time. Adequate length and size as a single piece can usually be obtained from either the occipital area or anywhere along a hemicoronal or scalp incision in the hair-bearing scalp.[5] The outer cortex is taken and reconstruction of the resultant defect is not usually necessary as it causes a minimal deformity. Some skill and experience are required in harvesting the graft to avoid the potential for inner cortex disruption and dural violation. Grafts are never harvested across suture lines due to the attachment of the underlying

dura and, in particular, the midline of the skull due to the presence of the underlying sagittal venous sinus. Sculpting the graft requires a powered burr and irrigation to obtain a desirable boat-like shape for dorsal augmentation. Many cranial bone grafts, due to their size and length, may benefit from some form of fixation. When placed through an open approach, securing the distal graft end to the upper or lower alar cartilages may be adequate (Fig. 26.8). Screw fixation to the frontonasal junction is most easily done through a coronal incision and is most commonly performed in reconstruction of more severely impacted or NOE-type injuries (Figs 26.9, 26.10). The main drawbacks of autogenous bone are the time required for harvest and sculpting, the need for fixation in some grafts and potential donor site morbidity, including a scalp scar.

Homograft cartilage or bone can also be used for dorsal augmentation. Use of banked cartilage and bone use is limited due to concerns about processing and potential disease transmission as well as the numerous available autogenous options. Improving methods of allogeneic tissue processing promise that this option may some day rival autogenous grafts. Irradiated cartilage is also currently available and provides a sterile as well as non-antigenic source of homograft cartilage but resorption potential is high.[1]

A variety of alloplastic materials have been used over the years to augment the nasal dorsum, including silicone rubber, Supramid, Mersilene mesh and Gore-Tex. Alloplasts offer the advantage of an unlimited supply and the avoidance of any donor site morbidity. Silicone rubber has been associated with an unreasonably high extrusion rate and is not widely used today. Although Supramid and Mersilene mesh have been reasonably well tolerated in the nasal dorsum, they have both been found to have a significant resorption rate over time and the occurrence of infection poses a potentially difficult problem. Gore-Tex is by the far the most commonly used alloplast placed in the nasal dorsum today (Fig. 26.11). There is considerable controversy over its use, with strong voices on both sides of the issue.[6,7] Its ease of use and effectiveness in dorsal augmentation are undeniable but the risks of an alloplast under only a cutaneous cover offer long-term concerns about infection, thinning of the nasal skin and potential extrusion.

In most cases, alloplasts are chosen due to their availability off the shelf and their favorable handling properties but the issue of lack of autogenous donor tissue is never justified given the many sites of availability of fascia, cartilage and bone in any individual. No patient lacks adequate autogenous tissue, only the surgeon's desire and experience to harvest it. The intensity of this controversy, however, has been waning with the more recent introduction of processed dermal grafts which offer a biologically safe and well-tolerated alternative without the need for autogenous harvest. They are very pliable, easy to cut and shape and have utility in rhinoplastic surgery as a dorsal camouflage of either underlying grafts or osteocartilaginous irregularities[8] (Fig. 26.12). Their long-term volume retention as a pure augmentative material, however, is not well characterized due to their recent clinical availability.

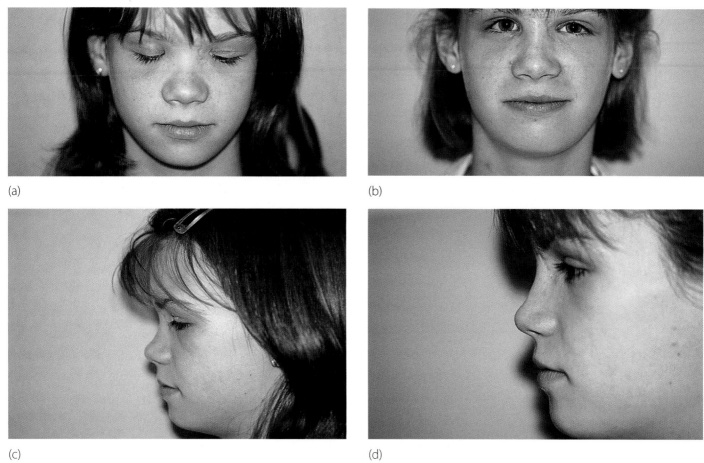

(a)

(b)

(c)

(d)

Fig. 26.9: Fourteen-year-old female who sustained an NOE-type facial fracture who was referred for treatment of her secondary deformities after primary facial fracture repair. She was treated with cranial bone graft augmentation and lag screw fixation, medial canthoplasties with transnasal wiring, removal of indwelling metal hardware and dacrocystorhinostomies (external incisions) through her previous coronal incision. **(a)** Preoperative frontal. **(b)** One year postoperative frontal. **(c)** Preoperative lateral. **(d)** One year postoperative lateral.

Osteotomies

Correction of deformities of the bony nasal vault is typically done with osteotomies. Nasal osteotomies can achieve closure of an open roof deformity, the straightening of a deviated nasal dorsum and narrowing of the nasal side walls. All osteotomy techniques essentially infracture one or both of the nasal bones. Widening of the nasal dorsum via out-fracturing of a nasal bone, while useful, is an inherently more unstable procedure.

Commonly used osteotomy techniques include lateral osteotomy, intermediate osteotomy, medial osteotomy, and superior osteotomy (Fig. 26.13). Lateral osteotomies are typically performed in a high-low-high fashion in a linear direction from an intranasal incision at the superior edge of the inferior turbinate. Starting osteotomies in this position will ensure preservation of the lateral and nasal suspensory ligament attachments to the pyriform aperture. Elevation of the inner lining of the nose is carried out with a freer elevator. The actual bony cuts are then made with a small 3 mm unguarded osteotome. The intermediate osteotomy is utilized when there is a marked height difference between the two nasal bones or

when there exists a marked convexity to one of the nasal bones. The position between the medial and the lateral osteotomy depends on the clinical situation. When utilized for correction of height, it should be placed close to the nasal facial groove. For correcting nasal convexity, a path through the area of convexity should be utilized. Medial osteotomies are required in the correction of the markedly deviated nose. The path of the medial osteotomy begins at the junction of the septum and the nasal bone and proceeds in an angulated fashion to meet either the back fracture site or the superior osteotomy site. If a saddle nose deformity or an open book deformity exists, a medial osteotomy should not be required.

The nose severely deviated to one side should be approached with osteotomies in a sequential fashion. The sequence is performed in the same fashion as opening a book (Fig. 26.14). The medialized nasal bone is first approached with a lateral osteotomy and then a medial osteotomy, allowing lateralization of the bone. Next a medial osteotomy is performed on the laterally deviated side, allowing return of the septum to the midline. Finally the laterally displaced bone is brought back towards the midline with a lateral osteotomy.

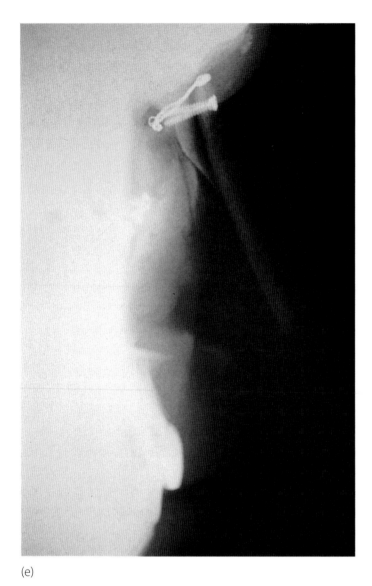

(e)

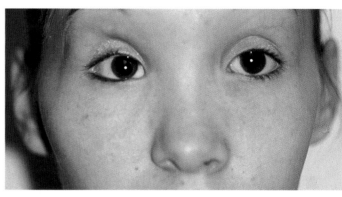

(a)

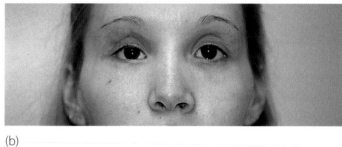

(b)

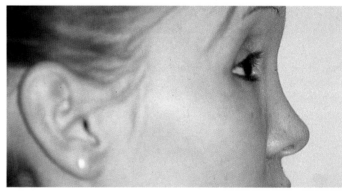

(c)

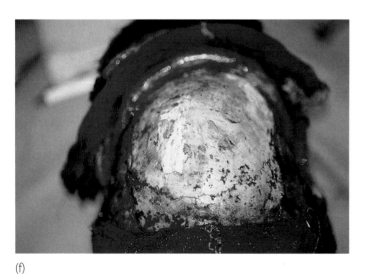

(f)

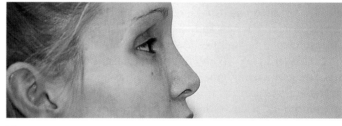

(d)

Fig. 26.9: (e) One year postoperative lateral X-ray. **(f)** Cranial bone graft donor site (upper frontal) was recontoured with hydroxyapatite bone substitute.

Fig. 26.10: Seventeen-year-old female who sustained an NOE-type facial fracture who sought secondary treatment for her residual deformities after an insufficient primary repair. She was treated with cranial bone graft augmentation and lag screw fixation, medial canthoplasties with transnasal wiring, small alloplastic malar augmentations and dacrocystorhinostomies. **(a)** Preoperative frontal. **(b)** One year postoperative frontal. **(c)** Preoperative lateral. **(d)** One year postoperative lateral.

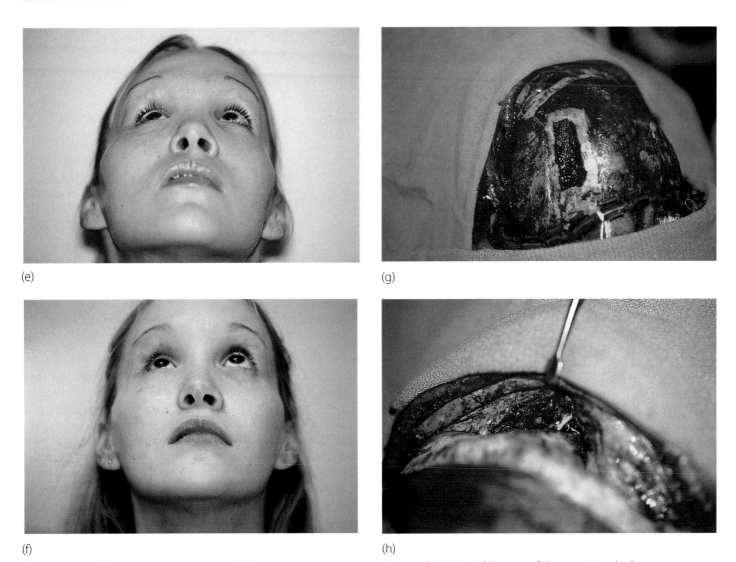

(e)

(g)

(f)

(h)

Fig. 26.10: (e) Preoperative submental. **(f)** One year postoperative submental. **(g)** Cranial bone graft harvest site which was reconstructed with hydroxyapatite bone putty. **(h)** Lag screw fixation of graft to dorsum with transnasal wiring of medial canthi.

Spreader grafts

Deformity of the middle nasal vault can lead to both nasal obstruction as well as airway obstruction due to collapse of the internal nasal valve (less than a 15° angle). Spreader grafts provide a solution to both of these problems and are one of the most important contributions to corrective rhinoplastic surgery introduced in the last two decades[9] (Fig. 26.15). With significant dorsal septal deflections, where scoring of the septum would be inadequate, spreader grafts can be used unilaterally to create the illusion of a straight middle nasal vault (Fig. 26.16). Bilateral middle nasal vault narrowing (i.e. inverted-V deformity) may be corrected with bilateral spreader graft placement.

The placement of spreader grafts can be done through either a closed or open approach but it is inherently easier for most surgeons to properly position and secure them through an external approach. After elevation of the skin envelope, a submucosal pocket is developed between the upper lateral cartilage and the septum. The pocket should span the entire length of the upper lateral cartilage. Spreader grafts can be fashioned from either septal cartilage, conchal cartilage or resected vomer. Some surgeons have even utilized grafts fashioned from resorbable polymers with good success, feeling that the residual scar is sufficient as a volumetric expander.[10] Length should allow extension from just under the nasal bones to the caudal edge of the upper lateral cartilage. Width is determined by the defect being repaired but typically varies between 1 and 3 mm. Grafts are secured in position with a 5–0 resorbable monofilament suture in a horizontal mattress fashion through upper lateral cartilage, graft, septum and opposite side graft if used (see Fig. 26.15).

Septoplasty

The nasal septum functions as the backbone of the nose and has a tremendous effect on the appearance of the dorsum. Deflections of the septum can make both the middle third and the lower third of the nose appear deviated. While septal deviation and deflections can exist in a wide variety of

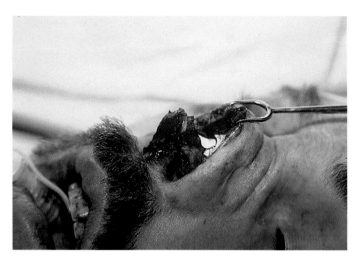

Fig. 26.11: Gore-tex (polytetrafluoroethylene) graft placed over the dorsum in reconstruction of a traumatic saddle nasal deformity through an open approach.

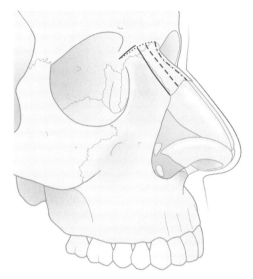

Fig. 26.13: Nasal osteotomy options (lateral = straight line, intermediate or midlevel = dashed line, medial = dotted line, superior = dot-dash line).

anatomical forms, the traumatized nose most frequently presents as an S-shaped or reverse S-shaped anteroposterior deformity due to buckling and fracture of the septum from oblique forces.[16] The S orientation will depend upon the initial direction of the traumatizing blow (Fig. 26.17a). With more severe superior or direct displacing forces on the nasal tip or dorsum, the septum fractures, telescopes and shortens onto itself.

Correction of the deviated septum is usually done through a hemitransfixion incision. Deviated portions of the septum are removed, preserving at least a 1 cm strut both dorsally and caudally (see Fig. 26.6b). When possible, removed cartilage is morselized and returned to the septum if not used as grafts. If minor deviations exist in this important preserved strut area, light vertical scoring may be utilized on the concave side of the septal deformity. For maximal septal cartilage preservation, the S-shaped deformity is corrected by removal of the posterior portion of the bone and cartilage,

bilateral cephalocaudal scoring on the concave areas, and osteotomy and repositioning of the nasal spine and vomer bone (Figs 26.17b, 26.18, 26.19). For more major deflections in which the caudal septum remains deviated, spreader grafts should be utilized with the upper lateral cartilage opposite the deviated side sewn differentially to the spreader graft–septal composite to pull it to the midline.[16] Intranasal extramucosal splints may also be used to improve cartilage memory if spreader grafts are not used.

Illusion of nasal lengthening

Traumatized noses that have only minimal shortening may be amenable to illusion techniques where a small amount of lengthening can be achieved. One such technique involves inferior rotation of the nasal tip.[11] This technique involves

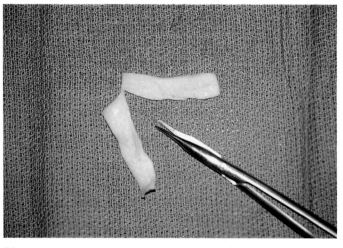

(a)

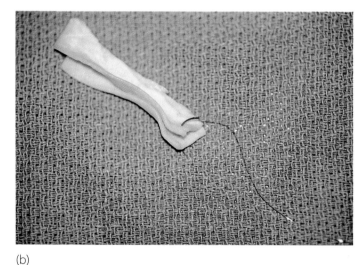

(b)

Fig. 26.12: Processed human dermis (acellular dermis) provides a soft and reasonably thick (0.75–1.5 mm) graft material for the nasal dorsum that can be easily cut **(a)** and securely sutured. **(b)** Its revascularization is rapid and assured but its ultimate volume retention is not well characterized.

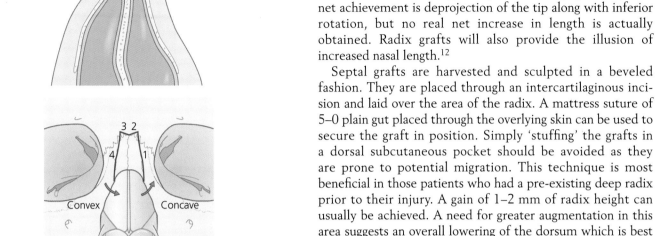

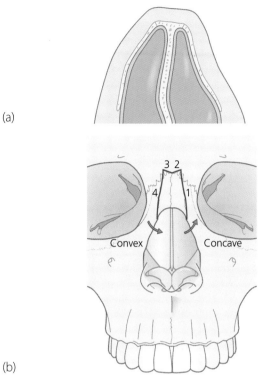

(a)

(b)

Fig. 26.14: Osteotomy technique for severe nasal pyramid deviation. **(a)** Typical deviated nose from trauma with convex/concave deformities of the bones and septal angulation. **(b)** Pattern and sequence of osteotomies for straightening of nasal bone asymmetry.

freeing the lower lateral cartilages from their surrounding attachments and rotating the tip downward (Fig. 26.20). The net achievement is deprojection of the tip along with inferior rotation, but no real net increase in length is actually obtained. Radix grafts will also provide the illusion of increased nasal length.[12]

Septal grafts are harvested and sculpted in a beveled fashion. They are placed through an intercartilaginous incision and laid over the area of the radix. A mattress suture of 5–0 plain gut placed through the overlying skin can be used to secure the graft in position. Simply 'stuffing' the grafts in a dorsal subcutaneous pocket should be avoided as they are prone to potential migration. This technique is most beneficial in those patients who had a pre-existing deep radix prior to their injury. A gain of 1–2 mm of radix height can usually be achieved. A need for greater augmentation in this area suggests an overall lowering of the dorsum which is best addressed by other techniques.

Nasal lengthening

A variety of surgical maneuvers may be used to create an actual increase in nasal length. In most nasal fracture deformities both increased nasal length and increased tip projection are needed. All techniques involve cartilage grafting and include tip grafts, columellar struts and septal extension grafts.

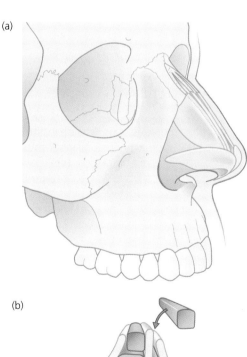

(a)

(b)

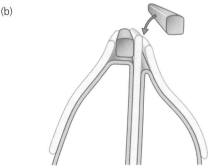

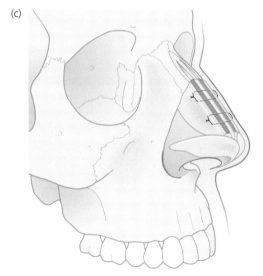

(c)

Fig. 26.15: Spreader graft placement technique. Narrowing of the middle vault due to medial collapse of the upper lateral cartilages. **(a)** Spreader grafts often extend from the osseous-cartiliganous junction to beneath the domes to open up the internal nasal valves. **(b)** Spreader (septum usually) grafts are placed into position between the upper lateral cartilage and the nasal septum. **(c)** The grafts are best secured by 5–0 resorbable horizontal mattress sutures.

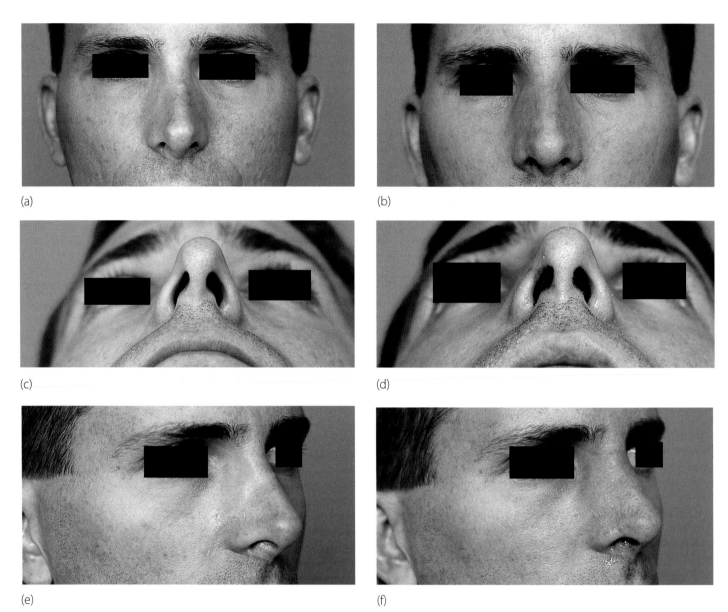

Fig. 26.16: Male patient with 2-year-old nasal fracture initially treated with closed reduction technique at an outside institution with airway obstructive symptoms and nasal asymmetry. Patient was treated through an endonasal approach with unilateral spreader graft and nasal side wall graft of septal cartilage. **(a)** Preoperative frontal view. **(b)** Two weeks postoperative frontal view. **(c)** Preoperative submental view. **(d)** Two weeks postoperative submental view. **(e)** Preoperative right oblique view. **(f)** Two weeks postoperative right oblique view. His airway obstructive symptoms were completely resolved and the right upper and middle vaults have been restored. The spreader graft has done a good job of opening the internal nasal valve and correcting the collapse of the right lower alar cartilage.

A very versatile method is the dynamic adjustable rotating tensioning technique (DARTT) that aims to achieve all of these in a single procedure.[13] Performed through an open rhinoplasty approach, multiple septal cartilage grafts are used and placed as a single columellar strut with two other grafts serving as septocolumellar interpositional grafts (Fig. 26.21). These three grafts are used to create a new tip complex which provides columellar support, allows repositioning of the nasal tip in an inferior direction and obtains an opening in the internal nasal valve. A wide arc of rotation is possible and the appropriate tip projection and rotation can easily be selected. This technique offers adaptability as well as maximal stability.

Another grafting technique is that of a two or three-tiered graft that is sutured to the caudal edge of the medial crura.[14] Using either septal or conchal cartilage, the graft is buttressed against the very stable medial crura and distal septum through an open approach (Fig. 26.22). The redraping of the skin over the graft creates an increased dorsal length although it is not as significant as that of the DARRT technique.

Columellar extension

Isolated retraction (impaction) of the columella can be corrected in a variety of ways. Composite auricular grafts added to the caudal end of the septum have been tradition-

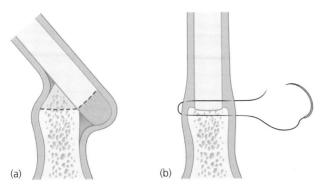

Fig. 26.17: **(a)** Correction of S-shaped anteroposterior deformity with removal of posterior bone and cartilage (dark area) and bilateral anteroposterior scoring on the concave side of the cartilage (straight and hatched lines). **(b)** Repositioning of the caudal end of the septum is almost always needed with removal of the overlapping portions of the septal cartilage and maxillary crest bone (lined areas) and fixation of the freed cartilage end to the bony anterior nasal spine area.

ally described as a method of creating columellar extension.[15] A more effective technique also employs a small auricular cartilage graft but staggered septal-columellar incisions are made, completely releasing the septal-columellar unit. The graft is then placed through the more caudal incision with the composite cartilage graft supported by the opposite mucosal flap. This extension of the membranous septum provides for a very real increase in columellar show.

Controversies

Timing of surgery and choice of grafting material would be the primary issues of debate. Some surgeons may advocate earlier intervention after the primary injury once the extent of the nasal problem is clear. Others prefer to wait until the nose is more 'stable' with healed cartilage and bone, when the tissues may handle better. There is no clearcut answer and the issue is often decided by the magnitude of the deformity, the degree of airway obstruction and the patient's desires. Now that the open approach is more widely accepted, earlier intervention can be more easily performed with higher assurances of postoperative stability due to the visibility provided and the ability to more securely fix grafts into the desired positions.

Graft materials are more hotly debated and there are advocates of both autogenous and alloplastic implants. Like elsewhere on the face, both can work successfully when good technique is used and skin and mucosal cover is of good quality. Autogenous materials clearly require more work to

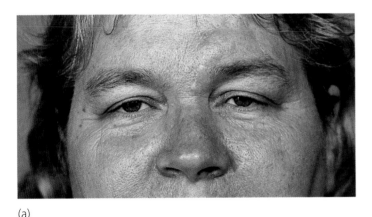
(a)

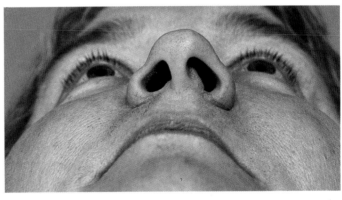
(b)

Fig. 26.18: Female patient with initial nasal fracture of 1 year ago inadequately treated by closed reduction techniques has resultant left-sided septal deviation, right middle and upper vault collapse and left nasal airway obstruction. She was treated through an endonasal approach with septoplasty and caudal septal fixation, left inferior turbinate reduction, septal spreader graft to right middle vault and septal graft to right nasal side wall. **(a)** Preoperative frontal view. **(b)** Preoperative submental view.

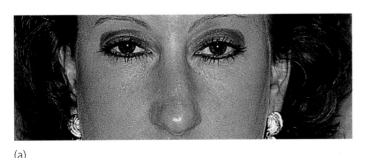
(a)

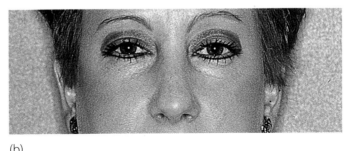
(b)

Fig. 26.19: Female patient with 12-year-old nasal deformity secondary to an untreated fracture as an adolescent. The resultant septal deformity is superimposed on a pre-existing dorsal hump and drooping tip deformity. She was treated with a simultaneous correction of the deviated septum through anteroposterior scoring, limited septal resection, dorsal hump reduction and superior tip rotation techniques. **(a)** Preoperative frontal view. **(b)** Six month postoperative frontal view.

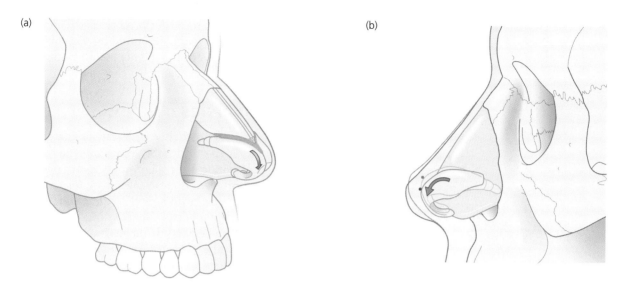

Fig. 26.20: Inferior tip rotation technique for lengthening an esthetically short nose. **(a)** Release of the lower lateral cartilages from their attachments to the upper lateral cartilages, suspensory ligaments and septum. **(b)** Direction of rotation of lower lateral cartilages and their effect on nasal length and tip position.

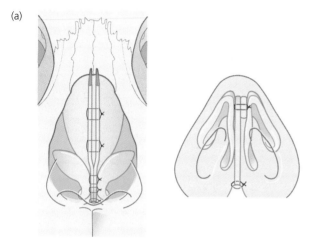

Fig. 26.21: Dynamic adjustable rotational tip tensioning (DARTT) technique. **(a)** Frontal and basal views. **(b)** Lateral view demonstrating the degree of tip rotation that can be achieved by adjusting the placement of the septocolumellar interpositional grafts.

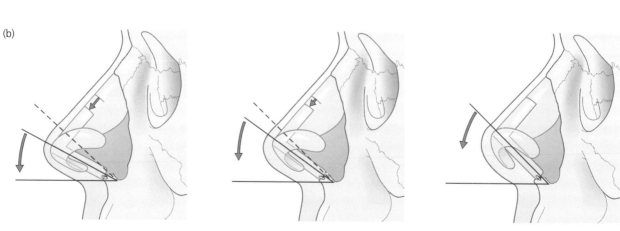

harvest, shape and place but their long-term benefits almost always justify the effort. This is particularly true in the secondary reconstruction of the traumatized nose where significant restructuring and grafting may be needed and the mucosal coverage may be scarred and less plentiful.

Conclusion

The posttraumatic nose can be a difficult problem to correct secondarily and involves an appreciation of the contributions of the nasal bones, septum and upper and lateral cartilages

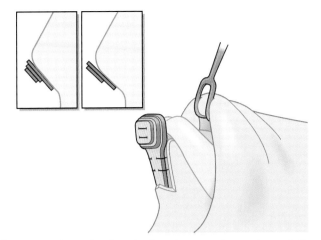

Fig. 26.22: Lengthening the foreshortened nose through tiered cartilage grafts placed on a primary columellar strut. A stack of two or three grafts can be used.

to both the esthetic and functional problems that the patient is experiencing. Optimal correction of the architectural deformities of the traumatized nasal framework, such as the saddle nose and short nose problems, requires accurate diagnosis and reconstruction which is best done through an open approach given the complexity of the anatomic changes. Stable long-term results depend on the surgeon's ability to restore a balance between the tensile and compressive forces of the nasal superstructure.

A wide variety of deformities can be encountered during the secondary treatment of these difficult nasal injuries. A thorough knowledge of the plethora of available techniques is required to achieve optimal results. Onlay and interpositional cartilage grafts, osteotomies, septal repositioning and the judicious use of alloplastic materials are the mainstays of treatment and most patients will require a combination of these techniques to either correct or camouflage the nasal problem. These techniques are applied to achieve nasal symmetry, elevation and straightening of the dorsal line and opening of the internal nasal valve. Improvements in breathing and appearance are almost always achieved but complete return of nasal morphology to its preinjury state may not be attainable in all patients.

References

1 Frodel Jr JL 1992 Primary and secondary nasal bone grafting after major facial trauma. Facial Plastic Surgery 8: 194
2 Stuzin JM, Kawamoto HK 1988 Saddle nasal deformity. Clinics in Plastic Surgery 15: 83
3 Rohrich RJ, Krueger JK, Adams Jr WP, Marple BF 2001 Rationale for submucous resection of hypertrophied inferior turbinates in rhinoplasty: an evaluation. Plastic and Reconstructive Surgery 108: 536–544
4 Collawn SS, Fix J, Moore JR, Vasconez LO 1997 Nasal cartilage grafts: more than a decade of experience. Plastic and Reconstructive Surgery 100: 1547
5 Posnick JC, Seagle MB, Armstrong D 1990 Nasal reconstruction with full-thickness cranial bone grafts and rigid internal skeletal fixation through a coronal incision. Plastic and Reconstructive Surgery 86: 894
6 Owsley TG, Taylor CO 1994 The use of Gore-tex for nasal augmentation. A retrospective analysis of 106 patients. Plastic and Reconstructive Surgery 94: 241
7 Daniel R 1996 Gore-tex for nasal augmentation (reply). Plastic and Reconstructive Surgery 96: 229
8 Gryskiewicz JM, Rohrich RJ, Reagan BJ 2001 The use of Alloderm for the correction of nasal contour deformities. Plastic and Reconstructive Surgery 107: 561
9 Sheen JH 2000 Spreader graft: a method of reconstructing the middle vault following rhinoplasty. Plastic and Reconstructive Surgery 106: 922
10 Stal S, Hollier L 2000 The use of resorbable spacers for nasal spreader grafts. Plastic and Reconstructive Surgery 106: 922
11 Gunter JP, Rohrich RJ 1989 Lengthening the aesthetically short nose. Plastic and Reconstructive Surgery 83: 793
12 Naficy S, Baker SR 1998 Lengthening the short nose. Archives of Otolaryngology Head and Neck Surgery 124: 809–813
13 Dyer II WK, Yune ME 1997 Structural grafting in rhinoplasty. Facial Plastic Surgery 13: 269–277
14 Hamra ST 2001 Lengthening the foreshortened nose. Plastic and Reconstructive Surgery 108: 547–549
15 Dingman RO, Walter C 1969 Use of composite ear grafts in correction of the short nose. Plastic and Reconstructive Surgery 43: 117–123
16 Guyuron B, Uzzo CD, Scull H 1999 A practical classification of septonasal deviation and an effective guide to septal surgery. Plastic and Reconstructive Surgery 104: 2202

27 Secondary Orbital Surgery

Kenneth J Sneddon

Introduction

Residual deformities in the orbital region arise for a number of reasons.

- Extent and severity of original injury
- Tissue loss
- Associated injuries
- Inadequate initial diagnosis
- Compromised initial management
- Complications of initial treatment

The severity of the initial facial injury may in itself make it impossible to achieve a good result after the initial surgical repair; this is particularly likely to be the case when there is extensive tissue loss resulting from the traumatic injury. Neurological damage, be it associated with a head injury or direct nerve damage, can result in deformities such as facial paralysis or ptosis. These generally are not repaired at the time of initial management and require secondary correction. The extent and severity of associated injuries may preclude the optimum management of the facial injuries in the immediate and early posttrauma period, leading to delayed or compromised primary surgery. Inadequate diagnosis of the true nature of the injury or poor initial management may lead to poor outcomes. These patients present with residual deformities giving rise to both cosmetic and functional implications (Fig. 27.1).

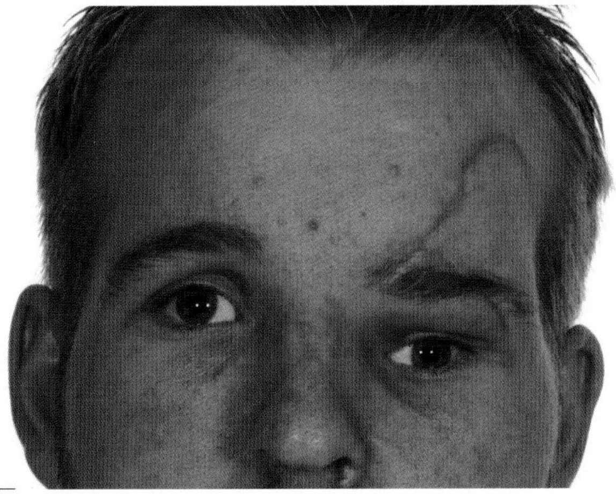

The typical secondary deformities which are seen can be split into those of an underlying skeletal nature or those relating to soft tissue problems.

Skeletal deformities include:

- loss of facial shape
- inadequate projection of normal cheek contour
- enophthalmos
- exophthalmos (rare)
- orbital dystopia
- traumatic telecanthus.

It is the zygomatic complex as a whole which is the key to the orbital skeleton and many of the deformities seen result from inadequate or misplaced reduction of zygomatic fractures. Both inadequately reduced zygomatic fractures and fractures of the orbital walls (the so-called 'blow-out' fractures) lead to changes in orbital volume and shape and in turn to enophthalmos and orbital dystopia.

Soft tissue deformities include:

- scarring
- tethering of skin
- pigmentary changes
- tissue loss
- eyelid problems: ectropion, entropion, ptosis
- medial canthal malposition
- epiphora – lacrimal drainage problems.

Fig. 27.1: Combined effect of both skeletal and soft-tissue elements, leading to scarring, orbital dystopia, enophthalmos and loss of cheek contour in a patient where there was no initial management due to the severity of the head injury.

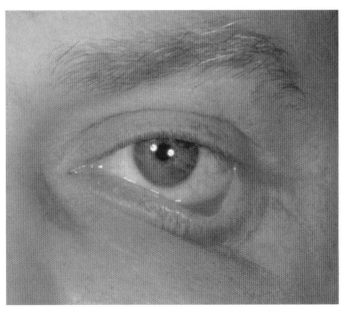

Fig. 27.2: Infection around an orbital rim plate has led to tethering of the overlying skin and an unsightly ectropion.

Scarring around the orbital region may have profound effects on the facial appearance. The presence of scars, even well healed, in this area is very obvious and difficult to camouflage. Scar contracture can have serious consequences leading to distortion of anatomical landmarks and in particular the lower eyelid, where it may result in unsightly ectropion (Fig. 27.2). Tethering of the relatively thin skin of the eyelid and the periorbital area to the underlying bone results in loss of the animation required for normal facial expression.

It is difficult and to an extent artificial to truly separate the bony and soft tissue elements of these injuries. Inadequate support of the soft tissues due to inadequate bony reduction further complicates the issue and difficulties in dealing with scarred thickened and fibrosed soft tissues may lead to poor cosmetic results even in the presence of perfect bony reconstruction. Finally, combinations of skeletal and soft tissue problems lead to such deformities as telecanthus and canthal malpositions.

The management of secondary deformities is requested by patients for many reasons. These injuries can result in very obvious and in some cases severe cosmetic defects and patients can suffer enormous psychological trauma as a result. They may lose self-confidence and previously outgoing personalities can become shy and retiring. In more extreme cases they may withdraw from society and find themselves unable to cope with their work or mix socially with their friends. Patients vary enormously in their perception of problems and the most serious psychological reactions are not necessarily seen in those with the most serious injuries. It is salutary to remember that the patient's and the clinician's perceptions of a deformity may be very different. Patients nowadays have increasingly high expectations and quite rightly feel that if they sustain an injury then it should be corrected and they be returned to their normal preinjury state. Sadly this is not always possible and one of the clinician's tasks in the management of these patients is to combine encouragement and support with realistic expectations of what can be achieved.

These are also important injuries from a medicolegal point of view.

Assessment

Much information can be gained from a thorough history and clinical examination. Careful clinical assessment leading to an accurate diagnosis of the deformity is essential to future management. Examination must assess facial shape and symmetry, the position of the globe in three dimensions and in comparison with the contralateral side. The eyelids, brows and position of the medial and lateral canthi must also be assessed. Measurements of the distance of the medial canthus from the facial midline and of the pupil to the lateral orbital rim should be taken and compared bilaterally for symmetry. The position of the malar fat pad over the cheek is crucial to the cosmetic appearance. As a result of trauma or previous subperiosteal dissections this may migrate inferomedially, accentuating the effect of posterior displacement of the zygomatic complex. There may be functional problems, of which perhaps the most common is diplopia. Evaluation of

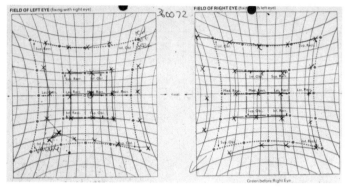

Fig. 27.3: Hess chart, showing tethering of inferior rectus.

diplopia is best achieved by means of the Hess chart (Fig. 27.3) or the 'prism bar' which allow objective assessment of ocular movements and an estimation of the degree of diplopia respectively.

Enophthalmos is commonly associated with orbital trauma. This 'sinking' of the eye back into the orbital cavity produces a characteristic clinical appearance of supratarsal hooding or a supratarsal sulcus deformity, which produces shadowing above the eye (Fig. 27.4). This clinical sign indicates loss of inferoposterior support of the globe. A true orbital dystopia may be associated. Clinically enophthalmos is best assessed by examining the patient from above and behind, looking down on the eyes and gently retracting the upper eyelids to reveal the globes. This means of clinical examination is surprisingly sensitive and enophthalmos of 2–3 mm can be detected by this method. More formal measurement of enophthalmos is carried out by using a Keeler frame or Hertel exophthalmometry; however, both these devices use the orbital rim as a reference point and are thus potentially inaccurate in patients in whom the orbital rim is not intact or displaced.

More accurate assessment of enophthalmos can now be obtained by means of surface scanning techniques. These use either laser surface scanning or three-dimensional stereophotographic techniques to produce scans from which accu-

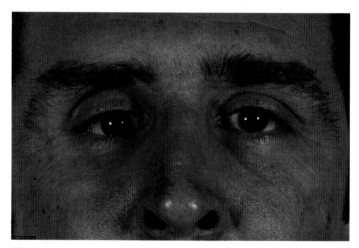

Fig. 27.4: Clinical signs of enophthalmos: supratarsal hooding with obvious shadowing above the left eye.

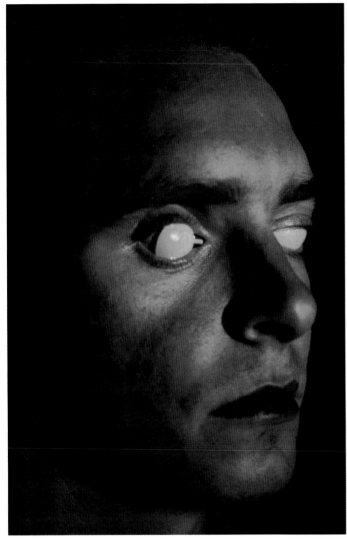

Fig. 27.5: 3D optical surface scan allows accurate measurement between two sides. Also shows contour defect and supratarsal hollowing. The eye shells were used in the development of the scanner to reduce reflection from the cornea but are no longer needed.

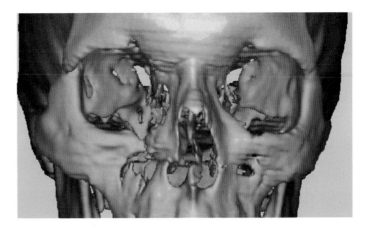

(a)

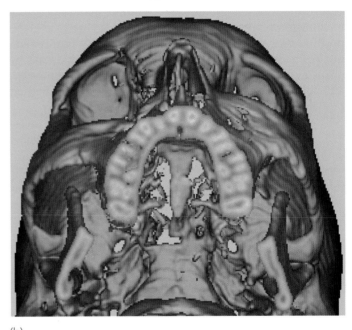

(b)

Fig. 27.6a&b: 3D reformatting of CT scan data allows ready visualization of skeletal anatomy and viewing from any angulation.

rate measurements can be made (Fig. 27.5). Using these techniques, differences of only 0.5 mm between the positions of the eyes can be identified. These surface scans can also be used to assess asymmetries in facial contour as a result of displacements of the underlying zygomatic complex. High-resolution CT scanning in both axial and coronal planes allows detailed visualization of the bony and soft tissue anatomy of the orbit. With recent developments in three-dimensional reformatting an easily visualized representation of the bony displacements is readily achieved (Fig. 27.6a&b). Measurements of orbital volume can also be made and related to the degree of enophthalmos. MRI scanning may also be of use, especially for assessing the extraocular muscles.

Enophthalmos

Before it is possible to determine a rational approach to the treatment of enophthalmos it is essential to have an under-

standing of the underlying pathophysiology. There are several mechanisms postulated for the development of post-traumatic enophthalmos.

- Increase in orbital volume
- Herniation of orbital fat
- Fat atrophy
- Herniation of extraocular muscles
- Soft tissue contraction
- Loss of ligamentous globe support

The relative contributions of these theories are controversial. What is clear is that posttraumatic enophthalmos represents an imbalance between orbital contents and orbital volume.

Manson et al[1] investigated the relationship between fat and ligaments in the provision of globe support. Orbital fat is traditionally separated into extramuscular and intramuscular compartments, fine ligaments dividing these compartments.[2]

The extramuscular fat compartment is present essentially in the anterior portion of the orbit whilst posteriorly almost all the fat is intraconal. Their investigations showed that removal of intraconal fat produced globe displacement similar to clinical enophthalmos. The removal of extramuscular fat on its own, whilst producing globe displacements, was of less significance than the loss of posterior intraconal fat. The average change in globe position in patients undergoing cosmetic blepharoplasty was noted to be less than 1 mm, suggesting that anterior extramuscular fat plays little part in globe position. It was clear that the ligamentous system on its own was incapable of maintaining the full forward projection of the globe for which the presence of intramuscular cone fat was required. That the ligamentous sling system of the orbit is important in maintaining globe position is evidenced by the observation that the removal of the orbital floor as part of a maxillectomy procedure does not lead to a change in globe position as long as the periosteum and sling system remain undisturbed. Removal of bone from multiple orbital walls by changing the mechanics of the sling system does, however, alter globe position and is partially the rationale behind orbital decompression for thyroid eye disease.

The advent of CT scanning allowed far more detailed investigation into the relationship between orbital volume changes and enophthalmos (Fig. 27.7). A number of authors have reported on the volumetric changes in orbital volume and soft tissue orbital volumes following injury.[3,4,5] Thin-slice CT scans can be used to assess orbital volume accurately. They showed a linear relationship between increased orbital volume and enophthalmos, with each 1 cm^3 increase in orbital volume leading to 0.47 mm of enophthalmos. Whitehouse and colleagues demonstrated an even greater degree of enophthalmos of 0.8 mm for each 1 cm^3 of orbital expansion.[22] These relationships are valid for fractures greater than 4 weeks old when initial post-traumatic oedema has settled. Manson and colleagues[5] investigated not only bony orbital volume changes but also soft tissue volumes within the orbit. These studies revealed slight (5%) increase in total soft tissue volume and also of retrobulbar volume (5%), whereas bony orbital volume was increased by up to 18%. Fat and globe volume changes were not significant. Fat atrophy was not a predominant feature in most patients. They went on to demonstrate that reconstruction of the bony orbit reversed these volume changes and restored globe position. Manson et al conclude that:

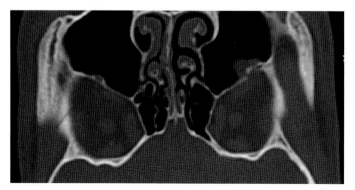

Fig. 27.7: Axial CT scan showing small orbital floor defect.

the principal mechanism of posttraumatic enophthalmos involves displacement of a relatively constant volume of orbital tissue into the enlarged bony orbit, Changes in the shape of the orbital soft tissue to a more spherical configuration allow posterior, inferior and medial globe displacement.

Although in this chapter we are strictly discussing the management of secondary deformities it is clear that early correction of enophthalmos gives superior results. From the data described above, the authors have identified criteria which they feel accurately predict the likelihood of enophthalmos developing and as such identify those cases where early surgical intervention would be beneficial. Raskin et al describe Group 1 fractures (less than 13% orbital expansion), which failed to demonstrate enophthalmos on follow-up examination, and Group 2 fractures (greater than 13% orbital expansion), which frequently demonstrated enophthalmos when managed conservatively.[23] On this basis they advocate the following algorithm.

Group 1 fractures are selected for surgical management if they display persistent motility defects after a 7-day course of steroid therapy. Patients with Group 2 fractures are managed surgically after a 5-day preoperative regimen on steroids, antibiotics and decongestants. Manson feels able to predict the development of enophthalmos in those cases where the orbital floor disruption exceeds a total area of 2 cm^2, where the bony orbital volume increase exceeds 1.5 cc or 5% and where significant fat and soft tissue displacement occur.

Treatment

When dealing with secondary corrections it is useful to distinguish those cases where the initial injury is confined to the internal orbit (generally referred to as orbital blow-out injuries although more accurately identified as orbital wall/floor defects) as separate from those in which there is disruption of the orbital framework. These latter cases in which there is discontinuity of the orbital frame result from previously untreated or inadequately treated zygomatic or nasoethmoid injuries. The sequence of treatment in these cases always involves initially correcting the orbital framework before moving on to correct any internal orbital damage.

Internal orbital injuries

In these cases the aim of treatment is to restore globe position and release any mechanical entrapment which may be contributing to diplopia. The orbital framework is intact and there is as such therefore no change in facial contour. The classically described pure blow-out fracture typically relates to an orbital floor defect of less than 2 cm^2, occurring in the anterior or middle part of the orbit. These defects are generally straightforward to repair. Following an approach to the orbital floor, which can be via either a cutaneous or a transconjunctival[6-9] route, the defect is reached by subperiosteal dissection of the orbital contents proceeding from the orbital rim backwards. Once the defect is outlined the herniated orbital contents are freed from the maxillary sinus and gently returned to the confines of the orbital cavity. Repair of the defect may be achieved by one of a number of different materials. A thin sheet of the chosen repair material is shaped to cover the defect and if it can be made to overlap the margins of the defect onto sound bone all around, generally does not require fixation (Fig. 27.8). The weight of the orbital contents resting upon it serves to stabilize the repair.

Sadly not all orbital floor defects are as simple or as straightforward to correct and this is more so the case with patients presenting for secondary reconstructions.

Complex orbital wall defects are defined as those where the defect extends to involve more than one of the orbital walls (most often the floor and medial wall but any combination is possible) and where the defect extends backwards into the posterior third of the orbit (Fig. 27.9). In these cases not only must the orbital volume be restored but in order to achieve satisfactory results the precise shape of the orbit must also be reconstructed.

It is worth briefly reviewing the shape of the orbit. The orbit is classically described as an open pyramid with its apex posteriorly; however, the walls of the pyramid are not flat! The orbital floor behind the orbital rim is initially concave until a point just behind the equator of the globe where it becomes convex upwards, inclining at around 30°, creating a retrobulbar constriction in the orbit. Combine this with a roughly 45° inclination of the floor from the lateral to the medial wall and one then sees a prominent posteromedial and inferomedial bulge. This bulge behind the globe and adjacent to and on the medial side of the posterior extent of the inferior orbital fissure is a critical area in orbital reconstruction. This posterior medial wall area is the region Hammer[10] describes as the 'key area' (Fig. 27.10) and its reconstruction is essential in gaining anterior projection of the globe.

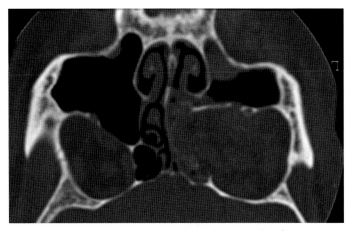

Fig. 27.9: Axial CT scan showing complex orbital defect. Large defect of floor and medial wall, disruption of orbitomaxillary plate and complete opacification of ethmoid sinuses.

Reconstruction of these complicated multiwall orbital defects is more difficult. Essential to a satisfactory repair is adequate exposure and dissection around the entire defect. Exposure in these cases is rarely sufficient via a lower lid approach on its own. A transconjunctival incision with the addition of a lateral canthotomy allows far greater exposure of the orbital cavity, while a transcaruncular extension medially gives even greater exposure of the medial wall. Even these two extensions of the standard transconjunctival incision still only give access to about two-thirds of the circumference of the orbit. To allow full 360° dissection of the orbit as advocated by Hammer, a lower lid incision has to be combined with a coronal approach. This certainly gives by far the best exposure of the medial wall and is the only incision to give adequate exposure of the nasoethmoid complex. In order to maximize the nasoethmoid exposure it is necessary to incise the periosteum on the deep side of the flap in the region of the nasal bridge.

Subperiosteal orbital dissection can be more difficult in secondary corrections due to dense scarring and an adherence of orbital tissue to periorbital structures. As in all surgery it is

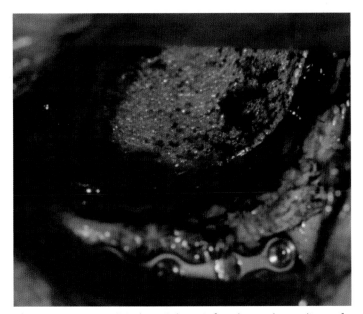

Fig. 27.8: A 1 mm 'Medpore' sheet is fitted over the outlines of an orbital floor defect.

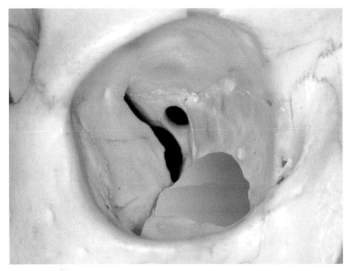

Fig. 27.10: Hammer's 'key area' the inferomedial bulge shown coloured orange.

important to establish the correct plane of dissection and this is most easily accomplished by starting from an uninjured part of the orbit and approaching the defect from all sides. To gain complete exposure of the orbital cavity a number of structures have to be divided. There are a number of small vessels, which run from the infraorbital bundle to the periorbita, which have to be divided. The division of the anterior ethmoidal artery high on the medial wall significantly improves access in this area. Finally as one dissects back along the orbital floor one comes across the contents of the inferior orbital fissure which prevent further dissection in a posterior direction. There are no anatomical structures of importance running through the inferior orbital fissure and its contents should be divided after careful coagulation with bipolar diathermy. To further hamper visibility when the periorbita has been perforated, orbital fat herniates through and bulges over the retractors on both the medial and lateral sides. The use of two retractors is often of more use than one larger malleable strip. Two simple homemade retractors can be of great help, however, a simply reshaped teaspoon being a useful instrument. The second and perhaps most useful of all is to cut a sheet of silastic to the approximate dimensions of the orbit and use this as a retractor placed underneath normal malleable strips, thus preventing herniation of fat over the edge of the retractor.

Once the defect has been identified the key element is to free and return herniated orbital contents to the confines of the orbital cavity. Whilst in the acute setting this can usually be achieved with little difficulty this task is much less readily accomplished in secondary reconstruction. Often one has to resort to careful sharp dissection to release the orbital contents from the margins of the defect and adjacent periorbital tissues. This tissue can be surprisingly vascular and thorough bipolar coagulation is required as one dissects.

After the displaced orbital contents have been released the true nature and extent of the orbital wall defects become apparent. When difficulty is experienced in freeing the defect extra access can be gained by orbitotomies. Removing a portion of the orbital rim improves both visualization of the defect and access to it (Fig. 27.11), especially for posteriorly placed defects. A suitable plate is first shaped and temporarily fixed to the orbital rim so as to allow accurate repositioning of the segment at the end of the procedure. Using either a fine saw or burr, a portion of the orbital rim is then removed. Once identified and fully exposed, several features of these defects become apparent. Firstly the defect is often extensive and of a complicated three-dimensional shape. It is clear that a single graft would be difficult to shape and often too large to insert through the available access. Also it is worthy of note that the posterior extent of the defect often means that it is not possible to provide a suitable ledge posteriorly on which to rest a graft.

In these large and complex defects bone is the material of choice for reconstruction. Generally more than one graft is required. Hammer places great emphasis on the reconstruction of his 'key area' of the posteromedial wall and begins his reconstruction using a single sheet of calvarial bone cantilevered off an anterior plate to reconstruct this area. He

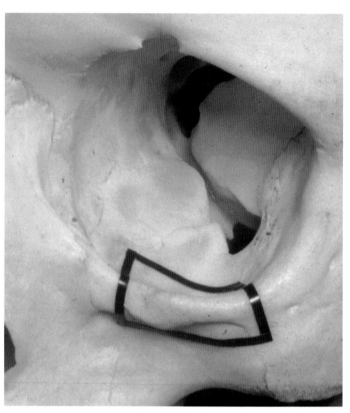

Fig. 27.11: Illustration of inferior orbitotomy. Removing a section of rim from the inferior, lateral or superior aspect affords greater access and visibility to posterior defects.

makes no attempt to overlap the margins of the defect with this graft but orientates it in such a way as to restore the posteromedial bulge. This graft then acts as a support for further grafts. It is this restoration of the shape of the posteromedial orbit which provides the anterior projection of the globe. Other authors place a sheet of bone in the orbital floor and a further separate graft in a more vertical orientation to restore the medial orbital wall. These grafts often do not need to be rigidly fixed as they can be wedged into position.

When restoring the orbit in this fashion, it remains essential, however, to place graft material behind the equator of the orbit to provide anterior projection of the globe. Bone graft placed too anteriorly in the orbit simply elevates the globe without correcting enophthalmos. It is generally stated that in the correction of enophthalmos, overcorrection is the key to long-term success. It is clear that globe position does change following reconstruction. It is assumed that this relapse, for want of a better term, is related to resorption of bone graft material generally considered to be in the region of 30%, although it is likely that there is also some minor reduction in soft tissue volume after reconstruction. Perioperative edema at the time of reconstruction can be misleading and result in an underestimate of the degree of enophthalmos correction that has actually been achieved.

Orbital frame injuries (zygomatic fractures)

In all cases of orbital trauma repair, the first stage of treatment is the reconstruction of the orbital skeleton. This concept is no different in secondary repair although there are some added difficulties compared with the early management of such injuries. First and foremost amongst these is the very fact that the fractures have healed and bony continuity has been re-established. Osteotomies of the zygomatic complex are therefore required to mobilize the bony fragments and allow repositioning. The situation varies slightly between cases where there has been no previous surgery and those in which there has been inadequate reduction in the past. In those cases where there has been no previous surgery there may be gross dislocations of large fragments resulting in significant deformities of the zygomatic complex. There may be bony union or there may be areas of fibrous union with soft tissues interspersed between bone fragments. In cases where there have been previous attempts at surgical correction there is generally better bony contact and good bone healing.

The principal problem with these cases is one of inaccurate reduction of the original bony injury; generally it is one of rotation around the vertical axis of the zygomatic complex. Very small rotational discrepancies around this axis can lead to significant changes in the orbital volume. This can best be visualized by looking at the lateral orbital wall behind the lateral rim. This is a substantial piece of bone and generally reduces well. Steps seen at this area indicate rotational discrepancies and inaccurate reduction. The other common problem relates to the zygomatic arch. This is an area where mistakes are often made. It is generally assumed that the arch is indeed an arch form and is therefore fixed with a nice gentle curve. This on closer inspection is not the case; the zygomatic arch projects in a relatively straight line and is often fixed with too much of a curve. This shortening and overbending of the arch leads to outward rotation of the zygoma, creating a defect in the lateral orbital wall, lack of anterior projection of the maxilla and an increase in facial width.

With fracture repair the reconstruction is essentially a jigsaw puzzle with all bony fragments present. Once they have been adequately reduced they tend to fit nicely together and can be fixed in position to give a true anatomical reduction. This generally is not the case with secondary or delayed reconstruction. Relatively early after injury the bone ends round off and change slightly in shape. Small fragments may devitalize and subsequently resorb. The net effect of these changes is that simple reduction of the fragments as in early fracture repair does not lead to restoration of the original preinjury state; indeed, this may not be possible. In such a scenario the best possible orbital framework that can be achieved is produced by realignment of the fragments. This often results in small gaps which can be spanned by plates or filled with bone graft to restore continuity.

Exposure

Even more so than in primary repair, in secondary corrections wide exposure is essential to allow accurate three-dimensional reconstruction. Although in some simpler cases a zygomatic osteotomy can be successfully achieved through local incisions alone, almost invariably to gain adequate exposure a coronal flap is required. This must be brought down sufficiently to fully expose subperiosteally the whole of the area involved in the original injury, exposing the whole of the zygomatic arch and the body of the zygoma. It is argued by some that in order to achieve the greatest accuracy in reconstruction and to gauge symmetry, the coronal flap should be reflected sufficiently to expose also the contralateral zygoma for comparison. In addition to the coronal flap, access is required to the area of the zygomatic buttress via an incision intraorally in the buccal sulcus and also an incision to expose the infraorbital rim.

Careful planning of the approach to the orbital rim is required in secondary corrections. The choice of incision may be predicated by incisions used at previous surgery or there may be scars resulting from the original injury which can be utilized and revised at the same time. There may be existing problems of lower eyelid position as a result of the original injury and some degree of shortening of the lower eyelid may already be present. The incision used must take these factors into account and must on no account risk worsening the situation. For these reasons very high subciliary or 'blepharoplasty' incisions are often best avoided in the secondary situation. Transconjunctival approaches are often indicated. It is often more satisfactory to complete the approach to the infraorbital rim before raising the coronal flap. Subperiosteal exposure of the zygomatic complex is required and this may be more difficult than normal in areas where there is tethering of the overlying soft tissue to underlying fracture lines or plates. Also areas where the overlying soft tissues have been damaged by the original injury may make elevation more difficult.

Reduction

After full exposure of the injured area, the site and extent of the deformity are usually obvious. Even when there has been good bony healing the original fracture lines are usually apparent. The fractures have to be recreated to allow repositioning of the fragments. Very often bony repair is not fully consolidated and it is often possible to open these fracture lines by prising them apart with an osteotome. Where this is not the case a combination of chisels or a surgical saw are used. Separation is achieved at the FZ suture, the zygomatic arch and the infraorbital rim. The cut at the infraorbital rim is extended downwards to pass through the area of the zygomatic buttress being accessed at this point via the intraoral incision. The only area that remains to gain full freedom is to join the cuts at the infraorbital rim and the FZ suture. This is best achieved some 4–5 mm inside the orbital margin by means of a fine burr or osteotome.

Particularly in cases where there has not been previous surgery and there is significant displacement, following the recreation of the fracture lines and completion of the osteotomies it is often necessary to remove bone to allow the correct realignment of the fragments. The zygoma is repositioned using the lateral orbital wall as a guide to avoiding rotations and the FZ suture to assess the correct vertical dimension. Straightening out the zygomatic arch and comparing with the contralateral side also help to achieve good position. The fragments are rigidly fixed with plates. Generally microplates are sufficient across the infraorbital rim where there is considerable advantage in their small size whilst heavier plates are placed at the FZ suture, the zygomatic buttress and across the zygomatic arch. To achieve stable fixation in three dimensions it is generally necessary to place fixation at least at three points.

By the nature of these injuries there are often gaps between the bone ends and although these can be bridged by plates, they should if possible be filled with bone graft to ensure a smooth postoperative contour. Small negative contour deformities often remain after repositioning of the zygoma and these can be filled out with bone chips or small onlays. Positive deformities can be burred down to smooth them off.

Nasoethmoid fractures

The nasoethmoid area poses some of the biggest challenges in secondary reconstruction. Small degrees of deformity, if symmetrical, may be acceptable but any degree of asymmetry is usually disfiguring and unacceptable to the patient. Although many patterns of fracture may present they are traditionally classified according to the size of the central canthal-bearing fragment.[11]

- *Type I*: these fractures exhibit a large central fragment consisting of the entire medial portion of the orbital rim with the medial canthal ligament attached to it.
- *Type II*: show disruption of the inner orbital frame into several pieces but with the ligament attached to a piece of bone of sufficient dimensions to allow direct fixation.
- *Type III*: the central fragment in these injuries is severely comminuted. There may be either complete avulsion of the canthal ligament or more usually it remains attached to a very small fragment of bone which is, however, too small to allow direct fixation.

There is some doubt as to the correlation of this classification with clinical outcomes and it is not frequently used. In secondary corrections the classification is also of less clinical relevance as the fractures have often by and large united.

Secondary deformity of the nasoethmoid region presents as flattening and foreshortening of the nose resulting in an upturned appearance to the nostrils. Traumatic telecanthus (Fig. 27.12) is cosmetically unacceptable not only because of the increased spacing of the eyes but also due to the blunting of the canthal angle at the medial end of the palpebral fissure. There may be associated injuries to the frontal sinus or the lacrimal drainage system. A dacrocystogram[12] is often a useful additional investigation in the assessment of these injuries.

In principle the approach to secondary correction is straightforward: mobilize or refracture the fragments and fix them in the correct position after reduction. Needless to say, the practice is very much less straightforward than the theory. The first step is to mobilize the bony nasal skeleton, including the lacrimal crest and, thus including the canthal

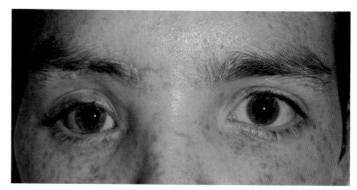

Fig. 27.12: Traumatic telecanthus.

attachment. It is imperative that if it remains attached, the canthal insertion is not stripped during the subperiosteal exposure, as it is rare to be able to perfectly recreate the normal anatomical configuration. The nasal complex tends to telescope inside the frontonasal region and reduction requires that the central nasal fragment is pulled out to length. Fixation of the nasal root to the frontal bone can be achieved by means of miniplates; an inverted Y plate often works well in this region (Fig. 27.13). If there are associated fractures of the frontal sinus these have to be repaired first.

The nasal bones at the time of secondary repair often appear to have healed well but are in fact often splayed. Simple fixation of the central fragment therefore would result in increased nasal width, militating against complete correction of telecanthus. This nasal widening is accentuated by the often significantly increased soft tissue thickness in this area as a result of previous injury. To combat these problems it is important to obtain as much skeletal narrowing as possible. In cases where there has been extensive comminution healing can result in the production of considerable

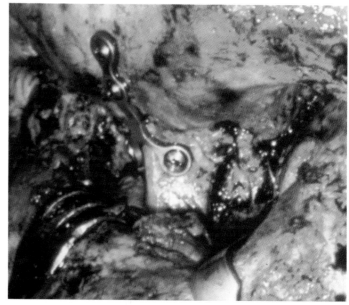

Fig. 27.13: Y plate used to stabilize nasal bridge. The inferior limbs of the Y can be compressed to give narrowing of the nasal bone and if sufficiently posterior the screw hole can anchor a suture passed through the medial canthus.

callus, which widens the nasal bridge. This needs to be reduced with a burr. The placement of a small plate horizontally across the bridge of the nose to compress the two sides into an acceptable shape is a useful maneuver. It is generally claimed that it is almost impossible to overcorrect traumatic telecanthus. When there is not a large central nasal fragment present bone grafting may be required to recontour the nasal bridge or to recreate the nasofrontal angle. Bone graft may also be required to reconstruct the medial orbital wall and to give a site to which the medial canthal ligament may be reattached. Calvarial bone grafts harvested from either the outer or inner table of the parietal skull are ideal for these purposes and are available via the surgical approach.

If there has been extensive comminution or loss of bone from the nasal area this is reconstructed by using a strut graft cantilevered off the frontal bone. In cases of secondary reconstruction scarring and contraction of the overlying skin may render the placement of a sufficiently large graft to give the required contour difficult. There is always a danger of too large a graft perforating through the overlying skin and care must be taken to avoid this complication.

Medial canthus

The reattachment of the medial canthus in those cases where it has been detached is one of the most demanding parts of any secondary reconstruction. Proper reduction of telecanthus depends critically on accurate repositioning of the medial canthal ligament. An understanding of the anatomy of the canthal ligament is crucial.[13] The medial canthal ligament is a complex three-dimensional structure and not a simple single ligament, as is often imagined. The key to optimal canthal reattachment is an appreciation of the fact that the true anatomical attachment is indeed more posteriorly placed than is often realized. When, as is often the case, the reattachment is placed too anteriorly a disappointing cosmetic result is obtained with the medial palpebral angle distracted from the globe. This produces an unsightly asymmetry even though the true intercanthal distance may be correct.

The nature of the canthal detachment determines the technique used for reattachment. Generally the canthus remains attached to a small fragment of bone and with the microplates available today, it is generally possible to obtain fixation of this canthal-bearing fragment to its anatomical position.[14] When this can be achieved with a good degree of solidity, a stable result can be expected. Rarely the canthus is avulsed from the bone and has no bony fragment attached to it. This situation makes identification of the canthus difficult, let alone reattachment. To aid in the identification of the canthal ligament the deep aspect of the inner canthal angle can be picked up with a fine pair of dissecting forceps. When traction is placed on the forceps in a medial direction the canthal angle is seen to move freely if the canthus has been correctly identified. If the medial end of the detached canthus remains elusive it can be located to the lacrimal sac by passing a needle through the canthal angle and identifying it on the deep surface posterior to the lacrimal sac. A fine wire suture is passed through the canthus and if properly identified, pulling on this wire should pull the canthal angle in the desired direction and reduce the telecanthus.

If this test is satisfactory some form of canthopexy must now be performed. It may be possible to perform a direct canthopexy, attaching the canthus to plates placed in the region of the anterior and posterior lacrimal crests. If there is a sufficiently substantial piece of bone in the correct position, 'tendon anchors'[15] may be used to attach the canthus. Both these means of direct canthopexy do have the advantage over the more traditional transnasal canthopexy of making it somewhat easier to obtain posterior positioning of the canthal attachment. When there is insufficient bone a transnasal canthopexy must be performed. The wire suture attached to the canthus is passed across the nasal skeleton and fixation achieved on the contralateral side.

Correct positioning of the holes to allow the passage of the wires through the nose is essential in order to obtain the desired direction of pull on the medial canthus. Placement of the holes is aided if there is any identifiable lacrimal crest or by reference to the contralateral side. The holes are made with a drill burr or nasal awl. As stated previously, it is important to place the holes further posteriorly than is often imagined. This can be technically quite challenging as it is often difficult to obtain the correct angulation of the drill to place these holes without interference from the globe.

After being passed through the nose the canthopexy wires are fixed to a small plate or screw on the opposite nasal bone. Where bilateral canthopexy is required wires are passed from either side of the nose. Fixation in these patients was always difficult and it used to be the practice to pass the wires back over the nasal bridge and twist the right and left wires together, thus producing a circumferential wire. With modern microplates this is rarely required and adequate fixation can usually be achieved. Tightening of the canthopexy wires is continued whilst measuring the intercanthal distance in order to achieve correct reduction. It is wise to overcorrect somewhat to allow for some relapse. Final tightening of the canthopexy is the last step in a secondary correction as once the canthal attachment has been re-established access to the medial orbital wall and lacrimal system is impeded.

It is often prudent to support the canthopexy from the cutaneous surface. This can be achieved by the use of clear acrylic buttons. It is important not to overtighten the button, as there is a risk of skin necrosis. This must be watched for and clear acrylic makes this more easily achieved.

Lacrimal system

The lacrimal system is often damaged in midfacial and especially nasoethmoid trauma. Obviously it is best if this is repaired early as the lacrimal system can become encased in dense scar tissue, making secondary repair very much more difficult. Problems can also arise with lacrimal drainage in the presence of a patent system. This problem arises when the medial eyelid is not in proper relationship to the lacus. Eyelid contraction and canthal malposition can be responsible for this problem. Investigation of the lacrimal system should be by means of a dacrocystogram.[10] Secondary repair by dacrocystorhinostomy is indicated but is technically challenging in the presence of often considerable scar tissue. The use of Lester Jones tubes is an alternative.

Technological Developments

Accurate reconstruction of the orbital volume and shape of the orbital floor in particular is essential for the correction of enophthalmos, as has been discussed previously. The advent of reformatted three-dimensional imaging, along with computer-generated modeling and CAD/CAM technology, has exciting possibilities for orbital reconstruction.[16,17] These techniques have been found to be particularly useful in some cases of secondary correction and also in cases of fibrous dysplasia of the orbit.

The process begins by obtaining CT data using either conventional thin-slice CT or helical scanning. The benefits of helical scanning are considerable in so much as it allows finer detail in 3D by effectively producing more slices for a given radiation dose. Imaging of the thin orbital walls demands the highest possible resolution to avoid the production of artefactual defects. A medical imaging workstation can reconstruct 3D representations from the data. Surface or contour displays of the soft tissue or bony surfaces may be visualized. Images can be viewed from any direction by simple manipulation of the on-screen image and accurate point-to-point measurements can be made. A second type of image can be obtained which provides three orthogonal slices (coronal, sagittal and transverse) at any selected point. The orientation of these slices is not fixed with respect to the original acquired slices which allows for rotation to correct for imprecise alignment of the patient in the scanner. Bilateral comparisons useful for orbital reconstruction are therefore feasible. Accurate orbital volume measurements can be made, arbitrarily shaped pieces can be isolated and subsequently moved around and operations can be simulated. Portions of the normal orbital anatomy can be isolated, duplicated, mirrored and transposed to the affected side to facilitate planned reconstruction.

Even without any further application of technology, the detail that can be gained from images of this quality greatly facilitates an accurate diagnosis and formulation of a treatment plan. As an example, accurate measurement of the posterior limit of orbital floor defects from the inferior orbital rim gives one far greater confidence in continuing with a posterior dissection without fear of coming across the optic foramen. It is worrying to see just how close the posterior edges of some large floor defects come to the optic foramen which is generally about 44 mm behind the orbital rim.

The development of computer-aided manufacture of models has greatly extended the scope of this technology. In the early days modeling was achieved using a removal process whereby, with a computer-guided milling machine, models were manufactured out of expanded polyurethane. Reproduction of undercuts was limited, with the more widely available machines with only three degrees of freedom, but more

expensive five-axis machines were capable of more accurate reproduction. The cost of such machinery was a serious limiting factor. The other main form of model construction under development was stereolithography. In contrast to milling, this is a constructive process where layer-by-layer polymerization of a curable resin is achieved by a computer-driven laser. This technology was capable of producing models of stunning accuracy but was both a lengthy and expensive process. More recently a wider range of model manufacturing processes have been developed, including surface deposition modeling, which have reduced the costs significantly. We have used this technology to manufacture custom-fabricated implants for enophthalmos correction and secondary orbital reconstructions.

Case 1: correction of late enophthalmos

A 37-year-old man had been involved in a skiing accident, sustaining an orbital floor injury, which had not been diagnosed at the time of injury. He subsequently presented with unsightly enophthalmos seeking secondary correction (Fig. 27.14a&b). Three-dimensional optical surface scanning clearly demonstrated the degree of enophthlamos.

Having obtained the appropriate data from helical CT scans, an examination of the images on the workstation allowed accurate identification of the defect in the orbital skeleton. A model of the affected region was manufactured. Using the computer, a mirror image of the normal side was obtained. Making the assumption, which is generally valid, of symmetry between the two orbits, the mirror image of the normal side is taken to represent the preinjury state of the affected orbit. By comparing the two models a custom-fabricated titanium implant (Fig. 27.15) was made to not

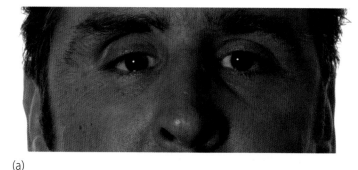

(a)

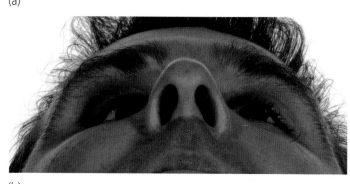

(b)

Fig. 27.14a&b: Full face and inferior view showing supratarsal hooding, enophthalmos and orbital dystopia.

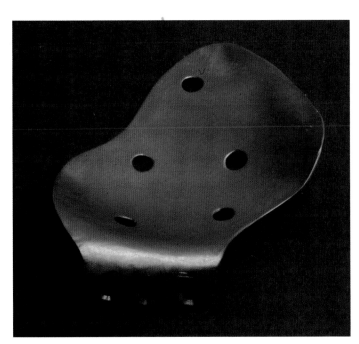

Fig. 27.15: A custom made titanium implant, perforated to allow screw fixation.

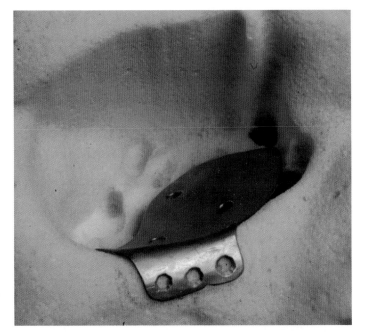

Fig. 27.16: The implant is seen on the computer generated model. It extends to cover the defect, is shaped to recreate the inferomedial bulge and the flange allows accurate localization and screw fixation to the orbital rim.

only reconstruct the defect but also to accurately recreate the normal contour of the orbital floor anatomy (Fig. 27.16). Using a standard transconjunctival approach with a lateral canthotomy, the orbital defect was identified. After freeing of the herniated orbital contents it was a simple matter to insert the prefabricated implant and secure it to the orbital rim. In addition to the greater accuracy of the orbital reconstruction achieved, a significant saving in theater time was also obtained (Fig. 27.17).

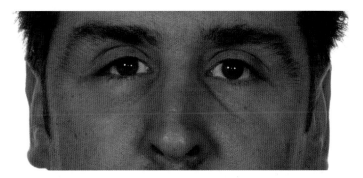

(a)

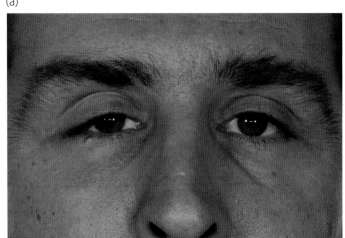

(b)

Fig. 27.17a&b: Postoperative view showing correction of orbital dystopia and significant improvement in enophthalmos. The slight ptosis seen in this image resolved fully about eight weeks postoperatively.

Case 2: orbital reconstruction

A 37-year-old woman presented for secondary orbital reconstruction of an orbital deformity (Fig. 27.18, 27.19 & 27.20). She had sustained an injury many years ago when as a teenager she had been kicked by a horse, sustaining a severe fracture of the right zygoma and loss of the right eye. She

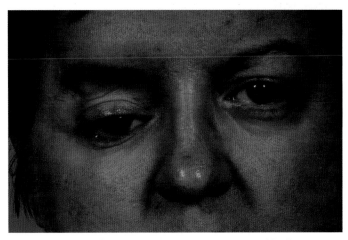

Fig. 27.18: Significant orbital dystopia, supratarsal hollowing and loss of cheek prominence.

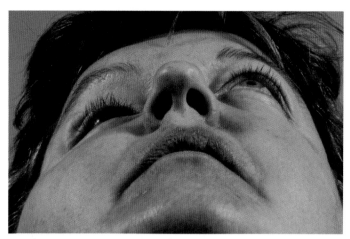

Fig. 27.19: Inferior view shows degree of enophthalmos, loss of malar projection and over-reduction of the zygomatic arch.

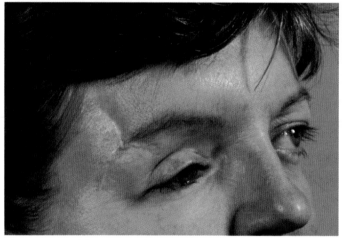

Fig. 27.20: Oblique view shows scarring and tethering of lateral canthus to retropositioned lateral orbital rim.

wore an orbital prosthesis and had had one previous attempt at orbital reconstruction by means of zygomatic osteotomy which had been unsatisfactory. This was due to overreduction of the zygoma with bowing of the zygomatic arch and inadequate projection of the right cheek.

It was decided to carry out a further zygomatic osteotomy but this time using a custom-fabricated titanium implant (Fig. 27.21 a&b) to recontour the right zygoma and reconstruct the orbital floor with the subsequent placement of a 'Medpore' sphere to give a dynamic ocular prosthesis. Three-dimensional images were obtained and a suitable model manufactured. This quite clearly identified the problems with the previous reconstruction. A zygomatic osteotomy is clearly required to reconstruct the correct contours of the orbital framework and in order to support an ocular prosthesis it is necessary to reconstruct the orbital floor.

A custom-fabricated titanium implant was fashioned by mirror-imaging the normal orbit; it had an orbital rim component and an extension to restore the orbital floor (Fig. 27.22 & 27.23). It was inserted via a coronal flap and an infraorbital incision. The zygomatic bone was osteotomized. The implant had been created to fit the normal bony contours of the orbital rim at the extent of the defect. It was fixed in position at these points and the osteotomized orbital rim advanced and fixed to it. By this means the implant acts as a template to reposition the zygomatic bone as closely as possible to its normal preinjury position (Fig. 27.24, 27.25 & 27.26).

Alternative applications

There is great flexibility in the application of this technology to orbital reconstruction. In the case described above an implant was manufactured to act as a template for repositioning of the orbital rim and also to reconstruct the orbital floor. It is not always necessary to osteotomize the orbital rim as it is possible to construct an implant that fits perfectly onto the

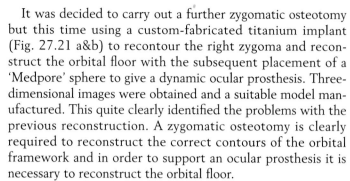

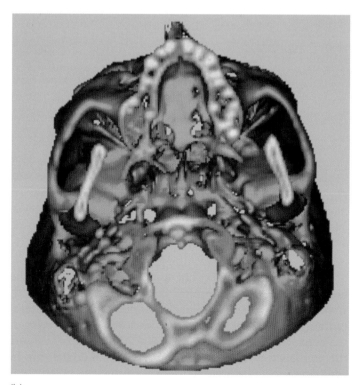

(a)

(b)

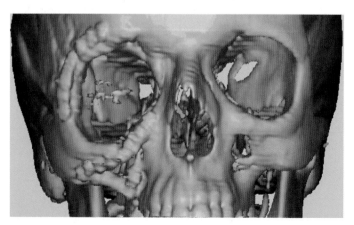

Fig. 27.21a&b: 3D reconstructions reveal underlying skeletal deformity.

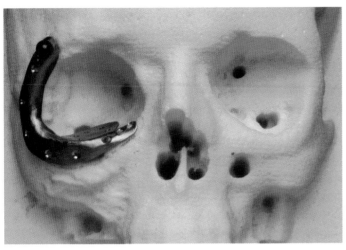

Fig. 27.22: Custom titanium implant extending from uninjured bone medially on the inferior rim to a correctly positioned rim above the FZ suture. An orbital floor extension reconstructs the defect.

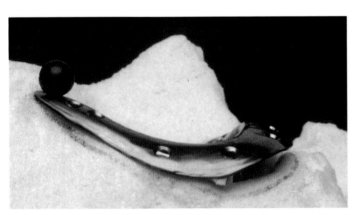

Fig. 27.23: The lateral view shows the degree of retroposition of the zygomatic complex. Advancement of the osteotomized zygomatic complex to this template ensures correct positioning.

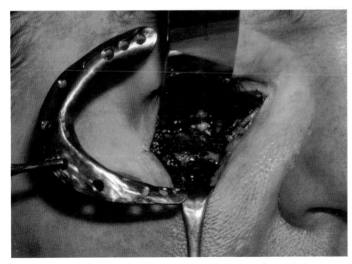

Fig. 27.24: Inferior orbital rim exposed via an infraorbital incision. The implant is visualized and the gap in the inferior rim after osteotomy can be seen.

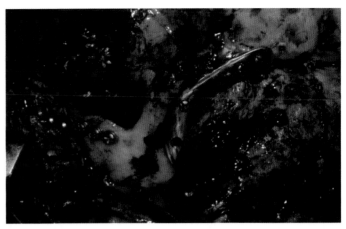

Fig. 27.25: The implant inserted and fixed via a coronal flap approach. The mobilized zygomatic complex has been advanced to the implant, the extent of which is demonstrated by the gap in the zygomatic arch.

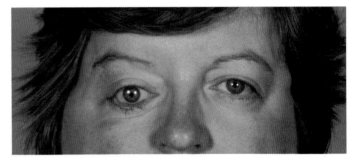

Fig. 27.26: Postoperative view.

existing bony contours and is itself shaped to reconstruct the normal anatomy, although in this scenario a much larger prosthesis is required. Alternatively it is possible to perform a mock osteotomy of the zygoma and orbital skeleton on a plastic model, marking the site of the bone cuts required. It is obviously straightforward on the model to reposition the bones to restore perfect symmetry. Suitable plates required to obtain fixation can be pre-bent on this mock-up and subsequently sterilized prior to surgery. This technique allows much greater precision in performing the required reconstruction and saves considerably in theater time as much of the work has been done preoperatively.

Soft Tissue Considerations

Accurate repositioning of the bony elements of the zygoma and orbital rim does not, sadly, on its own lead to uniformly successful results. This is largely due to the overlying soft tissue drape. The soft tissue changes associated with severe bony injuries are often underestimated and militate against good results in secondary reconstruction. Soft tissue injury may be evident at the time with extensive lacerations or degloving-type injuries. These types of injuries obviously leave scars but it is the more subtle soft tissue injuries which often contribute to secondary deformity. Tethering of the overlying soft tissue to areas of underlying bony injury may give very obvious deformity. Displacement of the cheek fat pad produces an obvious sagging of the face with accentuation of the nasolabial fold and apparent flattening in the infraorbital area.

For esthetic reconstruction the soft tissue elements must also be fully considered and after the completion of the bony skeletal reconstruction, the soft tissues must be redraped across the cheek. For the soft tissues to be mobilized sufficiently to allow redraping, extensive subperiosteal dissection is required to release any tethering. Deep plane face lift techniques are used to resuspend the soft tissue in their correct position. Subperiosteal sutures are used anteriorly to anchor the cheek fat pads to the inferior orbital rim and laterally a SMAS plication gives support to the tissue over the lateral cheek. If a coronal flap has been raised to gain access, excess skin can be excised to tighten the soft tissues when final suturing takes place as per a standard face lift.

Particular attention must be paid to the correct canthal position. The medial canthal position has been discussed above in terms of nasoethmoid injuries but the lateral canthal position is also of importance.

Unlike the medial canthal ligament whose attachment is generally preserved if at all possible, the lateral canthal ligament is routinely detached when raising a coronal flap. This is done as it significantly increases exposure whilst being relatively straightforward to reattach.

The lateral canthal ligament should be reattached to the lateral orbital rim in a slightly overcorrected position. This is best achieved by drilling a small hole at an appropriate point in the lateral orbital wall and suturing the ligament to it with a non-resorbable suture.

Minor contour irregularities often remain after bony reconstruction and are best managed by small onlay grafts.

Eyelids

Following orbital trauma asymmetry of the eyes is one of the most obvious deformities. Changes in the width of the palpebral fissure, canthal malpositions and lid abnormalities are immediately obvious. Ectropion is one of the more frequently seen lid problems. There are a number of possible etiologies of ectropion but in the posttraumatic scenario cicatricial ectropion is the most likely. Apart from the obvious esthetic deformity a number of functional problems may arise. These include drying of the eyes with corneal irritation and epiphora if the punctum is no longer in contact with the tear pool. There are six elements of pathology that may be present in an ectropic eyelid: horizontal lid laxity, medial canthal tendon laxity, punctal malposition, vertical tightness of the skin, orbicularis paresis and disinsertion of the lower eyelid retractors. One or more of these features may be present in any one lid. Accurate identification of the underlying anatomical abnormality allows selection of the appropriate procedure for surgical correction.

Post trauma, perhaps the most common cause of ectropion is vertical shortening of the anterior lamella, which pulls the eyelid away from the globe. Vertical shortening may arise from a single vertical scar crossing the lid margin. In these cases scar contraction leads to ectropion and there is often associated notching of the lower lid. Alternatively vertical tightness results simply from contraction of surgical approaches to the lower lid. Infraorbital incisions are more prone to late ectropion than transconjunctival approaches. Overenthusiastic suturing of the deeper layers is often responsible. It is recommended that only the periosteum over the orbital rim is closed and then the overlying skin.

Vertical shortening is best treated by either Z-plasty or skin grafting.

Z-plasty

By the utilization of a Z-plasty the tension in a scar can be released and the limbs of the scar reorientated in a more appropriate direction. The Z-plasty works by the principle of the transfer of tissue to reduce pull in one direction at the expense of a line perpendicular to it.

In the case of a vertical scar running across the lower eyelid, this releases the downward pull leading to ectropion and converts the scar to run parallel to the lid margin. The linear margins of the scar are outlined. A line is drawn from both the superior and inferior ends of the scar at 60° and in opposite directions. These lines should be equal to the vertical length of the scar. The old scar is excised by cutting round the markings and the lines drawn are incised. The resultant skin flaps when raised produce two equal triangles. These are undermined widely until they can be transposed with ease and without undue tension. The delicate skin flaps must be handled with care to avoid damage to the skin margin. The flaps are sutured in position with 6/0 nylon sutures. The lower lid should be supported and placed under some tension either by a temporary tarsorrhaphy or, more comfortably, by using a 'Frost' suture taped to the brow. For longer vertical scars two or more Zs can be placed along the vertical limb.

Skin grafting

Where the vertical shortening extends over a more diffuse area skin grafting is the treatment of choice. Both in terms of the functional result and for better esthetics, full-thickness grafts are preferable to split-thickness skin in the lower lid area. The skin can be harvested with relative ease from the postauricular area. A horizontal incision is made parallel to and some 2–4 mm below the lid margin. The incision is carried down to whatever depth is necessary to release all the scar bands and allow the eyelid to return to its normal position. A Frost suture is again used to place gentle upward traction on the lower lid. A template is fashioned from a suture packet and a full-thickness graft harvested from the post-auricular region. The graft must be thoroughly defatted before application. Meticulous hemostasis is required before placing the graft, as any hematoma beneath it will jeopardize survival. The graft is best secured using 6/0 silk sutures spaced evenly around the margins of the defect. Alternate sutures are left long to secure a proflavine bolus tie-over dressing, which should remain in situ for one week. As before, it is prudent to support the lower lid with a Frost suture for the first postoperative week.

Horizontal laxity

Horizontal laxity of the lower lid may manifest either medially or laterally (Fig. 27.27). It is the result of stretching of the medial or lateral canthal ligaments rather than elongation of the tarsal plate itself. A number of procedures are available for correction of this problem and include a full-thickness wedge excision of the lower lid with primary closure. Rather than excision of a simple wedge, resection of a pentagon of tissue gives better results. A criticism of this procedure is that it can lead to blunting of the lateral canthal angle and does not in itself address the underlying pathology of stretching of the lateral canthal tendon. The lateral canthal sling or tarsal strip procedure is most appropriate for these cases.

The procedure begins by making a lateral canthotomy with sharp scissors. This is deepened through the orbicularis till the lateral orbital rim is reached. The tip of a Freer elevator is placed just inside the lateral orbital rim and the periosteum is exposed but not incised. By pulling the lower lid in a medial direction the lower limb of the lateral canthal ligament can be felt as a tight band. The ligament is exposed and then divided. Once the cantholysis has been performed the whole lower lid becomes mobile. The ligament is grasped and put under tension, pulling laterally. Scissors are passed subconjunctivally and the lower lid divided along the gray line into anterior and posterior lamellae. The length of this incision in the gray line is determined by the amount of horizontal laxity that requires correction. Skin, orbicularis and conjunctiva are excised to the point where the new lateral canthus is to be fashioned. The newly fashioned lateral canthus is passed deep to the upper limb of the lateral canthus and reattached to the periosteum of the lateral orbital rim with a non-resorbable suture. There should be sufficient tension to slightly over-correct the horizontal laxity. The ligament should also be placed in a slightly more superior position than normal to allow for some minor degree of stretching. The lateral canthotomy is closed with 6/0 nylon sutures (Fig. 27.28).

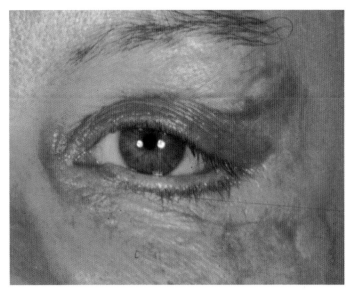

Fig. 27.28: Postoperative view showing tightening of the lower lid and elevation of the lateral canthus.

Materials for Orbital Reconstruction

Many materials have been described for use in the repair of bony orbital wall defects and whilst almost every material has some theoretical advantages or disadvantages, it remains fair to say that none of the available materials fulfill all the requirements of the ideal graft material.

- The material should be strong enough to support the orbital contents, without herniation into the defect.
- It should be available in thin sheets to bridge defects or be able to provide bulk for volume expansion.
- It should be easily shaped and molded to the complex anatomical shape required and should retain that shape without memory.
- It should remain dimensionally stable in the long term.
- It should be biocompatible.
- It should be resistant to infection.
- It should be radio-opaque whilst not producing scatter artefact, impairing future radiological investigations.

Autologous materials

- Bone (multiple donor sites)
- Septal cartilage
- Periosteum
- Fascia lata

Alloplastic materials

- Silastic
- Hydroxyapatite
- PTFE
- Coral
- Titanium
- PDS sheet
- PLLA

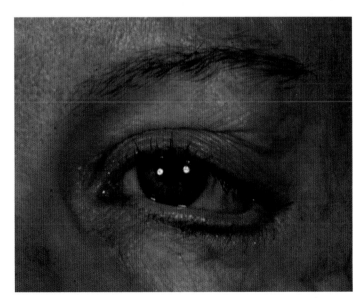

Fig. 27.27: Lateral ectropion and inferior displacement of the lateral canthus.

Working on the principle of replacing like with like then autogenous bone would be the obvious choice. Bone can be harvested from a number of sites; for small floor defects the contralateral antral wall[18] provides a suitably shaped and thin piece of bone. The morbidity associated with the harvest of such a graft is the least of the available donor sites. For larger grafts the calvarium and iliac crest are the most commonly used.

The calvarium has much to recommend it as a donor site for orbital reconstruction. If a coronal flap has been raised as part of the access for the reconstruction then the graft can be harvested without the need for any further incisions and negligible added morbidity. Even if the orbital floor is approached via a lid incision then only a small hemicoronal flap is required to harvest a suitable piece of bone. The calvarium produces sheets of graft of around 2–3 mm in thickness. After repair of the overlying scalp there is a barely noticeable defect in the skull. If for any reason a craniotomy is required as part of the reconstructive process then the calvarium can be split and the inner table used as graft before replacing the craniotomy. Calvarial bone is, however, very dense and there is a limit to the extent to which it can be shaped. Leaving the periosteum attached to the outer surface, however, allows the bone to be sectioned through its full thickness to give essentially a flexible sheet of bone and periosteum. The very dense nature of this bone is thought to be the reason why this appears to be the most dimensionally stable of the available grafts, particularly when rigidly fixed.

Iliac crest is a useful source of bone grafting material and can provide large quantities of bone. The bone is somewhat easier to shape than calvarial bone but does exhibit greater resorption. The donor site morbidity is higher and requires a second distant operative site.

In spite of the problems of donor site morbidity and lack of dimensional stability due to resorption, autogenous bone remains the material of choice for the reconstruction of large defects. It is less liable to infection and more tolerant of it should it arise. Septal cartilage offers a useful autologous alternative to bone;[19] it is easily accessible, relatively abundant and provides adequate support to the orbital floor. Donor site morbidity is negligible.

In a desire to avoid a donor site and overcome some of the problems associated with the use of autogenous bone, many alloplastic materials have been used in orbital reconstruction. Silastic (medical grade silicone polymer) was available in a range of thicknesses and in reinforced and plain forms. It was easy to cut to size and shape and was of sufficient strength to support the orbital contents, certainly in small and medium-sized defects, and as such became popular. As with all alloplastic materials, it was susceptible to infection and rates varying between 0.4% and 7% were quoted. Silastic promotes a foreign body reaction around it, taking the form of encapsulation of the implants in a dense non-adherent fibrous capsule. This fibrous capsule accounts for a number of problems that have been reported late after surgery (up to 20 years) of extrusion of the implants and chronic sinus formation.[20] As a result silastic has fallen out of favor and can no longer be recommended as a material for orbital reconstruction.

Titanium has been widely used in orbital reconstruction and has several advantages: it is generally presented in the form of a mesh and is available in sheets of varying thickness. It is malleable and therefore easily adapted to the shape of the orbital defect and yet has sufficient strength to be able to support the orbital contents when bridging relatively large defects. It is the most biocompatible of all the available materials. Because of the mesh structure, connective tissue can grow around and through the implant, thus preventing migration. This does, however, have the potential disadvantage of making the implant very difficult to remove should this ever be required. Titanium produces relatively little artefact on CT scanning and does not therefore preclude subsequent radiological assessment. The mesh structure allows for relatively straightforward fixation by placing screws through the mesh. Titanium can also be used in solid sheets and perhaps has its greatest potential when used in conjunction with modern CAD/CAM custom-fabricated implants.

Of the non-metallic alloplastic materials, Medpore (expanded PTFE) is perhaps the most commonly used. As with titanium, it is available in a number of thicknesses to offer varying degrees of support to the orbital contents. The thicker sheets, although having more strength, are more difficult to shape and the material has a degree of memory, tending to return to its original shape after placement. A useful presentation of Medpore is in a sheet form with channels incorporated in the material into which can be inserted plates to anchor and secure the material. This is generally achieved by cantilevering the sheet off the inferior orbital rim. Medpore has a rough surface into which connective tissue can grow to stabilize the implant. There are, however, a number of reported cases of infection and displacement and as with titanium mesh, removal can be difficult.

The appeal of a resorbable material, that would provide sufficient rigidity and support until bony healing followed by total resorption, is obvious. The advent of PDS sheet generated much excitement, as it initially appeared to offer these desired properties. As research results were published, however, a number of complications became apparent. Postoperative sequelae were common, including sensory disturbance, restriction of globe motility and enophthalmos developing after orbital repair. PDS is resorbed by a process of hydrolytic dissolution. Early loss of support after a period of only 4 weeks has been demonstrated which was not sufficient to allow adequate bony healing of the orbital defect. This study also demonstrated cyst-like 'lakes' associated with the implant material and so-called sterile sinus formation. It is now generally accepted that this material is not suitable for the repair of large defects.

Poly L-lactic acid/polyglycolic acid co-polymer (Lactosorb) has been investigated and shown to have potential for orbital floor repair.[21]

Conclusion

Secondary orbital deformities present some of the greatest challenges in the management of facial trauma. Advances in imaging and modeling have allowed a greater understanding of the anatomy of these injuries and, together with developments in plating technology and materials, have aided more accurate skeletal reconstructions. In spite of this, however, results are often disappointing for both the patient and surgeon. These limitations arise largely due to problems with the overlying soft tissues which may have shrunk, fibrosed and tethered. The challenges for the future are to better manage the skin integument to reflect the more accurate underlying reconstruction.

References

1 Manson PN, Clifford CM, Su CT, Iliff NT, Morgan R 1986 Mechanisms of global support and post-traumatic enophthalmos: 1 The anatomy of the ligament sling and its relation to intra-muscular cone orbital fat. Plastic and Reconstructive Surgery 77(2):193–202

2 Koorneef L 1977 Spatial aspects of the orbital fibro-muscular tissue in man. Swets and Zeitlinger, Amsterdam

3 Kreipke DL, Moss JJ, Franco JM et al 1982 Computed tomography and thin sectioned tomography in facial trauma. Plastic and Reconstructive Surgery 69:423

4 Bite U, Jackson I, Forbes G, Gehring D 1985 Orbital volume measurements in enophthalmos using three dimensional CT imaging. Plastic and Reconstructive Surgery 75:502–507

5 Manson PN, Grivas A, Rosenbaum A, Vannier M, Zinreich J, Iliff N 1986 Studies on enophthalmos: II Measurement of orbital injuries by quantitative computed tomography. Plastic and Reconstructive Surgery 77(2):203–214

6 Eppley BL, Custer PI, Sadove AM 1990 Cutaneous approaches to the orbital skeleton and periorbital structures. Journal of Oral and Maxillofacial Surgery 48:842–854

7 Ilankovan V 1991 Transconjunctival approach to the infraorbital region. A cadaveric and clinical study. British Journal of Oral and Maxillofacial Surgery 29:169–173

8 Appling WD, Patrinely JR, Salzer TA 1993 Transconjunctival approach vs subciliary skin-muscle flap approach for orbital fracture repair. Archives of Otolaryngology Head and Neck Surgery 119: 1000–1006

9 Wesley RE 1998 Transconjunctival approaches to the lower lid and orbit. Journal of Oral and Maxillofacial Surgery 56:1

10 Hammer B 1995 Orbital fractures: diagnosis, operative treatment, secondary corrections. Hogrefe and Huber, Seattle

11 Markowitz BL, Manson PN, Sargent L et al 1991 Management of the medial canthal tendon in nasoethmoidal fractures: the importance of the central fragment in classification and treatment. Plastic and Reconstructive Surgery 87:843

12 Gruss JS, Hurwitz JJ, Nik NA, Kassell E 1985 The pattern and incidence of nasolacrimal injury in nasoethmoid orbital fractures: the role of delayed assessment and dacrocystorhinostomy. British Journal of Plastic Surgery 38:116

13 Zide BM, McCarthy JG 1983 The medial canthus revisited – an anatomical basis for canthopexy. Annals of Plastic Surgery 11(1):1–9

14 Shore JW, Rubin PA, Bilyk JR 1992 Repair of telecanthus by anterior fixation of cantilevered miniplates. Ophthalmology 99(7):1133–1138

15 Okazaki M, Akizuki T, Ohmori K 1997 Medial canthopexy with the Mitek anchor system. Annals of Plastic Surgery 38(2):124–128

16 Zooneveld F, Van der Dussen M 1992 Three dimensional imaging and model fabrication in oral and maxillofacial surgery. Contemporary Maxillofacial Imaging 4:19–33

17 Perry M, Banks P, Richards R, Friedman EP, Shaw P 1998 The use of computer generated three-dimensional models in orbital reconstruction. British Journal of Oral and Maxillofacial Surgery 36(4):275–284

18 Lee HH, Alcaraz N, Reino A, Lawson W 1998 Reconstruction of orbital floor fractures with maxillary bone. Archives of Otolaryngology Head and Neck Surgery 124(1):56–59

19 Lai A, Gilklich RE, Rubin PA 1998 Repair of orbital blow-out fractures with nasoseptal cartilage. Laryngoscope 108(5):645–650

20 Sewall SR, Pernoud FG, Pernoud MJ 1986 Late reaction to silastic following orbital floor fracture. Journal of Oral and Maxillofacial Surgery 42:821

21 Cordewener FW, Bos RR, Rozema FR, Houtman WA 1996 Poly(l-lactide) implants for repair of human orbital floor defects: clinical and magnetic resonance imaging evaluation of long term results. Journal of Oral and Maxillofacial Surgery 54(1):9–13

22 Whitehouse RW, Battenbury M, Jackson A, Noble JL 1994 Prediction of enophthalmos by computed tomography after 'blow-out' orbital fracture. British Journal of Ophthalmology 78:618–620

23 Raskin EM, Millman AL, Lubkin V et al 1998 Prediction of late enophthalmos by volumetric analysis of orbital fractures. Ophthalmic Plastic and Reconstructive Surgery 14(1):19–26

28 Facial Nerve Injuries: Reconstruction, Reanimation and Masking Procedures

Rainer Schmelzeisen

Introduction

Aims

After facial nerve injuries the aim must be to provide the patient with a normal esthetic appearance of the face at rest and during animation. This aim can only be achieved with current techniques of micronerve reconstruction and/or muscle transposition and transplantation. Static procedures aim at an improved appearance of the patient's face at rest but fail to rehabilitate the patient during function as, for example, when expressing emotions and for swallowing and speaking. Most static procedures improve the patient's situation for a defined time period. However, decisions for treatment and selection of surgical procedures have to be made with regard to the individual patient's situation and his expectations, taking into account factors like general condition, age and type and degree of injury. The patient must be provided with the best possible individualized treatment.

Anatomy of the facial nerve

Injuries of the facial nerve not only cause a paresis of the target muscle. As the facial nerve is responsible for the range of facial expressions, injuries to the nerve cause serious disturbances in social life, since the translation of emotions to others is impaired.

As a mixed motor and sensory nerve with the main function of innervation of the muscles of voluntary facial expression, the facial nerve originates from the homolateral facial nucleus in the caudal pons. Cortical projections to the facial nuclei pass through the internal capsule into the pons where they diverge, innervating both the contralateral and homolateral nucleus.

Autonomic fibers from the greater petrosal nerve reach the sphenopalatine ganglion supplying the lacrimal and nasal minor salivary glands. Next within the facial canal, the nerve to the stapedius muscle exits, followed by the chorda tympani nerve providing taste efference from the anterior tongue as well as secretor motor efference to the submandibular gland approximately 5 mm proximal to the stylomastoid foramen.

As the facial nerve travels through the labyrinthine segment of the facial canal and the greater petrosal nerve (exiting anteriorly) and the geniculate ganglion resides anterior to the somatic motor fibers, turning at the first genoposteriorly into the tympanic or horizontal segment, the facial canal is smallest in diameter in this segment. Over 90%

of facial nerve injuries from blunt temporal bone trauma may occur in this region, resulting from the traction forces exerted by three branches.[1–3]

Whereas lesions proximal to the meatus and within segments of the fallopian canal cause disturbances of tear and saliva production, taste sensation, impairment of the stapedius muscle and different patterns of facial paralysis. Lesions distal to the stylomastoid foramen result in selective dysfunction of the facial muscles.

At the exit from the stylomastoid foramen, the facial nerve divides into the temporofacial and the cervicofacial branches. At the pes anserinus, five classic distal branches arise as the temporal, zygomatic, buccal, mandibular and cervical branches. The temporofacial branch anastomoses with the auriculotemporal nerve (V[3]) and divides into branches destined for the cutaneous muscles of the skull and face. It leaves as:

- superior buccal branches (buccinator, upper part of the orbicularis oris muscles)
- infraorbital branches (greater and lesser zygomatic muscles, levators of the upper lip and nasal alae, transverse and dilator nasal muscles)
- frontal and palpebral branches (palpebral part of the orbicularis oculi, frontal part of the epicranius muscles)
- temporal branches (muscles of the outer aspect of the external ear).

After the anastomosis of the cervicofacial branch with the auricular branch of the cervical plexus, the branch divides into several others in the region of the mandibular angle:

- inferior buccal branches (lower half of the orbicularis oris muscle)
- cervical branch (platysma) (Fig. 28.1).

Functional Problems

Causes of injuries

Unilateral palsy or paralysis of the face can generally be divided into damage above the upper motor neuron or damage involving the lower motor neuron and its distal termination upon the facial musculature. Supranuclear palsy spares the frontalis muscle because of the bilateral innervation of the nucleus from both cerebral hemispheres. In these supranuclear palsies, the facial involvement is often the most minor part of the patient's problem.

Lesions of the lower motor neuron usually involve the entire face. Nuclear lesions usually involve adjacent brainstem structures (abducens/trigeminal nerve). The part of the

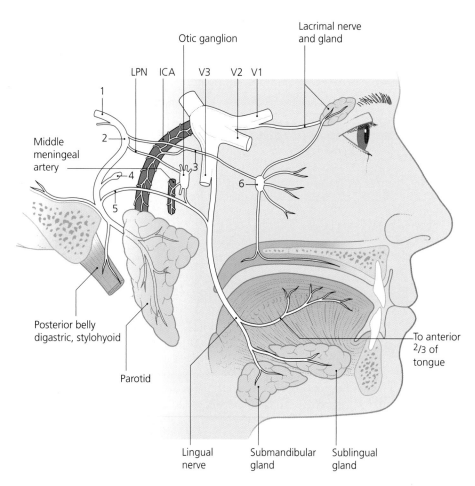

Otic ganglion

Lacrimal nerve
and gland

LPN ICA   V3   V2 V1

Middle
meningeal
artery

Posterior belly
digastric, stylohyoid

Parotid

Lingual
nerve

Submandibular
gland

Sublingual
gland

To anterior
2/3 of
tongue

Fig. 28.1: Schematic drawing of the facial nerve. 1. Facial nerve. 2. Geniculate ganglion. 3. Greater petrosal nerve. 4. Stapedius branch. 5. Chorda tympani. 6. Sphenopalatine ganglion.

nerve most commonly damaged appears to lie within the facial canal and at each end of the canal.

The largest etiological category of facial palsy is idiopathic facial ('Bell's') palsy, often diagnosed by exclusion of other etiologies.[3] It is characterized by a rapid onset of unilateral facial palsy including movements of the forehead, orbicularis oculi, perioral muscles and platysma. Defective taste sense (anterior two-thirds of the tongue) and hyperacusis may additionally be present. The etiology of Bell's palsy is still unknown. There are a number of other causes of facial nerve palsies which are listed in Box 28.1.

Central upper facial nerve injuries may occur due to tumor surgery at the cerebellopontine angle or result from skull base fractures or trauma.[4,5] In its extracranial course, the facial nerve is most often injured by sharp lacerations. However, the most frequent cause of injury is iatrogenic during resection of tumors in the parotid gland. Under these conditions, immediate microsurgical repair, including the use of grafts, is indicated. Resecting malignant parotid gland or skull base tumors may necessitate the resection of branches of the facial nerve or the nerve itself. It must be decided on an individual basis whether a primary reconstruction of the facial nerve using nerve grafts is indicated.

Investigation of facial nerve functions

In clinical investigation of a patient with a facial palsy, determination of onset characteristics is very important. In

patients with Bell's palsy, an acute onset, such as on waking up in the morning after normal facial motion the night before, is typical. Sudden onset may also be present in infectious or inflammatory problems (i.e. herpes zoster oticus, multiple sclerosis). Patients with tumors usually demonstrate progressive paresis over long periods with initial mild symptoms (such as weakness of labial depressor muscle).

In trauma patients, a delayed onset of facial palsy has a significantly better prognosis than in patients with immediate onset.[2] Associated symptoms may also indicate certain diseases. Oral pain, respiratory infections and hearing loss may accompany acute otitis media, whereas initial fever, arthritis and neuropathies may be indicative of Lyme disease. Also herpes zoster oticus shows typical additional symptoms (vesicular eruptions, severe pain).

Temporal bone neoplasms may cause other cranial nerve involvements (cochlear/vestibular nerves, ninth, 10th, 11th nerves → jugular foramen, fifth, sixth and seventh nerves → temporal bone). Lesions of the second, third, fourth and sixth cranial nerves may suggest multiple sclerosis.[2]

First, a careful observation of voluntary facial movements is undertaken. The symmetry of forehead wrinkling is investigated when the patient is asked to raise the brows. A functioning orbicularis oculi muscle allows for a complete closure of the eyelids and absence of visible upward rotation and exposure of sclera (Bell's phenomenon).

A forced wide smile distinguishes symmetries of the perioral muscles depending on the buccal and marginal mandi-

Box 28.1 Causes of facial nerve palsy

Congenital	Moebius syndrome (congenital nuclear aplasia) (possibly + palsy of external rectus muscles)
	Myotonic dystrophy
	Melkersson–Rosenthal syndrome + lingua plicata, swelling of the face/upper lip
	Congenital cholesteatoma/congenital facial nerve palsy
Neurologic	Myasthenia gravis
	Multiple sclerosis
	Guillain–Barré syndrome
Neoplastic	Facial nerve tumors (schwannoma, neurofibroma, neurogenic sarcoma)
	Glomus tumors (glomus jugulare/-tympanicum)
	Others (meningioma, acoustic neuroma)
	Parotid tumors
	Temporal bone/external auditory canal tumors
Infectious	Otitis media
	Bacterial causes (diphtheria, tuberculosis)
	Viral causes (herpes zoster oticus, mumps, infectious mononucleosis)
Other causes	Toxic
	Metabolic
	Idiopathic
Iatrogenic	Parotidectomy
	Rhytidectomy
	Lateral skull base surgery
Traumatic	Temporal bone fractures (longitudinal, transverse)
	Penetrating trauma (gunshot)
	Facial lacerations
	High altitude palsy

bular branches. Comparison of the depth of the nasolabial fold and the symmetrical contraction of the platysma muscle is also important. The Schirmer test measures tear production over a 5-minute period.

Objective methods of determining the secretory function of the parotid and submandibular glands exist. Pure taste sensation may be investigated by using samples of sweet, bitter, acid and salty substances on the anterior tongue. An audiologic investigation may reveal the dysacusis caused by a non-functional stapedius muscle which usually moves the tympanic membrane inwards for sound absorption. Laboratory tests of sedimentation rate, treponemal antibody titer and Lyme disease titer are scheduled. High-resolution CT is indicated in patients where temporal bone diseases, as for example skull base fractures, are suspected. MR is indicated in order to detect lesions at the cerebellopontine angle. The

typical symptoms of different facial nerve injuries are demonstrated in Box 28.2.

The House–Brackman classification is usually used for rating of facial palsy. Grade I refers to normal function without weakness while slight facial asymmetry with a minor degree of synkinesis is classified as grade II. Obvious but not disfiguring asymmetry, for example with contracture and/or hemifacial spasm but residual forehead movement, is judged as grade III. Grade IV represents obvious, disfiguring asymmetry with lack of forehead motion and incomplete eye closure. Asymmetry at rest and only slight facial movement is rated as grade V. Complete absence of tone or motion is grade VI.[6]

Today, routinely electromyography (EMG) and electroneurography are employed. In cases of acute injury, nerve excitability tests are used but normal results are less reliable than abnormal results, as functional deficits may also occur at a later time. Electromyography analyzes the function of the muscles during needle insertion and gives information on the existence of spontaneous activity/action potentials from voluntary muscle contraction. Spontaneous activity indicates a pathologic process within the nerve while fibrillation potentials may be a sign of nerve disruption.

During evoked electromyography a supramaximal stimulus is applied at the skin surface near the stylomastoid foramen. Intact axons will provide action potentials recorded distally. In facial nerve injury the amplitude of the action potential is defined as a percentage of the normal side. Magnetic transcranial and electrical stylomastoid stimulation allow for differentiation of lesions and distinction between central and peripheral facial nerve palsy.[7,8]

Principles

State of the art in surgical management

When the distal facial nerve branches and musculature are intact, reinnervation from the proximal facial nerve is ideal. Reinnervation using another motor nerve may be indicated if the proximal facial nerve cannot be identified. Cases with partial return of nerve function are always problematic. The danger of destroying functional nerve branches by a surgical procedure must be weighed against the possible advantages of reconstructive procedures.

Four basic strategies are applied for surgical correction of facial paralysis:

- direct micronerve reconstruction in given indications
- transfer of 12th nerve to the stump of the facial nerve
- cross-face nerve graft from facial branches on the normal side to the paralyzed side
- free vascularized muscle grafts.

According to the types of nerve injury and the general chance of a spontaneous regeneration in neuropraxia and axonotmesis, exact information about the mechanism of facial nerve injury is mandatory. In cases of a sharp transection in the absence of significant adjacent soft tissue trauma or infection, immediate primary management by a well-trained operating team may be indicated.

Box 28.2 Typical symptoms of different facial nerve injuries

Complete peripheral facial paralysis	Ipsilateral forehead: absence of frontalis function Brow ptosis No closure of upper eyelid Drooping of lower eyelid In closing the eyelids, the globe rotates upwards, resulting in a visible sclera (Bell's phenomenon) Absence of nasolabial fold, corner of mouth droops downward Generalized flattening of the face
Central facial paralysis (cerebral vascular accident; tumor above the level of the facial nucleus)	Function of both frontalis muscles and orbicularis oculi preserved (uncrossed fibers will maintain innervation to the upper face) Bell's phenomenon not present Involuntary emotion expression often preserved
Lesion of the facial nucleus in the pons	Symptoms like peripheral paralysis Tear and saliva production preserved Taste sensation of the anterior two-thirds of the tongue preserved (intermedial nerve enters the facial nerve caudally)
Facial nerve lesions at the cerebellopontine angle cephalad to internal auditory meatus (i.e. acoustic neuroma)	Complete peripheral facial paralysis Tearing, salivation and taste often abnormal (intermedial nerve approaches the internal auditory meatus) Stapedius muscle function impaired
Facial nerve lesion caudal to the geniculate ganglion/cephalad to the stapedial branch	Complete peripheral facial paralysis (e.g. lesion at the internal auditory meatus) Exception: lacrimal gland production preserved (greater petrosal nerve an sphenopalatine ganglion) Lesions between the stapedial nerve and the chorda tympani: normal tear production, normal stapedial muscle function with complete peripheral facial paralysis Lesions caudal to the chorda tympani: peripheral extracranial paralysis
Facial nerve lesion at the stylomastoid foramen	Complete peripheral nerve paralysis (no disturbance of tear/saliva production, taste, stapedius muscle function)
Lesions occurring within the confines of the parotid gland	Selective paralysis of voluntary motor functions Paralysis of temporal branch: asymmetric motion to the forehead, some dysfunction of the upper and possibly the lower eyelids Paralysis of zygomatic branch: paralysis of the muscles zygomatic major, minor, levator anguli oris, levator superioris: impairment of smile Paralysis of buccal branch: buccinator muscle, orbicularis oris muscle distortion: buccozygomatic connections make complete branch dysfunction rare Paralysis of mandibular branch: innervates muscles triangularis, risorius, quadratus labii inferiores, mentalis, orbicularis oris: asymmetry of smile, affected commissure pulled upward and internally rotated Paralysis of cervical branch: innervation of platysma, little functional loss in cases of injury

Often, it is not known what type of nerve injury is present. Although peripheral dissected facial nerve branches are identified under magnification or with electric stimulation, the clinical consequences of these injuries often cannot be judged immediately. Therefore, in primary wound closure, suspected branches of the facial nerve are marked with non-resorbable sutures. The suture material is positioned at the external wound surface in order to identify the nerve fibers at a later stage. This allows judgment of the clinical consequences of a nerve injury and performance of micronerve anastomosis in sterile conditions. Primary nerve grafting procedures are avoided.

Nerve reconstruction in general is performed 3–4 weeks following the injury by using direct nerve anastomosis or placement of a nerve graft.

Reconstructions of the facial nerve are limited by the atrophy of the musculature which occurs approximately 6–12 months following the injury. Reanimation procedures like faciofacial and seventh to 12th nerve anastomosis are performed not earlier than 6–12 months following the trauma. In long-standing facial nerve palsy, muscle grafts are often necessary due to the increasing atrophy of the facial muscles.

Microsurgical techniques

In all microsurgical techniques for facial nerve reconstruction, attempts should always be made to get impulses from the ipsilateral facial nerve, for example by a surgical preparation of the nerve out of the tumor or by the use of nerve grafts. If these possibilities do not exist, other procedures (i.e. 12th to seventh procedures) may be considered.

In cases of primary or early secondary nerve reconstruction following a defined injury, direct identification and preparation of the nerve stumps in general are possible. Coaptation or grafting techniques can then be performed easily.

In secondary microsurgical nerve repair, exploration of the site of the lesion and the stumps of the facial nerve always follows a certain order, especially in cases of peripheral facial nerve palsies in which the injury or the extent of the injury is uncertain.

It is easy to identify the facial nerve stumps which have been marked with sutures beforehand. In older secondary lesions, this is not possible and in these cases, the first step is the systematic preparation of the extratemporal course of the central facial nerve.[10–12,20] The identification of the nerve at the stylomastoid foramen has to be regarded as the approach of choice and tracing the nerve back from the periphery should be attempted only where the central approach is not possible.

The skin incision runs in an anteriorly curved fashion into the submandibular neck fold. The skin can then be dissected away from the fascia of the parotid gland. The cartilaginous auditory canal and the pointer, an anterior extension of the cartilage, are identified. The main trunk of the facial nerve lies approximately 1 cm caudal to that pointer at the transition level between the cartilaginous and osseous auditory canal. If the origin of the sternocleidomastoid muscle at the mastoid and the biventer muscle are additionally prepared, the facial nerve trunk lies cranial to the angle created by these two muscles (Fig. 28.2).

For further preparation, the fibrous tissue fibers between the parotid gland and osseous auditory canal are separated step by step and crossing vessels are coagulated. Fatty tissue cranial to the facial nerve is mobilized anteriorly. Then the approximately 2 mm thick facial nerve stump is identified with the help of a nerve stimulator. The division into its main branches usually occurs after 1 cm. With a small trunk scissors, the tissue overlying the nerve is dissected away from the nerve and elevated. With a second scissors this tissue is transsected. In this manner, the branches are traced into the periphery of the gland. For peripheral branches, the marginal branch may be identified best. It lies lateral to the superficial neck fascia and crosses the facial artery and vein. Via the submandibular skin incision, it can be identified at the lateral surface of the submandibular gland and then traced dorsally.

At the superior border of the parotid gland, the temporal and zygomatic branches leave the parotid gland and are iden-

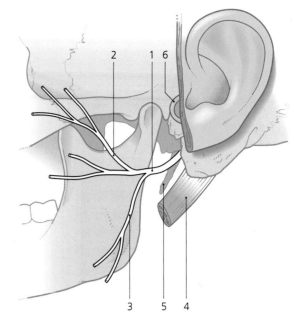

Fig. 28.2: Identification of the facial nerve. 1. Facial nerve. 2. Temporofacial branch. 3. Cervicofacial branch. 4. Digastric muscle. 5. Styloid process. 6. Cartilaginous pointer.

tified below the zygomatic arch in the subcutaneous tissue. The buccal branches are found cranial to Stensen's duct.

After identification of the nerve branches, the first procedure in surgical intervention is external neurolysis with preparation of the tissue surrounding the nerve and resection of the scarred perineurium. If the nerve itself is scarred, intraneural neurolysis is performed in order to remove cicatricial compression of the nerve fiber bundles caused by an epineural or paraneural scar. Healthy perineurium is left intact in order not to interrupt blood supply to the individual nerve bundles and the exchange of fibers between the various fascicles.

Following neurolysis, the nerve is moved away from the scar tissue bed and placed into healthy tissue to avoid further scar formation.

Direct nerve suture nerve grafts

When the nerve is interrupted, a direct suture of the nerve stumps may be performed without tension. As the facial nerve is mono- or oligofascicular at its central aspect with polyfascicular branches, we do not perform an interfascicular preparation and suture. The main trunk of the facial nerve and small distal branches are repaired by epineural sutures that are technically easier and provide less surgical trauma to the inner nerve structures. Depending on the nerve diameter, two, four or six 10.0 nylon sutures are applied.

In nerve coaptation, fibrous tissue proliferation at the sutured area may endanger axons arising from the central nerve stump and may impair penetration of the axons into the distal stump. Secondarily, already regenerated axons may be compromised by scar formation. Fibrous tissue formation may be initiated by traumatization of the nerve ends, interpositioning of blood clots between the nerve stumps and application of tension.

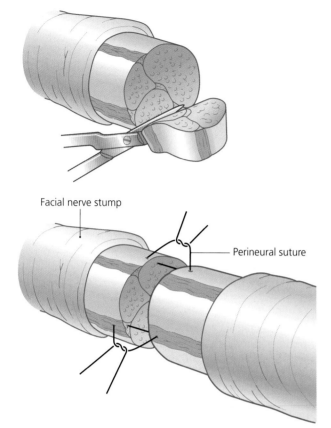

Facial nerve stump

Perineural suture

Fig. 28.3: Perineural suture technique. If an epineural suture technique is chosen, the epineurium is not stripped back. Before suturing, the fascicles are trimmed, before the anastomosis is performed.

As the epineural fibroblasts proliferate faster than the fibroblasts in the Schwann cells of the endoneural space, the epineurium at the central nerve stump may be carefully diminished. In order to have a smooth nerve surface, the protruding axons are cut to facilitate adaptation of the stumps.

With a (saw-type) scissors, the nerve is cut in a definitively uninjured area and existing central neuroma is resected. The epineurium is shortened and after further trimming of the axons, the needle is passed superficially through the fibrous tissue sheath (epi-/perineurium). The knots are cut short in order to avoid foreign material reactions in the vicinity of the sutures. Torsions of the nerve stumps must be avoided (Fig. 28.3).

Nerve grafts

End-to-end coaptation can only be performed following sharp injury of the facial nerve. Following tumor resection of malign parotid tumors, larger nerve defects necessitate nerve grafting as well as in secondary posttraumatic defects following resection of neuromas. Appropriate donor sites must be easily accessible and cause minimal donor site morbidity.

The great auricular nerve can easily be found below the auricle on the external surface of the sternocleidomastoid muscle.

The sural nerve can be exposed by an oblique incision behind the lateral malleolus. After exposing the sural nerve, its further

course is identified by pulling the nerve and palpation in the proximal direction. By additional horizontal incisions at 6–8 cm distances the nerve can be followed up to below the knee. The proximal end is cut and the nerve is mobilized at its distal side. Thereby long grafts which are also suitable for cross-face grafts can be harvested (Figs 28.4, 28.5).

The technique of aligning the stumps of the recipient nerve and the transplanted nerve is similar to end-to-end suturing. If the cross-sections of the stumps of the recipient and transplanted nerve do not fit with each other in size, it is possible to use two or even more grafts for bridging. Particularly in reconstruction of the branches of the facial nerve, the distal diversions of the sural and great auricular nerves allow for one central nerve anastomosis and several anastomoses in the periphery to the distal branches of the facial nerve (Fig. 28.6).

Table 28.1 Functional results following microneurosurgical reconstruction of the facial nerve performed at the Department of Oral and Maxillofacial Surgery, Medical University, Hanover. Results were evaluated according to the modified method of Fisch & Rouleau[40]

Patient no.	Int. T/R	t (months)	T	Outcome (points)
1	2 months	77	Graft	75
2	–	58	Graft	100
3	48 months	66	Graft	60
4	5 days	105	Graft	72
5	5 days	24	End-to-end	83
6	–	48	Graft	75
7	36 months	104	Graft	30
8	12 months	18	VII–XIIn	72
9	7 months	51	VII–XIIn	30

Int. T/R = interval between trauma and reconstruction
t (months) = follow-up investigation after n months following reconstruction
T = technique
Outcome (points): 30–50 points = poor result
        51–70 points = moderate result
        71–90 points = good result
        91–100 points = normal facial nerve function

Table 28.2 Photographic evaluation following reconstruction of the facial nerve (n = 9)

Score	No. of patients	%
91–100 excellent (normal)	1	11.1
71–90 very good	5	55.6
51–70 good	1	11.1
30–50 moderate	2	22.2
≤29 bad	0	0
Total	9	100

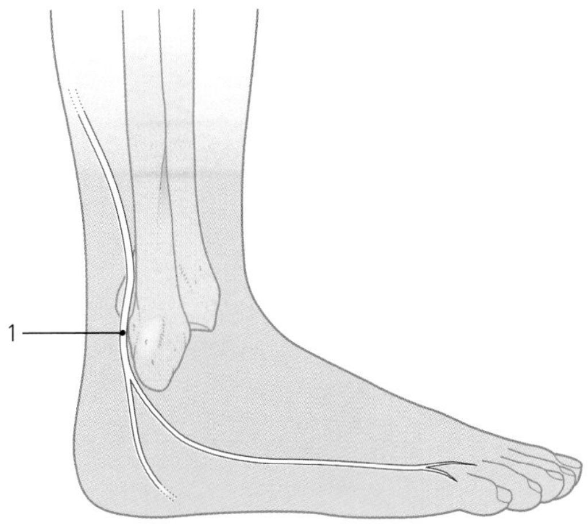

Fig. 28.4: (a,b) Harvesting of a sural nerve graft. Incision of the skin at the external surface of the lower leg 1 cm dorsal to the lateral malleolus. After identification of the sural nerve medial to the peroneal artery, the nerve is traced cranially. According to the length of the graft required, several additional horizontal incisions are performed. 1. Sural nerve. 2. Short saphenous vein. 3. Peroneal artery.

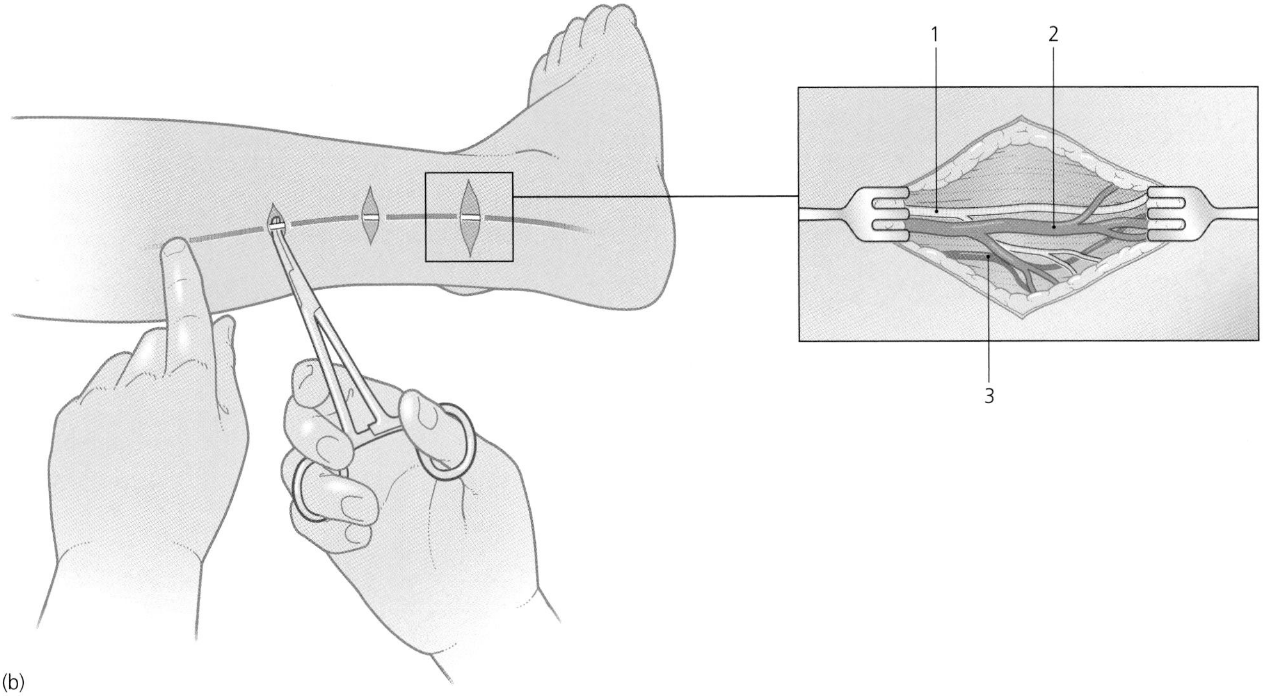

From the main trunk three grafts may be placed to the main distal branches. Also two grafts may be coapted to the upper and lower branches bypassing the central branches in order to prevent mass movements of the midface.[9] In cases with potential malignant neural invasion the contralateral greater auricular nerve may be used.

Immediate nerve grafting gives the best functional results.[10] The postoperative results following facial nerve reconstruction correlate with the delay between trauma and reconstruction (Tables 28.1, 28.2).

Reanimation techniques

Anastomosis of 12th to seventh nerves

If the proximal facial nerve cannot be used for anastomosis, nerve crossover techniques are indicated in general not earlier than 9–12 months after the injury. Young patients seem to demonstrate less nerve and muscle atrophy, allowing for late crossover procedures even after several years.[11]

In cases when a direct nerve suture is not indicated, another motor nerve may be chosen as a donor motor nerve. In most cases, the hypoglossal nerve is selected which can easily be detected underneath the intermediate tendon of the biventer muscle. The nerve is traced dorsally onto the surface of the carotid artery. Classic techniques recommend a total resection of the nerve distal to the descending branch. The complete hypoglossal nerve stump is then coapted to the peripheral facial nerve stump (Fig. 28.7).

The hypoglossal/facial nerve anastomosis may cause additional functional problems for the patient. Tongue atrophy with functional disturbance of swallowing, speech and mastication may occur following complete interruption of the hypoglossal nerve. Therefore a modified coaptation technique using the descending branch or by splitting the hypoglossal nerve is favored. The hypoglossal nerve may only be partially severed so that only one-third or one-half of the nerve is coapted with the nerve graft.[12–16]

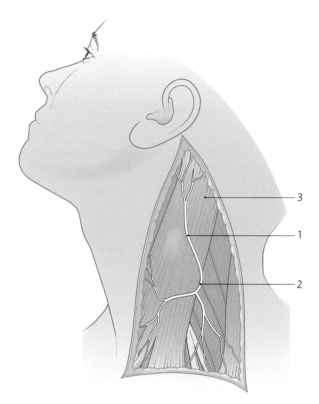

Fig. 28.5: Harvesting of a great auricular nerve graft. Vertical incision lateral to the sternocleidomastoid muscle. 1. Great auricular nerve. 2. Transverse cervical nerve. 3. Sternocleidomastoid muscle.

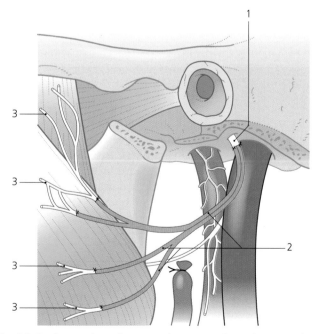

Fig. 28.6: Coaptation of two sural nerve grafts at the central stump of the facial nerve with peripheral splitting of the grafts for anastomosis with the facial nerve branches. 1. Central stump of the facial nerve. 2. Grafts. 3. Peripheral branches of the facial nerve.

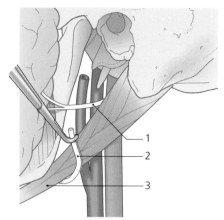

Fig. 28.7: Schematic drawing of hypoglossal–facial nerve anastomosis. First the anterior border of the sternocleidomastoid muscle is identified. The hypoglossal nerve is identified underneath the biventer muscle; its proximal segment crosses the carotid artery. The hypoglossal nerve is sectioned after extending the parotidectomy approach into the submandibular fold. 1. Facial nerve. 2. Hypoglossal nerve. 3. Biventer muscle.

Cross-face grafts

Reinnervation of the paralyzed side with a cross-face nerve graft requires division of facial nerve branches on the undisturbed side to serve as axon donors. The donor branches are chosen from the buccozygomatic region which has extensive crossbranching, as opposed to the single temporal or marginal mandibular branches. Careful selection of redundant buccozygomatic branches of the facial nerve on the normal side does not ultimately impair the motions of eye closure, smile or pucker.

Thirty to forty percent of the healthy facial nerve branches are severed and coapted to corresponding peripheral branches of the paralyzed side with sural nerve grafts of adequate length. The advantage of the procedure is the emotional correlation of both sides of the face.

The cross-face procedure may be performed with the grafting procedure on the healthy side and a coaptation to the paralyzed facial nerve branches 4 months afterwards. However, more often the procedure is performed as one stage.

Following cross-facial nerve grafts, transient weakness of the risorius and zygomatic muscles on the healthy side is observed but movement of the normal hemiface does not appear to be permanently affected.[17] Particularly in cross-face grafts, the degree of recovery is critically dependent on time after onset of the facial palsy.[18] However, clinical experience shows that not all expectations about ideal symmetrical function co-ordinated with the healthy side are fulfilled, probably also due to a progressive atrophy of the mimic musculature.

Following cross-facial nerve grafting which was performed prior to transplantation of a pectoralis minor muscle graft, the number of regenerating axons was not correlated with age, nor with regeneration time. Lack of a distal connection does not appear to lead to secondary degeneration of the regenerated myelinated fibers which stayed in an immature state for months.[19–21]

Free vascularized muscle grafts

The main indication for microneurovascular free muscle transplantation is in cases of facial paralysis in which primary or secondary nerve repair will probably not produce a successful result, for example in cases where the facial muscles have severely degenerated. Other indications are primarily unsuccessful procedures with nerve grafting or local muscle transposition.

The first clinical application of vascularized gracilis muscle grafts was described by Harii et al in 1976.[22] A great variety of muscle grafts, including the pectoralis minor, latissimus dorsi, rectus abdominis, extensor digitorum brevis and abductor hallucis longis, were described for reconstruction in longstanding facial palsies. These muscle grafts also allow for complex reanimation procedures of the face. The latissimus dorsi muscle is used for substitution of the zygomatic and levator labii muscles, whereas the serratus anterior segment is used for substitution of the depressor labii muscles. Today, the gracilis muscle is regarded as one of the muscle grafts of choice because it is relatively easy to harvest, has great versatility and leaves no donor site problems. The main indication for (gracilis) muscle transplantation is the recovery of the smile which requires relatively strong muscle power and good excursion.[22–26]

The gracilis muscle originates from the inferior ramus of the pubic bone and inserts at the medial aspect of the tuberosity of the tibia (pes anserinus). Proximally, the muscle is located superficial to the adductor longus and magnus muscles and distally it is located in the vicinity of the sartorius and the semimembranosus and semitendinosus muscles. The vascular supply is via the medial circumflex femoris artery originating from the deep femoral artery. The average diameter of the artery is 1.5 mm and it is generally accompanied by two veins. The muscle is innervated by the obturatorius branch lying proximally to the vascular pedicle (Fig. 28.8).

Prior to the operation, the position of the nasolabial fold on the healthy side as well as the direction and amount of excursion of the corner of the mouth is transferred and marked on the paralyzed cheek. With these permanent markings, the patient enters the operating room.

The paralyzed cheek is widely undermined through a pre-auricular facelift incision extending into the submandibular fold where suitable recipient vessels are identified. As the temporal vessels and especially the superficial temporal vein are often very fragile, in general they are not used for vascular anastomosis.

The undermining starts just above the superficial parotid fascia and extends slightly into the upper and lower lip where the lateral portion of the remnants of the orbicularis oris muscles is exposed. Stay sutures are placed at the orbicularis oris muscle in the upper and lower lips as well as in the modiolus. Then additional sutures are placed in these three positions described above for later fixation of the distal portion of the muscle. The effect of the fixation sutures has to be repeatedly tested by pulling the sutures cranially. These sutures determine the effect of the muscle pull later applied. Care has to be taken not to fix the sutures too superficially underneath the skin to avoid creating unnatural folds.

Harvesting of the gracilis muscle

Usually the muscle is harvested from the side contralateral to the palsy. The surgeon stands opposite to the leg. The patient is placed in a supine position with the knee flexed and the hip abducted. A line is drawn between the pubic tubercle and the medial condyle of the tibia, the gracilis muscle being positioned posterior to that line. At the proximal upper leg, a 10 cm incision is made along the posterior border of the adductor longus muscle. After separation of the fascia overlying the adductor longus and gracilis muscles, that can be identified by the straight orientation of the muscle fibers, the vascular pedicle is approached beneath the adductor longus muscle. The vascular pedicle enters the muscle approximately 8–10 cm distal to the pubic tubercle and runs on the surface of the adductor brevis muscle. When the pedicle is traced to its origin at the deep femoral vessels, several small vascular branches, which enter the adductor longus muscle, have to be clipped carefully. The motor nerve originating from the obturator nerve enters the muscle in the vicinity of the vascular pedicle but then runs more proximally in an oblique fashion towards the hip.

With a nerve stimulator, a muscle segment of adequate length and contractility can be identified. In order to avoid too much muscle bulk, the anterior segment of the muscle can be separated from the residual gracilis muscle. The epimysium should be left intact on the muscle surface in order to allow the muscle later to glide within that epimysium (Figs 28.9, 28.10).

After harvesting of the muscle, the distal portion is split to insert muscle parts into the lateral aspects of the upper and lower lip. Before securing the muscle with the stay sutures previously placed, the proximal and distal muscle ends are reinforced with resorbable mattress sutures in order to prevent ruptures of the stay sutures within the muscle. Then the cranial fixation of the muscle to the zygoma is performed (Fig. 28.11). The neurovascular repair is performed under the operating microscope.

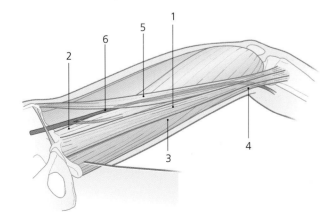

Fig. 28.8: Anatomy of the gracilis muscle. 1. Gracilis muscle. 2. Adductor longus muscle. 3. Adductor magnus muscle. 4. Semitendinosus muscle. 5. Sartorius muscle. 6. Deep femoral artery/vein and entrance of the neurovascular bundle.

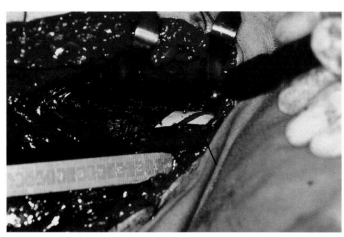

Fig. 28.9: Harvesting procedure for a gracilis muscle graft. Intraoperative situation after identification of the motor branch of the gracilis muscle (arrow). The corresponding contractile region is identified with a nerve stimulator.

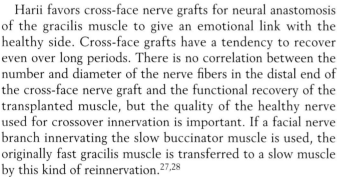

Fig. 28.10: Anterior segment of the gracilis muscle with vascular pedicle (arrow head) and motor branch (arrow).

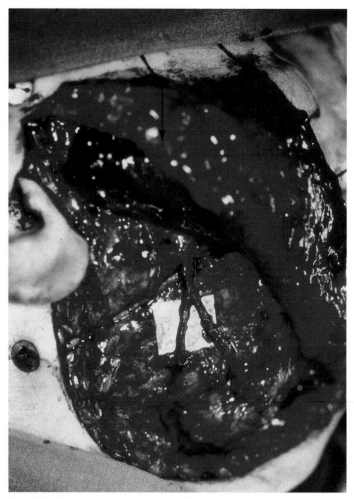

Fig. 28.11: Intraoperative aspect following neurovascular anastomosis and fixation of the muscle at the zygoma (arrow).

Harii favors cross-face nerve grafts for neural anastomosis of the gracilis muscle to give an emotional link with the healthy side. Cross-face grafts have a tendency to recover even over long periods. There is no correlation between the number and diameter of the nerve fibers in the distal end of the cross-face nerve graft and the functional recovery of the transplanted muscle, but the quality of the healthy nerve used for crossover innervation is important. If a facial nerve branch innervating the slow buccinator muscle is used, the originally fast gracilis muscle is transferred to a slow muscle by this kind of reinnervation.[27,28]

It is recommended that the hypoglossal nerve is chosen as a recipient motor nerve in patients for whom muscle transplantation combined with a cross-face nerve graft cannot be performed because of bilateral facial paralysis or previous surgery at the healthy side. As in 12th to seventh nerve anastomosis, we prefer the technique of hypoglossal nerve sectioning in contrast to separation of the whole nerve. Ueda et al recommend use of the bundle of the hypoglossal nerve diverging inferiorly to innervate the suprahyoid muscles as the recipient motor nerve to permit natural movements of the grafted muscle without functional disability of the tongue.[29]

The masseteric branch can also be used for neurosurgical anastomosis of the gracilis muscle nerve. It can be identified at the sigmoid notch penetrating the medial pterygoid muscle.

Surgical correction of the eyelid

Medical treatment for protection of the cornea (ointment or taping) often fails and surgical procedures such as tarsorrhaphy, magnetic implants, gold weights and springs may be associated with infections or the need for revisional procedures. Sophisticated load techniques may provide good esthetic and functional results with high stability.

Muscle transposition for treating paralytic lagophthalmos is difficult and the results are often hard to predict. Ueda et al have observed superior functional results of temporalis muscle transfer for closure of the eye compared to lid loading with gold implants. However, cornea protection was also given in the loading procedures used in combination with other procedures. Muscle transposition for ocular protection may impose an increased strain on the patient for re-education.

In our hands, good results were obtained with the insertion of gold weight implants, in accordance with other authors.

(a) 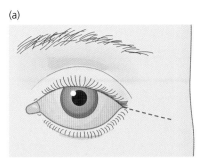 (b) 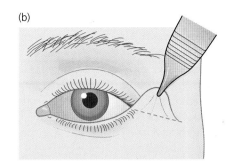 (c)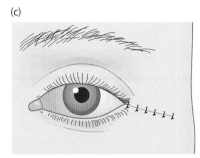

Fig. 28.12: (a, b) Determination of skin excess before full-thickness skin excision of the lid. **(c)** Reconstruction of the muscle with absorbable sutures followed by skin closure.

The weight is usually temporarily fixed on the skin of the eyelid prior to surgery. The weight should not impair opening of the eyelid but closure should be complete at rest. The weight is usually about 1–1.4 g.

Using an upper eyelid incision, the curved weight is fixed to the tarsal plate. Additionally, the levator aponeurosis may be advanced over the implant and the final eyelid height may be adjusted with levator myotomies.

A circumscribed procedure such as isolated corrections of the upper or lower eyelid may also give a good improvement of the patient's situation.

More often lower eyelid techniques are used with wedge resections combined with rotations of the lower lid skin. During that procedure the lateral canthal tendon may also be repositioned (Fig. 28.12).

In some patients a composite skin/cartilage graft may be useful for supporting the lower lid. In our hands, this procedure has not been helpful in poorly vascularized surroundings as, for example, following midface trauma with multiple scarring.[30–34]

Outcomes

In central lesions, no statistical correlation between the length of the graft used and the degree or timing of the clinical recovery was found.[11]

Facial nerve reconstruction in cases of nerve discontinuity, or as reanimation procedures with the contralateral facial or ipsilateral hypoglossal nerve as the donor nerve, gives overall satisfactory results with symmetry at rest and complete eye closure equivalent to a House–Brackmann grade III in 69%.

Green et al reported that no patient with a neural repair (direct anastomosis or cable graft) had better results than a House–Brackmann grade III. Patients undergoing direct anastomosis of the nerve obtained a House–Brackmann grade III. Most often in patients undergoing cable nerve grafting, a House–Brackmann grade IV was obtained. Patients with normal or nearly normal facial nerve function (grades I–II) had only undergone decompression of the facial nerve.[20,21] Hypoglossal/facial nerve anastomosis gave excellent results in 56% of the patients (n=32) and 66% of the patients would have repeated the operation. The procedure is most effective when used as soon as possible after the palsy has developed.

The results of crossover techniques depend on the grade of atrophy of the facial nerve, giving better results if the atrophy is less than 50% of the normal nerve. Even after 2–7 years following the nerve injury, good results may be obtainable. Combinations of hypoglossal/facial anastomosis with transposition of temporal or masseter muscles are also possible.[14]

Table 28.3 Postoperative results of vascularized muscle grafts

| Patient no. | Age at surgery (years) | Interval surgery/ follow-up (months) | Nerve | Objective (investigator) | | Subjective (self-estimation) | | Acceptance |
				Stat.	Smile	Stat.	Smile	Situation improved, patient would have procedure again?
1	16	67	X	+++	++	++	++	Yes
2	53	65	X	++	++	+	+	Yes
3	47	59	Cross-face	+++	++	++	+	Yes
4	40	55	Cross-face	++	++	++	+	Yes
5	36	29	R. masticatorius	++	+	+	+	No
6	60	24	XII	++	++	++	+	Yes

+++ = results correlate with healthy side
++ = significant improvement
+   = minor improvement

In the Clinics of Oral-Maxillofacial Surgery at Freiburg and Hanover, 20 gracilis muscle grafts have been performed. All patients showed significant improvement of face symmetry at rest after the operation. The simplified semiquantitative evaluation of our long-term results in six patients is shown in Table 28.3. Besides the functional results demonstrated via photography, we regard the subjective estimation of the patient as very important. All patients explained that they would have had the surgical procedure again and that the muscle transfer was a significant contribution to better self-esteem and an important basis for improved social contacts. One patient did not rate the result as good because he expected a normal function of the mimic musculature postoperatively despite an extensive preoperative informed consent.

Additionally, in a postoperative CT scan investigation for determination of muscle volume a significant volume overshoot was demonstrated in another six patients after an average follow-up time of 1.5 years (Figs 28.13, 28.14).[22,27,35–37]

Controversies

In some patients in selected indications, static procedures may be beneficial for an esthetic improvement. Fascia lata or foreign materials can be used for correcting the static position of the angle of the mouth. Various techniques have been described for elevation of the angle of the mouth. Most often, the soft tissue is suspended with fascia lata, towards the zygomatic arch. Most static procedures only show a temporary effect (Fig. 28.15).

As an alternative to microvascular procedures or in patients whose general status or previous operations do not allow for microvascular surgery, regional muscle transpositions with the temporal muscle, the masseter or the platysma may be considered.[38,39]

The temporalis muscle is approached via a temporal/pre-auricular vertical incision that can be extended cranially to include the deep fascia, which may be based superiorly. Alternatively, fascia lata may be fixed to extend the muscle insertion. Although the zygomatic arch may be removed in order to gain additional length, the force of contraction may be diminished due to the loss of the fulcrum. The temporalis fascia flap may be split into two slips that are passed through incisions in the lip/cheek groove and then sutured to the dermis. Overcorrection is always necessary.

Besides muscle bulk lateral to the zygomatic arch, a visible volume defect in the region of the temporal muscle often occurs postoperatively (Fig. 28.16).

Masseter muscle transfer can be performed extraorally as transfer of the whole muscle belly or as the transposition of the anterior half of the muscle via an intraoral approach. The blood and nerve supply to the muscle enters from the infratemporal fossa through the coronoid notch. The muscle is removed sharply with its tendinous insertion and bluntly elevated from the periosteum to the coronoid process. The inferior tendon is used for anterior fixation

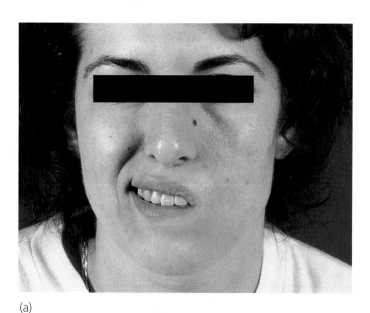

(a)

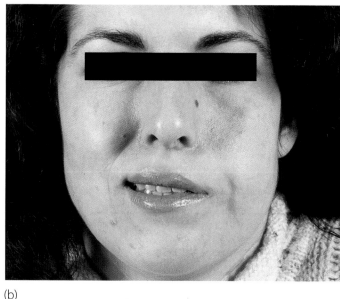

(b)

Fig. 28.13: **(a)** Twenty-year-old female patient with facial nerve paralysis on the left side. **(b)** Postoperative result 3 years after surgery with improved balance of the mouth and lateral pull of the gracilis muscle (anastomosis to hypoglossal nerve).

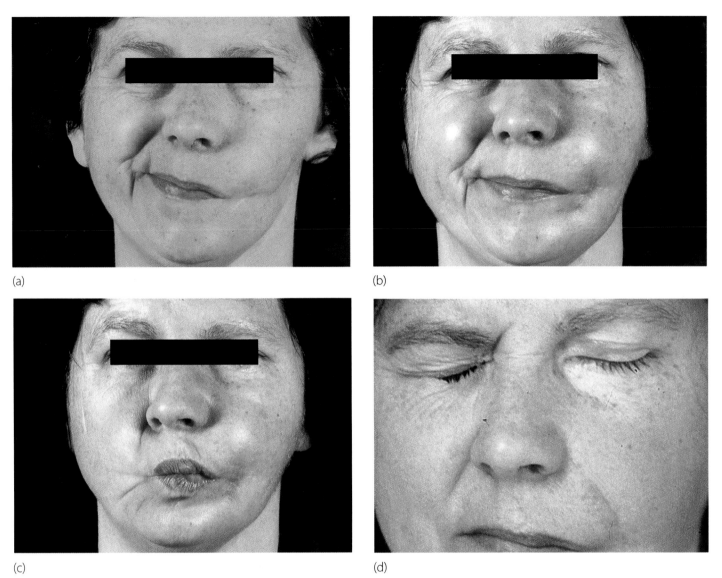

Fig. 28.14: (a) Left facial nerve palsy preoperatively following surgery for an acoustic neuroma. **(b)** Postoperative result one year after gracilis muscle transplantation with the nerve coaptation to a cross-face graft 9 months before. **(c)** Gold weight implantation with a weight of 1.5 g inserted into the upper eyelid. **(d)** Postoperative result with complete eye closure.

of the muscle. As in the temporalis muscle procedure, the muscle is split at the anterior portion in order to preserve the nerve supply to both muscle slips. Again, these muscle slips are fixed with non-absorbable sutures to the underlying dermis. Overcorrection is performed. Disadvantages of the procedure are the volume deficit in the angle of the mandible and the lateralized direction of pull (Fig. 28.17).

Often the success of the transfer of masticatory muscles is limited by a complex re-education process for the patient and a failure of these muscles to reach sufficient large areas. In

these cases, for example extending the temporal muscle flap with galea allows more extended rotation.

Temporalis muscle transposition may also be used for early temporary treatment of complete facial palsy when recovery of the nerve function is predicted to be extended and incomplete, as the procedure does not interfere with neural regeneration.

An interesting alternative for a reanimation procedure using a vascularized muscle graft is the transfer of the free rectus femoris muscle, as the long motor nerve is led through the upper lip and sutured to the contralateral facial nerve without the need for a two-stage procedure.

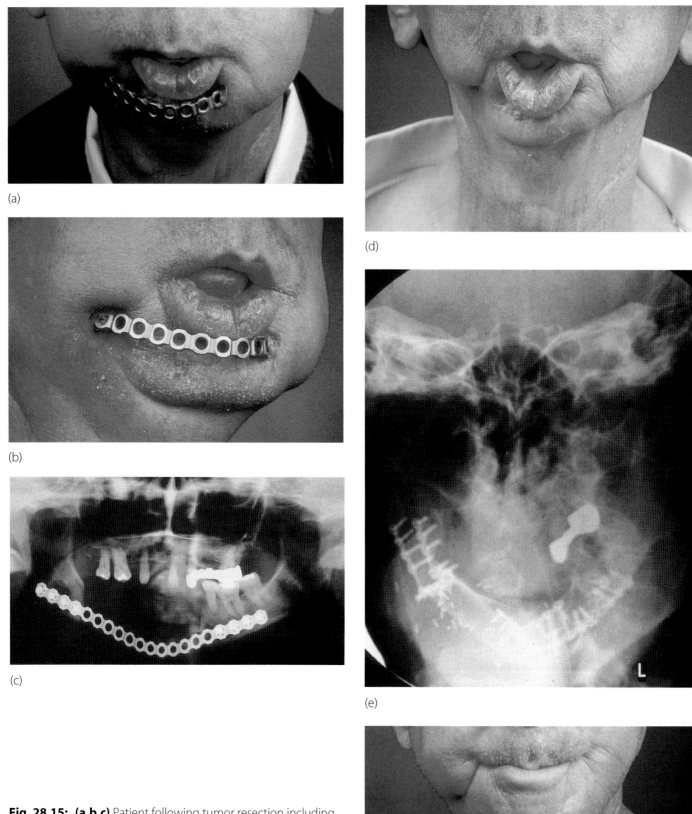

Fig. 28.15: (a,b,c) Patient following tumor resection including continuity resection of the mandible with plate exposure. **(d)** Lip incompetence with liquid drooling and difficulties in speech. **(e,f)** Transfer of osteocutaneous parascapular graft for bony reconstruction and chin reconstruction.

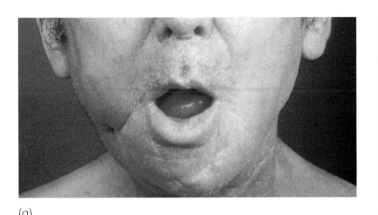
(g)

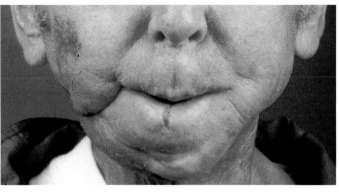
(h)

Fig. 28.15: (g) Soft tissue shrinkage and scarring cause reappearance of lip incompetence. **(h)** Postoperative aspect of patient following insertion of a fascia lata strip fixed at the zygomatic arch on both sides.

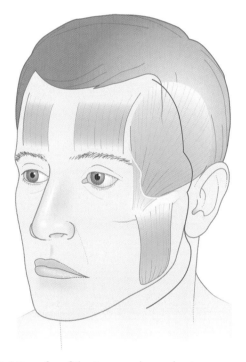
(a)

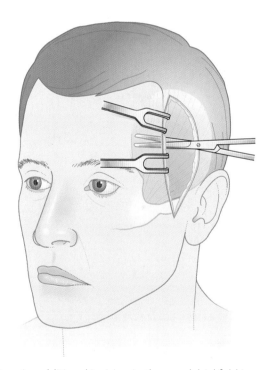
(b)

Fig. 28.16: (a) Transfer of the temporal muscle via a pre-auricular/coronal incision. An additional incision in the nasolabial fold is performed. **(b)** The temporal fascia is identified.

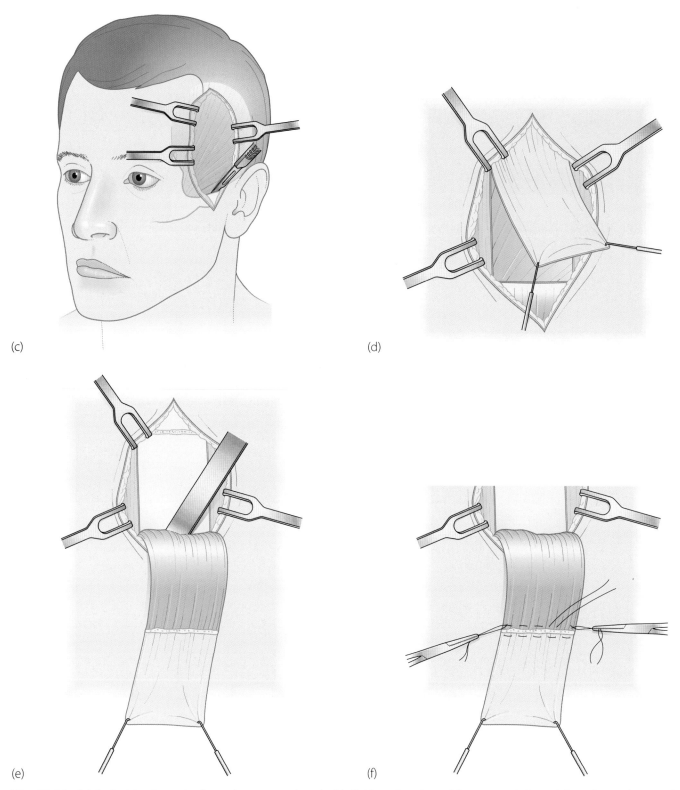

(c)

(d)

(e)

(f)

Fig. 28.16: (c) An incision is made above the zygomatic arch. **(d–f)** After elevation of the superiorly based deep fascia, the muscle is incised cranially leaving the temporal fascia attached to the muscle.

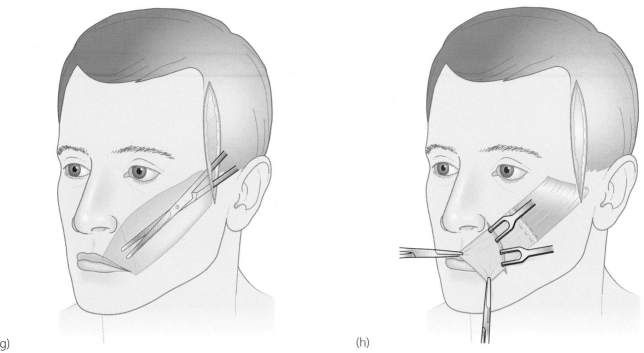

(g)

(h)

Fig. 28.16: (g,h) The ends of the fascia are fixed in the upper and lower lip. The muscle border is located in the level of the nasolabial fold.

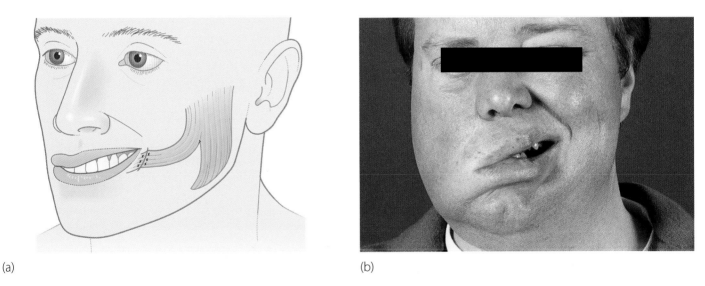

(a)

(b)

Fig. 28.17: (a) Schematic drawing of a masseter muscle transfer showing the anterior split of the muscle. **(b)** Preoperative aspect of a patient with facial nerve palsy on the right side.

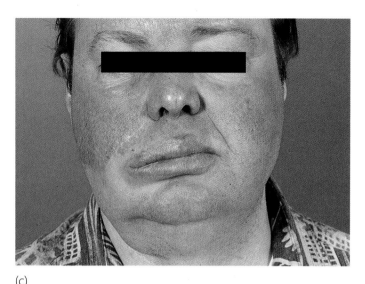

(c)

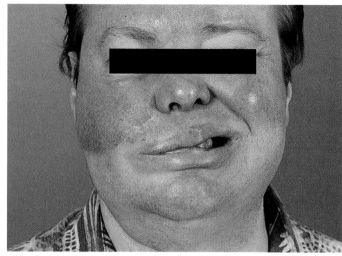

(d)

Fig. 28.17: (c) Static result 2 years after masseter muscle transfer. **(d)** Dynamic result postoperatively.

Key points

- Exact knowledge of the anatomy of the facial nerve is necessary.

- Precise clinical and electrophysiological investigation of facial nerve functions.

- Establishment of a treatment plan according to:
  —patient's expectations
  —general conditions of the patient
  —best possibility in the individual outcome.

- Planning of procedure with regard to type of lesion and interval between trauma and repair.

- Hypoglossal–facial nerve anastomosis is probably the most reliable procedure for micronerve reconstruction.

- In long-standing facial palsies neurovascular anastomosed muscle grafts are the method of choice.

References

1 Wang RC, Barrow H, Weiss MH, Parisier SC 1991 Diagnosis of disorders within the temporal bone causing facial paralysis. In: Rubin LR (ed) The paralyzed face. Mosby-Year Book, St Louis, pp 91–100

2 Leblanc A 1992 Anatomy and imaging of the cranial nerves: facial nerve, Springer Verlag, Berlin, pp 171–210

3 Louis SM, McKnight P 1991 Medical causes of facial paralysis, including Bell's palsy. In: Rubin LR (ed) The paralyzed face. Mosby-Year Book, St Louis, pp 87–90

4 Roland JT Jr, Hammerschlag PE, Lewis WS, Choi I, Berenstein A 1994 Management of traumatic facial nerve paralysis with carotid artery cavernous sinus fistula. European Archives of Otorhinolaryngology 251(1): 57–60

5 Tatagiba M, Matthies C, Samii M 1994 Facial nerve reconstruction in neurofibromatosis 2. Acta Neurochirurgica 126(2–4): 72–75

6 House J 1983 Facial nerve grading systems. Laryngoscope 93: 1056–1069

7 Glocker FX, Magistris MR, Rösler KM, Hess CW 1994 Magnetic transcranial and electrical stylomastoidal stimulation of the facial motor pathways in Bell's palsy: time course and relevance of electrophysiological parameters. Electroencephalography and Clinical Neurophysiology 93: 113–120

8 Rösler KM, Magistris MR, Glocker FX, Kohler, A, Deuschl G, Hess CW 1995 Electrophysiological characteristics of lesions in facial palsies of different etiologies. A study using electrical and magnetic stimulation techniques, in: Electroencephalography and Clinical Neurophysiology 97: 355–368

9 Fisch U, Lanser MJ 1991 Facial nerve grafting. Otolaryngology Clinics of North America 24: 691–708

10 Vaughan ED, Richardson D 1993 Facial nerve reconstruction following ablative parotid surgery. British Journal of Oral and Maxillofacial Surgery 31(5): 274–280

11 Stephanian E, Sekhar LN, Janecka IP, Hirsch B 1992 Facial nerve repair by interposition nerve graft: results in 22 patients. Neurosurgery 31(1): 73–76

12 Cusimano MD, Sekhar L 1994 Partial hypoglossal to facial nerve anastomosis for reinnervation of the paralyzed face in patients with lower cranial nerve palsies: technical note. Neurosurgery 35(3): 532–533

13 Linnet J, Madsen FF 1995 Hypoglosso-facial nerve anastomosis. Acta Neurochirurgica 133(3–4): 112–115

14 Kunihiro T, Kanzaki J, Yoshihara S, Satoh Y 1994 Analysis of the prognosis and the recovery process of profound facial nerve paralysis secondary to acoustic neuroma resection. Otorhinolaryngology 56(6): 331–333

15 Arai H, Sato K, Yanai A 1995 Hemihypoglossal-facial nerve anastomosis in treating unilateral facial palsy after acoustic neurinoma resection. Journal of Neurosurgery 82(1): 51–54

16 Kukwa A, Marchel A, Pietniczka M, Rakowicz M, Krajewski R 1994 Reanimation of the face after facial nerve palsy resulting from resection of a cerebellopontine angle tumour. British Journal of Neurosurgery 8(3): 327–332

17 Cooper TM, McMahon B, Lex C, Lenert JJ, Johnson PC 1996 Cross-facial nerve grafting for facial reanimation: effect on normal hemiface motion. Journal of Reconstructive Microsurgery 12(2): 99–103

18 Inigo F, Ysunza A, Rojo P, Trigos I 1994 Recovery of facial palsy after crossed facial nerve grafts. British Journal of Plastic Surgery 47(5): 312–317

19 Jacobs JM, Laing JH, Harrison DH 1996 Regeneration through a long nerve graft used in the correction of facial palsy. A qualitative and quantitative study. Brain 119: 271–279

20 Samii M, Matthies C 1994 Indication, technique and results of facial nerve reconstruction. Acta Neurochirurgica 130(1–4): 125–139

21 Green JD Jr, Shelton C, Brackmann DE 1994 Surgical management of iatrogenic facial nerve injuries. Otolaryngology Head and Neck Surgery 111(5): 606–610

22 Harii K 1991 Microneurovascular free muscle transplantation. In: Rubin LR (ed) The paralyzed face. Mosby-Year Book, St Louis, pp 178–200

23 O'Brien B, Kumar V 1991 Cross-face nerve grafting with free vascularized muscle grafts. In: Rubin LR (ed) The paralyzed face. Mosby-Year Book, St Louis, pp 201–212

24 Jiang H, Guo ET, Ji ZL, Zhang ML, Lu V 1995 One-stage microneuro-vascular free abductor hallucis muscle transplantation for reanimation of facial paralysis. Plastic and Reconstructive Surgery 96(1): 78–85

25 Zhao L, Miao H, Wang W, Zhang D 1994 The anatomy of the segmental latissimus dorsi flap for reconstruction of facial paralysis. Surgical and Radiologic Anatomy 16(3): 239–243

26 Ueda K, Harii K, Yamada A 1995 Free vascularized double muscle transplantation for the treatment of facial paralysis. Plastic and Reconstructive Surgery 95(7): 1288–1296

27 Ueda K, Harii K, Yamada A 1994 Long-term follow-up of nerve conduction velocity in cross-face nerve grafting for the treatment of facial paralysis. Plastic and Reconstructive Surgery 93(6): 1146–1149

28 Frey M, Happak W, Girsch W, Bittner RE, Gruber H 1991 Histomorphometric studies in patients with facial palsy treated by functional muscle transplantation: new aspects for the surgical concept. Annals of Plastic Surgery 26(4): 370–379

29 Ueda K, Harii K, Yamada A 1994 Free neurovascular muscle transplantation for the treatment of facial paralysis using the hypoglossal nerve as a recipient motor source. Plastic and Reconstructive Surgery 94(6): 808–817

30 De Min G, Babighian S, Babighian G, Van Hellemont V 1995 Early management of the paralyzed upper eyelid using a gold implant. Acta Otorhinolaryngolica Belgica 49(3): 269–274

31 Meyer-Schwickerath R, Radtke JH 1994 Paralytisches Ektropium: Unterlidsuspension am Oberlid. (Paralytic ectropion: Lower lid suspension to the upper eyelid.) Klinische Monatsblatter fur Augenheilkunde 205(2): 93–97

32 Ueda K, Harii K, Yamada A, Asato H 1995 A comparison of temporal muscle transfer and lid loading in the treatment of paralytic lagophthalmos. Scandinavian Journal of Plastic and Reconstructive Surgery and Hand Surgery 29(1): 45–49

33 Catalano PJ, Bergstein MJ, Sen C, Post K 1994 Management of the eye after iatrogenic facial paralysis. Neurosurgery 35(2): 259–262

34 Gladstone GJ, Nesi FA 1996 Management of paralytic lagophthalmos with a modified gold-weight implantation technique. Ophthalmic Plastic and Reconstructive Surgery 12(1): 38–44

35 Eppley BL, Kalenderian E, Winkelmann T, Delfino JJ 1989 Facial nerve graft repair. Suture versus laser-assisted anastomosis. International Journal of Oral Maxillofacial Surgery 18: 50–54

36 Schliephake H, Schmelzeisen R, Tröger M 2000 Revascularized muscle transfer for facial reanimation after long standing facial paralysis. International Journal of Oral and Maxillofacial Surgery 29: 243–249

37 Schmelzeisen R, Neukam FW, Reich RH, Schliephake H 1993 Neurovasculär reanastomosierte Muskeltransplantate bei der Behandlung langbestehender N.-facialis-Paresen. [Neurovascular reanastomosed muscle grafts for the treatment of long-standing facial nerve palsy.] Deutsche Zeitschrift für Mund-, Kiefer- und Gesichtschirurgie 18: 145–149

38 May M, Drucker C 1993 Temporalis muscle for facial reanimation. A 13-year experience with 224 procedures. Archives of Otolaryngology Head and Neck Surgery 119: 378–382

39 Cheney ML, McKenna MH, Megerian CA, Ojemann RG 1995 Early temporalis muscle transposition for the management of facial paralysis. Laryngoscope 105(9): 993–1000

40 Fisch U, Rouleau M 1980 Facial nerve reconstruction. Journal of Otolaryngology 9(6): 487–492

29 Psychological Support

Alex Clarke, Lisa Alexander

The aim of this chapter is to provide a brief overview of research into the psychosocial impact of facial trauma for adults and children, summarize the problems encountered by these patients, and describe effective psychological management. Brief case histories will be used as illustrations throughout.

Introduction

As biomedical techniques become increasingly sophisticated, patients who might in the past have had a poor prognosis are successfully completing treatment. However, those who undergo treatment are often left with impaired function and/or appearance and the process of treatment may last months or years with no clear guarantees about outcome. This applies across the many different conditions included under the maxillofacial heading from head and neck cancers to severe burn injuries.

Although the importance of psychological rehabilitation has been acknowledged since the pioneering work of McIndoe and his team at East Grinstead during the 1940s, there is an increasing interest in the psychological problems that patients experience and the psychological predictors of good long-term outcome. Unfortunately, much of the research in this area is confined to description of the problems and although many reports summarize their findings with a call for counseling or 'psychological support', this often sounds vague, ill defined, time consuming and expensive and lacks specific goals.

Social psychology and the face

The study of the face has received an enormous amount of attention from psychologists. The neurological basis of face perception and recognition is a fascinating area of research whose complexity highlights the importance of the face in the social context. We are all unique, although the transfer of facial characteristics to our offspring ensures family and race characteristics, which underpin cohesiveness in social groups. The face is an important determinant of our internalized sense of who we are. Just as all of us are instantly recognized by friends and family, we each have an internalized body image that is highly resistant to change. Accepting a change in appearance is not the same thing as habituating to it and patients often describe the experience of shock at catching sight of themselves in a shop window or in a photograph many years after the initial trauma. Adapting to any disfiguring condition, even where change is very minor, can therefore be a very long process, often described as one of bereavement, with a clear focus on grieving for lost looks.[1]

Physical attractiveness is judged to a significant extent on facial characteristics such as skin texture, size and shape of eyes and facial symmetry, with vast amounts being spent each year on cosmetics which enhance these features. Disfiguring conditions have a huge personal impact in terms of perceived attractiveness with interesting sex differences; whereas facial scarring for example can exaggerate the sexual stereotype for men (more macho, aggressive, willing to take risks), for a woman the stereotype is weakened and she may appear less feminine as well as less attractive. This does not mean that disfigurement is less of an issue for men. Young men in particular describe the perception of themselves as 'being hard' as a major problem in social encounters where it may elicit unwelcome aggressive behaviors from their peer group.

A young man with 'minotaur' syndrome who appeared excessively 'macho' opted for elective surgery to soften his face and lessen the hostile interaction he perceived from those around him as a result of his macho appearance.[2]

Similarly, a number of young men contacting the charity Changing Faces have described the problems caused by facial scarring that either arises from or resembles the 'Glasgow smile' resulting from glass and bottle injuries to the face. This kind of injury can incite aggression in other young men anxious to test themselves against a 'hard' protagonist.

Simple barriers to sexual activity such as altered facial sensation and the ability to kiss a partner can cause enormous distress and yet have received very little attention in terms of investigating psychosocial sequelae and/or support.

Kissing is not simply important in sexual relationships. The inability to kiss not only his wife but also his grandchildren was the major source of distress for a patient in his 70s with trauma to his jaw, for whom the appearance-related concerns were far less significant.

The head, neck and face also provide us with the basis of communication. Laryngectomy and removal of the vocal chords will remove the ability to speak permanently, future 'speech' being achieved through a variety of alternative

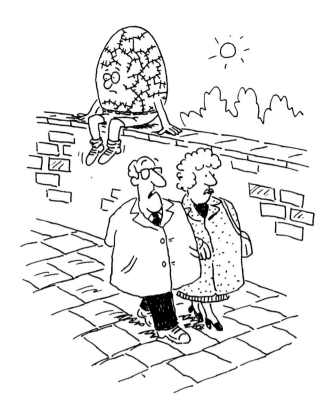

"It's remarkable what modern Surgery can do..."

Fig. 29.1 Reproduced with permission of Changing Faces, London.

mechanical means. Cancer and the treatment for invasive disease can therefore have a major impact on what the voice sounds like or whether the individual can speak at all, with psychological factors playing an important part in whether the individual re-establishes communication through esophageal or other prosthetic speech mechanisms.[3]

In addition to providing the neural and muscular basis of speech production, non-verbal signaling such as eye contact, facial gesture and blushing depend on facial structure. These non-verbal behaviors support verbal exchanges, helping to pace and structure conversation as well as allowing us to express emotion and to indicate personal attitudes.[4] Interruption of these mechanisms, often because patients will try to avoid eye contact or smiling where there is a facial palsy, can add to the awkwardness of social encounters.

Problems may also occur with swallowing. Ingestion of food, chewing, swallowing and salivation are frequently affected following maxillofacial trauma, with profound implications for ensuring optimum nutrition but also impacting dramatically on the social aspects of eating. Patients can be embarrassed about the difficulties of drooling or spilling food, using special utensils or straws. The interruption of what is an important social activity might be expected to impact on self-esteem. Indeed, the inability to express personality through speech and the social exclusion from activities such as having a drink or a meal with friends can have as great an impact on self-image as objective change in

physical appearance.[5] For those patients who experience accidental trauma or major surgery to the face, the psychological impact of facial dysfunction may impact in any or all of these areas.

Methodological issues in the psychology of maxillofacial trauma

Research studies examining the psychological impact of maxillofacial trauma utilize a range of different methodological approaches. Early reports share with many other areas of medical research a reliance on anecdotal or case history approaches and retrospective survey of a clinical cohort. Prospective studies provide more reliable information, but do not always include standardized measures of psychological distress. Much of the evidence of psychological issues in maxillofacial research is based on simple non-standardized interview techniques and clinical observation.

More recent studies in the last decade have used a more sophisticated research framework, conducting prospective studies with carefully constructed research protocols based on psychological models or frameworks with associated standardized measures. Studies measuring the incidence of psychiatric symptoms fall into this category, together with studies based on quality of life models and coping research. Body image, although a popular descriptive term, is beset by measurement problems. Used in many studies to refer to objective physical changes in appearance, it is often confused with the internalized representation of the self as measured, for example, in studies of obesity and anorexia nervosa. For the purposes of maxillofacial research, and in the absence of any way of measuring this internalized representation in this area, the term 'facial disfigurement' is preferred as a less ambiguous means of describing altered physical appearance.

A further interesting methodological issue arises in the integration of the work that has been done on individual conditions such as head and neck cancer and burns injury, with generic studies of facial disfigurement, which investigate psychological impact of disfigurement across conditions. This facial disfigurement literature is worth reviewing, partly because of the obvious relevance to maxillofacial patients but also because of its grounding in well-designed and controlled social psychological research. It will therefore be briefly described before moving on to consider research on specific conditions within maxillofacial trauma.

The psychosocial impact of facial disfigurement

Research studies are remarkably consistent in describing the problems that people with a disfigurement encounter. The predominant difficulties lie within the area of social interaction, with people being subjected to unwanted intrusions such as staring or comments. Macgregor's classic study has not been bettered in terms of summarizing patient self-report data:

> In their attempts to go about their daily lives, people are subjected to visual and verbal assaults and a level of

familiarity from strangers . . . (including) naked stares, startled reactions, 'double takes', whispering, remarks, furtive looks, curiosity, personal questions, advice, manifestations of pity or aversion, laughter, ridicule and outright avoidance.[6]

First impressions are important in our image-conscious society and adapting to disfigurement, even when minor, can be profoundly difficult.[7] First encounters are particularly stressful, staring and intrusions are commonplace and social avoidance can rapidly develop as the simplest means of survival. As in other anxiety disorders, the avoidance of the feared situation provides only temporary relief and removes the opportunity to 'learn by experience' or build up a repertoire of coping strategies. Confronting social situations thus becomes increasingly difficult.

Not surprisingly, this group of people may have very low self-esteem and expectation about life chances. For example,

> A child with severe scarring was perceived by his school as very aggressive and having severe behavior problems. In an attempt to 'normalize' his experience, his parents had offered no explanation of his accident and given him no skills with which to deal with his peers' inevitable curiosity. Individual sessions with the child, together with a school visit in which an assembly on diversity was run, resulted in a positive behavior record and improved school performance.

many believe that they need to make compromises in terms of relationships, 'you have to take what you can get', or believe that they have low employment prospects.[8] For children, all the problems of chronic illness, such as repeated hospitalization, time off school and disruption of peer relationships and education, may be compounded by bullying at school and lowered teacher and parental expectation.[9]

Although this perceived hostility from other people has led to the description of facial disfigurement as 'the last bastion of discrimination' in the UK,[10] the situation is not completely one sided. The increased uncertainty, embarrassment and self-consciousness that people experience when their appearance changes can often result in changes in behavior which elicit a negative response from other people. Altered posture, avoidance of eye contact, hiding the face

with the hand and hair and even overzealous use of cosmetic camouflage and clothing, especially hats, can elicit the very responses that the individual is trying to avoid.

Whilst it is easy to see how repeated exposure to negative events can lead to behavior change, particularly the increasing avoidance of social situations, the role of individual beliefs is also important. In addition to the evidence that people behave differently in response to someone who is visibly different, the *expectation* of a negative response is enough for the visibly different person to report events differently. Social psychologists have examined the impact of these beliefs about disfigurement. Actors were made up to look disfigured, but under the guise of having fixative added, and unknown to them, the experimental group had that make-up removed before being exposed to the experimental situation.[11] Subjects who believed themselves to be scarred reported stronger reactions from other people than the control group. This finding could be due to heightened sensitivity leading to the misinterpretation of events or to subtle alterations in the subject's behavior – poor posture, eye contact, etc. – producing genuinely stronger reactions from the onlooker. However, sensitivity to the disfigurement and the tendency to attribute all negative experiences to facial appearance, even where unrelated, is a commonly reported problem[1] and a possible explanation for the significance to the individual of apparently only minor disfigurement.

From the clinical perspective, these findings are important because the modification of inappropriate cognitions (beliefs) and the introduction of more appropriate cognitions and behavior form the basis of effective psychological intervention in this group. Social anxiety and avoidance can be very effectively targeted using this well-established approach.

Relatively few studies have attempted to look beyond the description of psychosocial problems in the target population to the factors associated with good adjustment in the long term. An exception has been Macgregor,[6] who identified coping style as important. Those who cope well and report fewer problems tend to use 'positive' coping strategies summarized in Box 29.1, all of which allow them to manage social situations; 'negative' coping strategies are those that facilitate the avoidance response.

Recent measures of the effectiveness of the first specialist Disfigurement Guidance Unit funded by the NHS report the number of effective coping strategies used by an individual to be a better predictor of good outcome than a particular kind of strategy per se; in other words, those who managed their

---

Box 29.1   Coping style as a predictor of good long-term adjustment after facial disfigurement[1,7,12]

'Positive' coping strategies	'Negative' coping strategies
Good social skills	Poor social skills
Assertive	Aggressive
Taking the initiative in new situations	Avoidance or withdrawal from new situations
	Use of alcohol
	Unrealistic pursuit of surgical solutions

disfigurement most effectively and reported fewer problems were those who had developed a variety of different responses that they could use.[13]

In summary, then, this research is important to those working within the maxillofacial trauma field, primarily because it identifies individual behavior as a determinant of successful long-term outcome rather than appearance per se. This is very encouraging because behavior is learned and can be modified; thus there is a very clear basis for psychological management of patients with altered appearance and this is not, therefore, a group who have to rely solely on biomedical solutions aimed at restoring appearance.

Psychological Aspects of Maxillofacial Trauma

Anxiety, depression and posttraumatic stress disorder (PTSD)

It seems almost too obvious that these areas are important in the context of maxillofacial trauma. As described in the previous sections, disfigurement exposes individuals to a range of social stressors and psychological stresses which are predisposing factors in the development of this trio of disorders. The relevant literature in this area indicates that depression, anxiety and PTSD are the most commonly reported psychological sequelae of burn injury or other types of trauma. The three often exist together and high levels of co-morbidity are expected. Many individuals who suffer burn injury or trauma already show a range of behaviors which place them at risk for developing mental illness, substance abuse, social problems or previously existing psychiatric problems being those most often cited. The challenges of dealing with facial injury and disfigurement add to the psychological difficulties that may already be present. The degree to which an individual feels responsible for his injury may affect his attitude to asking for help.

Psychiatric assessment and management

Studies based on psychiatric models measure symptoms of mental distress such as depression and anxiety and PTSD, which are clearly defined within DSM-IV criteria[14] and measured using standardized scales such as the Hospital Anxiety and Depression Scale.[15] Brief descriptions of anxiety and depression are given below, with a summary of relevant data regarding the development of these symptoms in this population. PTSD is described with more detail, since it is covered in less depth in the rest of this chapter.

Definitions

Depression

Depression is a concept that can be understood in many ways. Readers will be familiar with the concept of depressed mood, in terms of a subjective feeling of unhappiness, encompassing feelings of guilt, worthlessness, feeling listless or apathetic and putting oneself down. Depression can be associated with other medical problems, developing as a secondary reaction. Depressed mood can be seen as a reaction to circumstances which an individual can work through with assistance from others and which will dissipate over time. Readers will be familiar with the lowering of mood that many patients experience a few days post surgery. Clinical depression is more serious and more pervasive and often requires a formal intervention to be resolved.

To obtain a clinical diagnosis of depression an individual displays a cluster of symptoms that generally comprise 'depressed mood, loss of interest, anxiety, sleep disturbance, loss of appetite, lack of energy and suicidal thoughts'.[16] Additional symptoms may include 'weeping and slowness of speech and action . . . extreme withdrawal, hallucinations often of voices ridiculing them, and delusions that they have been responsible for a horrific catastrophe'. Thoughts of death, self-harm or suicide can occur.[16]

Depression can also be further classified in a psychiatric framework, depending on history and symptoms, into the following subdivisions:

- bipolar (manic-depressive)
- endogenous
- reactive
- neurotic
- psychotic.[14]

Classification may influence choice of medical treatment. A psychiatrist generally makes the diagnosis. It is more difficult to recognize depression in someone who is physically unwell or who has been injured; many of the physical symptoms described above (and below in the section on anxiety) can overlap with symptoms of physical illness, e.g. appetite loss is to be expected if an individual has difficulties eating. An instrument such as the Hospital Anxiety and Depression Scale (HADS),[15] which was designed to detect depression and anxiety whilst disregarding ambiguous physical symptoms, can be very useful in screening patients at risk of developing anxiety and/or depression.

Anxiety disorders

Fear is a natural response to anything perceived as threatening. Responses occur on a number of levels – behavioral, cognitive (thoughts), affective (emotional) and physiological. Social fears and anxiety in relation to disfigurement are common. Much of this chapter discusses approaches that can be used in helping individuals to overcome these fears and anxieties. Anxiety disorders can severely impair an individual's ability to engage in his chosen lifestyle. Common anxiety disorders are outlined here as classified in the DSM-IV.[14]

- *Anxiety states*: including generalized panic disorder in which many aspects of the environment are interpreted as potentially threatening, even if there are no grounds for anticipating danger. A moderate level of anxiety is experienced over a protracted time period.
- *Phobic disorders*: includes social phobias (fear of situations in which a person can be watched), simple phobia (of specific objects or situations, e.g. the dentist or dogs),

Miss X was extremely concerned about the results of surgery to correct a minor disfigurement in her mandible. She became preoccupied with how she was viewed by others and began to suffer panic attacks in public places and over time began to avoid all situations which she feared would entail exposure to public scrutiny. She was unable to complete her course of study and severely curtailed her social life. She became very low in mood and took an overdose of sleep medication and cut her arms with a razor.

By learning anxiety management techniques, managing her panic attacks and challenging her beliefs about how others judged her she was able to increase her activity levels and improve her self-esteem. Medication helped her mood to lift and she was able to re-engage in the activities that she enjoyed.

Mr Y suffered a serious compression fracture to his skull with associated skin loss and disfigurement to his brow area. He was seen with his wife when they were experiencing some problems adjusting to the trauma of the accident. Mr Y was coping with his disfigurement by wearing a hat in public although he was able to leave his scars uncovered around the home. It became apparent that he was becoming more anxious about revealing his scars when he discussed putting his hat on at home if anyone outside the family was visiting and whenever the doorbell rang. He realized that his avoidance was growing when he found he had put on his hat in response to a doorbell ringing on the television. Discussion helped him to begin to tackle his avoidance and develop strategies to control his anxiety.

agoraphobia (the fear of being alone in public places with no route of escape).
- *Panic disorders*: experiencing intense, overwhelming terror ('panic attacks') for no apparent reason. Often certain situations are avoided for fear of suffering an attack. Individuals can believe that their symptoms of panic are life threatening, e.g. chest pains and breathlessness = heart attack.
- *Obsessive-compulsive disorders*: experiencing obsessions (repeated intrusive thoughts that cause distress and anxiety) and/or compulsions (rituals such as hand washing/checking behaviors which an individual goes through in an attempt to reduce anxiety)
- *Posttraumatic stress disorder*: described in detail below.

Many people are apprehensive about the reactions of other people to some aspect of themselves. Someone with social phobia or severe anxiety may avoid social situations or behave in a way that they feel helps them to 'hide', e.g. holding up a newspaper. Many of the fears and behaviors associated with anxiety can happen out of the conscious awareness of the individual, who becomes conditioned to avoiding anxiety-provoking situations.

Medical treatment is often associated with pervasive anxiety. An anxious patient will be particularly tuned into threatening stimuli and is more likely to interpret information as threatening.

Treatment

Effective treatment comprises a combination of approaches. Outcome studies show that with serious depression a combination of psychological therapy and medication is most efficacious.[17] The principal medications used in treating depressive illness are cyclic antidepressants, MAO inhibitors and newer 'third generation' medications. Medication takes up to 6 weeks to be effective and due to side effects is not suitable for all patients. Psychological treatment (particularly cognitive-behavioral approaches which have been found to have the best outcomes) ensures more marked improvements of longer duration and generalizability and may also prevent lapses.[17]

Depression can be seen as due to negative thinking styles and biases in perception and cognitive functioning. The negative outlook encompasses the self, the world and the future, resulting in the characteristic picture of depression. The therapist and patient work together to change this worldview using cognitive approaches and behavioral tasks in the context of a warm, empathic and genuine relationship. Anxiety disorders generally react well to a combination of psychological therapy (again, cognitive-behavioral approaches have been shown to have the best outcomes) and medication. Cognitive-behavioral approaches comprise:

- exposure to feared stimulus: both external (through behavior) and internal (thoughts), plus extinction of the anxiety response
- education: understanding what is happening and why
- increasing skills in relevant areas: relaxation and breathing, cognitive strategies such as challenging negative thoughts, social skills
- reducing use of anxiogenic substances

These principles of treatment are described in later sections of this chapter when discussing anxiety management with reference to those with facial disfigurement.

Prevalence of problems

Much research has looked at the associations between disfigurement and mental health but the reservations outlined earlier in this chapter apply here. Of course, common sense tells us that those with unusual faces have to contend with prejudice from those around them and associated problems with social interactions. Consistent social rejection and/or isolation would appear to place individuals at risk of at least the milder forms of depression and social anxiety. Low self-esteem resulting from feelings of rejection and not looking 'acceptable' and thus worthwhile would also seem to predispose to depression. Anticipation of negative reactions from others can lead to behaviors such as withdrawal, shyness or aggression which can themselves invite negative reactions from others. All of these factors increase the likelihood of isolation, low self-esteem and lack of positive experiences.

Intimate relationships

Research has shown that those coping with disfigurement can also have problems in their closest relationships. Feeling ashamed of one's physical appearance can lead to inhibitions. One study found that 9% of women would not reveal their birthmarks to anyone, not even their husbands.[18] Another looked at sexual satisfaction rates in burn victims.[19] Out of a maximum possible 100% satisfaction level, men rated their satisfaction with their sex life as 82.5%, women as 52%. In the female subjects, sexual satisfaction was strongly and negatively correlated with physical dysfunction and body image, not burn size or location.

Grieving process

Many professionals in this area suggested that an individual needs to go through some form of grieving for the 'lost self' to be able to then generate helpful coping strategies. This process can often appear similar to depression. Careful assessment needs to be made to identify the underlying processes.

Research in this area tends to look at different populations with different degrees of disfigurement. The most widely studied group of subjects are those who have been burned. Research indicates that levels of anxiety and depression, which are high in the period immediately post burn, do not diminish over time but indeed may even rise. A widely cited study found that levels of depression in burns patients on discharge was 12.5%, rising to over 20% at 2-year follow-up.[20] Thirty-one percent of subjects were significantly anxious on discharge from a burns unit and at 2-year follow-up 26% still fell into this category.[20]

Social anxiety was measured in one study looking at young adults with partial-thickness facial burns who were interviewed an average of 12 months post burn. The interviewers noted that no significant scarring was noticeable. Out of 28 patients, three did not return to their job, 16 decreased social activities and over half consumed more alcohol than before. Seven out of 28 had grown a beard or changed hairstyle to cover a perceived change in appearance. The authors suggest that this is indicative of high levels of anxiety.[21]

A review of the literature on psychological outcomes for the burn injured[22] comments on the lack of consistent measures used when looking at the burns population, but describes a number of studies which indicate an increased rate of depression in this population (up to 30% severe depression) which is related to other psychosocial problems such as family support, levels of resting pain and medical setbacks. The same review comments on the positive relationship between premorbid psychopathology and post-burn depression, suggesting the presence of a chronic condition. Further longitudinal research in this area needs to be carried out before definite conclusions can be drawn.

Body image changes can also be linked to depression. Severity and site of injury in the burn population do not seem to predict post-injury adjustment, so a more complex process is once again occurring.

Children

Children who have experienced trauma present a special challenge in terms of assessment and treatment. Their adjust-

ment needs to be seen as part of a family process. Parents and teachers may become overprotective or have overly low expectations of the child, a pattern that has been found consistently in the cleft lip and palate population.[23] An important review article of the psychosocial sequelae of pediatric burn injury[24] concludes that there is little consensus on the adjustment of children following burn injury. Difficulties with study design (small samples, lack of control groups and standardized measures) make conclusions difficult. Some studies show significant levels of depression, withdrawal, delinquency and aggressiveness, whereas other studies (generally those using standardized measures) report only a minority of children showing significant problems at follow-up. Location of burn injury and degree of visible disfigurement have been found to be related to depression and lowered ambitions for the future or, conversely, to have no significant relationship to adjustment. Family/maternal adjustment is also an important factor in the adjustment of burned children. A tenuous relationship between maternal and child adjustment has been found, as well as family functioning prior to the burn injury. There is a need to assess the whole family and support system, e.g. teachers, siblings, and not focus on just the injured patient. One review suggests rates of child psychopathology following burn injury in the order of 15–20%. The conclusions are as follows.

> Antecedent conditions that predate the injury (e.g. family discord) and parental and family reactions (e.g. guilt) to the child's injury and during the recovery process likely interact with a variety of child organismic (e.g. personality traits), developmental (e.g. age, cognitive level of functioning) and biological (e.g. burn severity) variables to mediate psychological outcome.[24]

Psychosocial support

One of the most important protective factors related to the development of these problems is psychosocial support, whether from family members or some other source. Quality of support as well as number of those offering support would seem to be important and often the supporters themselves will need some assistance to enable them to continue to provide difficult and emotionally draining support to their family member. Many patients express a desire for ongoing support and in the head and neck cancer field ongoing support groups have been very successful. Specialized psychological support is rare in this field but teams can develop approaches to identify those at risk of psychological adjustment problems (see Box 29.4) and use of screening instruments such as the HADS[15] can also be incorporated into a care package.

Hierarchy of interventions

A tiered approach to psychological support enables a team to offer interventions as appropriate within the existing service or to identify deficits. A hierarchy for interventions has been designed for treating mental health problems in a medical setting,[25] which is applicable to those receiving treatment for maxillofacial trauma.

1. If a patient becomes 'stuck' in his depression/anxiety or his mental state is compromising his treatment then he should be referred to a specialist. The medical team should always be aware of the stigma associated with referral to psychiatric services, so problems should be managed by the team as appropriate.
2. Counseling, either by the medical professional personally or by a counselor working as part of the team, is the next level of intervention. Counseling is helpful in working through the process of adjustment.
3. Clinical management entails ensuring that a patient is sufficiently supported to progress through his psychological adjustment. This may mean in turn supporting a patient's support system, ensuring good patient–professional communication and encouraging problem-focused coping. In this way mastery can be developed which helps to overcome depression.

To conclude, the best treatment is maximizing the coping mechanisms that an individual already has and in that way encouraging mastery. If this process starts from the first point of contact then problems can be swiftly identified and managed appropriately by the team.

Posttraumatic stress disorder

Introduction

The majority of patients being treated for maxillofacial trauma have sustained their injury through a traumatic incident. This section will look at the possible consequences of exposure to trauma, the effects on psychological functioning and then describe some of the treatment approaches. Obviously this is not intended to be a comprehensive review of this vast area and readers who wish to look at this area in further depth are referred to other texts.[26]

Human beings are in a continual state of homeostasis: as our environment changes so we try to adapt to the adjusting demands. This applies to everyday occurrences and also to extraordinary experiences. As we age, we learn to make sense of what has been encountered and to place it into context. When an event occurs which is far outside ordinary expectations, a major process of adjustment may have to take place. Feelings at these times may be unique, powerful and unfamiliar. When we are threatened or frightened, the body and brain are programmed to ensure our survival (fight, freeze or flight reactions).

If exposed to threat, the individual will generally try to deal effectively with the event by thinking about that threat and thus attempt to learn how to cope better with that threat should it occur again in the future. However, if thinking about the threat causes intensely unpleasant feelings, the individual may attempt to push it out of his mind, so that it does not get processed emotionally and continues to emerge into consciousness.

Maxillofacial trauma implies, by its name, an exposure to some type of trauma which results in injury to the face. Interpersonal violence is becoming the most common cause of maxillofacial trauma to adults in Western society (see the section below on risk factors for maxillofacial injury). Being exposed to violence from another individual can be seriously challenging to our beliefs regarding the world as a safe, benevolent place to be. The result may be the knock-on effect of making the whole world, or at least the people in it, seen malevolent. Other causes of injury can also challenge the view of the world as a predictable safe place, for example, car crashes, accidents in the home or at work. Resulting injuries and disfigurement can compound the challenge to healthy psychological functioning.

Definition of PTSD

The syndrome of PTSD was first officially recognized in 1983 by the American Psychiatric Association. After a number of updates and revisions, the current definitions in DSM-IV[14] and ICD-10[27] are those in common circulation. They are outlined in Box 29.2.

Facial disfigurement can compound many of the symptoms shown in Box 29.2 by giving constant reminders of the trauma and increasing feelings of social isolation. Thus many individuals with maxillofacial trauma have experienced events which would lead them to be predisposed to PTSD.

The proportion of individuals who develop PTSD depends on both the nature and severity of the trauma and also other predisposing factors. In the worst cases of trauma, up to 100% of those exposed have developed symptoms of PTSD. Research in burns units indicate that between 7% and 41% of patients with burns develop posttraumatic anxiety and up to 45% will go on to develop PTSD.[22,28] A recent study showed that 32% of road traffic accident victims showed symptoms of PTSD after a year.[29] Those individuals who showed more severe symptoms in the week following trauma were more likely to go on to develop PTSD and this is a pattern that occurs throughout the literature.

Who is more likely to develop PTSD?

Factors affecting the likelihood of developing severe PTSD reactions are listed below.[30] All the following relate in a linear fashion to the likelihood of developing PTSD.

- Severity of trauma (more severe <PTSD)
- Length of trauma (longer trauma <PTSD)
- How close to the trauma an individual was (proximity <PTSD)
- How dangerous the trauma was (more dangerous <PTSD)
- The number of traumas experienced by an individual (more <PTSD)
- Negative reactions from others following the trauma (increased negativity <PTSD)
- If the trauma was inflicted by others (increased risk if trauma was)
- History of psychological problems and substance misuse in premorbid history also increase the possibility of developing PTSD

PTSD in children

Children are affected by trauma in many different ways. As with adults, their reactions depend on many factors including

For a person to suffer from PTSD he must have been exposed to a traumatic event of exceptional severity.

To be diagnosed with PTSD, symptoms that fall into the following three main areas must be present.

■ Re-experiencing that event in recollections/memories, dreams/nightmares and daytime imagery/flashbacks.

■ Avoidance and emotional numbing shown by emotional detachment/numbing/avoidance of the stimulus associated with trauma. Examples could be activities previously enjoyed, places or people and feelings of detachment from others.

■ Increased arousal evidenced by sleep disturbance, anger outbursts, hypervigilance, exaggerated startle response, difficulties concentrating.

Generally the above should arise within 6 months of trauma. An acute stress disorder is diagnosed if the symptoms persist less than 3 months, acute PTSD if the symptoms last 1–3 months and chronic PTSD if the symptoms persist longer than this.

As well as these three main areas, other problems may also commonly arise, including the following.

■ Panic attacks. These may occur upon exposure to something that reminds an individual of the trauma, e.g. seeing a person who looks like their attacker, a similar car to that in which their accident occurred, flames etc.

■ Severe avoidant behaviors. This arises from avoidance of reminders of the trauma, but can generalize to the point that, for example, a person stops leaving the house.

■ Depression. This has already been discussed, but in the context of trauma can manifest as a lack of interest in previously enjoyed activities and feelings of guilt and self-blame even if the accident was not the fault of the individual.

■ Suicidal thoughts. Increased likelihood of suicide.

■ Substance abuse. This can result from attempts to relieve the symptoms of PTSD, as an escape, but will only give short-term relief and exaggerate psychological responses over time and make recovery and progress difficult.

■ Feelings of isolation. A person who has experienced trauma has been through a unique experience and can feel that 'no-one else can understand'. Their symptoms can result in isolation and marital/family problems.

■ Feelings of mistrust and betrayal towards the world and others.

■ Anger and irritability. This can make it difficult to obtain support from others.

personality, family support, sex, age and coping strategies of the child and the severity of the trauma. Many children show short-term disturbance following trauma, in particular in sleep patterns, eating and unwillingness to be away from their loved ones.

In the longer term a child may develop avoidance as a way of coping with his memories and feelings. Avoidance is an important factor in the development of longer term problems, so it is important that the child is helped to deal with some of the things that he is avoiding.[26,31] Although avoidance may help in the short term, over time it can impact on a child's ability to cope with what has happened and may affect his ability to integrate the trauma into a new worldview.

Following the traumatic event, the stimuli which are avoided by the youngster are both external and internalized.

■ The external stimuli may include people, places, objects and events that remind the child of the trauma.
■ Repetitive intrusive memories, thoughts, images and emotions when awake, and trauma-related nightmares during sleep, are the main anxiety-provoking stimuli. These may cause the child to suffer from hyperarousal and attempts at avoidance.
■ The child may try to exclude trauma-related images from consciousness through suppression (just don't think about it) or distraction (thinking about something else). At times he can appear distracted or very 'flat' and emotionless; this is related to attempts at avoiding thinking about the trauma.
■ In terms of behavior, children may avoid anything that reminds them of the traumatic event. They also attempt to avoid situations that will lead to trauma-related memories or thoughts. For example, some children will not go to bed for fear of having nightmares. Others will not separate from their parents or caregivers or sleep alone.

A central concern for many traumatized children (and often adults as well) who subsequently experience intrusions is the degree to which PTSD symptoms reflect the onset of 'madness'. Young people and their parents therefore benefit from talking to a professional who is experienced in this field to educate them about their reactions.

Children with PTSD engage in an ongoing approach–avoidance struggle with respect to stimuli that remind them of the trauma. The child feels pulled in two directions at once and can get caught in an unhelpful cycle of thoughts and behaviors.

■ Older children experience a pressure to talk about the trauma but have difficulty doing so.
■ Younger children, while they may avoid talking about the trauma or other things on the outside related to it, often engage in play activities such as drawing or make-believe games in which they repeatedly re-enact the trauma situation. This conflict probably reflects their wishes to avoid danger but also to think things through and to absorb and process what has happened to them.[31]

It is important that children are given a chance to work through and express their emotions in a safe environment. It is quite normal for children to talk repeatedly about what has happened to them or to play the same trauma-related game over and over again. By doing this they are helping their mind to come to terms with what has happened to them.

Identification of PTSD

Normal reactions and symptoms

It is common for those who have been exposed to trauma to experience, at least briefly, some of the previously described symptoms. Generally they pass quickly without treatment. Those who have been traumatically injured often thought that they were going to die. Re-experiencing the traumatic event in 'flashbacks' or nightmares is common and generally passes with time. Being reminded of the accident can cause a recurrence of symptoms and this can be true of seeing the disfiguring injury itself. This can lead to avoidance of the feared stimulus that can bring back these disturbing images.

Support in the first month

Input from involved professionals generally involves support and education. Through reassurance, explanation and normalization, individuals and their families can learn about their reactions. It is common, in the authors' experience, for individuals to believe that they are 'going mad' and are unable to control any of their symptoms. Simple anxiety management strategies focused around controlled breathing and distraction can be helpful at this time.

If symptoms persist for more than a month then professional help should be sought.

Treatment of PTSD

If an individual appears to be suffering from the symptoms described above and these symptoms persist for longer than the initial phase of adjustment post injury, assistance from other sources should be sought.

Treatment strategies fall into two main areas:

- psychological interventions
- medication.

Psychological interventions encompass four main areas summarized below.

Anxiety management

- Relaxation training
- Controlled breathing
- Positive thinking/self-talk
- Assertiveness training
- Thought stopping

Cognitive therapy

This involves identifying unhelpful beliefs, which can disturb emotions and behaviors, and learning ways to challenge these beliefs and develop more realistic and helpful beliefs. For example:

> The way that I am feeling indicates that I am going mad and have no control over my emotions.

replaced by:

> My feelings are due to reactions to trauma and I can control some of the symptoms.

Exposure therapy

In essence this involves confronting the feared stimulus that is a reminder of the trauma and evokes anxiety, e.g. gas fire, car journeys. This can be in therapy or with supportive others, in reality or imagined. This mode of therapy works by extinguishing the fear response through repeated exposure and associated anxiety management strategies.

Play therapy

Play therapy can be useful for children. Games can be a way to tackle topics that would be too difficult to tackle directly. Playing with children also gives them a way to express themselves that would be too difficult with words.

Medication

Evidence-based drug treatment for PTSD centers on antidepressant drugs. Generally medication needs at least 8 weeks to take effect and drug therapy needs to be long term. Combination with psychological treatment brings the best outcome.[30]

Mood disturbance is also common following trauma, in particular irritability, tearfulness and poor concentration. This can be compounded in the short term by high doses of painkillers, which can depress mood and disinhibit. Also prolonged periods of boredom, uncertainty and worry about treatment and financial concerns can impact on mood.

Mr X was referred for psychological help due to his low mood. Following severe burn injuries at work he had spent several weeks in intensive care, but was now recovering. He was able to describe vivid dreams during the period when he was sedated when he believed that other family members had been killed in an accident. These dreams were so vivid that he thought that his relatives were dead and the staff were not telling him the truth. In addition, he felt that he was 'going mad' since he was suffering from acute anxiety symptoms which he was unable to control. Psychoeducation about reactions following trauma, anxiety management strategies and a chance to explore his feelings regarding his injuries and being disfigured helped him to begin to focus on his recovery and accommodate his feelings of grief at the injuries he had received.

Support for the family of an injured individual is also often essential at the time of early treatment. Family reactions can have a huge impact on longer term functioning and, for example, preparing relatives for the appearance of their injured loved one so that they do not appear shocked or horrified can have a positive impact on self-acceptance. Also, those close to the individual may have also been exposed to the traumatic event and may themselves be suffering from PTSD. If their functioning is compromised this can impact on the psychological recovery of the injured party.

Monitoring of symptoms

It is important for staff to ensure that there is time to talk in a quiet and unthreatening way. Often individuals are frightened or ashamed to admit their fears and symptoms. Referral to relevant resources should be implemented if symptoms persist. It is important, in the psychological interventions of PTSD, that early identification and treatment of this problem is undertaken. Chronic PTSD can seriously impact on the quality of life and functioning of an individual.

Factors contributing to exposure to trauma

A review of the epidemiology of maxillofacial trauma was recently produced[32] and will not be replicated here. In summary, the authors conclude that worldwide, assaults and road traffic accidents provide the majority of cases of this type of trauma. Other categories such as sports injuries, gunshot wounds, falls and industrial accidents contribute to a minority of cases. Injuries resultant from interpersonal assault are increasing in Western cultures and becoming the primary cause of maxillofacial trauma. Levels of interpersonal violence are rising, particularly in young males aged 18–25. Alcohol use is also correlated with such assaults, fights between young male strangers who had consumed excessive amounts of alcohol comprised the majority of occurrences of interpersonal violence in a study of attendees at an inner-city British hospital.[33] Interpersonal violence towards women was usually what is commonly known as 'domestic violence', assaults by partners or those known to them.

A group of patients that have been studied extensively are those who have been burned. A large minority of patients admitted to hospital due to burn injuries fall into the category of 'sensory impairment' whether through drug or alcohol use, age (very young or very old) or psychiatric illness. Premorbid psychopathology in those who sustain burn injuries severe enough to warrant hospitalization includes depression, personality disorders and alcohol and drug abuse.[22] In addition, dementia or 'neurological disorders' are commonly reported and individuals from lower socioeconomic groups are disproportionately represented. Estimates of previous psychiatric illness range from 28% to 75%. Individuals who have suffered burn injury also seem to have a high frequency of risk-taking behavior: those with psychiatric illness may be careless, actively self-harming, disturbed or have reduced levels of competence.[28] Certain personality characteristics may increase an individual's level of risk due to participation in dangerous activities or sport or disregard for personal safety.

Premorbid factors and risk behaviors

An important early review paper[34] identified the contribution of premorbid psychological traits in predicting outcome after head and neck cancer. In particular, the evidence linking heavy alcohol use and smoking with neoplasms of the aerodigestive tract suggests that alcoholics are disproportionately represented within this patient group. This in turn has an impact on psychiatric disorder in the postoperative population since depression and suicide are higher in the alcoholic population than in other groups. Although relatively few cancer patients commit suicide, this is a population at greatly increased risk.[35]

Implications for treatment

Prevention is better than cure. Many interventions have been developed to tackle alcohol and drug misuse, interpersonal violence and risk-taking behaviors, e.g. not wearing seat-belts in cars. A review of interventions designed to prevent injuries in problem drinkers[36] concluded that there is some evidence for a variety of medical and psychological interventions reducing injuries including falls, drinking-related injuries, domestic violence and suicide. Interventions included education, medication, cue exposure, brief interventions and motivational interviewing. The authors caution that more research is needed before conclusions can be drawn. However, by offering support, education and referral to specialist services it seems likely that professionals working in the trauma field can assist their patients in reducing their risk behaviors and thus the likelihood of repeat injury. Patients who are identified as drinking in a dependent or problem fashion should be counseled appropriately and offered the chance to be referred to local alcohol services for specialized help.

Conventional programmes of risk reduction, e.g. smoke alarms, education, only minimally impacted in psychologically disturbed subgroups. Interventions need to be on a wide scale, addressing complex social problems.

Do untreated psychological problems resolve over time?

The popular lay idea that 'time is the best healer' is not supported by the evidence in the maxillofacial setting. A study looking at the change in outcomes for the head and neck cancer population over time reports that whilst medical problems decrease with time following surgery, psychosocial problems increase.[37] Although using only a small clinical sample (n=55), its findings are very significant. Patients seem to lack the appropriate coping skills to manage the profound change that they have experienced and the study suggests that this pattern might be prevented with better clinical input. This has also been found in the long-term follow-up of patients who have had severe burns.[20,38,39]

This finding, that whilst medical problems may resolve, psychosocial problems remain and may get worse with time, is significant for several reasons. In the first instance, it stimulates the ethical arguments about the moderation of procedures that have this devastating impact and in doing so supports a more comprehensive approach to the study of outcomes – the quality of life model (see below). It also provides support to those researchers working within a coping skills framework, who are not only attempting to discover those factors which predict successful coping but who are beginning to develop models for clinical intervention.

The 'quality of life' approach

The value of using a quality of life framework for investigating the long-term impact of medical conditions lies in the intrinsic acknowledgment of the patient as a person with life roles beyond those of a sick patient. The model includes the basic premise that the value of a procedure will be determined not only in terms of the impact on the course and progress of the disease but also in terms of its effect on the individual. As such, medical issues such as side effects of drugs, measurement of anxiety and depression, etc. are important but social issues such as ability to continue with employment also become key indicators of the value of a procedure. It is not difficult to see that this model provides not only a comprehensive picture of outcome within conditions, but also has the potential for comparing across conditions and treatment modalities.

The definition of quality of life has proved challenging. A widely adopted definition is: 'Quality of life refers to patients' appraisal of and satisfaction with their current level of functioning as compared to what they perceive to be possible or ideal'.[40] The WHO Quality of Life group defined quality of life as 'An individual's perception of their position in life in the context of culture and value systems in which they live, and in relation to their goals, expectations, standards and concerns'.[41] Whilst this definition seems comprehensive, others have suggested that quality of life is simply 'what the patient says it is'.[42] As the model has been developed, issues such as religious beliefs have been added to it and a large number of researchers have been involved in devising, validating and measuring quality of life scales. Self-report has become a contentious issue, with some suggestion that a large part of the literature on quality of life is redundant because it is based on health professional assessment of what is essentially an individual issue. Self-report is today considered vital if the measure is to have any meaning. As scales have become more and more precisely validated on specific populations, other researchers have stressed the artificiality of imposing set categories on questionnaires and the need for people to generate their own categories has been stressed.[42] Despite all these difficulties, the quality of life literature has grown enormously and within many medical settings has produced perhaps the most useful approach to measuring outcome. This can be illustrated with reference to research on head and neck cancer.

Using the quality of life scales developed by the European Organization for Research and Treatment of Cancer (EORTC),[43,44,45] a comparison was made between 204 long-term surviving head and neck cancer patients and a matched control group.[46] Reduced quality of life was noted in the experimental group, prompting suggestion that clinicians need to be aware of continuing psychosocial morbidity in the 'cured' group. This is one of the first papers to suggest the potential for psychological interventions to make an impact on quality of life and that this patient group is one that would potentially benefit from this kind of support. In a second paper,[47] patient-rated quality of life scores were compared with physician ratings. Patients consistently rated their quality of life as lower than that rated by the clinicians. This study once again stresses the importance of self-report and the need for interventions which attempt to improve patients' coping strategies and meet their rehabilitation needs. Finally, in a paper examining outcome between 7 and 11 years after treatment, considerable psychological distress was detected on both the General Health Questionnaire and the EORTC questionnaire.[48] This again indicates that psychological distress should be treated, ideally in the form of teaching coping strategies which might impact on quality of life.

A further advantage of the quality of life approach has been the development of measuring tools. From a point 20 years ago when psychological concepts were measured in an ad hoc way in this field, there are now a number of well-validated research tools that can be used to describe the head and neck cancer population and other populations with similar difficulties. Few longitudinal studies have been reported so far and those that have been done follow the natural progression of outcomes rather than evaluating the effectiveness of particular psychological interventions. However, this work has led to an exciting stage in the field where having outlined the problems and developed appropriate research tools, the next logical step is the development of appropriate intervention programs. This is an approach that is still being developed in other areas of facial trauma, but the multidisciplinary nature of the concept, with social and psychological factors weighed alongside more traditional surgical outcomes, has clear advantages in providing the basis for long-term evaluation of conditions and treatment impact.

Coping theories and interventions

'Coping' theories have generated much work in clinical and health psychology and in particular on cancer. These studies have an a priori model within which they attempt to describe psychological issues and how patients manage them. Some studies then go on to suggest or investigate potential intervention strategies within this coping framework. For example, in a study investigating the effects of nursing care guided by self-regulation theory on coping with radiation therapy, by preparing patients carefully pretreatment, less disruption to life activities was found both during and after treatment.[49] Although this is a study of breast and prostate patients, it is well designed and controlled and has a clear practical application for the way in which nurses can prepare patients for invasive procedures in other conditions.

Another approach to rehabilitation after head and neck cancer surgery is in the context of Lazarus's cognitive transactional theory of stress.[50] This approach proposes that a patient will respond to the stress of surgery by trying to identify and develop an appropriate coping response. From this approach developed the Stress-Coping model, known as the 'Dropkin' model (after the author), which allowed the exploration of the process of rehabilitation and the prediction of those aspects of behavior which facilitate good outcome. This model can apply to many groups of patients whose disfigurements may place them at a social disadvantage.

Box 29.3 Behavioral observation and action plan for maxillofacial patients based on Dropkin's plan for head and neck cancer patients

	Postoperative days						
	1	2	3	4	5	6	7
Motor activities							
Lying in bed					A		A
Sitting in chair in room					S		S
Ambulation in room					S		S
Ambulation out of room					E		E
Ambulation beyond ward					S		S
					S		S
Self-care behaviors					M		M
Wash face (mirror)					E		E
Brush hair					N		N
Dressed unaided					T		T
Assist with dressings							
					P		P
Social interaction					O		O
Ambulation out of room					I		I
Eye contact?					N		N
Posture?					T		T
Interaction with staff							
Eye contact?					O		T
Posture?					N		W
Verbal?					E		O
Interaction with other patients							
Eye contact?							
Posture?							
Verbal?							

Action plan

Days 1–7   Monitor and assist

Day 5   Review and prompt ambulation attempt if not out of room

Day 7   All items should have been achieved. Discuss targets with patient reviewing particular concerns. Consider specialist referral.

(NB: Postoperative dates illustrated are for head and neck cancer patients. Target dates for other conditions should be determined by reference to relevant cohort.)

The Dropkin model has been translated into a very practical care plan with specific objectives defined for each postoperative day (Box 29.3). For example, early socialization is identified as a predictor of good long-term outcome, therefore patients are encouraged to leave their rooms and use the whole ward during early ambulation. Immediate postoperative care includes early confrontation of the facial disfigurement by looking in the mirror. Although attempted avoidance may be common this is vigorously challenged and patients are also encouraged to take part in self-care, for example helping with dressings, from the earliest possible stage. It is suggested that postoperative day 5 is an important watershed, with patients who are still having difficulty in taking part in their care more likely to have long-term problems. By day 7, very active clinical intervention from an experienced nurse is indicated for those patients who still have problems in the area of socialization and early ambulation. This intervention takes the form of challenging unhelpful beliefs and emphasizing the importance of surgery; essentially, a cognitive intervention aimed at encouraging the patient to develop a behavioral response. This is one of the first studies to introduce the idea of 'coping' into the literature and it is an extremely effective piece of applied research, using psychological theory to generate and test very practical outcomes. However, there is clearly scope to develop more creative and innovative forms of intervention.

The goals of rehabilitation can thus be summarized in terms of reintegration into social and work settings. The importance of a rehabilitation program that starts early, preferably preoperatively, should be stressed and include strategies such as those outlined above to ensure that the potential for healthy psychosocial recovery is maximized.

Together with the research on quality of life in head and neck cancer, those papers using a coping model to underpin their work consistently stress the need for patients to be offered some kind of support following surgery. Dropkin[50] stands out in specifying the very practical ways in which support can be offered but this work is confined to presurgical preparation and inpatient management: long-term support has so far received less attention.

Programs that work

One of the exceptions to this rule is the work being developed with patients who contacted the charity Changing Faces in the UK, for help with the long-term management of maxillofacial conditions.[51] This work uses a cognitive-behavioral framework to challenge unhelpful cognitions about the condition and its impact and provides a very practical training in coping strategies.

The impact of this kind of approach has been examined using a group format and measured very positive outcomes in terms of lowered social anxiety and avoidance behavior after an intervention of only 2 days.[12] More recently, a program has been developed that can be delivered successfully by head and neck cancer nurse specialists.[52] This approach is based on a model for understanding much of the dysfunction following treatment of head and neck cancer in terms of social embarrassment. Patients may not only look different but also sound different and report problems in eating in public. Using a coping skills approach, patients can learn different strategies for managing these difficulties in the same way as they manage social interaction problems associated with disfigurement, with positive impact on social functioning and quality of life.

A similar approach, delivered in both group and individual settings, has been used at the first NHS-sponsored Disfigurement Support Unit.[13] Patients who had been disfigured as a result of maxillofacial trauma showed benefits in their cognitive evaluation of the noticeability and importance of their change in appearance, improvement in social anxiety and appearance-related distress and also in behavioral measures such as the development of positive coping strategies. Greater number and variety of alternative coping strategies were associated with better outcome.

Given the number of papers that have suggested the importance of coping strategies and of teaching effective management strategies to patients, it is encouraging that this approach is gradually beginning to receive more attention with patients who have maxillofacial trauma, particularly since it is increasingly used in the management of other chronic conditions.

It is also important to note that problems associated with dysfunction as well as disfigurement, including chronic pain, can be modified using psychological as well as biomedical approaches, particularly as level of dysfunction is such a strong predictor of good long-term outcome on quality of life measures. Psychological intervention that impacts on the beliefs and behavior of a given population aims not to remove the problem or to make individuals 'feel better' about the problem but to actively change the way in which they manage and control it.

Patient and family perspectives

A further source of information about psychosocial aspects of maxillofacial trauma is based on focus groups or discussion with patient organizations. The conclusions can be summarized by reference to the recent study of head and neck cancer.[53]

Quality of life was extremely important to patients and they stressed that head and neck cancer has a major impact on both patients and their families. Some of the most striking findings of this study were concerned with deceptively simple issues, such as kindness and patience from medical staff, and someone available to really listen to their concerns, and advise. This suggests that counseling might have a role and many of the patients in this study were aware that counseling has become an important part of rehabilitation after conditions such as breast cancer. Many people wished that it had been offered and felt that they were unable to ask unless it was offered. Some felt that counselors would not understand unless they had undergone a similar experience, suggesting that there might be a role for group interventions and peer support. Similarly, the numbers of patients contacting the lay-led charities which work with maxillofacial patients, such as Changing Faces and Let's Face it, are an indication that lay-led groups can act as an important resource in the long-term psychological support of these patients (see[51] for review).

Long-term support from an informed professional has been highlighted as important in other studies. Patients may discover that they knew more about the management of a tracheostomy or other aspect of their condition than their GP or district nurse. The opportunity to access very practical help such as how to get hold of portable suction equipment is important. Facilitating the skills of health professionals in the community by providing training for district nurses and inviting them to meet patients before discharge can considerably enhance rehabilitation.[54]

Summary of psychological impact of maxillofacial trauma

Taken as a body of work, research confirms that maxillofacial trauma may have a major impact on the individual. Patients represent a high-risk group for severe psychiatric illness especially given the high incidence of premorbid conditions such as alcoholism and substance abuse, which increase the probability of severe depression, anxiety and potential suicide postoperatively.

Psychosocial problems may persist and get worse over time even where medical problems resolve. Measurable psychiatric symptoms may persist months or years after the traumatic event with a resulting breakdown in lifestyle. Where avoidant coping strategies are used, individuals do not have the opportunity to develop a repertoire of positive coping responses and social avoidance may develop into complete social isolation. Length of time since trauma is not therefore a useful predictor of outcome without considering the patient's coping style.

The impact of change of appearance on psychological distress has produced equivocal findings. For many maxillofacial patients, separating the relative impact of disfigurement and dysfunction is difficult to do, but it is intriguing that studies of other conditions in which there is no associated dysfunction, e.g. dermatological conditions, find no relationship between severity (usually size or noticeability) of the lesion and psychological distress. This counterintuitive finding has been repeatedly reported.[7,51] Work with burn-injured adults has found no relationship between *objective* severity of the burn and psychological distress, but a significant relationship between *perceived* severity and distress.[39] Given this evidence, it is important to consider the psychological impact of *any* change of appearance after trauma; there is no basis for assuming that patients with minor scarring are at less risk for psychological distress than those with severe scarring. Similarly, following surgery for head and neck cancer, patients with a severe disfigurement may adapt as well as patients with a much less obvious defect. Clearly there is a psychological dimension to adaptation which involves the cognitive appraisal of the outcome in the light of other issues. A good working understanding of the ways in which these factors combine is in terms of 'the impact of the disease on the individual'.[54] In other words, how well can this person adapt to changes caused by trauma or treatment given their lifestyle and the extent of their social support?

The importance of social interaction is highlighted in the literature on disfigurement across conditions and re-emerges in the quality of life literature as a major determinant of long-term outcome after maxillofacial trauma. The use of prostheses, pressure garments for burns injury and the exposure of the individual to situations which are perceived as socially embarrassing are particularly highlighted. Speech and eating difficulties can impact on the individual because of their social effect rather than because of the day-to-day management in practical terms. Interventions aimed at facilitating a patient's ability to maintain social function within the family, at school and at work are a logical development from these findings and a few successful studies have been reported.

Social support, as in many studies of adaptation after major surgery or disease, is important in predicting good outcome. This is a challenging finding given the premorbid characteristics of patients who experience burns, trauma and head and neck cancer, with the very factors that increase risk of injury or disease also predicting poor social support. Maximizing support is an important goal for rehabilitation nevertheless, with relatives involved in planning long-term care where possible and where support is not necessarily evident in close family attachments, introduction to lay-led support groups.

Impact of age, gender and ethnicity must also be considered. Research studies on disfigurement across conditions find no effect for these variables but this may be because there has been relatively little research on large populations, and particularly within ethnic populations. Given the importance of the face in reinforcing feminine stereotypes,

however, there is an assumption that facial injuries for girls and women are linked with poorer outcome, but any effect is likely to be diminished as society increases the pressure for perfection for men too.

Planning and Managing Psychological Support after Maxillofacial Trauma

Given the number of different approaches to psychological research outlined in the previous section, it follows that psychosocial support could be defined differently according to the background and theoretical orientation of whomever is providing it. In practice, the most pragmatic way of understanding what psychosocial support might be is to look at the two main ways in which it is delivered to patients.

Psychological support as an integral part of routine patient care

Psychological support can be described as part of the routine management of all patients. Patient care therefore includes a psychosocial component in the same way that all patients are offered analgesia, routine physiotherapy, wound care management, etc. This process may be designed and managed by one designated person, but will be delivered by all members of the multidisciplinary team. The aim is to ensure that treatment outcomes are maximized by providing appropriate information to ensure compliance, reduction of anxiety, promotion of self-care and development of appropriate coping strategies in the short and long term. In essence, this approach provides a patient-centered environment that looks beyond the condition to the individual, his needs and the needs of his family. This is psychological support as patients commonly refer to it in self-report studies. Their experience is characterized by staff attitudes, time available to talk through issues that concern them, information available when they need it, etc. This may be experienced as relative informality, but in fact depends on careful management to ensure that protocols of care are in place; the inclusion of the term 'psychological support' as part of the nursing process is not enough without ensuring that all staff are appropriately trained and that psychological issues are not dismissed as secondary to physical aspects of care.

In some units, psychologists may be central in organizing this support but in others mental health professionals may not be involved at all; indeed, it can be difficult for a ward team who offer this standard of care to understand what a liaison psychiatrist or clinical psychologist can add. 'We do all our own psychological support' is not an uncommon view.

Problem-focused psychological support

Mental health professionals are more commonly involved in the second category of psychological support and this can be defined as problem-focused support. Rather than offer intervention to all patients undergoing treatment, patients are selected on the basis of problems encountered in their management. These may occur at any stage in treatment; for example, patients may need to be assessed for substance misuse prior to surgery and appropriate smoking or alcohol cessation programs instigated. Problems may be identified postoperatively in terms of poor coping or socialization in line with a Dropkin-style protocol or patients may have increased anxiety or depression, flashbacks or other symptoms requiring treatment. Long-term follow-up can disclose failure to re-engage in day-to-day activities, social avoidance and isolation, poor compliance with treatment, e.g. use of pressure garments, or for children, school refusal or failure. Problem-focused psychological support is usually managed and delivered by a designated mental health professional.

The way in which these two kinds of support are integrated is obviously very important. A problem-focused approach is only as good as the screening process that identifies problems in the first place. At the inpatient stage, careful monitoring of progress with early socialization, monitoring of mood and self-care behaviors or an apparent lack of social support can be important indicators in identifying who needs further help. Standardized measures such as screening instruments for anxiety and depression and quality of life measures can be useful in assessing long-term outcome, but a good clinical interview can be equally important. Many psychological issues, particularly problems such as poor sexual function, will rarely be volunteered by the patient and will not be picked up at all unless there are clear protocols for psychological assessment included in routine follow-up. Box 29.4 gives an example of questions developed to identify psychosocial issues by the organization Changing Faces. Raising questions about appearance and disfigurement is notoriously difficult. These have been selected from a pilot study with medical registrars, on the basis that they are questions that medical personnel feel comfortable asking.

Children are particularly difficult to assess, either denying their problems completely or rating them as much worse than the ratings given by their parents. A specialist assessment is indicated wherever there are signs of problems, often first evident as a breakdown in behavior routines.

In practice, a problem-focused approach will only work effectively in settings where psychological support is a routine part of the treatment package, where appropriate assessment procedures are in place and where pathways to appropriate referral are both available and properly understood.

Building psychosocial support into routine patient care

Patient advocacy

Increasingly, in specialist services, a multidisciplinary team will manage patients with representation from many different specialisms. From the patient perspective, this translates into a lot of different people to see, often at one visit and frequently in one room (the 'goldfish bowl' effect). This is a daunting prospect for anybody and the efficiency with which

---

Box 29.4 Example of a simple psychological screening process for identifying patients' appearance-related concerns[55]

STEP ONE

Q1 How do you think that the change in your appearance will affect your life, if at all? (Record response)

If patient indicates no impact, confirm with a statement:
So there is nothing that you think you will feel uncomfortable about when you first go home?
If yes, go on to step 2. If no, go on to step 3.

STEP TWO

Q2 What are the specific things that you feel less comfortable about?
(list 3 examples)   1
                     2
                     3

STEP THREE

Q3 Sometimes patients ask what to do when other people ask questions about their (use patient's condition as the example). I'd be interested to hear what kind of thing you think that you might do.
(record response)

STEP FOUR: Observation of behaviour during the assessment
Did the patient avoid making eye contact with you?   **Y/N**
Did the patient try to conceal his face by turning to one side or covering his face with his hand?   **Y/N**

STEP FIVE: Action planning
Based on the patient's verbal and non-verbal responses to your questions, do you think there are any social or emotional consequences of the change in his appearance due to maxillofacial trauma?

Yes   No   Maybe   (please circle one)
If your answer is 'yes' or 'maybe' will you:

- suggest that he speaks to the psychologist
- ask the psychologist to speak to him
- offer him relevant information
- suggest a coping strategy yourself.

---

information exchange takes place will be reduced by patient anxiety. For children, there may be concerns that have not even been shared with parents.

One way of overcoming these problems is through advocacy. An initial interview with the patient by one member of the team can both explain procedures and elicit any particular questions and concerns. This member of the team then takes responsibility for ensuring that everything that is of importance to the patient is discussed with the relevant team member. A second review session in a one-to-one setting can ensure that all advice is clearly understood and any outstanding issues dealt with. In practice, this role can be filled by a designated nurse or clinical nurse specialist or member of the medical team. This is a particularly helpful model for managing large ward rounds.

Although the process of using tissue expanders was explained to a 10-year-old boy undergoing reconstructive surgery after burns, he became increasingly withdrawn and tearful at home. Assessment with a child psychologist using drawing and modeling materials demonstrated that he assumed that his head was going to become enormous and that he might eventually be unable to move. This misperception was managed by encouraging him to prepare his own questions and alerting his consultant to prompt him at an early appointment.

Information

The request for information is a consistent finding in research into patient satisfaction with diagnosis and treatment, in studies of quality of life during rehabilitation and throughout the health psychology literature. Most patients want to be adequately and honestly informed at each stage of treatment, although it is important to respect the subgroup of patients who prefer to leave all decision making in the hands of their medical team.

However, balanced against this desire for information, patients sometimes complain of being bombarded with information at certain points in the treatment course, for example at diagnosis, and of feeling bewildered and unable to take all of it in. Information given verbally at any stage may not be remembered accurately, the patient may lack the appropriate framework for asking questions and information may be poorly understood. The same problems are reported by relatives and carers, even if present during consultation, who may remain uninformed or misinformed and therefore unable to offer the optimum level of appropriate support both during treatment and when the patient goes home. Given the evidence of the importance of social support in health outcomes generally, they can be seen as a huge untapped or wasted resource.

Whilst health professionals recognize that patients need information to manage their working and social lives, they have been slower to recognize the role of the individual in actively managing the condition. Despite the evidence that an informed and knowledgeable patient can expect a better outcome, patients can still be viewed with suspicion if they ask for a second opinion, want to read professional literature or even take notes in the consultation. Access to information via the Internet which has no efficient quality control is becoming a problem in medical settings. There remains a problem in providing the kind of information the patients are asking for, which facilitates rather than challenges the working arrangement between health professional and patient.

In some units, patients are routinely offered a folder of information relating to various aspects of their care or invited to hold their own care plans, building up information on each aspect of their care as it becomes relevant. An example of this is the Teamwork project currently being evaluated with cancer patients in the UK, in association with the National Cancer Alliance. However, the principle applies equally well in other conditions, particularly where there is a long time course, frequent investigations and management by multidisciplinary teams. Patient-led organizations such as CancerBacup and Changing Faces produce a variety of different publications that can be made available routinely. Perhaps a more patient-centered approach, and certainly a cheaper one, is to provide details of what exactly is available, when the patient is most likely to find it helpful and which member of the team is the appropriate person to ask. This allows the individual to pace the process of information gathering and reduces the chances of misinformation gathered from the least experienced member of the team. This also allows the patient to take the lead in eliciting information. Whether communicating directly with a patient or designing written material for them to take away, the following are useful guidelines.[56]

All written material offered to patients should have the source attributed and be dated to ensure quality control standards. A small ward or outpatient library can be easily assembled and accessed and makes good use of time spent waiting for appointments.

Planning for elective surgery

Modification of risk behaviors

Clearly, the nature of maxillofacial trauma means that many patients are treated as an emergency. However, for some conditions where a series of surgical procedures is planned as part of reconstructive surgery, psychological assessment can be very helpful. In addition to screening for PTSD or other psychiatric symptoms that require treatment, psychological support may target risk behaviors. A smoking cessation program can provide real benefits in terms of lung function and wound healing even where the patient stops smoking just a few days or weeks prior to surgery. Alcohol intake should be carefully assessed since detoxification over a few days can prevent problems of acute confusional states postoperatively. Protocols for managing substance abuse range from early admission of patients (by a few days), so that alcohol can be withdrawn and appropriate medication substituted, to individual sessions supporting smoking withdrawal.[54]

Looking in the mirror and early socialization

Most specialist units remove mirrors so that the introduction to a new appearance can be planned (although in practice, most patients catch sight of themselves in reflective surfaces anyway). It clearly makes sense to ensure that appearance is optimized as much as possible, e.g. to wait until the immediate edema is reduced. However, it is important that protocols do not, however unwittingly, promote a policy of avoidance. The key to successful rehabilitation is the confrontation and

Patient recall is influenced by the following.

- Intellectual level has a low but constant correlation to recall levels.
- More medical knowledge generally means higher rates of recall.
- Primacy effect – material presented first is recalled better.
- Statements perceived as important are recalled better.
- What patient recalls short term tends to be recalled for some time.
- Patients' understanding, memory, satisfaction and their levels of compliance are all linked.

Implications for consultations.

- Use the primacy effect.
- Stress importance.
- Simplify.
- Categorize.
- Repeat.
- Follow-up to ensure understanding.
- Written material – needs to be noticed, read, understood, believed and remembered.
- Keep it simple!

management of change and this approach should begin as soon as possible.

The first step is education. In this phase, the patient needs to understand that appearance will continue to change dramatically and that this is not the end of the process. Questions should be answered frankly and uncertainty about outcome should be framed as far as possible in terms of the control that the individual can exert. For example, the long-term presence of disfigurement or scars can be discussed in terms of the use of pressure garments.

Understanding responses to altered appearance in terms of the framework in Fig. 29.2 is helpful in planning support for the patient at this stage. This framework, developed for working with patients at Changing Faces, focuses on the patient's feelings, beliefs (cognitions) and behavior. It can be used both to understand the issues confronting patients and to form the basis of therapeutic interventions.

However well prepared, patients will experience shock and need time to talk about their feelings. They may choose to talk about how they feel, they may wish to have time before talking or they may choose not to disclose their feelings at all. Managing this process at a time when the patient is assured of the opportunity for contemplation, rather than just before visitors are due, etc, is of obvious importance. This process has been likened to bereavement or grieving for the lost self and the emphasis is on the chance for someone to talk about his feelings rather than offering management strategies at this stage.

Beliefs about the future are likely to be confused. For all the reasons discussed earlier in this chapter, people may feel that their plans and hopes about the future have suddenly all vanished. Catastrophizing or magnifying negative events may lead to a situation where the patient believes that he will never work again, never have friends, never form relationships, etc. Acknowledging this pattern of thinking without necessarily probing too far is a helpful intervention at this stage. Talking in general terms about these patterns of thinking, particularly when changing dressings or helping patients with self-care activities, will help to acknowledge these thoughts as a normal part of the response to trauma. This is also a chance for extreme reactions or altered mood to be picked up.

As the initial shock of the trauma becomes less extreme, focusing on behavior becomes a key intervention. Involving patients in their own self-care such as dressings, encouraging relatives to ask whether cutting up food, doing up buttons, etc. is helpful before assuming the care role, all help to promote independence from the outset. Early mobilization around the unit provides the earliest opportunities for social interaction and the basis for building key non-verbal strategies. Encouraging patients to stand up with a good posture, to maintain eye contact, to nod, to stop and talk to other patients and discouraging behaviors like covering the face with the hand or trying to let hair fall forward over the face are important.

Gradually building on this behavior each day will not only provide the foundations of effective coping but will impact on patients' beliefs and feelings about themselves and their opportunities for the future. Verbal coping strategies can be supported by written information, but learning to answer simple questions about appearance is a very helpful skill. Anyone who has obviously sustained a facial injury will be questioned and giving a simple answer to the question 'What happened to your face?' is something that everyone should be prepared for and feel confident about responding to.

This early socialization can be set down as a protocol with assessment at key stages and planned intervention where problems arise. In practice, this is exactly the same process as wound management where stitches are inspected for signs of infection, removed on a set day and where a remedial process – antibiotic therapy – is triggered where problems arise. For example, the patient who is particularly tearful or reluctant to leave his room by the end of the first week might be referred for specialist help from the psychologist.

A three-point standard for all patients who have altered appearance at the point of discharge is set out in Box 29.5.

Planning future care

The importance of this moment for the patient cannot be overemphasized. All the patient's concerns, once the immediate life-threatening phase is over, are in terms of the uncertainty of the future and what can be done in terms of medical and surgical input.

The uncertainty of outcome after maxillofacial trauma is compounded by the length of time involved in waiting to see how well reconstructive techniques have worked before planning the next phase. Understanding that the medical team does not yet know precisely what further surgery will be needed can be hard for people to take in. Similarly, it is frustrating for the medical team to be framing their responses

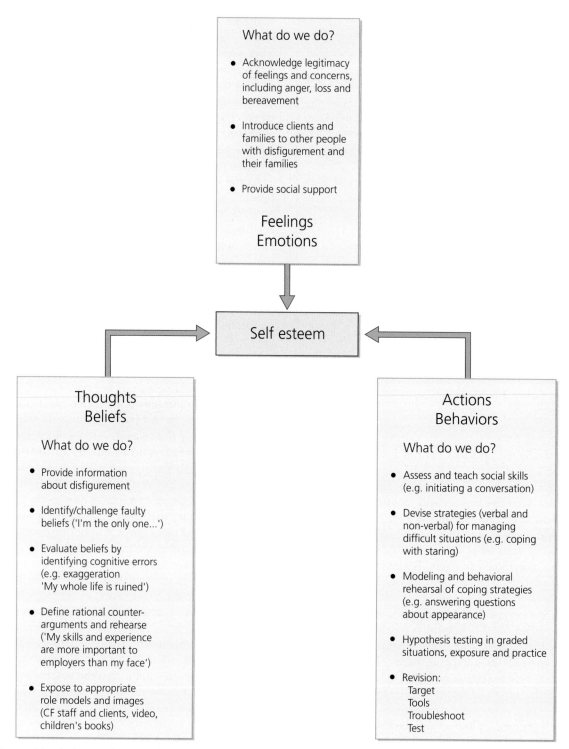

Fig. 29.2: A cognitive-behavioral approach to managing disfigurement (reproduced with permission from reference 51).

in a way that can come across as evasive. Putting a time frame on decisions, preferably within a written care plan, is of great value to the patient. A clear indication of how frequently appointments will be planned and the kinds of decisions that will be made at each one is very reassuring. Structuring the time between decisions in terms of patients' and relatives' roles also turns what is effectively a 'wait and see' process into one of active management and control. For example, diary keeping, both of significant personal events and treatment compliance (wearing of pressure garments, taking medication, etc.) and the use of photographs pasted in to record change are ways in which the family can measure progress. These kinds of approaches are especially helpful with children who have less understanding of time. It is also important to stress that physical and psychological recovery may proceed at different rates. Patients have not necessarily recovered or 'got over it' just because the wound has healed. Relatives can find this very difficult to absorb and lay-led organizations or support groups can be very helpful in supporting people through this stage.

Box 29.5   A three-point standard for patients who have altered appearance, at the point of discharge[58]

Patients should:

- have the name of the appropriate patient support group

- have access to relevant information about their condition and its management

- be able to answer simple questions about their condition.

Psychological issues in reconstructive surgery

Whilst there is a clear and logical imperative towards surgery which aims to restore function, techniques aimed at restoring appearance stimulate a wider debate. Both the medical team and the patient can find psychological support useful in the process of decision making. Reconstructive surgery can continue forever in the sense that there is always the opportunity to revise a scar and to make minor improvements to appearance. Sometimes it is the patient who seeks additional surgery and sometimes surgeons feel a responsibility to suggest further revision if improvement is possible. Both groups may find it difficult to work out the cost–benefit analysis, which focuses on the individual and the likely improvement in his lifestyle and self-esteem rather than simply on the surgical result. In this decision it is vital to base decisions on the evidence that it is *perceived noticeability and importance to the patient* of any altered appearance that is important rather than objective assessment. Psychological assessment can help to understand the benefits of surgery in this context, to allow patients to examine their motivation and to decide the point at which they feel comfortable about stopping the search for surgical solutions. Intervention can also be useful where there are unrealistic expectations about what surgery can achieve and where the motivation for surgery is principally about self-confidence, psychologists can help to clarify the relationship between objective physical appearance and self-esteem.

The evidence for the psychological benefits of reconstructive surgery is more compelling in esthetic surgery than for surgery following trauma. This may in part result from the mismatch between the patients' expectations of surgery and what can realistically be achieved or from the differences in the perceived value of appearance to the two different populations, but is also certainly due to the paucity of good controlled research studies. This is a field in which reliable instruments for measuring the change in appearance, the patients' perception of that change and the impact on relevant psychological variables have not been available. The recent publication of the Derriford Appearance Scale[57] and the body image module of the EORTC scales[45] will allow some of this important work to take place.

Problem-focused support

The process of routine care described above is provided largely by the multidisciplinary team. Psychological issues are acknowledged as part of the expected response to trauma and managed by facilitating coping responses, maximizing patients' sense of self-efficacy and perceived control in order to promote a good quality of life. Built into these standard care protocols are assessment stages in which problems are identified which require more focused input; this is the stage at which problems are viewed as either different from or more severe than the usual problems encountered by patients experiencing maxillofacial trauma and this is where referral to mental health professionals is appropriate. Typical problems will include PTSD, family problems, severe mood disorders such as depression and anxiety, poor social skills and social withdrawal, sexual anxiety and dysfunction. For children, problems encountered with bullying and poor school performance can be exacerbated into school refusal or phobia.

Who can provide problem-focused support?

One of the difficulties for the medical team working in this area is to fully understand the difference between the many different disciplines offering psychological support. A referral to a clinical psychologist, a psychiatrist, a psychotherapist or a counselor may result in quite different goals for the patients and different approaches to their management. Even within these disciplines, different therapists have preferred models for understanding behavior. 'What works for whom' is clearly important and although a detailed review of the different merits of various psychological therapies is clearly not within the scope of this chapter, a brief outline of these different approaches and their appropriateness in different situations will be given in order to facilitate effective clinical referral, service planning and delivery.

Psychiatrists

Doctors who work within a medical model, understanding psychiatric symptoms, for example depression, in terms of illness. (Psychologists, in contrast, would understand depression more in terms of a response to a set of maladaptive thoughts, beliefs and behaviors.) Some psychiatrists offer psychotherapy, others refer to other health professionals if they feel that psychotherapy would be helpful, but only psychiatrists are qualified to treat patients using medication.

> A woman in her late 30s developed a depressive illness and became socially withdrawn following a dogbite to her face. Treated with antidepressant medication, her mood improved but she remained phobic about going out. A cognitive – behavioral program run by a clinical psychologist allowed her to build a series of coping strategies and gradual exposure on a graded regime resulted in her successful recovery and return to work.

Clinical psychologists

Qualified psychologists who have undergone a postgraduate training. They are essentially problem solvers, drawing heavily on their knowledge of research to help their clients understand the nature of their difficulties and designing and testing effective solutions. Clinical psychologists may use a number of different approaches in their work, but they usually set clear targets and measure outcomes.

A man in his late 20s who had lost an eye in a traffic accident was referred for help with his social anxiety and difficulty in forming relationships with prospective partners. Work with the psychologist focused on his discomfort with eye contact and anxiety in large groups. Cognitive techniques were used to challenge his perception of how he thought people perceived him and behavioral strategies were taught to help him cope with staring, comments and questions and to take the initiative in conversation. His social anxiety fell and he increased his social activity, beginning to have successful relationships with girlfriends.

Counselors

May have between one and many years training. They use the relationship between themselves and their clients to provide an environment in which the client can work towards living more resourcefully and successfully. The counselor's role is to listen and to help the client to clarify and organize his thoughts; a counselor does not give advice in the sense of suggesting solutions. Counselors may not have a degree in psychology or use the scientific understanding of behavior in their work, but they often have specialist expertise in working in a specific area, e.g. cancer, bereavement and disfigurement.

Psychotherapists

Perhaps most easily defined by comparing what they do with counselors. There is much overlap between counseling and psychotherapy, with many counselors arguing that what they do is in fact psychotherapy. In practical terms, though, counseling can be seen to be rather more about what is happening here and now, whilst psychotherapy is about the way in which patterns of behavior from the past repeat themselves in the relationship between the therapist and the client. This means that counselors are generally working with their clients on a specific problem, whilst psychotherapists are working on a more general approach to managing any problem in a different way.

Any or all of these specialists might have a role in maxillofacial trauma. There is a clear role for a liaison psychiatrist in managing PTSD, anxiety and depression with appropriate medication. Clinical psychologists often work with psychiatrists in the management of anxiety and depression, using a cognitive-behavioral approach to help patients to challenge unhelpful beliefs and develop more appropriate behavior. Clinical psychologists might also work within a coping framework to help patients develop more positive coping strategies

---

A woman in her 30s who had severe burn injuries dating from childhood referred herself for counseling to help her with her depressed mood and social isolation. Having been hospitalized for over a year as a child she had been educated in a special needs school although she was of above average intelligence. Counseling allowed her to identify areas of her life that she wanted to change. She moved out of the house she shared with her mother and increased her independent social activities. During the course of the sessions, it became clear that she had many questions about limits imposed by her injuries, e.g. her ability to have children, although she had been too frightened to consider medical referral. Counseling helped her to prioritize her concerns and she was reassured about the legitimacy of referral. She was encouraged to seek further surgical assessment and successfully underwent surgery to release contracted scar tissue.

A patient who had been markedly disfigured following maxillofacial trauma as a child did not have his disfigurement repaired until adulthood, when surgery was completely successful. Psychotherapy referral was arranged to allow him to explore his feelings of anger, primarily towards his parents who he blamed both for the injury and for their failure to discuss it with him or seek reconstructive surgery despite his evident unhappiness throughout his childhood.

---

by a process of anxiety management and graded exposure aimed to overcome social avoidance. With children, they may work together with schools to ensure that the child's needs are fully understood and that there are recognized procedures in place to manage any discrimination. Most psychologists would work in a similar way.

Both psychiatrists and clinical psychologists offer forms of therapy that are highly structured and directive. Patients are either prescribed a course of treatment or consent to a series of therapeutic sessions in which the focus of intervention is behavior change. Targets are set and outcomes are measured. In contrast, psychotherapy and (usually) counseling are non-directive, with the therapist following the lead of the patient.

Although there has been very little research into what works for this population, there is more evidence for the directive approach to management. Coping skills training has been demonstrated to be effective in both individual and group settings. Counselors employed in health settings often, in practice, take a more solution-focused approach to treatment than in other settings, but long-term individual psychotherapy is probably indicated only when, as in the example above, there are long-standing emotional difficulties. Long-term psychotherapeutic groups have not been evaluated with this population.

This distinction between directive and non-directive approaches is also important in considering lay-led support groups. The stereotype support group, a collection of people sympathizing with each other about their problems, is not helpful. However, good patient-led support groups adhere much more closely to a coping model, promoting self-management, inviting speakers to talk to them about the specialized aspects of their condition and providing focused and informed support to their members. They are an increasingly important resource in the long-term management of all chronic medical conditions.

Conclusion

This chapter has reviewed the main principles of psychological support for patients who have undergone maxillofacial trauma, with particular emphasis given to the management of appearance-related concerns. A distinction has been drawn between the process of psychological support delivered as part of the routine process of care and clinical interventions provided for those patients who develop specific psychological problems.

Providing a supportive environment for patients is important both in preventing long-term problems and in providing for the early identification of problems that require more focused input. The principles of effective support have been discussed and it is important to note that this is delivered by the whole multidisciplinary team rather than exclusively by mental health professionals. Changing Faces is only one organization that can provide training and support in the form of study days and access to relevant resources.

Access to relevant mental health specialists varies in different units. Liaison psychiatry may be more easily accessed than help from psychologists, although this direct help is also available through the lay-led routes. The important message is that psychological support is more than simply providing a listening ear and clinical intervention using the kind of directive approaches that have been outlined provides patients with both surgical and psychological alternatives for managing the impact of maxillofacial trauma.

References

1 Partridge J 1994 Changing faces: the challenge of facial disfigurement. Penguin Books, London

2 Morselli PG 1993 The minotaur syndrome: plastic surgery of the facial skeleton. Aesthetic Plastic Surgery 17: 99–102

3 Stam HJ, Koopmans JP, Mathieson CM 1991 The psychosocial impact of a laryngectomy: a comprehensive assessment. Journal of Psychosocial Oncology 9(3): 37–58

4 Argyle M 1994 The psychology of interpersonal behavior. Penguin, New York

5 Diamond J 1999 C – because cowards get cancer too. Vermillion, London

6 Macgregor F 1974 Transformation and identity: the face and plastic surgery. Quadrangle/New York Times Book Company, New York

7 Lansdown R, Rumsey N, Bradbury E, Carr T, Partridge J 1997 Visibly different: coping with disfigurement. Butterworth-Heinemann, London

8 Partridge J 1998 Changing faces: taking up Macgregor's challenge. Journal of Burn Care and Rehabilitation 19(2): 174–180

9 Bradbury E 1996 Counselling people with disfigurement. British Psychological Society Books, Leicester

10 McGrouther DA 1997 Facial disfigurement: the last bastion of discrimination. British Medical Journal 314: 991

11 Strenta F, Kleck R 1985 Physical disability and the attribution dilemma: perceiving the causes of social behaviour. Journal of Social and Clinical Psychology 3: 129–142

12 Robinson E, Rumsey N, Partridge J 1996 An evaluation of the impact of social interaction skills training for facially disfigured people. British Journal of Plastic Surgery 49: 281–289

13 Kleve L, Rumsey N, Wyn-Williams M, White P 2002 The effectiveness of cognitive behavioural interventions at Outlook: a disfigurement support unit. Journal of Evaluation in Clinical Practice 8(4): 387–395

14 American Psychiatric Association 1994 Diagnostic and statistical manual of mental disorders, 4th edn. American Psychiatric Association, Washington DC

15 Zigmond A, Snaith R 1983 The hospital anxiety and depression scale. Acta Psychiatrica Scandinavica 67: 361–370

16 Rippere V 1994 Depression: investigation. In: Lindsay SJE, Powell GE (eds) The handbook of adult clinical psychology, 2nd edn. Routledge, London

17 Bradley BP 1994 Depression: treatment. In: Lindsay SJE, Powell GE (eds) The handbook of adult clinical psychology, 2nd edn. Routledge, London

18 Lanigan S, Cotterill J 1989 Psychological disabilities amongst patients with port wine stains. British Journal of Dermatology 121: 209–215

19 Tudahl LA, Blades BC, Munster AM 1987 Sexual satisfaction in burns patients. Journal of Burn Care and Rehabilitation 8: 292–293

20 Wallace I, Lees J 1988 A psychological follow-up study of adult patients discharged from a British burn unit. Burns 14(1): 39–45

21 Balakrishnan C, Hashim M, Gao D 1999 The effect of partial thickness facial burns on social functioning. Journal of Burn Care and Rehabilitation 20(3): 224–225

22 Patterson DR, Everett JJ, Bombardier CH, Quested KA, Lee VK, Marvin JA 1993 Psychological effects of severe burn injuries. Psychological Bulletin 113(2): 362–378

23 Walters E 1997 Problems faced by children and families living with visible difference. In: Lansdown R et al (eds) Visibly different: coping with disfigurement. Butterworth-Heinemann, London

24 Tarnowski KJ, Rasnake LK, Garvaghan-Jones MP, Smith L 1991 Psychosocial sequelae of pediatric burns injuries: a review. Clinical Psychology Review 11: 371–398

25 Salmon P 2000 Psychology of medicine and surgery. John Wiley, Chichester

26 Yule W (ed) 1999 Post traumatic stress disorders. Concepts and therapy. John Wiley, Chichester

27 WHO 1993 The ICD-10 classification of mental and behavioural disorders: clinical descriptions and diagnostic guidelines. World Health Organization, Geneva

28 Tarrier N 1995 Psychological morbidity in adult burns patients: Prevalence and treatment. Journal of Mental Health 1: 51–62

29 Koren D, Arnon I, Klein E 1999 Acute stress and post traumatic stress disorder in traffic accident victims: a one year prospective follow-up study. American Journal of Psychiatry 156(3): 367–373

30 Foa EB, Davidson JRT, Frances A, Ross R 1999 Expert consensus treatment guidelines for post traumatic stress disorder. Journal of Clinical Psychiatry 60 (suppl 16)

31 Carr A 1999 The handbook of child and adolescent clinical psychology. A contextual approach. Routledge, London

32 Breitbart W, Holland J 1988 Psychosocial aspects of head and neck cancer. Seminars in Oncology 151: 61–69

33 Henderson JM, Ord RA 1997 Suicide in head and neck cancer patients. Journal of Oral and Maxillofacial Surgery 55: 1217–1221

34 Thomas DW, Hill CM 1999 Etiology and changing patterns of maxillofacial trauma. In: Ward-Booth P, Schendel SA, Hausamen JE (eds) Maxillofacial surgery. Churchill Livingstone, London

35 Hussain K, Wijetunge DB, Grubnic S, Jackson IT 1994 A comprehensive analysis of craniofacial trauma. Journal of Trauma 36: 34–47

36 Dinh-Zarr T, DiGuiseppi C, Heitman E, Roberts I 2000 Interventions for preventing injuries in problem drinkers (review). The Cochrane Library, issue 1. Update Software, Oxford

37 Rapaport Y, Kreitler S, Chaiklick S, Algor R, Weissler, K 1993 Psychosocial problems in head and neck cancer patients and their change with time since diagnosis. Annals of Oncology 4: 69–73

38 Baur KM, Hardy PE, Van Dorten B 1998 Post-traumatic stress disorder in burn populations: a critical review of the literature. Journal of Burn Care and Rehabilitation 19(3): 230–240

39 Kleve L, Robinson E 1999 A survey of psychological need amongst adult burn-injured patients. Burns 25: 575–579

40 Cella DF, Tulsky DS 1990 Measuring quality of life today: methodological aspects. Oncology 4(5): 29–38

41 WHO 1997 Measuring quality of life. World Health Organization, Geneva

42 O'Boyle CA, McGee H, Hickey A, Joyce CRB, Browne J, O'Malley K 1993 The schedule for the evaluation of individual quality of life. Administration manual. Department of Psychology, Royal College of Surgeons in Ireland, Dublin, Ireland

43 Aaronson NK, Ahmedzai S, Bergman B et al 1993 The European Organisation for Research and Treatment of Cancer QLQ-C30: a quality of life instrument for use in international clinical trials in oncology. Journal of the National Cancer Institute 85: 365–367

44 Bjordal K, Kaasa S 1992 Psychometric validation of the EORTC core quality of life questionnaire 30 item version and a diagnosis-specific module for head and neck cancer patients. Acta Otolaryngolica (Stockholm) 32: 311–321

45 Bjordal K, Ahlner-Elmquist M, Tolleson E et al 1994 Development of a European Organisation for Research and Treatment of Cancer (EORTC) questionnaire module to be used in quality of life assessments in head and neck cancer patients. EORTC Quality of Life Group. Acta Oncologica 33(8): 879–885

46 Bjordal K, Freng A, Thorvik J, Kaasa S 1995 Patient reported and clinician rated quality of life in head and neck patients: a cross-sectional study. European Journal of Cancer, Part B, Oral Oncology 31B(4): 235–241

47 Bjordal K, Mastekaasa A, Kaasa S 1995 Self reported satisfaction with life and physical health in long-term cancer survivors and a matched control group. European Journal of Cancer. Part B, Oral Oncology 31B(4): 340–345

48 Bjordal K, Kaasa S 1995 Psychological distress in head and neck cancer patients 7–11 years after curative treatment. British Journal of Cancer 71(3): 592–597

49 Johnson JE, Fieler VK, Wlasowicz GS, Mitchell ML, Jones LS 1997 The effects of nursing care guided by self-regulation theory on coping with radiation therapy. Oncology Nursing Forum 24(6): 1041–1050

50 Dropkin MJ 1989 Coping with disfigurement and dysfunction after head and neck cancer surgery: a conceptual framework. Seminars in Oncological Nursing 5(3): 213–219

51 Clarke A 1999 Psychosocial aspects of facial disfigurement: problems, management and the role of a lay-led organisation. Psychology, Health and Medicine 4(2): 127–142

52 Clarke A 2000 Resourcing and training head and neck cancer nurse specialists to deliver a social rehabilitation programme to patients. Unpublished DPsychol thesis, University of London

53 Edwards D 1997 Face to face. Patient, family and professional perspectives of head and neck cancer care. King's Fund, London

54 Feber T (ed) 2000 Head and neck oncology nursing. Whurr, London

55 Coughlan GM 2000 Personal communication

56 Ley P, Llewelyn S 1995 Improving patients' understanding, recall, satisfaction and compliance. In: Broome A, Llewelyn S (eds) Health psychology, processes and applications, 2nd edn. Chapman and Hall, London

57 Carr T, Harris D, James C 2000 The Derriford Appearance Scale (DAS-59). A new scale to measure individual responses to living with problems of appearance. British Journal of Health Psychology 5(2): 201–215

Section 4

Innovations

30 Biomaterials in Craniomaxillofacial Surgery

Rudolf R M Bos, Henk J Busscher

Introduction

Materials used to support or replace diseased tissues, collectively called 'biomaterials', play an important role in craniomaxillofacial surgery. Collaboration between material scientists, biomaterial engineers, clinicians and clinical investigators has accelerated the understanding of the requirements and potentials of different implant materials. Alloplastic materials play an essential part in the reconstruction of function and contour in craniomaxillofacial surgery. Many different polymers, metals, ceramics and composites are used as biomaterials. Some have to achieve a temporary goal such as, for instance, osteosynthesis materials, others should function for a lifetime such as, for instance, artificial joints. There are many requirements that biomaterials must meet if they are to form either a temporary or a lasting union with the part of the body being treated. Adequate strength or, more probably, suitable mechanical behavior is a necessary but not sufficient condition since chemical and electrical factors as well as biologic responses all contribute to success or failure.[1]

Very often, the primary requirement is mechanical strength and biocompatibility is considered as a secondary requirement, despite the fact that many biomaterials applications in the human eventually fail due to infection. In his *Science* paper, the famous biomaterial scientist Antony G Cristina went as far as to call biomaterials in the human body a 'microbial time bomb', as they seem to have a magnetic action on infectious micro-organisms. Whether or not a biomaterial becomes infected depends in part on what is described as a 'race for the surface' between tissue cells and micro-organisms.[2] The 'wettability' of a biomaterial's surface, dictates the race for the surface and controls full integration of an implant (a race won by tissue cells) or infection (a race won by micro-organisms) (Fig. 30.1).

This chapter reviews the most commonly used biomaterials in craniomaxillofacial surgery.

Bone Substitutes

Over the years the need to graft bone has increased due to trauma, tumor surgery, congenital absence or hypoplasia and for strictly esthetic purposes. Many surgeons prefer the use of autogenous bone grafts to reconstruct bony defects. Autogenous bone grafts have disadvantages including shortage of donor sites, donor site morbidity, growth deformity and unpredictable resorption. The favorite donor sites for craniomaxillofacial reconstruction are calvarium, rib and iliac bone. It seems that there is less resorption of cranial bone than with rib or iliac bone.[3] Over the past 20 years all kinds of bio-

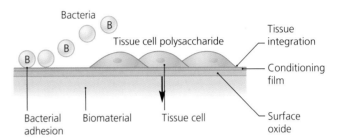

Fig. 30.1: The 'race for the surface'. If the race is won by tissue cells, a stable implant is achieved. If infecting organisms are able to colonize an implant prior to the arrival of the first tissue cells, failure is imminent.

materials have been developed that can be used as bone graft substitutes. They have demonstrated their usefulness in craniomaxillofacial reconstruction with their ability to augment and replace portions of the craniofacial skeleton.

Demineralized bone

Demineralized bone can be used for reconstruction of craniomaxillofacial defects.[4] The advantages of using demineralized bone are that it is pliable, easy to shape and to fit and in limitless supply and that it is free from donor morbidity, which is particularly useful in children. Implantation of demineralized bone hardly affects tissue reaction and osteoclastic activity; 8–12 weeks after the implantation of demineralized bone, new bone formation was noticed in histologic evaluations. Fragmentation of the implanted demineralized bone was observed 12 weeks postoperatively, but in combination with new bone formation and without multinuclear cell activity. Hydrolytic enzymes may cause this fragmentation. Long-term evaluation, 4 years after implantation, shows that there are still large areas of non-vital bone without osteocytes in the bone lacunae and osteoblasts on the surface. Several areas show fragmentation of the autogenous bone matrix. Several areas contiguous with non-vital bone showed evidence of transformation into living bone and remodeling. Active resorption, osteoclasts and inflammation of fibrous changes were not observed in the long term.

Demineralized bone pastes have been developed over the last 20 years,[5] composed of living osteoblasts derived from homograft materials, theoretically providing osteogenic cells capable of inducing osteogenesis. Demineralized bone pastes can be used alone or in combination with, for instance, hydroxyapatites. The advantage of such a combination is that it provides a structural supporting matrix with cells that have osteogenic ability.

Hydroxyapatite

Hydroxyapatite (HA) is the principal mineral component of bone and determines 60% of the calcified human skeleton. It has been manufactured synthetically for over 30 years and has been in clinical use for at least 20 years.[6] Certain marine corals consist of HA and have a structure that is similar to that of human bone. There are two forms of HA: one is ceramic and the other non-ceramic. Non-ceramic HA is not sintered after the HA crystals have been formed and therefore is more absorbable in vivo than the ceramic form. Ceramic forms of HA have excellent biocompatibility and show osteoconduction and osteointegration when placed in direct contact with viable bone. Osteoinduction is not evident because of the absence of inductive growth factors.[7] Non-ceramic HA can also be formed into cements, whereas ceramic HA cannot.

Ceramic hydroxyapatite

Ceramic hydroxyapatite is synthesized in crystal form at low pH and then heated (sintered) at 700–1300°C to form a solid mass of HA. Ceramic HA is available in two forms: dense and porous. The dense form is completely synthetic, it has no pores and can be fabricated into blocks or granules, which are difficult to shape and do not permit tissue ingrowth. Granules have greater contour adaptability than the solid blocks but no intrinsic structural integrity and do not become mechanically stable until surrounded by fibro-osseous tissue. Dense HA granules are difficult to contain within the desired site of implantation and there is a possibility of migration to unwanted areas after several months or years.[8]

Porous HA can be produced synthetically or can be based on the skeletons of marine coral. The calcium carbonate skeleton of the coral is chemically converted to HA and the original porous structure of the coral retained.[9] Porous ceramic granules appear to be less prone to migration over time. Another possibility to prevent migration is to combine HA granules with resorbable carrier compounds. The very important advantage of porous HA is the ingrowth of fibro-osseous tissue so it becomes fixed to the surrounding bone within a few weeks. When fibro-osseous tissue ingrowth is

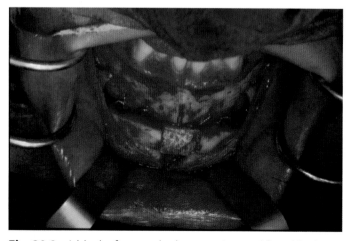

Fig. 30.2: A block of porous hydroxyapatite used for widening of the chin.

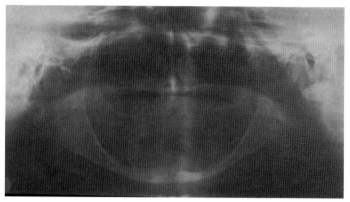

(a)

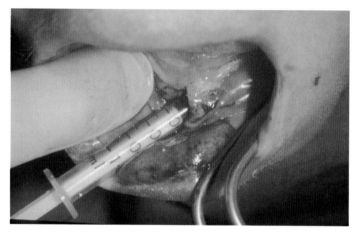

(b)

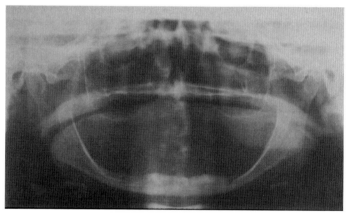

(c)

Fig. 30.3: (a) Orthopantomogram of a patient with an extremely resorbed mandible. **(b)** Subperiosteal injection of hydroxyapatite granules for augmentation of the mandible. **(c)** Orthopantomogram 12 weeks after augmentation with hydroxyapatite granules.

completed the implant consists of approximately 40% of residual HA implant and about 60% of fibro-osseous tissue. Porous HA in block form is rather fragile and very difficult to contour (Fig. 30.2). Its application therefore has been limited in craniomaxillofacial surgery. Application of porous HA for alveolar ridge augmentation (Fig. 30.3) has proved that HA is resistant to infection after fibro-osseous tissue ingrowth is completed but it easily becomes exposed especially when the overlying soft tissue is thin or compromised.[10]

Porous ceramic HA can be chemically combined with various biomaterials to improve its physical properties. It can also be used as a carrier of bioactive substances such as bone morphogenetic proteins which increase the ingrowth of bone into the pores.[11]

Non-ceramic hydroxyapatite

Tetracalcium phosphate cement (HA cement) is a form of non-ceramic hydroxyapatite. It is the only calcium phosphate cement that sets into a stable shape and is converted in vivo to pure HA. It can be produced by direct crystallization of HA at physiologic pH and temperature and does not require heating to form a structurally stable implant. The dry cement is composed of tetracalcium phosphate and dicalcium phosphate. It sets in approximately 15 minutes and converts to HA within 4 hours.[12] After conversion to HA it is no longer water soluble and it is slowly replaced by bone over time. Its contour is stable. Animal studies proved that 35% of implanted HA was replaced by fibro-osseous tissue and bone replaced 75% of this fibro-osseous tissue after 12 months implantation. Even in human clinical trials the cement was found to be functionally non-resorbable over 42 months on the basis of CT scans, and incidentally by direct intraoperative inspections during secondary surgery.

These biologically active forms of HA cement are especially useful in situations where contour is not an important factor or where bone replacement of the implant material is necessary, for instance in the reconstruction of skull base defects, in orthopedic applications and pediatric cranio-maxillofacial surgery. HA cement can be used in the growing skull as it was observed to have no adverse effects on development.[13] HA has no toxic reactions and it has a low rate of infection of about 4% even when the HA implant is in contact with the paranasal sinuses or oral cavity.[14] An important disadvantage of HA cement is that it is very difficult to give it the desired contour because it tends to settle with gravity during the setting process. HA granules can also be mixed with fibrocollagen and autogenous blood to form a paste that can be injected into subperiosteal pockets. It becomes firmly fixed by fibrous tissue ingrowth from the surrounding tissues. It has been used to augment the malar bone, premaxilla, nasal dorsum and glabella area. Large volumes of this paste have been used to fill cranial defects in children. The infection rate was about 3%.

Recently, a mixture came on the market consisting of type I bovine dermal fibrillar collagen (PFC) and a mixture of 65% ceramic HA and 35% β-tricalcium phosphate (TCP) granules. The HA-TCP granules and the PFC are separately packed, to be mixed on the operating table to form a granular non-setting paste. Autogenous bone marrow can be added to the mixture which gives it more osteoinductive and osteogenic properties. This mixture allows bony ingrowth and rapid vascularization. Its disadvantage is that this non-setting mixture can be easily deformed before fibro-osseous tissue ingrowth has occurred. The disadvantage is that there would be contour change and volume loss because of the resorption of both the collagen and the tricalcium phosphate components, which amount to about 40% of the total mixture. It is interesting that adding autogenous bone marrow to the mixture decreases the infection rate from 5% to 2.5%.[15]

Polymers

In general we think of polymers as being plastics. These polymers are relatively weak solid materials that soften as temperature increases. They are all around us, more and more so as new and improved polymers begin to displace metals and ceramics from traditional applications. Polymers and polymer-based composites represent one of the most exciting areas of modern materials science. They combine moderate strength, low cost and easy raw material availability with the ability to regulate physical properties by design of composition, internal structural arrangement and processing. Nowhere has the impact of modern polymeric materials been greater than in medicine, with the resulting wide use of polymeric disposable supplies, dressings and sutures and the incorporation of polymers into medical devices, surgical instruments and implants.[1] The most widely used will be discussed in this chapter.[16,17]

Polydimethylsiloxane

Polydimethylsiloxane, better known as silicone, is widely used in craniomaxillofacial surgery. It has proved to be highly compatible with soft tissues, it is easy to shape, resistant to the physiologic environment and can be produced with a wide range of mechanical properties. Its surface is hydrophobic (see Table 30.1). Depending on the number and nature of side chains and crosslinks and on the average

Table 30.1 Chemical structure of various polymeric biomaterials, including chemical functionalities, and metals, together with their water contact angles

Polymer name	Chemical functionality	Water contact angle (degrees)
Silicone rubber	-(O-SI-CH3)-	111
Polyethylene	=C-H$_2$, -C-H$_3$	95–100
Polypropylene		94
Polytetrafluoroethylene	=C-F$_2$, -C-F$_3$	104
Polymethylmethacrylate		70–80
Polylactide		
Titanium(oxide)		35–45
Stainless steel		65–75

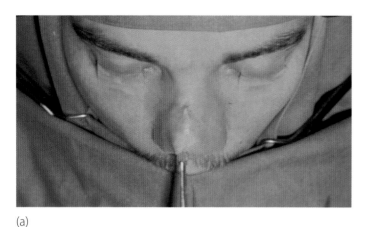

(a)

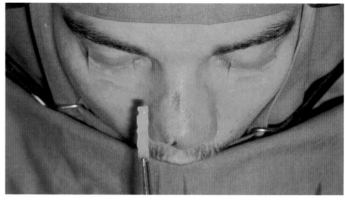

(b)

Fig. 30.4: (a) Dehiscence of a silicone implant used for cosmetic reconstruction of the nasal dorsum. **(b)** The silicone implant after removal from the nose.

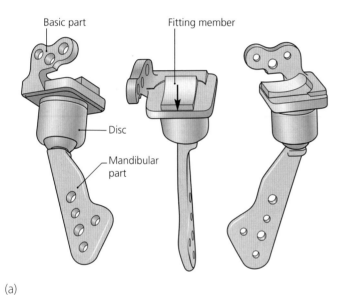

(a)

Fig. 30.5: (a) Schematic drawing of the Groningen temporomandibular joint prosthesis with its polyethylene disc. **(b)** Intraoperative view of the polyethylene disc during insertion of the Groningen TMJ prosthesis.

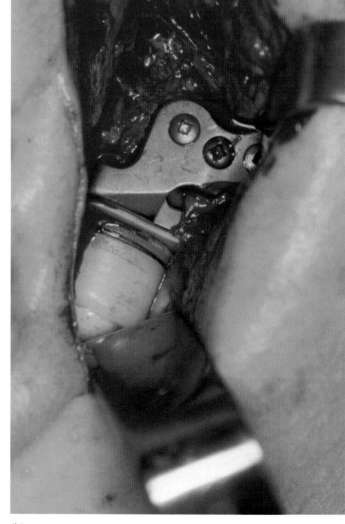

(b)

molecular weight, the resulting material may be liquid or solid, rubbery or brittle. They may be produced as thermoplastics or as two-part thermoset materials: the latter are used to manufacture a custom mould either before implantation or in situ. The natural host response to the smooth surface of silicone is a fibrous encapsulation. To prevent extrusion of silicone implants, the overlying soft tissues should not be thin, unstable or under tension (Fig. 30.4). Injections of large amounts of liquid silicone for purposes such as breast augmentation may induce systemic toxicity.

The poor abrasion resistance of silicone rubbers prevents their use in weight-bearing applications. Abrasion of silicone rubbers will cause a granulomatous inflammatory reaction, locally as well as in regional lymph nodes. There is an ongoing controversy that silicone breast implants may cause connective tissue disease.[18] Silicone blocks are widely used for craniofacial augmentation purposes, for instance malar bones, chin and nasal dorsum. Using these blocks one should be careful to prevent migration of the blocks and erosion of the underlying bones as well as perforation of the compromised overlying skin.[16]

Polyethylene

Polyethylene (PE) is one of the most commonly used biomaterials.[1] It is the base polymer for other materials such as polypropylene and polytetrafluoroethylene. It elicits a minimal tissue reaction, especially when manufactured in a high-density, high molecular weight form. In this form it serves as a reference standard to other materials because of its minimal tissue reaction. Ultra high molecular weight polyethylene (UHMWPE) has proven to date to be the best polymer for load-bearing applications in metal–polymer wear pairs such as artificial joints. Artificial temporomandibular joints have been developed in which UHMWPE serves as an artificial disc in between a metal fossa part and a ceramic condylar head[19] (Fig. 30.5).

PE is also available in a porous form. The porous structure of this implant material allows ingrowth of soft tissues 1 week after implantation and bony ingrowth 3 weeks after implantation. The porous PE is easy to shape but difficult to remove after ingrowth.[20] A porous polyethylene reinforced with titanium is available to reconstruct bony defects of the skull after tumor ablation or trauma. Excellent craniofacial symmetry and stability are achievable. Many implant forms are commercially available, including malar, chin, mandible, nasal bone and orbital floor implants. Flexible porous polyethylene blocks can be ideally suited to repair small to medium-sized cranial defects. Host response to polyethylene is mild and complications are rare. Porous PE has advantages over autogenous bone in that it is not susceptible to contour change and it has proved to be a safe and effective bone substitute for contouring the facial skeleton.

Polymethyl methacrylate

Polymethyl methacrylate (PMMA) has been used as bone cement for the past 40 years and is an acceptable space filler without resorption.[1] Its mechanical properties are excellent to serve as a bone replacement in the craniofacial area and its surface is moderately hydrophobic (see Table 30.1).

Methyl methacrylate has two different components, mixing powder polymer and a liquid monomer. The chemical reaction is exothermic and the associated toxicity is related to the free monomer component. A cardiovascular collapse and even death, which has been described in patients undergoing a total hip replacement with freshly mixed methyl methacrylate, has not been reported after use in craniofacial surgery. The free methyl methacrylate monomer may cause asthmatic reactions.

PMMA has been used for reconstruction of skull defects for many years, in cement form as well as in a presurgically shaped and polymerized solid implant form (Fig. 30.6).

Patients with isolated cranioplasty rarely experience infections but the infection rate increases considerably in those patients undergoing a cranioplasty simultaneously with the reconstruction of the orbital wall or nose, in whom the infection rate was about 23%. When the facial contour requirement is important, especially preshaped PMMA delivers a predictable contour without any resorption.[21] PMMA can be used in the adult patient with healthy overlying soft tissues and no infection. It is not an adequate implant material for reconstruction of craniofacial bones in the growing child.

Polytetrafluoroethylene

Polytetrafluoroethylene (PTFE) is used as a base material for different implants.[1] It is nowadays frequently used for so-called guided tissue regeneration of dental alveolar bone in dental implantology (Fig. 30.7) and periodontology. The PTFE sheets sold under the name Gore-Tex prevent fibrous tissue ingrowth and allow bony regeneration of a blood clot covered by the Gore-Tex fabric.

A composite of PTFE reinforced with carbon fibers or later aluminum oxide, sold under the name Proplast, has been widely used for malar (Fig. 30.8) and chin augmentation. Proplast is a microporous material and does not allow fibrous or bony ingrowth. It was initially reported that Proplast did not give rise to many complications. It seemed to have a low infection rate of about 4%, displacement was rare (3.5%) and implant removal had to take place in about 8%. However, this implant material is no longer manufactured. This may be due to a high incidence of infection and displacement in the long run.[22] It is our own experience that of a series of 10 patients operated on at the beginning of the 1980s in whom Proplast was used for bilateral malar augmentation, 19 out of 20 implants had to be removed because of chronic fistulae or even chronic sinusitis due to migration of the Proplast implants into the maxillary sinus. Proplast has also been used as lining of the fossa part of the Vitek temporomandibular joint prosthesis. However, rapid wear and, more importantly, an aggressive foreign body response to the wear debris has rendered this material unusable in implant applications in which wear phenomena are possible.[23]

Resorbable Polymers

The polymers discussed so far are intended to retain their shape and their essential properties after implantation. However, there are a number of applications in which it would be desirable to have properties change or even to have the material completely disappear with time. This principle has been long recognized in the use of resorbable sutures in subcutaneous tissue sites. One of the most challenging of these potential applications is in internal fixation of fractures and osteotomies (Fig. 30.9).[9] It would be ideal to have a device that would slowly weaken and eventually disappear, transferring load to the healing bone and encouraging maximal Wolff's Law remodeling.

In the last three decades much progress has been made in the development of biodegradable osteosyntheses. The vast

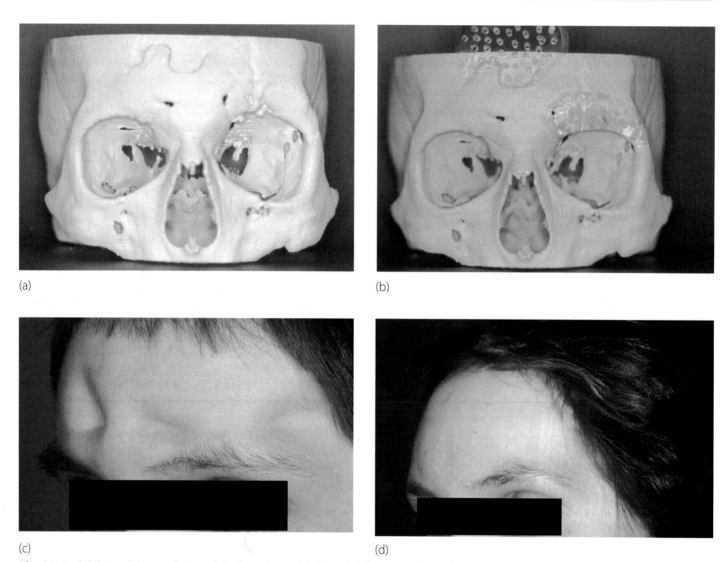

(a)

(b)

(c)

(d)

Fig. 30.6: **(a)** Stereolithographic model of a patient with frontal deformities after a firework accident. **(b)** Polymethyl methacrylate implants on the stereolithographic model. **(c)** Preoperative view of a patient with frontal defects after a car accident. **(d)** Postoperative view after implantation of polymethyl methacrylate implants through a coronal incision.

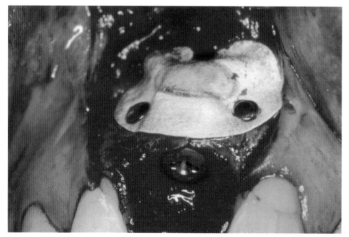

Fig. 30.7: A Teflon sheet used for guided tissue regeneration of a bony dehiscence along a dental implant.

majority of bioresorbable osteosyntheses used today are produced from synthetic semicrystalline poly 4 (α-hydroxy acid) polymers.[24] Polylactide (PLA) is the material which is most often used as it is most suitable to produce implants with acceptable mechanical properties (Fig. 30.10). Polyglycolide (PGA) is another material often used; it degrades faster and is used primarily in applications where high strength is not the most important factor. Polymer blends of PLA and PGA are also often used to tailor the properties of a polymer to a specific application. Besides PLA, PGA and PLA/PLG co-polymers, a number of other aliphatic polyesters such as poly(p-dioxanone) (PDS) and poly(ε-caprolactone)(PCL) have also been investigated for use as bioresorbable osteo-syntheses. PDS is used to make pins (Orthosorb®) and orbital floor implants. However, PDS and PCL are primarily used for the production of bioresorbable sutures such as Monocryl®, a PCL/PGA monofilament suture, and in PDS monofilament suture.

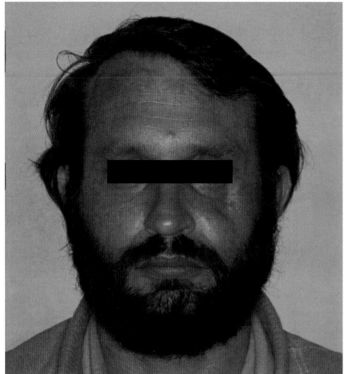

(a)

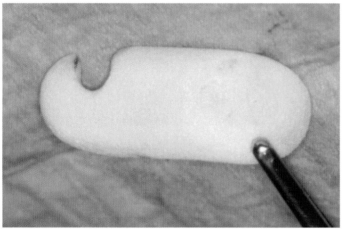

(b)

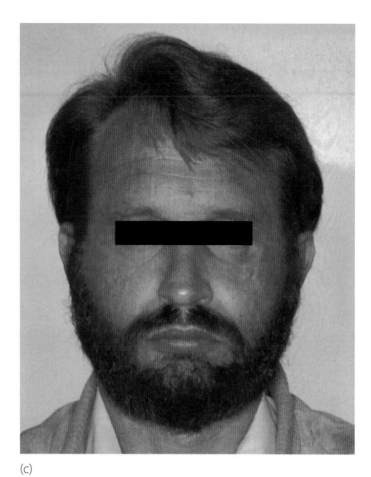

(c)

Fig. 30.8: (a) Preoperative view of malformation of the left malar bone due to untreated trauma. **(b)** Example of a Proplast-Teflon malar implant, to be inserted around and lateral to the infraorbital nerve. **(c)** Postoperative view 3 months after transcutaneous implantation of the Proplast-Teflon malar implant.

At the present time, there are a number of aspects in which biodegradable osteosyntheses perform rather satisfactorily. In other aspects, however, considerable problems are encountered that stand in the way of their general clinical use. The mechanical properties of the resorbable materials are still not as good as those of metallic ones. Besides, the perioperative handling of resorbable devices is far more critical and difficult. The mechanical properties of resorbable plates and screws or pins are easily destroyed during bending or by torsional forces during insertion. Another main problem area in the development of bioresorbable osteosyntheses is the issue of biocompatibility. For a long time the biocompatibility of bioresorbable PLA and PGA polymers has been considered to be beyond reproach. Degradation of these polymers occurs primarily by hydrolysis; enzymatic activity is thought to play a contributing

role in the later stages of degradation. Free radicals, in particular hydroxy radicals, also appear to play a role in the degradation process. The end products of degradation of PLA and PGA, lactic acid and glycolic acid are hypothesized to be eliminated from the body as carbon dioxide and water and a small portion by excretion in the urine and feces. Homo polymers of PLA and PGA give rise to a clinically detectable foreign body reaction. Blending co-polymerization or crosslinking seem to be a solution to limit or even avoid foreign body reactions during degradation. However, a recent study documented the presence of very persistent nano- and microparticles in the degradation pathway of a PLA-PGA co-polymer in use as a so-called bioresorbable implant material.[25] This study indicates that poly (α-hydroxy acid) implants may not completely degrade within 15–20 years. At present, it seems prudent to assume that

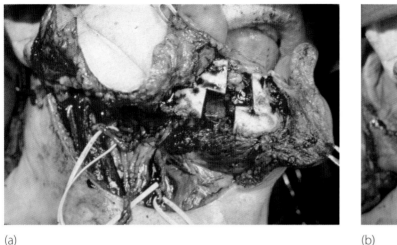

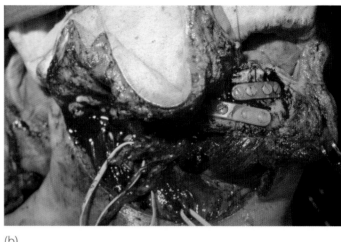

(a)   (b)

Fig. 30.9: **(a)** Lateral swing osteotomy of the mandible in a patient with a planocellular carcinoma of the oropharynx. **(b)** Fixation of the osteotomy with two resorbable PLA plates and screws.

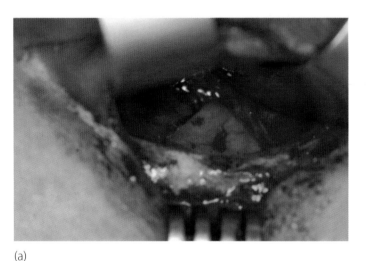

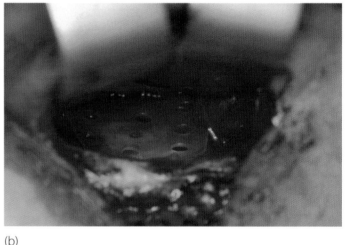

(a)   (b)

Fig. 30.10: **(a)** Interoperative view of a blow-out fracture of the orbital floor. **(b)** Reconstruction of the orbital floor with a resorbable PLA sheet (0.4 mm thickness).

crystalline debris from poly (α-hydroxy acid) implants will remain present in the recipient indefinitely with the potential for the development of unforeseen complications. Especially where use of multiple or large implants is considered, such remnants may pose a long-term health risk. These problems need to be solved so that bioresorbable osteosyntheses can perform to their full potential and thus, eventually, make their general clinical application routine.

Another routine application of biodegradable materials could be as a scaffold for bone reconstruction. An ideal bone substitute would be a biomaterial that has osteoconductive and inductive properties and will be replaced by regenerating host bone. Biodegradable meshes have been produced already that can be filled with particulate bone marrow or mixtures of bone marrow and hydroxyapatite. These measures have been used already in experimental studies for mandibular reconstruction.

Biodegradable foams have also been used in experimental studies, loaded with bone morphogenetic proteins, platelet-

derived growth factor or transforming growth factor or with osteoblasts or chondroblasts. All these studies are so far experimental.[26] Only some meshes are available for clinical use.

Metals

Metals enjoy wide application in craniomaxillofacial surgery as structural, load-bearing materials in devices for fracture fixation, partial and total joint replacement devices (see Fig. 30.5), instruments and external splints. The principal reasons for this broad popularity are excellent mechanical properties and biocompatibility. Today one principally uses metals such as stainless steel, chromium-molybdenum alloys or commercially pure titanium.[1] The metal of choice in craniomaxillofacial surgery was stainless steel until approximately 1986. For the maxillofacial field, however, titanium is now looked upon as the material of choice. The superior biocompatibility of titanium is conveyed by its oxide skin that forms spontaneously upon exposure to an oxygen-containing environment, including air.

Internal fixation with different systems of plates and screws is a widely accepted method in craniomaxillofacial trauma (Fig. 30.11), orthopedic surgery and reconstruction after tumor surgery. Many surgeons prefer not to remove metallic plates and screws. One of the reasons may be that the removal of plates and screws used for fixation means an additional surgical intervention with all its risks and socio-economic and psychological disadvantages. In respect of biocompatibility, commercially pure titanium is thought to be superior in comparison to stainless steel products due to its completely inert oxide skin. Although titanium is more expensive than steel it may be cost effective in the long run because of its favorable characteristics. It is thought to be non-allergenic and completely inert and biocompatible. That means that a second intervention to remove titanium plates and screws is not necessary.[27] This means that for internal fixation in the maxillofacial area, titanium is now almost exclusively the material of choice. The coincidental finding that titanium has a more or less exclusive property of osseo-integration means that titanium is used worldwide as a dental implant material and as an osseous implant to fix maxillofacial prosthetics. Computer-designed titanium implants can also be used for cranial reconstruction after trauma or tumor surgery. The infection rate of titanium implants is extremely low.

Biofilm Formation

The formation of a biofilm on the surface of biomaterials in the human body results from adsorption of macromolecular components such as salivary proteins and the adhesion of infectious micro-organisms. The biofilm mode of growth protects the organisms against the host defense and environmental attacks, such as antibiotic treatment. Consequently, very often infection of biomaterials applications necessitates removal of an implant.[21,28]

Interactions of biomaterials with bacteria and tissue cells are directed not only by specific receptors and outer membrane molecules on the cell surface, but also by the atomic

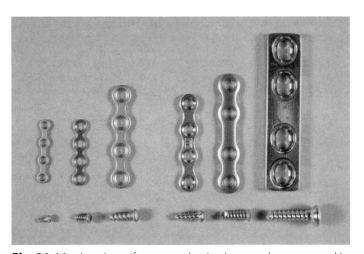

Fig. 30.11: A variety of osteosynthesis plates and screws used in craniomaxillofacial surgery.

geometry and electronic state of the biomaterial surface. Understanding these mechanisms is important to all fields of medicine and is derived from and relevant to studies in microbiology, biochemistry and physics. Modifications to biomaterial surfaces at an atomic level will allow the programming of cell-to-substratum events, thereby diminishing infection by enhancing tissue compatibility or integration or by directly inhibiting bacterial adhesion.

The Bränemark implant system consists of an endosteal titanium screw and a transmucosal abutment, prone to biofilm formation. The abutment surface properties dictate the amount of biofilm formed and roughened abutment surfaces harboured 25 times more bacteria than smooth abutment surfaces after 3 months. Influences of surface hydrophobicity on biofilm formation are generally more evident in situations of more fluctuating shear conditions than in a pocket. In vivo studies over a 9-day period in human volunteers have demonstrated far less biofilm formation on hydrophobic Teflon strips glued on the front incisors of human volunteers than on native, more hydrophilic tooth surfaces[29] (Fig. 30.12).

Conclusion

Biomaterials are being used with increasing frequency for tissue substitution. The major barriers to the use of biomaterials are the possibility of bacterial adhesion to biomaterials, which causes biomaterial-centered infection, and the lack of successful tissue integration or biocompatibility with biomaterial surfaces.

When looking for suitable biomaterials, one should critically examine scientific papers on that material. The fact that bony ingrowth in hydroxyapatite granules occurs in young rabbits does not automatically mean that bony ingrowth also occurs in elderly people who need filling out of bony defects or augmentations before inserting dental implants. When looking for so-called resorbable materials, one should read carefully how hard investigators looked for remnants of material to discriminate between real resorption and degradation or disintegration only.

Many articles report that some biomaterials present higher complication rates than autogenous tissue. It is difficult to attribute many of the complication rates solely to the implant material itself. Many factors such as surgical techniques, host response and potential toxicity of the implant itself may influence such complication rates. For example, the variation of antibiotic regimen, varying attention to aseptic techniques, differences in the normal flora, susceptibility to antibiotics and variations in the method of mechanical fixation can influence infection rates for a given material. Modern biomaterials produce a very low level of acute local or systemic host response in patients. However, mechanisms are known for a variety of immunologic responses, including neoplastic transformation. Increasing periods of implantation, secondary to earlier surgical intervention, and increased surface areas of implants, as required for fixation by biologic ingrowth, may be placing patients at increasing risk. It is to be hoped that, as material researchers and clinicians become more sensitive to

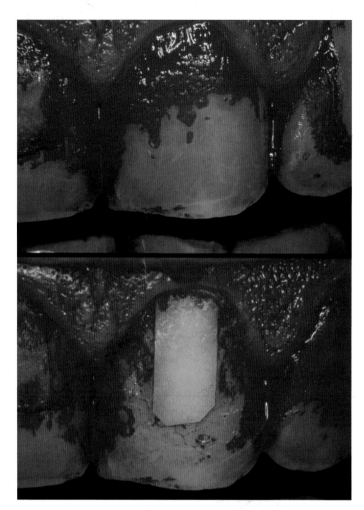

Fig. 30.12: The amount of biofilm formed on a hydrophobic material glued to the front incisor of a human volunteer is considerably less than that formed on a more hydrophilic tooth surface in the absence of tooth brushing over a period of 9 days.

the biologic response implications of the biomaterials that they use, patient analyses will clarify the situation and provide upper boundaries on the prevalence of such effects.

References

1 Black J 1988 Orthopedic biomaterials in research and practice. Churchill Livingstone, Edinburgh

2 Cristina AG 1987 Biomaterials-centered infection: microbial adhesion versus tissue integration. Science 237: 1588–1595

3 Zins JE, Whitaker LA 1983 Membranous versus enchondral bone: implications for craniofacial reconstruction. Plastic and Reconstructive Surgery 72: 778–785

4 Neigel JM, Ruzicka PO 1996 Use of demineralized bone implant in orbital and craniofacial reconstruction and a review of the literature. Ophthalmic Plastic and Reconstructive Surgery 12: 108–120

5 Glowacki J, Kaban CB, Murray JE 1981 Application of the biological principle of induced osteogenesis for craniofacial defect. Lancet 1: 959–962

6 Jarcho M 1981 Calcium phosphate ceramics as hard tissue prosthesis. Clinical Orthopaedics and Related Research 157: 259–278

7 Ono I, Takheiko O, Murata M 1992 A study on bone induction in hydroxyapatite combined with bone morphogenic protein. Plastic and Reconstructive Surgery 90: 870–879

8 Harvey WK, Pincock JL, Matukas VJ, Lemons JE 1985 Evaluation of subcutaneous implanted hydroxyapatite-Avitene mixture in rabbits. Journal of Oral and Maxillofacial Surgery 43: 277–280

9 Cottrell DA, Wolford LM 1998 Long-term evaluation of the use of coralline hydroxyapatite in orthognathic surgery. Journal of Oral and Maxillofacial Surgery 56: 935–941

10 Salyer KE, Hall CD 1989 Porous hydroxyapatite as an onlay graft substitute for maxillofacial surgery. Plastic and Reconstructive Surgery 84: 236–244

11 Ripamonti U, Ramoshebi LN, Matsaba T, Tasker J, Crooks J, Teare J 2001 Bone induction by BMPs/OPs and related family members in primates. Journal of Bone and Joint Surgery of America 83 (suppl 1 (P+2)): 116–127

12 Jackson IT, Yavuzer R 2000 Hydroxyapatite cement: an alternative for craniofacial skeletal contour refinements. British Journal of Plastic Surgery 53: 24–29

13 Lykins CL, Friedman CD, Costanino PD, Horioglu R 1998 Hydroxyapatite cement in craniofacial skeletal reconstruction and its effects on the developing craniofacial. Archives of Otolaryngology Head and Neck Surgery 124: 153–159

14 Costantino PD, Chaplin JM, Wolpoe ME, Catalano PJ, Sen C 2000 Application of fast setting hydroxyapatite cement: cranioplasty. Otolaryngololy Head and Neck Surgery 123: 409–512

15 Cornell CN 1992 Initial clinical experience with use of Collagraft as bone graft substitute. Techniques in Orthopedics 7: 55–63

16 Rubin JP, Yaremchuck MJ 1997 Complications and toxicities of implantable biomaterials used in facial reconstructive and aesthetic surgery: a comprehensive review of literature. Plastic and Reconstructive Surgery 100: 1336–1353

17 Homsy CA 1998 Complication and toxicities of implantable biomaterials for facial aesthetic and reconstructive surgery. Plastic and Reconstructive Surgery 102(5) 1766–1768

18 Sanchez-Guerrero J, Colditz GA, Karlson E, Hunter DJ, Speizer FE, Liang MH 1995 Silicone breast implants and the risk of connective tissue disease and symptom. New England Journal of Medicine 332: 1666–1670

19 Van Loon JP, Bont LGM, Stegenga B, Verkerke GJ 2002 Groningen temporomandibular joint prosthesis. Development and first clinical application. International Journal of Oral and Maxillofacial Surgery 31(1): 44–52

20 Odum BC, Bussard GM, Lewis RP, Lara WC, Edlich RF, Gampper TJ 1998 High-density porous polyethylene for facial bone augmentation. Journal of the Long-Term Effects of Medical Implants 8(1): 3–17

21 Gosain AK, Persing JA 1999 Biomaterials in the face: benefits and risks. Journal of Craniofacial Surgery 10(5): 404–414

22 Moos KF, Jackson IT, Henderson D, Gibbs PM 1979 The use of Proplast in oral and maxillofacial surgery. British Journal of Oral Surgery 16(3): 187–197

23 Mercuri LG 1999 Considering total temporomandibular joint replacement. Cranio 17(1): 44–48

24 Suuronen R, Haers PE, Lindqvist C, Sailer HF 1999 Update on bioresorbable plates in maxillofacial surgery. Facial Plastic Surgery 15(1): 61–72

25 Cordewener FW, Schmitz JP 2000 The future of biodegradable osteosyntheses. Tissue Engineering 6(4): 413–424

26 Stock UA, Vacanti JP 2001 Tissue engineering: current state and prospects. Annual Review of Medicine 52: 443–451

27 Meningaud JP, Poupon J, Bertrand JC, Chenevier C, Galliot-Guilley M, Guilbert F 2001 Dynamic study about metal release from titanium miniplates in maxillofacial surgery. International Journal of Oral and Maxillofacial Surgery 30(3): 185–188

28 Donlan RM, Costerton JW 2002 Biofilms: survival mechanisms of clinically relevant micoorganisms. Clinical Microbiology Review 15(2): 167–193

29 Quirijnen M, Marechal M, Busscher HJ, Weerkamp AH, Arends J, Van Steenberghe D 1989 The influence of surface free energy on planimetric plaque growth in man. Journal of Dental Research 68: 796–799

31 Minimally Invasive Surgery

Ralf Schön, Rainer Schmelzeisen

Introduction

Experience of TMJ arthroscopy and endoscopic sinus and skull base surgery equips the oral and maxillofacial surgeon for the endoscopic-assisted treatment of maxillofacial trauma. The endoscopic-assisted management of maxillofacial trauma has been described for the treatment of mandibular condyle fractures, fractures of the zygomatic complex, the orbit and the frontal sinus.[1–4] The repositioning and fixation strategy of open fracture treatment with osteosynthesis has not changed. However, by using endoscopic-assisted techniques, incisions, especially when extraoral approaches are indicated, can be limited and intraoperative control after fracture reduction in areas of limited exposure and visibility can be performed endoscopically.[5] Nevertheless, there is no influence on the indication for surgical treatment when using endoscopic techniques.

State-of-the-Art

Mandible

Mandibular condyle fractures

Fractures of the mandibular condyle are common and account for 9–45% of all mandibular fractures.[6,7] Closed reduction is the method most widely employed for the treatment of displaced condylar fractures.[7] Anatomic reduction is rarely achieved and the rehabilitation and TMJ function depend on forced adaptation of the altered condylar morphology or formation of a new joint. With precise fracture reduction by pre-auricular, retromolar or submandibular approaches, damage to the facial nerve and the creation of visible scars are described.[8] Due to these possible complications, the indications for open reduction or closed treatment are still in debate.[9,10]

The risk of facial nerve damage and extensive visible scars can be reduced by minimally invasive endoscopic techniques.[1,5,11] In selected cases a transoral approach is applied to minimize the risk of facial nerve damage and to avoid visible scars.[5,12,13] However, in severely displaced fractures the extraoral approach seems to be advantageous for the endoscopic-assisted reduction of mandibular condyle fractures.[5]

Mandible fractures in other locations

In mandiblar fractures of other locations, such as the mandibular angle and ramus, the transoral approach is prefer-

ably used to avoid visible scars and possible facial nerve damage. The transoral approach is indicated when there is no comminution. However, via an enoral approach the inferior and posterior aspects of the fracture and possible lingual gaps cannot be controlled. Endoscopic control of the fracture site after transoral reduction and fixation of fractures provides further information about the accuracy of the fracture reduction. The alignment of the posterior and inferior aspects of angle fractures and the presence of a lingual gap in ramus fractures can be detected endoscopically and if necessary corrected intraoperatively.

Midfacial and frontal sinus fractures

Endoscopic-assisted techniques for the treatment of fractures of the zygoma, the midface and the orbit have been reported.[2,3,14,15] In fractures of the zygomatic complex the orbital floor and infraorbital rim are often inspected by transconjunctival or mid lower eyelid incisions. Non-displaced fractures of the orbital floor without the need for treatment are often noted. Furthermore, inadequate results after repositioning may occur due to rotation of the fragment if the repositioning at the sphenozygomatic buttress is not controlled.

The inspection of the lateral orbital wall in displaced fractures of the zygomatic complex is performed endoscopically by a limited blepharoplasty incision.[2] In zygoma fractures the orbital floor can be endoscopically inspected transorally via the maxillary sinus. The result after fracture reduction can also be evaluated at the infraorbital rim and the lateral orbital wall. Additional transconjunctival or infraorbital incisions can be avoided when there is no displaced fracture of the orbital floor or displacement of the fragments at the infraorbital rim after repositioning. When indicated, osteosynthesis of the infraorbital rim can be performed endoscopically by the transoral approach.

The endoscopic treatment of comminuted fractures of the zygomatic arch is reported to avoid open reduction via coronal incisions.[3]

Frontal sinus fractures of the anterior wall may be reduced using minimally invasive techniques.[4] At least two incisions posterior to the hair line are needed for the insertion of the endoscope and instruments for the repositioning of fractures. Stab incisions may be needed for the direct manipulation of the fragments. The indication for minimally invasive endoscopic surgery of the frontal sinus may be limited to single fragment fractures of the anterior table of the frontal sinus.

Surgical technique

Endoscopic equipment

Initially a prototype of an endoscopic plate application device (Synthes Paoli, PA, USA) with a 30° angle 4 mm diameter endoscope (Karl Storz, Tuttlingen, Germany) was used via an extraoral approach.[1] Due to the limitation of angulation at the time of plate insertion using the plate application device and the need for transbuccal incisions, the device was successfully used in selected cases when the submandibular approach was performed. In selected cases 45° and 70° angle endoscopes are used, which are more difficult to employ as there is limited straightforward vision when inserting the endoscope. A suction and irrigation device allows irrigation of the endoscope tip in limited optical cavities, when blurred vision of the lens is caused by blood.

The monitor and the endoscopic equipment should be placed in the operating room facing the surgeon and the assistant. Intraoperatively watching the endoscopic picture on the monitor while sitting in a comfortable position is important. The light source and the camera should be close to the patient's head to avoid limitations of movement of the endoscope. A second suction device is recommended when an endoscope with a suction and irrigation device is in used.

Mandibular condyle fractures

In 43 patients endoscopic-assisted open reduction of mandibular condyle fractures was performed. Thirty-six condyle fractures were treated by endoscopic transoral approach. Thirteen out of 17 mandibular condyle fractures had additional mandibular fractures (Tables 31.1, 31.2).[5] The type of fracture, degree of displacement and result of reduction were evaluated intraoperatively using the endoscope and preoperatively and postoperatively by Towne's and panoramic radiographs (Figs 31.1–31.4).

Submandibular approach

The ascending ramus of the mandible was approached submandibularly. After incision of the platysma the masseter muscle was dissected at the inferior aspect of the mandibular angle. Then the periosteal tissue on the ascending mandibular ramus was elevated and the endoscope inserted subperiostally and advanced cranially until the fracture gap became visible in the endoscope (Fig. 31.3).

Transoral approach

The transoral incision was similar to the surgical approach for sagittal split osteotomies of the mandible in orthognathic surgery. Local anesthetics were injected 8–10 minutes prior to incision to control bleeding. To create the optical cavity the periosteal tissue on the ascending mandibular ramus was elevated, freeing the posterior aspect of the ascending ramus and the mandibular angle. Additionally the inferior inserting fibers of the temporalis muscle were stripped from the lower aspect of the muscular process. The endoscope was inserted subperiosteally and advanced cranially towards the fracture without incision of the masseter muscle to avoid bleeding and damage to the facial nerve (see Fig. 31.8).

Table 31.1 Patients and type of mandiblar condyle fractures: extraoral approach (n=9)

Patient no.	# Location	Dislocation	Transbuccal	Age	Mand. #*
1	Subcondylar	No	Yes	32	Yes
2	Condylar neck	Yes	Yes	30	Yes
3	Subcondylar	Yes	Yes	42	Yes
4	Condylar neck	No	Yes	55	No
5	Condylar neck	Yes	Yes	33	Yes
6	Subcondylar	No	Yes	29	No
7	Condylar neck	Yes	Yes	29	Yes
8	Condylar neck bilateral	Yes	Yes	41	Yes
9	Condylar neck	Yes	Yes	23	Yes

* Mand. # = additional mandibular fractures

Table 31.2 Patients and type of mandibular condyle fractures: transoral approach (n=8)

Patient no.	# Location	Dislocation	Transbuccal	Age	Mand. #*
1	Condylar neck	Yes	Yes	37	No
2	Subcondylar	No	No	33	Yes
3	Condylar neck	Yes	Yes	38	Yes
4	Subcondylar	Yes	No	51	Yes
5	Condylar neck	No	Yes	29	Yes
6	Subcondylar	No	No	28	No
7	Subcondylar	No	Yes	28	Yes
8	Subcondylar	Yes	No	25	Yes

* Mand. # = additional mandibular fractures

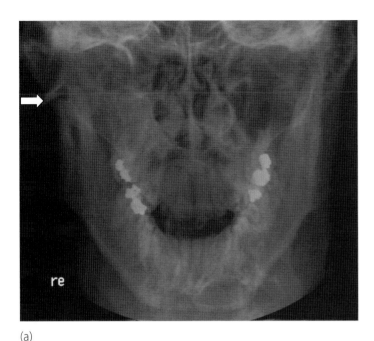
(a)

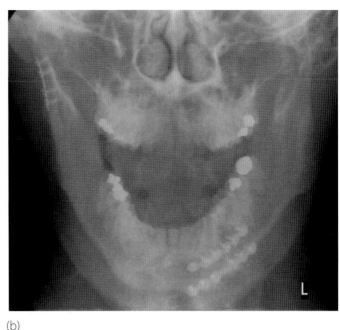
(b)

Fig. 31.1: Panoramic and Towne's radiographs preoperatively **(a)** and postoperatively **(b)** after endoscopic-assisted transoral reduction and fixation of a displaced condyle fracture with lateral override (arrow).

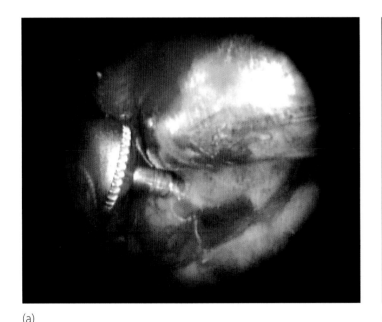
(a)

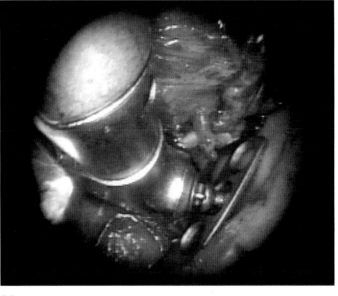
(b)

Fig. 31.2: Intraoperative view of angulated drill **(a)** and screwdriver **(b)** during transoral fixation of a displaced condylar fracture without transbuccal step incision.

Repositioning and fixation

Distraction of the TMJ region using a reduction forceps at the mandibular angle when using the submandibular approach and pressure onto the mandibular molars when using the transoral approach were administered to facilitate the repositioning of the condylar fragment. The periosteum and the soft tissues in the vicinity of the proximal fragment were removed carefully to allow the placement of miniplates.

Special instruments were inserted for the reduction of the condylar fragment. Stab incisions in the condylar region were made for the transbuccal insertion of the screws. After insertion of the first screw in the condylar fragment the fracture reduction was facilitated by pulling the miniplate using modified nerve hooks. The second screw was then inserted next to the fracture in the mandibular fragment. Osteosynthesis was performed using a 2.0 mm AO/ASIF DC-miniplate (Synthes Paoli, PA, USA) with at least two screws at each side of the fracture. After fracture reduction and fixation using two screws, the alignment at the posterior border of the ascending ramus was controlled endoscopically before osteosynthesis was completed (see Figs 31.4, 31.8).

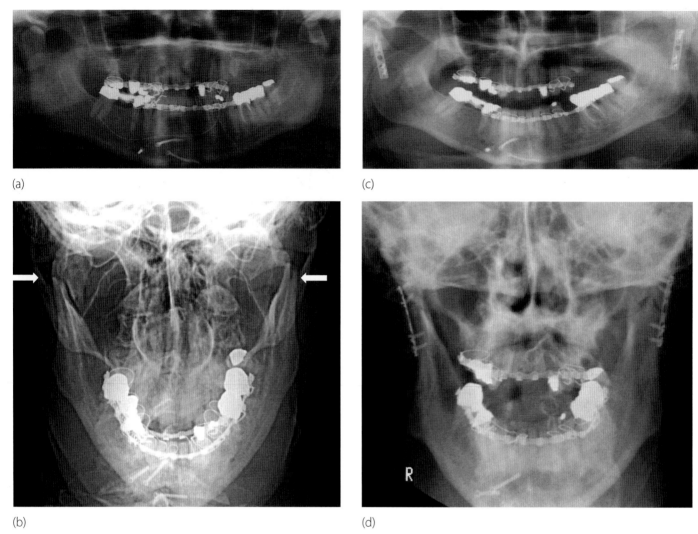

(a)

(c)

(b)

(d)

Fig. 31.3: (a) Preoperative and **(b)** postoperative. **(c,d)** radiographs after endoscopic-assisted reduction and fixation of a severely displaced bilateral condyle fracture via the submandibular approach. Lag screw fixation of the median mandibular fracture was performed previously at another clinic. Note the severely displaced fragments with medial override on the left and medial displacement with shortening of the ascending ramus on the right (arrows).

Angulated drills and screw drivers were used under endoscopic vision by a transoral approach to avoid transbuccal stab incisions (see Fig. 31.2).

Mandible fractures in other locations

In 21 patients with mandible fractures, endoscopic-assisted control after transoral fracture reduction was performed in areas of limited vision such as the inferior and posterior aspects of the ascending ramus in mandibular angle fractures (Box 31.1). The result after fracture reduction was controlled endoscopically in areas of limited visibility when the transoral approach was performed to avoid displacement at the inferior and posterior aspect of the fracture and prevent lingual gaps before osteosynthesis was completed.

The endoscopic-assisted technique was also used for the removal of osteosynthesis material via limited intraoral incisions. Osteosynthesis material at the mandibular angle, the ascending ramus and the mandibular condyle inserted via

Box 31.1 Indications for endoscopically assisted trauma procedure (66 patients between April 1997 and May 2002)

Condylar fractures	n = 45
Investigation/treatment of midface fractures with additional orbital injury (e.g. orbital floor)	n = 49
Decompression of optic nerve	n = 3
Fixation of distraction devices in the mandible	n = 2
Treatment of mandibular fractures/plate removals	n = 21
Revisions of frontal sinus	n = 7
Others (e.g. exploration of skull base; treatment of lesions in combination with conventional surgical procedures)	n = 14

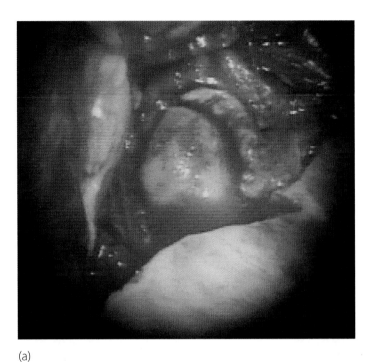

(a)

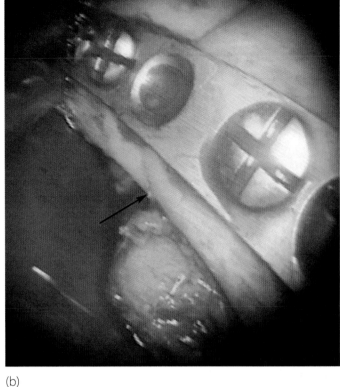

(b)

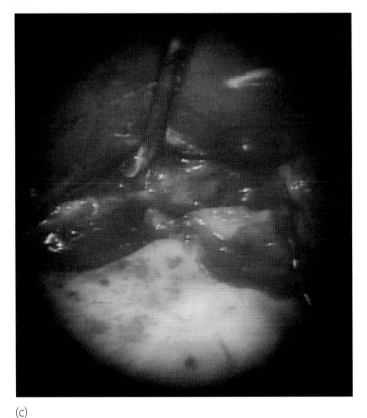

(c)

Fig. 31.4: Displaced condyle fracture of the same patient as in Fig. 32.3. The right fragment was severely dislocated with medial override. **(a)** Intraoperative endoscopic view by 30° angle endoscope before osteosynthesis. **(b)** View after osteosynthesis with 2 mm AO/ASIF titanium zygoma miniplate. Alignment of the fragments was controlled endoscopically at the posterior aspect of the ascending ramus (arrow). The left fragment was difficult to find due to the severe displacement. **(c)** Intraoperative endoscopic view of the displaced fracture via a 30° endoscope.

extraoral and intraoral approaches was removed transorally using an angulated screwdriver in selected cases.

Midfacial and frontal sinus fractures

In 49 patients with fractures of the zygomatic complex and the orbit, endoscopic-assisted treatment was undertaken. Limited incisions were performed and due to the superior visibility using endoscopic techniques, further incisions such

as a transconjunctival approach could be avoided in selected cases.

Zygoma fractures

Due to possible rotation of the zygomatic bone, the result after repositioning has to be evaluated intraoperatively before osteosynthesis is performed. The repositioning cannot be determined precisely from the lateral orbital wall and the intraoral approach. An additional extraoral approach for the exploration of the orbital floor and the infraorbital rim is recommended when displaced zygoma fractures are suspected. Using these additional incisions, often non-displaced fractures without the need for treatment at the orbital floor and infraorbital rim are noted.

In zygoma fractures the endoscope is inserted via a limited blepharoplasty incision to control the fracture dislocation at the sphenozygomatic buttress at the lateral orbital wall (Figs 31.5, 31.6). In displaced zygoma fractures defects of the facial wall of the maxillary sinus often exist and can be used to insert the endoscope for the transoral inspection of the orbital floor (Fig. 31.7). Mobility of the orbital floor is noted endoscopically when pressure is applied to the orbital content. Fractures of the infraorbital rim can also be investigated transorally. After fracture reduction evaluation of the alignment of the infraorbital rim, the sphenozygomatic buttress and the zygomaticomaxillary buttress is performed. Following temporary osteosynthesis at the lateral orbital aspect and the zygomaticomaxillary buttress with two screws for each plate, the result of repositioning and fixation is evaluated before osteosynthesis is completed. Moderate displacement of the infraorbital rim can be treated transorally. In selected cases osteosynthesis at the infraorbital rim can be performed endoscopically via the transoral approach. When there is no displacement of the orbital floor further investigation via transconjunctival or infraorbital incisions can be avoided.

When displaced orbital floor fractures are present the endoscopic-assisted repositioning of orbital soft tissues into maxillary sinus and orbital floor fractures can be performed transorally (Fig. 31.7). In comminuted fractures of the orbital floor and infraorbital rim open reduction and insertion of resorbable foils, bone grafts or titanium mesh may be indicated to stabilize the result of fracture reduction or to reconstruct the orbital floor and infraorbital rim. In those cases exposure of the fracture site by the transconjunctival or mid lower eyelid incision is indicated (Fig. 31.9). The result of repositioning of the orbital soft tissue and reconstruction of the orbital floor can be controlled via the maxillary sinus (Figs 31.7, 31.9).

Fractures of the anterior wall of the frontal sinus may be reduced using minimally invasive techniques when the fracture is not comminuted. Two or three limited incisions in the scalp for the insertion of the endoscope, suction and instruments such as the elevator can be used for the reduction of the fracture similar to endoscopic brow lift surgery. Fixation without further stab incisions is difficult. Impressed fragments may be elevated using single screws inserted via stab incision under endoscopic control. This technique may be indicated when the fracture is not comminuted. When displaced fractures of the posterior table are present open treatment via a coronal incision is indicated.

Other authors describe the endoscopic-assisted injection of bone substitute to fill contour defects of the forehead secondarily after frontal sinus fractures without impairment of frontal sinus function.

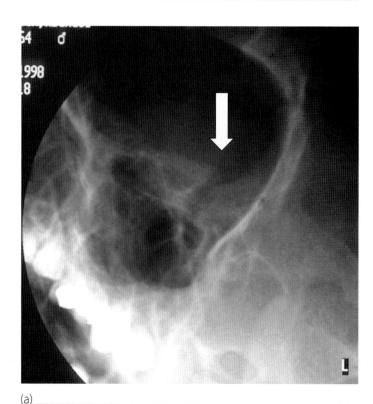

(a)

(b)

Fig. 31.5: Towne's radiographs preoperatively **(a)** and postoperatively **(b)** after endoscopically assisted reduction and fixation of a dislocated zygoma fracture (arrow), carried out via a laceration in the upper left eyelid (see Fig. 32.6).

Outcome

Mandible

Mandibular condyle

An endoscopic-assisted reduction of fractures of the condylar process was performed in 43 patients, using a submandibular

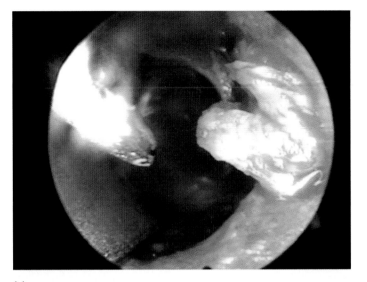

(a)

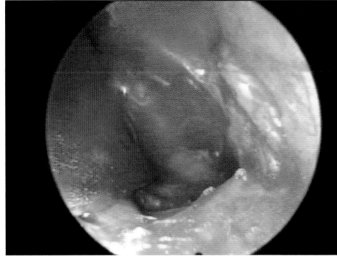

(b)

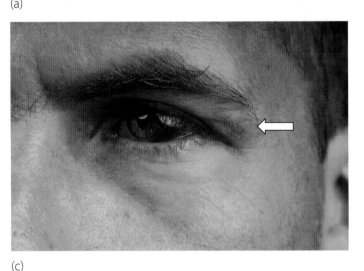

(c)

Fig. 31.6: (a,b) Intraoperative endoscopic views of the lateral orbital wall. A displaced fragment was detected and endoscopically replaced via a limited laceration in the upper eyelid. **(c)** Clinical view of the patient and the limited scar at the left upper eyelid (arrow) 10 days after surgery.

approach in nine patients and a transoral approach in 34 patients. The nine patients treated by extraoral approach demonstrated six condylar neck fractures, two subcondylar fractures and two comminuted fractures of the subcondylar region. One patient suffered from a severely displaced bilateral condylar neck fracture (see Fig. 31.3). Thirty-four patients treated by a transoral approach showed condylar neck fractures (n = 14) and subcondylar fractures (n = 22). Seven out of 10 fractures were displaced and exposed via the extraoral approach. Thirty-two out of 36 fractures were displaced when transorally explored. Two patients demonstrated bilateral condylar fractures, nine condylar fractures were displaced medially, and 27 laterally.

Plate fixation and control of reduction was facilitated endoscopically (see Figs 31.3, 31.8). Transbuccal stab incisions for the insertion of the screws were performed in all patients with the submandibular approach and in 30 patients with the transoral approach. In the patients with the transoral approach, angulated drills and screwdrivers facilitated the fixation of the fractures without transbuccal incisions (see Fig. 31.2).

Temporary weakness of the mandibular branch of the facial nerve was observed in two patients with the submandibular approach. The impairment subsided within 6 months after surgery in both patients.

After 6 months the mouth opening in all patients exceeded 40 mm interincisal distance without significant deviation. There were no signs of temporomandibular joint dysfunction, none of the patients suffered from pain in the temporomandibular joint area and there were no signs of facial nerve damage 6 months postoperatively. The average length of the submandibular scar was 4–5 cm. The scars were esthetically acceptable in all nine patients.

Mandibular fractures in other locations

Precise fracture repositioning was achieved by transoral endoscopic control after fractures of the mandibular angle and ramus. In 21 patients the control after fracture reduction was obtained endoscopically in areas of limited vision. Initially only two screws were fixed temporarily and evaluated before

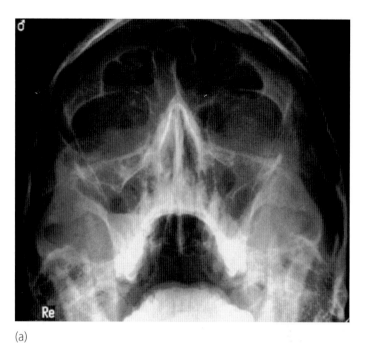

(a)

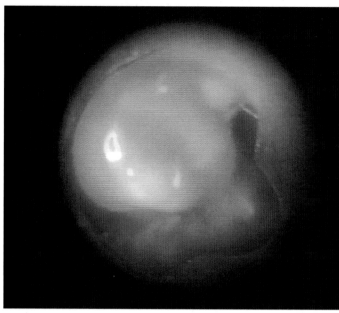

(b)

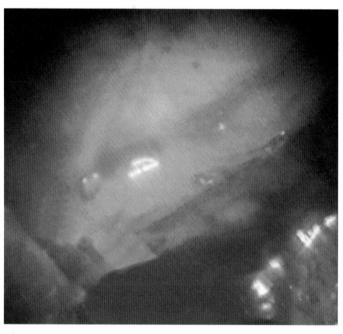

(c)

Fig. 31.7: (a) Preoperative Towne's view of medial midface fracture. Displacement of the orbital floor was not detected on radiographs. **(b)** An endoscopic inspection of the orbital floor transorally via a defect in the facial wall of the maxillary sinus demonstrated dislocation of orbital soft tissue into the maxillary sinus. **(c)** Note the orbital floor following endoscopically controlled reduction via the maxillary sinus with a transconjunctival approach.

the osteosynthesis was completed. In three out of 21 patients the fixation had to be corrected because of inadequate positioning not noted prior to the endoscopic control. Postoperatively a good result of repositioning and fixation was noted, without signs of malocclusion, in all patients.

Midface and frontal sinus fractures

Intraoperatively the degree of dislocation of zygoma fractures and the result after reduction were controlled endoscopically in 49 patients via limited incisions. Fractures of the lateral orbital wall were endoscopically inspected via blepharoplasty incisions (see Figs 31.5, 31.6). The orbital floor and the infraorbital rim were visualized via the transoral approach (see Figs 31.7, 31.9). For the treatment of non-displaced orbital floor fractures endoscopically assisted techniques were used to avoid additional mid lower eyelid or transconjunctival incisions in 31 patients. Postoperative images demonstrated good results after endoscopic-assisted treatment. None of the patients presented with diplopia.

Dislocation of orbital soft tissues into the maxillary sinus was detected in eight patients with comminuted fractures of the orbital floor (see Figs 31.7, 31.9). Transconjunctival or mid lower eyelid incisions are indicated in comminuted fractures of the orbital floor to allow for adequate fracture reduction, stabilization or reconstruction of the orbital floor using resorbable foils, bone grafts and titanium mesh under complete visual control.

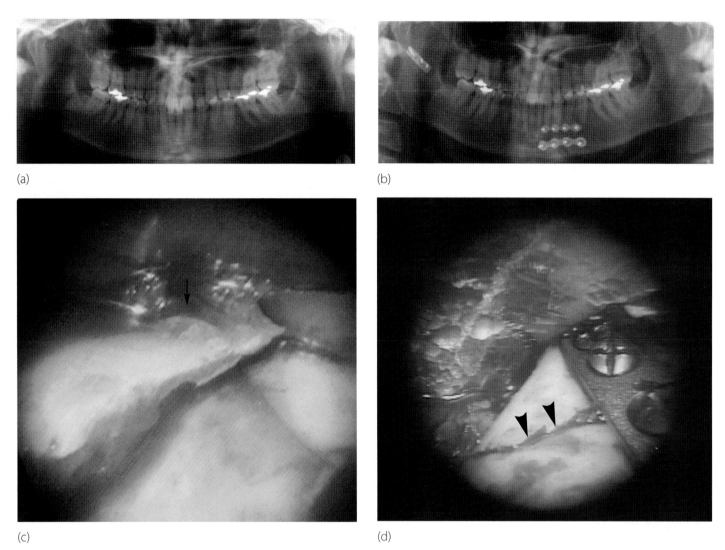

(a)

(b)

(c)

(d)

Fig. 31.8: Displaced mandibular condyle fracture and paramedian fracture of the mandible from footballing accident. **(a,b)** Pre- and postoperative panoramic radiographs. **(c,d)** Intraoperative transoral views of the mandibular condyle fracture with lateral override using a 30° angle endoscope, before (arrow) and after osteosynthesis (arrowheads) .

In four patients fractures of the anterior wall of the frontal sinus were reduced using minimally invasive techniques when there were no signs of a comminuted fracture. However, due to the limited bone thickness of the frontal sinus, the injury was underestimated in high-resolution CT scans in two out of the four patients prior to surgery. After elevation of the periosteal tissue multiple fragments were noted and the treatment strategy had to be changed to an open reduction via coronal incision. The endoscopic-assisted treatment of frontal sinus fractures is indicated when there is no comminution or involvement of the posterior table.

Controversies

Minimally invasive endoscopic procedures have been described for various indications in the craniomaxillo-facial area.[2,3,4,14] To minimize the risk of damage to the facial nerve

and visible scars, endoscopic-assisted techniques via limited or transoral incisions were demonstrated (Box 31.1).[1,5,9–13]

In oral and maxillofacial trauma, adequate exposure for comminuted fractures is mandatory to allow for precise three-dimensional fracture reduction. The indication for endoscopic-assisted treatment is limited to fractures which can be treated without wide exposure. The creation of an optical cavity is required to obtain endoscopic vision of the fracture site by limited incisions. The extension of the incision depends also on the type of fracture and treatment planned. However, the volume of the optical cavity has to allow the handling of instruments. Special instruments designed for endoscopic repositioning and fixation have been developed. Due to the concept of working in an optical cavity, incisions in inconspicuous areas can be used as surgical ports.

The endoscopic-assisted treatment of oral and maxillofacial surgery trauma proved to be helpful to obtain good

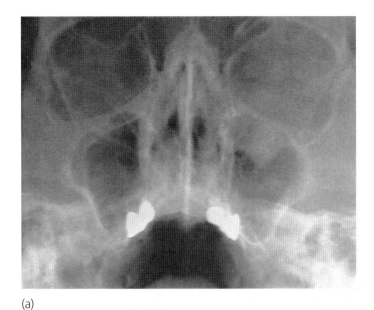

(a)

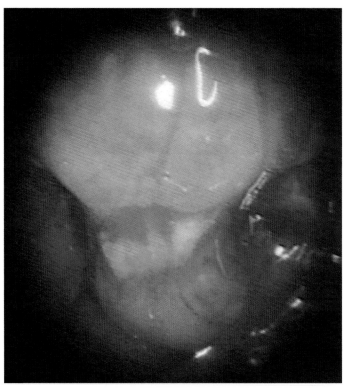

(b)

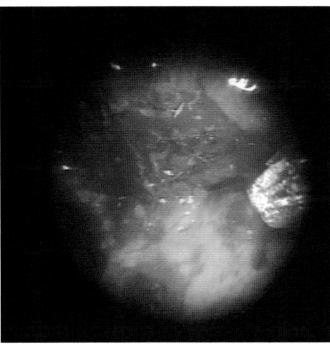

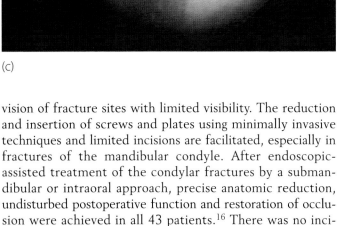

(c)

Fig. 31.9: (a) Radiograph demonstrating orbital floor fracture. **(b)** Intraoperative endoscopic view via the maxillary sinus demonstrates a comminuted orbital floor fracture with displacement of orbital soft tissue into the maxillary sinus. **(c)** Replacement of the orbital soft tissue and reconstruction of the orbital floor was performed by a transconjunctival approach with transoral endoscopic control following repositioning of the orbital soft tissue via the maxillary sinus.

vision of fracture sites with limited visibility. The reduction and insertion of screws and plates using minimally invasive techniques and limited incisions are facilitated, especially in fractures of the mandibular condyle. After endoscopic-assisted treatment of the condylar fractures by a submandibular or intraoral approach, precise anatomic reduction, undisturbed postoperative function and restoration of occlusion were achieved in all 43 patients.[16] There was no incidence of damage to the facial nerve after 6 months and all extraoral scars were esthetically satisfying in all patients.

Different approaches for the treatment of displaced condylar fractures have been demonstrated. The surgical approach is chosen according to the type and location of the fracture. The extraoral approach was preferably selected for displaced fractures with medial override and for comminuted

or condylar neck fractures from April 1998 to December 1999. Superior visibility of the fracture site and easier handling of instruments for the endoscopic-assisted reduction and manipulation of the fragment were advantages of the submandibular approach.[1,5,11]

The transoral approach was used for endoscopic treatment of subcondylar fractures and condylar fractures which were not severely displaced or for fractures with lateral override. Angulated drills and screwdrivers facilitated the transoral management of condylar fractures without the need for transfacial stab incisions.[5,16]

Compared to the submandibular approach, the endoscopically assisted transoral approach is less time consuming, intraoral scars are invisible and the risk of facial nerve damage is minimal. Direct vision can be limited by the coronoid process of the mandible but in selected cases using angulated scopes, superior vision was achieved posterior to the coronoid process.

The transoral use of endoscopes for control after fracture reduction in areas of limited vision such as the posterior aspect of the ascending ramus and the inferior aspect of the mandible provided further information about the quality of fracture reduction and may help to improve surgical results.[16] The transoral endoscopic approach for condyle fractures was a new method four years ago and became routine procedure in our clinic. We now adopt the transoral endoscopic approach for all fractures where an open procedure is indicated, even when severe displacement is present.

The transoral endoscopic removal of osteosynthesis materials, such as after fixation of condylar fractures or angle fractures treated extraorally, was performed. The transoral use of endoscopes for the removal of plates, even in areas such as mandibular condyle fractures or angle fractures treated extraorally, was possible without extraoral incisions. The endoscopic-assisted removal of osteosynthesis material inserted by an extraoral approach allowed limited intraoral incisions in the previously operated site to avoid facial nerve damage.

The aim of minimally invasive management of midfacial trauma is to minimize the operative trauma. However, as in mandibular fractures, the indication may be limited in the midfacial area, when comminution and multiple displaced fragments may require wide exposure. Fractures of the zygomatic complex are often inspected by transconjunctival and infraorbital incisions to evaluate fractures of the orbital floor and infraorbital rim. The endoscopic inspection of the lateral orbital wall and sphenozygomatic buttress by limited blepharoplasty incision proved to be helpful for the evaluation of suspected displaced zygoma fractures before and after repositioning fracture reduction. Often non-displaced fractures are seen without need for further treatment. To avoid incisions that serve a diagnostic purpose only, the endoscopic control of the orbital floor can be performed transorally via the maxillary sinus.

The endoscopic-assisted reduction of comminuted zygomatic arch fractures has been reported using pre-auricular and transconjunctival incisions with lateral canthotomy.[3] Due to multiple fragments, wide exposure is often required and extracorporeal realignment of the arch fragments may be indicated. For fixation with a long 2.0 mm osteosynthesis plate in the anterior aspect, incisions in the visible area by lateral canthotomy are reported. These incisions leave visible scars in an exposed area of the face.[3] In severely comminuted fractures of the zygomatic complex open reduction via coronal incision provides better exposure for a safer reduction without visible scars. Furthermore, comparison with the unaffected side can be performed to allow for precise anatomical reduction as those fractures often occur in panfacial trauma.

The endoscopic endonasal approach for the reduction of medial orbital wall fractures has been described.[15] In fractures of the medial orbital wall with orbital soft tissue displaced into the ethmoid area, the placement of bone grafts or resorbable foils may be indicated for the reconstruction of the orbital volume to prevent enophthalmos formation. Bone grafts or resorbable foils which are indicated for the reconstruction of the medial orbital wall in extended fractures cannot be inserted transnasally. Medial orbital wall fractures without displacement of orbital soft tissue into the ethmoid area and without signs of double vision should not be treated. In frontal sinus fractures minimally invasive techniques can be applied in selected cases.[4]

When comminuted fractures or involvement of the posterior table of the frontal sinus or the anterior skull base are present with suspected CSF leakage, open treatment via a coronal incision with wide exposure of the fracture site is indicated and endoscopic techniques should not be performed. Due to the limited thickness of the bone involved in frontal sinus fractures, the degree of comminution is often misjudged by CT scans. This may cause difficulties in reduction by limited incisions as the degree of comminution and displacement can often only be appreciated after elevation of the periosteal tissue and exposure of the fragments. Therefore the indications for endoscopically assisted fracture reduction of the frontal sinus area may be limited.

Contour defects of the forehead can be treated using minimally invasive techniques. Bone substitutes can be injected under endoscopic control after a frontal sinus wall has healed in dislocation. Furthermore, esthetically compromising contour defects often present following craniotomy for neurosurgical treatment can be evened out.

Conclusion

Future perspectives for widening the indications for minimally invasive surgery are based on the combination of endoscopic techniques and computer-assisted surgery. The endoscope position can be monitored using the computer-assisted techniques which allow endoscopic-assisted surgery of the anterior skull base or next to anatomical structures such as the optical nerve and the internal carotid artery. Further developments of bone cements or bone glues may lead to other indications and new treatment strategies for endoscopic surgery in craniofacial trauma. The repair of contour defects and fixation of non-displaced fractures may be carried out using those bone cements and glues.

Furthermore, intraoperative imaging using CT may allow for immediate quality control after minimally invasive procedures for the repositioning of craniomaxillofacial fractures.

An intensive training in endoscopic techniques and the handling of special instruments is mandatory before the endoscopic-assisted treatment of oral and maxillofacial fractures is performed. Due to a steep learning curve, the operation time of the initially time-consuming endoscopic-assisted procedures can be reduced significantly.

References

1 Lauer G, Schmelzeisen R 1999 Endoscope-assisted fixation of mandibular condylar process fractures. Journal of Oral and Maxillofacial Surgery 57: 36–39

2 Schön R, Gellrich N-C, Schramm A, Schmelzeisen R 2000 Endoskopische Chirurgie im Mund-, Kiefer- und Gesichtsbereich –

Video demonstration einer endoskopisch assistierten Versorgung einer dislozierten Jochbeinfraktur [Endoscopic oral and maxillofacial surgery – video demonstration of the endoscopic assisted treatment of a displaced zygoma fracture]. Journal der Deutschen Gesellschaft fur Plastische und Wiederherstellungschirurgie 12: 21

3 Lee CH, Lee C, Trabulsy PP 1996 Endoscopic-assisted repair of a malar fracture. Annals of Plastic Surgery 37: 178

4 Graham HD, Spring P 1996 Endoscopic repair of frontal sinus fracture: case report. Journal of Craniomaxillofacial Trauma 2(4): 52–55

5 Schön R, Gutwald R, Schramm A, Gellrich N-C, Schmelzeisen R 2002 Endoscopic assisted treatment of condylar fractures. Extraoral vs. intraoral approach. International Journal of Oral and Maxillofacial Surgery 31: 237–243

6 Schön R, Roveda SIL, Carter B 2001 Mandibular fractures in Townsville, Australia. Incidence, etiology and treatment using the 2.0 AO/ASIF miniplate system. British Journal of Oral and Maxillofacial Surgery 39: 145–148

7 Walker RV 1994 Condylar fractures: nonsurgical management. Journal of Oral and Maxillofacial Surgery 52: 1185

8 Weinberg MJ, Merx P, Antonynshyn O, Farb R 1995 Facial nerve palsy after mandibular fractures. Annals of Plastic Surgery 34: 546

9 Ellis E III, Dean J 1993 Rigid fixation of mandibular condyle fractures. Oral Surgery, Oral Medicine, Oral Pathology 76: 6

10 Hall MB 1994 Condylar fractures: surgical management. Journal of Oral and Maxillofacial Surgery 52: 1189

11 Lauer G, Schmelzeisen R, Wichmann U 1998 2. Endoskopgestützte. Fixation von Gelenkfortsatzfrakturen des Unterkiefers [Endoscopic assisted fixation of condylar fractures of the mandible]. Deutsche Zeitschrift fur Mund-, Kiefer- und Gesichtschirurgie 2S: 168–170

12 Chen C-T, Lai J-P, Tung T-C, Chen Y-R 1998 Endoscopically assisted mandibular subcondylar fracture repair. Plastic and Reconstructive Surgery 103: 160–165

13 Jacobovicz J, Lee C, Trabulsky PP 1998 Endoscopic repair of mandibular subcondylar fracture. Plastic and Reconstructive Surgery 101: 160–165

14 Vasconez LO, Core GB, Oslin B 1995 Endoscopy in plastic surgery: an overview. Clinics in Plastic Surgery 22: 585

15 Michel O 1993 Isolierte mediale Orbitawandfrakturen: Ergebnisse einer minimalen invasiven endoskopisch-kontrollierten endonasalen Operationstechnik [Isolated fractures of medial orbital wall: results using a minimal invasive endoscopic controlled endonasal operation technique]. Laryngo-Rhino-Otologie 72: 450–454

16 Schön R, Schramm A, Gellrich N-C, Schmelzeisen R 2003 Follow up of condylar fractures of the mandible is 8 patients in 18 months after transoral endoscopic-assisted open treatment. Journal of Maxillofacial Surgery 61(1) 49–54

32 Computer-Assisted Oral and Maxillofacial Surgery: Technology and Clinical Developments

Stefan Hassfeld, Joachim Mühling

Introduction

Computers are used increasingly as a supportive tool for diagnosis, operative planning and treatment in medicine and dentistry. They are used in connection with modern digital imaging techniques such as computed tomography (CT) and magnetic resonance imaging (MRI), as well as ultrasound to improve the visualization of anatomical and physiological conditions in keeping with the human imagination. Almost every medical specialty shows a tendency towards less invasive procedures. At the same time, we strive to overcome the limits of conventional surgical methods. Within our own specialty this extends into all areas ranging from dental implantology to the treatment of craniofacial malformations and advanced tumors within this anatomically complex region.

Whereas in diagnostic imaging enormous progress has been made, the intraoperative use of imaging techniques has been, until now, relatively restricted. Intraoperative three-dimensional (3D) imaging with ultrasound, CT and MRI is still costly and only available at an experimental level. Computer-assisted surgery will be a help in this field in the future and techniques of virtual reality (VR) will become increasingly important in relation to medical appliances.

The goal of the interactive, intraoperative application of 3D image data has been realized in part through instrument navigation systems. For the first time, navigation systems enable the surgeon to show the actual instrument position in the operation site on the 3D reconstructed image data set of the patient. Conversely, it is also possible to focus on the position of a pathological or anatomical structure of the patient within the operative field.

Diagnostic imaging

Three-dimensional imaging techniques such as CT, MRI and ultrasound can present almost every anatomical and pathological structure with a high resolution and quality. Present developments concentrate on artefact reduction as well as the automatic fusion of the various imaging modalities. A further automatic segmentation of anatomical structures based on image data to facilitate the graphic operation simulation is still in a developmental stage.

Planning and simulation

The automated generation of the proposed operation as well as the simulation of surgical procedures and the presentation of their effects are partly applicable within the framework of virtual surgery. For the simulation of operational results, i.e. for the virtual 3D graphic simulation of various treatment alternatives on the computer, software has to be developed to allow for interactive manipulation, including viewing from various angles, cutting, palpating, insertion of implants, etc., in real time within the 3D visualization. Here the user's interaction has to be brought into line with the usual surgical actions. In the future, input media with power feedback (haptical interfaces from the field of VR technologies) will offer options for intuitive controlling of complex 3D simulation environments through the surgeon.

Intraoperative support

The image data acquired preoperatively during diagnosis should be available for interactive use by the surgeons at all times. Modern techniques of computer-assisted surgery can thereby help to decrease the operational risk and postoperative morbidity rate even further. Future interactive support for the surgeon can be characterized within the following areas.

Passive tools for support of the intraoperative orientation will allow for the routine transmission of the preoperative plan to the patient. These tools include, for example, projection techniques, head-mounted displays and instrument navigation systems.

Guiding systems (semiactive manipulator systems) will show the surgeon a risk-free path for the operation instruments in connection with the operation plan. Thus, operation strategies can be transferred to the operation site precisely and safely.

Surgical robots will execute specific operation steps completely autonomously. In this case the surgeon leaves control to the robot for certain parts of the operation. The best-known example is the highly precise milling of the femur shaft for the adaptation of a hip joint endoprosthesis which is already in routine clinical use.

Postoperative evaluation

Postoperatively, a comparison between the control image data and the original image data for the evaluation of the real surgical result will permit scientific studies using the follow-up controls. The resulting data can be used for the optimization of operational strategies using the software tools to improve prediction of the surgical outcome.

Diagnostic Imaging

The existence of suitable image data in the form of two- and three-dimensional data sets is critical for successful preoperative planning and intraoperative navigation. In many cases, we use several, partly complementary image-producing methods in the same anatomical area in order to obtain detailed, supplementary information of the clinical image.

CT offers the advantages of a precise reproducible local presentation as well as the high-contrast presentation of osseous structures. The image quality of CTs is diminished through patient movement and metal artefacts, as well as the limited soft tissue contrast. Advantages of MRI are the excellent soft tissue presentation and the free choice of image planes, as well as the possibility of functional imaging (diffusion- and perfusion-weighted acquisitions, MR angiography). Additionally, the patient is not subjected to radiation. Disadvantages are especially the various artefacts, for example distortion, both appliance specific or patient induced, the chemical shift, susceptibility artefacts, movement and metal artefacts.

Sonography offers the advantages of quick access, a high local resolution, the free choice of image planes and especially the possibility to track anatomical structures and determine functional parameters (circulation, vascular support).

Disadvantages are the dependence on the examiner and geometrical distortions, as well as the associated noise. The use of 3D sonography now allows for an even more widespread application of sonography, with the possibility of reconstruction of the image layers parallel to the CT or MRI images which in addition may be aligned to the view of the surgeon, resulting in improved orientation.

The possibility of intraoperative use offers an additional advantage of sonography and, to a lesser extent, of CT and MRI.[1] Imaging must be considered not only with respect to diagnosis but also in connection with operational planning and other methods based on these image data. Especially important are the imaging parameters chosen by the surgeon in cooperation with the radiologist, for example the parameters of the cutting plane, layer spacing and thickness or the use of contrast medium.

Due to the increasing necessity to include image information in treatment planning, it is desirable to combine the different information from various sources to achieve a fused image data set (Fig. 32.1). For this purpose, an automated fusion of the various image modalities as well as an automated segmentation of the anatomical and pathological structures should be achievable. With the present state of the art, this is not yet possible. So far only bones and skin surfaces can be segmented automatically based on CT data. However, knowl-

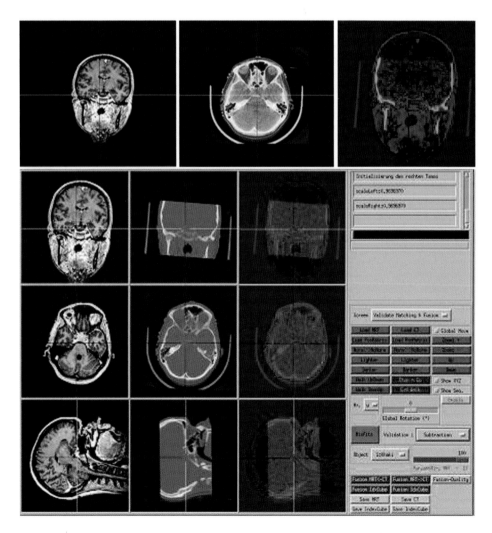

Fig. 32.1: Registration and fusion put the different image data sets (MRT, above left, and CT, above middle) into a common geometrical context (fused image data set MRT red and CT green, above right). The software makes it possible to represent the individual data sets and the fused data set in different frames on the monitor.

edge of the exact position of at-risk structures, such as vessels and nerves, is especially important for the use of, for example, robots in order to avoid a collision during the planning phase of the operational steps to be performed by the robot.

For example, many implantologists wish to have a 3D representation of the bone conditions for the planning of complex cases. Not least because of radiation, however, so far CT has been used infrequently as a diagnostic aid. Since dental implantology is interested primarily in bony structures and high soft tissue resolution is not necessary, a dose reduction seems promising. Dose-reduced CT allows exact metric measurements in the range of 1 mm or less as well as the 3D representation of the jawbone, facilitating a precise 3D implantation plan with justifiable radiation. Thus we consider CT-assisted planning to be indicated before dental implantations with reduced bone volume, especially near the maxillary antrum and the mandibular canal, as well as when multiple implants are planned.

Due to technical developments 3D X-ray techniques are expected to become increasingly important in dental surgery. Cone-beam CT scanners produce a 3D image data record without having to move the patient table. With the cone-beam technique, dedicated devices can be built especially for dentistry which, in design, could be similar to conventional devices (Fig. 32.2). It seems to be a realistic possibility that very soon further devices will be available whose costs can be compared to those of current orthopantomography devices.

Planning and Simulation

In contrast to the rapid progress in diagnostic imaging, the development and clinical use of new technologies for planning and performing therapy are still lagging behind. This can clearly be seen from the fact that the patient's 3D CT image data are still exposed as two-dimensional images on the X-ray film. An analysis is mostly restricted to general statements or a few metric measurements. Planning is carried out mentally by the treating physicians and thus depends very much on their experience and powers of imagination.

The aim of operation planning in oral and maxillofacial surgery is the optimization of the surgical result with regard to functional and esthetic aspects. The prerequisite for successful operation planning is the preparation of preoperative patient image data. For the segmentation of the original image data, individual pixels or voxels are assigned to certain classifications such as skin, bones, at-risk structures, tumors, etc. Powerful graphic workstations are necessary for an interactive manipulation with a commitment to detail.

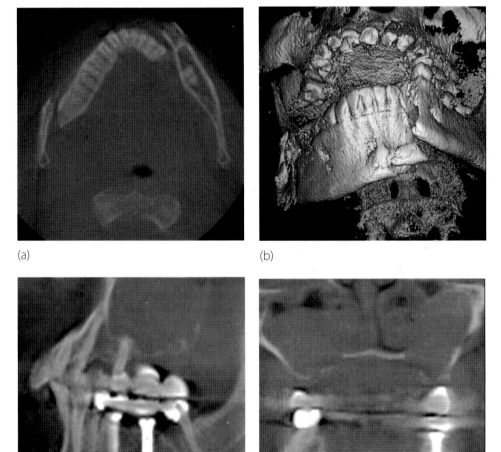

(a)

(b)

(c)

(d)

Fig. 32.2: Image examples from cone-beam CT (NewTom QR-DVT 9000). Axial **(a)** and 3D representation **(b)** of a mandibular angle and a paramedian fracture with free basal fragment. Sagittal **(c)** and coronal reformats **(d)** for demonstrating bone volume in vicinity of implant.

With the aid of the patient model generated from the original image data, the definition of the operation goal and the planning can be performed. However, one must be aware that the model is only an approximation of the patient. Certain information, for example that between the layers of the image data, is missing, so the precision is limited by the layer thickness.

At the present time, there is a serious discrepancy between the scientific development of tools with often very complex software systems and the simple handling requirements of the surgeon. This problem poses an obstacle to the introduction of theory to practical application because, at the moment, the interactive planning of a complex bone-shifting operation requires more than one hour.

In order to use new technologies optimally and safely plan and carry out surgical interventions, an operation planning system is necessary that the surgeon may consult during preoperative planning as well as during intraoperative intervention and postoperative evaluation. During preoperative planning firstly the operative aim has to be defined. As an example, the bone segments to be translocated have to be specified and virtually sawed, deformed and positioned.

Two application areas will highlight the clinical importance of preoperative planning and simulation.

Computer-assisted planning in dental implantology

Conventional preimplant planning is usually conducted with a two-dimensional panoramic radiograph. This method cannot supply an assessment of the actual bone volume in a buccolingual dimension. Often, it becomes apparent during surgery that the bone is too narrow or is not suitable for an implant due to concave border surfaces. For safety reasons, large distances have to be left between implants and neighboring structures in cases where the third dimension is unknown. Thus, the use of the available bone cannot be optimized. Within the past several years, CT-based planning systems for dental implantology have been introduced with the goal of overcoming these limitations. To choose the most suitable implant insertion locality, it is possible to 'move through' an almost unlimited succession of finely graduated cross- and panoramic sections. At any time, the treating physician can thus reconstruct exactly the right type of information according to the respective requirements for the treatment planning without having to examine the patient yet again. For the first time, these software-generated secondary sections from the CT data set of a jaw now allow for an overlay-free presentation and evaluation of the vestibulo-oral dimension of the alveolar process as well as the immediate metric registration directly on the screen. However, most software systems commercially available today have one serious disadvantage: real 3D visualization is not possible.[2]

Software programs for interactive 3D planning of dental implantations have only lately become available. Apart from a highly resolved, detail-corresponding visualization of the patient's volume data, therapy planning additionally requires the representation of artificial objects such as implants, drills and saws which can more precisely be shaped in the form of surface objects. For operator convenience, frame rates of several images per second are necessary; only in this case is intuitive and interactive positioning of the implants possible.

A system for interactive 3D planning for dental implantology, developed at our hospital (Fig. 32.3), allows the 3D positioning of implants with high image quality. The representation of the mandibular canal requires only the identification of the mandibular foramen and the mental foramen; from that the software automatically performs an analysis of the most probable course of the mandibular canal within the CT image data. According to bone availability, the distance to critical structures and planned prosthetic superstructures the dentist decides on the implant's position.[3]

From a prosthetic view, in order to prevent interferences between the optimal number, localization, angulation and type of implants and the existing anatomical preconditions, it is necessary to match the preoperatively obtained data (bone quality and bone quantity) with prosthetic demands (statics, dynamics and esthetics) during the planning. Thus the successful result of an implant superstructure can be optimized and guaranteed for the long term. Future developments in this area also encompass the integration of a 3D simulation of prosthetic superstructures and their esthetic effect into the planning software environment. Thus, a synoptic virtual implantation from a prosthetic and surgical view could be achieved for the first time.

The above advantages of CT-based implantation planning do have to be considered in relation to the disadvantages of the availability of scanners, higher costs and higher radiation for the patient. In this respect many authors consider it better to apply standard orthopantomography techniques for routine examinations and to use the CT-based implantation planning in particularly complex cases with reduced bone volume, especially near the maxillary sinus and mandibular canal, as well as when the insertion of multiple implants is planned.

The decisive step to an exact implant insertion, however, has not yet been achieved. In the simplest case 3D planning data can be used to produce individual drill guides with titanium tubes to guide the drill. Also, connection to intraoperative navigation systems used for implant insertion is possible. From a technical view point, medical robots can also be used for implant insertion. Many things are still at the developmental or prototype stage but significant effects on surgical routine are already foreseeable.

Computer-assisted planning for the correction of malformations

New software and hardware technologies have led to successful surgical navigation systems being used in many disciplines, e.g. removing foreign bodies and tumors. In order to use these new technologies optimally and safely to plan and carry out a surgical intervention operation, planning systems are necessary which support the surgeon during preoperative planning as well as intraoperatively.

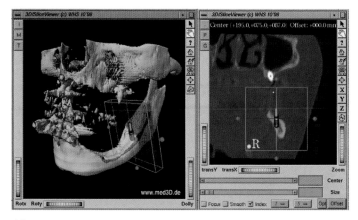

(a)

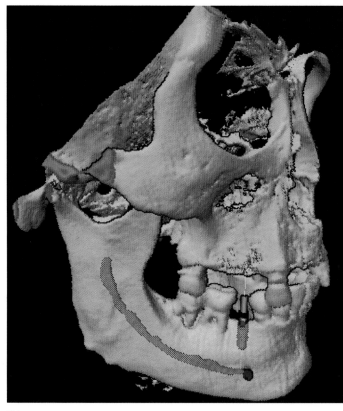

(b)

Fig. 32.3: (a) Positioning of an implant on the monitor. The implant's position and orientation can be interactively changed in the 2D layer or 3D visualization. In the semitransparent representation on the left the 3D relation of the implant to the mandibular canal is obvious (Courtesy of Dr W Stein, Heidelberg, Germany, www.med3D.de). **(b)** Semi-automatic segmentation of the mandibular canal. For user interaction it is merely necessary to click the mandibular foramen mandibulae and the mental foramen.

Software developments for the virtual cutting and shifting of bone parts now allow a patient-specific simulation of complex bone-shifting interventions.[4–7] Through collision detection, it becomes apparent which bone parts must be remodeled further. For a better graphic quality, the individual bone segments are differentiated through the use of different colors. After determination of the optimal shifting distance on the computer screen, the calculated data can be applied precisely to the operation site (that is, to the patient), e.g. with the aid of the navigation systems, thus ensuring optimal precision of the surgery (Figs 32.4, 32.5).

The simulation of the surgical outcome, i.e. the 3D graphic representation of the various osteotomies on the computer, supports the surgeon in the planning and choice of the best operation. The 3D visualization facilitates the assessment of the planned operation and permits discussion with colleagues. Conventional limits with regard to imaginative power are overcome and this method also allows the patient to anticipate the results of the operation. Another goal to achieve is that the 3D simulation of the results of a planned intervention includes the soft tissue changes.[8] The patient would then be able to decide upon the surgical method together with the treating physician, which would strengthen the relationship between physician and patient.

The use of the term 'operation planning' varies in the literature. With most operation planning systems, only a simulation of the postoperative image can be carried out and only a few systems also support the intraoperative realization of the preoperative planning. The individual planning systems can be classified into three categories.

1. *Systems without technical support*: these carry out above all a previsualization of the postoperative state.
2. *Systems with passive navigation support for intraoperative navigation*: with these systems, for example, a preoperatively planned access path can be run through by the surgeon using visual control. Apart from the access path, many systems show also objects such as tumors or foreign bodies and tissue at risk that has to be avoided.
3. *Systems with active support*: by a surgical robot, for example.

In complex surgical interventions, such as the preoperative planning of a fronto-orbital advancement (FOA), the increase in intracranial volume achieved by the bone shift can be visualized. In order to simulate interventions of this kind computer geometric models have to be produced from the CT images; these models clearly represent the anatomical structures as well as simulating the interventions relevant for the operation, such as drilling, sawing or deformation. Methods for interaction have to be made available which guarantee an exact and intuitive input of the surgical actions on the computer.

Future of surgery simulation

Tools for 3D interaction with the image data (human–machine interface) require the selection of points or partial volumes in the 3D scene. Generally a 2D mouse is used for this task but 3D input devices can accelerate the processing as well as increase the precision of the whole procedure. By including the sense of touch in this interaction another improvement may be made and for this reason force feedback devices are increasingly integrated as part of the human–

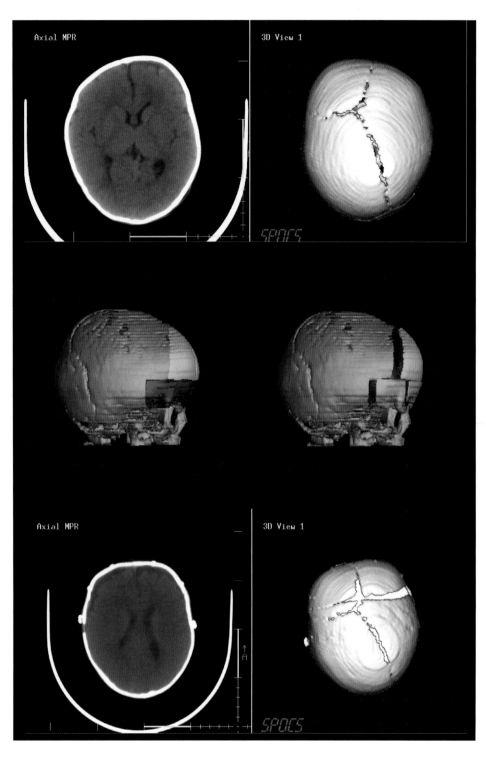

Fig. 32.4: Simulation of correction of a plagiocephaly through fronto-orbital bone advancement. A postoperative comparison of the control CT image data with the basic CT image data for evaluation of the operative real result is shown below (above pre-, below postoperative, images in the middle left simulation pre, on the right simulation post).

machine interface. Surgeons performing the planning feel as if they have actually made an incision into the skin or bone surface[5,9] (Fig. 32.6).

Intraoperative Support

Projection of the operative plan onto the patient

Anatomically and pathologically relevant structures or planning data such as the incision line could be directly projected on to the patient or virtually mirrored into 3D glasses (Fig. 32.7). Such see-through devices or head-mounted displays (HMD) are already available for military use. For medical use, however, they will have to be modified. Apart from simple handling problems (the surgeon standing at the table cannot put on and take off the glasses and might possibly have to refocus them or look above or below them to see well), there are technical problems regarding the resolution and frequency of the image representation.

The alternative would be the direct projection of the desired information onto the patient. This requires exact

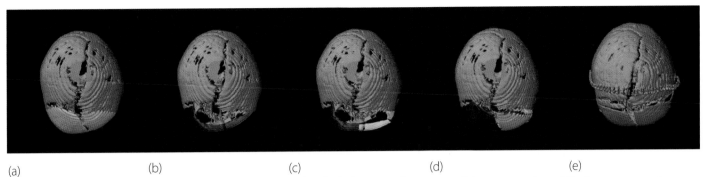

(a)   (b)   (c)   (d)   (e)

Fig. 32.5: Simulation of correction of a plagiocephaly – detailed planning of segments: **(a)** segmentation of the bone segments; **(b)** temporary removal of the frontal bone; **(c)** shaping and foreshifting of the orbital segment; **(d)** reorientation of the frontal bone; **(e)** postoperative situation.

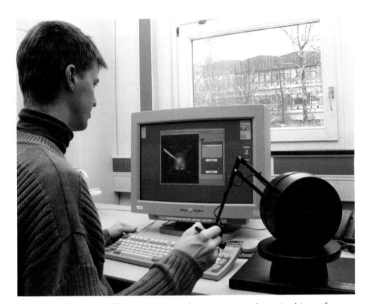

Fig. 32.6: Input of the incision planning via a haptical interface.

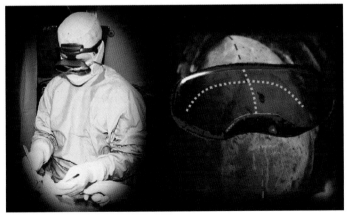

Fig. 32.7: Semitransparent glasses to overlap the computer simulation with the real operation area.

planning and a co-ordination of the patient's head, the eyes of the observer and the projector. As objects in a lower position cannot be projected correctly with respect to their position, their interface with the surface has to be visualized and the surface position must therefore be known at all times. Technically this is already possible, but it requires a great deal of effort.[10] The above-mentioned augmented reality techniques will facilitate a much easier interactive use of diagnostic images and planning data intraoperatively.

Intraoperative support by instrument navigation

As a universal tool for operations in the areas of neurosurgery, ENT, orthopedics and oral and maxillofacial surgery, intraoperative instrument navigation is already routinely used in many hospitals and clinics. The navigation system records the spatial position and orientation of a probe or a surgical instrument. After the registration has been completed, the preoperatively acquired image data of the patient is faded into the actual position of the instrument through 2D and 3D visualization. During intraoperative navigation (Fig. 32.8c) the spatial position data of the navigation instrument are permanently presented on the CT and/or MRI data set of the patient. Simultaneously, the instrument tip position is shown as a crosshair in the original layers as well as in two vertical, secondary computed levels on the screen (in axial original layers, for example, additional sagittal and frontal views are shown). The 3D reconstruction of the CT data is shown in a fourth screen window displaying the position and orientation of the whole instrument (e.g. a probe) and a projected virtual extension of the instrument axis (Fig. 32.8b).

Assessment of navigation technology and accuracy

The intraoperative use of operation planning data on the basis of X-ray pictures was first performed in neurosurgery with stereotactic systems firmly attached to the skull. These systems allow for the localization of deep-seated intracranial structures and are still used today for neurosurgical operations due to their good precision and well-tried handling.[11]

By transition from the computer-assisted plan to the operation phase based on frameless navigation and localization techniques, surgeons can see their actual instrument position

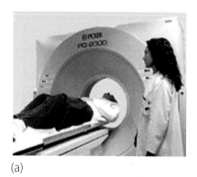
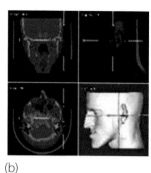

(a)   (b)

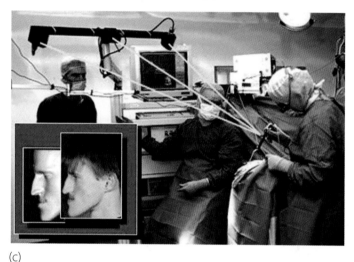

(c)

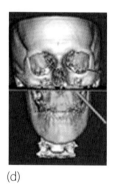
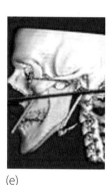
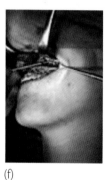

(d)   (e)   (f)

Fig. 32.8: Principle of intraoperative instrument navigation. **(a)** CT or MRI data, **(b)** 3D visualization, **(c)** optoelectronic navigation system for registration of image data to patient position, **(d–f)** 3D visualization of image date and instruments corresponding to actual clinical position.

for the first time on the 3D reconstructed image data set of the patient. Conversely, it is also possible to determine the position of a pathological or anatomical structure shown in the images of the individual patient's anatomy. The precision of such navigation systems is generally reported to be in the range of 2–5 mm.[11-15] Naturally, the accuracy of these systems is substantially higher in rigid structures such as bones and osseous areas than in soft tissue areas.

From a technical point of view, instrument navigation in medical surroundings is possible:

- *mechanically* through position calculation with a gear of movable angles

- *electromagnetically* through detection of field changes with coils
- *based on ultrasound* through real-time measurements of the sound signals
- *video-optically* through position calculation with infrared diodes or recognition of patterns with CCD cameras.

The *mechanical systems* offer the advantages of good technical precision (about 1 mm), low susceptibility to failure and easy sterile covering with a tube. The disadvantages are the unwieldy handling, restricted range and mobility as well as their space requirement at the operating table.[13]

Electromagnetic systems offer the advantages that very small detector coils can be used, no visual contact between instrument and sensor system is required as well as a rapid computation of the signals and easy sterilization. However, their disadvantages are susceptibility to interference through magnetic fields and metal objects and the subsequent possible limited accuracy. Incorrect position sensing of up to 4 mm may occur.[4,15-17]

The *ultrasound-based systems* offer the advantages of a technically acceptable precision in the range of 1–5 mm, convenient handling and easy sterilization. Nevertheless, the systems are subject to interference through reflection, Dopplers' effect, air movement, background noise and obstructions in the sound path so they are rarely used today.

Systems with *optical coupling* are used increasingly in intraoperative navigation.[14-18] Optical navigation systems offer the advantages of a high technical precision in the range of 0.1–0.4 mm, convenient handling and easy sterilization. The disadvantages lie in the necessity for constant visual contact between cameras and instruments and the susceptibility to interference through light reflexes on metallic surfaces in the operating environment.

The resolution of CT data is very high. Our team, for example, experimentally determined the precision to be between 0.3 mm and 0.5 mm.[19] This is so small that we can safely assume that, with regard to the interactive use of the image data, the limiting factor is the precision of the intraoperative realization, not the image generation.

The resolution of MRI data achieves similar results but problems may occur with some cases due to massive irregular geometrical deviations in the examination volume. The combination of CT data and MRI data on a geometrical basis of the CT data sets offers a viable solution.

Possible errors exist with the segmentation and 3D reconstruction of the data sets. Flaws in the respective calculation algorithm, for example, may lead to inaccuracies of the 3D object (enlargement, reduction, distortion). Another possibility is the incorporation of image parts which were not supposed to be part of the structure to be reconstructed and, conversely, necessary parts might also possibly be excluded.

Registration

The basic requirement of any navigation technique is the registration of the patient's position in relation to the image data set, which can be performed according to various principles.

In the case of frame-based stereotaxy, this is accomplished by attaching the frame to the patient's head before taking the required images. For frameless navigation techniques generally anatomical landmarks or artificial markers are utilized. Subsequently they are marked with the mouse (or automatically) on the image data set in the operating room and traced on the patient with the navigation system. The workstation then computes the correlation between actual patient position and image data set. This procedure requires the absolute fixation of the patient or a permanently high precision measurement of the patient's movements since every relative movement of the patient's co-ordinate system within this process alters the results of the implemented correlation of patient position and image data set.

The choice of the registration procedure itself has a decisive influence on the navigation accuracy. Registration with anatomical landmarks is not precise enough, with divergences of 2–5 mm being described. Adhesive markers are described as being sufficiently exact. The markers should be attached to skin portions which do not tend to shift too much and are not expected to experience a change (such as swelling, distortion through draping, etc.) during the time period between CT scan and operation. Nevertheless, problems with lost or, even more critical, slightly displaced skin markers can occur due to the time lapse between tomography and operation (often more than 24 hours).

Miniscrews inserted preoperatively into the bone are substantially more precise.

Recently, surface-based concepts for the automatic registration of the patient position are increasingly mentioned. With these systems, the patient surface is traced by laser scanners or illuminated by a structured light and the resulting data set is then matched with the preoperatively obtained diagnostic image data of the patient.

Additional *reference frames* utilizing infrared diodes such as the operating instruments make it possible to move the operating table together with the fixated patient without the surgeon having to repeat the registration.[13] However, these reference frames are often blocked by or hidden behind the surgeon. Referencing systems fixated directly on the patient are supposed to permit patient movements and to recognize and adjust to unnoticed shifts automatically. The patient does not necessarily need to be immobilized. Such systems supply a firm mechanical fixation but should also be removable and not too invasive and flexible in their handling (Fig. 32.9). Non-invasive constructions with support in the auditory canals and a nasion support can cause an error of approximately 1 mm between the frame's position during the preoperative image production and its attachment in the operating room. Hauser et al[20] describe the intraoperative accuracy of this kind of system combining a facial bow with an optical navigation system of ≤2 mm.

We currently prefer the use of intraosseous fixated screws[13] since this method eliminates a number of problems associated with adhesive markers or surface scan registration. The quality of registration is independent of the application pressure of the probe, the positioning of the probe tip on the marker is unmistakable and the danger of a shift of the markers between scan and operation is eliminated. The temporary insertion of screws into the cranial bones of the

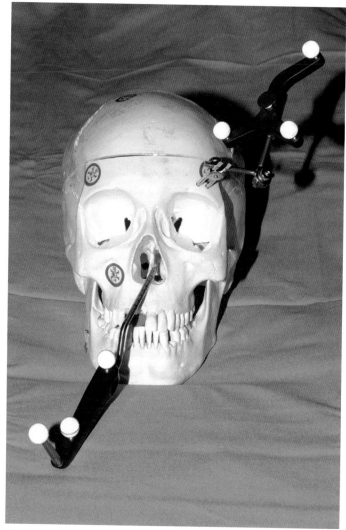

Fig. 32.9: Instrument set for passive optical navigation. Pointer and reference frame, rigidly fixed to supraorbital rim, for registering patient's movements.

patient can certainly be justified in the case of tumor resection, but this procedure seems to be somewhat excessive for elective surgery. In these cases the fixation of adequately formed markers to the remaining teeth of the patient through an acid-etching technique or by positioning a plastic dental splint would be a possible alternative. This method also provides absolute stability, is non-invasive and is associated with easy postoperative removal.

Only a few comparable studies regarding the precision of navigation and measurement of intraoperative navigation systems can be found in the literature. They describe experiences gained through clinical applications and test series on various phantoms and state navigation accuracy values in the range of 1–5 mm and 1–3 mm in bony structures.[19] This shows that an error, defined as the divergence of the imaged position from that of reality, is always possible in computer-aided surgery. An accumulation of errors ranging from the image reproduction to the actual surgery with navigation is unavoidable. Today the intraoperative accuracy of the navigation systems in bones and soft tissue in the vicinity of bone is usually less than 3 mm.

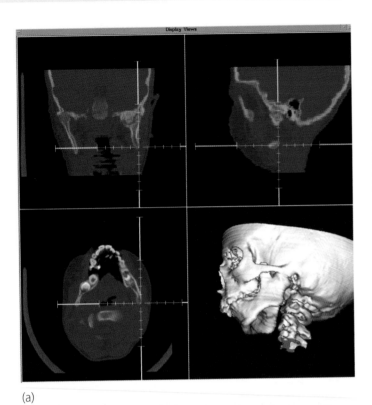

(a)

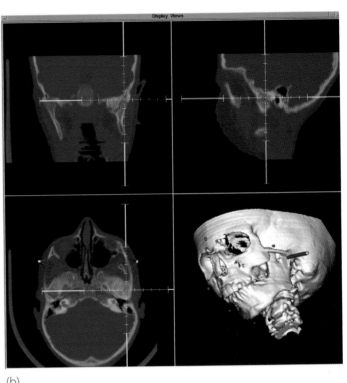

(b)

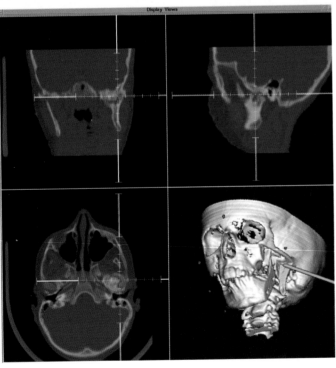

(c)

Fig. 32.10: (a) Screen view: visualization of the mandibular joint ankylosis on the left side. 3D view (right below) and orthogonal incisions. **(b)** Intraoperative use of the navigation system. Operative removal of the mandibular joint ankylosis. The crosshairs correspond to the actual position of the tip of the navigation probe. The actual position of the navigation probe is visualized as a green stick. (Note the representation of the skin markings correlating to the head position on the CT data record.) **(c)** During resection of the ankylosis. Cube-shaped cutting of the data record in the 3D view corresponding to the actual position of the tip of the navigation probe.

According to our own experience, CT-based navigation can achieve an accuracy of ≤3 mm in bones and in soft tissue areas in the vicinity of bones. Registering the patient position with preoperatively inserted screw markers, thus eliminating skin shifts, achieved accuracy values of ≤2 mm.[13,19] Using the MR scan as a navigation basis, application accuracy values of ≤4 mm were achieved in the soft tissue regions surrounding the skull base. In pure soft tissue surgery the flexibility of the tissue can render the preoperatively obtained data obsolete.

Two clinical cases will be presented to demonstrate the advantages of intraoperative instrument navigation technology.

Clinical application of navigation systems

Between the autumn of 1993 and mid 2001 more than 200 clinical applications of navigation technology took place at the Department of Maxillofacial and Craniofacial Surgery, University of Heidelberg, using mainly CT data (layer thickness ≤2 mm). Some of the surgical episodes were performed in interdisciplinary co-operation with the Heidelberg University Clinic Department of Neurosurgery, ENT Department and Department of Ophthalmology.

Orientation in complex surgical situations

A 10-year-old patient suffering from a left temporomandibular ankylosis, with severely restricted mouth opening following trauma in early childhood, underwent surgery. During the operation planning the system facilitated a precise 3D analysis of the changes in the temporomandibular joint (Fig. 32.10a). In the operative revision the navigation system contributed to the precise and safe orientation near the severely altered lateral cranial base (Fig. 32.10b,c).

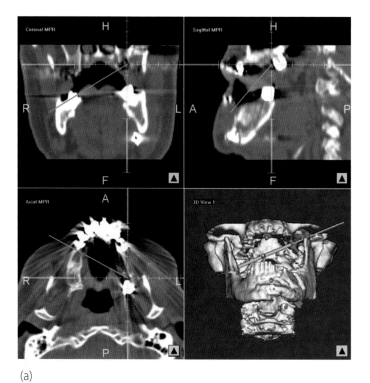

(a)

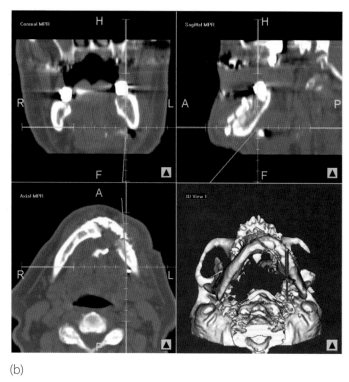

(b)

Fig. 32.11: Visualization of a gunshot wound with multiple bullet fragments scattered in maxillary and mandibular regions. Navigation is used for localizing and removing fragments. **(a)** Intraoperative use of the navigation system for localizing and removing bullet fragments in the left submandibular region. The crosshairs correspond to the actual position of the tip of the navigation probe. The actual position of the navigation probe is visualized as a green stick. 3D view (right below) and orthogonal images. **(b)** Intraoperative use of the navigation system for localizing and removing bullet fragments in left retromaxillary region.

Localization of foreign bodies

The second patient had been shot in the face. Multiple bullet fragments were scattered in the maxillary and mandibular regions. After using the system for detailed visualization and analysis of the positions of the fragments and the bony fractures, the navigation technique was used intraoperatively for precisely localizing and removing the bullet fragments in the left pterygopalatinal and submandibular regions (Fig. 32.11a,b).

Clinical evaluation of navigation technology

Based on literature review and our own experience, instrument navigation techniques have proved to be very advantageous for:

- localization of anatomical and pathological structures (e.g. foreign bodies, tumors) in the operative field
- planning surgical access
- precise intraoperative realization of the individual 3D plan in jaw asymmetries and craniofacial malformations
- protection of essential structures
- control of resection borders in tumor surgery
- planning and insertion of implants
- teaching purposes and postgraduate medical education.

Using these techniques the spatial orientation of surgeons operating in complex anatomical regions may be improved considerably. The possibility of checking resection borders opens up new perspectives in tumor surgery and osteotomies and tumor resections may be carried out faster and more-precisely but due to the time-consuming registration of the patient's position, the total operation time can as yet not be reduced.

In our extensive clinical evaluation of the instrumental navigation technique, however, we have found the following deficiencies.

- At the moment there are no navigation systems with an intraoperative accuracy of less than 2 mm, as desired by surgeons.
- There are no reliable details referring to the actual accuracy during the surgical intervention.
- The systems are time-consuming due to fault-prone registration procedures when correlating the system's co-ordinates and the patient's location. Software operation is not particularly well integrated ergonomically into the operation procedure and visualization on the monitor is not adapted to the surgeon's view of the operation site.
- The connection of motor-driven instruments (drills, milling cutters, saws, etc.) is not yet possible due to the lack of real-time visualization.
- With increasing operation time the preoperative image data no longer correspond to the actual operation status.

Intraoperative imaging

Fundamental problems of intraoperative instrument navigation techniques can arise from the possible deviation of the preoperatively obtained image data from the actual operation situation. This can be caused by changes due to swelling and distortions as a result of the removal of bone parts, etc. Inaccuracies during the phases of data acquisition, data preparation, registration of patient position and the navigation technique itself may also produce problems. Due to the stability of the structures, deviations during surgery involving osseous structures are considerably less than during operations involving soft tissues alone. A possible solution for these deviations is the use of intraoperatively applicable image data procedures such as ultrasound, CT and open MRI.[1]

Further concepts aim at using the ultrasound, CT and MRI techniques applicable in the operating theater in order to validate the preoperatively obtained patient data, to update them if necessary and then to visually pass them on to the operating surgeon in their updated form.

Finally we also have to think of an intraoperative 4D technique, i.e. moving pictures, for example in order to be able to include functional aspects in joint areas in the planning, simulation and operation.

Intraoperative support by medical robots

Rapid technological progress in hardware, falling prices and the rapid development of planning and controller software increasingly allow the use of robots in the operating theater. Medical robotic systems are being tested or are already in commercial use in stereotactic neurosurgical interventions, orthopedic surgery of the hip or knee and in active endoscopic systems for minimally invasive surgery. Robots in the operating theater are the last link in the chain of efforts to give the surgeon comprehensive technical support. They make it possible to carry out precise incisions in large bony structures after preoperative planning, e.g. for the optimal administering of implants and transplants.[21]

With the autonomous use of robots the surgeon permits the robot to perform certain parts of the operation completely by itself. After finishing the procedure the robot arm goes back to its base and will be removed from the operation table as the surgeon continues the operation. Thus the robot should be considered as a tool that relieves the surgeon of certain tasks requiring high precision but the development of such systems is a relatively large challenge as the precision and safe handling are extremely important in surgical interventions.

The development of semiactive systems, where the operation plan supplies the surgeon with a corridor for the direction of the surgical instrumentation, seems promising. This could be realized, for example, by a manipulative computer-controlled arm which guides the surgeon's instrument on the calculated osteotomy track, thus serving as a remote-controlled guide for the surgeon. The surgeon controls the instrument while it is connected to the manipulative arm and in doing so each devia-

tion from the planned operative procedure will be announced or even avoided by the system utilizing active power feedback systems in order to protect at-risk areas such as nerves and vessels. A robot of this kind could, for instance, support an inexperienced surgeon by preventing penetration into high-risk areas. We have already tested a prototype system of this kind with phantom and animal experiments and further clinical use is already planned (Fig. 32.12).

Present surgical interventions with robotic assistance distinguish themselves by the following characteristics.

- The robot-assisted intervention itself is relatively simple but no surgeon is capable of manually working with the same high precision as the robot.
- Complex interventions, such as cardiac surgery or laparoscopic operations, can only be performed under direct control by the surgeon, i.e. by telemanipulation.

In contrast to robots previously used in orthopedics and neurosurgery, a robotic system for craniomaxillofacial surgery makes higher demands on the system's conception. The bone structures involved are more complex and there are more vital structures such as nerves and vessels in the operative area.

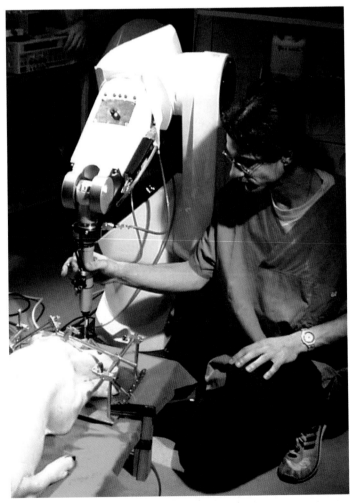

Fig. 32.12: Test of the interaction between surgeon and robot in the semiactive mode with a pig preparation.

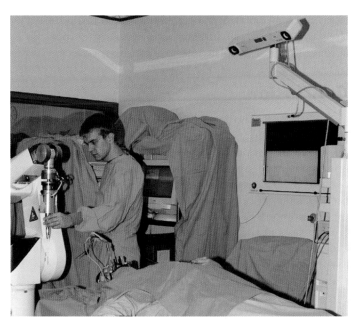

Fig. 32.13: Preclinical tests with a surgical robot painting incision lines on a volunteer's skin.

The central precondition for successful intervention with a robotic system is an adapted patient model containing all relevant information. This relies on data obtained from the imaging techniques which are used to define the patient's individual anatomical and pathological characteristics.

The Maxillofacial and Craniofacial Surgery Unit of the University of Heidelberg, in co-operation with the Institute of Real-Time Computer Systems and Robotics at the Faculty of Computer Science, University of Karlsruhe, is working on a robotic system to be used in maxillofacial and craniofacial surgery (Fig. 32.13). The robot is a modified industrial model with six degrees of freedom and a load of 6 kg. The robot, which is installed on the rollable foot of an operating table, is run in an upright configuration. During the operation the foot is lowered onto the floor in order to keep the surgical robot's base in a firm position. The following system components are included:

- Robot Unimation RX90 with control software.
- End effector, consisting of bone milling machine and bone drill, force/torque sensor (facilitates power-controlled manual guidance of the robot) and overload protection.
- Infrared navigation system for positional determination, registration and control of the patient, the robot and other tools.
- Co-ordination processor for the sensory data.
- Planning and simulation data processor.

In an extensive accuracy analysis with phantoms and animal cadavers, the precision of this prototype robotic system was tested. Clinical use of this system is planned soon.

At present we are also testing the realization of preoperative 3D planning for dental implantology through a smaller assisting robot. In this case the robot positions an instrument for guidance of the surgical handpiece (Fig. 32.14). The initial drilling is carried out manually by the physician during which the position, drilling direction and depth are specified by the robot-assisted guide. As a result, the surgeon can transfer the implant's position, which has been optimally defined previously on the computer, exactly onto the patient.

Future robotic techniques in oral and maxillofacial surgery could include:

- drilling of holes with an automatic stop after penetrating the bone in order to protect the tissue lying deep to the bone
- milling of bone surfaces in plastic surgery according to a 3D operation plan
- performing deep saw cuts for osteotomies and allowing for the precise 3D transposition of the subsequent bone segments
- defined drilling of the implant bed for positioning of dental or surgical implants
- preoperative automatic selection of the necessary osteosynthesis plates, their bending by a special machine and their intraoperative positioning in defined positions.

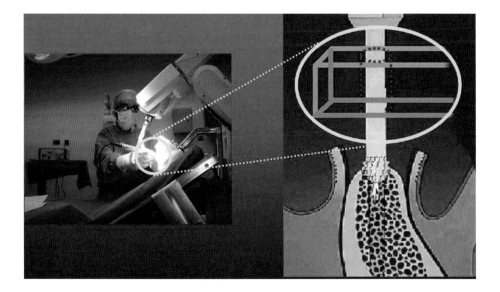

Fig. 32.14: Interaction between surgeon and robot during tests on a phantom. The robot is serving as a 3D interactive drill guide for the precise insertion of dental implants (Courtesy Dr R Boesecke, Medical Robotics, Schwabmünchen, Germany).

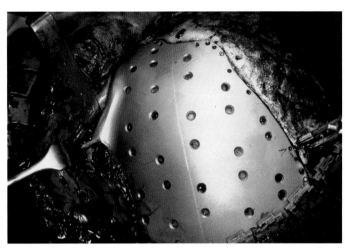

Fig. 32.15: Secondary skull reconstruction after extended trauma with CAD-CAM technology-based direct fabrication of a titanium implant (implant planning and fabrication by Prof Dr H Eufinger, Maxillofacial Surgery Unit, University of Bochum, Germany, www.cranioconstruct.de/2001/index.htm).

Integration of computer-assisted design

Applications of the computer-aided design and manufacturing (CAD-CAM) technique are also used in surgery, with the main focus being the computer-assisted construction and manufacture of individual spatially dimension-fitting implants. Titanium implants for the precise replacement of osseous defects of the skull,[22] for example, may now be produced directly and not indirectly, using physical models or templates, as has previously been necessary. Figure 32.15 demonstrates a skull reconstruction with CAD-CAM technology-based direct fabrication of a titanium implant.

Evaluation of Surgical Outcome

Rapid progress in the field of Internet technology means that the routine use of teleradiology and telemedicine will become a reality in oral and maxillofacial surgery. Clinical and image data of all stages of treatment will be available to all referring physicians associated with the patient's management. Smart cards will enable patients to carry their relevant medical data with them. Multicenter and multidisciplinary databases will enable new research options. This, however, raises the question of data safety and security which will have to be discussed thoroughly by the medical community.

Postoperative computer-assisted assessment of 3D morphology can be achieved by surface scanning technologies. In doing so, the operation's success may be checked and the data obtained may be used for the planning and operation simulation for future procedures, thus improving the likely operative outcome. Further work should be aimed at developing tools for the semi-automatic generation of operation plans in a virtual surgical environment. In craniofacial surgery, for example, a proposal with individually optimized bone cuts and 3D repositioning of bone segments could be presented by the computer to the surgeon who would then be able to accept or change the plan before performing surgery.

Conclusion

Computer and robotic techniques may optimize operation planning and help to improve the precision and quality of the operative performance. Through improved control of the operational risks pre-existing limits may be disregarded and completely new operations may be performed. The following prerequisites are required from any future integrated system for computer-assisted oral and maxillofacial surgery.

All phases of the treatment – preoperative diagnostic procedures, operational planning, performance of the operation and evaluation of the results – must be integrated. The system should be capable of supporting the surgeon with conventional operations without technical aids as well as with technically supported operations involving passive navigation, and ultimately with active robotic assistance.

Today the instrument navigation technique, with its interactive use of patient image data, already supports surgeons precisely and reliably. It is a substantial improvement in the area of orientation and safety in complex anatomical regions, for the localization of pathological changes or foreign objects and for the surgical correction of distinct malformations. Osteotomies and resections in the area of tumor surgery, especially at the skull base, and for reconstructive surgery may now be performed faster and more precisely. We do have to emphasize that, from a surgical perspective, a system accuracy of less than 2 mm is highly desirable. However, in spite of the described deficiencies, these 'prototype' navigation systems can already be successfully used for the benefit of the patient and the support of the surgeon as described above. In the near future, as a result of the techniques of computer-assisted surgery and their associated quality improvements and reduced operative risks, there may well be a considerable decline in patient-related stress. Nonetheless, the total operation time may not yet be reduced due to set-up time and sometimes complex registration procedure requirements The economic consequences of such high-technology surgical applications should always be discussed but there are already reports of decreased hospitalization time as a result of using navigation systems in neurosurgery.

Many authors consider instrument navigation systems to be the future standard procedure in the case of complex operations.[1,14,17,18] In some fields, especially in osseous surgical interventions with high demands on precision, operative robots have already proved their worth in routine clinical practice.[21] General limitations on the intraoperative use of navigation and robotic systems emerge from the fact that the preoperative image data become increasingly inexact due to changes in the patient's data caused by the operative procedure itself. It is here that we must work on the integration of intraoperative image data (ultrasound, MRI, CT, conventional X-ray) into the planning, simulation and navigation system.[1] Considerable limitations in the field of image generation, computer hardware and software have as yet prevented the routine use of such intraoperative 'Imaging updates'.

As the initial feasibility has now been proven, it is our aim to produce an economic operation system with handling as simple and intuitive as possible. This will encourage a broad clinical use of computer-assisted oral and maxillofacial surgery.

Acknowledgements

Figures 32.1, 32.6, 32.12 and 32.13 are based on a collaboration with the Institute for Process Control and Robotics, Prof Dr H Woern, Faculty of Computer Science, University of Karlsruhe, Germany. Figure 32.7 is based on a collaboration with the Institute for Process Control and Robotics, Prof Dr R Dillmann, Faculty of Computer Science, University of Karlsruhe, Germany. Both projects are being funded by the Sonderforschungsbereich 414 'Information Technology in Medicine – Computer and Sensor Supported Surgery' of the Deutsche Forschungsgemeinschaft.

References

1 Wirtz CR, Knauth M, Staubert A et al 2000 Clinical evaluation and follow-up results for intraoperative magnetic resonance imaging in neurosurgery. Neurosurgery 46: 1112–1120

2 Verstreken K, van Cleynenbreugel J, Martens K et al 1998 An image-guided planning system for endosseous oral implants. IEEE Transactions on Medical Imaging 17: 842–852

3 Hassfeld S, Stein W 2000 Dreidimensionale Planung für die dentale Implantologie anhand computertomographischer Daten. [3D-planning in dental implantology based on CT data.] Dtsch Zahnärztl Z 55: 313–325

4 Kikinis R, Gleason PL, Moriarty TM et al 1996 Computer-assisted interactive three-dimensional planning for neurosurgical procedures. Neurosurgery 38: 640–649

5 Neumann P, Siebert D, Faulkner G et al 1999 Virtual 3D cutting for bone segment extraction in maxillofacial surgery planning. Studies of Health Technology Information 62: 235–241

6 Robb RA, Aharon S, Cameron BM et al 1997 Patient-specific anatomic models from three dimensional medical image data for clinical applications in surgery and endoscopy. Journal of Digital Imaging 10(suppl 1): 31–35

7 Vannier MW, Marsh JL 1996 Three-dimensional imaging, surgical planning, and image-guided therapy. Radiologic Clinics of North America 34: 545–563

8 Keeve E, Girod S, Kikinis R et al 1998 Deformable modeling of facial tissue for craniofacial surgery simulation. Computer Aided Surgery 3: 228–238

9 Munchenberg J, Woern H, Brief J et al 2000 Intuitive operation planning based on force feedback. Studies of Health Technology Information 70: 220–226

10 Xia J, Ip HH, Samman N et al 2000 Computer-assisted three-dimensional surgical planning and simulation: 3D virtual osteotomy. International Journal of Oral Maxillofacial Surgery 29: 11–17

11 Zamorano L, Jiang Z, Kadi AM 1994 Computer-assisted neurosurgery system: Wayne State University hardware and software configuration. Computerized Medical Imaging and Graphics 18: 257–271

12 Birkfellner W, Watzinger F, Wanschitz F et al 1998 Systematic distortions in magnetic position digitizers. Medical Physics 25: 2242–2248

13 Hassfeld S, Zoeller J, Albert FK et al 1998 Preoperative planning and intraoperative navigation in skull base surgery. Journal of Craniomaxillofacial Surgery 26: 220–225

14 Hauser R, Westermann B 1999 Optical tracking of a microscope for image-guided intranasal sinus surgery. Annals of Otology, Rhinology and Laryngology 108: 54–62

15 Marmulla R, Hilbert M, Niederdellmann H 1997 Inherent precision of mechanical, infrared and laser-guided navigation systems for computer-assisted surgery. Journal of Craniomaxillofacial Surgery 25: 192–197

16 Gunkel AR, Freysinger W, Thumfart WF 2000 Experience with various 3-dimensional navigation systems in head and neck surgery. Archives of Otolaryngology Head and Neck Surgery 126: 390–395

17 Watzinger F, Birkfellner W, Wanschitz F et al 1999 Positioning of dental implants using computer-aided navigation and an optical tracking system: case report and presentation of a new method. Journal of Craniomaxillofacial Surgery 27: 77–81

18 Reinhardt HF, Trippel M, Westermann B et al 1996 Computer assisted brain surgery for small lesions in the central sensorimotor region. Acta Neurochirurgica Wien 138: 200–205

19 Hassfeld S, Mühling J 2000 Comparative examination of the accuracy of a mechanical and an optical system in CT and MRT based instrument navigation. International Journal of Oral and Maxillofacial Surgery 29: 400–407

20 Hauser R, Westermann B, Probst R 1997 Noninvasive tracking of patient's head movements during computer-assisted intranasal microscopic surgery [published erratum in Laryngoscope 107: 1000–1001]. Laryngoscope 107: 491–499

21 Taylor RH, Joskowicz L, Williamson B et al 1999 Computer-integrated revision total hip replacement surgery: concept and preliminary results. Medical Image Analysis 3: 301–319

22 Eufinger H, Wehmoeller M 1998 Individual prefabricated titanium implants in reconstructive craniofacial surgery: clinical and technical aspects of the first 22 cases. Plastic and Reconstructive Surgery 102: 300–308

33 Clinical Application of Computer-Assisted Reconstruction in Complex Posttraumatic Deformities

Nils-Claudius Gellrich, Alexander Schramm, Rainer Schmelzeisen

Correcting complex posttraumatic deformities remains a challenge firstly in the diagnostic evaluation of the deformity, secondly in setting up the therapeutic schedule and thirdly in the surgical correction itself. Until now, computer-assisted preoperative planning (CAPP) and surgery (CAS) has not been practiced as part of the surgical routine in the field of posttraumatic deformities.[1-5] The aim of this chapter is to demonstrate the value of modern computer-assisted analysis, simulation and especially intraoperative navigation by using optical navigation systems in the field of posttraumatic reconstructive craniomaxillofacial surgery. In our experience the promotion of a conventional navigation system in a 'multifunctional-planning-navigation-control-unit' direction sets new standards in craniofacial plastic and reconstructive surgery.

Introduction

Primary diagnostics are indispensable in assessing the mostly combined bony and soft tissue deformities in major craniofacial posttraumatic disorders. Advances in imaging techniques (spiral CT with multiplanar reconstruction and 3D imaging) and associated technologies (i.e. stereolithographic models) have led within recent years to improved preoperative planning for the craniomaxillofacial surgeon.[6-11] Stereolithographic models provide an idea of the 3D situation only of hard tissue defects and permit, to some degree, the pre- or intraoperative manufacturing of individual prostheses, but they do not fulfill further requirements of reconstructive surgery. Stereolithographic models reflect just one segment within the gray scale of the acquired spiral CT data set. Their use carries the risk of mistakenly reproducing pseudoforamina instead of minuscule, thin bony structures, which are widely present especially around the midfacial skeleton (Fig. 33.1).

On the other hand, a spiral CT data set provides information on a variety of both soft and hard tissue questions, which is only limited in the transmission of information from the radiologist to the surgeon.[10] To obtain sufficient information about the preoperative situation, surgeons must familiarize themselves with the patient's individual anatomy. However, modern navigation systems make it possible to increase the amount of CT/MRI information and to handle it easily. The surgeon can adjust the gray scale and reconstructions to current demands.[12-15] In cases of posttraumatic enophthalmos this is particularly important to assess precisely the displacement of orbital contents before surgery (Fig. 33.2). The features of CAS/CAPP are listed in Box 33.1.

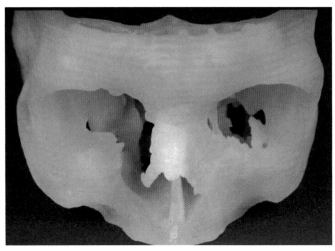

Fig. 33.1: Stereolithographic model with a right midfacial defect. Pseudoforamina are widely present in the normal left orbit.

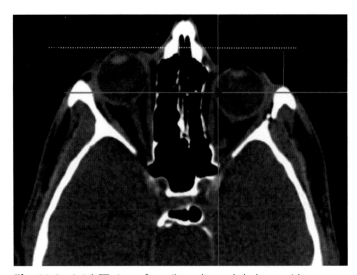

Fig. 33.2: Axial CT view of a unilateral enophthalmos with a retruded left malar bone. The interrupted horizontal white line shows the intended projection for the left globe, the perpendicular yellow line demonstrates the CT-based Hertel's index.

Proper assessment of asymmetry is the first and most important step before setting up the reconstructive plan. The correct measurement of distances between anatomic structures helps to determine the severity of deformation, e.g. if bony prominences are displaced or deviations from the original midline or occlusal plane are concerned. Sometimes even well-established clinical measurements like the Hertel's

Box 33.1   Advantages of CAPP and CAS in posttraumatic reconstruction

- Measurement of distances

- Volume measuring of, for example, orbital contents

- Mirroring parts of the data set to an individually created plane with virtual reconstruction of form in definable ranges

- Virtual insertion and positioning of autologous bone grafts, realizing preoperative simulation of augmenting deficient bony contours

- Outlining of endangered structures like the optic nerve

- Intraoperative navigation which allows checking of the individual anatomy online and comparing preoperatively planned contour changes

- Assessment of changes between the preceding and the actual CT/MR in cases where postoperative spiral CT/MR is performed for control

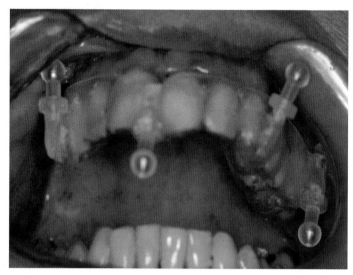

Fig. 33.3: Non-invasive system: upper occlusal splint with four markers.

index come to their limit and must be regarded with great skepticism because they do not take into account the amount of bony dislocation at the lateral orbital rim. However, this is often present in severe midface fractures. In this case objective computer-based measurement technique is advantageous: the CT-based corrected Hertel's index – the perpendicular between projection of the corneal surface and the lateral orbital rim – allows for the quantification of globe projection, including the additive effect of bony displacement (Fig. 33.2).[16] Further transverse, craniocaudal and posterior–anterior measurements within the orbit suggest where the problem is situated and how much bone grafting or reconfiguration of periorbital bone is necessary.[17] Using this planning procedure, the surgeon becomes familiar with the individual deformity in a three-dimensional manner.

Among a total of 125 patients (posttraumatic midface and skull base deformities, severe ankyloses of the TMJ, optic nerve decompression, complex craniosynostoses cases, midface and skull base tumor resections with primary and secondary reconstructions and complex dental implant insertion) being treated with CAPP and CAS, six fields of computer-based craniofacial reconstruction were highlighted.

1. Secondary correction of a panfacial fracture
2. Posttraumatic enophthalmos with and without reosteotomy and advancement of the malar bone
3. Optic nerve decompression in therapy of traumatic optic neuropathy
4. Navigated endoscopic frontal sinus revision following severe skull base comminution
5. Combined periorbital autologous bone grafting with CAD/CAM titanium implants
6. Recontouring of severe bone and soft tissue deformities by augmenting the contours with calcium phosphate cement

Spiral CT datasets (Somatom Plus 4 scanner, 1 mm collimation/slice thickness, 2 mm table feed, 1 mm increment) were acquired to serve for CAPP and CAS on the STN navigation system (Stryker-Leibinger) with STP 4.0 software.

Due to the insufficient accuracy of commercially available non-invasive registration systems, the combination of CAPP with virtual correction, intraoperative navigation and postoperative control has not yet become a routine procedure in the treatment of orbital deformities. We overcame this problem by using an individual non-invasive registration system developed by the authors (Fig. 33.3).[18,19] These thermoplastic splints are fabricated individually by a dental technician, permitting reuse in the same patient. Occlusal splints were routinely used in the upper jaw with four

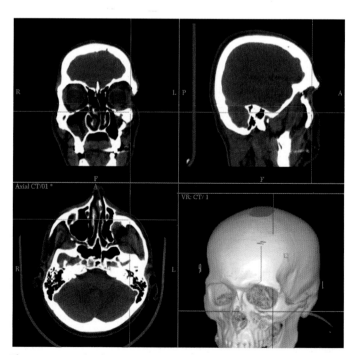

Fig. 33.4: Multiplanar and 3D view of a patient following severe left midface trauma.

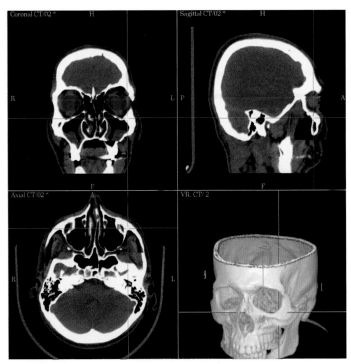

Fig. 33.5: Simulation of an ideal virtual correction of the patient in Fig. 33.4 by mirroring a subvolume from the unaffected right onto the left side.

markers in different XYZ axes. All four markers are kept out of artefact zones such as prosthodontic restorations (Fig. 33.3). The markers can be alternated according to the demands of the selected imaging modality (MRI, CT) and of intraoperative use. The major advantage of this registration system is its easy reproduction but it is limited in emergency cases where quick assessment of a spiral CT dataset is mandatory, such as in cases of traumatic optic neuropathy, or in edentulous patients. In such cases either temporary inserted bone markers or surface matching are used.

At the workstation itself, the full dataset can be adapted to the surgeon's requirements regarding gray scale, i.e. whether the hard or soft tissues are to be weighed. On the workstation the patient's individual anatomy is assessed in multiplanar (axial, coronal, sagittal) and 3D views (Fig. 33.4). Virtual correction can be made either by drawing new contours or designing virtual implants at the workstation (Fig. 33.2). In unilateral deformities that do not cross the midline, the mirror tool developed by the authors in co-operation with the Stryker-Leibinger company permits an ideal reconstruction by superimposing the unaffected over the affected and/or deformed side, thus creating a new dataset (Fig. 33.5).[20] The majority of traumatic or tumor-related orbital deformities are unilateral, so that many cases can be approached by a side-to-side comparison. In reconstructive surgery cases the surgeon must define the individual plane to which the selected range of dataset should be mirrored from the unaffected to the deformed side. The software guides the surgeon exactly through this procedure. Intraoperatively, either the native CT dataset can be referred to or, alternatively, the modified CT dataset, so that navigation of intraoperatively achieved reconstruction in comparison to preoperative virtual correction is possible at any step of the operation. The time required for intraoperative navigation, once mastered, is an extra 30 minutes, whereas the preoperative planning takes about 1 hour.

The precision of intraoperative navigation between the virtual patient on the workstation and the actual patient on the operating table is around 1 mm. This can be achieved by using the above-mentioned individually made occlusal thermoplastic splint with four reference markers in different XYZ positions. Experimental and clinical evaluation of this system proved this overall accuracy of 1 mm.[18]

Intraoperative navigation was done using frameless stereotaxy (Fig. 33.6). Three infrared cameras controlled the pointer (P) via integrated LEDs and the patient's position

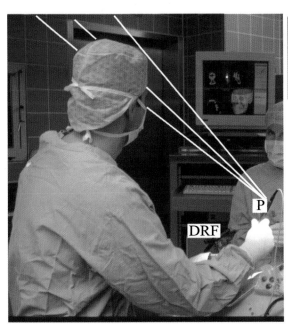

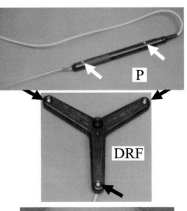

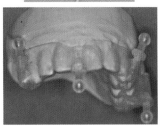

Fig. 33.6: Set-up for intraoperative navigation. The dynamic reference frame (DRF) is firmly attached to the Mayfield clamp by which the patient's position is controlled. Instrument and/or pointer position is monitored via integrated LEDs (P). The maxillary occlusal splint with four markers in different XYZ axes allows for non-invasive referencing.

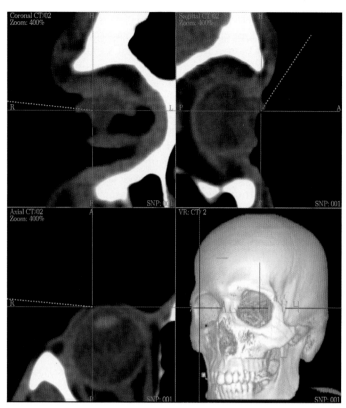

Fig. 33.7: Screenshot during navigated surgery with the virtually reconstructed CT dataset in multiplanar, i.e. coronal, sagittal and axial, 3D views. The pointer (dotted lines) monitors the virtually reconstructed CT dataset as to whether the advanced left globe matches the computer-assisted preplanned contour.

was controlled via a dynamic reference frame (DRF) fixed rigidly to the Mayfield's clamp.

Intraoperative pointer-based navigation with the STN workstation was used not only to navigate the present bony contours but also to check on new contours, e.g. surfaces augmented with autologous bone grafts, bone substitutes or advanced facial bones (Fig. 33.7). The augmentation procedure was finished when the intraoperative situation matched the preoperatively planned virtual contours on the workstation.

Clinical Application of CAPP and CAS

Correction of a panfacial fracture

Following a major traffic accident with a panfacial fracture that was treated in another institution, the patient in Figure 33.8a underwent, as a first step, bilateral orbital reconstruction with autologous calvarial split-bone grafting and telecanthus correction according to the Hammer method.[1] The second step in secondary reconstruction was to perform correction of the displaced mandibulo-maxillary complex by bimaxillary reosteotomy. CAPP was used to define the repositioning in respect to the overall asymmetry. Firstly vectors for the ideal correction of the maxilla were defined (Fig. 33.9) and followed during later surgery with navigational control. The bony result of the bimaxillary correction is demonstrated in Figure 33.10b. Figure 33.11 demonstrates a

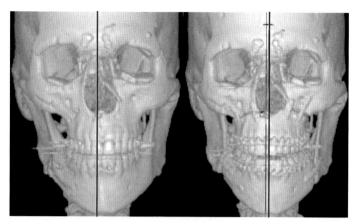

Fig. 33.8: 3D view of a patient after secondary enophthalmos and telecanthus correction following a traffic accident before **(a)** and after **(b)** repositioning of the bimaxillary complex.

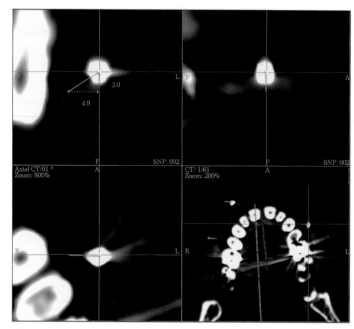

Fig. 33.9: Planning of the vectors for ideal maxillary shifting. The light-blue lines in the multiplanar view resemble the amount of movement of defined points (center of referencing points).

clinical frontal view before orbital correction and after bimaxillary surgery.

Posttraumatic enophthalmos with and without reosteotomy and advancement of the malar bone

Symmetry in orbital reconstruction is important for functional and esthetic reasons.[21] Orbital asymmetry mostly results from a combined soft and hard tissue deformity including the orbital contents, the bony orbit and the periorbital soft tissues, including the canthal ligaments.

Enophthalmos due to the enlargement of orbital volume is a severe complication in posttraumatic orbital deformities, if primary reconstruction could not be correctly achieved.[22]

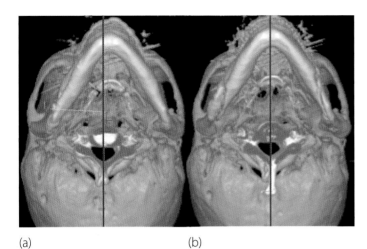

(a)   (b)

Fig. 33.10: Pre- **(a)** and postoperative **(b)** view from below showing the corrected left shift of the maxillo-mandibular complex.

Particularly in posttraumatic orbital deformities, measurement of sagittal globe projection can be done in the same position at the workstation as if the patient is on the operating table.[23] The sagittal projection of the globe can be virtually marked and corrected (see Fig. 33.2). The globe projection changes can be measured in reference to the corneal surface and optic canal entrance, because the latter is the most reliable landmark in posttraumatic patients as far as quantifying sagittal changes in orbital contents is concerned (Fig. 33.12). In addition to measuring functions, the software permits the 3D evaluation of orbital contents with individual figures (Fig. 33.12). With this method the orbits can be directly compared to each other and the postoperative outcome can be objectively quantified.

The average decrease following single orbital reconstruction in a group of 18 secondary posttraumatic enophthalmos corrections was 4.0 ± 1.9 cm^3 or 65% of an average adult eye-globe volume; the average overcorrection of sagittal globe projection was 2.7 mm.[16] However, the clinical outcome, which was achieved in all patients by only one operation, seems to justify this temporary excess in sagittal globe projection, because there is always a certain relapse in globe projection following enophthalmos corrections. Figure 33.13a shows a patient with right enophthalmos due to a midface trauma 2 years earlier. The right malar bone and orbital frame were retruded. Additionally, the patient showed right temporal hollowing, eyebrow displacement, telecanthus and a displaced lateral canthal ligament. The right malar bone with the superior-lateral periorbital frame was advanced via a coronal approach. Hollowing due to temporalis muscle atrophy was reconstructed by augmenting the right temporal region with a calvarial split-bone graft. The orbit was recontoured using calvarial split-bone grafts. The right medial and lateral canthal ligament were repositioned. Figure 33.13b shows the postoperative result after reconstruction of the enlarged orbit with autologous split-bone grafts. During the operation the bone graft position can be checked by navigation at any moment as can the distance to highly vulnerable structures like the optic nerve (Fig. 33.14).[23] For intraoperative navigation the mirrored dataset was used as a virtual model for the intended ideal reconstruction. The individually mirrored plane and the extension of vertical, sagittal and transverse ranges to be

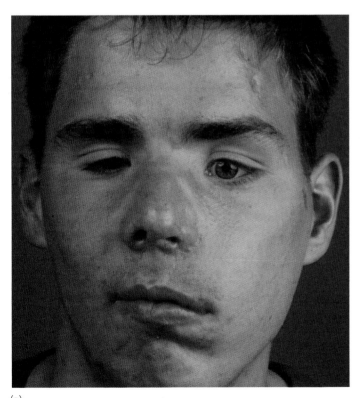

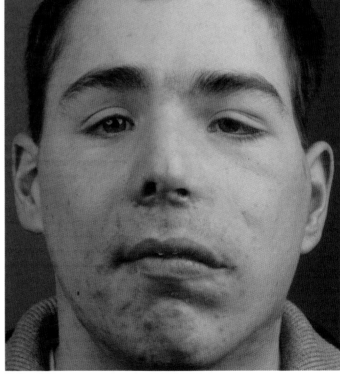

(a)   (b)

Fig. 33.11: Clinical view of the patient in Figs 33.8–33.10 **(a)** before orbital correction and **(b)** after bimaxillary surgery.

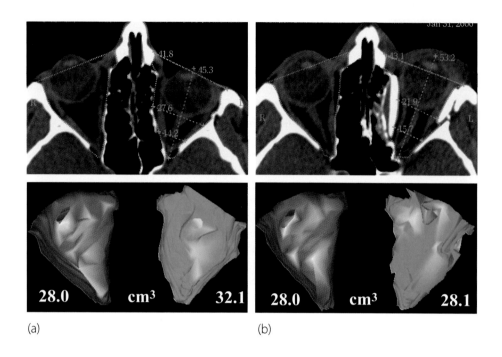

(a) (b)

Fig. 33.12: Axial CT images from a patient with left enophthalmos **(a)** before and **(b)** after correction with corresponding bilateral orbital volumes. The figures show a 4.0 cm³ reduction in orbital enlargement on the left side.

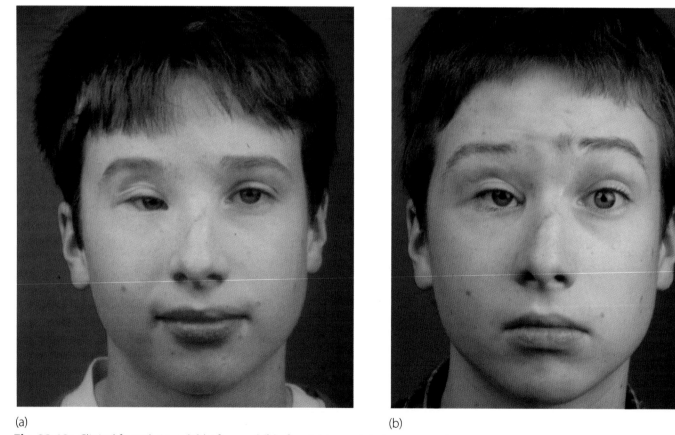

(a) (b)

Fig. 33.13: Clinical frontal views **(a)** before and **(b)** after right enophthalmos correction.

mirrored have to be selected at the workstation. This method of superimposing a contour by mirroring results in a virtual template that can serve directly for intraoperative navigation and postoperative control is an easy way to achieve symmetry. The postoperative evaluation of the orbital volumes showed a clear improvement on the corrected side: the decrease in orbital volume in this patient equals 80% of an average adult globe volume (Fig. 33.15).

All patients with secondary enophthalmos corrections were operated on using a coronal combined with a transconjunctival approach. In patients with additional malar bone advancement an intraoral incision is added.

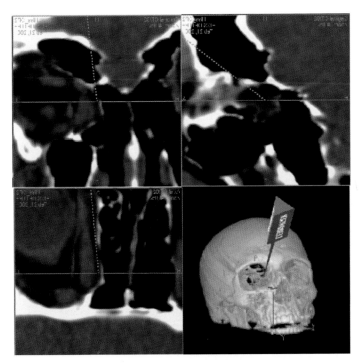

Fig. 33.14: Intraoperative screenshot during navigated orbital reconstruction from the patient in Fig. 33.13. With the pointer-based navigated surgery (dotted line) the virtually reconstructed CT dataset can be used for control as to whether, for example, the intraoperatively augmented medial orbital wall matches the computer-assisted preplanned contour.

In Figure 33.16 a screenshot during navigational control for reconstruction of the left medial orbital wall is shown, in which the mirrored dataset from the patient in Figures 33.4, 33.5 and 33.7 was used intraoperatively. The surgical plan included advancement of the retruded left malar bone and augmentation of the left orbit. Figures 33.17 and 33.18 show different 3D views for preoperative planning and simulation and postoperative control.

In primary unilateral orbital reconstructions with severe destruction of the bony frame and orbital cone, navigated surgery can be performed on the basis of an online side-to-side comparison. Figure 33.19 shows a screenshot during reconstruction of the left orbital floor in a comminuted midface fracture. The tip of the dotted line equals the tip of the pointer checking on the primarily reconstructed orbital floor by using autologous calvarial split-bone grafts. During the operation the bone graft position can be checked by navigation at any moment as can the distance to highly vulnerable structures like the optic nerve (Fig. 33.20). Figure 33.21 demonstrates multiple 3D plus multiplanar views to control the pre- (Fig. 33.21a) and postoperative (Fig. 33.21b) CT scans. In addition to the craniomaxillofacial reconstruction, neurosurgical colleagues performed a left anterior skull base revision via a frontal osteoplastic approach.

Optic nerve decompression in therapy of traumatic optic neuropathy

Among different therapeutic options in the treatment of traumatic optic neuropathy, surgical optic nerve decompression is an important option especially if there is evidence of fractures in the posterior third of the orbit and/or optic canal. In addition to clinical ophthalmological findings, the decision to decompress or not can be based on electro-physiological evidence, i.e. flash visual evoked potentials.[23] The operation is performed with a surgical microscope. Preoperative planning of the surgical approach can be transferred to the visual field of the microscope to guide the surgeon to the optic canal (Figure 33.22). The focus of the microscope is correlated to the CT dataset, so the surgeon is able to identify the anatomic structures visualized through the microscope by watching the CT scan at any time (Fig. 33.23). Using frameless stereotaxy the decompression of the optic nerve in trauma or tumor cases becomes a safe as well as a minimally invasive procedure. The multiplanar

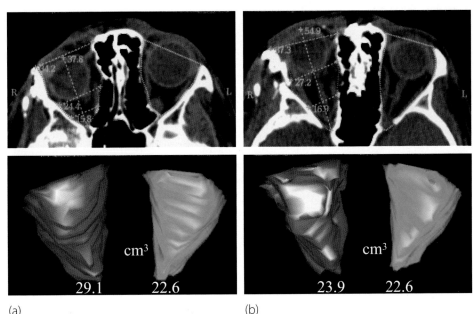

(a)   (b)

Fig. 33.15: Axial CT images from the patient in Fig. 33.13 showing the orbital region, with corresponding bilateral orbital volumes **(a)** pre- and **(b)** postoperative. Right orbital volume was decreased by 5.2 cm³.

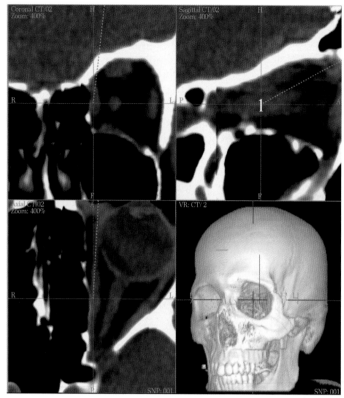

Fig. 33.16: Multiplanar and 3D view screenshot during navigated control of medial orbital wall augmentation. The tip of the pointer (dotted line) shows the correct reconstructed contour of the medial orbital wall compared to the mirrored dataset, resembling the ideal reconstruction. New position on top of the augmented calvarial grafts (1).

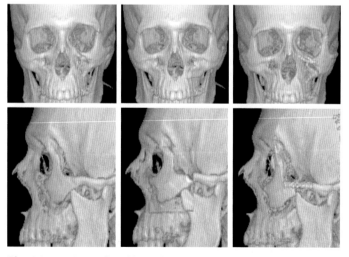

Fig. 33.17: Frontal and lateral 3D CT views from the patient in Figs 33.4, 33.5, 33.7 and 33.16 preoperatively, following simulation and postoperatively.

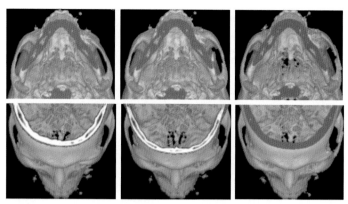

Fig. 33.18: Bird's and worm's eye 3D CT views from the patient in Figs 33.4, 33.5, 33.7, 33.16, and 33.17 preoperatively, following simulation and postoperatively.

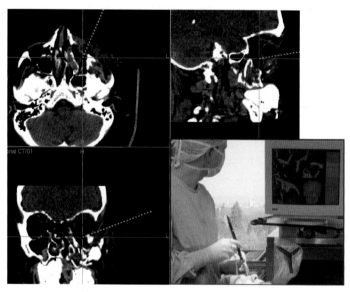

Fig. 33.19: Screenshot from a patient with a comminuted left orbital fracture undergoing navigation-controlled primary orbital reconstruction. The pointer (dotted line) marks the intended position of the orbital floor to be reconstructed (i.e. side-by-side either split grafts or titanium mesh can be contoured).

CT shows a fracture in the bony optic canal as the radiological correlate for a bony lesion as being the pathophysiological mechanism for the optic nerve injury. The identical CT dataset which was scanned for the primary craniofacial diag-

nostic work-up could be used for intraoperative navigation. The only prerequisite is that during the CT scanning process a registration system has to be applied to the patient. In this emergency situation a prefabricated upper occlusal splint, mounted with the above-mentioned four markers, was used, filled with a silicone-based impression material. Intraoperatively the CT dataset and the patient on the operating table could be easily matched by using the scanned four reference points.

Figure 33.23 shows an intraoperative screen shot in a multiplanar view during transnasal/transethmoidal optic nerve decompression. Figures 33.24a and 33.24b compare the matched pre- and postoperative views in the coronal and axial planes.

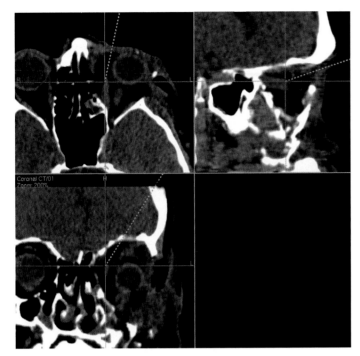

Fig. 33.20: Screenshot from the patient in Fig. 33.19 during reconstruction of the left medial orbital wall. The dotted line represents the pointer – the tip of the pointer checks for the contour of the inserted calvarial split bone grafts.

Navigated endoscopic frontal sinus revision following severe skull base comminution

Following a car accident a male adult patient lost his frontal bones due to major infection in the comminuted frontal sinus and ethmoidal area (Fig. 33.25a). Prior to reconstruction of the neurocranium the severely deformed frontoethmoidal region was operated on with tracked endoscopic minimally invasive surgery (Figs 33.26, 33.27). The axis and the tip of the endoscope are indicated by a dotted line (Fig. 33.27b). Figures 33.26 and 33.27a show the clinical view and Figure 33.27b demonstrates a screen shot during tracked endoscopic surgery. Secondarily, a CAD/CAM-titanium (CranioConstructBochum, Germany) implant was inserted to reconstruct the major frontal defect. Figure 33.28 shows the intraoperative lateral view, Figure 33.25b demonstrates the clinical view 10 days after reconstruction.

Combined malar bone advancement with custom-made titanium implant

Following a close gunshot injury the patient corresponding to the CT scan in Figure 33.29 suffered from gross mid- and upper face deformity and was admitted for secondary reconstruction to our department. Figure 33.29 shows the eye

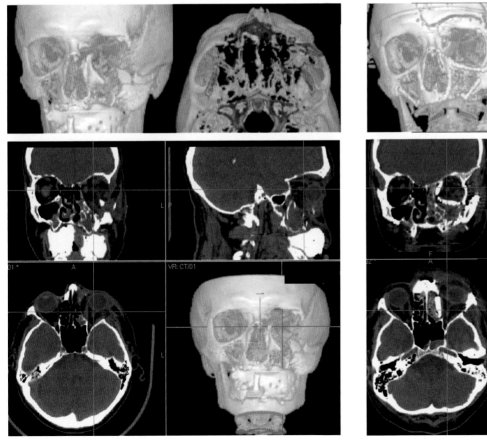

(a)

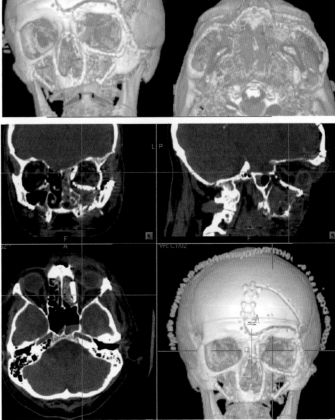

(b)

Fig. 33.21: Control of pre- **(a)** and postoperative **(b)** 3D and multiplanar views from the patient in Figs 33.19 and 33.20.

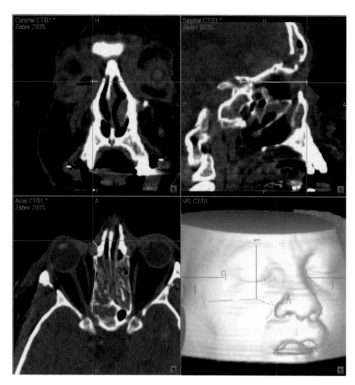

Fig. 33.22: Computer-assisted preoperative planning of the approach for optic nerve decompression in multiplanar and 3D views of a patient with a right traumatic optic nerve lesion.

prosthesis in place in the left deformed orbit. Prior to surgery a custom-made titanium implant was CNC-milled on the basis of a virtually ideally reconstructed subvolume of the CT dataset (CranioConstructBochum, Germany). The first step was to position the individual titanium implant in the left bifrontotemporal region and the second step was the reosteotomy of the left malar bone and the navigationally controlled advancement and fixation of the bone segment. For better control the mirror tool was preoperatively applied again to achieve an ideal reconstructed virtual model.[16] The latter (Fig. 33.30) served intraoperatively for navigated control of the advancement of the left malar bone segment prior to rigid fixation. In a third step an additional autologous calvarial split-bone graft was used to augment the left temporal hollowing, which was due to severe muscle loss. The mirrored dataset was used again to check on the preplanned contours in the temporal region. Figures 33.31 and 33.32 show postoperative multiplanar and 3D views, whereas Figure 33.32 demonstrates the correct reconstruction of the deficient left temporal region.

Recontouring of severe bone and soft tissue deformities by augmenting contours with calcium phosphate cement

The preoperative CT scan in a multiplanar view shows a left periorbital and temporal bony and soft tissue defect following an osteoplastic trepanation without osseous reintegration of the temporal bone (Fig. 33.33). The first step

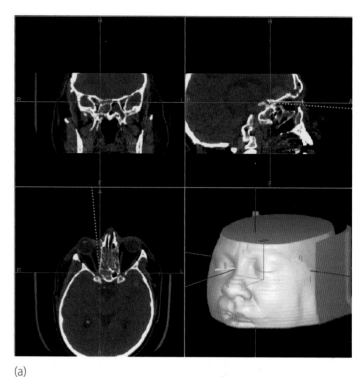

(a)

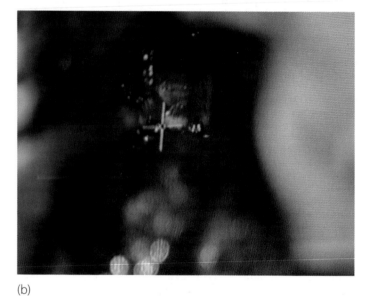

(b)

Fig. 33.23: (a) Intraoperative multiplanar and 3D views (screenshot) during navigated optic nerve decompression. The tip of the dotted line is correlated with the focus of the microscope, **(b)** in which the optic nerve (cross-marked in the microscopic view) can be seen.

was to virtually ideally reconstruct the patient prior to operation by mirroring a subvolume of the CT dataset from the unaffected right onto the left side (Fig. 33.34). Intraoperatively (Fig. 33.35) autologous calvarial split-bone grafts were used to recontour the left orbit and calcium phosphate cement served for recontouring of the severe left temporal hollowing. Figure 33.36 shows a screenshot during navigation with the mirrored dataset, where the pointer checks on the contour during reconstruction. To

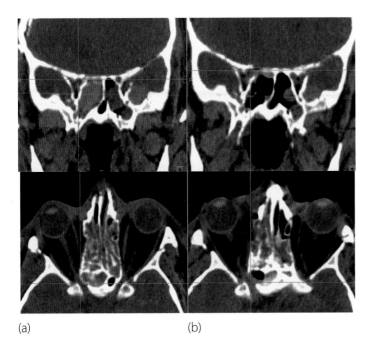

(a)   (b)

Fig. 33.24: Matched pre- **(a)** and postoperative **(b)** axial and coronal view of the patient in Figs 33.22 and 33.23. Following transethmoidal optic nerve decompression the bony ring of the optic canal has been opened.

reduce the amount of calcium phosphate cement a calvarial split-bone graft was used as an onlay graft to the forehead. The augmentation was stopped when the preplanned contours matched with the intraoperative achieved augmentation (Fig. 33.37). Figure 33.38 shows a postoperative CT in a multiplanar and 3D view following recontouring of the periorbital and temporal left defect. Figure 33.39 shows matching of lateral 3D views of the preoperative, ideally virtually reconstructed and postoperative CT datasets of the same patient on the workstation of the STN navigation system.

The non-invasive registration system marked by the radio-opaque spheres is patented by the authors.

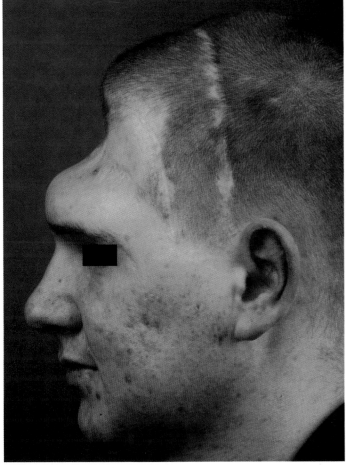
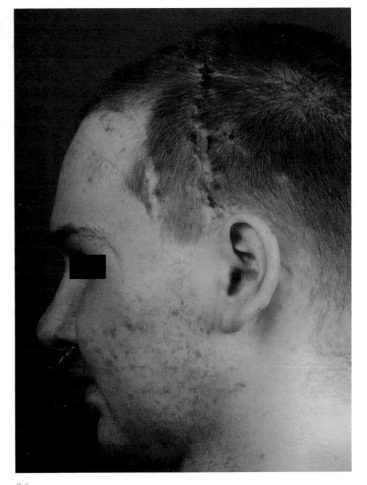

(a)   (b)

Fig. 33.25: Pre- **(a)** and 10 days postoperative **(b)** lateral view of a patient with an extended bifrontal defect following a car accident.

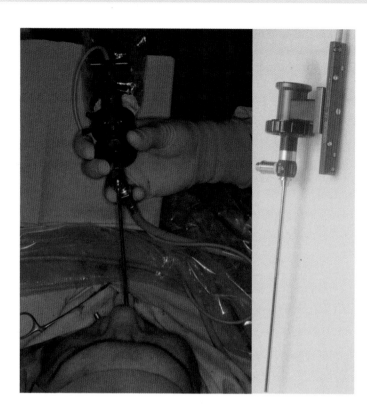

Fig. 33.26: Bird's eye view during navigated endoscopic surgery on the patient in Fig. 33.25 with a tracked endoscope (right).

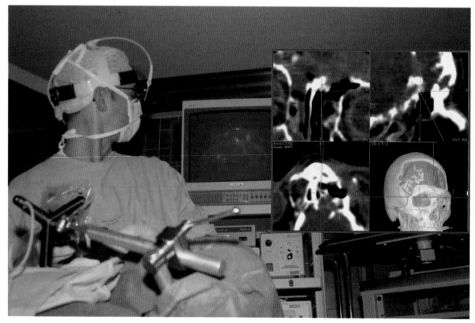

Fig. 33.27: Intraoperative overview during computer-assisted endoscopic surgery showing a multiplanar and 3D view of the same patient (inset), which is available to the surgeon in realtime, in which the tip of the dotted green line marks the tip of the tracked endoscope.

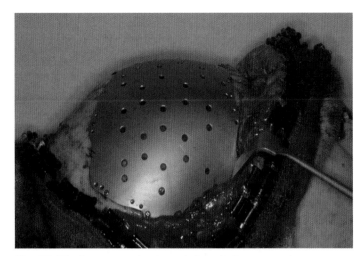

Fig. 33.28: Intraoperative lateral view during secondary bifrontal reconstruction with a commercially available custom-made titanium implant (CCB, Bochum, Germany).

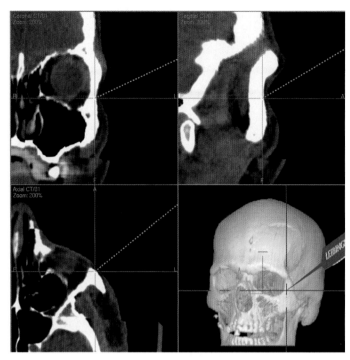

Fig. 33.30: Intraoperative screenshot during navigated control of repositioning the advanced left malar bone complex. The tip of the dotted line indicates the pointer tip, showing that the correct position for the lateral orbital rim is achieved according to the virtually reconstructed dataset demonstrated here.

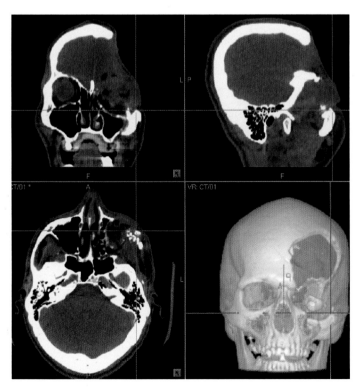

Fig. 33.29: Multiplanar and 3D view of a patient's CT dataset following a closely fired gunshot wound showing extended left soft and hard tissue loss.

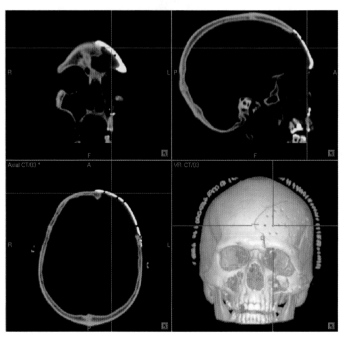

Fig. 33.31: Postoperative multiplanar and 3D view from the patient in Figs 33.29 and 33.30.

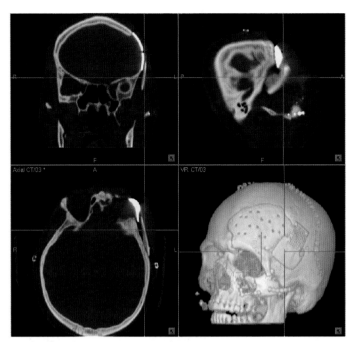

Fig. 33.32: Postoperative multiplanar and 3D view from the patient in Figs 33.29–31 showing additional bone grafting to overcome the temporal hollowing.

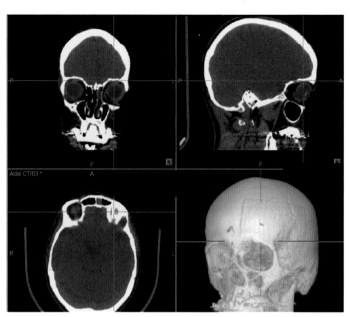

Fig. 33.34: Corresponding views to Fig. 33.33 following virtual reconstruction by applying the mirror tool.

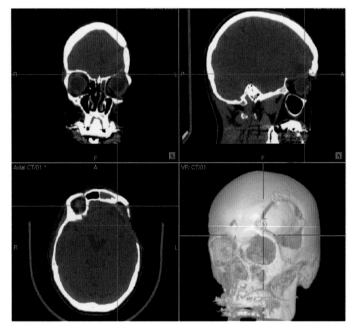

Fig. 33.33: Preoperative multiplanar and 3D view from a patient with left temporo-orbital soft and hard tissue loss.

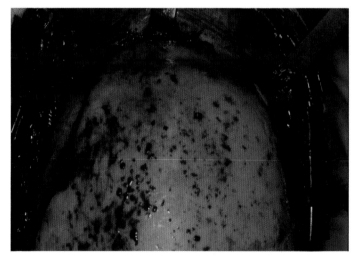

Fig. 33.35: Clinical view from above after exposing the deficient left temporo-orbital region via a bicoronal approach.

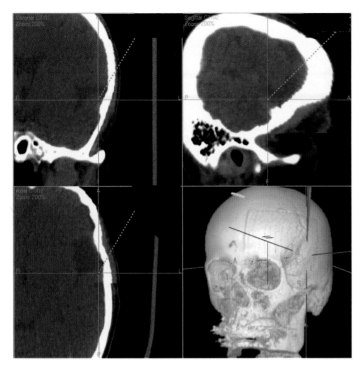

Fig. 33.36: Intraoperative screenshot from the patient in Figs 33.33–35 pointing at the surface of the deficient temporal region (tip of the dotted line) in the virtually ideally reconstructed CT dataset.

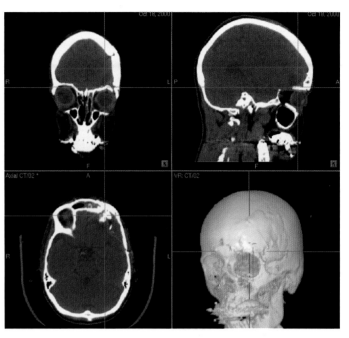

Fig. 33.38: Postoperative multiplanar and 3D view from the patient in Figs 33.33–37 corresponding to Fig. 33.33 (preoperative) and Fig. 33.34 (virtually reconstructed).

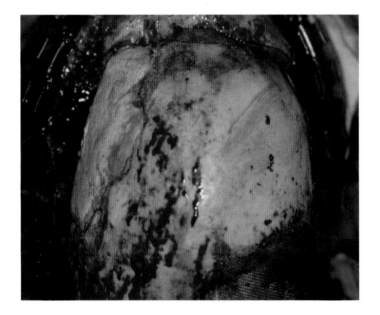

Fig. 33.37: Clinical view corresponding to Fig. 33.35 following augmentation of the left frontotemporo-orbital region with calcium phosphate cement.

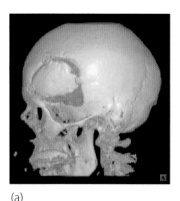

(a)

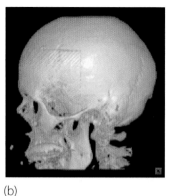

(b)

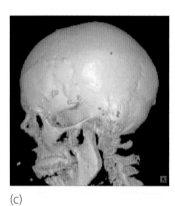

(c)

Fig. 33.39: Matched lateral pre- **(a)**, simulated **(b)** and postoperative **(c)** 3D CT views of the patient in Figs 33.33–38.

References

1 Hammer B, Prein J 1995 Correction of post-traumatic orbital deformities: operative techniques and review of 26 patients. Journal of Craniomaxillofacial Surgery 23(2): 81

2 Howard G, Osguthorpe JD 1997 Concepts in orbital reconstruction. Otolaryngology Clinics of North America 30(4): 541

3 Kawamoto HK Jr 1982 Late posttraumatic enophthalmos: a correctable deformity? Plastic and Reconstructive Surgery 69(3): 423

4 Manson PN, Grivas A, Rosenbaum A, Vannier M, Zinreich J, Iliff N 1985 Studies on enophthalmos: II. The measurement of orbital injuries and their treatment by quantitative computed tomography. Plastic and Reconstructive Surgery 77(2): 203

5 Schmelzeisen R, Husstedt H, Zumkeller M, Rittierodt M 1997 Profilerhalt und Verbesserung bei primärer und sekundärer Orbitare-konstruktion. Mund, Kiefer und Gesichtschirurgie 1 (suppl 1): 87

6 Eufinger H, Wittkampf AR, Wehmoller M, Zonneveld FW 1998 Single-step fronto-orbital resection and reconstruction with individual resection template and corresponding titanium implant: a new method of computer-aided surgery. Journal of Craniomaxillofacial Surgery 26(6): 373

7 Heissler E, Fischer FS, Bolouri S et al 1998 Custom-made cast titanium implants produced with CAD/CAM for the reconstruction of cranium defects. International Journal of Oral and Maxillofacial Surgery 27(5): 334

8 Hoffmann J, Cornelius CP, Groten M, Probster L, Pfannenberg C, Schwenzer N 1998 Orbital reconstruction with individually copy-milled ceramic implants. Plastic and Reconstructive Surgery 101(3): 604–612

9 Holck DE, Boyd EM Jr, Mauffray RO 1999 Benefits of stereolithography in orbital reconstruction. Ophthalmology 106(6): 1214–1218

10 Luka B, Brechtelsbauer D, Gellrich NC, König M 1995 2-D and 3-D reconstructions of the facial skeleton: an unnecessary option or a diagnostic pearl? International Journal of Oral and Maxillofacial Surgery 21: 99–103

11 Perry M, Banks P, Richards R, Friedman EP, Shaw P 1998 The use of computer-generated three-dimensional models in orbital reconstruction. British Journal of Oral and Maxillofacial Surgery 36: 275–284

12 Haβfeld S, Mühling J, Zöller J 1995 Intraoperative navigation in oral and maxillofacial surgery. International Journal of Oral and Maxillofacial Surgery 24: 111–119

13 Marmulla R, Niederdellmann H 1998 Computer-aided navigation in secondary reconstruction of post-traumatic deformities of the zygoma. Journal of Craniomaxillofacial Surgery 26(1): 68–69

14 Watzinger F, Wanschitz F, Wagner A, Enislidis G, Millesi W, Baumann A, Ewers R 1997 Computer-aided navigation in secondary reconstruction of post-traumatic deformities of the zygoma. Journal of Craniomaxillofacial Surgery 25(4): 198–202

15 Wirtz CR, Knauth M, Haβfeld S, Tronnier, VM, Albert FK, Bonsanto MM, Kunze S 1998 Neuronavigation – first experiences with three different commercially available systems. Zentralblatt fur Neurochirurgie 59(1): 14–22

16 Gellrich NC, Schramm A, Hammer B, Rojas S, Cufi D, Lagrèze W, Schmelzeisen R 2002 Computer-assisted secondary reconstructions of unilateral posttraumatic orbital deformities. Plastic and Reconstructive Surgery 110(6): 1417–1429

17 Ilankovan V, Jackson IT 1992 Experience in the use of calvarial bone grafts in orbital reconstruction. British Journal of Oral and Maxillofacial Surgery 30(2): 92–96

18 Schramm A, Gellrich NC, Naumann S, Bühner U, Schön R, Schmelzeisen R 1999 Non-invasive referencing in computer assisted surgery. Medical and Biological Engineering and Computing 644 (suppl)

19 Schramm A, Gellrich NC, Schimming R, Schmelzeisen R 2000 Rechnergestützte Insertion von Zygomaticus-Implantaten (Brånemark System®) nach ablativer Tumorchirurgie. Mund, Kiefer und Gesichtschirurgie 4: 292

20 Gellrich NC, Schramm A, Hammer B, Schmelzeisen R 1999 The value of computer-aided planning and intraoperative navigation in orbital reconstruction. International Journal of Oral and Maxillofacial Surgery 28 (suppl 1): 52

21 Gruss JS 1985 Naso-ethmoid-orbital fractures: classification and role of primary bone-grafting. Plastic and Reconstructive Surgery 75(3): 303

22 Manson PN, Ruas EJ, Iliff NT 1987 Deep orbital reconstruction for correction of post-traumatic enophthalmos. Clinics in Plastic Surgery 14(1): 113

23 Gellrich NC 1999 Controversies and state of the art in therapy of optic nerve lesions in craniofacial traumatology and surgery. Mund, Kiefer und Gesichtschirurgie 3: 176

Index

Note:
All index entries refer to maxillofacial (or facial) features unless otherwise noted. Page numbers in **bold** refer to major discussions in the text. Page numbers in *italics* refer to figures/boxes or tables. *vs* denotes comparisons

Abbreviations:
CT – computed tomography
MRI – magnetic resonance imaging
PTSD – posttraumatic stress disorder
RSTL – relaxed skin tension lines

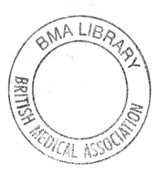